The Laboratory Rat

The Handbook of Experimental Animals

Editors-in-Chief

Gillian Bullock
University Hospital
Department of Pathology
Ghent
Belgium

Tracie E Bunton
DuPont Pharmaceuticals Company
Department of Research and Development
Stine-Haskell Research Center
Newark, DE
USA

List of Editorial Advisory Board

The Laboratory Rat

Edited by

Georg J Krinke

Novartis Crop Protection AG

Stein

Switzerland

ACADEMIC PRESS

A Harcourt Science and Technology Company

San Diego   San Francisco   New York
Boston   London   Sydney   Tokyo

Academic Press
32 Jamestown Road, London, NW1 7BY, UK
http://www.academicpress.com

Academic Press
A Harcourt Science and Technology Company
525 B Street, Stuie 1900, San Diego, California 92101-4495, USA
http://www.academicpress.com

ISBN 0-12-426400-X

Library of Congress Catalog Card Number: 99-63118
A catalogue for this book is available from the British Library

Access for a limited period to an on-line version of The Laboratory Rat is included in the purchase price of the print edition.
This on-line version has been uniquely and persistently identified by the Digital Object Identifier (DOI)

10.1006/bklr.2000

By following the link

http://dx.doi.org/10.1006/bklr.2000

from any Web Browser, buyers of The Laboratory Rat will find instructions on how to register for access.

Typeset by Bibliocraft, Scotland, UK
Printed in Slovenia by Midas Printing Ltd

00 01 02 03 04 MD 9 8 7 6 5 4 3 2 1

Contents

List of Contributors

Allegrini, P R
Novartis Pharma AG
Basel
Switzerland

Allmann-Iselin, I
Swiss Federal Institute of Technology
Schwerzenbach–Zürich
Switzerland

Ballam, G C
Purina Mills Inc.
St. Louis
MO
USA

Barrow, P
Phoenix International Preclinical Services
Europe (Chrysalis)
Les Oncins
L'Arbresle
France

Bolon, B
Amgen Inc.
Thousand Oaks
CA
USA

Bono, C D
Experimental Pathology Laboratories
Herndon
VA
USA

Classen, W
Novartis Crop Protection AG
Stein
Switzerland

Clifford, C B
Charles River Laboratories Inc.
Wilmington
MA
USA

Elwell, M R
Covance Laboratories
Vienna
VA
USA

Gaillard, E T
Experimental Pathology Laboratories Inc.
Research Triangle Park
NC
USA

Galbreath, E
Eli Lilly & Co.
Indianapolis
IN
USA

Gassmann, M
Institute of Physiology
University of Zürich-Irchel
Zürich
Switzerland

Gembardt, C
BASF AG
Ludwigshafen
Germany

Haught, D G
Purina Mills Inc.
St. Louis
MO
USA

Hedrich, H J
Hannover Medical School
Hannover
Germany

Itakura, A
Department of Veterinary Clinic
Tokyo University of Agriculture and Technology
Tokyo
Japan

Kaufmann, W
BASF AG
Ludwigshafen
Germany

Keenan, K P
Department of Safety Assessment
Merck Research Laboratories
West Point
PA
USA

Kei-ichiro, M
Graduate School of Bioagricultural Sciences
Nagoya University
Nagoya 484–8601
Japan

Kemp, R W
Astra Zeneca
Macclesfield
Cheshire
UK

Kilo, J
Institute of Physiology
University of Zürich-Irchel
Zürich
Switzerland

Komárek, V
Agricultural University
Prague
Czech Republic

Krinke, A
PATHEV
Frenkendorf
Switzerland

Kunstýr, I
Medizinische Hochschule Hannover
Hannover
Germany

Laroque, P
Laboratories MSD-Chibret
Riom
Clermont-Ferrand
France

Lüscher, T F
Cardiology
University Hospital
Zürich
Switzerland

Maeda, K
Graduate School of Bioagricultural
Sciences
Nagoya University
Nagoya
Japan

Mahrous, T A
Novartis Crop Protection AG
Stein
Switzerland

Matsuda, H
Department of Veterinary Clinic
Tokyo University of Agriculture and
   Technology
Tokyo
Japan

Muhle, H
Fraunhofer Institute
Hannover
Germany

Mutai, M
Toxicology Laboratory
Yokohama Research Center
Mitsubishi Chemical Corporation
Yokohama
Japan

Nebendahl, K
University of Göttingen
Göttingen
Germany

Nicklas, W
Deutsches Krebsforschungszentrum
Heidelberg
Germany

Ohkura, S
Primate Research Institute
Kyoto University
Aichi
Japan

Reifenberg, K
Laboratory Animal Research Unit
University Ulm
Germany

Remie, R
Department of Laboratory Animal Science
Solvay Pharmaceuticals
Weesp and University Center for Pharmacy
Groningen University
Groningen
The Netherlands

Rogers, K
Experimental Pathology Laboratories
Herndon
VA
USA

Sargent, L
National Institute of Occupational
   Safety and Health
Morgantown
WV
USA

Schaetti, P
Novartis Crop Protection AG
Stein
Switzerland

Schulz, H
GSF – National Research Center for
   Environment and Health
Institute for Inhalation Biology
Munich
Germany

Senoo, H
Department of Anatomy
Akita University School of Medicine
Akita
Japan

Shibutani, M
National Institute of Health Sciences
Tokyo
Japan

Tanaka, A
Department of Veterinary Clinic
Tokyo University of Agriculture and
   Technology
Tokyo
Japan

Taylor, G R
University of Missouri-St. Louis
St. Louis
MO
USA

Tsukamura, H
Graduate School of Bioagricultural
    Sciences
Nagoya University
Nagoya
Japan

d'Uscio, L V
Institute of Physiology
University of Zürich-Irchel
Zürich
Switzerland

Weiss, J
Transgene Laboratory and Animal Facility
Center for Molecular Biology
University Heidelberg
Germany

Whittaker, D
Huntingdon Life Sciences
Alconbury
Huntingdon
Cambridgeshire
UK

Wüthrich, R P
Physiological Institute
University Zürich-Irchel
Zürich
Switzerland

Zimmermann, F
Transgene Laboratory and Animal Facility
Center for Molecular Biology
University Heidelberg
Germany

Foreword

THE gestation period for this new series actually took several years. The original ideas spanned fundamental atlases, encyclopedias and hosts of others. Finally, after consulting many people, the outstanding comment was, "We are fed up with looking for important data which is scattered throughout the literature". And so, this compendium of knowledge covering a range of laboratory animals came into being.

During this development period, the publishing world also changed. Having thought originally about the book format, then about a CD-ROM, we are now producing an online version. We decided to keep the book format for those who do not have access to the internet or who still like to turn pages. The electronic version has allowed us to experiment with style, content and presentation, and we are still in the learning process. With this, the first volume in the series, we would like to thank the Volume Editor with whom we have had fantastic co-operation. By popular request we chose "The Laboratory Rat" to start as it has such widespread use in research and toxicology but the "The Laboratory Fish", very important for environmentalists and researcher alike, will not be far behind.

We would like to express our appreciation for the support, moral and other, we have had from the Editorial Advisory Board members. Finally, without the help and encouragement of Carey Chapman, Lorraine Parry, Emma Parkinson and other members of Academic Press, we would not be in the happy position of launching "The Laboratory Rat" today.

Gillian Bullock
Tracie E Bunton
Editors-in-Chief
The Handbook of Experimental Animals

Preface

*T*HIS publication aims to provide accessible practical information for researchers and technicians backed by sound theoretical wisdom. The authors have thus been chosen from both universities and applied research organisations. To achieve a global, well-balanced approach they come from a wide range of countries from three continents.

Toxicological aspects represent an immensely important part of the coverage. As toxicology research is extremely firmly regulated, much attention was paid to the content dealing with toxicology with special comments and specific chapters.

Experimental medicine was considered especially in the section dealing with procedures, and a special section was devoted to genetic engineering and molecular technology.

For practical reasons the extent of data presented had to be restricted. For instance, anatomical aspects could not be described in the finest detail. However, to provide added value for the reader, potentially confusing differences in anatomical terminology used by different authors were compared and explained. It was decided that selected anatomical features of aging organs and tissues would be demonstrated.

Neither rat histopathology nor clinical medicine is a primary topic in this work. Nevertheless, the section dealing with rat pathogens includes unique examples of experimental infections that are essential to know but rare to see in appropriately health-controlled colonies.

The Editor of this work has learned a great deal during the editing of the contributors' manuscripts and would like to express his gratitude to all authors for their worthy efforts. Behind the scenes, invaluable support was provided by those who helped to identify and recruit the authors: Dr Jerry F Hardisty (Research Triangle Park, USA), Professor Ulrich Mohr (Hanover, Germany), Professor Peter Thomann (Zürich, Switzerland). Dr Christian Gembardt (Ludwigshafen, Germany) provided material for histology illustrations, and Mrs Christina Würmlin (Stein, Switzerland) checked organ anatomy and topography. Last but not least, for the publisher, Ms Lorraine Parry, associate editor, provided a driving spirit to realise this endeavour.

Georg J Krinke

PART 1

The History and Development of the Rat as a Laboratory Model

Contents

CHAPTER 1

History, Strains and Models

Hans J Hedrich
Hannover Medical School, Institute for Laboratory Sciences,
Hannover, Germany

Introduction

The laboratory, or Norway, rat (*Rattus norvegicus*) is one of the most commonly used experimental animals, offering as it does the best 'functionally' characterized mammalian model system. The rat serves as a model organism for the analysis of a number of important biomedical traits, such as cardiovascular diseases, metabolic disorders (lipid metabolism, diabetes mellitus), neurological disorders (such as epilepsy, parkinsonism), neurobehavioural studies, organ transplantation, autoimmune diseases (such as arthritis, experimental allergic encephalomyelitis, etc.), cancer susceptibility and renal diseases. It offers a number of unique advantages for modelling human diseases, developing new therapeutic agents, and in studying responses to environmental agents. The size of the rat, in contrast to the other commonly used experimental animal, the laboratory mouse, makes it ideal for certain physiological manipulations. Another field of clinical research, toxicology,

also has traditionally relied on the rat as an important test species, as can be seen from the extensive literature of chemical exposure on this species. In addition, the recent development of genetic and genomic tools for the rat now provides an unprecedented opportunity to take advantage of the rich and robust history of experimental studies utilizing this species to study human disease. It is this wealth of past and recent information available on the rat and the multiplicity of strains available with different characteristics that turn the laboratory rat into an indispensable tool for biomedical research.

Historical Foundations

Rat is the common name for any large member of a family of rodents (see Table 1.1), mostly with

Table 1.1 Taxonomy

Phylum:	Chordata
Class:	Mammalia
Order:	Rodentia
Suborder:	Myomorpha
Family:	Muridae
Subfamily:	Murinae
Genus:	Rattus
Species:	R. norvegicus (Berkenhout, 1769)
	R. rattus (Linné, 1758)

While there is no subspecies to *Rattus norvegicus*, for the black rat (*Rattus rattus*) several subspecies have been described which do not interbreed within the species nor with the Norway rat (see Yoshida, 1980).

dull-coloured, coarse fur, long tails, relatively large ears and pointed snouts. They are known for their powerful incisor teeth, which enable them to gnaw through hard materials.

The original geographical distribution of rats prevailing before the influence of human travel cannot be established with certainty since most parts of the world have now been occupied by the Norway rat (*Rattus norvegicus*) as well as the various subspecies of the black, roof or house rat (*Rattus rattus*). Meng et al. (1994) state that 'Rodents were first known through the localities of the latest Palaeocene-earliest Eocene age in Asia and North America. They are widely considered to have originated in Asia based on the occurrence there of erymylids, their perceived nearest relatives.' It is considered as certain that large parts of the Mediterranean countries, the Middle East, India, China, Japan, all of Southeast Asia, including the Philippines, New Guinea and Australia are the natural habitat of genus *Rattus* (Figure 1.1). The original natural habitat of the Norway rat is the vast plains of Asia, probably northern China and Mongolia, where rats still live in burrows, and that of the black rat (*Rattus rattus*) is the Indo-Malayan region. From this region rats spread to other parts of the world during the Middle Ages according to mammalian taxonomists (Tate, 1936; Silver, 1941; Southern, 1964). They have spread from this original natural habitat throughout the entire world, always keeping in close association with humans.

It still remains unclear at what time the Norway rat became commensal with humans. This event may have taken place as long as some thousand years or just several hundred years ago. This commensalism with human beings and the tendency to settle in association with routes of human migration is common to both rat species (Yoshida, 1980).

According to Thenius, who described the phylogenesis of rats in the *Encyclopaedia of the Animal Kingdom* by Grzimek (1968), the Norway rat had appeared in Central Europe by 1553. This assumption was based on an illustration (Figure 1.2) of a rat thought to be a Norway rat depicted by the famous Swiss naturalist Conrad Gesner in his *Historiae animalium* (1551–1558, German edition, 1669). The text could easily be describing the black rat, however, although Gesner mentions the appearance of a considerable proportion of white rats with red eyes.

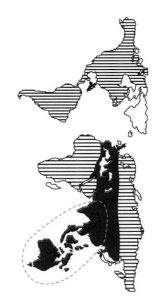

Figure 1.1 Worldwide distribution of rats. The encircled area indicates the approximate preglacial distribution of genus *Rattus*. The black area indicates the distribution of genus *Rattus* before this genus conquered the world (hatched).

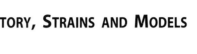

Figure 1.2 Historical picture of the rat by Conrad Gesner 1553. Picture of 'De Mure domestico majore, commonly called rat' as depicted in C. Gesner's *Historiae animalium*, originally published in 1553, partial German edition printed in 1669, reprinted 1980 by Schlütersche Verlagsanstalt, Hannover; reprinted with kind permission of the publisher.

Another common idea supports the fact that Norway rats may have crossed the River Volga in south Russia no earlier than 1727 in a huge migratory event and inhabited Western Europe. There is little evidence to support the assumption by Castle (1947) that the brown rat (*Rattus norvegicus*) entered Western Europe via the Norwegian peninsula.

Historically reliable accounts of the presence of the Norway rat in Europe date back to the eighteenth century (e.g. England 1730, France 1735, Eastern Germany 1750, Spain 1800) when it is reported as competing with and displacing the smaller and less aggressive black rat species in most parts of Europe, and also in the United States. As early as 1755 the Norway rat arrived in North America via the ships of new settlers (see Grzimek, 1968), while Lantz (1909) reported the first arrival on the eastern seaboard of the United States as being in around 1775.

In the eighteenth and nineteenth centuries, rats were trapped, killed, sold for food especially in times of famine in Europe, or used for rat-baiting contests, originally in Europe and later in America as late as the end of the last century. In this era albino, black, piebald (hooded) coloured Norway rats were captured or selected from offspring of captive rats and tamed for baiting contests due to their distinct and attractive appearance. Albino mutants were first brought into laboratories early in the nineteenth century to serve as objects of physiological studies, for example in fasting studies as early as 1828 (McCay, 1973), in attempts to measure the quality of proteins (Savory, 1863) or in studies on the

importance of the adrenal glands (Philipeaux, 1856). It is thus safe to state that the Norway rat was the first animal species to be domesticated for strictly scientific purposes (Richter, 1954). The first breeding experiments recorded are those by Crampe (1877, 1883, 1884, 1885) who shortly after Mendel and long before the rediscovery of Mendel's laws in 1900 reported on the laws of coat colour inheritance, describing albino, non-agouti black and hooded offspring obtained from different breeding experiments.

It is generally believed that the first inbred rat strain to be bred was the PA strain. Helen Dean King began inbreeding of albino rats at the Wistar Institute in Philadelphia as early as 1909 (King, 1918a,b,c, 1919) at the same time as Clarence Cook Little's initial efforts to develop the oldest inbred mouse strain dba, now known as DBA/1 and DBA/2. However, there is evidence that an earlier strain existed and should be considered as the oldest rat stock or strain. According to a report in the *Magasin Pittoresque*, a black hooded rat colony existed in the Jardin des Plantes in 1856 (Bazin, 1988). This institution, founded in 1635, was turned into a museum of natural history in 1793 with plants and live animals on exhibit. The rat colony was still present 132 years after first being reported and still served as a source of food for reptiles. A colony, now definitely inbred PAR/Lou has been derived from this original source.

The early history of the renowned Wistar Institute of Anatomy and Biology in Philadelphia, which served as one of the first laboratory animal breeding and research facilities, of further research institutions and their renowned scientists in the United States devoted to research in nutrition, biochemistry, physiology, endocrinology, cancer, behaviour and genetics have been thoroughly reviewed by Lindsey (1979). Most of the rat colonies in these early times were maintained as random bred stocks. It was the 'Wistar rat' and to a lesser extent the 'Sprague-Dawley rat' that overtook all others in animal laboratories throughout the world and that served as founders of many of the rat strains today. Since the early attempts more than a century ago the Norway rat has become a major laboratory tool in biomedical research. This fact is reflected by the wealth of scientific literature dealing with rats published since 1966. Until recently, publications using rats have outnumbered publications using the mouse by at least two to one. With the advent of molecular biology and since mouse strains can be tailored more successfully by molecular genetic techniques (targeted mutations), the ratio has been reduced to approximately 1.5:1. Publications reporting the use of inbred rats have occurred as frequently as those using inbred mice, even though standardized rat genetic models may not be readily available to researchers.

As described previously, the Norway rat was the first mammalian species to be domesticated primarily for scientific purposes. From these early times the rat has become the most widely studied experimental animal in biomedical research and the wealth of knowledge that is now available, primarily in physiology, and the abundance of 'genetically defined' strains displaying different characteristics have made this species an extremely valuable scientific tool (Jacob et al., 1995). Certain disciplines, such as immunology, and experimental medicine focusing on transplantation, autoimmunity and other immune dysfunctions, or cancer, arthritis, hypertension, diabetes (type I and II) and neurological disorders extensively use rat models. Some of the genetically defined rat models have been defined by comparing the aetiology and pathophysiology of the respective disorders in rat and humans. Other disciplines that have extensively used the rat as an experimental model include nutrition research (relying on a ~0.98 correlation between rat and human in digestibility of nutrients), and neurophysiology and behavioural biology. More recently, pharmacology and toxicology are increasingly recognizing the importance of genetics on xenometabolism. As transplantation research and immunobiology

established the rat as one of their favourite research tools, a group of scientists keen to unravel the immunogenetic systems of the species, namely the major histocompatibility complex (MHC), AgB or H-1, now called RT1, decided in the sixties to meet regularly to discuss urgent problems, such as the organization of the rat MHC, to exchange reagents and to resolve fundamental nomenclature problems. As a result of the efforts of this 'Old Rat Gang' with Drs G. Butcher (Cambridge), E. Günther (Freiburg), T.J. Gill III (Pittsburgh), J. Howard (Cambridge), H. Kunz (Pittsburgh), O. Stark (Prague), a series of regular workshops on 'Alloantigenic Systems in the Rat' were initiated. Today the rat group, supported by the publication of these workshops in *Transplantation Proceedings*, still come together every 2 years, although with the development of rat genetics the scope has broadened from immunogenetics to all aspects of the use of inbred strains, Independent of this group, Dr M. Festing, a strict proponent of the use of inbred strains, founded *Rat News Letter*, a biannual journal devoted to all aspects of the laboratory rat. The journal recently evolved into *Rat Genome* as a printed communication tool for the scientific rat community, with H. Kunz (Pittsburgh), T. Natori (Sapporo), and G. Levan (Göteborg) serving as editors.

Until recently, there have been two main drawbacks with the rat as a model organism. The rat gene map has been poorly developed and there have been very few polymorphic markers available. Both of these factors have severely hampered high-level genetic research in the rat. During the last few years both of these problems have been largely overcome. It is now possible to fully exploit the potential of the rat as a model organism in biomedical research. Microsatellite markers have been shown to greatly facilitate genetic mapping approaches in the rat and resulted in the composition of linkage maps covering all chromosomes by means of simple sequence length polymorphisms. These microsatellite framework maps do not only assist in assigning known classical genetic markers (including pathophysiological deviants), but also provide the resources for identifying genes involved in complex genetic traits. While almost no reliable chromosomal assignment was available 15 years ago, currently more than 6000 'anonymous' markers cover the majority of the genome (Pravenec et al., 1996; Bihoreau et al., 1997; Brown et al., 1998; Walder et al., 1998; for URL see Table 1.2). These markers assigned to linkage groups have been chromosomally mapped and oriented (Andoh et al., 1998; Szpirer et al., 1998). Some 650

Table 1.2 Information, mapping and source sites for the rat on the World Wide Web

Site	Data and displays	URL
RATMAP[a]	Anonymous and expressed rat loci Linkage information Cytogenic maps Genetic nomenclature Meetings and conferences	http://ratmap.gen.gu.se
MGI[b]	Genetic markers Polymorphisms Maps Mammalian homology Inbred strain characteristics	http://www.informatics.jax.org/rat/
Wox[c]	Linkage maps Polymorphisms	http://www.well.ox.ac.uk/~bihoreau
WIBR/MIT[d]	Linkage maps	http://www.genome.wi.mit.edu/rat/public
ARB[e]	Linkage maps Primers	http://www.nih.gov/niams/scientific/ratbase/index.htm
Encyclopaedia of the Rat[f]	Strains/markers	http://www.mh-hannover.de/institut/tierlabor/genearchiv.htm
ILAR	Animal models and genetic stocks International Index of Laboratory Animals Laboratory Code Registry Related publications	http://www2.nas.edu/ilarhome/

[a] Displays MIT maps by chromosome.
[b] M. Festing's List of Inbred Strains of Mice and Rats (MGD).
[c] The Wellcome Trust Centre for Human Genetics.
[d] Rat Genome Project at the Whitehead Institute/MIT Center for Genome Research.
[e] National Institute of Arthritis and Musculoskeletal and Skin Diseases (NIH/NIAMS).
[f] This database is still under construction. It presently allows one to check for characteristics of the strains maintained in Hannover, but will soon provide genetic marker descriptions based on Hedrich (1990).

presently known genes are also placed within this framework. Many of the microsatellite alleles have been characterized for several inbred strains (for URL see Table 1.2). A Rat Expressed Sequence Tag (EST) Project has been initiated developing full-length cDNA libraries with greater than 50 000 ESTs sequenced, and a gene-based EST map. In addition to these new genomic tools, transgenic rats are being produced by genetic manipulation in many laboratories and several commercial settings. These transgenic rats are used to study hypertension, autoimmune diseases, neoplasia, etc.

Rat Strains and Stocks

Recent developments in rat genomics and the availability of genetically defined strains will certainly allow the functions of genes to be established not only by linking clinical phenotypes, physiology and genetics but also by using comparative mapping techniques switching between rat, mouse and human. All of the present rat colonies originate from a random bred or outbred stock. The major colonies, like Wistar, Sprague-Dawley, Osborne-Mendel, Long-Evans, Holtzman, Slonaker, Albany, etc. still exist as so-called sublines, but rather as independent colonies due to founder effects and genetic drift, with similar or new names mostly adhering to the nomenclature rules (Lindsey, 1979). The stocks derived from Wistar and Sprague-Dawley are among the most popular rats used experimentally, irrespective of the fact that their genetic make-up is often extremely variable. Indeed they have served over a long period of time as the major source in animal experimentation, primarily in toxicity studies.

As it is important to control the variables that influence animal experimentation, such as environmental and experimental variables as well as the genetic make-up of the animals used, the use of 'genetically defined' laboratory animals is to be advised. Inbred strains allow for a much better standardization of the test conditions and improve the quality of results. Certain scientific disciplines (e.g. immunology) exclusively use genetically defined animals. Other research disciplines minimize variability by selecting an appropriate genetic model such that the extent of analyses can be reduced or kept at a minimum. This approach has the added advantage that it is in line with animal welfare legislation, which calls for reduction and refinement. Geneticists can provide not only homogeneous populations, but also, over longer periods of time, genetically heterogeneous populations with specific characters from isogenic strains. Each resynthesized population is essentially identical to the preceding ones.

Experimentation based on laboratory animals depends to a large extent on the genetic uniformity and constancy of the animals. Therefore, standard inbred, congenic, consomic or recombinant inbred strains are usually used. A detailed knowledge of the various categories of inbred strains is required

for the selection of the inbred strain or combination of inbred strains that is best suited for the task at hand (see Chapter 10). The history of rat strains used for critical research on human diseases is impressive in its breadth and depth. Today there are a large number of strains producing highly valuable insights into the pathogenesis of disease, with major public health implications, including more than 220 inbred strains and many more substrains as well as a growing list of congenic, consomic, recombinant inbred and transgenic strains. A first listing of rat strains was published by Billingham and Silvers (1959), and there have been subsequent listings by Festing and Staats (1973) and by Greenhouse *et al.* (1990). Festing (1979) and Table 1.3 lists most of the inbred strains known. The selection of strains on the basis of genetic diversity may be facilitated by a genealogic tree (see Figure 1.3) calculated on the basis of published genetic and biochemical marker typings ($N = 995$) of 63 major strains and 214 substrains (Canzian, 1997). The calculation clearly shows the extreme genetic distance between BN substrains, the PAR strain and most of the other strains, which are arranged in clusters (subtrees) of relationship. However, not all assignments to clusters must be assumed to reflect a relationship because of diverse and apparent independent origins. The relationship of strains based on biochemical genetic markers produced by Festing and Bender (1984) was similar but did not arrive at the precision of the above study, mainly due to the lesser number of markers available at that time.

In a joint effort by several groups on two occasions, large sets of rat strains and substrains have been typed for biochemical genetic and immunogenetic markers (Bender *et al.*, 1984, 1994). The results of the latter study provided a strain distribution pattern of 39 markers for 156 strains and substrains. It is interesting to note that the data by Canzian (1997) clearly indicate that the genetic diversity among inbred strains of rats is higher than that of the mouse, although, for example, the polymorphism of the major histocompatibility complex of the rat is much lower than that of mouse, human and several other species. More than 600 expressed genes have been described and mapped in the rat. Variants for some of these loci are presently not known.

Extracted from RATMAP (see Table 1.2) and in conjunction with a consolidated short report by the Rat Chromosome Committee (1999), these

Table 1.3 Table list of inbred rat strains

Strain	Description	Strain	Description
AAW		BH	(Black hooded)
AB		BI	
AB/1		BIL	
AB/2		BIRMA	(Birmingham A)
ABH		BIRMB	(Birmingham B)
ACH	(AxC 9935 Piebald)	BLK	
ACI	(AxC 9935 Irish)	BN	(Brown Norway)
ACP	(ACP9935 Irish piebald)	BP	(Brown Praha)
AD		BROFO	
AGA		BS	
AGUS		BUF	(Buffalo)
AHAR		C	
AHH/R		CAP	
ALB	(Albany)	CAR	(Hunt's caries resistant)
AM		CAS	(Hunt's caries susceptible)
AMDIL		CBH	
ANOP		CF	
AO		CFHB	
AP		CFY	
APR		CHB	
AS		COP	(Copenhagen 2331)
AS2		CPBB	(BC)
AUG	(August)	CRDH	
AVN		CRT	
AXC		CWS	
A990	(August 1990)	DA	
A7322	(August 7322)	DB	
A28807	(August 28807)	DEBR	
A35322	(August 35322)	DONRYU	(YOS)
B		DSS/3N	
BB		EXBH	
BBZ		E3	
BC	(CPB-B, CPBB)	FCH	
BDE		FH	(Fawn hooded)
BDI	(Berlin Druckrey I)	FHH	(Fawn hooded hypertensive)
BDII	(Berlin Druckrey II)	FHL	
BDIII	(Berlin Druckrey III)	FNL	
BDIV	(Berlin Druckrey IV)	F344	(Fischer 344)
BDV	(Berlin Druckrey V)	F6R	
BDVI	(Berlin Druckrey VI)	G	(CPB-G)
BDVII	(Berlin Druckrey VII)	GEPR/3	
BDVIII	(Berlin Druckrey VIII)	GH	(Genetic hypertension)
BDIX	(Berlin Druckrey IX)	GHA	
BDX	(Berlin Druckrey X)	GK	
BEG		HCS	(Harvard caries susceptible)

Abbreviation	Description
HMT	
HS	
IIM	
INR	(Iowa nonreactive)
IR	(Iowa reactive)
IS	
JC	
K	
KDP	
KGH	
KIRBY	
KX	
KYN	(Kyoto notched)
LA	
LE	(Long Evans)
LEA	
LEC	
LEJ	
LEM	
LEO	
LEP	(Long Evans Praha)
LER	(Lewis resistant)
LET	
LETL	
LEW	(Lewis)
LH	(Lyon hypertensive)
LIH	(Liverpool hooded)
LIS	(Lister hooded)
LL	(Lyon low blood pressure)
LN	(Lyon normotensive)
LOU	(Louvain)
LUDW	
MAXX	
MHS	(Milano hypertensive)
MLCS	
MNR	(Maudsley nonreactive)
MNRA	
MNS	(Milano normotensive)
MR	(Maudsley reactive)
MSUBL	
MW	
MWF	(Munich Wistar Froemter)
M14	
M17	
M520	(Marshall 520)
NBL	(Noble or Nb)
NBR	(NIH black)
NEDH	(Slonaker)
NER	
NIG-III	
NSD	
NZR	
ODU	
OKA	
OLETF	
OM	(Osborne-Mendel)
OXYR	
OXYS	
PA	
PAR	
PETH	
PVG	(King albino)
P77PMC	
R	(HO)
RCS	
RHA	
RII/1	
RLA	
RP	
S5B	
SBH	
SBN	
SC	
SD	
SDJ	
SDNK	
SEL	(Selfed 36670)
SHHF	
SHR	(Okamoto hypertensive)
SHRSP	
SPRD	
SR	(Dahl R)
SS	(Dahl S)
TA	
TE	
TF	
THA	
THE	
TLE	
TM	
TMB	(Tryon maze bright or Berkeley S1)
TMD	(Tryon maze dull or Berkeley S3)
TO	(Tokyo)
TOM	
TS1	

TS3		WKA	(Wistar King A)
TT		WKAH	
TU		WKAM	
TW		WKHA	
TX		WKHT	
U		WKS	
W		WKY	(Wistar Kyoto)
WA		WKYO	
WAB	(Wistar albino Boots)	WM	
WAG	(Wistar albino Glaxo)	WMS	
WBB		WN	
WBN		WOKA	
WCF		WR	
WDF		WST	
WE	(CPB-WE)	YA	
WEC		YO	
WEK	(WEchoc)	Y59	
WELS		ZDF	
WF	(Wistar Furth)	ZI	(Zitter)
WIN		Z61	(Zimmerman)
WIST	(Wistar)		

The data have been collected from the literature and databases (Festing, 1979; Greenhouse et al., 1990). For further information on strains as well as sources see

http://www.informatics.jax.org/bin/strains/search
http://www.mh-hannover.de/institut/tierlabor/genearchiv.htm
http://www2.nas.edu/amgs/rats.html

markers are listed in Appendix 1, separately for each chromosome. Specific disease genes or genetic disorders are:

- on chromosome 1 (RNO1): blood pressure, *Bpfb1*; collagen-induced arthritis, *Cia2*; rat haematoma, *be*; ichthyosis, *Ic*, noninsulin-dependent diabetes mellitus QTLs, *Nidd/gk1* and *Niddm1*; renal disease susceptibility QTLs, *Rf1* and *Rf2*; warfarin resistance, *Rw*; tail anomaly lethal, *Tal2*; thymus enlargement gene, *Ten1*

- on RNO2: several blood pressure controlling QTLs; mammary carcinoma susceptibility QTL, *Mcs1*; noninsulin-dependent diabetes mellitus QTLs, *Nidd/gk2* and *Niddm2*

- on RNO3: diabetes insipidus, *Avp* (*di*); blood pressure QTLs, *Bp15*, *Bp20* and *Bp37*; retinal dystrophy, *rdy*; tubular basement membrane antigen, *Tbm2*; Wilm's tumour, *wt1*; zitter, *zi*;

- on RNO4: blood pressure QTLs, *Bp21*, *Bp33*;

collagen-induced arthritis, *Cia3*; insulin-dependent diabetes mellitus, *Iddm1*, identical with lymphopenia, *Lyp* (*l*); lipid level QTL, *Lil2*; noninsulin-dependent diabetes mellitus QTL, *Nidd/gk3*; alloreactivity, *Nka*; oil-induced arthritis QTLs, *Oia2*, *Oia3*; sensitivity to stroke QTL, *Str3*

- on RNO5: blood pressure QTLs, *Bp7*, *Bp49*; obesity (fatty/corpulent), *fa*; hypodactyly, *Hd*; jerker (deafness) *je*; leptin receptor (fatty), *Lepr*; NIDDM, *Nidd/gk4*; incisorless, *in*; sensitivity to stroke QTL, *Str2*

- on RNO7: blood pressure QTL, *Bp38*; collagen-induced arthritis QTL, *Cia4*; mammary carcinoma susceptibility QTL, *Mcs2*

- on RNO8: blood pressure QTLs, *Bp22*, *Bp35*, *Bp39*; polydactyly-luxate syndrome, *Lx*; mammary carcinoma susceptibility QTL, *Mcs4*; mixed-lineage leukaemia, *Mll*; noninsulin-dependent diabetes mellitus QTL, *Nidd/gk5*

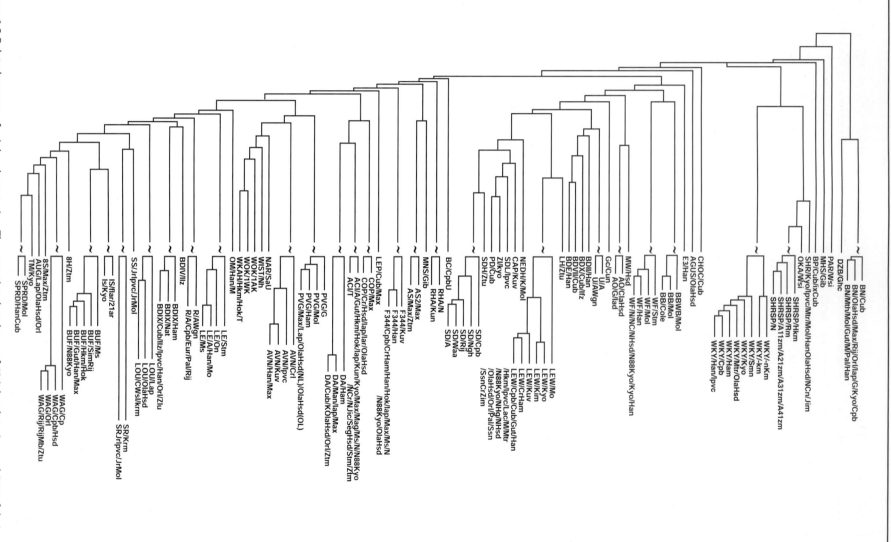

Figure 1.3 Relatedness tree for inbred rat strains. The genetic relatedness of 63 inbred strains and 214 of their substrains are shown. Reprinted with kind permission of the author and publisher.

strain is characterized by a very high incidence (>90%) of endometrial carcinomas (Deerberg and Kaspareit, 1987), arising in virgin females. The Eker rat on the other hand is an interesting model of renal cancer. It carries a known insertional mutation (Tsc2) that, in the heterozygous state, is associated with spontaneous renal cell carcinoma, uterine leiomyoma, and haemangiomas, while in the homozygous state the mutation acts as an embryonic lethal. Other important research fields that have successfully made use of specific characters of certain rat strains are psychobiology, neurophysiology and neuroendocrinology. Studies on autoimmune diseases and induced complex diseases, including many neurodegenerative diseases, have made extensive use of inbred rat strains. Apart from the strain used and whether it is susceptible or resistant, the inducing agent also plays an important role (Table 1.5).

The analysis of polymorphic genetic variables that affect biological functions depends on the availability of inbred and in particular of congenic or consomic strains. The use of this type of strain has increased in biomedical research in recent years mainly in conjunction with the identification of genes (quantitative trait loci, QTL) involved in multifactorial diseases. Since congenic strains differ only in a short chromosomal segment from their background strain, it is possible to investigate the phenotypic effect of this differential locus isolated from distracting effects caused by other loci of the genetic background. On the other hand it is also possible to determine whether background effects modify gene function, and if so, the nature of these effects. These approaches have played an important role in experimental immunology and in transplantation biology for decades. The same approach is also being used to verify the function of specific alleles or of transgenes, e.g. in hypertension research, where several groups have developed congenic and consomic strains, either with a single differentiating locus affecting blood pressure, respectively with a putative hypertension modifying locus, or several loci on a large chromosomal region (Pravenec and Rapp, personal communication).

In order to further promote the rat as a tool for biomedical research, it is crucial that specific tools are developed to genetically modify rats in the same manner as is now possible in the mouse. A particularly cogent research application of the rat will definitely be the study of QTLs in a variety of diseases. The first few decades of the twenty-first

- on RNO10: several blood pressure QTLs; collagen-induced arthritis, *Cia5*; collagen-induced antibody, *Ciaa2*; athymic nude (HNF-3/forkhead homologue 11; winged helix), *Hfh11* (*whn*); NIDDM, *Niddm3*; polycystic kidney disease, *Pkd1*; tremor, *tw*; tuberous sclerosis (renal carcinoma), *Tsc2*
- on RNO12: breast cancer, *Brca2*; ; noninsulin-dependent diabetes mellitus QTL, *Niddm5*
- on RNO13: several blood pressure QTLs; thymus enlargement gene, *Ten2*
- on RNO14: noninsulin-dependent diabetes mellitus QTL (OLETF), *Dmo3*; noninsulin-dependent diabetes mellitus QTL (OLETF), *Odb2*
- on RNO16: blood pressure QTL, *Bp23*, *Bp40*
- on RNO17: blood pressure QTL, *Bp8*; demyelination, *dmy*
- on RNO18: several blood pressure QTLs
- on RNO19: blood pressure QTL, *Bp32*; lipid level QTL, *Lil1*
- on RNO20: aurothiopropanolsulphonate-induced autoimmune glomerulonephritis, *Atps1*; collagen-induced arthritis, *Cia1*; dwarfism, *dw3*; fertility, *ft*; insulin-dependent diabetes mellitus (MHC-associated), *Iddm2*; oil-induced arthritis, *Oia1*; resistance to chemical carcinogenesis, *Rcc*
- on RNOX: blood pressure QTL, *Bp3*; noninsulin-dependent diabetes mellitus QTL, (OLETF), *Obd1*; testicular feminization, *Tfm*.

This impressive list of polymorphic genes further demonstrates the value of the laboratory rat as an important experimental animal model. Aside from these single locus effects, which may be modified by the genetic background, quite a number of rat strains are self-functioning as spontaneous complex disease models, and thus provide valuable insights into the pathogenesis of disease (see Table 1.4). For cardiovascular diseases several inbred strains or sets of strains are available, with SHR and SHRSP being known most widely. Actually, the same holds true for metabolic disorders, like IDDM, NIDDM, metabolic X syndrome, familial dyslipidaemic hypertension, disorders of glucose and fatty acid metabolism. In cancer research, several rat strains have proven valuable in various studies, particularly with respect to precancerous lesions. While F 344 rats develop spontaneous leukaemia and prostate cancers, Sprague-Dawley derived strains, like SPRD-*Cu3*, develop mammary tumours spontaneously at a high rate and with almost 100% within 60 days when given dimethyl benzanthracene (DMBA). The BDII

Table 1.4 Selected spontaneous complex disease models

Disease type	Susceptible strains	Control strains
Hypertension	SHR	WKY
	SS	SR
	DSS	
	LH	
	MHS	LN, LL
	FHH	MNS
	GH	FHL
	SBH	SBN
	TGR(mRen2)27	
Stroke	SHRSP	
Metabolic disorders		
IDDM	BBDP	BBDR
	LETL	
	LEW.1AR1-*Iddm*	
NIDDM	GK	
	OLETF	
	BHE/cdb	
	CRDH	
	SHHF	
Behavioural and neurological disorders	MR	MNR
	RHA	RLA
	ZI	
	GEPR/3	
	WF/Ztm	
Spontaneous tumours	BUF/Mha	
	BDII	
	Eker rat	
Arthritis	TgN(HLA-B27 hB2m)	
Wilson's disease	LEC	

century are likely to be dominated by assigning function to the complete genomic sequence, particularly with respect to those regions involved in common human diseases. While the paradigm for ascribing function to the genome is not well defined, it is clear that investigators will use comparative mapping strategies and multiple species platforms to accomplish this goal. Toward this end, the rat offers the best 'functionally' characterized mammalian model system.

Table 1.5 Induced complex diseases

Autoimmune disease	Rat strains		Inducing agent
	Susceptible	Resistant	
Adjuvant arthritis	DA, LEW	WF	CFA
Oil-induced arthritis (OIA)	DA	LEW.1A	Oil
Avridine-induced arthritis[a]	DA, LEW	E3	Avridine
Collagen-induced arthritis (CIA)[b]	BB, DA	F344	Collagen type II
Experimental immune glomerulonephritis (EAG)[c]	BN, PVG	LEW, WAG	GBM
Autoimmune complex nephritis (AIC)	LEW	BN	Tubulus antigen
Autoimmune tubulointerstitial nephritis	BN	LEW	TBM
Systemic autoimmunity glomerulonephritis	BN	LEW.1AV1	ATPS
Experimental allergic encephalomyelitis (EAE)	LEW	BN	MBP
Chronic relapsing EAE (CREAE)[d]	DA		MOG
Experimental autoimmune myasthenia gravis[e]	F344	COP, WF	AChR
Experimental allergic neuritis (EAN)[f]	LEW		MBP (PNS)
Experimental autoimmune uveitis (EAU)[g]	LEW	TO	IRBP, S-Ag

[a] Vingsbo et al. (1995).
[b] Breban et al. (1993); Knoerzer et al. (1997).
[c] Pusey et al. (1991).
[d] Lorentzen et al. (1995).
[e] Biesecker et al. (1988).
[f] Brosnan et al. (1988).
[g] Sasamoto et al. (1994).

References

Andoh, Y., Kuramoto, T., Yokoi, N., Maihara, T., Kitada, K. and Serikawa, T. (1998) *Mamm. Genome* **9**, 287–293.

Bazin, H. (1988) *Rat News Lett.* **20**, 14.

Bender, K., Adams, M., Baverstock, P.R. *et al.* (1984) *Immunogenetics* **19**, 257–266.

Bender, K., Balogh, P., Bertrand, M.F. *et al.* (1994) *J. Exp. Anim. Sci.* **36**, 151–165.

Biesecker, G. and Koffler, D. (1988) *J. Immunol.* **140**, 3406–3410.

Bihoreau, M.T., Gaugier, D., Kato, N. *et al.* (1997) *Genome Res.* **7**, 434–440.

Billingham, R.E. and Silvers, W.K. (1959) *Transplant. Bull.* **6**, 399–406.

Breban, M.A., Moreau, M.C., Fournier, C., Ducluzeau, R. and Kahn, M.F. (1993). *J. Clin. Exp. Rheumatol.* **11**, 61–64.

Brosnan, J.V., King, R.H., Thomas, P.K. and Craggs, R.I. (1988) *J. Neurol. Sci.* **88**, 261–276.

Brown, D.M., Matise, T.C., Koike, G., *et al.* (1998) *Mamm. Genome* **9**, 521–530.

Canzian, F. (1997) *Genome Res.* **7**, 262–267.

Castle, W.E. (1947) *Proc. Natl Acad. Sci. USA* **33**, 109–117.

Crampe, H. (1877) *Landwirtsch. Jahrb.* **6**, 385–395.

Crampe, H. (1883) *Landwirtsch. Jahrb.* **12**, 389–449.

Crampe, H. (1884) *Landwirtsch. Jahrb.* **13**, 699–754.

Crampe, H. (1885) *Landwirtsch. Jahrb.* **14**, 539–619.

Deerberg, F. and Kaspareit, J. (1987) *J. Natl Cancer Inst.* **78**, 1245–1250.

Festing, M.F.W. (1979) *Inbred Strains in Biomedical Research.* London: Macmillan Press.

Festing, M.F. and Bender, K. (1984) *Genet. Res.* **44:3**, 271–281.

Festing, M.F.W. and Staats, J. (1973) *Transplantation* **16**, 221–245.

Gesner, C. (1669) *Thier-Buch* (partial edition of *Historiae animalium* in German), reprinted 1980 by Schlütersche Verlagsanstalt, Hannover.

Greenhouse, D.D., Festing, M.F.W., Hasan, S. and Cohen, A.L. (1990) In: Hedrich, H.J. (ed.) *Genetic Monitoring of Inbred Strains of Rats*, pp. 410–480. Stuttgart: Gustav Fischer.

Grzimek, B. (ed.) (1968) *Enzyklopädie des Tierreiches*, Vol. 11. Zurich: Kindler Verlag.

Hedrich, H.J. (ed.) (1990) *Genetic Monitoring of Inbred Strains of Rats.* Stuttgart: Gustav Fischer.

ILAR Committee on Rat Nomenclature (1992) *ILAR News* **34**: 7–24.

Jacob, H.J., Brown, D.M., Bunker, R.K. *et al.* (1995) *Nature Genet.* **9**, 63–69.

King, H.D. (1918a) *J. Exp. Zool.* **26**, 1–54.

King, H.D. (1918b) *J. Exp. Zool.* **26**, 335–378.

King, H.D. (1918c) *J. Exp. Zool.* **27**, 1–35.

King, H.D. (1919) *J. Exp. Zool.* **29**, 135–175.

Knoerzer, D.B., Donovan, M.G., Schwartz, B.D. and Mengle-Gaw, L.J. (1997) *J. Toxicol. Pathol.* **25**, 13–19.

Lantz, D.E. (1909) *US Dept of Agriculture, Biol. Survey, Bull.* **33**, 9–54.

Lindsey, J.R (1979) In: Baker, H.J., Lindsey, J.R. and Weisbroth, S.H. (eds) *The Laboratory Rat,* Vol. 1, pp. 1–36. New York: Academic Press.

Lorentzen, J.C., Issazadeh, S., Storch, M. *et al.* (1995) *J. Neuroimmunol.* **63**, 193–205.

McCay, C.M. (1973) In: Verzár, F. (ed) *Notes on the History of Nutrition Research,* p. 109. Berne: Hans Huber.

Meng, J., Wyss, A.R., Dawson, M.R. and Zhai, R. (1994) *Nature* **370**, 134–136.

Philipeaux (1856) *C. R. Hebd. Séances Acad. Sci.* **43**, 904–906.

Pravenec, M., Gauguier, D., Schott, J.J. *et al.* (1996) *Mamm. Genome* **7**, 117–127.

Pusey, C.D., Holland, M.J., Cashman, S.J. *et al.* (1991) *J. Nephrol. Dial. Transplant.* **6**, 457–465.

Rat Chromosome Committee (1999) *J. Exp. Anim. Sci.* 1/2.

Richter, C.P. (1954) *J. Natl Cancer Inst.* **15**, 727–738.

Sasamoto, Y., Kotake, S., Yoshikawa, K., Wiggert, B., Gery, I. and Matsuda, H. (1994) *J. Curr. Eye Res.* **13**, 845–849.

Savory, W.S. (1863) *Lancet* **2**, 381–383.

Silver, J. (1941) *Wildlife Circ.* **6**, 1–18.

Southern, H.N. (1964) *The Handbook of British Mammals.* Oxford: Blackwell Scientific.

Szpirer C., Szpirer, J., van Vooren, P. *et al.* (1998) *Mamm. Genome* **9**, 721–734.

Tate, G.H.H. (1936) *Bull. Am. Museum Nat. Hist.* **72**, 501–728.

Vingsbo, C., Jonsson, R. and Holmdahl, R. (1995) *J. Clin. Exp. Immunol.* **99**, 359–363.

Walder, R.Y., Garrett, M.R., McClain, A.M. *et al.* (1998) *Mamm. Genome* **9**, 1013–1021.

Yoshida, T.H. (1980) *Cytogenetics of the Black Rat.* Tokyo: University of Tokyo Press.

CHAPTER 2

National and International Guidelines for the Conduct of Chemical Safety Studies: Choice of Strains

Mamoru Mutai
Toxicology Laboratory, Yokohama Research Center,
Mitsubishi Chemical Corporation, Yokohama, Japan

The Rat as an Experimental Animal in Chemical Safety Studies

Chemical safety studies are performed in order to assess the risk posed by certain chemicals to humans and the environment. These chemicals include medical drugs, agricultural chemicals, food additives and a diversity of other synthetic or naturally occurring substances, which sometimes include not only end-use products but also raw materials or synthetic intermediates. Most of the regulatory authorities in developed countries require safety studies to be conducted as far as the manufacturing stage so as to predict any safety problems with the new product.

Various *in vitro* and *in vivo* testing methods have been established as part of such safety studies. In

Table 2.1 Major chemical safety studies using rats

Acute toxicity study

Subacute (synonymous with subchronic) toxicity study

Chronic toxicity study

Reproductive and developmental toxicity studies (including teratogenicity study)

Carcinogenicity (synonymous with oncogenicity or tumorigenicity) study

Neurotoxicity study

Mutagenicity (synonymous with genotoxicity) studies

Metabolism (pharmacokinetic/toxicokinetic) studies

Pharmacological studies

order to standardize the experimental design and criteria for the choice of studies, most safety studies submitted to the regulatory authorities are subject to the requirements of test guidelines together with the requirements of Good Laboratory Practice (GLP) regulations.

Historically, rats have been used in the area of medical science and experimental biology, and are well known to be sensitive to a number of toxicants. Thus, the rat is the principal mammalian species recommended in the guidelines of *in vivo* chemical safety studies listed in Table 2.1.

Those safety studies using mammalian species are intended to reproduce the situation in which a test agent will be exposed to humans. Thus, they are required to assess the multiple endpoints, such as observations of behavior, body weight, food and water intake, blood and urine analysis as well as histopathology for the assessment of the test agent.

In consideration of the above, rats have the following strong advantages. They can be easily handled with practice. They are relatively small in size but 8–10 times larger than the mouse, which allow them to be treated with a test article via a variety of routes such as gavage, mixed in the diet, intravenous, subcutaneous as well as intraperitoneal. Small amounts of blood can be repeatedly withdrawn with ease, and surgical operations for obtaining blood and other body fluids, and to remove small organs, such as pituitaries and adrenals at necropsy are not a problem. Rats can be housed in large numbers in a restricted animal room, and they breed easily and continuously during their normal reproductive lifespan. The latter is not only an advantage for obtaining and maintaining an economical supply of the animals but is also useful for the safety assessment of chemicals on their reproductive performance.

However, the results of these safety studies are frequently complicated by various factors such as species differences in sensitivity between the experimental animal and humans, which may result in differences in anatomical, physiological, reproductive and behavioral features. Together with the latter knowledge of exposure/metabolism differences as well as data from *in vitro* experiments, toxicologists can evaluate the data from chemical safety studies, and extrapolate these results to humans with care in their interpretation.

Guidelines for Chemical Safety Studies Using Rats

International Guidelines

There are two major international guidelines for chemical safety studies. The *OECD Guidelines for Testing of Chemicals* provide procedures for the laboratory testing of health effects (chemical safety studies), as well as physico-chemical properties, effects on biotic systems (ecotoxicology) and degradation/accumulation. Table 2.2 shows the list of major OECD guidelines for *in vivo* safety studies featuring the use of rats. Since the OECD guidelines cover all industrial chemicals, most of the chemical safety studies that are generally used in the OECD member countries are included in these guidelines. Most of these guidelines became effective in 1981

Table 2.2 Major OECD testing guidelines recommending the use of rats

Guideline number	Title
401	Acute Oral Toxicity
402	Acute Dermal Toxicity
403	Acute Inhalation Toxicity
407	Repeated Dose Oral Toxicity – Rodent: 28/14-day
408	Subchronic Oral Toxicity – Rodent: 90-day
410	Repeated Dose Dermal Toxicity: 21/28-day
411	Subchronic Dermal Toxicity: 90-day
412	Repeated Dose Inhalation Toxicity: 28/14-day
413	Subchronic Inhalation Toxicity: 90-day
414	Teratogenicity
415	One-generation Reproduction Toxicity
416	Two-generation Reproduction Toxicity
417	Toxicokinetics
424	Neurotoxicity Study in Rodents
451	Carcinogenicity Studies
452	Chronic Toxicity Studies
453	Combined Chronic Toxicity/Carcinogenicity Studies
474	Mammalian Erythrocyte Micronucleus Test
486	Unscheduled DNA Synthesis (UDS) Test with Mammalian Liver Cells *In Vivo*

and additions or changes have been made when necessary.

In the pharmaceutical industry, the respective regulatory authorities and industries in Japan, the European Union and the USA organized the International Conference on Harmonization of Technical Requirements for Registration of Pharmaceuticals for Human Use (ICH). These six parties discussed ways in which to harmonize the requirements for registration in these areas. Most of the harmonized tripartite guideline documents regarding safety studies were published in 1997. Table 2.3 shows those ICH guidelines for safety studies using rats. They are expected to become internationally effective for registration of new pharmaceuticals in other countries and regions.

Table 2.4 lists their fields and the corresponding regulatory authorities. Among these national guidelines, the guideline for toxicity studies on drugs was first established in 1984 by the Ministry of Health and Welfare (MHW). Additions or revisions have been made when necessary. Studies using rats are also the major component of safety assessments in these national guidelines.

Their recommendations for testing standards are either directly based on or carefully coordinated with the OECD guidelines. Thus, foreign data generated under the OECD guidelines are considered acceptable by the Japanese authorities for the submission/registration of new chemical products.

In pharmaceuticals, official translations of the ICH harmonized guidelines are successively published by the MHW and become effective immediately. Thus, for a transition period these ICH guidelines will coexist with the existing MHW guidelines. In order to unify the comprehensive national guideline that introduces the ICH recommendations, the MHW will publish the fully revised guidelines in 1999.

National Guidelines in Japan

In Japan, the two international guidelines above are effective and widely used in the corresponding chemical classes. In addition, Japan has seven national guidelines for chemical safety studies.

Table 2.3 ICH harmonized tripartite guidelines regarding safety topics (finalized)

Title	ICH topic code
Guideline on the Need for Carcinogenicity Studies of Pharmaceuticals	S1A
Testing for Carcinogenicity of Pharmaceuticals	S1B
Dose Selection for Carcinogenicity Studies of Pharmaceuticals	S1C
Addendum to "Guideline on Dose Selection for Carcinogenicity Studies of Pharmaceuticals": Addition of a Limit Dose and Related Notes	S1C/R
Guidance on Specific Aspects of Regulatory Genotoxicity Tests for Pharmaceuticals	S2A
Genotoxicity: A Standard Battery for Genotoxicity Testing of Pharmaceuticals	S2B
Note for Guidance on Toxicokinetics: the Assessment of Systemic Exposure in Toxicity Studies	S3A
Pharmacokinetics: Guidance for Repeated Dose Tissue Distribution Studies	S3B
Detection of Toxicity to Reproduction for Medicinal Products	S5A
An Addendum on Toxicity to Male Fertility: An Addendum to the ICH Tripartite Guideline on Detection of Toxicity to Reproduction for Medical Products	S5B
Preclinical: Safety Evaluation of Biotechnology-derived Products	S6
Guideline for the Timing of Non-clinical Safety Studies for the Conduct of Human Clinical Trial for Pharmaceuticals	M3

Table 2.4 Japanese national guidelines for chemical safety studies

Effective fields	Corresponding authority	Year established or revised
Pharmaceuticals	MHW	Revised 1993
Food additives	MHW	Revised 1996
Animal drugs	MAFF	1988
Feed additives	MAFF	1992
Agricultural chemicals	MAFF	1985 (will be revised at 1999)
Industrial chemicals	MHW	1986 and 1987
Labor's hygiene	ML	1988

MHW, Ministry of Health and Welfare; MAFF, Ministry of Agriculture, Forestry and Fishery; ML, Ministry of Labor.

General Recommendations for Safety Studies in the Guidelines

Route of Exposure

The route of treatment is to be selected based on the expected human exposure, whenever possible. The most common routes are oral. These include gavage treatment using a gastric tube and the dietary route where the test agent is mixed in with the diet. In case of pharmaceuticals, the use of the respective clinical route (oral, intravenous, intramuscular or subcutaneous, etc.) is recommended by the regulatory authorities. For environmental chemicals where there is a chance of exposure by other routes, inhalation or dermal routes are also recommended as secondary routes for acute and/or subacute toxicity studies.

Age of the Rats

Recommendations regarding the age of rats do not differ between these guidelines. For acute toxicity studies, so-called young or young adult rats, up to approximately 8 weeks old, are usually recommended. Since prolonged experiments are required in subacute and chronic toxicity studies as well as carcinogenicity studies, starting the test chemical treatment from the age following weaning up to 6 weeks old is preferred. However, the guidelines for dermal route studies indicate a body weight range of 200–300 g as an alternative to these age recommendations in order to provide an adequate body surface area.

For reproductive and developmental toxicity studies, the age of the rats depends on the study design. In principle, the animals should be at the reproductive age i.e. at the beginning of mating.

Choice of Studies

The strategy needed for each safety study is reflected in the chemical class concerned and mode of human exposure, and differs between the guidelines. For pharmaceuticals, the ICH M3 guideline defines the timing and the type of safety studies required.

Acute studies and data from safety pharmacology and toxicokinetic/pharmacokinetic experiments are generally required for all pharmaceuticals before human clinical trials are started. The length required for subacute and chronic toxicity studies depends on the duration of treatment in the clinical trials. On the other hand, the need for reproductive and developmental toxicity studies depends on the patient population to be exposed or cause for concern resulting from other toxicity studies.

In the case of carcinogenicity studies, the ICH issued a harmonized tripartite guideline 'Guideline on the Need for Carcinogenicity Studies of Pharmaceuticals (S1A)' in 1995. This states that all pharmaceuticals that will be continuously administered over a substantial period of time (six months or more) are generally required to have their carcinogenicity assessed before submission to the regulatory authorities. In addition, those agents where carcinogenicity is suspected either from their chemical structure, their pharmacological effects or from other toxicity studies are also required to assess their carcinogenic potential.

For agricultural chemicals most of the safety studies listed in the guidelines are required to be carried out. However, in the case of agricultural chemicals for nonedible crops, assessment of chronic toxicity, reproductive and developmental toxicity (except for teratogenicity) and carcinogenicity studies are not generally required.

For animal drugs, feed additives as well as food additives, the Japanese Ministry of Agriculture, Forestry and Fishery (MAFF) and MHW have listed the same safety studies as for other chemical classes in their guidelines. In practical use, which safety studies should be conducted is decided on a case-by-case approach. Clearly the most important issue for safety assessment of these chemicals for domestic animals is whether there is any residue of the chemicals or their derivatives in meat, milk or eggs, as most food additives are digested in the alimentary canal.

In the guideline for industrial chemicals issued by the MHW, screening toxicity tests including the 28-day repeated dose oral toxicity study in rats, two in vitro mutagenicity studies as well as ecotoxicity studies, are recommended to be carried out first. When the results of these studies suggest a certain toxicity, mutagenic potential, nonbiodegradability or a high degree of bioaccumulation, then the expanded safety assessments are required. These assessments include chronic toxicity studies, reproductive and developmental toxicity studies, carcinogenicity studies as well as metabolic and pharmacological studies. These evaluation procedures are also advised in the Minimum Premarketing Sets of Data issued by the OECD in 1983.

Choice of Strains

Acute, subacute and chronic toxicity studies

The choice of strain to be used in acute, subacute and chronic toxicity studies is made on the basis of a knowledge of the lifespan, spontaneous disease rates as well as any sensitivity to known toxic substances. Acute toxicity studies in rats are usually performed in strains that are bred and maintained in closed colonies, like the Sprague-Dawley or Wistar strains. Subacute and chronic toxicity studies as well as acute toxicity studies are sometimes considered for inclusion in a series of experiments in order to evaluate the 'general toxicity' of test agents. Thus, some guidelines recommend using the same species in these studies.

In Japan, the most common rat strain used in these studies is the Sprague-Dawley. The Wistar rat is also used by those restricted facilities which maintain the historical background data for this strain. For pharmaceuticals, the selection of the strain sometimes depends on the strain used in the experiments that supported the efficacy of those particular pharmaceuticals. In the case of agricultural chemicals, a chronic toxicity study is often combined with a carcinogenicity study. The Fischer rat is the major strain for carcinogenicity studies in Japanese facilities. Thus in series of subacute to chronic toxicity and carcinogenicity studies on agricultural chemicals, the Fischer rat is usually the rat of choice in Japan.

Reproductive and developmental toxicity studies

The strain used in reproductive and developmental toxicity studies is selected following consideration of its reproductive performance, such as fertility, rate of spontaneous malformation, and sensitivity to known toxicants. The guidelines recommend that the preliminary and main study should be done on the same strain of animal. In the ICH guideline for medical drugs, reproductive and developmental toxicity studies are usually divided into three series of studies, which include the male and female fertility study, the embryo–fetal study and the pre- and postnatal development study. In this case, the same strain is recommended for use throughout the series.

In Japan, the most popular strains for use in reproductive and developmental toxicity studies are the Sprague-Dawley and the Wistar, for both of which there exist abundant historical background data on reproduction and fetal development. Their high pregnancy rate and the number of fetuses per litter are considered appropriate for assessing the effects of test agents.

Carcinogenicity studies

Carcinogenicity studies are the most long-term experiments among those safety studies using rats. Almost all guidelines for these studies recommend selecting the strain in relation to a long lifespan, the known spontaneous tumor rate, as well as the sensitivity to known carcinogens. In general, Sprague-Dawley and Wistar rats have become the common strains in the US industries and European countries, respectively (Weatherholtz, 1997). Experimental research by the US governments tends to favor Fischer rats (Solleveld et al., 1984).

In Japan, the favored strain for carcinogenicity studies is the Fischer rat. This might be related to the fact that the procedures and knowledge for carcinogenicity studies were introduced from the US national institutes. Thus, the historical background data for carcinogenicity studies in Japanese facilities consist of those of the Fischer rat; those of the Wistar and the Sprague-Dawley rats are limited. However, a survey of carcinogenicity studies carried out in Japanese pharmaceutical companies suggests that the Fischer rat and the Sprague-Dawley may be used equally (Mutai et al., 1998). This is because half of these studies were conducted by laboratories in the EU or the USA as contract research for Japanese companies or were incorporated from other foreign companies. These data suggest that the preference for the Fischer rat in Japanese facilities may be based on the availability of historical background data alone. The above survey also suggests that there is no disadvantage in using other strains, i.e. the Sprague-Dawley and the Wistar rats, for application to and registration with the Japanese authorities.

Other studies

For neurotoxicity studies, Sprague-Dawley rats are generally considered preferable. Pharmacological and pharmacokinetic/toxicokinetic studies are usually performed using strains derived from closed colonies. The results of these studies are sometimes evaluated together with the results from acute, subacute or chronic toxicity studies. Thus, the use of the same strain, which has already been used in these toxicity studies, is desirable.

Outlines of the Various Safety Studies

Acute Toxicity Studies

Acute studies are conducted in order to clarify any adverse effects immediately after exposure to test agents. Often, these studies provide the first information for characterizing any such toxicity. Most of the studies consist of an exposure to the test agent during a restricted short period and a subsequent observation period.

The duration of exposure can be defined as a single dose of the test agent or as multiple or continuous doses given within 24 hours. To examine lethal and toxic symptoms and their reversibility, careful cage-side observations are required immediately after dosing and at subsequent appropriate times during the recovery period of 14 days. In order to clarify the dose–response relationship, several lethal doses between the approximately 100% lethal dose and the nonlethal dose are included.

Endpoints of acute toxicity studies in rodents are lethality, measurement of body weight, cage-side observation as well as necropsy. Histopathological examinations are also performed if necessary.

As an index of lethality, calculated values of 50% of the lethal dose or concentration (LD_{50} or LC_{50}) have been widely accepted. Historically, the establishment of LD_{50} values using large number of animals (i.e. 10 animals/group/sex) was the endpoint for acute studies. However, doubts about the reproducibility of LD_{50} values have been expressed by an international corroborative study (Hunter *et al.*, 1979; Zbinden and Flury-Roversi, 1981) and the use of large numbers of animals has been criticized by animal welfare groups. Exact LD_{50} determination is no longer recommended by any authorities. As an alternative, rough estimates of LD_{50} values or the approximate lethal dose (ALD) using small numbers of animals (usually five animal/group/sex) is currently adopted. Some improved methods for acute toxicity studies such as the 'fixed dose method' and 'toxic class method' have been issued by the OECD (Guidelines 420 and 423, respectively). Additionally, several guidelines have set the upper dose limit as 2000 mg/kg for oral or subcutaneous routes and 5 mg/L for the inhalation route.

Lethal dose values are often used for categorizing chemicals with regard to their 'toxicological hazard classification'. These classifications define the relative toxicity of the chemicals as shown in Table 2.5

Table 2.5 Toxic hazard classification of acute toxicity

Japan[a]	US-EPA[b]
Toxic substance	Danger
Oral LD_{50} <30 mg/kg	Oral LD_{50} <50 mg/kg
Dermal LD_{50} <100 mg/kg	Dermal LD_{50} <200 mg/kg
Inhalation LC_{50} <200 ppm (1 h)	Inhalation LC_{50} <0.05 mg/L
Deleterious substance	Warning
Oral LD_{50} 30–300 mg/kg	Oral LD_{50} 50–500 mg/kg
Dermal LD_{50} 100–1000 mg/kg	Dermal LD_{50} 200–2000 mg/kg
Inhalation LC_{50} 200–2000 ppm (1 h)	Inhalation LC_{50} 0.05–0.5 mg/L
	Caution
	Oral LD_{50} 500–5000 mg/kg
	Dermal LD_{50} 2000–5000 mg/kg
	Inhalation LC_{50} 0.5–5.0 mg/L

[a] Toxic and Deleterious Substance Control Law, Japanese MHW.
[b] Data requirements for pesticide registration, US Environmental Protection Agency.

and are used for product labeling or preparing the precautions such as the Material Safety Data Sheet (MSDS). Data from acute studies are also necessary for selection of dose levels for subsequent subacute studies.

Subacute and Chronic Toxicity Studies

Subacute (2–13 weeks) and chronic (26–104 weeks) toxicity studies are carried out to clarify the toxicity of a test agent by continuous exposure, and to provide basic information on the target organs. In addition, the establishment of the no observable effect level (NOEL) or the no observable adverse effect level (NOAEL), is required in these studies. These important concepts, the NOEL/NOAEL, are designed to define the dose level which produces no biologically (adverse) significant differences between the group of chemically exposed animals and the unexposed control group.

In these toxicity studies, a 2- or 4-week recovery period is commonly included in the study design in order to investigate the reversibility of any toxic effects.

At least three dose levels and a control group of both sexes are recommended. Ideally, the highest dose level should be selected to produce clear evidence of toxicity without lethality. The lowest dose is intended to exhibit no toxic signs and to establish the NOEL or the NOAEL. Thus, the middle doses are selected to produce slight or minimal signs of toxicity with a dose–response relationship. The number of rats to be subjected to these studies differs between the guidelines, and depends on the duration of exposure. Most guidelines recommend a minimum of 5–10 animals/group/sex for subacute studies and 10–20 animals/group/sex for chronic toxicity studies.

The common parameters used in subacute and chronic toxicity studies are as follows: daily cage-side observation of animals; body weight and food consumption measurements; hematology, blood clinical chemistry, and urinalysis; ophthalmologic examination; gross necropsy and organ weight measurements; histopathological examination. In some cases, especially for pharmaceuticals, determination of the circulating blood level of the test agent is made using satellite animals. Other examinations, such as electrocardiograph, auditory or visual examinations, are also performed if necessary.

With these dose levels and endpoints, subacute and chronic toxicity studies can define the toxicity profile of test agents and the NOEL/NOAEL. Based on these results, safety factors or therapeutic windows for determining acceptable prolonged exposure levels to humans can be established.

Reproductive and Developmental Toxicity Studies

Reproductive and developmental toxicity consists of a wide variety of endpoints. These include effects on mating or fertility of parents, maternal or embryo–fetal toxicity, including embryo anomalies, effects on lactation and weaning, the growth and development of pups.

The assessment of these toxicity endpoints depends on the actual conditions of exposure of humans to these chemicals. In general, people may be exposed to chemicals, including agricultural chemicals, animal drugs and food additives, continuously over their entire lifespan. For the assessment of reproductive and developmental toxicity of these chemicals, guidelines recommend multigeneration (usually two-generation) reproductive and developmental toxicity studies using rats. A two-generation study is defined as that exposing the test agent directly to the F0 generation, indirectly (via maternal placenta or milk) as well as direct exposure of the F1 generation and indirect exposure of the F2 generation. The study is usually terminated at weaning of the F2 generation. The endpoints of multigeneration studies consist of the following measurable parameters and calculated indices: the number of pups; stillbirths; live births and the presence of gross anomalies; the growth parameters and physical/behavioral abnormalities of pups; the indices of mating, pregnancy, parturition and viability of pups. From these results, the NOEL or the NOAEL dose levels are defined in each generation.

In addition to multigeneration studies, teratogenicity studies including detailed anatomical examination of embryos is also recommended. The exposure period of the test agent in teratogenicity studies is recommended to cover the major period of organogenesis (in case of rats 7–17 days of gestation) as defined by the guidelines. The endpoints of teratogenicity studies are maternal toxicity, fetal toxicity and teratogenicity parameters. The latter two include embryo–fetal death, the number of viable fetuses, and the number of corpora lutea, the ratio of fetus sex to fetus weight, external examination of fetuses, detailed anatomical examination for skeletal and soft-tissue anomalies. The establishment of the NOEL or NOAEL is also expected in the teratogenicity study.

Pharmaceuticals are usually intended for use in medical treatment over a restricted time span and are given to the patient at a therapeutic dose. Assessment of reproductive and development toxicity for pharmaceuticals is divided into three segments covering the span from before mating of parents to weaning of the offspring. The ICH harmonized tripartite guideline (S5A) defines these three segments as the study of fertility and early embryonic development to implantation, the study for effects on pre- and postnatal development including maternal function and the study for effects on embryo–fetal development. The ICH guideline also accepts single-study designs combining the fertility study and the pre- and postnatal development study into a single investigation, or two-study designs consisting of the fertility study together with the pre- and postnatal development study under certain circumstances.

In general, each guideline requires at least three dosage groups and one control in which 20 virgin young adults are subjected to reproductive and developmental toxicity studies. The high dose is required to produce minimal toxicity in the parent generation based on the data from all available studies.

Carcinogenicity Studies

Carcinogenicity studies are the largest scale safety studies, consisting of not less than 50 males and 50 females for at least three dose levels and a control group. Chemical carcinogenicity is evaluated by a lifespan study using two rodent species (usually rats and mice) for chemicals to which people are likely to be exposed chronically. Historically, the rat and the mouse are the commonly used animal species for carcinogenicity studies, since the type and incidence of spontaneously occurring tumors are well documented in these species. The duration of any experiment is recommended as being not less than 24 months in rats, and between 18 and 24 months in mice.

Generally, the test agent is given via a dietary admixture. However, the gavage, subcutaneous, intravenous or inhalation routes may also be selected based on the human exposure route.

The highest dose level is selected based on the criteria of the maximum tolerated dose (MTD; Haseman, 1985). The highest dose used via the dietary route is usually limited to 5% w/w in consideration of nutritional conditions. New criteria for the upper limit dose concentration of equivalent doses of 1000 and 1500 mg/kg/day have been adopted by the OECD and the ICH, respectively. For pharmaceuticals, the new methodologies for high dose selection, such as consideration of systemic exposure of the test agent, have also been issued by the ICH.

The major endpoints of carcinogenicity studies are the incidence of benign and malignant tumors, mortality, and the cause of death in moribund animals as well as the incidence of preneoplastic lesions. To identify time-to-tumor relationships and to apply life-table analyses of tumor incidences, palpation of cutaneous or subcutaneous tissue mass is also important. In these endpoints, the histopathological examination of tissues and organs by an experienced pathologist is critical in the evaluation of carcinogenicity. The guidelines recommend examination of all tissues and organs of the control and highest dose groups and all unscheduled death animals in any group, as well as all tissue masses found in any animals.

Careful consideration should be paid to the interpretation of the results. These include the comparison of the spontaneous tumor rate, the latency of tumors, age-adjusted analysis, combination of benign and malignant tumors that have the same origin, as well as the mode of action of carcinogenesis (Haseman et al., 1984; National Toxicology Program, 1984).

Neurotoxicity Studies

Methods for the assessment of chemical neurotoxicity using mammalian species have included functional behavior, electrophysiological, biochemical or neuropathological examinations. The systematization and standardization of these examinations has progressed considerably in recent years. In the US, the Environmental Protection Agency published its guidelines for the assessment of neurotoxicity in pesticides in 1991 (US-EPA, 1991). The OECD has also established testing guideline 424 for neurotoxicity. In these two guidelines, the rat is named as the principal mammalian species.

Current Japanese guidelines do not include neurotoxicity assessment. However, the recommendations for such an assessment, equivalent to the OECD guideline, will be included in a revision of the guideline for agricultural chemicals by Japanese MAFF.

The principle of these neurotoxicity guidelines is to examine toxic effects by chemicals, based on the observation of behavior and neuropathological changes, and to clarify the dose–response relationship, reversibility, as well as NOAEL. The guidelines cover acute, subacute (28-day and 90-day) and chronic (52-week) studies using rats. The following special examinations are required in these studies: detailed clinical observations at the cage side and open-field, known as the 'functional observation battery' (FOB); quantitative motor activity assessment; and neuropathological examination in which whole-body perfusion for fixation and special staining are recommended.

Mutagenicity Studies

For mutagenicity assessment, *in vivo* studies are considered to play an important role in support of *in vitro* studies. However, rats are not clearly recommended for the mutagenicity assessment battery that is currently used in any international or Japanese national guidelines. With regard to the micronucleus test in rodents, which is a widely used *in vivo* study, the rat is an acceptable species. However, the mouse is generally recommended as a principle rodent species in the guidelines.

The OECD established the guideline for the *in vivo* unscheduled DNA synthesis (UDS) assay using rats. The ICH S2B guideline also points out the usefulness of the UDS assay using rats as a second *in vivo* study which will be chosen when any *in vitro* assay shows a positive result.

Pharmacology Studies

In Japan, pharmacological studies are required on agricultural chemicals and general industrial chemicals. For pharmaceuticals, the Japanese MHW has also issued a guideline for general pharmacology studies. Internationally, pharmacological studies are not established in the guidelines of safety studies. In the EU and the USA, 'safety pharmacology' studies should be conducted. However, the standardization of such testing recommendations has not yet been achieved. Recently, the ICH has started to discuss a guideline for safety pharmacology.

The data from pharmacological studies are useful for assessing acute toxic reactions by chemical substances, especially their functional aspects. These studies provide valuable information for the prediction and characterization of possible acute poisonings and give directions for detoxication treatment.

Japanese guidelines recommend assessing the pharmacological effects on the central nervous system, autonomic nervous system, digestive organs, skeletal muscles and blood using appropriate pharmacological testing methods. In these studies, rats are a commonly used species as well as mice and rabbits.

Metabolism/Pharmacokinetics and Toxicokinetics Studies

Metabolism/pharmacokinetics studies

The toxic reaction caused by a chemical substance is closely related to its pharmacokinetic properties. Kinetic data are indispensable in the risk assessment of chemicals. The OECD and Japanese guidelines for agricultural chemicals, animal drugs, feed additives and industrial chemicals indicate the outline of these studies. For pharmaceuticals, the Japanese MHW has established guidelines for pharmacokinetic studies.

The purpose of pharmacokinetic studies is to obtain information on the pharmacokinetics of the test agent in order to consider the mode of its toxic action and to assess the risk of testing the chemical on humans. The phases of the kinetics of a test agent and its derivatives to be assessed are its absorption, distribution, accumulation, metabolism and excretion. Suitable doses for these studies are generally lower than those used in other toxicity studies. In the case of pharmaceuticals, the doses are selected from the range of pharmacological doses.

The guidelines recommend using one or more species of mammals. This type of study requires repeated sampling of body specimens (blood, urine, feces, bile, etc.). The data are often evaluated with other toxicology studies. Thus, the rat is a very common species for use in metabolism studies.

Toxicokinetics studies

On the other hand, toxicokinetic studies are focused on the kinetics of a test agent within the toxicological dose range. These studies are conducted in order to clarify the systemic exposure of test agents, and to provide an interpretation of the toxicity findings. The ICH guideline recommends measuring the plasma concentration of the test agent or its metabolite using the satellite animals from concurrent toxicity studies.

animals and humans at a single organ, cellular or intercellular level. Ultimately, the toxicologist will need the results of *in vivo* experiments that reflect the relationship between toxic reactions and systemic exposure for the prediction of quantitative risk estimation of chemicals in relation to human health. Thus, the rat will, without doubt, maintain an important position in *in vivo* safety studies in the future.

Considerations

The rat is the most widely recommended mammalian species in *in vivo* chemical safety studies in the international and Japanese national guidelines. Movements towards the harmonization of requirements for chemical safety studies in pharmaceuticals were started in 1991 between Japan, the EU and the USA in the form of the ICH. Recent refinements of the OECD guidelines will be expected to promote international harmonization of safety testing in other chemical classes. In Japan, the revision of the guidelines for agricultural chemicals has now progressed with careful consultation as far as the OECD guidelines. This harmonization will reduce not only the total cost of new chemical product development, but also the unnecessary use of animals in safety testing.

There are some differences between the choice of rat strains between regions. However, these differences seem to be largely based on historical reasons, and are not based on the recommendations of the guidelines. Thus, these differences do not appear to be a serious barrier for introducing foreign safety data into Japan. In most cases, the most suitable strain for certain tests is scientifically inconclusive. To facilitate the common use of chemical safety study data between nations, the establishment of a uniform strain suitable for the estimation of health hazards for humans is expected as well as the harmonization of guidelines.

Recently, the examination of *in vitro* tests as replacements or additional mechanistic studies for *in vivo* experiments has been encouraged. From these results, the mechanisms for toxic reactions can often be elucidated. However, these experiments can only support an extrapolation between experimental

References

Haseman, J.K. (1985) *Fundam. Appl. Toxicol.* **5**, 66–78

Haseman, J.K, Huff, J. and Boorman, G.A. (1984) *Toxicol. Pathol.* **12**, 126–135.

Hunter, W.J., Lingk, W. and Recht, P. (1979) *Assoc. Off. Anal. Chem.* **62**, 864–873.

ICH Harmonised Tripartite Guideline (1993) Detection of toxicity to reproduction for medicinal products.

ICH Harmonised Tripartite Guideline (1995) Guidance on the need for carcinogenicity studies of pharmaceuticals.

ICH Harmonised Tripartite Guidelines (1997) In: D'Arcy, D.F. and Hannon, D.W.G. (eds) Proceedings of the Fourth International Conference on Harmonisation, Brussels, 1997. pp. 941–1066. The Queen's University of Belfast.

Mutai, M., Aoki, T., Irimura, K. *et al.* (1998) *Jpn J. Toxicol. Sci.* **23**, 341.

National Toxicology Program (NTP) (1984) *Report of the NTP Ad Hoc Panel on Chemical Carcinogenesis Testing and Evaluation*, pp. 165–280. PB-84-244565.

OECD Guideline for testing of chemicals.

Solleveld, H.A., Haseman, J.K. and McConnell, E.E. (1984) *J. Natl Cancer Inst.* **72**, 929–940.

US-EPA (US Environmental Protection Agency) (1991) *Pesticide Assessment Guidelines Subdivision F. Hazard Evaluation; Human and Domestic Animals, Neurotoxicity*. PB-91-154617.

Weatherholtz, W.M. (1997) In: Williams, P.D. and Hottendorf, G.H. (eds) *Comprehensive Toxicology*, Vol. 2, pp. 101–120. Pergamon.

Zbinden, G. and Flury-Roversi, M. (1981) *Arch. Toxicol.* **47**, 77–99.

PART 2

Housing and Maintenance

Contents

CHAPTER 3

Handling and Restraint

Robert W Kemp
Astra Zeneca, Macclesfield,
Cheshire, UK

Introduction

The laboratory rat, like its wild counterpart, is an extremely intelligent animal, probably more so than the other rodents commonly used for biomedical research. This is reflected in its behaviour and, when treated properly and sympathetically, its tolerance to handling and restraint. Although feared by many novice animal scientists and technicians, outbred rats of either sex are usually docile and tractable, particularly if handled regularly and from early in their life. Some inbred strains, however, can be a little more fractious than their outbred cousins and these will need to be treated with more respect. The rat does not suffer fools gladly and if handled incompetently and with a lack of confidence or not afforded due respect will express its feelings quickly, decisively and in a way the handler is unlikely to misinterpret or forget!

It is imperative that all animals, irrespective of species, are handled and restrained in the correct manner, first and foremost to prevent any possibility of injury to those animals. Our primary concern

when performing any form of manipulation must be for the health and welfare of the animal. A good handling or restraining technique will not only eliminate the risk of physical injury to the animal but will also reduce the level of stress caused by the manipulation. Although the welfare of the animal must be paramount we must also consider the safety of the individual carrying out the procedure in order to minimize the risk of injury through bites or scratches. Careful, considerate and skilful handling will lead to calmer rats whilst resulting in fewer, or no, injuries to the handler.

Safety

Although the risk of bites appears uppermost in the minds of many people working with laboratory rats, the incidence should be low and the damage caused extremely small. Rats will not usually make an un-provoked attack on the handler. Something he or she did incorrectly will have triggered the attack and an investigation into the cause will clearly implicate the person performing the handling. The handling/restraining technique of any member of staff bitten on a frequent basis should be reviewed by a more experienced colleague. Undoubtedly this investigation will highlight poor or incorrect technique or, perhaps, a lack of confidence, at which time the appropriate action must be taken. This may involve retraining or an attempt made to build or restore the confidence of the handler, perhaps by using younger animals, for example those that are newly weaned.

Some workers are known to favour the wearing of 'antibite' gloves when handling or restraining laboratory rats. They are usually worn because of a lack of confidence in the handler accompanied by a lack of experience or inadequate training. In my experience there are no gloves commercially available which offer protection from a rat bite whilst still providing the necessary sensitivity of touch that will allow the animal to be restrained correctly. Whilst offering adequate protection to the handler this lack of sensitivity could pose a risk of injury to the animal either through crushing or being dropped on to the floor of the animal room. Their use should not be encouraged and this type of personal protection should not be seen as a substitute for correct handling, particularly as the animal's health and welfare could be put at stake.

The greatest risk to human health through working with laboratory rodents, and rats in particular, is the development of an allergy to them. At some establishments the incidence of animal allergy in staff working with animals has been reported to be as high as 37% (Davies et al., 1983). This may be manifested initially as a mild rhinitis, conjunctivitis, tightness of the chest or the development of rashes or weals on the skin. In some individuals the respiratory symptoms may lead to asthmatic attacks. In many instances the reaction of individuals to the allergens can become so severe that redeployment of the affected individual to non-animal work may be the only option (Davies and McArdle, 1981). Rare cases of anaphylactic shock as a result of a rat bite have been reported (Teasdale et al., 1983). Contracting an allergy is not just restricted to those new to animal work. Although a significant proportion of staff become sensitized within their first year of contact there are recorded cases of animal workers with up to 20 years' exposure to a particular species developing an allergy (Lutsky and Neuman, 1975).

The main source of allergens appears to be from the urine of prepubescent male rats but the prepubescent female is also implicated to a lesser extent (Longbottom, 1984). In the warm conditions to be found within an animal unit the urine-soaked bedding dries and then, due to the activity of both humans and animals, the allergen becomes airborne. Whilst working in animal rooms containing rats, care must be taken to minimize the generation of airborne particles. Staff must be provided with high-quality respiratory protection. Those who refuse to wear this protection, wear it incorrectly or use a design which offers insufficient protection, are particularly vulnerable to laboratory animal allergens.

To greatly reduce the risk of developing an allergy to rats there are a few simple rules to observe when working in the animal facility. It is important to wear good protective clothing – gown or boilersuit, hat and gloves – and adequate respiratory protection at all times. Masks should be changed regularly as their efficiency becomes impaired and damaged gloves should be replaced immediately with a new pair. Reusable respiratory protection should be cleaned and stored correctly. Care must be taken with the storage of used protective clothing, possibly contaminated with dust or urine, to eliminate contact with outdoor clothing. Hands must always be washed when leaving the animal area. The housing of rats in filter-top boxes, isolators and ventilated or laminar flow racks are effective ways of reducing the level of allergen in the working environment.

Wild rats act as a reservoir for several zoonotic agents. Whilst there are reported cases of laboratory and animal technicians contracting disease from laboratory rats these are relatively rare and most of them occurred several years ago before the introduction of the high-quality disease-free animals which are widely available for use today.

Handling and Restraint of the Rat

A definition of both handling and restraint will serve to eliminate any confusion over these two terms in the text that follows. Handling is seen as the manipulation of an animal by hand for the purposes of removing it from the cage and transferring it to another cage, onto the pan of a balance for weighing or onto another surface such as a benchtop for

Training – the Individual and the Animal

restraint purposes. Restraint is defined as the immobilization of a conscious animal by keeping it, or part of its body, in a fixed position for a significant period of time while an examination or procedure is carried out (Biological Council, 1992). It may also be necessary to partially restrain an animal to prevent interference and/or damage to an operative site following surgery if, for example, blood vessels or ducts have been cannulated. This will be discussed briefly towards the end of this chapter but if restraint for this purpose is contemplated reference should be made to Chapter 27 or the publication by Waynforth and Flecknell (1992) in which this topic is covered in much greater detail.

It is possible for a researcher to carry out many different types of procedure on the rat with one hand whilst restraining the animal in the other. Some procedures, however, will require the cooperation of two people, one providing the restraint whilst the other performs the technique. Longer term restraint will require the use of a specialized restraining device. This latter type of restraint may also be used if an assistant is not available or to reduce a two-person task into one which may be performed alone.

Successful hand restraint employs sufficient firmness to prevent movement and possible injury to the rat whilst a procedure is performed. Some procedures, for example injections, may cause some momentary pain or discomfort, resulting in the rat attempting to take avoidance action. It is important that the degree of restraint is such that it is capable of counteracting this movement but is not so firm as to risk physical injury to the animal.

Any form of restraint can be stressful to the animal, with the degree of stress often increasing over time. Its duration, therefore, should be kept to an absolute minimum. It has been shown that even the briefest handling procedure, lasting for as little as 30 seconds, can act as a stressor as measured by a rise in the plasma glucocorticoid levels (Kvetansky et al., 1978). Barclay et al. (1988) found that restraint produced significant values of their 'Disturbance Index' and that this increased with the duration of restraint.

The degree of stress can, however, be reduced. Kant et al. (1985) concluded that rats subjected to repeated restraint become habituated to the procedure which was then no longer perceived as stressful. Familiarization of animals to the techniques to which they are later to be exposed should, therefore, be seen as an important part of the acclimatization period leading up to the actual experimental work.

Perhaps the most common problem leading to a high risk of accidental injury to the rat is incorrect and inadequate restraint. This is usually a lack of firmness, allowing the animal too much freedom of movement. In this situation there is a realization on the part of the rat that escape is a distinct possibility and on the handler that his or her fingers are in danger of being bitten! At such times it is not unknown for an individual to panic, dropping the animal rather than carefully replacing it back in the cage and trying a second time.

Before performing any type of handling or hand restraining technique on the rat it is essential that the individual who is to perform the procedure is both properly trained and aware of the effect his or her actions will have on the animal. Although it may be possible to follow the instructions in the following text, this should not be viewed as a substitute for proper and thorough training by a more experienced member of staff. This training should be carefully structured, ample time allowed and, of course, be followed by some form of assessment. Initially, compliant animals that are fully familiar with the technique in which training is to be given should be used. Once the trainee has mastered the technique using these animals, he or she may then be allowed to progress to more naïve animals.

Following delivery to the animal facility all animals should undergo a period of acclimatization. This should last for approximately 7 days but may be reduced to 3 days depending on the type of procedure that is to be performed. During this time the animals should be handled regularly and fully familiarized with the methods of restraint to be used later. Rats respond to considerate and skilful handling and time and effort spent here will pay dividends during the course of the experiment in the form of more relaxed animals and in some cases better and more reproducible experimental results. When handled initially there will undoubtedly be some apprehension and tension within the animal coupled with a strong urge to escape. If this is the case the rat should be held around its upper body and gently shaken. This will have a temporary calming effect on the animal, which then can be restrained using one of the methods described later. This and a compassionate and skilful approach to handling will help to overcome any fear or resistance. Barclay et al. (1988)

Anticipating the Animal's Behaviour

Before attempting to handle or restrain a rat it is prudent to make a quick assessment of its likely response to what may be either a novel experience or one which may be resented. In certain circumstances rats may be more difficult to handle and this can lead to an increased risk of injury to either the handler or the animal. Some of these are described below.

- Animals that have just arrived in the animal facility should be treated with greater care. Stress incurred during the transportation, by their new surroundings and by changes in personnel will undoubtedly affect behaviour. It is also unlikely the newly delivered animals will be familiar with the types of restraining and handling methods used in the new facility. There will undoubtedly be some apprehension on their part and a reluctance to be caught and restrained. It is at this time that more patience and consideration is required on the part of the handler. Once settled into their new environment time must be spent on the familiarization process described above.

- Many nursing females will show little or no reaction to the removal or handling of their young but some may perceive a threat to their offspring and take appropriate defensive action to counter that threat.

- An animal which is sick or injured is often more likely to take exception to handling and restraint.

- A rat exposed to a repeated traumatic experience, no matter how mild, will quickly associate removal from the cage or the method of restraint with the unpleasant procedure and take appropriate evasive action.

- Rats are gregarious animals and react strongly to isolation over prolonged periods. They can become destructive in the absence of environmental stimuli and often aggressive towards the handler or to new cage mates if regrouped. If there is a sound scientific requirement to single house a rat it is advisable to provide some form of environmental enrichment or, failing that, to ensure the animals are handled frequently. Failure to observe these simple measures will inevitably be to the detriment of the handler. In cases where rats are to be segregated, for example following surgery, where there is a need to protect a wound or an indwelling catheter, consideration should be given

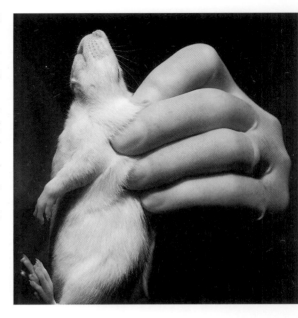

Figure 3.1 The typical 'relaxed rat' position.

showed that handling by an experienced person could lead to a reduction of activity in rats and later confirmed these findings by demonstrating that the behaviour of rats was significantly disturbed when animals were restrained by an inexperienced handler.

Rats, like many other animals, do appear to recognize individuals and will act accordingly when handled by unfamiliar staff. The acclimatization period is, therefore, an important part of experimental work, allowing time for animals to adjust to their new environment, the staff who will be working with them and the handling/restraining techniques which they will experience. It is important to overcome the rats' initial fear or trepidation to handling or restraint by taking the time and trouble to relax them. The typical 'relaxed rat' position is easily recognizable as the animal tucks up both rear legs and extends one, or both, front legs down its side (Figure 3.1). To reach this relaxed state the animal should be handled in the manner described below. The rat is gripped gently but firmly by placing the hand over its back and with the thumb and second finger placed over the shoulders. The index finger is placed on the head and the three digits then closed together, dragging a fold of skin with them. After performing this simple relaxing technique the animal will prove to be more compliant and much easier to handle. The effects on the rat's behaviour are long lasting and will be obvious for several days even if no additional handling is given in that time. An alternative, but slightly less effective, way is to lift the animal by the loose skin extending from the neck along its back. This technique will be described later.

to single housing the animal for several days prior to the surgical procedure. This will avoid the 'double stress', on regaining consciousness, of postoperative recovery coupled with isolation. During the preoperative period the rat can be provided with some form of environmental enrichment to ease the stress of segregation, but if this is not possible the animal should receive additional sympathetic handling. These minor precautions will not only be to the benefit of the animal but help to ensure that it remains docile and easy to handle.

Approach to the Rat

The approach to handling rats is no different to that used for most laboratory animals. Confidence, or at least an outward show of it, is a key factor. Hesitation on the part of the handler is likely to alarm the animal(s). On the other hand, the approach should not be rushed as this may well frighten the rats, making them more difficult to handle or, possibly, aggressive. Ensure the animals are aware of the handler's presence by confidently placing the gloved hand into the cage and allowing the rats to become used to it. (Although this approach will work with the majority of animals, remember to assess the situation and anticipate what their likely behaviour will be.) An attempt can then be made to capture an animal prior to its removal from the cage.

It is permissible to use the tail to lift a rat from the cage providing it is gripped at its base (Figure 3.2). Handling the rat by the base of its tail is

only useful for moving the animal from one location to another close by or for a cursory inspection of the animal's condition. Transferring the rat from cage to cage by this method or from the cage to an adjacent balance pan for weighing is quick and the animal will suffer no harmful effects. If, however, the rat is to be suspended in this manner for more than 2 or 3 seconds, the weight of its body must be supported by using the other hand, the arm or by placing the animal on a flat surface. On no account must an animal be pulled by its tail if, for example, it is using its front feet to grip onto the cage, nor must a rat be swung by its tail as has been described in some publications when discussing euthanasia by concussion of the brain. This is because the force exerted on the tail can result in the overlying skin becoming detached from the body (thought to be a defence mechanism). If the rat holds on to the cage its grip should be carefully broken using the other hand before an attempt is made to lift it. When euthanasing a rat by concussion the animal should be held on its back by gripping around the pelvis with one hand, with the other hand supporting the weight of the animal and controlling its upper body.

Neonates should on no account be held by the tail as this can lead to injury. Young of up to 5 or 6 days of age may be carefully scooped out of the nest and supported in the cupped palm of the hand (Figure 3.3). In this position they can easily be examined or their sex determined. Alternatively, they may be picked up from the cage and held gently between the thumb and first two fingers (Figure 3.4). This method of restraint can be used as the young grow older and become more mobile

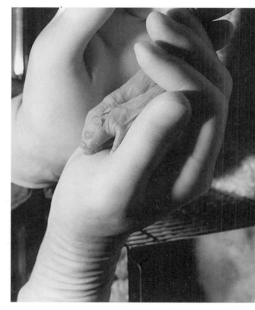

Figure 3.3 Holding neonates in the cupped hand.

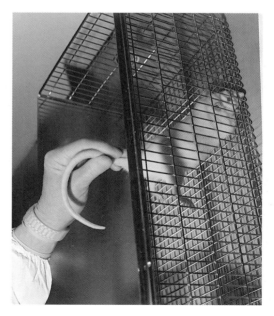

Figure 3.2 Removing a rat from the cage by the base of its tail.

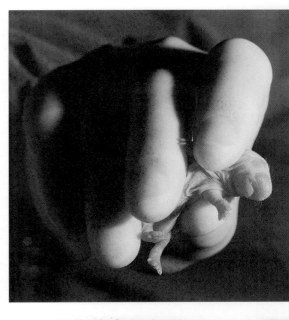

Figure 3.4 Restraining a neonate between thumb and fingers.

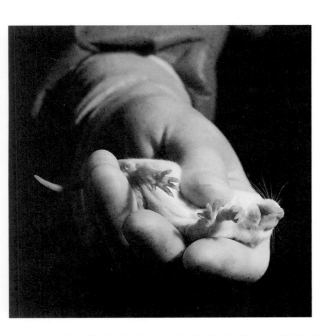

Figure 3.5 Restraint of preweaner.

but it may require the use of all the fingers to prevent them from escaping (Figure 3.5). Once the young reach 2 weeks of age the method of handling described in the next paragraphs for adult animals can be employed, although at this age the risks of bites are low and the head control, therefore, less critical. It is permissible to lift young rats of this age by the base of the tail as described previously. The sex of newly weaned animals can easily be determined by holding the base of the tail and lifting the animal's rear legs off the floor of the cage to expose the genitalia (Figure 3.6).

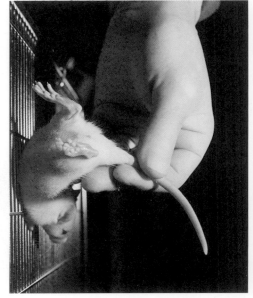

Figure 3.6 Using the tail method of restraint to sex a rat.

Methods of Restraint by Hand

For more detailed inspection purposes or to perform a procedure on the animal, some form of restraint will be required in order to immobilize the animal or part of it. Some procedures, for example injections, can be performed by a single individual – restraining the rat with one hand whilst the other is used to manipulate the hypodermic needle and syringe; other procedures may require the assistance of a colleague to hold the rat. Alternatively, it may be possible to use a restraining device which will in effect mean the procedure can be carried out by a single member of staff. The use of restraining devices will be discussed later in this chapter.

Both young and adult rats can be lifted from the cage by placing one's hand over the back of the rat and sliding the thumb underneath the animal and between its front legs until it rests on the lower side of the jaw (Figure 3.7). It is the thumb which will give the important control of the animal's head, restricting movement and preventing any possibility of a bite. Care must be taken to apply only sufficient pressure with the thumb to control head movement without impairing the animal's ability to breathe (Figure 3.8). Alternatively, control of the head may be achieved by again placing the hand over the back of the rat as described previously but on this occasion using the thumb and fingers to apply gentle pressure in order to cross the front legs, again providing that important restriction of head movement (Figure 3.9). Once lifted from its cage, additional support may be provided by taking the weight of the rat's lower body in the other hand.

These methods of restraint are suitable for holding an animal whilst performing a minor procedure.

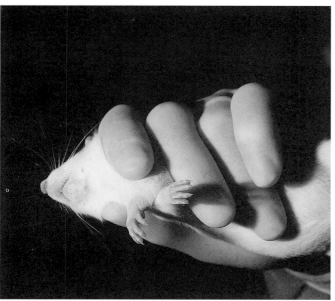

Figure 3.9 Head control by crossing the front legs.

its ears. The closeness of the grip to the ears is important as this will prevent excessive head movement. The hand is pressed down gently and the loose skin from the left and right dorsal surface is pulled into the palm of the hand by using the whole of the thumb on one side and the remaining fingers on the other. A tent of skin, extending from the neck region to as far down the animal's back as hand size will allow, is trapped in the palm of the hand, effectively immobilizing the animal. This method of restraint can be used to remove an animal directly from the cage, providing it has a solid floor with some sort of bedding material to act as a cushion or, alternatively, the rat should be removed from the cage by the tail and repositioned on the front of the handler's body and restrained from this point (Figure 3.10). Once a rat becomes accustomed to this method of restraint it will usually assume the 'relaxed rat' position with hind legs tucked up and one or both front legs extended down the side of the body. Not only can this method of restraint be used for a detailed examination of the animal but it is also used for immobilizing animals for the single-handed administration of a substance by several routes.

Before attempting any procedure, and in particular those involving hypodermic needles or metal cannula for oral dosing, it is vital to ensure the rat is properly and comfortably restrained, i.e. comfortable for both the rat and the handler. Given the opportunity, an animal will attempt to escape during

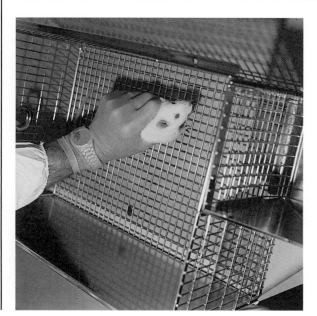

Figure 3.7 Grasping a rat around its body to remove it from the cage.

This would include, for example, a thorough health examination or a simple technique such as the application of a substance to the eyes of the animal. If the animal is to be restrained for a more involved procedure the following method should be used.

The rat has an ample supply of loose skin extending from the rear of the neck along the back. This provides an excellent and painless point to grip and restrain the animal. The rat is captured by gripping the base of the tail and the other hand placed over the back of the animal with the thumb and forefinger positioned over the neck and close to

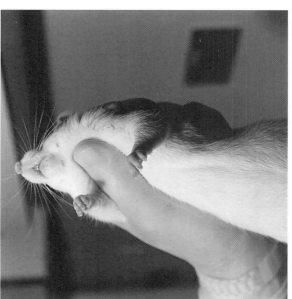

Figure 3.8 Head control using the thumb.

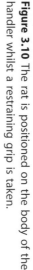

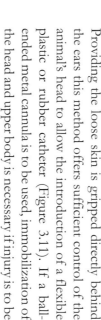

Figure 3.10 The rat is positioned on the body of the handler whilst a restraining grip is taken.

a procedure it perceives as unpleasant. This may result in injury to the animal, a misplaced injection or, occasionally, injury to the person dosing the animal, e.g. needle puncture.

Oral administration

Providing the loose skin is gripped directly behind the ears this method offers sufficient control of the animal's head to allow the introduction of a flexible plastic or rubber catheter (Figure 3.11). If a ball-ended metal cannula is to be used, immobilization of the head and upper body is necessary if injury is to be

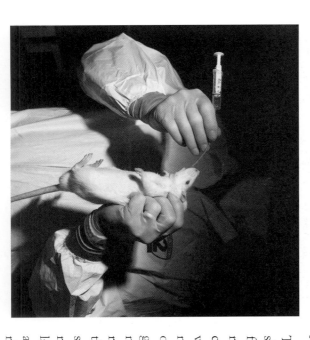

Figure 3.11 Oral dosing using a flexible plastic catheter.

avoided. Whilst this method of restraint should be sufficient to prevent movement, the position of the rat's head will necessitate the use of a curved cannula to allow easy passage down the oesophagus. If, however, the rat is restrained in the manner described previously for relaxing the animal (Figure 3.12) it will enable the head to be pulled gently backwards, presenting a straight passage from the mouth to the cardiac sphincter. This will allow the insertion of a straight metal ball-ended cannula into the mouth and unrestricted passage into the oesophagus.

Figure 3.12 Oral dosing using a metal cannula. Note the use of the index finger to pull back the animal's head.

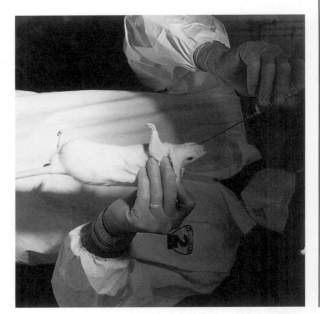

Intraperitoneal administration

The rat is held ventral side uppermost with the head slightly lower than the body, allowing the viscera to fall slightly forward towards the diaphragm and reducing the risk of the needle puncturing the caecum or intestines (Figure 3.13). It is good practice when giving an intraperitoneal injection to insert the needle subcutaneously into the abdomen at an angle of 20–30° and then lift the syringe to 45°, pushing gently through the muscle layer and into the peritoneal cavity. Employing this technique will greatly reduce the number of misdirected injections. Although it is acceptable to perform this technique single-handedly for young animals, the degree of restraint achieved may not be sufficient for older and larger rats. It is advisable with these animals to use an assistant to restrain the animal, thus eliminating the risk of accidental injury to the rat and/or a misplaced injection.

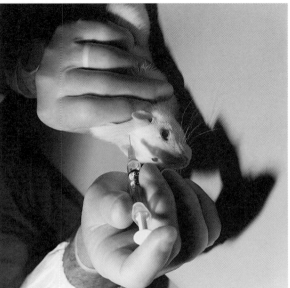

Figure 3.13 Scruff restraint while administering via the intraperitoneal route.

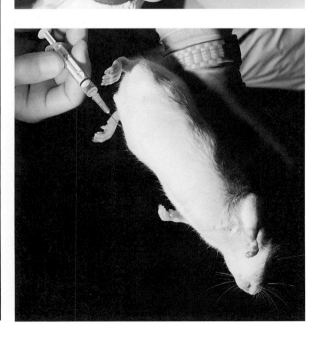

Figure 3.15 An alternative method of restraint for subcutaneous injection.

Intramuscular administration

Although the type of restraint will be similar to the previously described methods, administration by this route will require two people – one to restrain the animal whilst the second person extends the rat's rear leg with one hand to expose the muscle mass and uses the other hand to deliver the injection (Figure 3.16).

The subject of administration routes will be discussed in more greater detail in Chapter 24.

Subcutaneous administration

It is possible to slide the needle between the thumb and first finger and into the subcutaneous space in the animal's scruff. Care must be taken to avoid puncturing either digit with the needle (Figure 3.14) and it might be found to be safer and more convenient if the animal is placed on a horizontal surface and gentle pressure exerted from above whilst the injection is performed (Figure 3.15).

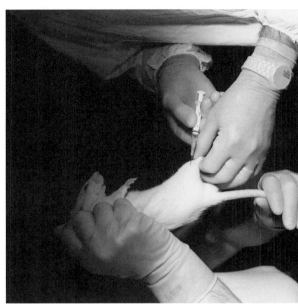

Figure 3.16 Restraint for intramuscular injection using two people.

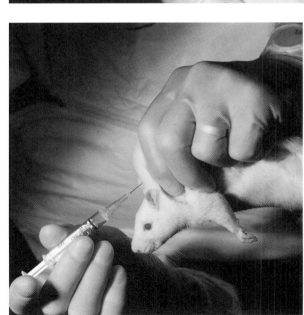

Figure 3.14 Scruff restraint while administering a subcutaneous injection.

Restraining Devices

The use of some form of restraining device will be necessary for longer term immobilization or for administration techniques requiring the use of both hands. There are numerous types and designs of restraining devices, some available commercially whilst others have been successfully designed and fabricated within the laboratory. One of the commonest reasons for using a restrainer is to allow easy access to the rat's tail for either intravenous administration or tail vein bleeding. Some restrainers are, however, designed to give access to other parts of the animal's body.

Simple injections, for example intraperitoneal or intravenous into a superficial vein, only require short-term restraint usually lasting less than one minute. This duration of restraint should cause little stress to the animals, particularly if they are allowed to become accustomed to the method of restraint beforehand. It may, however, be necessary to restrain a rat for longer periods of time, in which case serious thought should be given to the reason why restraint is necessary, the length of time the animal must be restrained and the various methods that are available. The least stressful method of immobilization is by chemical means using an anaesthetic or, perhaps, a combination of a sedative or a tranquillizing agent with some form of physical restraint. If the experimental requirements preclude the use of chemical agents, the rat will have to be physically immobilized by confining it within some form of restraining tube or cage. The use of these devices can be extremely stressful to rats of all ages. In fact one of the most commonly used methods of inducing gastric ulcers in rats is by restraint over a period of several hours. Restraint time must, therefore, be kept to an absolute minimum and time devoted to accustoming the rats to the device before the procedure commences will help reduce the degree of stress the animal is exposed to.

The simplest method of short-term restraint is to wrap the animal in a piece of fabric. This method is cheap but, importantly, readily acceptable to the animal whilst also providing effective restraint for minor procedures. Muslin is an ideal material as it is fairly soft and will give a little as the animal moves. This small amount of movement, whilst appearing to contribute to the comfort of the rat, should not normally cause any problems and minor procedures may be performed successfully. The rat is placed on the muslin, a fold of material cast over its back and

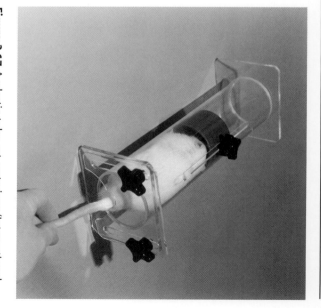

Figure 3.17 A plastic tube rat restrainer (International Market Supply, Congleton, Cheshire, UK).

tucked beneath it and the animal then gently rolled over once or twice, wrapping it in the material but leaving its head and tail free. This method of restraint provides easy access to the tail for bleeding or intravenous administration but it is advisable to enlist the help of an assistant, who can carry out the wrapping and unwrapping process and also place a hand over the wrapped animal whilst the procedure is carried out. Following the procedure the animal can easily be removed, taking care to ensure the legs or feet do not become entangled in the material. Waynforth and Flecknell (1992) describe a similar method of restraint using the DecapiCone. This is a triangular-shaped polyethylene sleeve designed for restraint prior to euthanasia by decapitation. They state that DecapiCones can be used to immobilize rats for both subcutaneous and intraperitoneal injections with the needle being inserted through the polyethylene membrane and into the injection site. The use of these sleeves allows these techniques to be performed by a single person.

Tubular clear plastic restrainers are commonly used for immobilizing rats for tail vein administration or bleeding. Many types are available but the design principle is similar. In the restrainer shown here (Figure 3.17) the rat, held by the base of the tail, is encouraged to crawl inside the restraining tube and the vertically sliding backplate lowered and locked into place. Care must be taken not to physically trap the tail. Whilst still holding the rat's tail, the adjustable head ring is slid down the tube to restrict any forward movement and is also locked into place.

differing sizes. Some restrainers are designed to allow access to other parts of the rat's body in addition to the tail and with some designs it is possible to administer both subcutaneous and intraperitoneal injections through an appropriate opening in the tube wall. Tube restrainers are only ideal for immobilization over short periods as heat dissipation can be a problem. Longer periods of restraint can lead to increased discomfort in the animal.

Owen *et al.* (1984) reported some agitation amongst rats whilst being persuaded to enter plastic restraining tubes and a high degree of stress in animals maintained there for upwards of one hour. They describe an alternative, simple method of restraint which they showed to be less stressful. Their restrainer comprised a base board on which a piece of cloth is held between two wooden bars. Each bar is fastened to the board by two wingnuts. The rat enters a tent of material between the two bars and the fabric is then pulled tight to fit snugly around its back. The wingnuts are then tightened to secure the animal (Figure 3.18). The animals readily entered the cloth restrainer and remained there for several hours at a time with no outward signs of discomfort. Rats housed in plastic tubes for an hour, however, were extremely agitated, showing gnawing and scratching behaviour and often vocalization. A commercially available restrainer operating on a similar principle to their version is now available. In this design the rat is restrained between two layers of nylon netting which are held on a fully adjustable stainless steel frame (Figure 3.19). Rat restraining harnessess are also available. Fitted with adjustable Velcro sides these can be used for rats of different sizes and can then be attached to an adjustable holding frame (Figure 3.20).

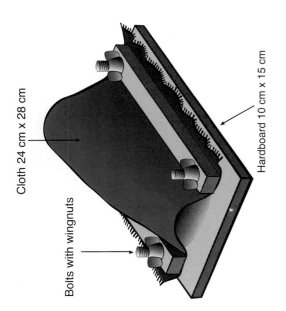

Cloth 24 cm × 28 cm

Bolts with wingnuts

Hardboard 10 cm × 15 cm

Figure 3.18 A simple 'home-made' restrainer for longer term restraint.

The head ring is perforated so as not to inhibit the captive animal's breathing. By mounting the restrainer in a retort stand the height and angle of the tube can be adjusted, making the subsequent procedure easier to perform and, therefore, more comfortable for the operator. This is particularly important if the procedure is to be performed on a large batch of animals. It is unlikely that problems will be encountered in persuading the animal to enter the tube as this is a natural rat behaviour that appears to have been retained from their wild predecessors. In fact it is often more difficult to entice the rat into leaving the tube once the procedure has been completed! The diameter of the restrainer tube should be sized so as not to allow the animal sufficient space to turn once inside. It is advisable to have a range of tubes with different diameters to cater for animals of

Long-term Restraint

The problems of long duration restraint and its effect on the rat have already been discussed in this chapter. Historically much of this type of restraint followed surgical intervention and was necessary to protect a wound or prevent interference with an indwelling infusion line. The development and use of tethering equipment has now made other forms of restraint for these purposes obsolete. The rat is fitted with a jacket that is then fastened with hooks and Velcro. The catheter is protected by a stainless steel tether attached to a swivel device. This allows the rat ample movement within the cage but,

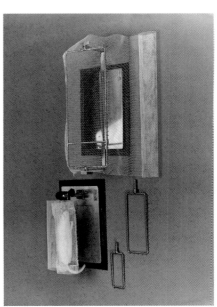

Figure 3.19 Nylon net restrainer and stand (Scanbur, Koge, Denmark).

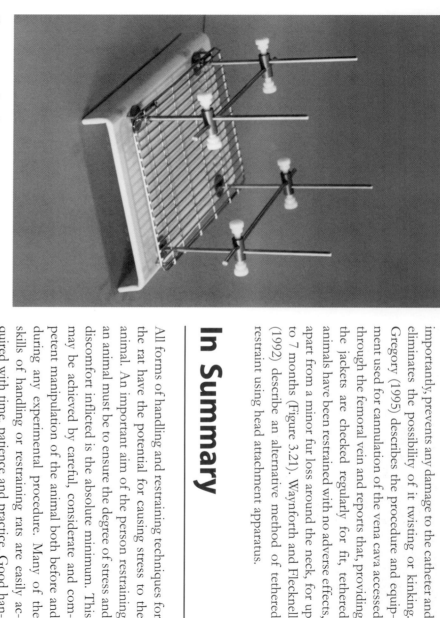

Figure 3.20 Rodent harness holding frame (International Market Supply, Congleton, Cheshire, UK).

In Summary

All forms of handling and restraining techniques for the rat have the potential for causing stress to the animal. An important aim of the person restraining an animal must be to ensure the degree of stress and discomfort inflicted is the absolute minimum. This may be achieved by careful, considerate and competent manipulation of the animal both before and during any experimental procedure. Many of the skills of handling or restraining rats are easily acquired with time, patience and practice. Good handling and restraint should take into consideration the following points:

- Assess the effect the technique is likely to have on the rat.
- Anticipate its likely reaction to the method of handling or restraint.
- Approach the animal confidently and in a way that will cause least alarm to it or any cage mates.
- Act positively and firmly.

Providing these criteria feature in all handling interactions with the laboratory rat the investigator can be assured the animal will be subjected to the least possible inconvenience, stress will be kept to minimal levels and this will be reflected in greater validity of experimental results.

References

Barclay, R.J., Herbert, W.J. and Poole T.B. (1988) *UFAW Animal Welfare Research Report 2*. Potters Bar, Herts: Universities Federation For Animal Welfare.

Biological Council (1992) *Guidelines on the Handling and Training of Laboratory Animals*. Potters Bar, Herts: Universities Federation of Animal Welfare.

importantly, prevents any damage to the catheter and eliminates the possibility of it twisting or kinking. Gregory (1995) describes the procedure and equipment used for cannulation of the vena cava accessed through the femoral vein and reports that, providing the jackets are checked regularly for fit, tethered animals have been restrained with no adverse effects, apart from a minor fur loss around the neck, for up to 7 months (Figure 3.21). Waynforth and Flecknell (1992) describe an alternative method of tethered restraint using head attachment apparatus.

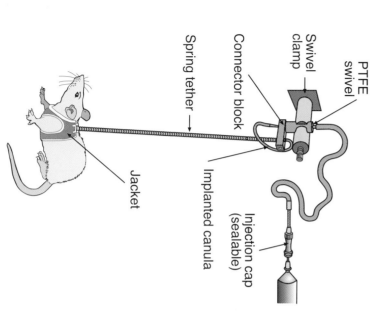

PTFE swivel

Swivel clamp

Connector block

Spring tether

Implanted canula

Injection cap (sealable)

Jacket

Figure 3.21 Catherized rat showing tether and swivel arrangement.

Botham, P.A., Davies, G.E. and Teasdale, E.L. (1987) *Br. J. Ind. Med.* **44**, 627–632.

Davies, G.E. and McArdle, L.A. (1981) *Int. Arch. Allergy Appl. Immunol.* **64**, 302–307.

Davies, G.E., Thompson, A.V., Niewola, Z., Burrows, G.E., Teasdale, E.L. and Bird, D.J. (1983) *Br. J. Ind. Med.* **40**, 442–449.

Gregory, D.J. (1995) *J. Anim. Technol.* **46**, 115–130.

Kant, C.J., Egglestone, T, Landman-Roberts, L., Kenion, C.C., Driver, G.C. and Meyerhoff, J.L. (1985) *Pharmacol. Biochem. Behav.* **22**, 631–634.

Kvetansky, R., Sun, C.L., Lake, C.R., Thoa, N., Torda, T. and Koplin, I.J. (1978) *Endocrinology* **103**, 1868–1874.

Longbottom, J.L. (1984) *Clin. Immunol. Allergy* **4**, 19–36.

Lutsky, I. and Neuman, I. (1975) *Ann. Allergy* **35**, 201–205.

Owen, J.A., Tasker, R.A.R. and Nakatsu, K. (1984) *Experientia* **40**, 306–308.

Teasdale, E.L., Davies, G.E. and Slovak, A.J.M. (1983) *BMJ* **286**, 1480.

Waynforth, H.B. and Flecknell, P.A. (1992) *Experimental and Surgical Technique in the Rat.* London: Academic Press.

CHAPTER 4

Husbandry

Isabelle Allmann-Iselin
Institute of Toxicology of the Swiss Federal Institute of Technology,
Schwerzenbach-Zürich, Switzerland

Introduction

For a laboratory animal facility, proper housing, husbandry and management are essential to animal well-being, to the quality of research and teaching for which the animals are used, and to the health and safety of personnel.

In animal research many parameters will influence the results of an experiment. Beside the animal itself (strain, health) external stimuli will affect the experimental outcome. It is therefore of utmost importance to be aware that there are such effects and that they can be minimized. To reproduce data from animal experimentation the same environment must be used in different laboratories. This can be achieved by following the advice published in standard reference books in various countries (e.g. Van Zutphen *et al.*, 1993; ILAR, 1996).

It is also important to follow the recommended guidelines based on animal welfare laws. Animals should be housed with the goal of maximizing species-specific behaviour and minimizing stress-induced behaviours.

Microenvironment and Macroenvironment

The microenvironment is the physical environment directly surrounding the animal. In general, it is located within a macroenvironment, such as an animal room. These two environments are interdependent, but the two compartments might be of different environmental quality due to their different size, content, material and enclosure. The environmental differences between the cage and the animal room must be recognized as these differences may influence experimental results.

Macroenvironment

Housing

Housing refers to the macroenvironment. It is important to maintain optimal conditions in the colony

Table 4.1 Environmental requirements of rats

Temperature (°C)	20–24
Relative humidity (%)	60
Ventilation (air change/h)	10–15
Light/dark (hours)	12–14/12–10
Minimum cage floor size	
One individually housed adult (cm²)	350
Breeding animal with pups (cm²)	800
Group (cm² adult)	250
Minimum cage height (cm)	14
Water intake (mL/100 g/day)	10–12
Food intake (g/100 g/day)	5–50 during the night mainly

Reproduced with permission from Van Zutphen et al. (1993).

room, given that these impinge directly on the metabolism in the animal. A temperature change may induce a direct or indirect influence on the experiment, as described by Fox et al. (1984).

The regulation of body temperature within the normal range is essential for the well-being of homeotherms. If temperatures go outside the thermoneutral zone (over 29°C or below 4°C) adaptive mechanisms will be induced. These include peripheral vascular contraction, **piloerection** or even increased metabolic activity and adaptive behaviour such as huddling or posture to reduce body heat loss. Thermoregulation in the laboratory rat has been reviewed by Gordon (1990), who states that the temperature range that allows optimal growth in the rat (20–26°C) coincides with that of its behavioural preferences.

The normal temperature in a rat room should be 20–24°C (Table 4.1). High temperature and air humidity influence susceptibility to infectious agents. Low humidity induces 'mechanical' changes in rats (e.g. ring tail) (Fox et al., 1984). The normal humidity in a rat room should not be below 50% (Table 4.1).

Ventilation

The purpose of ventilation is to supply adequate oxygen, remove thermal heat, adjust temperature and humidity. It can also be used to create an air pressure difference between adjacent rooms.

Ventilation must be adjusted to the size of the room, the layout of the room and the number of animals. An exact evaluation during the design of an

experiment due to increased or decreased activity or microenvironment. Recommended environmental requirements for rats are listed in Table 4.1.

The housing conditions may be conventional (i.e. with no barrier), optimal hygienic conditions (OHC) (i.e. clean working conditions with gloves, lab coat and shoe covers) or specified pathogen free (SPF), where the barrier consists of autoclave and showering.

Space recommendations

The standard animal room is of a defined size and layout and is suitable for holding or breeding, while also affording the possibility of performing experimental procedures (GV-SOLAS, 1989). The recommended size of the animal room is 20 m² effective floor area and the maximum holding capacity of a standard room of 20 m² is 1000 rats. This is calculated for rats with 200 g body weight in cages with a floor area of 810 cm² (Makrolon Type III). The advantage of this room size is its flexibility. Species can be kept separately and the risk of infections spreading is minimized due to the number of rooms and small number of animals per room.

Temperature and humidity

Environmental temperature and relative humidity can depend on husbandry and housing design and have to be thoroughly evaluated when planning and managing an animal facility. Changes in temperature and humidity can have undesirable effects on an

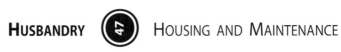

animal facility can be carried out using a computerized system as shown by Hughes *et al.* (1996). It is important to optimize the air flow to avoid unnecessary stagnation of air, recirculation of contaminated air in the room or induction of drafts. All of these can exert a detrimental influence on animal well-being. A frequency of 10–15 fresh air changes per hour is accepted as a general standard.

Illumination

Light can influence the physiology, morphology and behaviour of animals. In general, lighting should be diffused throughout an animal holding room, providing sufficient illumination for animal well-being, allowing good housekeeping practices and safe working conditions. There should be no windows and the light timer should be controlled for a diurnal cycle, to support a normal animal biology. The light/dark cycle can be normal (light on during daytime) or reversed (light on during night), depending on the experimental procedures. The light and dark hour phases have to be in an equally proportional relation. The normal light/dark cycle should be 12–14/12–10 hours.

Experimental rats are very often albino rats, which are sensitive to light and develop **retinopathy** with acute exposure to light (high lux level) or cumulative chronic exposure to light, as shown by Bellhorn (1980). It is therefore important to measure the light quality and quantity in the animal rooms and in the cages and to consider different possible locations of the cages.

The accepted light level in the room is 325–400 lux at 1 m above floor level for routine care duties. At the cage level it should be a maximum of 130 lux according to ILAR (1996) and Semple-Rowland and Dawson (1987).

It is important to check that the light cycle is operating correctly on a daily basis, as very low light can induce retinal degeneration, whereas minor deviations in the intensity duration of environmental light at a given time of day may cause disruptions in **chronobiologic rhythms** (Dauchy *et al.*, 1997). Therefore a proper monitoring procedure is an essential part of the control system.

Noise

Exposure to intense noise can lead to a wide variety of functional and structural changes in laboratory animals. Although little information regarding noise effects at moderate levels is available, the range of intensities at which such effects begin to be manifested in humans seems also to pertain in animals. Peterson (1980) mentions that the level and patterning of noise can induce either auditory effects (e.g. hearing loss) or nonauditory effects in the form of a variety of illnesses, dysfunctions and structural changes resulting from intense noise exposure. The separation of human and animal areas minimizes disturbances to both the human and animal occupants of the facility. Nonetheless, radio music sound will habituate the animals to the variability of sound or noise.

The recommended noise level not to be exceeded is 85 dB. It is important to remember, though, that rats can hear sounds of high frequency (60–80 kHz) and ultravocalization plays an important role in social interactions. These sounds are not audible to humans, but can be emitted by equipment such as video recorders and should be taken into consideration. In contrast, rats are less sensitive than humans or other laboratory animals to noises below 1000 Hz and will be less affected by these noises (e.g. air conditioning noise) (Peterson, 1980).

Microenvironment
Caging for rats

Air quality within the animal cage is of equal importance to the quality of the air in the macroenvironment. The two most common contaminants, as derived from the intracage accumulation of animal waste, are ammonia and carbon dioxide. An acceptable ammonia level should not exceed 25 ppm. The principal adverse effect of ammonia is irritation of the respiratory tract as shown histologically by Gamble and Clough (1976). It may be an important pathogenic factor and a potential coirritant in toxicology studies.

The temperature and humidity of the animal's microenvironment is dependent on a number of factors, including the temperature, humidity and ventilation of the macroenvironment, cage design, cage material and presence of a cage filter top, number of animals per cage and bedding material. More extensive factors and details are described by Woods (1980). These environmental variables can be controlled within the primary enclosure and maintained by proper control of the associated variables within the secondary environment (Besch, 1980).

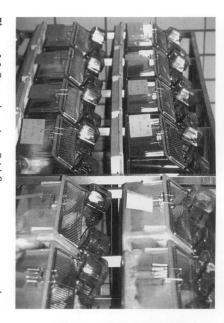

Figure 4.1 Group housing. Grid-floor cages versus sawdust in full-bodied cages.

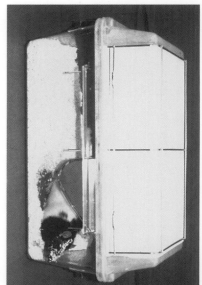

Figure 4.3 Microisolator cage with filter top.

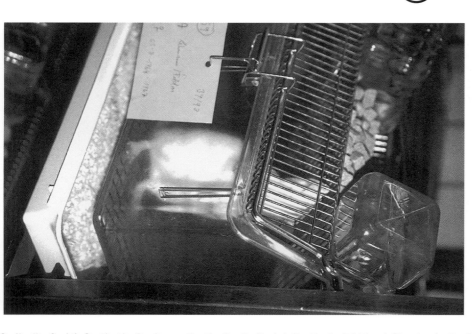

Figure 4.2 Group housing on grid floor cages. Notice sawdust in the tray beneath the cage.

The cage can be either a full-bodied cage, open on the top and covered with a rod lid, or covered with a filter top, depending on the status conditions of the housing. The filter top functions as a barrier permeable to air, preventing infectious agents from either entering or leaving the cage area. Grid-floor cages are also used. The ILAR recommends solid-bottomed cages based on evidence suggesting that solid-bottomed cages with bedding are preferred by rats in a free choice situation. However, firm conclusions on the importance of housing rats on solid floors cannot be drawn without studying the strength of preference for a solid floor. The evidence from the study by Manser et al. (1995) suggests that housing rats on solid plastic floors with bedding is beneficial for animal welfare and that unless there are compelling reasons for using grid-floor cages they should not be used. An advantage of housing rats in grid-floor cages compared to solid-floor bedded cages is that ammonia levels build up much more rapidly in the latter, other things being equal (Raynor et al., 1983). Extensive research to evaluate different housing conditions have been reviewed by Blom (1993). Research currently in progress is investigating animal preference as well as the effect of the cage type on performance in cognitive tests. Knowledge of housing conditions and behaviour may be used to reformulate existing guidelines on housing conditions if deemed desirable (Figures 4.1 and 4.2).

In filter-top cages tight control of the microclimate is necessary (Figure 4.3). The cover of the microcages will inhibit the release of gaseous decomposition products building up from faeces and urine; therefore an increase in ammonia (NH_3) and carbon dioxide (CO_2) levels as well as temperature and humidity, can be expected (Serrano, 1971). Direct effects on the animals might be found, as demonstrated by Baer et al. (1997), as well as indirect effects such as higher susceptibility to experimental stress. Corning and Lipman (1991) showed that different filter tops have different effects on the levels of NH_3, CO_2 and on relative humidity, but no effect on the temperature within the cage. The numbers of animals per cage should therefore be restricted and the number of changes of cages per week should remain constant. A simple test is that when ammonia can be smelled on opening the cage the levels are too high. This indicates that either the number of animals or the frequency of cage cleaning or both will have to be adapted.

Lipman et al., (1992) evaluated the differences in intracage carbon dioxide, ammonia and relative humidity level in filter-top cages with or without individual ventilation, open-air cages and the air of the room in all four situations. The temperature was the same. CO_2, NH_3 and relative humidity were highest in the unventilated cages, followed by the ventilated cages, then the open cages, and lowest in the colony room.

Space recommendations

The minimum cage size for keeping rats (and other laboratory animals) is specified in the laws of different countries and in the guidelines of relevant organizations. The dimensions and the number of animals per cage are listed in, for example the Guidelines for Minimum Cage Size per Animal by the EU, GV-SOLAS (1989) and ILAR (1996) (in USA). Dimensions and numbers of animals per cage are comparable in these examples. At a minimum, an animal must have sufficient space to turn around and to express normal postural adjustments, must have ready access to food and water, and must have sufficient clean bedded or unobstructed area to move and rest.

The minimum cage size for a single caged rat of 120–500 g body weight is 350 cm²; the floor area for adult rats in small groups should be $350 \text{ cm}^2 + 1 \text{ cm}^2$ per g body weight; and the floor area for weaned rats in small groups should be $350 \text{ cm}^2 + 0.6 \text{ cm}^2$ per g body weight.

Caging material

The caging material should be chosen carefully to avoid any negative influence on the animals. It should be free of any material which could harm the animal or which could influence its susceptibility to disease. Cages should be constructed of material which cannot be ingested and which does not react with waste products. Cages should be of heat-resistant material so that they can be autoclaved for use in an SPF or isolator unit.

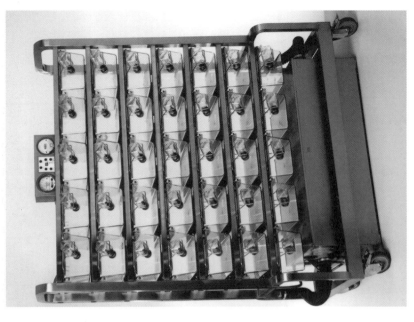

Figure 4.4 Ventilated rack Type 3 (VR-3035ms/AHV-39) with an air handler unit (BioZone, Margate, UK).

Rack-containment of cages

Cages can be placed in a rack, in a ventilated rack, or in a cubicle. In the 1980s ventilated rack systems were created to reduce intracage levels of carbon dioxide, ammonia and relative humidity, especially in filter-top cages. The idea was to achieve the environmental uniformity necessary for consistent experimental results. Wu et al. (1985) presented a novel forced-air system for rodent cages where the air velocity measurements in the cages did not exceed 8 m/min at the rat level (three air changes/min) (Figure 4.4).

Individual versus grouped caging

Whenever it is appropriate, social animals should be housed in pairs or larger groups, rather than individually, provided that such housing does not interfere with experimental results nor poses an undue risk to any animal (Figures 4.5 and 4.6).

Bedding material

Criteria for the evaluation of laboratory animal bedding materials are quite precise. Bedding should provide a surface that is hygienic and that fulfils both physical and chemical requirements essential to the health and well-being of the animals. It should be chosen in view of its absorbent capacity, its availability and low dust content. Based on the findings of Wirth (1983), wood appears to be the most suitable raw material for laboratory animal bedding. Hardwoods contain high levels of tannins and alkaloids, therefore softwoods are to be preferred. Of the softwoods, pine is not usable because of its high resin content. Weichbrod et al. (1988) demonstrated some interesting changes in microsomal oxidative enzyme activity in the rat depending on the bedding and housing conditions The monooxygenase activity can be either increased if cedar chip bedding is used or decreased if pinewood bedding is used. Fir, birch and spruce seem to be the best sources. However, based on the findings of Kraft (1980), white pine shavings seem to be the most widely used laboratory animal bedding.

Apart from the possible effects of the bedding on metabolism, the content of toxic substances should also be taken into consideration. For toxicological studies the levels of toxic contaminants in the bedding must be controlled. The choice of the wood and the defined composition of the sawdust are sometimes stated by the manufacturer. Some companies also try to minimize contamination by preservatives during production. The choice of supplier should be as important as the bedding itself. All contact bedding should be sterilized before use, although under certain circumstances (conventional rats) this may be dispensed with.

Based on preference testing, Blom et al. (1996) showed that the size and/or the shape might be the major factor in the suitability of bedding particles for laboratory rats. Bedding consisting of large fibres seems to be preferred. Bedding preference might also be dependent on factors such as strain, age, sex and reproductive condition, although this issue remains to be investigated. Bedding has to be evaluated carefully depending on the experiment. Sterilization is recommended.

Feeding

Food can be given either *ad libitum* or restricted depending on the experimental protocol. For further details see Chapter 5.

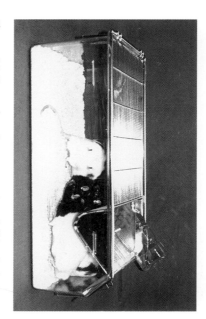

Figure 4.6 Group housing on sawdust; full-bodied cage.

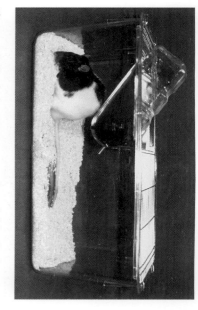

Figure 4.5 Single housing on sawdust; full-bodied cage.

Watering

Ideally, drinking water should be clear, colourless, tasteless and odourless. It should contain no pathogenic microorganisms and should be free from biological forms or chemicals which may be harmful to health or aesthetically objectionable. The water should not be corrosive or leave deposits on water-conveying structures, and it should be adequately treated to ensure consistency and quality as stated by, for example, the American Water Works Association or equivalent bodies. This definition is for human consumption, but the concept can be applied to water for laboratory rats as well.

Organic chemicals or microorganisms in the water can be eliminated by water treatment as described by Newell (1980). Filtration will eliminate solid particles; reverse osmosis, deionization and microfiltration or a combination of the three will eliminate dissolved minerals as well as organics.

Chlorination of water has been used and is still used to eliminate enteric vegetative bacteria. Cystic forms of intestinal protozoa and spore-forming bacteria are resistant to chlorine, however. There are two methods of chlorinating water, either by introducing chlorine gas into aqueous solution to obtain a concentration of 12–16 ppm, or by adding hydrochloric acid to water to obtain a pH of 2.5. The drawbacks of chlorination are the corrosive effects, the breakdown of rubber material and the production of chlorinated hydrocarbons in water with organic chemicals. Some of the chlorinated hydrocarbons are known carcinogens (IARC, 1991; Komulainen et al., 1997).

Water can be administered either using a bottle or with a programmed water-supply system, depending on the population size and the experimental procedure. The water bottles must be checked on a daily basis for leakage. A water bottle filled with coloured fluid is a good indicator for leakage due to air pressure system problems. The supply systems must be checked for bacterial and fungal production as well as for obstruction of the valve (i.e. sawdust, calcareous sediment). Monitoring of the water supply should be part of the husbandry. Biological bacteria, fungi and viruses) and chemical (pH, hardness, inorganic and organic chemicals) contaminants should be monitored carefully.

Predictability

It is the degree to which a stressor can be controlled or predicted and not the stressor itself that will determine the severity of stress symptoms, as demonstrated by Tsuda et al. (1983). Such predictability as well as controllability in terms of time of day and times per week might help to avoid stress (see Wiepkema and Koolhaas, 1993). If an event is not controllable it is important that it is predictable so as to diminish stress. Changing of the bedding, feeding and watering should always be carried out on a regular basis.

An animal will experience chronic stress when relevant environmental aspects have a low predictability and/or are not very well controlled over a long period of time. Animals can predict the delivery of food, but this event may be outside the control of the animal. In most laboratories, food availability is not controlled by the animal and therefore its predictability should be high, via a regular, stress-minimizing schedule.

Sanitation

All components of the animal facility, including animal rooms and support spaces, should be cleaned regularly and disinfected as appropriate to the circumstances. The temperature of cage cleaning should be high enough to remove microorganisms. When hot water is used alone it is the combined effect of the temperature and the length of time that a given material is exposed to the surface of the item that disinfects. This is called the cumulative heat factor. Detergents and chemicals can be added to the washing process to enhance the disinfecting effectiveness of hot water, but chemicals and detergents have to be rinsed off thoroughly. The recommended cleaning temperature with water only is 82°C for a minimum of 30 minutes. If appropriate detergents and chemicals are used, the duration of the procedure can be reduced. Depending on the housing conditions (optimal hygienic conditions or conventional), husbandry material (cages, water bottles, etc.) can be autoclaved, i.e. sterilized (Table 4.2).

Cage Cleaning

Bedding Changes

Bedding should be changed at a frequency which keeps the animals dry and clean. It is a matter of professional judgement to decide on the frequency. In some circumstances, frequent changes can be counterproductive, for example during the peripartum period when pheromones are essential for reproduction and when daily change can stress the animal due to lack of consistent odour, or due to inhibition of stable hierarchy formation. Based on the findings of Lipman et al. (1992) and Wu et al. (1985) in unventilated polycarbonate filter lid systems with rats (two rats of 250 g per cage 450 × 230 × 165 mm), ammonia levels were detectable on day 3 and exceeded 200 ppm on day 5. Cages with unventilated microisolator filter tops should therefore be cleaned twice a week due to the build up of ammonia, if the macroenvironment is in accordance with the guidelines given in ILAR (1996). Cages with ventilated microisolator filter tops or open cages can be changed once a week based on the findings of Lipman et al. (1992) and Wu et al. (1985).

Acid or alkaline cleaning

Detergent solutions are based on the acidic or alkaline principle. Acidic compounds are corrosive and it is important to check that they are compatible

Table 4.2 Conditions for the sterilization or disinfection of husbandry materials

Material	Pressure (kPa)	Temperature (°C)	Sterilization time (min)	Comments
Cages	100 (1 bar)	105	20	Disinfects. Heat resistance needs to be checked
	200 (2 bar)	121	30	Sterilizes. Heat resistance needs to be checked
Racks (metal)	200 (2 bar)	121	30	Sterilizes. Heat resistance of the wheels needs to be checked
Water	200 (2 bar)	121	45	Cool slowly
Sawdust	300 (3 bar)	135	30	

Disinfection

Disinfection of the cages as well as the animal room must be carried out on a regular basis. There are various disinfecting solutions and the biologically active substance should be changed on a regular basis. The active chemical should be changed with regular bacteriological controls. In choosing the appropriate soap and detergents, besides biological activity such factors as toxicity should also be taken into consideration (Burek and Schwetz, 1980). It is particularly important to ensure that the surfaces are rinsed free of residual chemicals and that the personnel have appropriate equipment to protect themselves from exposure to chemical agents used in the process.

Identification

Noninvasive

Coloration: tail-hair

The tails of rats can be coloured with water-proof coloured pencils as well as special animal identification method.

with the washing system, including any tubing. Acidic procedures are preferred when working with rabbits, guinea-pigs and hamsters to eliminate the high urea build-up produced in the urine of these species. With rats, the alkaline process is most frequently used. It is important to eliminate any residues of acidic or alkaline detergents with ample flushing with neutral clear water. After the cleaning process, the pH of the material surface can be checked with pH indicator paper.

identification pencils. Coloration of the hair can be achieved with normal hair dye used by humans. Most have probably been tested on rodents at some stage of their production and should not have any negative effects on the animal (Figure 4.7).

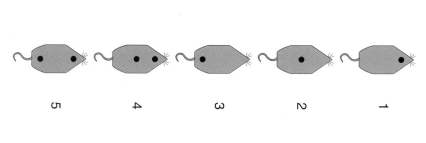

Colour coding system

Figure 4.7 Colour coding system for hair coloration identification method.

Invasive

Punching holes in ears

The standard ear punch code can be found in books such as that by Harkness and Wagner (1995) (Figure 4.8).

Ear tags

Ear tags allow a large variety of numbers, but there have been doubts expressed about sensitivity to the metals used. The weight of the tags must also be taken into consideration (Figure 4.9).

Toes

Toe-clipping as a method of permanent (>1 year) identification has been used for wild rodents in field research. Field biologists have argued that alternative methods are either too expensive (e.g. implantable **transponders**) or lead to reduced survival over

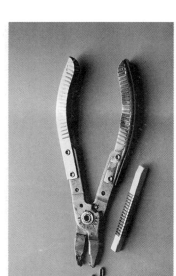

Figure 4.9 Miniature ear tag system for identification method (International Market Supply, Congleton, Cheshire, UK).

time (newly collected data regarding ear tags). This method should only be chosen if all other methods fail.

Tattoos

There are manual as well as electronic tattoo units. Any number and letter combination can be used. In rats, tails and ears can be used for this purpose. A good practice with professional tattooers (as some animal tattooing companies advertise and offer) is of excellent value and will improve the quality and therefore the readability of the tattoos.

Transponders

Many companies advertise transponders for animals. The size of the transponders are ideally suited for rats. Other information besides the identification number can be recorded, as direct computerized recording. The advantage is the unique identification of each animal. The disadvantages are the cost and the need to remove the chips before disposing of the cadaver.

Enrichment

It is possible to improve the quality of life for captive animals by enriching their environment so that they are able to perform more of their species-specific behaviour. Besides the cage structure, the influence of social interactions with humans must not be underestimated.

Captive environments may be chronically stressful to animals if there is no or only limited opportunity for active behavioural responses. Well-designed housing systems allow for effective coping

Ear notch-punch code   Single units right
Units of ten left   (e.g. 1, 2, 3 . . .)
(e.g. 10, 20, 30 . . .)

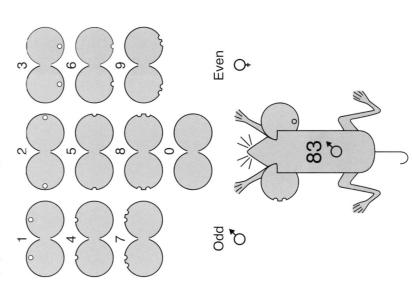

Figure 4.8 Ear notch punch code as identification method.

behaviour, which may enhance welfare. Environmental enrichment is not an **anthropomorphic** tool, it must be thoroughly evaluated. Van de Weerd *et al.* (1997) showed that in mice the nesting material has a positive physiological influence, producing effects on body weight and food intake, and also influences certain measured behaviour (including open field test, aluminium foil test) in the different housing conditions. In rats, the results are still rather contradictory and therefore a critical evaluation of any environmental enrichment for rats should be performed before implementing measures. Nesting boxes and nesting material to enhance the environment of rats were evaluated with preference testing by Manser *et al.* (1998a, b). It was demonstrated that laboratory rats prefer cages furnished with either a nest box, nesting material or both, to empty cages. Among the nest boxes tested was a purpose-built opaque black perspex nest box, based on the observation that rats sleep under foodhoppers and/or in the dark; this was found to be the preferred box for the rats.

Extensive research into environmental enrichment (Benefiel and Greenough, 1998) has been carried out and effects of the environment on brain and behaviour have been published. It is of uttermost importance to know and understand the influence of enrichment on the animal before applying it, but this effort is worth while if enrichment improves the well-being of laboratory animals and, therefore, the scientific quality of the data they provide.

Acknowledgements

I am extremely grateful to Professor P. Thomann for providing me with the opportunity to write this chapter and for his constructive criticism of earlier drafts of the manuscript; and to Dr C. Pryce for his linguistic assistance.

References

Baer, L.A., Corbin, B.J., Vasques, M.F. and Grindeland, R.E. (1997) *Lab. Anim. Sci.* **47**: 327–329.

Bellhorn, R.W. (1980) *Lab. Anim. Sci.* **30**: 440–450.

Benefiel, A.C. and Greenough, W.T. (1998) *ILAR J.* **39**: 5–11.

Besch, E.L. (1980) *Lab. Anim. Sci.* **30**: 386–406.

Blom, H. (1993) Evaluation of housing conditions for laboratory mice and rats, the use of preference tests for studying choice behaviour. Enschede: Offsetdrukkerij Febodruk. ISBN 90-393-0216-2.

Blom, H.J.M., Van Tintelen, G., Van Vorstenbosch, C.J.A.H.V., Baumans, V. and Beynen, A.C. (1996) *Lab. Anim.* **30**: 234–244.

Burek, J.D. and Schwetz, B.A. (1980) *Lab. Anim. Sci.* **30**: 414–421.

Corning, B.F. and Lipman, N.S. (1991) *Lab. Anim. Sci.* **41**: 498–503.

Council Directive 86/609/EEC of 24 November 1986 on the approximation of laws, regulations and administrative provisions of the Member States regarding the protection of animals used for experimental and other scientific purposes, *Official Journal L* 358, **386L0609**, pp. 1–28.

Dauchy, T.R., Sauer, L.A., Blask, D.E. and Vaughan, G.M. (1997) *Lab Anim Sci.* **47**: 511–518.

FELASA (Federation of European Laboratory Animal Science Association) (1997) *Harmonisation of Laboratory Animal Husbandry – Proceedings of the Sixth FELASA Symposium*, June 1996, Basle, Switzerland.

Fox, G.J., Cohen, B.J. and Loew, F.M. (1984) Laboratory animal medicine, chapter 23, American College of laboratory animal Medicine Series, Academic Press, Inc. Florida. ISBN 0-12-263620-1.

Gamble, M.R. and Clough, G. (1976) *Lab. Anim.* **10**: 93–104.

Gordon, J.J.C. (1990) *Physiol. Behav.* **47**: 963–991.

GV-SOLAS (Society for Laboratory Animal Science-Gesellschaft für Versuchstierkunde) (1989) *Publication on the Planning and Structure of Animal Facilities for Institutes Performing Animal Experiments.* Switzerland: Offsetdruck Gert Emminger.

Harkness, J.E. and Wagner, J.E. (1995) *The Biology and Medicine of Rabbits and Rodents.* Philadelphia: Lea & Febiger. ISBN 0-8121-11-76-1.

Hughes, H.C., Reynolds, S. and Rodriguez, M. (1996) *Pharmaceutical Engineering* March/April: 44–65.

IARC (International Agency for Research on Cancer) (1991) *Monographs on the Evaluation of Carcinogenic Risks to Human*, Vol. 52. Geneva: World Health Organization. ISBN 92-832-1252-5.

ILAR (Institute for Laboratory Animal Research) (1996) *Guide for the Care and Use of Laboratory Animals.* NRC. Komulainen, H., Kosma, V.M., Vaittinen, S.L. *et al.* (1997) *J. Natl Cancer Inst.* **89**: 848–856.

Kraft, L.M. (1980) *Lab. Anim.* **30**: 366–376.

Lipman, N.S., Corning, B.F. and Coiro, M.A. Sr. (1992) *Lab. Anim.* **26**: 206–210.

Manser, C.E., Morris, T.H. and Broom, D.M. (1995) *Lab. Anim.* **29**: 353–363.

Manser, C.E., Broom, D.M., Overend P. and Morris, T.H. (1998a) *Lab Anim.* **32**: 36–41.

Manser, C.E., Broom, D.M., Overend P. and Morris, T.H. (1998b) *Lab. Anim.* **32**: 23–35.

Newell, G.W. (1980) *Lab. Anim. Sci.* **30**: 377–384.

Peterson, E.A. (1980) *Lab. Anim. Sci.* **30**: 422–439.

Raynor, T.H., Steinhagen, W.H. and Hamm, T.E. Jr. (1983) *Lab. Anim.* **17**: 85–89.

Semple-Rowland, S.L. and Dawson W.W. (1987) *Lab. Anim. Sci.* **37**: 296–298.

Serrano, J.L. (1971) *Lab. Anim. Sci.* **21**: 75–85.

Tsuda, A., Tanaka, M. Hirai, H. and Pare, W.P. (1983) *Jpn. Psychol. Res.* **25**: 9–15.

Van de Weerd, H.A., Van Loo, P.L.P., Van Zutphen, L.F.M., Koolhaas, J.M. and Baumans V. (1997) *Physiol. Behav.* **62**: 1019–1028.

Van Zutphen, L.F.M., Baumans, V. and Beynen, A.C. (1993) *Principles of Laboratory Animal Science*. Amsterdam: Elsevier. ISBN 0-444-81487-6.

Weichbrod, R.H., Cisar, C.F., Miller, J.G., Simmonds, R.C., Alvares, A.P. and Tzuu, H.U. (1988) *Lab. Anim. Sci.* **38**: 289–298.

Wiepkema, P.R. and Koolhaas, J.M. (1993) *Anim. Welfare* **2**: 195–218.

Wirth, H. (1983) *Lab. Anim.* **17**: 81–84.

Woods, J.E. (1980) *Lab. Anim. Sci.* **30**: 407–413.

Wu, D., Joiner, G.N. and McFarland, A.R. (1985) *Lab. Anim. Sci.* **35**: 407–413.

CHAPTER 5

Nutrition

Kevin P Keenan
Department of Safety Assessment,
Merck Research Laboratories,
West Point, PA USA

**Gordon C Ballam and
Dorrance G Haught**
Purina Mills Inc., St. Louis, MO USA

Phillippe Laroque
Laboratories MSD-Chibret, Riom,
Clermont-Ferrand, France

Introduction

The laboratory rat (*Rattus norvegicus*) has been successfully used as an experimental model in nutritional research due to its moderate size, excellent reproduction, tractable behavior and omnivorous dietary habits. One of the first nutritional discoveries using the rat was that of McCullum and Davis (1913) and Osborne and Mendel (1913), who observed that a substance found in butter or the fat from eggs was required for long-term health and survival. This substance eventually was identified as vitamin A. Over the ensuing 85 years, the laboratory rat has become one of the most important animal models for biological and biomedical research. The origins of the major strains and stocks of laboratory rats were reviewed by Lindsey (1979) and nutritional recommendations through the late 1970s reviewed by Rogers (1979).

Factors Affecting Nutrient Requirements

At least 40 nutrients are required in the diet of the laboratory rat. Water and diet are the most complex mixture of exogenous organic and inorganic chemicals to which rats are exposed. The diet needs to be controlled and optimized for the sex, physiological condition (i.e. maintenance versus reproduction/lactation) and age-specific needs of the rat, because dietary composition and manner of feeding can significantly affect the animal's physiology, metabolism and alter the effects of test substances on experimental endpoints (Baker, 1986; Hart *et al*, 1995; Masoro, 1995; Roe *et al*, 1995; K.P. Keenan *et al*, 1998).

The principal indicators of dietary adequacy have been growth and reproductive performance. Most of the scientific basis for nutritional recommendations for growth and maintenance have focused on the growth of weanling rats as an indicator of optimal nutrition. Typically the maximum growth rate (body weight) is compared in young, growing animals fed diets *ad libitum* with various concentrations of a specific nutrient while keeping the concentrations of all other nutrients constant for one or two months (McDonald, 1997). The optimal concentration of a nutrient is then defined at the point where increasing concentrations in the diet did not significantly increase maximal growth. This index of growth analysis in establishing nutritional requirements in weanling rats is limited because it does not address the nutritional requirements of full-grown adult rodents. As a result, the nutritional maintenance requirements for mature rodents used in long-term studies are virtually unknown (McDonald, 1997).

The most authoritative source of information on nutritional requirements in the rat can be found in the publication *Nutrient Requirements of Laboratory Animals* (National Research Council, 1995) which was written by a subcommittee of the National Research Council. This report supersedes an earlier report published in 1978 (National Research Council, 1978). Readers interested in the absolute minimal requirements may wish to consult both reports as well as the original literature cited in those documents. The National Research Council (NRC) publication should only be used as a starting point for establishing nutritional requirements, because the NRC requirements are estimates of the minimal nutrient levels required, with no margin of safety. The following factors that influence nutrient requirements must be considered when establishing dietary nutrient concentrations.

Genetic differences

Genetic differences among rat strains, stocks, sexes and individuals may affect nutrient requirements (National Research Council, 1995). For example, genetic differences in growth potential among different strains and sexes influence the daily requirements for amino acids and other nutrients (Fenton, 1957; Goodrick, 1973).

Sex

The sex of the animal may also affect nutritional requirements. Male rats grow faster than females and have a body composition that is higher in protein (Ballam, unpublished data). Maximum tissue protein deposition requires higher amino acid levels than that required for maximum growth (Benevenga et al., 1994). Therefore, it is likely that there are many differences in the nutrient requirements of male and female rats that change during life.

Physiological stage

Physiological stage of life has a profound effect on the nutrient requirements of the rat. Nutrient requirements change with growth and reproductive status. Growing rats have greater protein and amino acid requirements than older rats in a state of maintenance (Mitchell et al., 1956; Sheehan et al., 1981; Baldwin and Mitchell, 1952; Hartsook and Grimminger, 1985). The nutrient requirements for reproduction and lactation are similar to those of growing animals (National Research Council, 1995), except for energy (which is higher for lactation); but relatively few studies have been conducted to elucidate them. With the exception of protein (Benevenga et al., 1994), the nutrient requirements for maintenance of the adult rat have not been carefully studied (McDonald, 1997). Adult rats that are not breeding or lactating require less dietary protein than growing animals.

Dietary energy, vitamin and mineral concentrations adequate for growing animals have been generally recommended to meet the requirements of adult rats in the maintenance state (National Research Council, 1995). Within the research community, rats are fed diets designed for growth and not for maintenance. Since most investigators prefer to feed a single diet throughout a study, the adult rat is usually overfed protein, energy, vitamins and minerals. The complications of overfeeding these nutrients, other than energy, in long-term toxicology studies are not well defined. Overfeeding protein has been thought to enhance **nephropathy**, a common diet-related disease in Sprague-Dawley, Wistar and F-344 rats. However, researchers have shown that restricting protein intake without restriction of calories had only minor effects on renal disease and longevity (Maeda et al., 1985; Iwaskai et al., 1988; Masoro et al., 1989; Gumprecht et al., 1993; Keenan et al., 1994b, 1995b; Roe et al., 1995).

Feed intake variation

Variation in feed intake affects total nutrient intake, which in turn, influences the ability of the diet to meet the nutrient requirements of the animal. Feed intake can be influenced by the energy content of the diet, environmental factors such as temperature, light cycle or by other management practices. Rats exposed to temperatures below their **thermal neutral zone** increase feed intake to satisfy their increased energy requirement to maintain a constant body temperature. In some cases, the greater feed intake may lead to overconsumption of the other nutrients. Conversely, factors that reduce feed intake, such as elevated temperatures, group housing, restrictive feeders and cage design or additional stresses, may require a greater nutrient density in the diet to meet the nutrient needs of the animal.

Nutrient bioavailability

Nutrient bioavailability must be considered in providing the proper amount of nutrients for rats (Coates, 1987). Nutrients found in natural feed ingredients are not 100% bioavailable to the animal. In addition, there are various constituents such as tannins, phytate and lignin contained in natural ingredients that can decrease nutrient availability. Nutrient interactions can also occur, making some nutrients less available. Therefore, care must be taken to account for the bioavailability of nutrients from the feed ingredients when formulating diets for laboratory animals.

Microbiology

The microbiological status of the rat is a key factor when considering the proper level of water-soluble vitamins, vitamin K and amino acids. Many of the microbially produced nutrients found in rat feces will not be available to the animals if **coprophagy** is reduced by management practices or cage design. Specific pathogen free (SPF) animals and germ-free animals also have an altered microbial nutrient synthesis, resulting in higher dietary nutrient requirements. Therefore, adjustments may be required in formulating diets for SPF or germ-free animals (Wostmann, 1975).

Statistics and chosen endpoints

The statistical methodology employed and the choice of the physiological endpoints can influence the determination of a nutrient requirement. The amino acid requirements of growing rats obtained by different statistical approaches will result in

different estimates of the nutritional requirement. For example, the growth response curve to an increased amino acid level is frequently in the shape of an asymptotic curve, with each increase of the nutrient giving a diminished response. The point where there is a 'break' in the curve and the growth response approximates a plateau is generally chosen as the requirement. An alternative procedure, is to use statistical calculations to set the requirement as the level at which 95% of the maximal effect would be seen if increasing levels of the nutrient were fed. Therefore, requirements estimated from the same data set by different statistical methods will be different. This point has been discussed extensively by Baker (1986) and Robbins *et al.* (1979).

Nutrient requirements may differ, depending upon the parameter chosen to evaluate the requirement. Dietary nutrient concentrations to maximize growth may be different from those to maximize feed efficiency, tissue protein or fat concentrations or immune function (Robbins *et al.*, 1977). For example, maximum tissue protein deposition in rats requires higher concentrations of amino acids than those required for maximum body growth (Benevenga *et al.*, 1994).

Nutritional Requirements

The following section contains a general discussion of some of the key nutrient groups: protein, carbohydrates, lipids, vitamins, minerals, and energy.

Protein and Amino Acids

Minimum dietary concentrations of protein required for growth, reproduction and maintenance have been estimated to be 15%, 15% and 5%, respectively (National Research Council, 1995). However, these optimum dietary protein concentrations are based on studies with purified diets with highly digestible protein such as lactalbumin. These protein concentrations are too low for animals fed commercial diets with natural ingredients such as corn, wheat and soybean meal. The bioavailability of nutrients in purified diets is usually greater than in diets composed of natural feed ingredients and, therefore, the nutrient content of diets containing natural ingredients needs to be higher. The total protein and indispensable or essential amino acid requirements have been estimated for growing rats and are assumed to meet the needs of adult animals (National Research Council, 1995). Most commercial natural-ingredient diets for rats fed in North America contain between 18% and 23% protein, support high rates of postweaning growth and are customarily fed during all stages of the rodent's life.

In some European laboratories, it is customary to feed diets containing 15% protein to rats in chronic toxicology studies. When animals are fed such diets, growth rates are initially reduced because the protein content of the diet is less than that necessary for maximum growth. However, as the animals grow older and become adults, these natural-product diets more closely meet the animal's adult protein needs.

The optimal dietary protein concentration of adult rats, consuming readily digestible, protein diets such as egg protein or lactalbumin as a balanced source of amino acids, has been estimated to be 5% of the diet (National Research Council, 1995). The protein requirement of rats fed diets composed of natural ingredients such as soybean meal is likely to be greater than 5%, but less than 12% suggested for maximal growth by the 1978 NRC report. Since most natural product diets contain between 18% and 23% protein, consumption of protein generally exceeds the amount necessary for adult rats in a physiological state of maintenance.

The rat's dietary requirements for amino acids actually requirements for amino acids contained in the dietary protein. There are 22 amino acids in body tissues that are physiologically essential. These amino acids can be nutritionally divided into essential amino acids (those that the rat cannot synthesize, or synthesize rapidly enough to meet metabolic requirements) and nonessential amino acids (those that can be synthesized from other amino acids). The essential amino acids that are indispensable or required in the diet of the growing rat are arginine, histidine, isoleucine, leucine, lysine, methionine, phenylalanine, threonine, tryptophan and valine (National Research Council, 1995). The essential amino acid requirements for maintenance, growth and reproduction are summarized by the most recent NRC committee (National Research Council, 1995).

Modifying or limiting dietary protein intake has been reported to decrease renal disease, without reducing body weight (Rao et al., 1993) in Fischer 344 rats. Iwasaki et al. (1988) demonstrated that replacing casein with soybean as a source of dietary protein retarded the progression of chronic nephropathy in Fischer 344 rats when caloric intake and body weights were similar between study groups. However, the restriction of protein intake by 40% without the restriction of calories had only minor effects on longevity, because few other aging processes were altered (Iwasaki et al., 1988; Masoro et al., 1989). Moreover, a 40% caloric restriction without protein restriction was as effective as caloric restriction with protein restriction in increasing Fischer 344 rat survival. Similar carefully balanced studies in Fischer 344 rats with the restriction of dietary fat or minerals without caloric restriction demonstrated no survival benefit (Maeda et al., 1985; Masoro et al., 1991). Studies with Sprague-Dawley rats (Keenan et al., 1992, 1994a,b, 1995b; Gumprecht et al., 1993; Laroque et al., 1997) and Wistar rats (Roe et al., 1995) fed natural-product diets with reduced protein content and increased fiber content have led to similar conclusions. These modifications had only a small effect on renal disease and did not consistently improve survival if the rats were allowed *ad libitum* food intake of the diets compared to controlled restricted food intake (Roe et al., 1995; K.P. Keenan et al., 1998). These data indicate that controlling caloric intake is more important than controlling protein intake to prevent renal disease and increase survival of rats in long-term studies. The protein requirements are influenced by total energy intake and dietary energy concentrations as well as the bioavailability and amino acid composition of the diet (National Research Council, 1995).

Carbohydrate and Fiber

No definitive carbohydrate requirement has been established for rats, although they need carbohydrates for successful reproduction and lactation. Carbohydrates such as sugars, starch and fiber, contribute to the gross energy in the diet. Rats do not have the enzyme systems to digest fiber, therefore, any caloric value obtained from fiber occurs as a result of bacterial fermentation in the cecum and colon and subsequent ingestion of feces by the animal (i.e. coprophagy). Purified diets frequently utilize starch, glucose and sucrose that can be well utilized by rats as the only form of digestible carbohydrate. However, some carbohydrates, such as fructose (and sucrose as a source of fructose) can lead to metabolic abnormalities compared to feeding glucose and starches in semipurified diets. Fructose or sucrose feeding will increase rat liver weight, liver lipid and glycogen content, liver lipogenic enzyme activity and result in hypertriglyceridemia. Fructose feeding has also been associated with increased **nephrocalcinosis** in female rats due to increased urinary phosphorus and magnesium and lower urinary pH (National Research Council, 1995). These potential problems can be avoided by using carbohydrates from natural sources. Carbohydrates in diets made from natural ingredients are derived principally from grain and grain by-products, such as corn, wheat, barley, oats, wheat middlings and molasses.

Requirements for dietary fiber have not been demonstrated in the rat, but fiber's effects may be beneficial. There are several different ways the fiber content of diets are described. The traditional measurement is 'crude fiber'. More sophisticated procedures measure fiber as **'acid detergent fiber'** and **'neutral detergent fiber'**. The effects of fiber depend on its source and properties (solubility, viscosity, fermentability). Fiber increases rats' fecal bulk and the size and weight of the cecum and colon (Keenan *et al.*, 1994a,b). Fiber is known to decrease gastrointestinal transit time, and fermentable fiber sources result in volatile fatty acid production, which are absorbed and used as an energy source. Increased fiber increases excretion of fecal nitrogen and decreases urinary nitrogen due to microbial fermentation and utilization of protein. Many fiber sources have been used and their metabolic effects can be predicted based on their physical properties and fermentabilities (National Research Council, 1995).

Increasing dietary fiber with insoluble, largely indigestible fiber sources such as cellulose, oat hulls, wheat bran and corn bran have been attempted to control nutrient intake in rats. Results have been mixed. Dilution of dietary energy content requires as much as 30–45% fiber to reduce the energy consumption of mature and weanling rats (Peterson and Baumgardt, 1971a,b). Lactating rats could not compensate for a 10% dilution in these studies. Keenan *et al.* (1994a,b) fed diets containing 15.7% crude fiber and 2.36 kcal/g to rats. The rats in this study compensated by eating 30% more food to maintain similar energy intakes as those fed a diet containing 4.1% crude fiber and 3.07 kcal/g of metabolizable energy.

Lipids

Lipids are a source of essential fatty acids, a concentrated source of energy, and an aid in the absorption of fat-soluble vitamins. The essential fatty acids can be divided into two types, omega-6 and omega-3. Linoleic acid, which is found in many plant feed ingredients, is the primary omega-6 fatty acid and is needed as a component of membranes, for membrane-bound enzyme function and as a precursor for prostaglandin formation. Requirements for linoleic acid have been determined to be 6.0 and 3.0 g/kg of diet for growth and reproduction, respectively (National Research Council, 1995). Linolenic acid is an omega-3 fatty acid commonly found in many feed ingredients. Rats also require linolenic acid, although a dietary requirement has not been quantified (National Research Council, 1995).

Most commercial laboratory rat diets contain 4–6% dietary fat and this level is adequate for growth and maintenance of rats. The National Research Council (1995) sets a requirement of 5% dietary fat. That requirement is based on a dietary concentration of fat that provides the maximum growth rate, which may not be appropriate for all situations. Data that support a total dietary fat requirement for growing and adult rats in excess of requirements for essential fatty acids are limited.

Vitamins

The literature on the vitamin requirements of rats, as reviewed by the most recent National Research Council committee (1995), is summarized in Table 5.1. Commercial diets usually contain levels equal to or in excess of the levels recommended. Some synthesis of the water-soluble vitamins and vitamin K occurs by microorganisms in the lower gastrointestinal tract, and provides the rat with a source of vitamins by recycling through coprophagy. Therefore, it is difficult to produce a deficiency of some vitamins such as folic acid, biotin and vitamin K without taking steps to reduce the intestinal bacterial population or prevent coprophagy. Conversely, if microbial synthesis and coprophagy are reduced, greater dietary concentrations of these vitamins are required.

Minerals

The National Research Council (1995) reviewed the requirements of rats for major minerals and trace minerals and their recommendations are summarized in Table 5.2. These recommendations are straightforward, but several factors need to be considered in long-term studies.

Table 5.1 Estimated requirements of the rat for vitamins[a]

Vitamin	Growth[b]	Reproduction
Vitamin A (IU/kg)	2300	2300
Vitamin D3[c] (IU/kg)	1000	1000
Vitamin E (IU/kg)	27.0	27.0
Vitamin K (mg/kg of phylloqinone)	1.0	1.0
Thiamin-HCl (mg/kg)	4.0	4.0
Riboflavin (mg/kg)	3.0	4.0
Niacin (mg/kg)	15.0	15.0
Pantothenic acid (mg/kg)	8.8	8.0
Vitamin B6 (pyridoxine) (mg/kg)	6.0	6.0
Folic Acid (mg/kg)	1.0	1.0
Vitamin B12[b] (mg/kg)	0.05	0.05
Biotin (mg/kg)	0.2	0.2
Choline (free base) (mg/kg)	750	750

[a] Expressed as on an as-fed basis for diets containing 10% moisture. Values taken or calculated from National Research Council (1995).

[b] Separate requirements for maintenance have not been determined; requirements for growth will meet maintenance requirements.

[c] Estimates adequate amount in diet; probably exceeds actual requirement.

The phosphorus levels in the diet are important. Much of the phosphorus in a natural-product diet is from plant products in the form of phytate phosphorus which is largely unavailable to the animal. The phosphorus requirement suggested by the National Research Council (1995) is based on highly available phosphorus such as that added to purified diets. When assessing the phosphorus levels in diets, one should consider the nonphytate phosphorus rather than the total dietary phosphorus concentrations.

The ratio of dietary calcium to phosphorus is a concern. When the nonphytate phosphorus levels exceed the calcium levels in the diet, nephrocalcinosis occurs with mineral deposits at the corticomedullary region (Clapp et al., 1982; Stonard et al., 1984; Ritskes-Hoitinga et al., 1989a,b, 1991). This process can lead to renal hypertrophy and degenerative renal tubular changes, especially in female rats. Generally, nephrocalcinosis is more common when rats are fed purified diets. The National Research Council (1995) suggests a calcium-to-phosphorus molar ratio of 1.3 to prevent nephrocalcinosis. This equates to a weight ratio of calcium to phosphorus of 1.68 to 1.

There have been suggestions that the elements chromium, arsenic, nickel, vanadium, silicon, tin, fluorine, lead, boron and cadmium may be required in rat diets. While there is some evidence these elements may have dietary requirements, the results are equivocal. Typical commercial laboratory diets, made from natural ingredients, contain these minerals at levels to meet the rat's nutritional requirements.

Energy

Energy has traditionally been stated in terms of kilocalories (also referred to as Calories). A kilocalorie (kcal) is equivalent to 1000 calories. A calorie is the amount of heat it takes to heat 1 gram of water 1 degree centigrade. The SI unit for energy is the joule (J), which is equivalent to 4.184 calories.

The energy content of food can be stated in four different ways: gross energy, digestible energy, metabolizable energy and net energy. Gross energy is the heat given off when an ingredient is burned to its ultimate oxidation products. Digestible energy is derived by subtracting the fecal energy of food

Nutrient	Growth[b]	Reproduction (females)
Calcium[c] (%)	0.50	0.63
Phosphorus[d] (%)	0.30	0.37
Magnesium (%)	0.05	0.06
Potassium (%)	0.36	0.36
Sodium (%)	0.005	0.005
Chloride (%)	0.005	0.005
Iron (mg/kg)	35.0	75.0
Copper (mg/kg)	5.0	8.0
Manganese (mg/kg)	10.0	10.0
Zinc[e] (mg/kg)	12.0	25.0
Iodine (mg/kg)	0.15	0.15
Molybdenum (mg/kg)	0.15	0.15
Selenium (mg/kg)	0.15	0.40

Table 5.2 Estimated requirements of rats for minerals[a]

[a] From National Research Council (1995).
[b] Separate requirements for maintenance have not been determined; requirements for growth will meet maintenance requirements.
[c] Calcium should exceed nonphytate phosphorus level by at least 68%; see text.
[d] Refers to level of nonphytate phosphorus; see text.
[e] Requirement in purified diets. The zinc required will be higher with diets composed of natural ingredients containing phytate (such as soybean meal and other plant products).

origin from the gross energy intake. When the energy lost in the gaseous products of digestion and that lost in the urine is subtracted from the apparent digestible energy, one arrives at the portion of total energy actually capable of transformation by the body. This value is called metabolizable energy. Net energy is obtained by subtracting the energy lost as heat from the metabolizable energy. This is the energy which is completely useful to the body. Most references to the energy content of feed refer to metabolizable energy. The metabolizable energy (ME) of many feed ingredients has been determined for domestic animals such as swine and poultry, but only limited studies have been conducted with rats. Consequently, the amount of metabolizable energy in rat diets is usually an estimate (National Research Council, 1995).

The metabolizable energy content of rat diets is estimated in two different ways: (1) physiological fuel values based on mathematical calculations from the chemical composition of the feed ingredients and (2) metabolizable energy values, which use animal models in digestibility studies. Physiological fuel

values are estimated by multiplying the percentage protein and the percentage carbohydrate (excluding crude fiber) by 4kcal/g and the percentage fat by 9kcal/g (Maynard et al., 1979). These caloric values, called physiological fuel values, were developed to apply to human foods. These types of calculations are likely to overestimate the digestibility of feed ingredients used in diets for laboratory rats (Maynard et al., 1979).

Metabolizable energy values are more accurately determined by conducting digestibility trials with monogastric animals. Commercial manufacturers of laboratory rodent diets offer metabolizable energy values calculated from a monogastric animal database (Purina Mills, 1996). Metabolizable energy values determined in this way will be about 90% of the physiological fuel values.

The metabolizable energy required by animals is an important consideration, particularly in studies where the amount of food is controlled or measured. Daily metabolizable energy requirements are determined by calculating the basal metabolic rate, and then adding the energy needed for activity, growth and reproduction. The maintenance metabolizable energy (ME) requirements of rats under most environmental conditions is described by the equation:

$$\text{ME for maintenance (kcal/day)} = 112 \times \text{body weight (in kg)}^{0.75}$$

(McCraken, 1975; National Research Council, 1995).

The minimum ME requirement for growth has been estimated to be approximately twice the ME needed for maintenance. While early gestation (up to gestation day 16) requires ME levels as high as 30% above maintenance, later gestation requires an ME as much as 2.5 times maintenance. The demands of lactation require 2–4 times the maintenance ME, depending upon the number of pups nursing the dam (National Research Council, 1995).

Energy Balance

Animals eat to meet their energy needs. Energy intake is regulated by a complex system involving both internal physiological controls and external clues. Gastric distention, response to sight, sound and smell of food, and changes in plasma concentrations of nutrients, hormones and peptides are some of the internal physiological controls that regulate energy intake. External clues include food availability, timing and size of meals, food composition and texture and diet palatability (Case et al., 1995).

Body weight appears to be physiologically regulated by balancing energy intake, expenditure and storage. A 'lipostatic theory' of body weight maintenance developed in the 1950s and 1960s proposed that a factor secreted from adipose tissue signaled the status of body energy stores to the brain and thus regulated feeding behavior and body fat mass (Kennedy, 1953; Coleman and Hummel, 1969). Recent studies investigating the effects of exogenous leptin administration to the leptin-deficient ob/ob mouse have led to the development of a simple model of leptin-initiated energy balance regulation that resembles the earlier theory (Houseknecht et al., 1998). Leptin is synthesized and secreted from white adipocytes into the blood and is transported to the brain where it acts to cause the release or inhibition of factors such as neuropeptide Y that ultimately result in a reduction in food intake, an increase in energy expenditure and increased physical activity (Halaas et al., 1995; Banis et al., 1996; Lynn et al., 1996; Malik and Young, 1996; Elmquist et al., 1997;

Jang and Romsos, 1998; Claycombe et al., 1998; Houseknecht et al., 1998). These subsequent reactions result in a reduction in adipose mass or the stimulation of other endocrine or auto/paracrine signals that inhibit leptin synthesis and secretion by adipocytes. Leptin may also directly affect the metabolism of peripheral tissues such as liver and skeletal muscle as well as adipocytes (Houseknecht et al., 1998).

It is now recognized that energy balance is the result of a complex, redundant and highly integrated neurohormonal system that controls homeostasis by several hormones secreted in proportion to adiposity, including leptin and insulin and the targets in the central nervous system on which they act (Woods et al., 1998; Flier and Maratos-Flier, 1998). Anabolic pathways that stimulate food intake and weight gain include the hypothalamic neuropeptide Y (NPY) axis, and catabolic pathways that reduce food intake and stimulate weight loss include the hypothalamic melanocortin system. Insulin and leptin are hormones that are regulated by adipose tissue, inhibit the anabolic pathways and stimulate the central catabolic pathways through an expanding list of central nervous system signaling molecules (Woods et al., 1998, Flier and Maratos-Flier, 1998).

It has been proposed that body weight is maintained by establishing a 'set point' at which body weight and fat mass are regulated. To maintain body weight, coordinated adjustments in both energy intake and expenditure serve to stabilize the weights of rats at a specified level and to resist their displacement from this level (Keesey and Hirvonen, 1997). However, the set point is a range, rather than a single point, which is governed by various factors such as hormonal status, age and genetics, and it is possible to shift the set point by a number of mechanisms (Wilding and Widdowson, 1997). The catabolic effects of leptin and insulin induce responses that lead to weight loss by loss of body fat stores. However, most obese mammals, including humans, have increased plasma leptin and insulin levels, except for the leptin-deficient obese (ob/ob) mouse. The leptin-resistant, genetically obese Zucker rat (fa/fa, mutated in the leptin receptor gene) does not reduce food intake or weight when given insulin centrally. Thus leptin and insulin act in complex ways that involve central nervous system peptide signaling and other hormonal systems. Glucocorticoid hormones are implicated in energy balances by their effects on NPY. Adrenalectomy decreases the effects of fasting to increase food intake and NPY gene expression and enhances the ability of insulin and leptin to induce anorexia and weight loss. These effects are reversed by glucocorticoid treatment and indicate that glucocorticoids are endogenous antagonists of leptin and insulin in the control of energy balance (Woods *et al.*, 1998). These and other studies demonstrate the complexity of the genetic, endogenous and exogenous factors controlling the hypothalmic-pituitary-adrenal-adipose axis and the way in which they could potentially result in changes in energy balance and the re-establishment of the set point (Wilding *et al.*, 1997).

Type and Form of Diet

Two types of diets are generally used when conducting experiments with rats: (1) purified (or semipurified) diets and (2) diets made from natural ingredients. There are several variations of purified or semipurified diets, although the usual components are casein, starch and/or sucrose, corn oil, purified wood pulp, and chemically pure minerals and vitamins. In diets made from natural ingredients, cereal grains such as corn, wheat and barley provide the carbohydrate while soybean meal and fish meal supply the protein. Minerals, vitamins and some amino acids may be added to these formulations.

Purified diets are suitable for investigating nutrient interactions because the nutrient concentrations are easier to control than in natural diets. However, purified diets are not as palatable as diets containing natural ingredients and rats fed purified diets have shorter lifespans and are more susceptible to degenerative diseases such as nephrocalcinosis and tumors than rats fed natural-ingredient diets (Silverstone *et al.*, 1952; Engle and Copeland, 1952; Fullerton *et al.*, 1992; Cohen *et al.*, 1994; Newberne and Sotnikov, 1996).

Diets containing natural ingredients should be formulated to a constant nutritional content basis because of the inherent nutrient variability contained in natural ingredients. Fixed formulations, where natural ingredients are kept at a constant concentration in the diet, are an unsuitable formulation strategy because this method does not take into account the variation in nutrient content which occurs in natural feed ingredients from batch to batch. Therefore nutrient content will differ between batches, when the formulation is fixed.

Diets for rats historically have been available in two forms: (1) meal (powder) and (2) pellets. Meal diets are manufactured by finely grinding all of the ingredients and mixing them uniformly. Under some circumstances, these diets become dusty and the animals separate and select the food particles they wish to consume.

Pelleted diets are manufactured by grinding all of the ingredients, blending them together, subjecting the blended meal to steam conditioning and forcing the meal through a metal pellet die to form a pellet. Pelleted diets have the practical advantage of delivering a more uniform nutrient package to the animal and producing less dust. Within the last few years, extruded diets have gained popularity. Extrusion is similar to pelleting except that the ingredients are more thoroughly cooked than in the pelleting process. Additionally, this technology enables the manufacturer to make particles of specific weights with greater uniformity and precision. These diets are ideal for restricting feed intake to control caloric intake and experimental variables in toxicity and carcinogenicity studies.

The Need to Control Dietary Intake

Improved laboratory animal husbandry and nutrition have succeeded in eliminating or controlling many of the confounding variables in rodent bioassays and have also reduced or eliminated many of the exogenous stressors that modify the animal's response to a test substance (Bhatt *et al.*, 1986; Hart *et al.*, 1995; Allaben *et al.*, 1996; Newberne and Sotnikov, 1996). However, reduction of these stressors has been offset by a steady increase in study-to-study variability, a lack of reproducibility and

A number of compounds in natural ingredients have been shown to be important in preventing the development of spontaneous and experimental tumors (He *et al.*, 1997; Anderson and Garner, 1997; Kurzer and Xu, 1997; World Cancer Research Fund/ American Institute for Cancer Research, 1997). While many of these chemopreventative compounds are yet to be identified, certain isoflavones and polyphenols appear to have important effects in preventing tumors.

increases in the onset and severity of spontaneous degenerative disease and tumors resulting in decreased rodent survival in chronic bioassays over the past two decades (Duffy et al., 1989; Rao et al., 1990; Fishbein, 1991; Lang, 1991; Haseman and Rao, 1992; Keenan et al., 1992, 1994a,b, 1995a,b, 1996a, 1997, 1998; Roe, 1994; Hart et al., 1995; Turturro et al., 1995; Allaben et al., 1996; Newberne and Sotnikov, 1996).

These adverse outcomes have been associated with overnutrition leading to increases in body weight in most of the rodents currently used in these bioassays (Rao et al., 1990; Lang, 1991; Haseman and Rao, 1992; Keenan et al., 1992; Roe, 1994; Hart et al., 1995; Turturro et al., 1995, 1996). While increased body weight appears to have been influenced by breeder selection and the expected genetic drift in any rodent population (Finch, 1990; Fishbein, 1991; Hart et al., 1995) most of these adverse events are clearly associated with a failure to control the animal's growth due to unlimited *ad libitum* (AL) overfeeding of otherwise nutritious food. The practice of AL overfeeding is largely one of caloric excess and is an example of massive nutritional overdosing.

The adverse phenomenon of AL caloric excess and its control by moderate dietary restriction (DR) has been well documented by nutritionists, toxicologists, pathologists and gerontologists (McCay et al., 1935; Ross, 1976; Weindruch and Walford, 1988; Klurfeld et al., 1989; Finch, 1990; Fishbein, 1991; Rose, 1991; Rogers et al., 1993; Merry and Holehan, 1994; Hart et al., 1995; Yu, 1995; Keenan et al., 1996b; Masoro and Austad, 1996; McDonald, 1997; Sohal and Weindruch, 1997; Weindruch, 1996; McDonald, 1997; Knight et al., 1998). In humans, caloric excess and decreased activity are the major nongenetic factors associated with morbidity and mortality after tobacco use (McGinnis and Foege, 1993; Manson et al., 1995; Björntorp, 1997; Rosenbaum et al., 1997). The human diseases associated with overeating include obesity, diabetes mellitus, the major cardiovascular diseases and cancers of the colon, uterus, ovaries, breast and prostate (McGinnis and Foege, 1993; Manson et al., 1995; Björntorp, 1997; Rosenbaum et al., 1997). Prevention and treatment of these human diseases requires the control and management of food intake. Many evolutionary biologists, nutritionists, gerontologists and medical scientists consider uncontrolled AL overnutrition to result in pathological aging and accelerated senescence that needs to be controlled by moderate restriction of

food intake (Finch, 1990; Rose, 1991; Hart et al., 1995; Masoro, 1995; Yu, 1995; Masoro and Austad 1996; McDonald, 1997; Weindruch, 1996; Rosenbaum et al., 1997). Over the past few years toxicologists and pathologists have recognized that AL overfeeding is the most important uncontrolled variable in the rodent bioassay (Allaben et al., 1996; Hart et al., 1995; Keenan et al., 1996a; C. Keenan et al., 1998; Newberne and Sotnikov, 1996). The effects of excessive AL caloric intake adversely affect every physiological process and anatomical structure at the molecular level. Several of these are described in more detail below.

Decreased Survival

Control rodent survival in carcinogenicity studies during the 1980s and 1990s has declined and become highly variable (Rao et al., 1990; Lang, 1991; Haseman and Rao, 1992; Keenan et al., 1992, 1994a, b, 1995a,b, 1996, 1997; Roe, 1994; Hart et al., 1995; Turturro et al., 1995, 1996; Allaben et al., 1996; Laroque et al., 1997; Knight et al., 1998). For example, male Sprague-Dawley rat 2-year survival during this period ranged from 7 to 73% (Lang, 1991, Keenan et al., 1994b), male Fischer 344 rats from 36 to 85%, male CD-1 mice from 20 to 80% and male B6C3F1 mice from 40 to 97% (Rao et al., 1990; Haseman and Rao, 1992; Hart et al., 1995; Turturro et al., 1995, 1996). In addition, the survival of these commonly used rodents was higher in the 1960s and 1970s than that seen presently under supposedly greater experimental control with the use of GLPs and the increased control of many exogenous infectious, nutritional and environmental stressors (McCay et al., 1935; Bhatt et al., 1986; Fishbein, 1991; Newberne and Sotnikov, 1996).

Excessive Body Weight

The relationship between AL overfeeding, excessive body weight and poor survival is now well established and has been demonstrated in every rodent strain and stock examined. For example, in some stocks of male Sprague-Dawley rats, average control body weight has risen from 550 g in the 1970s to over 900 g in the 1990s (Keenan et al., 1992, 1994a,b, 1997). An increase in average body weight has also been reported in Fischer 344 rats as well as CD-1 and B6C3F1 mice (Rao et al., 1990;

Table 5.3 Nutritional effects of *ad libitum* (AL) overfeeding or moderate (75% AL) and marked (50% AL) dietary restriction (DR) on Sprague-Dawley rats[a]

Parameter	AL		Moderate DR		Marked DR	
	Male	Female	Male	Female	Male	Female
Caloric intake (kcal/day)[b]	94±3.7	73±4.7	68±0.3	50±0.3	45±0.1	34±0.1
Body weight (g)	765±145	611±87	572±49	296±22	357±24	216±15
Body fat (%)	39	44	23	14	9	6
Tumor incidence (%)[c]	78	94	78	87	58	54
Benign tumors (%)	70	94	66	82	46	50
Malignant tumors (%)	26	30	22	40	16	10
Cardiomyopathy (grade)[d]	2.5	1.6	1.5	0.4	0.3	0.3
Nephropathy (grade)[d]	3.2	1.8	1.5	0.3	1.0	0.02
Oxidized liver lipid[e]						
4-HNE	–	–	82	48	60	66
MDA	–	–	26	14	41	57
Oxidized liver protein[e]						
Protein carbonyl	–	–	25	NC	49	19
Two-year survival (%)	18	18	68	56	78	82

[a] Sprague-Dawley rats: Crl:CD®(SD) IGS BR Charles River Laboratories, Raleigh, NC, USA, approximately 50/sex/group were studied for 106 weeks (112 weeks of age).

[b] PMI Lab Diet® Certified Rodent Diet 5002 (3.1 kcal/g of metabolizable energy, 21.4% protein, 5.7% fat and 4.1% crude fiber by analysis) was fed as pellets AL or by daily measured amounts to DR groups.

[c] Tumor incidence includes all tumor-bearing rats with benign and/or malignant neoplasms.

[d] Average lesion grade for all rats (grades of 0–5 for severity).

[e] Percentage decrease in total amount per liver relative to AL groups.

Abbreviations: 4-HNE, 4-hydroxy-2-E-nonenal; MDA, malondialdehyde; NC, no change from AL.

Modified with permission from K. P. Keenan et al. (1998).

Haseman and Rao, 1992; Allaben *et al.*, 1996; Turturro *et al.*, 1995, 1996). In addition to the increase in body weight over time, there has also been an increase in the variability between control group body weights.

Reports that the early weanling body weights of Sprague-Dawley rats correlated with tumor incidence and inversely with survival suggested that a genetically determined initial body weight would be the best predictor of longevity (McCay *et al.*, 1935; Ross, 1976). However, recent studies demonstrate that the weanling body weight of Sprague-Dawley rats does not correlate with survival in AL or DR-fed animals. Rather, the 12-month body weight following AL feeding correlates best with 24-month survival (Laroque *et al.*, 1997). Reports on Fischer 344 rats and B6C3F1 mice also show that initial body weight does not correlate with survival as well as 12-month body weights (Turturro *et al.*, 1995, 1996). These studies show that total adult food intake, but not initial weanling body weight, is the most important factor affecting adult body weight and survival. In addition, studies of adult onset food restriction in rats and mice suggest that factors affecting initial body size, early growth and development are neither necessary nor sufficient to explain the adverse effects of AL feeding or the positive effects of DR feeding on survival (Maeda *et al.*, 1985; Weindruch and Walford, 1988, Masoro, 1991; Yu, 1995).

The correlation between adult body weight, obesity and longevity has led to a tendency to extrapolate a mechanistic relationship between obesity and survival (Table 5.3). However, data on AL-fed

Fischer 344 rats demonstrated no correlation between adult body weight and longevity (Maeda et al., 1985; Masoro and Austad, 1996; Masoro, 1996). In contrast, DR-fed Fischer 344 rats had a positive correlation, that is the adult DR-fed rats with the most body weight lived the longest (Maeda et al., 1985; Masoro, 1995, 1996). Similar correlations have been drawn from studies with Wistar rats and with naturally lean and genetically obese (ob/ob) mice (Harrison and Archer, 1987; Masoro, 1996). These and other data led to the conclusion that increased body fat content may not be causally related to decrease in survival (K.P. Keenan et al., 1994b, 1995b, 1996, 1998; Turturro et al., 1995; Klinger et al., 1996; Masoro, 1996; Laroque et al., 1997; C. Keenan et al., 1998; Knight et al., 1998).

Metabolic Effects of Overnutrition

The normal metabolic use of nutritional fuel is essential for life but does have long-term, low-intensity negative consequences to the organism when caloric intake is excessive. The use of oxygen in oxidative metabolism of nutrients results in free radical production (Weindruch and Walford, 1988; Yu, 1995; Sohal and Weindruch, 1996; Weindruch, 1996; Weindruch and Sohal, 1997). In addition, glucose, like other reducing sugars, undergoes a nonenzymatic reaction with amino groups of proteins called the **glycation reaction** (Masoro et al., 1992; Yu, 1995). Thus, fuels such as glucose can become reactive molecules in their own right. Studies of these basic metabolic processes have led to several hypotheses that implicate free radicals, glycation reactions and/or Maillard reactions as causative factors in aging as a consequence of normal metabolism (Masoro et al., 1992; Yu, 1995; Masoro, 1995; Weindruch and Sohal, 1997).

The free radical theory of aging assumes that reactive oxygen molecules play an active role in aging processes and that low-intensity damage occurs throughout the lifespan of the organism. Mitochondria and microsomes, which contain the two electron transport systems of the cell, are the major physiological source of free radicals and can also become prime targets for free radical attack which in turn will compromise their functions. While free radical production is not reported to increase uniformly with age, the damage induced by oxidative metabolism, for example, lipid peroxidation, does increase with age (Table 5.3). In contrast, the antioxidant defense systems are depleted with age, particularly under conditions of AL overfeeding (Weindruch and Walford, 1988; Masoro, 1995; Yu, 1995; Sohal and Weindruch, 1996; Masoro, 1996; Weindruch and Sohal, 1997). The major repair functions, including DNA repair, as well as proteolytic and lipolytic enzymes that remove oxidatively damaged molecules, deteriorate most readily under AL feeding conditions, and are best maintained by moderate DR (Hart et al., 1995; Yu, 1995; Masoro, 1995, 1996; Weindruch, 1996; Weindruch and Sohal, 1997).

The glycation theory of aging proposes that glucose may serve as a mediator for aging by the nonenzymatic glycation of amino groups of proteins and the cross-linking of numerous proteins by modified glucose residues (Masoro et al., 1992; Masoro, 1995, 1996; Yu, 1995). The example of noninsulin-dependent diabetes mellitus shows the importance of nonenzymatic glycation inducing damage in numerous tissues with chronic elevations of plasma glucose levels and the resulting increased levels of numerous tissue glycated proteins. Glucose effectiveness or insulin sensitivity or both are diminished over time in AL-fed rats and are best maintained in moderate DR-fed rats (Masoro et al., 1992; Masoro, 1996). AL-fed rats characteristically have higher levels of circulating plasma glucose and insulin than their moderately DR-fed counterparts. The effects of moderate food restriction on lowering plasma glucose levels and increasing insulin efficiency may be a fundamental mechanism because it results in the efficient use of an important, but potentially toxic fuel (glucose) at sustained but lower concentrations that appear less damaging over the lifespan of the organism (Masoro et al., 1992; Masoro, 1995, 1996; Yu, 1995).

The combined free radical/glycation/Maillard reaction theory of aging links the metabolic consequences of AL overfeeding to excessive oxygen free radical production and glycation/Maillard reactions (Masoro, 1995; Yu, 1995). This theory postulates that the sources of damage, which may differ significantly in their reaction sites of generation and the primary tissue targets of these reactions, interact to cause the age-associated deterioration associated with AL overfeeding. This theory reflects metabolic mechanisms that are operative in the degenerative conditions induced by AL overfeeding as seen in studies of DR-fed animals that have reductions in oxygen free radical damage effects (Table 5.3) and have lower plasma glucose levels resulting in reductions of glycation/Maillard reaction end products in their tissues compared to their AL overfed counterparts (Weindruch and Walford, 1988; Duffy *et al.*, 1989; Hart *et al.*, 1995; Yu, 1995; Masoro, 1996; Weindruch, 1996; Weindruch and Sohal, 1997).

Effects of Overnutrition on Degenerative Disease and Tumorigenesis

Of the many nutritional factors that are known to be determinants of chronic degenerative disease and cancer, none is more profound or complex in its adverse effects than AL food (caloric) overconsumption. The proposed mechanisms for increased tumorigenesis and degenerative disease by AL overfeeding of calories to rodents have been the subject of several recent extensive reviews (Weindruch and Walford, 1988; Finch, 1990; Masoro *et al.*, 1991; Kritchevsky, 1993; Rogers *et al.*, 1993; Masoro, 1995; Yu, 1995; Keenan *et al.*, 1996). Many of the adverse effects of overnutrition seen in rodents are the result of increased growth of normal organs and neoplastic tissue (Tables 5.3 and 5.4). Absolute organ weights (except brain weight) are increased proportionally to body growth, but relative organ weights (as a percentage of body weight) are generally reduced in AL-fed groups and increased in DR-fed animals (Table 5.4). In AL-fed rats, these processes are enhanced by the early onset and excessive increases in growth-promoting hormones such as insulin, growth hormone, IGF-1, prolactin and other mammotrophic hormones and by decreases in growth-inhibiting adrenal corticoids (Rogers *et al.*, 1993; Merry and Holehan, 1994; Masoro, 1995; Yu, 1995). Alterations in the metabolism of carcinogens, other xenobiotics and steroids due to numerous enzyme and metabolic changes, particularly in the liver have been well documented (Fishbein *et al.*, 1991; Rogers *et al.*, 1993; Hart *et al.*, 1995; Masoro, 1995). These disease mechanisms are enhanced in AL-overfed rodents by increased oxidative free radical damage to DNA, proteins, enzymes and membranes and the loss of protective antioxidants and antioxidant enzyme systems (Table 5.3). In addition, glycation reactions due to increased plasma glucose levels and/or decreased insulin sensitivity lead to further damage of enzymes, proteins and DNA.

These hormonal and metabolic effects can lead to excessive organ growth (especially the metabolically active liver, kidneys and endocrine organs) with increased cell division and DNA synthesis, spontaneous DNA adduct formation, and alterations in DNA repair, which enhance the probability of spontaneous tumorigenesis (Finch, 1990; Keenan *et al.*, 1994a,b, 1995a,b; Hart *et al.*, 1995; Masoro, 1995; Yu, 1995; Sohal and Weindruch, 1996; Weindruch, 1996). AL-overfed rodents have decreased apoptosis of normal, aged and preneoplastic cells that further increases the likelihood of an early spontaneous tumorigenic event (Grasl-Kraupp *et al.*, 1994; James and Muskhelishvili, 1994). In addition, AL-overfed rodents also have increased expression of tumor virus genes or **proto-oncogenes**, a decreased immune response and an increase in autoimmune responses. These and other effects are observed in AL-fed rodents with all diets tested, including semipurified and natural-product diets (Weindruch and Walford, 1988; Finch, 1990; Hart *et al.*, 1995; Masoro, 1995). This list of the adverse effects of AL-overfeeding leading to chronic degenerative disease and tumors is not exhaustive. Conversely, there is not a more effective preventative measure to avoid the early onset of these spontaneous conditions than moderate food restriction (Weindruch and Walford, 1988; Finch, 1990; Fishbein, 1991; Keenan *et al.*, 1992, 1994a,b, 1995a,b, 1996, 1997; Hart *et al.*, 1995; Masoro *et al.*, 1996).

It is noteworthy that only laboratory rodents are currently allowed uncontrolled *ad libitum* overfeeding, whereas other laboratory animals, such as dogs, rabbits and primates, are carefully fed measured amounts of feed (Weindruch and Walford, 1988; Finch, 1990; Lane *et al.*, 1997; McDonald, 1997). To do otherwise with these species is considered poor veterinary and scientific practice. The use of DR, also referred to as dietary optimization, is becoming increasingly common in routine toxicology and carcinogenicity studies as it is known to result in healthier, more uniform (Table 5.4) animals than those maintained by traditional AL overfeeding methods (Lang, 1991; Roe, 1994; Laroque *et al.*, 1997; Giknis and Clifford, 1998; Keenan *et al.*, 1998; Knight *et al.*, 1998). This has been recognized by the National Research Council (1995) and is reflected in their current publications and recommendations for the nutritional requirements and husbandry procedures of laboratory animals (National Research Council, 1995; National Research Council, Committee on Rodents, 1996).

Table 5.4 Effects of *ad libitum* (AL) and moderate (75% AL) dietary restriction on body and selected organ weights of Sprague-Dawley rats[a]

Parameter	Age (weeks)	AL		Moderate DR	
		Male	Female	Male	Female
Body weight (g ± SD)	19	493±47	273±26	386±23	224±14
	32	620±73	348±39	462±27	252±19
	59	753±50	418±75	544±22	278±19
	112	720±108	606±56	551±46	296±17
Brain (g ± SD)	19	2.15±0.06	1.98±0.07	2.11±0.07	1.96±0.07
	32	2.31±0.10	2.04±0.06	2.17±0.10	2.05±0.10
	59	2.34±0.12	2.16±0.12	2.29±0.06	2.10±0.08
	112	2.35±0.08	2.20±0.13	2.37±0.11	2.16±0.08
Pituitary (g ± SD)	19	0.012±0.002	0.015±0.003	0.010±0.002	0.013±0.002
	32	0.013±0.001	0.020±0.004	0.013±0.001	0.015±0.002
	59	0.016±0.008	0.045±0.060	0.012±0.001	0.019±0.006
	112	0.090±0.095	0.091±0.081	0.018±0.009	0.081±0.072
Heart(g ± SD)	19	1.41±0.09	0.95±0.11	1.10±0.08	0.79±0.05
	32	1.66±0.16	1.10±0.09	1.30±0.10	0.87±0.08
	59	1.78±0.17	1.27±0.16	1.52±0.18	0.93±0.09
	112	2.12±0.20	1.61±0.17	1.73±0.16	1.06±0.09
Liver (g ± SD)	19	13.25±1.28	7.41±0.71	10.41±0.76	6.65±0.52
	32	16.22±2.49	9.06±0.92	12.35±1.07	7.62±1.02
	59	18.20±2.46	10.80±2.09	12.72±1.00	7.64±0.51
	112	17.61±2.18	14.29±2.99	12.63±1.39	8.20±0.77
Kidney (g ± SD)	19	3.19±0.33	1.79±0.18	2.50±0.27	1.54±0.11
	32	3.76±0.31	2.18±0.22	2.85±0.25	1.76±0.16
	59	4.42±0.44	2.83±0.42	3.44±0.32	2.17±0.18
	112	6.05±1.53	3.37±0.41	4.13±0.38	2.57±0.22

[a] Sprague-Dawley rats: Crl:CD®(SD) IGS BR Charles River Laboratories fed PMI Lab Diet® Certified Rodent Diet 5002 for 2 years.

Dietary Control of the Adverse Effects of AL Overnutrition

Control of Specific Nutrients and Contaminants

Total energy intake rather than a specific nutrient intake appears to be the main process accelerating aging and decreasing survival in AL-fed rodents. This is because DR-fed rodents have the same or slightly higher food intake per gram body weight and thus consume the same relative amounts of each nutrient as AL-fed rodents (Masoro *et al.,* 1991; Keenan *et al.,* 1992, 1994a,b, 1995a,b, 1996, 1997; Masoro, 1995, 1996). Many studies in different laboratories have shown conclusively that food (caloric) restriction *per se* rather than a specific nutrient restriction is the factor that improves survival and extends life in DR-fed rodents (Maeda *et al.,* 1985; Duffy *et al.,* 1989; K.P. Keenan *et al.,* 1992, 1994a,b, 1995a, 1996a, 1997, 1998; Gumprecht *et al.,* 1993; Merry and Holehan, 1994; Roe *et al.,* 1995; C. Keenan *et al.,* 1998; Knight *et al.,* 1998).

It has been speculated that food restriction may increase longevity by reducing the intake of toxic contaminants in the diet. However, this is highly unlikely considering the broad variety of semipurified diets and natural-product diets that have been used in DR studies and the extensive analyses and testing for contaminants applied to many of these diets (National Research Council, 1978; Newberne and Sotnikov, 1996; Purina Mills, 1996). The fact that DR-fed rodents consume approximately the same or slightly more food per gram body weight as AL-fed rodents means that they are exposed on a per gram body weight basis to the same levels of both nutrients and contaminants as their AL-fed counterparts. Thus research from many laboratories strongly rejects the idea that decreased survival is due to an excess of a specific nutrient or contaminant in AL-fed rats. All of the scientific evidence strongly points to the excessive total energy (calories) intake per animal as the main factor that decreases survival in AL-overfed rodents.

Control of Caloric Intake by Food Restriction

The relationship between AL overfeeding, excessive body weight, growth and poor survival is now well established and has been demonstrated in every rodent outbred stock, inbred strain and hybrid cross thus far examined (Weindruch and Walford, 1988; Finch, 1990; Fishbein, 1991; Hart *et al.,* 1995; Masoro, 1995; Yu, 1995). However, even under *ad libitum* feeding conditions there is still wide interlaboratory variability in food consumption, body weight, and 2-year survival reported for the same rodent stock or strain fed the same feed (Keenan *et al.,* 1994a,b; Turturro *et al.,* 1995, 1996; Laroque *et al.,* 1997). For example, data from 58 control groups of Charles River Sprague-Dawley rats fed PMI Lab Diet® Certified Rodent Diet 5002 on 2-year carcinogenicity studies performed by different North American laboratories during the 1980s demonstrated considerable variability in average food consumption, average body weights and 2-year survival (Keenan *et al.,* 1994b). But a strong correlation between food intake, body weight and survival was clearly established. The variability in AL food consumption was influenced by uncontrolled laboratory factors such as unintentional restrictive feeder construction and other limitations to food intake. Thus, many laboratories have been unintentionally conducting food restriction studies under so-called AL feeding conditions (Keenan *et al.,* 1994b).

The resulting decline in survival due to AL overfeeding lowers the statistical sensitivity to detect treatment-related tumors, particularly late occurring ones (Keenan *et al.,* 1994a, 1996a). Increasing the 2-year survival by DR can increase statistical sensitivity. Statistical analysis is simplified, and more importantly, there is a significant increase in exposure time to treatment. In some studies of Sprague-Dawley rats, 3–5 months of additional exposure time is gained during the course of a 2-year study (Keenan *et al.,* 1994a, 1996a).

Concern over the potential loss of the bioassay's carcinogenesis sensitivity with moderate DR has occurred since many published studies have shown that severe DR dramatically prevents both spontaneous tumors as well as those induced by a given dose of carcinogen (Pollard and Luckert, 1985; Klurfeld *et al.,* 1989; Kritchevsky, 1993; Rogers *et al.,* 1993). However, these studies usually use a more severe food restriction than is proposed and have shorter (5–12 month) endpoints. Studies performed in this way do not account for the marked delay of tumor onset induced by severe DR or the long-term confounding effects of AL overfeeding on the pathogenesis of these induced lesions. With moderate DR the 2-year spontaneous tumor incidence observed in Sprague-Dawley rats was in the range of AL-fed rats, but the tumors were found incidentally, most at a final necropsy, rather than at an unscheduled early necropsy (Table 5.3). Moderate DR appears to delay tumor onset time (16 weeks for spontaneous mammary gland tumors); but tumor progression does not appear to be altered as measured by tumor growth or tumor doubling times (Keenan et al., 1995a, 1996b). Moderate DR results in a delay in onset time of spontaneous endocrine and endocrine-related tumors, particularly those of the pituitary, pancreatic islet cells and mammary gland in Sprague-Dawley rats (K.P. Keenan et al., 1994, 1995a, 1998; Knight et al., 1998) in addition to other sites in Fischer 344 rats (Maeda et al., 1985; Masoro et al., 1991; Yu, 1995) and Wistar rats (Roe et al., 1995).

Another major factor that must be considered in studies of carcinogenesis with moderate and severe DR is the effect that different degrees of DR have on dose selection. Most investigators select arbitrary doses or determine doses in young, growing, AL-fed animals and then test them in adult DR-fed animals (Pollard and Luckert, 1985; Klurfeld et al., 1989; Kritchevsky, 1993; Rogers et al., 1993). The differences observed should not be surprising because DR-fed animals are more resistant to long-term metabolic injury and better able to handle the consequences of a given xenobiotic load. Therefore, it is necessary to determine doses of the test substance in the DR-fed model that will be used for the long-term bioassay. Moderate DR in the Sprague-Dawley rat does not significantly alter phase I and phase II drug metabolizing enzyme activities, fatty acyl CoA-oxidase activity or the qualitative toxicologic response to pharmaceuticals given at maximum tolerated doses (Keenan et al., 1994a, 1996a). Examination of pharmaceutical candidates in AL-overfed and moderate DR-fed Sprague-Dawley rats to determine maximum tolerated doses (**MTDs**), No Observable Effect (**NOEL**) doses and pharmacokinetic parameters (AUC and C_{max}) demonstrated that the DR-fed animals were healthier and thus better able to tolerate higher dosages of pharmaceuticals given by daily gavage (K.P. Keenan et al., 1996a, 1998). The high doses tested were better

tolerated by moderately DR-fed rats and the estimated oral MTDs and NOELs were approximately two- to four-fold higher under the moderate DR feeding conditions. In addition, toxicokinetic studies with these compounds demonstrated steady-state systemic drug and/or metabolic exposures (AUCs and C_{max}) that were either equal or higher in moderate DR-fed animals compared to their AL-fed counterparts (K.P. Keenan et al., 1996a, 1998).

When a test substance is administered in the diet, DR feeding allows exact dosing because DR-fed rats consume their entire daily allotment, and have the same or slightly higher food intake per gram of body weight as AL-fed rats. Therefore, DR-fed rats consume the same amount of energy, nutrients and test substances in the diet as AL-fed rats on a per gram of body weight basis (Masoro et al., 1991; K.P. Keenan et al., 1992, 1997, 1998; Masoro, 1995, 1996). Different diets can also be better compared if animals are fed isocaloric amounts in a controlled intake daily. This method has been used to demonstrate the relative roles of protein, fat, fiber and total energy intake on health and longevity (Iwasaki et al., 1988; Keenan et al., 1994b, 1995a,b; Maeda et al., 1985; Masoro et al., 1989, 1991; Roe et al., 1995). Manufacturers of laboratory rat diets have developed unique diet forms to facilitate the practical implementation of DR feeding on a large scale. Diets for toxicity and carcinogenicity studies are available in preweighed portion-controlled feeding packages. These diets are also available in particles of a uniform predetermined weight.

Conclusion: The Need for Nutritional Control

The environmental and nutritional conditions under which laboratory animals are maintained can powerfully influence the experimental results measured. Nutrition is of major importance in toxicological bioassays and research, because diet composition and the conditions under which it is fed can affect the metabolism and activity of xenobiotic test substances and alter the results and reproducibility of long-term studies. It is known that AL-overfed sedentary laboratory rodents suffer from an early onset of degenerative disease and diet-related tumors that lead to poor survival in chronic bioassays. AL-fed animals are not well-controlled subjects for any experimental studies. Examination of study-to-study variability in food consumption, body weight, organ weights and survival in carcinogenicity studies for the same strain or stock of rodents shows tremendous laboratory-to-laboratory variability (Keenan *et al.*, 1994a; Tables 5.3 and 5.4). However, a significant correlation between average food (calorie) consumption, adult body weight and survival has been clearly established (Laroque *et al.*, 1997). The use of moderate dietary restriction (DR) of a nutritionally balanced diet results in a better controlled rodent model with a lower incidence or delayed onset of spontaneous diseases and tumors. Operationally simple, moderate DR of balanced diets significantly improves survival, controls adult body weight and obesity, reduces age-related renal, endocrine and cardiac diseases, and reduces study-to-study variability, increases treatment exposure time, and increases the statistical sensitivity of these expensive, chronic bioassays to detect a true treatment effect. A severe dietary restriction such as a 40–50% reduction of the maximum AL intake of a given diet should not be recommended as an appropriate control method for toxicological studies. A moderate DR regimen of 25% restriction of the maximum unrestricted AL food intake of either a semi-purified or natural-product well-balanced diet is recommended as a nutritionally intelligent, well-established method in conducting well-controlled experimental studies with the laboratory rat.

Acknowledgements

Thanks to the following for support and suggestions: J.B. Coleman, K.A. Soper, C.-M. Hoe, B.A. Mattson, P. Duprat, D.L. Bokelman, M.J. van Zwieten, C.F. Hollander, S. Molon-Noblet, J.D. Burek and C.P. Peter. Thanks also to Ms Regina Foy for preparing this chapter.

References

Allaben, W.T., Turturro, A., Leakey, J.E.A., Seng, J.E. and Hart, R.W. (1996) *Toxicol. Pathol.* **24**, 776–781.

Anderson, J.J.B and Garner, S.C. (1997) *Nutrition Today* **32**, 232–239.

Baker, D.A. (1986) *J. Nutr.* **116**, 2339–2349.

Baldwin, J.K. and Griminger, P. (1985) *Exp. Gerontol.* **20**, 29–34.

Banjs, W.A., Kastin, A.J., Huang, W., Jaspan, J.B. and Maness, L.M. (1996) *Peptides* **17**, 305–311.

Benevenga, N.J., Gahl, M.J., Crenshaw, T.D. and Finke, M.D. (1994) *J. Nutr.* **124**, 451–453.

Bhatt, P.N., Jacoby, R.O., Morse, H.C. and New, A.E. (eds) (1986) Viral and Mycoplasmal Infections of Laboratory Rodents. New York: Academic Press.

Björntorp, P. (1997) *The Lancet* **350**, 423–426.

Case, L.P., Carey, D.P. and Hirakawa, D.A. (1995) Canine and Feline Nutrition. St. Louis, MO: Mosby-Year Book.

Clapp, M.J.L., Wade, J.D. and Samuels, D.M. (1982) *Lab. Anim.* **16**, 130–132.

Claycombe, K.J., Xue, B., Mynatt, R.L., Wilkison, W.O., Zemel, M.B. and Moustaid, N. (1998) *FASEB J.* **12**, A505. Abstr. 2934.

Coates, M.E. (ed.) (1987) *ICLAS Guidelines on the Selection and Formulation of Diets for Animals in Biomedical Research.* London: International Council for Laboratory Animal Science.

Cohen, L.A., Epstein, M., Saz-Pabon, V., Meschter, C. and Zang, E. (1994) *Nutr. Cancer* **21**, 271–283.

Coleman, D.L. and Hummel, K.P. (1969) *Am. J. Physiol.* **217**, 1298–1304.

Duffy, P.H., Feuers, R.J., Leakey, J.A., Nakamura, K.D., Turtuorro, A. and Hart, R.W. (1989) *Mech. Aging Dev.* **48**, 117–133.

Elmquist, J.K., Ahima, R.S., Maratos-Flier, E., Flier, J.S. and Saper, C.S. (1997) *Endocrinology* **138**, 839–842.

Engle, R.W. and Copeland, D.H. (1952) *Cancer Res.* **12**, 211–215.

Fenton, P.F. (1957) *Am. J. Clin. Nutr.* **5**, 663–665.

Finch, C.E. (1990) Longevity, Senescence and the Genome. Chicago, IL: The University of Chicago Press.

Fishbein, L. (ed.) (1991) Biological Effects of Dietary Restriction. New York: Springer-Verlag.

Flier, J.S. and Maratos-Flier, E. (1998) *Cell* **92**, 437–440.

Fullerton, F.R., Greenman, D.L. and Bucci, T.J. (1992) *Fundam. Appl. Toxicol.* **18**, 193–199.

Giknis, M.I. and Clifford, C.B. (1998) Spontaneous Neoplastic Lesions and Survival in Crl: CD® (SD) BRRats Maintained on Dietary Restriction. Wilmington, MA: Charles River Laboratories.

Goodrick, C.L. (1973) *Growth* **37**, 355–367.

Grasl-Kraupp, B., Bursch, W., Ruttkay-Nedecky, B., Wagner, A., Lauer, B. and Schulte-Hermann, R. (1994) *Proc. Natl Acad. Sci. USA* **91**, 9995–9999.

Gumprecht, L.A., Long, C.R., Soper, K.A., Smith, P.F., Hascheck-Hock, W.M. and Keenan, K.P. (1993) *Toxicol. Pathol.* **21**, 528–537.

Halaas, J.L., Gajiwala, K.S., Maffei, M., Cohen, S.L., Chait, B.T., Rabinowitz, D., Lallone, R.L., Burley, S.K. and Friedman, J.M. (1995) *Science* **269**, 543–546.

Harrison, D.E. and Archer, J.R. (1987) *J. Nutr.* **117**, 376–382.

Hart, R.W., Neumann, D.A. and Robertson, R.T. (eds) (1995) *Dietary Restriction: Implications for the Design and Interpretation of Toxicity and Carcinogenicity Studies.* Washington, DC: ILSI Press.

Hartsook, E.W. and Mitchell, H.H. (1956) *J. Nutr.* **60**, 173–195.

Haseman, J.K. and Rao, G.R.F. (1992) *Toxicol. Pathol.* **20**, 52–60.

He, L., Mo, H., Hadisusilo, S., Qureshi, A.A. and Elson, C.E. (1997) *J. Nutr.* **127**, 668–674.

Houseknecht, K.L., Baile, C.A., Matteri R.L. and Spurlock, M.E. (1998) *Rev. J. Anim. Sci.* **76**, 1405–1420.

Iwasaki, K., Gleiser, C.A., Masoro, E.J., McMahan, C.A., Seo, E.J. and Yu, B.P. (1988) *J. Gerontol.* **43**, B5–12.

James, S.J. and Muskhelishvili, L. (1994) *Cancer Res.* **54**, 5508–5510.

Jang, M. and Romsos, D.R. (1998) *FASEB J.* **12**, A504, Abstr. 2932.

Keenan, C., Barrett, D., Knight, E., Kimball, J., Smith, L. and Powers, W. (1998) *Toxicol. Sci.* **42**, 73.

Keenan, K.P., Smith, P.F., Ballam, G.C., Soper, K.A. and Bokelman, D.L. (1992) In: McAuslane, J.A.N., Lumley, C.F. and Walker, S.R. (eds) *Centre for Medicines Research Workshop. The Carcinogenicity Debate*, pp. 77–102. Lancaster: Quay Publishing.

Keenan, K.P., Smith, P.F., Hertzog, P., Soper, K.A., Ballam, G.C. and Clark, R.L. (1994b) *Toxicol. Pathol.* **22**, 300–315.

Keenan, K.P., Soper, K.A., Smith, P.F., Ballam, G.C. and Clark, R.L. (1995a) *Toxicol. Pathol.* **23**, 269–286.

Keenan, K.P., Soper, K.A., Hertzog, P.R. *et al.* (1995b) *Toxicol. Pathol.* **23**, 287–302.

Keenan, K.P., Laroque, P., Ballam, G.C. *et al.* (1996a) *Toxicol. Pathol.* **24**, 757–768.

Keenan, K.P., Laroque, P., Soper, K.A., Morrissey, R.E. and Dixit, R. (1996b) *Exp. Toxicol. Pathol.* **48**, 139–144.

Keenan, K.P., Ballam, G.C., Dixit, R. *et al.* (1997) *J. Nutr.* **127**, 851S–856S.

Keenan, K.P., Laroque, P. and Dixit, R. (1998) *J. Toxicol. Environ. Health Part B* **1**, 101–114.

Kennedy, G.C. (1953) *Proc. R. Soc.* **140**, 578–592.

Klinger, M.M., MacCarter, G.O. and Boozer, C.N. (1996) *Lab. Anim. Sci.* **46**, 67–70.

Klurfeld, D.M., Welch, C.B., Davis, M.J. and Kritchevsky, D. (1989) *J. Nutr.* **119**, 286–291.

Knight, E.V., Barrett, D.S., Keenan, C.M. *et al.* (1998) *Int. J. Toxicol.* **17** (suppl.2), 57–78.

Kritchevsky, D. (1993) *Food Res. Int.* **26**, 289–295.

Kurzer, M.S. and Xu, X. (1997) *Annu. Rev. Nutr.* **17**, 353–381.

Lane, M.A., Ingram, D.K. and Roth, G.S. (1997) *Age* **20**, 45–56.

Lang, P.L. (1991) *Chem. Reg. Reporter* **14**, 1518–1520.

Laroque, P., Keenan, K., Soper, K.A., Dorian, C., Hubert, M-F. and Duprat, P. (1997) *Exp. Toxicol. Pathol.* **49**, 459–465.

Lindsey, J.R. (1979) Historical foundations. In: Baker, H.J., Lindsey, J.R. and Weisbroth, S.H. (eds), *The Laboratory Rat*, Vol. 1, pp. 1–36. New York: Academic Press.

Lynn, R.B., Cao, G-Y., Considine, R.V., Hyde, T.M. and Caro, J.F. (1996) *Biochem. Biophys. Res. Commun.* **219**, 884–889.

McCay, C., Crowell, M. and Maynard, L. (1935) *J. Nutr.* **10**, 63–79.

McCracken, K.J. (1975) *Br. J. Nutr.* **33**, 277–289.

McCullum, E.V. and Davis, M. (1913) *J. Biol. Chem.* **15**, 167–175.

McDonald, R.B. (1997) *J. Nutr.* **127**, 847S–850S.

McGinnis, J.M. and Foege, W.H. (1993) *J. Am. Med. Assoc.* **270**, 2207–2212.

Maeda, H., Gleiser, C.A., Masoro, E.J., Murata, I, McMahan, C.A. and Yu, B.P. (1985) *J. Gerontol.* **40**, 671–688.

Malik, K.F. and Young, W.S. III. (1996) *Endocrinology* **137**, 1497–1500.

Manson, J.E., Willett, W.C., Stampfer, M.J. *et al.* (1995) *N. Engl. J. Med.* **333**, 677–685.

Masoro, E.J. (ed.) (1995) *Handbook of Physiology*, Section 11: *Aging.* New York: American Physiological Society; Oxford University Press.

Masoro, E.J. (1996) *Toxicol. Pathol.* **24**, 738–741.

Masoro, E.J. and Austad, S.D. (1996) *J. Gerontol.* **51A**, B387–B391.

Masoro, E.J., Iwasaki, K., Gleiser, C.A., McMahan, C.A., Seo, E.J. and Yu, B.P. (1989) *Am. J. Clin. Nutr.* **48**, 1217–1227.

Masoro, E.J., Shimokawa, I. and Yu, B.P. (1991) *Ann. N.Y. Acad. Sci.* **621**, 337–352.

Maynard, L.A., Loosli, J.K., Hintz, H.F. and Warner, R.G. (1979) In: *Animal Nutrition*, pp. 186–219. New York: McGraw-Hill.

Merry, B.J. and Holehan, A.M. (1994). In: Timiras, P.S. (ed.) *Physiological Basis of Aging and Geriatrics*, 2nd ed. pp. 285–310. Boca Raton, FL: CRC Press.

Mitchell, H.H. and Beadles, J.R. (1952) *J. Nutr.* **47**, 133–145.

National Research Council (1978) Nutrient Requirements of Laboratory Animals. 3rd revised edn, pp. 7–37. Washington, D.C.: National Academy Press.

National Research Council, Subcommittee of Laboratory Animal Nutrition (1995) In: *Nutrient Requirements of Laboratory Animals*, 4th revised edn, pp. 11–79. Washington, D.C.: National Academy Press.

National Research Council. Committee on Rodents (1996) Husbandry. In: *Laboratory Animal Management*, pp. 44–84. Washington, D.C.: National Academy Press.

Newberne, P.M. and Sotnikov, A.V. (1996) *Toxicol. Pathol.* **24**, 746–756.

Osborne, T.B. and Mendel, L.B. (1913) *J. Biol. Chem.* **15**, 311–326.

Peterson, A.D. and Baumgardt, B.R. (1971a) *J. Nutr.* **101**, 1057–1068.

Peterson, A.D. and Baumgardt, B.R. (1971b) *J. Nutr.* **101**, 1069–1074.

Pollard, M. and Luckert, P.H. (1985) *J. Natl Cancer Inst.* **74**, 1347–1349.

Purina Mills (1996) *The Animal Diet Reference Guide.* St. Louis, MO: Purina Mills Inc.

Rao, G.N., Hasemen, J.K., Grumbein, S., Crawford, D.D. and Eustis, S.L. (1990) *Toxicol. Pathol.* **18**, 61–70.

Rao, G.N., Edmondson, J. and Ewell, M.R. (1993) *Toxicol. Pathol.* **21**, 353–361.

Ritskes-Hoitinga, J., Lemmens, A.G. and Beynen, A.C. (1989a) *Lab. Anim.* **23**, 313–318.

Ritskes-Hoitinga, J., Lemmens, A.G., Danse, I.H.J.C. and Beynen, A.C. (1989b) *J. Nutr.* **119**, 1423–1431.

Ritskes-Hoitinga, J., Lemmens, A.G., Danse, I.H.J.C. and Beynen, A.C. (1991) *Lab. Anim.* **25**, 126–132.

Robbins, K.R., Baker, D.H. and Norton, H.W. (1977) *J. Nutr.* **107**, 2055–2061.

Robbins, K.R., Norton, H.N. and D.H. Baker (1979) *J. Nutr.* **109**, 1710–1714.

Roe, F.J.C. (1994) *Lab. Anim.* **28**, 148–154.

Roe, F.J.C, Lee, P.N., Conybeare, G. *et al.* (1995) *Food Chem. Toxicol.* **33** (suppl. 1): 1S–100S.

Rogers, A.E. (1979) Nutrition. In: Baker, H.J., Lindsay, J.R. and Welsbroth, S.H. (eds), The Laboratory Rat, Vol. 1, pp. 123–152. New York: Academic Press.

Rogers, A.E., Zeisel, S.H. and Groopman, J. (1993) *Carcinogenesis* **14**, 2205–2217.

Rose, M.R. (1991) Evolutionary Biology of Aging. New York: Oxford University Press.

Rosenbaum M., Leibel, R.L. and Hirsch, J. (1997) *N. Engl. J. Med.* **337**, 396–407.

Ross, M. (1976) In: Winick, M. (ed.) *Nutrition and Aging*, pp. 23–41. New York: J. Wiley.

Sheehan, P.M., Clevidence, B.A., Reynolds, L.K., Thye, F.W. and Ritchey, S.J. (1981) *J. Nutr.* **111**, 1224–1230.

Silverstone, H., Solomon A., and Tannenbaum, A. (1952) *Cancer Res.* **12**, 750–756.

Sohal, R.S. and Weindruch, R. (1996) *Science* **273**, 59–63.

Stonard, M.D., Samuels, D.M. and Lock, E.A. (1984) *Food Chem. Toxicol.* **22**, 139–146.

Turturro, A., Duffy, P. and Hart, R.W. (1995) In: Hart, R.W., Neumann, D.A. and Robertson, R.T. (eds) *Dietary Restriction: Implications for the design and interpretation of toxicity and carcinogenicity studies*, pp. 79–97. Washington, D.C.: ILSI Press.

Turturro, A., Duffy, P., Hart, R. and Allaben, W.T. (1996) *Toxicol. Pathol.* **24**, 769–775.

Weindruch, R (1996) *Toxicol. Pathol.* **24**, 742–745.

Weindruch, R. and Sohal, R.S. (1997) *N. Engl. J. Med.* **337**, 986–994.

Weindruch, R. and Walford, R.L. (1988) The Retardation of Aging and Disease by Dietary Restriction. Springfield, IL: Charles C. Thomas.

Wilding, J.P. and Widdowson, G.W. (1997) *Neurobiology. Br. Med. Bull.* **53**(2), 286–306.

Woods, S.C., Seeley, R.J., Porte, D. and Schwartz, M.W. (1998) *Science* **280**, 1378–1382.

World Cancer Research Fund/American Institute for Cancer Research (1997) *Food, Nutrition and the Prevention of Cancer: a Global Perspective.* Washington, D.C.: The American Institute for Cancer Research.

Wostmann, B.S. (1975) *World Rev. Nutr. Dietit.* **22**, 40–92.

Yu, B.P. (ed.) (1995) *Modulation of Aging Processes by Dietary Restriction.* Boca Raton, FL: CRC Press.

CHAPTER 6

Animal Welfare Laws and Regulations

David Whittaker
Huntingdon Life Sciences
Alconbury, Huntington, Cambridgeshire, UK

Introduction

It can be said that the ethics and culture of a society are the mothers of its laws. Put another way, the laws of a nation, state or union are the practical interpretations of its ethical and moral attitudes to life in general.

The international and national laws controlling the use of animals in experiments can be reviewed in just this light and in many cases provide excellent examples of the above definition. Whilst most people in the world could agree on the extremes of acceptability/unacceptability towards animals, there is still much diversity and divergence around many ethical issues relating to the use of animals in different societies. For instance, within the UK there is currently a significant public and political lobby to ban fox hunting as cruel and unnecessary, in contrast perhaps to bull fighting and ritual slaughter which are fully accepted within the countries they are practised. It is this diversity and divergence which perhaps leads to the different approaches taken with regard to controlling animal experimentation.

To fully understand and appreciate the origins of national laws relating to animals, one needs to study philosophy, especially the great philosophers and ence their thoughts have had well into the twentieth century and perhaps even into the twenty-first century. As an example, the concern expressed for 'over-sentimentality towards animals' by René Descartes in the early seventeenth Century was given Papal support by Pope Pius XII. He believed that the cries of animals should not arouse 'unreasonable compassion' and it is this predominance and legacy of the Catholic view of animals that goes some way to explaining the different moral and legal status afforded to animals in the southern states of Europe. This position also continues to cause current difficulties in framing pan European legislation on animal welfare, (Brookman and Legge, 1997).

Legal control of animal experimentation has a fine line to walk. It must be flexible and open enough to allow advances to be made in science, it must protect the scientist conducting legitimate research from prosecution under a miscellany of animal welfare laws and at the same time provide the animals the maximum protection against suffering that is possible. You might think this an impossible task. Yet current legislation in a large number of countries strikes just this balance. At the same time, the differences in these laws and regulations from nation to nation reflect the subtle differences in the cultural and ethical priorities that exist around the world. The UK is renowned as a nation 'of animal lovers' and this is reflected in the principal law and regulations controlling animal experimentation within that country. It is often said that few other nations afford animals the legal protection given to them in the UK.

As well as viewing the legislation on animal experimentation in isolation as instruments which reflect the considerations above, it must also be considered in context of other animal welfare legislation and legislation covering consumer protection. In this regard there are frequently, within a country, conflicting laws with respect to the use of animals in experiments. On the one hand there is a desire to reduce the number of animals used in experiments; on the other hand there are government bodies responsible for ensuring that products available to the public are inherently safe. Such safety testing still relies heavily on the use of animals.

There is sometimes a cascade of law which must be satisfied. This is exemplified within the European Union and Council of Europe, where member states must implement national legislation in order to satisfy European Directives and Conventions. In addition, the cascade may also extend downwards where within a country there exist autonomous or semi-autonomous states which have 'local' legislature in addition to any national laws. Good examples here are Germany and the USA. It is not difficult to imagine that within a three-tier legislative structure there is room for conflict and ambiguity of objectives.

We can now begin to see the big picture of legislation governing animal experimentation as dynamic, interfacing and frequently interacting with other law working sometimes 'for the animal', sometimes 'against it.'

The statute law in most countries is frequently supplemented with further guidelines and codes of practice. Such documents have two primary roles. First, they may be published to provide additional guidance on areas where the law itself is not explicit and where best practice may be an evolutionary process. They may also be published as an easy way to introduce change or ensure compliance in a particular area without having to change the instrument of law itself, which is usually a long and arduous process. Whatever the content of specific laws, those working with laboratory animals must always remember that the three objectives of that law provide for:

(1) The privilege to conduct research on live animals for the sake of protecting and promoting human and animal health.

(2) The opportunity and ability to advance science for the overall benefit of mankind.

(3) The highest achievable welfare standards compatible with the research objectives.

The remainder of this chapter will explore these concepts further by studying examples of specific national and international laws. Comparisons will be drawn to illustrate potential cultural differences. In order to bring structure to the considerations, individual aspects of the law will be considered separately (e.g. protocol control, procedural control, housing, statistics).

Finally, within this introduction it is best that the geographical scope of consideration is defined in order that the reader is not disappointed or misled into investigating the text for specific national references which are simply not there. Just as the author was commissioned to write this chapter, two new texts arrived on the desk: *Law Relating to Animals* (Brookman and Legge, 1997), which is some 460 pages and covers the subject from all parts of the world, and *Animal Welfare in Europe: European Legislation and Concerns* (Wilkins, 1997), which is over 400 pages and concentrates just on European animal welfare laws.

It is clear from just these two tomes that it would be impossible to cover even laboratory animal welfare legislation from around the world comprehensively in the space available. The author therefore concentrates on European legislation, making frequent direct comparisons to US law and other references and comparisons from the rest of the world as appropriate. Few references are made to the legal situation in South East Asia and Japan.

Likewise it is not possible, nor within the competence of the author, to consider 'intranational' control, as exists in the USA and Germany.

Finally it is vitally important to remember that the law is both an 'interpretative' and dynamic subject, constantly changing and developing. The reader must view this chapter merely as an overview, presenting an outline and structure to the legislature as it stands at the time of writing. The appropriate current law must always be referred to for exact and precise guidance on any matter.

Overall Structures and Frameworks

Within the general context of the 'European Community' there are two primary pieces of legislation which member states of the European Union and Council of Europe must consider. Taking the latter first, the Council of Europe (CoE) is made up at the time of writing of 43 member states, many of whom have joined very recently, following the break-up of the old Soviet Union. As a consequence, probably less than half of this membership is currently (1998) in a position to comply with CoE legislation governing the use of animals for experimental purposes.

The actual piece of legislation administered by the CoE is the European Convention for the Protection of Vertebrate Animals Used for Experimental and other Scientific Purposes, ETS 123 1986. Members of the CoE can choose to respond to the Convention in three ways. They can fail to recognize the Convention and in doing so recognize its existence but undertake no responsibility or obligation to comply in whole or part with it. A member state can *sign* the Convention and in doing so recognize its existence but undertake no obligation to satisfy in part or whole its content and intention. Finally, a member state may *ratify* the Convention and on doing so is said then to be a Party to the Convention. On ratification there is a moral obligation upon that state to comply with the Convention in full. There is, however, little legal enforcement of any Convention available to the CoE should a ratifying or signatory state fail to comply. The principle of effective implementation of a Convention works through a system of 'memorandums of understanding' or, put another way, agreement by a 'gentleman's handshake'. In practice this perhaps leads to variable compliance by those states signing and ratifying the Convention ETS 123.

This Convention is one of five appertaining to animal welfare. The other four are related to: Food Animals [transport] (No. 65), Animals kept for Farming Purposes (No. 87), Slaughter of Animals (No. 102) and Companion (pet) Animals (No. 125).

Those member states of the CoE which are also members of the European Union (EU) have been delayed in ratifying the Convention ETS 123 because of legal technicalities and conflicting requirements between the Convention and Directive 86/609, which is the legal instrument for controlling the use of animals in experiments within the EU framework. This legal technicality has not, however, in the main part impeded those countries which have wanted in spirit and intention to comply with both sets of regulations. Also it should be stressed that for the most part these two pieces of legislation mirror each other very closely and at the time of writing ratification of the Convention by the EU was anticipated in the very near future. Part of the Convention (Article 30) called for multilateral consultations by the parties within 5 years of its enforcement and every 5 years thereafter. The first multilateral consultation was held in 1993 and since then they have been held on a frequent basis, involving not only the competent authorities responsible for its implementation at national level but also all interested European and international organizations.

The multilateral consultations have been responsible for progressing many issues surrounding the Convention and also for accommodating new technologies and research methods which were either not invented at the time of drafting or perhaps not even considered as scientifically possible. A good example of such an issue is the introduction and rapid expansion of transgenic technology.

In addition, the multilateral consultations have been well placed to review progress on the development of welfare initiatives and introduce best practice through a number of nonlegal formats which negate the need to change the fundamental contents of the Convention requiring involvement of the European Parliament and inherent lengthy delays.

The Convention also contains, as appendices, guidance on the accommodation and care of animals as specified in Article 5 and on the collection of statistics as specified in Articles 27 and 28.

How does the Convention meet the three objectives laid out in the introduction? The preamble to the Convention is detailed in Box 6.1 and from this it is easily seen that its intention and spirit is to fulfil the objectives as described.

The Convention explicitly allows individual scientists to experiment on live animals in pursuit of knowledge, health and safety. At the same time it places an obligation on the scientific community to comprehensively embrace the '3R's' of Russell and Burch (refinement, reduction and replacement), (Russell and Burch 1992). How well these objectives are met is dependent on an infinite number of factors common to the success or failure of any legislature.

Finally, before leaving the Convention, it is worth while stating that many of the amendments and improvements made through the multilateral consultations have been also successfully integrated into the implementation and administration of the Directive 86/609.

BOX 6.1 Preamble

The Member States of the Council of Europe, signatory hereto,

Recalling that the aim of the Council of Europe is to achieve a greater unity between its members and that it wishes to co-operate with other States in the protection of live animals used for experimental and other scientific purposes;

Recognising that man has a moral obligation to respect all animals and to have due consideration for their capacity for suffering and memory;

Accepting nevertheless that man in his quest for knowledge, health and safety has a need to use animals where there is a reasonable expectation that the result will be to extend knowledge or be to the overall benefit of man or animal, just as he uses them for food, clothing and as beasts of burden;

Resolved to limit the use of animals for experimental and other scientific purposes, with the aim of replacing such use wherever practical, in particular by seeking alternative measures and encouraging the use of these alternative measures;

Desirous to adopt common provisions in order to protect animals used in those procedures which may possibly cause pain, suffering, distress or lasting harm and to ensure that where unavoidable they shall be kept to a minimum.

The European Union (EU) is a much smaller (currently 15 member states (1998) but again growing European community; The EU Directive 86/609 is a Council Directive on 'The approximation of laws, regulations and administrative provisions of the Member States regarding the protection of animals used for experimental and other scientific purposes'.

Given that both the Convention and Directive were implemented in the same year (1986) and had at least some common member states contributing to their development and establishment, it is not surprising that they closely mirror each other in content. For the author though, the Directive is distinctly different from the Convention in two major ways.

First, if we look at the aim (objectives) of the Directive it is 'less balanced' against those objectives in the introduction than the Convention and is more explicit in a fourth objective common to both but not listed in the introduction. The aim of the Directive (Article 1 of the Directive) is quoted in Box 6.2. For the author, the acknowledged necessity to use animals for experimental purposes appears to be only implicit in the Article. However, explicit within the Article are the facts that the animals' welfare will be protected by law and that these laws (national) will be harmonized so as to ensure a 'level playing field' across the member states (the fourth objective of both pieces of legislation).

BOX 6.2 Article 1

The aim of this Directive is to ensure that where animals are used for experimental or other scientific purposes the provisions laid down by law, regulation or administrative provisions in the Member States for their protection are approximated so as to avoid affecting the establishment and functioning of the common market, in particular by distortions of competition or barriers to trade.

The second major difference is the 'enforceability' of the Directive through national legislation compared with the Convention. On being a member state of the EU it is a mandatory requirement that the national legislation controlling the use of animals for experimental and other scientific purposes complies comprehensively with the Directive. Compare this to the 'gentleman's handshake' of the Convention.

However, even within this mandatory enforcement, history has provided us with an interesting anomaly. The UK attempted to comply with both the Convention and Directive from the outset and introduced in 1986 The Animals (Scientific Procedures) Act. Integral to the Act is Schedule 2 which lists animals to be obtained from designated breeding or supplying establishments. Schedule 2 is listed in full in Box 6.3.

BOX 6.3 Schedule 2: animals to be obtained only from designated breeding or supplying establishments

Mouse
Rat
Guinea Pig
Hamster
Rabbit
Dog
Cat
Primate

In 1993 the UK government received an infraction notice from Brussels which indicated that it was in breach of the Directive 86/609 as Schedule 2 of the Act did not include the common quail (*Coturnix coturnix*) as specified in Annex 1 (Article 21) of the Directive. At the other end of the scale, a project carried out for the Eurogroup for Animal Welfare in 1992 (Nab and Blom, 1993) reported how slowly some member states were reacting to the Directive. Belgium, Greece, Italy, Portugal and Spain were still in the process of *implementing* the Directive and poor and inadequate administrative support was also reported in Greece, Italy, Portugal and Spain.

In summary, the Convention and Directive attempt to harmonize the control of animals used in experimental and other scientific purposes across member states of the CoE and EU. The harmonization is achieved by setting standards for national legislation within those member states. The Convention attempts to bring about harmonization through general principles of agreement, having little recourse to enforcing law. On the other hand, the Directive is legally binding and failure to comply by member states can result in penalties.

National Legislation

It is appropriate now to move down the cascade of legislation to the national level. We now begin to

compare and contrast the controlling legislation of as many nations as we can, including the USA, Canada and Australia. In doing so it is imperative to remember that the legislation of all the European nations quoted should be at least striving to satisfy the Convention and the Directive as appropriate.

Consideration of the legislation nation by nation would perhaps be the easiest way to work through the subject. However, such a process can be tedious and in any case is available elsewhere (see Brookman and Legge, 1997). The task can also be performed by a process of comparison and contrast of the principle elements of the aims and objectives and how these are approached by the different countries. In this way the reader can begin to form an opinion how a nation approaches, in overall terms, the use of animals for experimental and other scientific purposes.

The remainder of the chapter will consider these elements in turn, examining how different nations approach the element through their legislation and regulations. To some extent, these elements have a loosely hierarchical structure to them and in reality frequently overlap, or are connected in a matrix manner. These aspects will be considered and addressed. For those interested in studying the legislation of any particular nation in more depth a comprehensive list is provided at the end of the chapter.

The elements to be considered are listed in Table 6.1.

The Work

The Scope of the Work

There is much variance between countries on what is included/excluded in the scope defined as 'experimental and other scientific procedures'. On the surface such a definition would appear to be self-explanatory, but what about clinical veterinary trials or wildlife investigations requiring the catching, tagging and release of birds, for example? What about catching and bleeding semidomesticated animals such as moose or reindeer for the purpose of zooepidemiology?

The European Convention and the Directive break the definition into two parts: acts or 'procedures' which constitute an experiment and the purpose(s) for which those acts or procedures were performed. In the author's opinion, in deciding whether or not work falls into this scope it is best to first consider the purpose or reason for the work. Considering the procedure or act in isolation or before the purpose can sometimes lead to confusion and even misinterpretation.

These definitions are detailed in Boxes 6.4 and 6.5 for the Convention and Directive respectively.

BOX 6.4 The Convention

Article 1 (c)

"*procedure*" means any experimental or other scientific use of an animal which may cause it pain, suffering or lasting harm, including any course of action intended to, or liable to, result in the birth of an animal in any such conditions, but excluding the least painful methods accepted in modern practice (that is, "humane" methods) of killing or marking an animal. A procedure starts when an animal is first prepared for use and ends when no further observations are to be made for that procedure; the elimination of pain, distress or lasting harm by the successful use of anaesthesia or analgesia or other methods does not place the use of the animal outside the scope of this definition.

Article 2

A procedure may be performed for one or more of the following purposes only and subject to the restrictions laid down in this Convention:

(a) (i) avoidance or prevention of disease, ill-health or other abnormality, or their effects, in man, vertebrate or invertebrate animals or plants, including the production and the quality, efficacy and safety testing of drugs, substances or products.

(ii) diagnosis or treatment of disease, ill-health or other abnormality, or their effects in man, vertebrate or invertebrate animals or plants;

(b) detection, assessment, regulation or modification of physiological conditions in man, vertebrate or invertebrate animals or plants;

(c) protection of the environment;

(d) scientific research;

(e) education and training;

(f) forensic inquiries.

Box 6.5 The Directive

Article 2 (d)

"*experiment*" means any use of an animal for experimental or other scientific purpose which may cause it pain, suffering, distress or lasting harm, including any course of action intended, or liable, to result in the birth of an animal in any such condition, but excluding the least painful methods accepted in modern practice (ie "humane" methods) of killing or marking an animal; an experiment starts when an animal is first prepared for use and ends when no further observations are to be made for that experiment; the elimination of pain, suffering, distress or lasting harm by the successful use of anaesthesia or analgesia or other methods does not place the use of the animal outside the scope of this definition. Non experimental, agricultural or veterinary practices are excluded.

Article 3

This Directive applies to the use of animals in experiments which are undertaken for one of the following purposes:

(a) The development, manufacture, quality, effectiveness and safety testing of drugs, foodstuffs and other substances or products:

(i) for the avoidance, prevention, diagnosis or treatment of disease, ill-health or other Abnormality or their effects in man, animals or plants;

(ii) for the assessment, detection, regulation or modification of physiological conditions in man, animals or plants;

(b) the protection of the natural environment in the interest of the health or welfare of man or animal.

Before exploring how the European states meet these requirements, some other countries will be considered for comparison.

USA

The defined scope of work meeting our criteria of 'experimental or other scientific purposes' can be found in Section 1 of the Animal Welfare Act 1996 (amended): 'the use of animals is instrumental in certain research and education for advancing knowledge of cures and treatment for disease and injuries

Table 6.1 Legislation controlling the use of animals for experimental and other scientific purposes (a common approach to interpretation of national legislature)

LEGISLATURE			
The work	**The facilities**	**The people**	**The administration**
Scope	Types	Categories	Competent authorities
Experimental	Definitions:	Management	Ministries
Other scientific species	User	Scientific	Departments
Authorization	Breeding	Veterinary	Interface
Cost/benefit analysis	Supplying	Technical	Statistics
Ethical review processes	Registration	Other	Legal
Severity banding	Inspection	Accountabilities	Technicalities
Reduction	Standards	Training	Infringements
Replacement	Guidelines		Penalties
Procedures	Codes of practice		Miscellaneous
Definitions			
Best practice			
Refinement			
Use of anaesthesia			
Reuse			
Euthanasia			
Post mortem tissue use			

which affect both humans and animals'. Within this, further definitions and guidance are provided in a variety of government and institutional documents, for example in the US government's Principles for the Utilisation and Care of Vertebrate Animals in Testing, Research and Training it states 'Procedures involving animals should be performed with due consideration of their relevance to human health, the advancement of knowledge or the good of society'.

From these quotes it would be fair to say that the US definition is less confined than those set in the European legislation. As will become clear later, however, a major regulating factor in the US system is the Institutional Animal Care and Use Committees (IACUCs).

Under scope of work, one interesting feature of the US legislation is that it excludes birds, rats of the genus *Rattus* and mice of the genus *Mus* from its definition of 'animal'. The author remains unclear as to why they should be defined out of the regulations, as they appear to be given adequate consideration in all other respects, but the numbers used presumably need not be recorded. This will be considered further under administration.

Australia

Australia lacks any national legislation controlling the use of animals for experimental and other scientific purposes. Each state has its own (different) law and codes to regulate experimentation. Australia (and New Zealand) rely heavily on the Australian and New Zealand Council for the Care of Animals in Research and Teaching (ANZCART) for leadership and guidance in the ethical and humane use of animals.

New Zealand

Work in New Zealand is conducted under Animals Protection (Codes of Ethical Conduct) Regulations 1987:

No person shall conduct any research, teaching, experimental, diagnostic, or toxicity or potency testing work, or work for the purposes of producing antisera or other biological agents involving the manipulation of live animals unless it is carried out in accordance with a code of ethical conduct approved by the Minister of Agriculture

Canada

Canada again has no national legislation controlling the scope of work and indeed employs a system of entirely 'voluntary, self regulation' administered at state level. The voluntary programme is administered by the Canadian Council on Animal Care (CCAC).

So it would seem that the US comes closest to Europe in providing some guidance on what constitutes 'experimental or other scientific purposes' through their national legislation.

Turning now to some of the European states we will see that the legislation reflects the requirements of the Convention and Directive with regard to controlling the scope of work permitted.

Sweden

The Animal Protection Act 1988, Section 19 (1) states

Animals must not without permission from the government or, where the government so decides from the National Board of Agriculture, be used for scientific research, education, the diagnosis of disease, the production of drugs or chemical products or for other comparable purposes if the animals are subjected to surgery, injections, bleeding or other suffering. Only animals bred for such purposes may be used. Such breeding may not take place without permission from the National Board of Agriculture.

So here we see the scope of the purpose defined by both goal (what the animals will be used for) and by those 'procedures' which are considered likely to cause pain, suffering, distress or lasting harm.

United Kingdom

The Animals [Scientific Procedures] Act 1986 takes a stepwise approach to scoping the work by first defining a protected species (Section 1), second by defining a 'regulated procedure' (Section 2), and then by specifying the purposes for which permission will be granted (Section 5.3).

The UK has perhaps the most detailed and constraining legislation with regard to what are permissible purposes, what is a protected species. Examples to support this view include:

• the exclusion of the use of animals for 'training purposes' except in the techniques of micro-surgery;

• the inclusion of the breeding of mutant strains (with harmful defects e.g. **athymic nude mice**, **obese and hypertensive rats**) and all **transgenic strains** (until proven not harmful over two generations kept for a natural lifespan) as a procedure;

• the inclusion of the common octopus (*Octopus vulgaris*) as a protected species under the Act; and in 1998 the UK government officially banned the use of the great apes, even though they had not been used for such purposes in the UK for over 30 years.

In summary, the more the legislation defines the scope of what constitutes 'experimental or other scientific purposes' the more likely it is to meet the aims and objectives of the regulations. The degree of constraint or flexibility around such scopes will to some extent reflect that nation's government's approach to central control and their moral approach to animals in society.

Switzerland

Section Six of the Swiss Animal Protection Act (1978) sets out conditions governing experiments on animals. Article 12 states 'experiments on animals' are to be construed as 'any procedures in which live animals are used for the purpose of testing a scientific hypothesis, acquiring knowledge, obtaining or testing a substance, or determining the effect of a particular procedure on the animal, as well as any use of animals in experimental behavioural research'.

Authorization of the Work

This, perhaps more than any other aspect of the use of animals, in experimental and other scientific purposes is currently under international scrutiny and can be best summarized in three words: cost/benefit analysis. In other words, if the proposal for the use of animals falls within the scope of the definition of experimental or scientific purpose, does the anticipated benefit to mankind (including benefit to animals) outweigh the intended or anticipated pain, suffering, distress or lasting harm to the animals in the study? National legislation frequently delegates this accountability to some form of local 'ethics' committee.

In Australia, Animal Experimentation Ethics Committees (AEECs) are overseen by the National

Health and Medical Research Council (NHMC) through the NHMC Animal Welfare Committee, which has a proactive role in advising local AEECs on ethical matters.

In Canada, institutions are required to have Animal Care Committees (ACCs), which receive guidance from the CCAC.

In Sweden the Animal Protection Act 1998 (Section 41–48) provides for the establishment and operation of local ethical committees which 'shall provide advisory services to those responsible for animal experiments'. Section 49 (1) states 'In considering a case the committee shall weigh the importance of the experiment against the suffering inflicted on the animal.'

In the USA this accountability for authorization lies clearly with the IACUC.

In the UK the cost/benefit analysis is the sole accountability of the Secretary of State. This accountability to decide on whether any particular work should be authorized is effectively delegated to the Home Office (Competent Authority) inspectors with only applications of special concern (e.g. work on cosmetics) being referred to the independent advisory body, the Animal Procedures Committee. Occasionally the Secretary of State may also request advice from expert external assessors. As from April 1999, however, it will be a requirement for all designated establishments under A[SP]A to have in place formal 'Ethical review processes' with strong advice that this should include a local ethics committee. After April 1999 the Home Office Inspectorate will not consider any applications for work to be authorized until it has been approved by the establishment's local ethical review.

Denmark's position is relatively aligned with the UK in that permits are issued by the Animal Experimentation Inspectorate, an administrative board set up by law and managed by the Council for Animal Experiments. The Chair of the Council and nine other members are appointed by the Minister of Justice.

Germany also provides for direct authorization of work from the Ministry of Food, Agriculture and Forestry.

In summary, there appear to be two systems working to perform cost/benefit analyses. One places the accountability on defined roles within a government organization. This places the onus on a few government officials to decide on the cost to the animals involved versus the likely gain to humanity. The other, probably more common system, provides

for cost/benefit analysis to be performed by local ethical committees, frequently with lay and or animal welfare interest membership. Each have their advantages and drawbacks. Much has been written on ethics committees and ethical review processes in recent times and the issue of cost/benefit analysis must be viewed as a dynamic and evolving subject.

Application of the 3R's

Even though a large number of nations delegate the cost/benefit analysis to local ethics committees, there is significant consistency and harmonization on the issue of the application of the 3R's. In all the national legislation reviewed by the author there is provision made for those conducting the experiment to ensure they apply the principles of the 3R's in designing their experiments. The extent to which this requirement is applied may vary according to the effectiveness of the ethical review process in operation.

Viewed another way, the cost/benefit analysis should aim to maximize the benefits by improved science, design, etc. and application of the 3R's should drive cost down to the minimum, i.e. the equation is not just about benefits outweighing cost, but that the costs are in addition minimized by the application of the 3R's!

Take three examples of the explicit requirement to consider the 3R's in national legislation:

UK, Section 5 (5) A[SP]A: 'The Secretary of State shall not grant a project licence unless he is satisfied that the applicant has given adequate consideration to the feasibility of achieving the purpose of the programme to be specified in the licence by means not involving the use of protected animals.'

US, Section 13 (3) B The Animal Welfare Act: 'that the principal investigator considers alternatives to any procedure likely to produce pain to or distress in an experimental animal.'

Sweden, The Animal Protection Act (1992) Section 49 (2): 'The committee shall also advise against the use of animals for such purposes where it is possible to acquire comparable information by other means.'

Whilst these quotes perhaps focus on the reduction and replacement aspects, the issue of refinement (reducing the pain, suffering, distress or lasting harm) must also be considered in any cost/benefit analysis. (Refinement also includes increasing the sensitivity and reliability of test systems so that fewer animals need to be used and repeat testing can be avoided.)

Procedures

We reviewed legislation around the scope of defining 'experimental and other scientific purposes', then we moved on to how the cost/benefit analysis of the work is controlled and the work ultimately authorized. An integral part of deciding if the work falls within the definition above and in performing the cost/benefit analysis is consideration of the 'procedures' to be performed upon the animals. Clearly if whatever is to be done to the animals does not constitute a 'procedure' under the national legislation then the work falls outside the scope of that legislation.

Also it is vital to remember, as explained earlier, that a veterinary technique (e.g. bleeding an animal) which is performed for a purpose outside the scope defined in the legislation is equally outside the control of that legislation, even though it may be performed on an animal inside the laboratory. Such a procedure would then be described as one of 'recognized husbandry' or as 'an act of veterinary surgery', depending upon specific national legislation.

Most nations now have a common understanding of what constitutes a 'procedure' and a common definition which is emerging is 'one which causes pain, suffering, distress or lasting harm equal to/or greater than the insertion of a hollow needle through the integument'. In considering definitions of procedure it must be remembered that it is the anticipated or potential consequences which affect the classification. For example, the feeding of diet containing a toxic or carcinogenic material will be immediately less painful than the insertion of a hollow needle into a body cavity. However, the ultimate anticipated effects of such a procedure will certainly be greater and therefore should be considered a procedure, bringing the work within the scope of the legislation.

It should be noted that the humane killing only (euthanasia) of an animal is not considered a procedure (see Boxes 6.4 and 6.5 for examples) under the European laws. The author is unaware of any national legislation which includes it as a recognized procedure.

However, the UK goes one step nearer to control by recognizing those methods of euthanasia which exempt killing of an animal in a laboratory, from procedural definition and inclusion. These methods are listed in a Code of Practice available as a supplement to the Act. The EU recently published guidelines on acceptable methods of killing (euthanasia) but to date have made no move to implement them as mandatory methods.

Animals euthanased without having procedures performed upon them but whose carcasses are used for tissue harvesting will be considered under statistics.

Under procedures, we must consider the issue of reuse. An animal can be considered to have been reused when more than one procedure is performed upon it for two or more unconnected experiments or other scientific purposes. This perhaps is an oversimplification of the term and the author is aware of the difficulties in reaching common international understanding. The issue is nevertheless an important one for a number of potential implications. The real moral dilemma around reuse is whether it is better to inflict repeated pain, suffering, distress or lasting harm on a single animal or to share that number of procedures amongst more animals. In reality, in those nations which allow reuse there are normally controls to ensure that animals which have already experienced more than minimal levels of suffering are prohibited from reuse.

The author understands that the legislation in a number of countries, Germany being one of them, absolutely forbids reuse of any description. Such an absolute ban leads to these nations being unable to agree to procedures such as the breeding of harmful mutant strains and the development and production of transgenic being classed as 'procedures' as they are in the UK. Such a classification of breeding *per se* would then make the use of these animals in the countries where reuse is banned impossible.

In the UK, reuse is strictly controlled through veterinary inspection and specific authorization procedures. Whilst reuse is clearly vulnerable to abuse if not strictly controlled, it clearly provides opportunities for effective use of the larger species such as dogs, cats and farm animals where the procedures are very minor but repetitive and have little welfare cost to the animals.

A good example of reuse would be repeated pharmacokinetic studies requiring oral dosing and repeat blood sampling in dogs for different classes of compounds. For instance, the repeat use for a number of drugs of the same class, e.g. cardiovascular, would not constitute reuse, but transfer of the animal to test drugs of the CNS class might be classed as reuse. The important issue is to ensure that the welfare of the animal is never jeopardized as a result of reuse. In some instances reuse may be allowed, providing the animal is terminally anaesthetized for the second or final study.

The Facilities

Facility Type

Three types or categories of facilities are generally recognized with regard to experimental animals. Control of the different categories and especially the degree of control frequently varies from country to country. The three categories can be defined as:

- Breeding establishment
- Supplying establishment
- Use or user establishment.

Frequently, a single research facility may actually have facilities which fall into at least two of these definitions. For instance, universities and large commercial research organizations frequently have in-house breeding as well as research laboratories and experimental animal facilities. In some countries (e.g. the UK), this may lead to the implementation of dual standards of housing and husbandry within the same perimeter fence.

The purpose and definition of breeding and use facilities are probably apparent and easily understood. Supplying establishments are less well understood both in terms of purpose and, in the 1990s, of need. A supplying establishment can be defined as an establishment which holds animals for a transitory period between the point of origin and final destination. Classically, supply establishments are best illustrated as those facilities which held wild-caught primates for some period (of quarantine) between their capture and shipment to end user.

In the past, such establishments performed a valuable function in providing a facility and resource for quarantining and treating newly caught animals before they were supplied for study purposes. In the 1990s the continued need for supplying establishments versus the emphasis on purpose-bred animals and reduction in transport stress must be questioned.

Facility Registration and Inspection

All types of facilities generally require some form of registration or designation under the European Convention and Directive and US Animal Welfare Act. The condition of registration or designation is usually consequent to meeting certain conditions and standards. The registration conditions and standards are usually monitored and enforced through a system of inspection by government-appointed agencies and representatives.

The agency responsible for such inspections and registration varies widely between countries and may or may not be the same agency controlling the work described earlier. The agency most often appointed to conduct such registrations and inspections is that with responsibility for agriculture and usually animal health and welfare, i.e. the Department of Agriculture in the USA. Other government departments and agencies are frequently also deployed in this area, e.g. Department of (Public) Health (in the Netherlands) and the Home Office (in the UK).

With regard to the conditions and standards that must be adhered to as part of the registration, there are a number of guidelines and codes of practice in operation at both international and national levels. The Articles of the Convention and Directive covering registration of the different establishment categories are given in Boxes 6.6 and 6.7.

BOX 6.6 Articles of the Convention and Directive covering registration of breeding or supplying establishments

Convention: Part V

Article 14

Breeding and supplying establishments shall be registered with the respective authority subject to the grant of an exemption under Article 21 or 22. Such registered establishments shall comply with the requirements of Article 5.

Directive

Article 15

Breeding and supplying establishments shall be approved by or registered with, the authority and comply with the requirements of Articles 5 and 14 unless an exemption is granted under Article 19 (4) or Article 21. A supplying establishment shall obtain animals only from a breeding or other supplying establishment unless the animal has been lawfully imported and is not a feral or stray animal. General or special exemption from this last provision may be granted to a supplying establishment under arrangements determined by the authority.

Other relevant Articles are 15, 16 and 17 of the Convention, which detail certain conditions of registration, and Articles 16, 17 and 18 of the Directive, which deal with breeding and supplying establishments.

BOX 6.7 Articles of the Convention and Directive covering registration of use/ user establishments

Convention: Part VI

Article 18

User establishments shall be registered with or otherwise approved by the responsible authority and shall comply with the conditions laid down in Article.

Article 19

Provisions shall be made at user establishments for installations and equipment approved for the species of animals used and the performance of the procedures conducted there. The design, construction and functioning of such installations and equipment shall be such as to ensure that the procedures are performed as effectively as possible, with the minimum degree of pain, suffering, distress or lasting harm.

Within the Convention, Articles 20–24 also lay down conditions for user establishments. Articles 19 (sections 2–5) and 21 of the Directive lay down further conditions of registration of user establishments.

Article 20 of the Directive makes provision for a single registration for establishments breeding animals for use in experiments on their own premises. However, the establishments shall comply with the relevant provisions of the Directive concerning breeding and user establishments.

With regard to the position in the US, user establishments are required to register under the Animal Welfare Act with the Secretary of Agriculture of the United States or his deputy. Federal research facilities are exempt from this requirement but must report through the IACUC to the head of the Federal Agency direct. The head of the Federal Agency conducting the research is responsible for all corrective action to be taken at the facility and for the granting of all exceptions to the inspection protocol. (Animal and Plant Health Inspection Service, USDA Subchapter A – Animal Welfare, Part 2 Subpart C – Research Facilities #2.30 Registration, and #2.37 Federal research facilities.) Breeding and supplying establishments in the US must hold a licence under Subpart A – Licensing of the above regulations.

Guidelines on Minimum Holding Conditions

Perhaps of greatest concern, if not of greatest importance, to those with accountabilities and responsibilities for 'establishments' are the minimum conditions which must be attained and maintained in order to retain registration. All too often in the past, those responsible and accountable for holding laboratory animals have regarded published guidelines on housing and care as the minimum they needed to instigate in order to comply with the regulations, rather than utilizing them as part of an overall assessment of what could be provided for the animals without compromising the science and within the resources available.

It is a disappointing fact that there is still great focus and emphasis on the minimum caging and environmental conditions which must be adhered to in order to remain in compliance. To a greater or lesser extent this attitude, at least in some quarters, is beginning to change to one of implementation of best practice which delivers optimum (known) welfare for the animals at a practicable cost and without compromise of the scientific objectives.

Those with accountabilities in this area are helped and guided by a number of international and national reference documents on caging, environmental and husbandry standards. These guidelines set out to ensure animals held for scientific purposes are provided with adequate comfort and care throughout their stay in the facilities. It should be noted that such guidelines and codes should never be used, interpreted or limited such as to prevent the introduction of innovative systems of housing designed to improve the welfare of animals.

Within Europe, national competent authorities and breeders/users are guided both by a policy statement in the Convention and Directive on the general care and accommodation of animals and by an Appendix/Annex respectively to the documents, specifying in more detail, the suggested standards.

The author finds the policy statement of both documents an archetypal piece of political drafting, aimed at keeping two parties with opposing and polarized views happy (i.e. the users versus the welfarists). These policy statements are presented as Article 5 of both the Convention and Directive and are reproduced in Box 6.8.

full extension from the ceiling without its feet touching the cage floor' would be of an adequate dimension to 'limit as far as is practicable the extent to which' or 'restrict to the absolute minimum the extent to which' (Ref. Appendix A Table 9 and Annex A Table 9).

As yet, these two documents remain the standard for the minimum caging dimensions for animals bred, held and used under the control of the Convention and/or Directive. However, under the auspices of the Council of Europe, Multilateral Consultation on the Convention, a working party has been set up to review Appendix A, with special reference to the report on *The Accommodation of Laboratory Animals In Accordance With Animal Welfare Requirements*, edited by P. N. O'Donoghue (commonly referred to as the Berlin Workshop 1993 (Report)).

It is anticipated by the Multilateral Consultation that the findings of the review will lead to an early amendment of Appendix A, incorporating the latest research findings on animal welfare, as well as established current best practice. Amendment to Annex A of the Directive is likely to follow shortly afterwards.

Similar guidance on housing and husbandry requirements can be found in most national legislation, usually following the model of separate guidelines. In the US the standards to be achieved are published by the Institute of Laboratory Animal Resources and can be found in the *Guide for the Care and Use of Laboratory Animals* (National Academic Press, 1996).

The UK produces two sets of codes of practice, one for user establishments and one for breeding establishments. Under UK law, a code of practice has greater legal enforcement than guidelines. Compliance with the codes forms part of the conditions of issue of a Certificate of Designation and failure to comply with codes may lead to revocation of the Certificate.

In summary, most if not all countries which provide for legislative control of animal experimentation include some form of registration of the establishments at which it is undertaken. Registration usually requires adherence to certain conditions and standards of accommodation, husbandry and care. These include statements around administrative detail, managerial control, the species of animals which may be held and the sources from which those animals may come. In particular, registration commonly requires adherence to specific caging and

---

BOX 6.8 Convention

Article 5 (Section 1)

Any animal used or intended for use in a procedure shall be provided with the accommodation, an environment, at least a minimum degree of freedom of movement, food, water and care appropriate to its health and well-being. Any restriction on the extent to which an animal can satisfy its physiological and ethological needs shall be limited as far as is practicable. In the implementation of this provision, regard should be paid to the guidelines for accommodation and care set out in appendix A to this Convention.

Directive

Article 5 (a) & (b)

(a) all experimental animals shall be provided with housing, an environment, at least some freedom of movement, food, water and care which are appropriate to their health and well being;

(b) any restriction on the extent to which experimental animal can satisfy its physiological and ethological needs shall be limited to the absolute minimum.

The author has yet to find anyone who can reconcile the provision of 'a minimum degree of freedom' with 'limiting as far as is practicable the extent to which it can satisfy its physiological and ethological needs'. Or even harder, the reconciliation of provision of 'at least some freedom of movement' with 'restricting the extent to which an animal can satisfy its physiological and ethological needs to the absolute minimum'.

These (conflicting) statements would seem to suggest that whoever dreamt them up believed that an animal's ethological needs could be entirely satisfied independently of the space provided. In other words, for each of the Articles above, only one of the two statements provided is really necessary. But each statement, read in isolation of the other, satisfies first the user and secondly the welfarist, respectively! Such broad, well-meaning statements become even harder to accept in the 1990s when their interpretation or conversion into the hard minimum standards of the appendix/annex are studied. For instance, did anyone seriously believe that a primate cage with a minimum height which allows the monkey to 'at least stand up erect', or 'swing in

The People

A common thread running through the use of animals in biomedical research across the world is the involvement of people. Their involvement comes through many varied roles and functions. Some are required explicitly under legislation and regulations, some are implied, and others which whilst being equally necessary and important perhaps receive no reference in the laws. The list of those involved covers the following areas:

- Scientific
- Technical
- Veterinary
- Management
- Others.

It has been the author's experience in discussing these roles at international level that confusion and misunderstanding can occur because of varied definitions of these categories. This is particularly so in defining scientific and technical roles. For the purposes of this chapter, those described as having a scientific role are those people accountable for the design and overall conduct of experiments. Technical roles primarily cover those people performing 'procedures' upon animals as defined in legislation and as discussed earlier in the chapter. There is also a more open consideration of technical roles to include staff whose primary job is to care for the animals without performing procedures upon them. Management and veterinary roles are self-explanatory. 'Others' may include competent authority

staff, including administrators and inspectors and members of any ethical or animal care and use committees.

The effectiveness of registration in setting and maintaining standards is most often a factor of the priority (and therefore resource) allocated to it by the government and relevant agency in question. In addition, it is now widely recognized that the minimum standards set in the 1970s and 1980s are woefully inadequate for some species and circumstances. This is especially true for the Old World and New World primates. Moreover, the concept of striving to implement 'best practice', rather than merely setting out to satisfy minimum legal requirements will hopefully be a driving force in the development of new guidelines.

environmental standards which are frequently the hub or focus of inspections by the controlling statutory body or competent authority.

The Federation of European Laboratory Animal Science Associations (FELASA) considered these roles in some depth and developed four categories commonly referred to as:

- Cat. A – Persons taking care of animals
- Cat. B – Persons carrying out animal experiments
- Cat. C – Persons responsible for directing animal experiments
- Cat. D – Laboratory animal specialists.

Details of these definitions can be found in *Laboratory Animals* (1995) **29**, 121–131. These basic definitions have been used by both the EU and CoE administration in developing education and training strategies for people involved in laboratory animal science.

FELASA based its recommendations on functions, which are common to all, rather than on nomenclature, which differs from country to country. Within the terms of the Council of Europe Convention the three Articles refer to appropriate definition and control of personnel involved (Box 6.9).

Part VI User establishments
Article 20

In user establishments:

(a) the person or persons who are administratively responsible for the care of the animals and the functioning of the equipment shall be identified;

(b) sufficient trained staff shall be provided

(c) adequate arrangements shall be made for the provision of veterinary advice and treatment;

(d) a veterinarian or other competent person should be charged with advisory duties in relation to the well-being of the animals.

These three important Articles of the Convention are closely mirrored in the European Union Directive under:

● Article 7 ('experiments shall be performed solely by competent authorised persons, or under the direct responsibility of such a person')

● Article 14 'Persons who carry out experiments or take part in them and persons who take care of animals used for experiments, including duties of a supervisory nature, shall have appropriate education and training.

● In particular, persons carrying out or supervising the conduct of experiments shall have received instruction in a scientific discipline relevant to the experimental work being undertaken and be capable of handling and taking care of laboratory animals; they shall also have satisfied the authority that they have attained a level of training sufficient for carrying out their tasks.'

● Article 16 mirrors Article 15 of the Convention (breeding and supplying establishments).

● Article 19.2 mirrors Article 20 of the Convention (user establishments).

It must be assumed that those European states who are signatory to the Convention and or a member of the EU are complying with these 'personnel requirements'.

In the USA, the Animal Welfare Act Subpart C – Research Facilities explicitly states under #2.30 Registration that 'an official who has legal authority to bind the parent organization shall sign the registration form.'

Section #2.32 Personal Qualifications explicitly states:

(a) It shall be the responsibility of the research facility to ensure that all scientists, research technicians, animal technicians and other personnel involved in animal care, treatment and use are qualified to perform their duties. This responsibility shall be fulfilled in part through the provision of training and instruction to those personnel.

(b) Training and instruction shall be made available and the qualifications of personnel reviewed, with sufficient frequency to fulfil the research facility's responsibilities under this section.

The text goes on to detail 14 points of training detail.

Section #2.33 Attending veterinarian and adequate veterinary care:

(a) Each research facility shall have an attending veterinarian who shall provide adequate veterinary care to its animals in compliance with this section.

(1) Each research facility shall employ an attending veterinarian under formal arrangements. In the case of a part time attending veterinarian or consultant arrangements, the formal arrangements shall include a written programme of veterinary care and regularly scheduled visits to the research facility.

(2) Each research facility shall assure that the attending veterinarian has appropriate authority to ensure the provision of adequate care and to oversee the adequacy of other respects of animal care and use.

Similar types of roles and accountabilities can be found in other countries, such as Australia and New Zealand.

On reading all of these regulations a number of common themes emerge:

● Accountability
● Authority
● Competence
● Education
● Training.

Each of these 'themes' is handled slightly differently at the national levels but there is general recognition that competency can only be achieved through education and training. Likewise, accountabilities can only be effectively discharged when those held in accountability are competent to be so. There has for a long time been a recognition that education and training are essential for those having a 'hands on' role in animal experimentation. There is also undoubtedly still room for development with regard to education and training for those with senior, more general, administrative accountabilities to ensure their accountabilities are fully understood and the consequences of failure highlighted.

Without exception, all countries with legislation regarding animal experimentation acknowledge the need to have trained, competent personnel to provide technical and veterinary care, as well as to ensure procedures are applied to a high standard of proficiency.

The Administration

Competent Authorities

As has already been discussed, there is a wide variety of authorities involved and responsible for controlling animal experimentation across the nations of the world. The more logical authorities include departments of health, animal health and welfare and agriculture. The situation in the UK is unique in that the controlling authority (the Home Office) has no other direct interest in human health or animal protection.

The level of control from the competent authority also varies widely and is reflected in the way the law is administered. In the UK, the competent authority has extremely tight control with little to no authority being delegated to people in overall administrative control of the facility. In other countries the competent authority play a very much more 'hands off', overseeing role, with most of the decisions surrounding the experimental work and its conduct delegated to the local ethical committee or (institutional) ACUC. Within the framework set out by the local committees, the facility management will then have the ability to conduct the research, adhering to the national legal requirements. In summary, the nominated national competent authority plays a vital role in interpreting and shaping national legislation and in deciding the degree of governmental involvement and control. Hence control can vary from an extremely tight central system with vigorous implementation to a largely delegated responsibility to individual research institutes with only nominal, central overview.

Statistics

The collection of statistics with regard to animal use continues to be a very contentious issue within and between the two European bodies (EU and CoE). The collection of statistics is a complex and resource-consuming task. The primary difficulties encountered in reaching agreement on collection have been agreement and common understanding of terms and definitions, together with frequency. Whilst the Convention makes provision for the collection of animal use statistics every year, the Directive only requires collection at intervals not exceeding 3 years. Failure to agree between the competent authorities on which time scale to use has been one of the issues delaying the EU from ratifying the Convention. The first attempt at collecting statistics for the EU member states took place in late 1992/1993 when information regarding animal use for 1991 was requested by the Commission (COM [94] 195 final). Straughan (1994) made some interesting observations on the report. There have been no further publications of European statistics since. Meanwhile many countries continue to publish their own national statistics following the European guidelines on tables to varying degrees. Recent moves within Europe are indicating a future requirement to not only report those animals used in 'procedures' but also those animals humanely killed for the purpose of harvesting tissues and body fluids and also the total numbers of animals bred for scientific purposes. Whilst there continues to be much debate amongst the competent authorities on the value of statistics, there can be no doubt that there is growing public and political pressure to publicize numbers as the first step in establishing milestones for reduction. Statistical reports for the US do not include rodents because they are not defined as animals under the appropriate legislation.

Legal Technicalities

In whichever country someone is performing animal experimentation they must be fully aware of the principles and technicalities of the law under which they are working. All too often they have a broad understanding of the principles but transgress on matters of administrative detail and technicalities. It behoves everyone to be sure they abide by the letter of the law at all times when it comes to animal experimentation: 'Not only must we care we must be seen to be caring'?

Conclusion

Whilst clearly there is now comprehensive recognition around the world of the need to provide legal protection for the use of animals in scientific research, it is neither absolute in terms of being global, nor uniform in principle, policy and implementation. In the introduction it was said that 'the ethics and culture of a society are the mother of its laws'. The discussion and examples set out in this chapter have provided evidence for this statement and have illustrated the importance of national, cultural differences in determining how both international and national legislation may be interpreted and implemented. Whilst it may be the vision of a few to bring about global harmonization with respect to the use of laboratory animals, in reality and probability this will never be the case given the immense diversity of cultural attitudes to animals and their exploitation for human need and benefit.

In formulating, developing and implementing legislation which controls both whether and how animals can be used for scientific purposes it is vital that the underpinning principles continue to be applied, i.e.

- It must continue to allow legitimate advancement of science and technology for the benefit of humanity.
- It must protect individual scientists conducting lawful and legitimate research from prosecution.
- It must provide the animals the maximum protection against unnecessary suffering.

As legislation, policies and procedures develop in some countries, it is also equally important that a fourth point is given consideration: legislation must provide a 'level playing field' in order to avoid implementing controls which then force certain types of scientific procedures out of one country and into another. A very good example of this at the time of writing is the (unilateral) virtual ban in the UK on the *in vivo* production of ascites monoclonal antibody production in mice. The reality of such a ban is the potential to merely drive such scientific procedures to a country where they are permitted. Such a move by the UK authority might be described as an effective implementation of replacement (one of the 3R's). However, such decisions may have negative consequences attached to them also. For instance, necessary *in vivo* ascites production work may be transferred from the UK to countries with lower welfare standards and controls. Also public pressure and action groups may force legislation to drive some and even, ultimately, all animal work from some countries

into others with distinctly different cultural attitudes and values towards animals. It then becomes debatable where the value of such legislative control lies.

In summary, whilst universal (global), standardization of laboratory animal legislation can never be possible, there are distinct advantages for all stakeholders to ensure that where possible there is harmonization in both principle and policy. Only in this way will improvements on a global scale be accomplished in the field of the 3R's, whilst at the same time maintaining a reasonable balance of scientific progress and commercial competitiveness at national level.

To this end, cooperation and consultation at multinational level are imperative and are to be encouraged. Positive examples of this are to be found in the CoE and EU. Also the current initiatives around harmonization of toxicity testing and collateral acceptance of regulatory studies must be applauded for their contribution to the reduced need for animal studies.

Finally, it is heartening to see attendance at the Council of Europe Multilateral Consultations not only of states which have yet to ratify the Convention but also of representatives from the US Department of Agriculture and from Japan.

References

Brookman, S. and Legge, D. (1997) In: *Law Relating to Animals*, Chapter 1. London: Cavendish Publishing.

Commission of the European Communities. First Report from the Commission to the Council and the European Parliament on the Statistics on the Number of Animals Used for Experimental and Other Scientific Purposes. COM (94) 195 final. Brussels, 27.05.1994.

FELASA (1995) *Lab. Anim.* **29**, 121–131.

Nab, J. and Blom, H.J.M. (1993) Implementation and Enforcement of EC Directive 86/609 on Animal Experimentation in Portugal, Italy, Greece and Spain. Final Report of a project initiated by Eurogroup for Animal Welfare and supported by the European Commission (out of print).

Russell, W.M.S. and Burch, R.L. (1992) (originally published 1959) *The Principles of Humane Experimental Technique*. Universities Federation of Animal Welfare, Wheathampstead, England.

Straughan, D.W. (1994) *Alternatives to Laboratory Animals* **22**, 289–292.

Further Reading

Brookman, S. and Legge, D (1997) *The Law Relating to Animals*. London: Cavendish Publishing.

Matfield, M. (1996) Laboratory animal welfare around the globe. *Lab. Anim.* **25**, 29–38.

Wilkins, D.B. (ed.) (1997) *Animal Welfare in Europe: European Legislation and Concerns*. London: Kluwer Law International.

Europe

Council Directive (86/609) of 24 November 1986 on the approximation of laws, regulations and administrative provisions of the member states regarding the protection of animals used for experimental and other scientific purposes. *Off. J. Eur. Commun.* L 358, Volume **29**, 18 December 1986.

European Convention for the Protection of Vertebrate Animals Used for Experimental and Other Scientific Purposes ETS 123 (1986). Council of Europe, Strasbourg. English and French translations.

Explanatory Report on the European Convention for the Protection of Vertebrate Animals Used for Experimental and Other Scientific Purposes (available with the Convention ETS 123, see above).

O' Donoghue, P.N. (ed.) (1994) *The Accommodation of Laboratory Animals in Accordance with Animal Welfare Requirements. Proceedings of an International Workshop held at the Bundesgesundheitsamt, Berlin, 17–19 May 1993.* Bonn: Bundesministerium fur Ernahrung, Land-wirtschaft und Forsten.

Recommendations for Euthanasia of Experimental Animals: Working Party Report for DGX1 of the European Commission to be used with Directive 86/609 (1996) *Lab. Anim.* **30**, 293–316 and *Lab. Anim.* (1997) **31**, 1–32.

United Kingdom

Animals (Scientific Procedures) Act 1986. Contained in: *Guidance on the Operation of the Animals (Scientific Procedures) Act 1986.* London: HMSO.

Code of Practice for the Housing and Care of Animals Used in Scientific Procedures. Reprinted 1996 (£7.25). London: HMSO.

Code of Practice for the Housing and Care of Animals in Designated Breeding and Supplying Establishments. Printed 1995. London: HMSO.

The Humane Killing of Animals under Schedule 1 to the Animals (Scientific Procedures) Act 1986. Code of Practice. Printed 1997. London: HMSO.

Sweden

The Swedish National Board for Laboratory Animals Ordinance Containing Regulations and General Recommendations concerning Ethical Examinations of the Use of Laboratory Animals for Scientific Purposes (1990). The Swedish National Board for Laboratory Animals (CFN), Ministry of Agriculture, 103 33 Stockholm, Sweden. *Provisions and General Recommendations Relating to the Use of Animals for Scientific Purposes* (1994). Available from address above.

Denmark

Statement Concerning Animal Experimentation (1992). The Ethical Council Concerning Animals, Danish Ministry of Justice, Slotshlmsgade 10, DK – 1216, Denmark.

Italy

Guaitani, A. and Bartosek, I. (1994) Regulatory aspects of animal experimentation in the biomedical sciences. *Forum (Trends in Experimental and Clinical Medicine)* **4.3**, 365–373.

Switzerland

Ethical Principles and Guidelines for Scientific Experiments on Animals (1995) Swiss Academy of Medical Sciences, Petersplatz 13, CH-4051, Basel.

United States of America

Animal and Plant Health Inspection Service, USDA. Subchapter A – Animal Welfare (#1.1 – #11.1). National Research Council (1996) *Guide for the Care and Use of Laboratory Animals.* Washington DC: National Academy Press.

DeHaven, W.R. (1998) The ins and outs of USDA's animal welfare act enforcement. *Contemporary Topics* **37**.

Canada

Canadian Council on Animal Care (1984) *Guide to the Care and Use of Experimental Animals*, Vols 1 and 2. Ottawa: CCAC.

Rowesell, H.C. (1991) The symbiosis of legislation and of voluntary control – the Canadian experience. *Anim. Technol.* **42**.

New Zealand

Code of Recommendations and Minimum Standards for the Care and Use of Animals for Scientific Purposes (1995) Code of Animal Welfare No. 17. Animal Welfare Advisory Committee, c/o Ministry of Agriculture, PO BOX 2526, Wellington, New Zealand.

Australia

Australian Code of Practice for Care and Use of Animals for Scientific Purposes (1990). NHMRC, CSIRO, Australian Agriculture Council, Australian Government Publishing Service, Canberra, Australia.

PART 3

Rat Pathogens

Contents

CHAPTER 7

Common Diseases

Elias T Gaillard
Experimental Pathology Laboratories Inc., Research Triangle Park, NC, USA

Charles B Clifford
Charles River Laboratories Inc., Wilmington, MA, USA

Introduction

Many pathogens have been reported to cause disease in the laboratory rat. In today's modern laboratories many of the pathogens that were commonplace in the past are only occasionally observed today. Much of this progress is due to improvements in husbandry, breeding or **rederivation methods,** and health surveillance tests used by the supplier and the users. However, the breeder and the users must be forever vigilant and cognizant of some of the more common pathogens and the disease they can cause, because infections can and will continue to occur.

This chapter will concentrate on the pathology of the more common pathogens of the laboratory rat. Although other ancillary tests (e.g. serological, bacteriological, etc.) will be mentioned briefly, the reader is encouraged to consult the listed references for details.

Viral Diseases

Parvoviruses

Based on serologic surveys, parvoviruses are some of the most common viral pathogens in wild and laboratory rats (Kilham and Margolis, 1966; Robey *et al.,* 1968; Gannon and Carthew, 1980; Lussier and Descoteaux, 1986; Gilioli *et al.,* 1996; Ueno *et al.,* 1996).

Recently, a classification scheme was proposed for rat parvoviruses (Jacoby *et al.,* 1996). In general, there are three main serogroups including *Rat virus* (RV), *H-1 virus* and *Rat parvovirus* (RPV). In the past, RPV was referred to as rat **orphan** parvovirus (Ueno *et al.,* 1996, 1997). Each of these different parvoviruses were fortuitous discoveries. RV and H-1 were discovered during experiments with rat tumors and transplantable human (Kilham and Oliver, 1959) and transplantable human tumors (Toolan et al., 1960), respectively; RPV was discovered during a pathogenesis experiment involving RV (Jacoby et al., 1987; Ball-Goodrich et al., 1998).

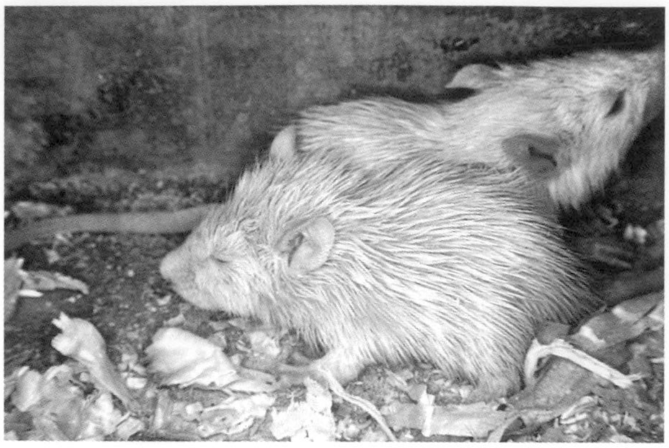

The rat is the natural host for RV; however, hamsters, mice and kittens have been experimentally infected with it (Kilham, 1961; Kilham and Margolis, 1965; ElDadah et al., 1967; Margolis and Kilham, 1972).

The natural host for H-1 is not clear since the virus was originally recovered from transplantable human tumors, tissues from cancer patients, human embryos and a spontaneous tumor in a rat (Toolan, 1960, 1961; Toolan et al., 1960, 1962). Hamsters and nonhuman primates have been experimentally infected with H-1 (Toolan, 1960, 1961, 1966; Kilham and Margolis, 1969). H-1 and RV share many of the same tissue tropisms and lesions (Margolis et al., 1968; Kilham and Margolis, 1969; Margolis and Kilham, 1970).

Like RV, the natural host for RPV is the rat. To the authors' knowledge there has only been one strain of RPV discovered and it is has been referred to as rat parvovirus type 1a (RPV-1a) (Ball-Goodrich et al., 1998). It appears that mice and hamsters are not susceptible (Ueno et al., 1997). Both RPV and RV are **tropic** for many of the same tissues and they both may result in a persistent infection. However, RPV is antigenically and genetically distinct from RV, and it apparently does not cause clinical signs or lesions in infant rats. It also seems that RPV may be more tropic for the small intestine and this site maybe the primary portal of entrance for RPV. The lung is believed to be the portal of entry and the site of initial replication for RV (Gaertner et al., 1993).

Since RV has probably been studied more extensively than any of the other parvoviruses of rats,

much of the information involving clinical signs, pathology, etc. refers to this virus.

Clinical signs and the disease outcome depend on viral factors and host factors (Kilham and Ferm, 1964; Kilham and Margolis, 1966; ElDadah et al., 1967; Robey et al., 1968; Cole et al., 1970; Margolis and Kilham, 1970; Nathanson et al., 1970; Jacoby et al., 1987; Gaertner et al., 1989, 1996). Viral factors include the viral strain, its virulence and tissue tropism. Host factors include the age and the immune status of the rat at the time of infection. For example, neonates may exhibit tremors, **ataxia**, jaundice, stunted growth, oily hair coats (Figure 7.1), diarrhea and sudden death, whereas rats infected as juveniles (4 weeks old) or adults usually have latent asymptomatic infections. However, if such latently infected rats become immunocompromised or stressed they may exhibit paralysis resulting from hemorrhage and necrosis in the brain and spinal cord. In addition, scrotal cyanosis and hemorrhage (Figure 7.2) may be observed in juvenile and adult male rats. There may also be a transient drop in breeding efficiency. Similar clinical signs may also be observed in naïve

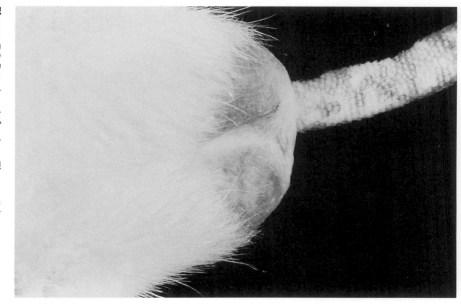

Figure 7.1 These rat pups' hair coats have an oily appearance.

Figure 7.2 Rat virus infection. The testicles appear cyanotic.

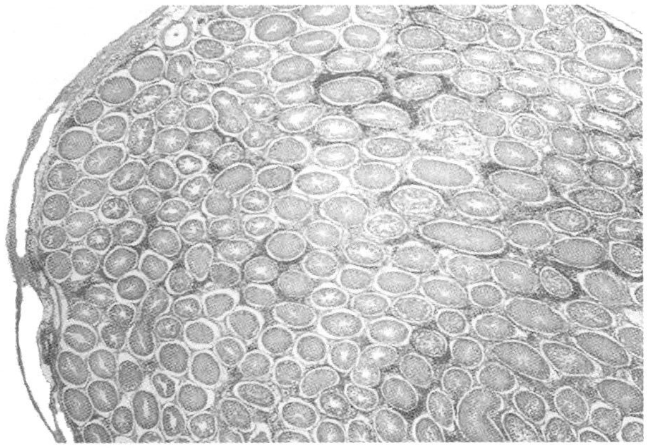

immune status (Jacoby *et al.*, 1987, 1991; Gaertner *et al.*, 1991, 1996). In addition, it seems that viral factors (e.g. the strain of RV) may also influence persistent infections.

RV can be shed in feces, milk and urine (Kilham and Ferm, 1964; Kilham and Margolis, 1966, 1974; Novotny and Hetrick, 1970; Lipton *et al.*, 1973; Jacoby *et al.*, 1987, 1991; Ball-Goodrich *et al.*, 1998). Similarly, RPV has also been detected in the feces, urine and saliva (Ueno *et al.*, 1997). Horizontal transmission of RV and RPV is thought to be primarily through direct animal-to-animal contact and fomites (Jacoby *et al.*, 1988; Yang *et al.*, 1995; Ueno *et al.*, 1996). Vertical or *in utero* transmission appears to be dependent on the virus strain, the route of inoculation and the inoculation dose (Jacoby *et al.*, 1988; Gaertner *et al.*, 1996). The duration of transmission after infection depends more on the age of the rat at the time of initial exposure than on the development of humoral immunity (Jacoby *et al.*, 1988). Experimentally infected neonates transmitted virus for 10 weeks after inoculation, whereas juvenile rats (4 weeks old) only transmitted RV for 3 weeks. In addition, Jacoby *et al.* also reported that the rats which had been experimentally infected as neonates continued to transmit virus for at least 7 weeks after **seroconversion.**

All parvoviruses are tropic for rapidly dividing cells and the clinical signs and lesions are the direct result of this tropism (Kilham and Margolis, 1966; Margolis *et al.*, 1968; Cole *et al.*, 1970; Margolis and Kilham, 1970, 1972; Baringer and Nathanson, 1972; Coleman *et al.*, 1983; Jacoby *et al.*, 1987; Gaertner *et al.*, 1993). RV attacks and destroys the cells in the external germinal cell layer of the cerebellar cortex of neonates, which results in granuloprival cerebellar hypoplasia and ataxia. Hepatocytes of the neonate and in some situations the adult are also targets for RV. Hepatic necrosis, hepatitis, fibrosis, nodular hyperplasia and jaundice result when the hepatocytes are targeted. The vascular endothelium and megakaryocytes are also attacked by RV and this along with the possible activation of the complement cascade may explain the hemorrhage observed in the testes (Figure 7.3), epididymis, central nervous system (Figures 7.4 and 7.5) and other tissues (Figures 7.4 and 7.5). The fetus is particularly vulnerable since a variety of tissues are mitotically active. In some *in utero* infections there are fetal deaths which result in decreased litter sizes and increased numbers of intrauterine resorption sites (Kilham and Margolis, 1966, 1969; Jacoby *et al.*, 1979).

Figure 7.3 Rat virus infection. Multifocal acute hemorrhage in a testicle. Hematoxylin and eosin. × 15.

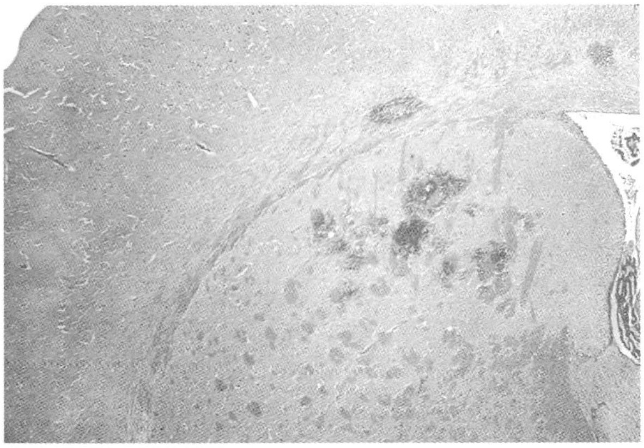

Figure 7.4 Rat virus infection. Multifocal hemorrhagic encephalopathy. Hematoxylin and eosin. × 15.

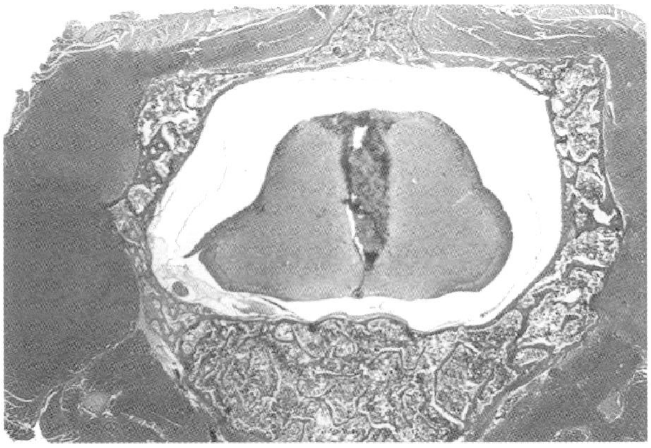

Figure 7.5 Rat virus infection. Hemorrhagic infarct in the spinal cord. Hematoxylin and eosin. × 15.

young adult rats which are introduced into an **enzootically infected** population of rats (Coleman *et al.*, 1983).

Persistent infections with parvoviruses are common, and the length of time in which virus can be detected in infected rats seems to depend on the rat's age at the time of infection and possibly its

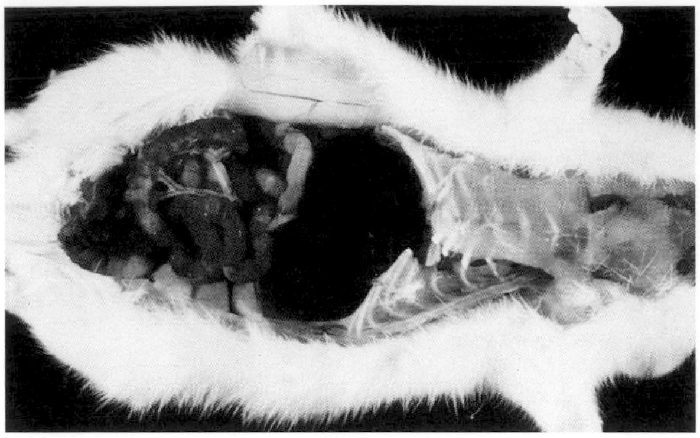

Parvoviruses of the rat are also tropic for many other tissues including lymphoid tissue (spleen, lymph nodes, Peyer's patches and thymus), smooth muscle (blood vessels, intestines and urogenital tract), heart (endocardium and myocardium), subependymal cells in the brain, erythropoietic cells, renal tubular epithelium, epididymal epithelium, uterine epithelium and bronchial epithelium (Margolis and Kilham, 1970; Jacoby et al., 1987; Gaertner et al., 1993, 1996; Ball-Goodrich et al., 1998). This may result in foci of necrosis at any of those sites. Hypocellularity in the spleen and lymph nodes may be observed during the chronic stages of infection.

Additional lesions which may be observed in the liver during the subacute to chronic phases of infection include postnecrotic parenchymal collapse, hepatic fibrosis (Figure 7.7), nodular regenerative hyperplasia, **hepatocytomegaly, karyomegaly,** multinucleated hepatocytes, increased mitotic figures, bile duct hyperplasia and peliosis hepatis (Margolis et al., 1968; Margolis and Kilham, 1970).

The diagnosis can be made with a variety of laboratory tests (Singh and Lang, 1984; ACLAD, 1991; Jacoby et al., 1996; Ball-Goodrich et al., 1998). The most commonly used serologic tests are the enzyme-linked immunosorbent assay **(ELISA)**, indirect immunofluorescence assay **(IFA)** and hemagglutination inhibition assay **(HAI)**. The ELISA and IFA can be used to identify antibodies to parvoviruses, and then the positive sera can be tested with the HAI assay to specifically identify whether or not the sera is reactive to either RV or H-1. There is currently no HAI test available to specifically identify RPV; however, negative results using the HAI test for both RV and H-1 is putative evidence of previous exposure to RPV (Ueno et al., 1996). Immunohistochemical staining of suspected tissues is also very useful if it is available. Additional

tests which are being investigated and which seem to have great potential are the **polymerase chain reaction (PCR)** and *in situ* hybridization techniques (Gaertner et al., 1993; Taylor and Copley, 1994a; Besselsen et al., 1995; Yagami et al., 1995; Ueno et al., 1996; Ball-Goodrich et al., 1998). Clinical signs, history and pathology may also be helpful in making the diagnosis. Histopathology is especially useful if intranuclear inclusion bodies are associated with lesions in the target tissues (e.g. cerebellar external germinal cells, hepatocytes, Kupffer cells, vascular endothelium, bile duct epithelium, etc.) (Kilham and Margolis, 1966; Ruffolo et al., 1966; Margolis et al., 1968; Cole et al., 1970; Margolis and Kilham, 1970; Baringer and Nathanson, 1972; Coleman et al., 1983).

Parvoviruses of rats have the potential to interfere with a variety of different types of research. Research utilizing cell cultures and transplantable tumors is especially vulnerable, as evidenced by the fact that some of the parvoviruses of rats were initially discovered as contaminants (Kilham and Oliver, 1959; Toolan et al., 1960). Toxicological studies and surgical experiments involving the liver may also be compromised by the activation of a latent parvovirus infection during hepatocyte regeneration or proliferation (Ruffolo et al., 1966; Margolis et al., 1968). There is also the possibility that a latent parvovirus infection could be activated when rats are immunocompromised by cytotoxic or immunosuppressive chemicals (Nathanson et al., 1970). In addition, it would not be too hard to imagine the problems which might be encountered by the pathologist and the toxicologist attempting to distinguish parvoviral lesions from toxic lesions. Similar problems also may be encountered with teratology studies. Parvoviruses may also interfere with carcinogenesis, oncology, cancer therapeutic and pathogenesis studies (Jacoby et al., 1987; Ball-Goodrich et al., 1998).

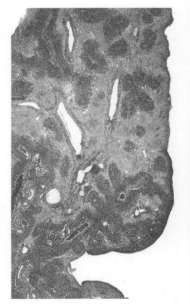

Figure 7.6 Rat virus infection. Note hemorrhage in the intestines and the cervical lymph nodes.

Figure 7.7 Chronic rat virus infection. There is extensive chronic inflammation in the hepatic parenchyma. Hematoxylin and eosin. × 15.

fact, Percy and Williams (1990) suggested that the term 'rat coronavirus group' may be a more appropriate designation until we know more about these coronaviruses.

The rat is the natural host for SDAV, RCV and CARS; however, mice have been experimentally infected with SDAV and CARS (Parker et al., 1970; Bhatt et al., 1977; Maru and Sato, 1982; Barthold et al., 1990; La Regina et al., 1992).

SDAV is transmitted through aerosol exposure, **fomites**, handling and close contact, and this may also be true for RCV and CARS (Thigpen and Ross, 1983; Percy and Wojcinski, 1986; La Regina et al., 1992). SDAV and CARS are highly tropic for the salivary glands; however, RCV's tropism for the salivary glands is relatively low (Bhatt and Jacoby, 1977; Maru and Sato, 1982; La Regina et al., 1992). In addition, SDAV and RCV also have an affinity for lacrimal glands and the respiratory tract (Percy and Williams, 1990). The respiratory tract is the first site of replication for SDAV and RCV, and from there the virus attacks the salivary and lacrimal glands (Bhatt and Jacoby, 1977; Wojcinski and Percy, 1986). SDAV also appears to have an affinity for the transitional epithelium of the kidney and urinary bladder of athymic rats (Weir et al., 1990).

The most common clinical sign associated with SDAV and CARS infections in rats is ventral cervical and/or intermandibular swelling (Figure 7.8) (Maru and Sato, 1982; Bhatt and Jacoby, 1985; Percy and Wojcinski, 1986; Bihun and Percy, 1995; Schunk et al., 1995). Ventral cervical swelling also has been reported with RCV infections (Macy et al., 1996). This particular clinical sign is very suggestive of a coronavirus infection; however, ventral cervical swelling can be caused by other things (e.g. tumors).

Additional nonspecific clinical signs which may be observed with coronaviruses of the rat include red tears **(chromodacryorrhea)** 7.9), red porphyrin staining of the front paws, respiratory disturbances (sneezing, rales, etc.), anorexia, decreased breeding efficiency and occasional ophthalmic signs (e.g. **blepharospasms;** photophobia, keratoconjunctivitis, etc.) (Parker et al., 1970; Lai et al., 1976; Fox, 1977; Weisbroth and Peress, 1977; Maru and Sato, 1982; Percy et al., 1984; Bhatt and Jacoby, 1985; Percy and Wojcinski, 1986; La Regina et al., 1992; Schunk et al., 1995; Macy et al., 1996).

Morbidity is usually high and mortality is usually low in uncomplicated cases of SDAV; however, mortality rates can be quite high in some rat strains infected with RCV (Parker et al., 1970; Weisbroth and

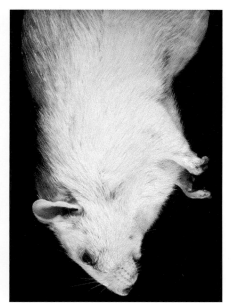

Figure 7.8 Experimental *Sialodacryoadenitis virus* (SDAV) infection. There is considerable ventral cervical swelling. (Charles River Laboratories, Technical Bulletin, 1983.)

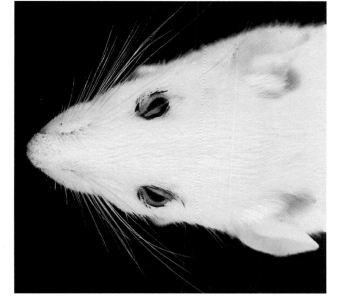

Figure 7.9 Experimental *Sialodacryoadenitis virus* (SDAV) infection. Note the red porphyrin staining around the eyes.

Coronaviruses

Infections with coronaviruses are very common in laboratory and wild rats (Parker et al., 1970; Gannon and Carthew, 1980; Lussier and Descoteaux, 1986; Rao et al., 1989; Gilioli et al., 1996). Several different coronaviruses have been discovered in rats including *Sialodacryoadenitis virus* (SDAV), *Rat coronavirus* (RCV) (Parker et al., 1970), and the *Causative agent of rat sialoadenitis virus* (CARS) (Maru and Sato, 1982). Since the diseases caused by each of these viruses are similar they will be considered together; however, significant differences will be noted. In

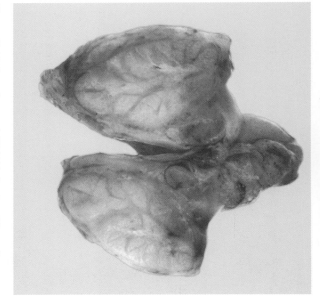

Figure 7.10 Experimental SDAV infection. There is an enormous amount of edema associated with the salivary glands. (Charles River Laboratories, Technical Bulletin, 1983)

Figure 7.11 Experimental SDAV infection. The salivary glands in Figure 7.10 were removed and incised. Note the widening of the interlobular connective tissue with edema.

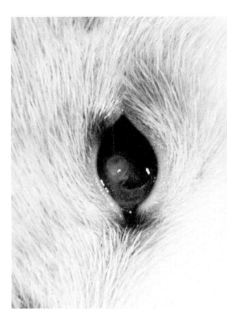

Figure 7.12 Chronic SDAV infection. This rat has ulcerative keratitis which was secondary to the inflammation and necrosis in the Harderian gland. (Charles River Laboratories, Technical Bulletin, 1983)

Peress, 1977; Percy and Wojcinski, 1986; Hajjar et al., 1991; Macy et al., 1996). Death may be observed in suckling rats infected as neonates with RCV (Parker et al., 1970; Macy et al., 1996). Otherwise the disease course is usually short and self-limiting with CARS, SDAV and older RCV-infected rats. However, SDAV and the disease it causes may persist for several months in athymic rats (Weir et al., 1990; Hajjar et al., 1991). It also seems that SDAV may have a synergistic relationship with *Myoplasma pulmonis* and this may also influence the disease expression and outcome (Schoeb and Lindsey, 1987).

Occasional chronic ophthalmologic problems may persist, probably as a result of the destructive effects on the Harderian gland and other lacrimal glands (Percy et al., 1989). It is believed that SDAV and RCV cause decreased lacrimation and this may leave the eye vulnerable to foreign bodies and opportunistic bacteria (e.g. *Pasteurella pneumotropica* and *Staphylococcus* spp). In spontaneous infections, secondary ophthalmic problems are most commonly seen in Lewis and **SHR** rats, and keratoconjunctivitis has resulted in experimentally infected athymic rats (Lai et al., 1976; Weisbroth and Peress, 1977; Weir et al., 1990).

Macroscopic lesions may include swollen and edematous salivary glands (Figures 7.10 and 7.11), with enlargement of the regional lymph nodes (Maru and Sato, 1982; Percy et al., 1984; Percy and Wojcinski, 1986; Percy and Williams, 1990; La Regina et al., 1992; Macy et al., 1996). Hyperemia

and exudation may be present at any location in the respiratory tract of rats infected with SDAV and RCV (Parker et al., 1970; La Regina et al., 1992). Occasional ophthalmic lesions include keratoconjunctivitis, corneal opacities and ulcers (Figure 7.12), megaloglobus, hypopyon (Figure 7.13), and **hyphema** (Lai et al., 1976; Fox, 1977; Weisbroth and Peress, 1977).

Histopathologic lesions are related to the virus strain, virus tropism, clinical signs and gross lesions (Parker et al., 1970; Bhatt and Jacoby, 1977; Maru and Sato, 1982; Percy et al., 1984, 1989; Percy and

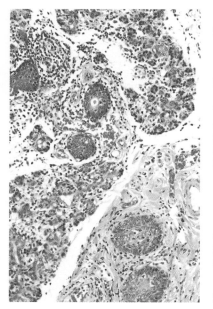

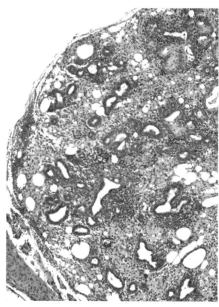

Figure 7.14 Spontaneous SDAV infection. The parotid salivary gland is mildly infiltrated with mononuclear cells and there is squamous metaplasia of intralobular and interlobular ducts. Hematoxylin and eosin. × 30.

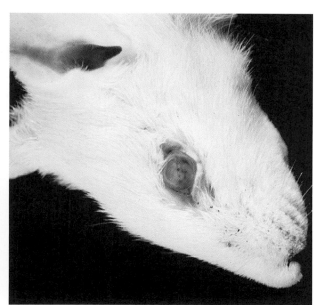

Figure 7.13 Chronic SDAV infection. This rat has both purulent exudate and blood in its eye.

Wojcinski, 1986; Wojcinski and Percy, 1986; Schoeb and Lindsey, 1987; Percy and Williams, 1990; La Regina *et al.*, 1992; Bihun and Percy, 1995; Liang *et al.*, 1995; Macy *et al.*, 1996; Compton *et al.*, 1998). All three coronaviruses cause inflammation and necrosis of the submaxillary (submandibular) salivary glands. Depending on the stage of the infection there may also be necrosis and/or squamous metaplasia of the ducts in the submaxillary salivary gland. Similar findings may be observed in the parotid salivary gland (Figure 7.14), Harderian gland (Figure 7.15) and other lacrimal glands of rats infected with SDAV or RCV. Lesions may also be observed in the respiratory tract with SDAV and RCV including interstitial pneumonia as well as inflammation, necrosis, and hyperplasia of the airways throughout the upper and lower respiratory tract. **Bronchiectasis** and squamous metaplasia of the bronchial epithelium have also been reported in persistently infected athymic rats (Weir *et al.*, 1990). Pulmonary atelectasis with compensatory **emphysema**, nonsuppurative perivasculitis and hyperplasia of the bronchial associated lymphoid tissue (BALT) may also be observed with RCV. Inflammation in the upper respiratory tract has been reported with CARS; however, there was apparently no involvement of the lower respiratory tract, parotid salivary gland or lacrimal glands (Maru and Sato, 1982). Enlargement of the lymph nodes in the neck is due to reactive hyperplasia and/or inflammation.

Figure 7.15 Chronic SDAV infection. This Harderian gland has chronic nonsuppurative inflammation. Hematoxylin and eosin. × 15

Ophthalmic lesions which may be seen include those observed at necropsy as well as lenticular degeneration, retinal degeneration and anterior **synechia** (Lai *et al.*, 1976; Weisbroth and Peress, 1977; Weir *et al.*, 1990).

Percy *et al.* (1986) observed a necrotizing encephalitis in rats which had been intranasally inoculated with SDAV during the first week of life. They speculated that similar lesions could possibly be seen in young suckling rats during natural epizootics; however, it appears that no cases have been reported in the literature. They also believed that the virus was probably carried to the brain via the blood, and not through the cribriform plate.

The clinical signs and lesions are not specific for coronaviruses of rats because similar findings can be observed with other viruses (Sendai virus, pneumonia virus of mice, papovavirus in athymic rats and cytomegalovirus), hypovitaminosis A, stress, dehydration and exposure to noxious gases (e.g. ammonia) (Eaton and Van Herick, 1944; Broderson et al., 1976; Fox, 1977; Rogers, 1979; Harkness and Ridgeway, 1980; Vogtsberger et al., 1982; Ward et al., 1984; Wojcinski and Percy, 1986; Percy and Barthold, 1993a; Liang et al., 1995).

The history, clinical signs and pathology may be very helpful in making a diagnosis; however, ancillary tests are needed for confirmation (ACLAD, 1991). Serologic tests (e.g. ELISA and IFA) can be used to confirm the diagnosis after the 7th to 10th day of infection. In addition, virus isolation, in situ hybridization, polymerase chain reaction (PCR), reverse transcriptase-PCR (RT-PCR) and immunofluorescent/immunohistochemical staining of tissues can also be used to arrive at a definitive diagnosis (Percy et al., 1984; Taylor and Copley, 1994b; Bihun and Percy, 1995; Macy et al., 1996; Compton et al., 1998). RT-PCR can also be used to detect rat coronaviruses using cage swabs (Compton and Vivas-Gonzalez, 1998).

Coronaviruses of rats have the potential to interfere with inhalatory research, respiratory disease research, reproductive research, nutritional research, toxicologic research, physiology research, tumor transplantation research and ophthalmologic research (Lai et al., 1976; Wojcinski and Percy, 1986; McDonald, 1988; Rao et al., 1989; Hajjar et al., 1991; Bihun and Percy, 1995; Macy et al., 1996).

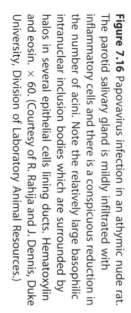

Figure 7.16 Papovavirus infection in an athymic nude rat. The parotid salivary gland is mildly infiltrated with inflammatory cells and there is a conspicuous reduction in the number of acini. Note the relatively large basophilic intranuclear inclusion bodies which are surrounded by halos in several epithelial cells lining ducts. Hematoxylin and eosin. × 60. (Courtesy of R. Rahija and J. Dennis, Duke University, Division of Laboratory Animal Resources.)

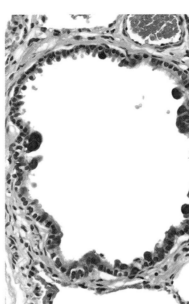

Figure 7.17 Papovavirus infection in an athymic nude rat. Note the large basophilic intranuclear inclusion bodies in several bronchiolar epithelial cells. × 60. (Courtesy of R. Rahija and J. Dennis, Duke University, Division of Laboratory Animal Resources.)

Papovavirus

In 1984, Ward et al. reported on a papovavirus which caused **parotid sialoadenitis** in athymic nude rats. There have been no other published reports of this virus causing disease in athymic rats; however, one of the authors of this chapter has seen the disease in three different cases, and the clinical disease and lesions were similar to those described by Ward and his colleagues (Gaillard, 1998, unpublished observation).

Ward et al. (1984) reported that approximately 10–15% of the athymic nude rats developed a wasting disease with respiratory **dyspnea**. The later clinical sign may have been due to opportunistic bacteria which had also been isolated from pneumonic lungs. A few of the rats died during that epizootic.

At necropsy the rats were emaciated and many of the rats' parotid salivary glands were atrophic and dark. In addition, some of the parotid salivary glands contained small white foci.

Microscopically, the parotid salivary glands had necrosis of acinar cells and ductular epithelium. The parotid salivary glands were also infiltrated with mononuclear cells (Figure 7.16). In some rats there was also epithelial hyperplasia in the ducts. Large basophilic intranuclear inclusion bodies, surrounded by a clear halo, were common in the affected cells in the parotid salivary gland (Figure 7.16), but were also occasionally observed in the laryngeal glands, bronchial/bronchiolar epithelium (Figure 7.17), and the Harderian gland. Intranuclear inclusion bodies also have been observed in alveolar epithelial cells (Figure 7.18) (Gaillard, 1998, unpublished observation). Ward and his colleagues also reported that tracheitis, bronchitis, **bronchiolitis** and secondary bacterial pneumonias were common findings.

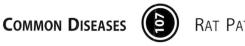

1977; Ishida and Homma, 1978; Gannon and Carthew, 1980; Lussier and Descoteaux, 1986; Rao *et al*., 1989; Gilioli *et al*., 1996). The mouse is particularly susceptible and acute **epizootic** and **enzootic** infections have been reported. In addition, there is evidence that hamsters, guinea pigs, rabbits and marmosets are also susceptible to infection with SV; however, some apparently seropositive guinea pigs may in fact be seropositive to other parainfluenza viruses instead of *Sendai virus* (Parker *et al*., 1966; Profeta *et al*., 1969; Hawthorne *et al*., 1982; Machii *et al*., 1989; Percy and Palmer, 1997).

Natural infections in rats are usually asymptomatic (Burek *et al*., 1977). However, nonspecific clinical signs referable to the respiratory tract have been reported in experimental infections (Carthew and Sparrow, 1980a; Castleman, 1983). Those clinical signs included moist nasal sounds, wheezing, snuffling and increased respiratory rates. Additional clinical signs which have been reported in experimental and in some natural infections are decreased weight gain/weight loss, decreased breeding efficiency, anorexia and lowered activity (Coid and Wardman, 1971, 1972; Castleman, 1983; Carthew and Aldred, 1988; Rao *et al*., 1989). Morbidity may be quite high but there may be little or no increases in the mortality rates in rats (Burek *et al*., 1977; Castleman, 1983).

The results from experiments conducted by Thigpen and Ross (1983) suggested that SV can be transmitted via the airborne route in rats. In mice, SV appears to be primarily transmitted by direct animal contact or by contact with contaminated **fomites** (Tennant *et al*., 1966; Parker and Reynolds, 1968; Carthew and Aldred, 1988). It is likely that these same methods of transmission also apply to the rat.

SV is tropic for the epithelium lining the nasal cavity, bronchi/bronchioles, alveoli and alveolar macrophages (Carthew and Sparrow, 1980a; Castleman, 1984; Castleman *et al*., 1987; Giddens *et al*., 1987). The epithelium in the trachea is probably also a target since lesions are frequently present at that location (Castleman, 1983).

Similar to other viruses which infect rodents, host factors may influence the disease patterns observed in rats infected with SV. The host's genotype, immune status and age are important factors (Burek *et al*., 1977; Carthew and Sparrow, 1980a; Castleman *et al*., 1987; Liang *et al*., 1995). For example, in one epizootic with SV the disease was more severe in Sprague-Dawley, BN/Bi and (WAG × BN) F1 rats, whereas WAG/Rij rats had a relatively milder disease (Burek *et al*., 1977). In this same epizootic, rats younger than

Figure 7.18 Papovavirus infection in an athymic nude rat. This is a photomicrograph of a different area of the same lung lobe as that in Figure 7.17. Several alveolar pneumocytes have large basophilic intranuclear inclusion bodies. A modicum of inflammatory cells are also present. Hematoxylin and eosin. × 95. (Courtesy of R. Rahija and J. Dennis, Duke University, Division of Laboratory Animal Resources.)

The prevalence of papovavirus infections in rats is not known, since there apparently are no serologic tests available at the present time. The clinical signs and lesions can be very suggestive and can be useful in making a presumptive diagnosis. If available, electron microscopy and immunoperoxidase tests can be used to make a definitive diagnosis (Ward *et al*., 1984). Initial attempts at virus isolation were unsuccessful.

The list of differential diagnoses includes coronaviruses of rats, cytomegalovirus and Sendai virus. Coronaviruses may cause similar lesions in the parotid salivary glands and lung, but intranuclear inclusion bodies are not a characteristic since they are RNA viruses. In addition, coronaviruses of rat may also cause lesions in the submaxillary salivary gland, whereas that salivary gland does not appear to be a target of papovavirus. The rat cytomegalovirus can cause similar lesions and intranuclear inclusion bodies in the salivary and lacrimal glands; however, it also causes cytomegaly and intracytoplasmic inclusion bodies (Percy and Barthold, 1993a). Although Sendai virus can cause lesions in the respiratory tract, it does not cause a sialoadenitis.

Sendai Virus

Sendai virus (SV) is a paramyxovirus (parainfluenza virus type 1) and infections of rats and mice are relatively common (Parker *et al*., 1966; Tennant *et al*., 1966; Parker and Reynolds, 1968; Zurcher *et al*., eight months had relatively more severe lung lesions than older rats. In addition, the infection is more severe and the virus persists for a longer time in **athymic nude rats**, compared with euthymic rats. The microbial status of the host is also important, since the disease outcome can be significantly affected by secondary opportunistic bacteria and mycoplasma (Burek et al., 1977; Schoeb et al., 1985).

Macroscopic lesions are frequently absent, but when present there may be small red to gray randomly distributed foci on the surface of the lungs or the lungs may be diffusely reddened (Castleman, 1983). In addition, the lungs may fail to collapse when the thoracic cavity is opened. Purulent exudate within the airways, ventral consolidation or abscesses in the lungs, as well as bronchiectasis would be suggestive of a possible infection with opportunistic bacteria and/or mycoplasma (Burek et al., 1977; Schoeb et al., 1985; Carthew and Aldred, 1988).

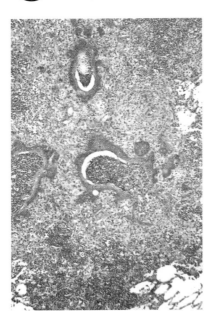

Figure 7.20 Intercurrent infection with Sendai virus and Streptococcus pneumoniae. Note the chronic active inflammation in the interstitium and the squamous metaplasia of the bronchiolar epithelium. Hematoxylin and eosin. × 15.

Histopathologic lesions are variable and depend on the stage of the infection (Burek et al., 1977; Carthew and Sparrow, 1980a; Castleman, 1983, 1984; Schoeb et al., 1985; Castleman et al., 1987, 1988; Giddens et al., 1987; Liang et al., 1995). During the acute stage the lesions include epithelial necrosis and inflammation in the nasal cavity, trachea, larynx, airways in the lung (Figure 7.19), and alveoli. The inflammatory cell infiltrates in these locations include variable numbers of mononuclear cells (lymphocytes and plasma cells) and neutrophils. Increased numbers of alveolar macrophages may also be present in the alveoli. In general, the lesions in the lung are centered around the airways, especially the terminal bronchioles, and the adjacent alveoli; therefore, these lesions can be collectively referred to as a necrotizing bronchointerstitial pneumonia. During the reparative stage there may be hyperplasia and squamous metaplasia of the epithelium in the nasal cavity, bronchi, bronchioles (Figure 7.20), and alveoli. Multinucleated syncytial epithelial cells may also be present in the bronchiolar epithelium and alveoli during the early and chronic stages of infection. In some lungs there may be collections of inflammatory cells and fibroblasts in the lumina of bronchioles, and presumably these structures may develop into epithelial covered polypoid structures (Figure 7.21). This finding is referred to as **bronchiolitis obliterans**. The lungs may completely return

In pregnant females there may be a bloody vaginal discharge, retarded embryonic development and increased resorption sites in the uterus (Coid and Wardman, 1971; Carthew and Aldred, 1988).

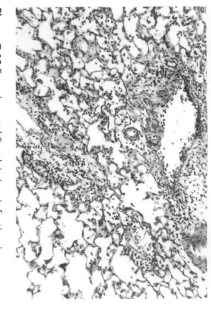

Figure 7.19 Experimental Sendai virus infection in a young Lewis rat. There is acute necrosis and inflammation of the bronchiole (top) and adjacent alveoli. Hematoxylin and eosin. (Courtesy of S. Botts.)

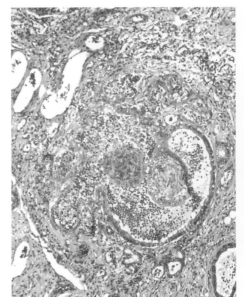

Figure 7.21 Intercurrent infection with Sendai virus and Streptococcus pneumoniae. Bronchiolitis obliterans which is characterized by the epithelial covered polypoid structure in the lumen of an inflamed bronchiole. Hematoxylin and eosin. × 20.

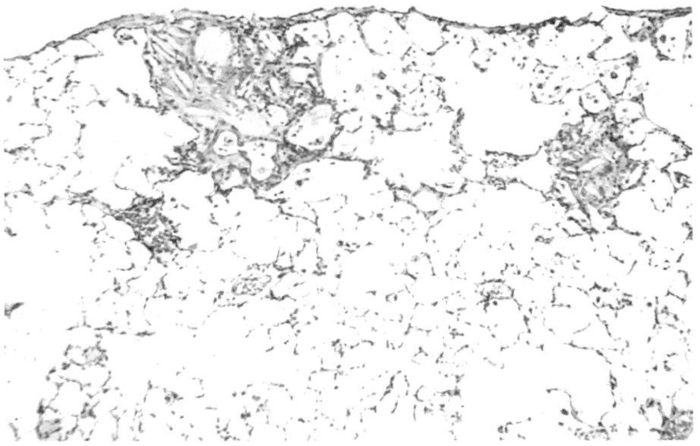

Figure 7.22 Focal scar from a previous infection with *Sendai virus*. Note the fibrosis, cholesterol clefts and alveolar macrophages. Hematoxylin and eosin. × 20.

to normal or there may be residual scars (Figure 7.22) including interstitial fibrosis, cholesterol clefts, and peribronchial and perivascular mononuclear cell cuffs. This later lesion may be the only lesion observed in aged rats during any stage of infection.

The lesions are suggestive of a possible SV infection but they are not **pathognomonic** since similar lesions may be caused by coronaviruses of rats and less likely *pneumonia virus of mice* (Eaton and Van Herick, 1944; Vogtsberger et al., 1982; Liang et al., 1995).

A definitive diagnosis can be made with serology (ELISA or IFA), virology and immunohistochemistry (Rottinghaus et al., 1986; Castleman et al., 1987; ACLAD, 1991). Immunohistochemistry and virology are useful in making a diagnosis during the acute stage of infection, but are less helpful after the second week of infection because the virus may have been eliminated from the tissues at that time (Castleman et al., 1987; Giddens et al., 1987; ACLAD, 1991). However, serology is useful for a much longer time, in that antibodies can be detected from about the first to second week of infection and remain detectable long after virus has been eliminated from the tissues. Taylor and Copley (1994b) have also evaluated a polymerase chain reaction (PCR) test as a diagnostic technique for SV infections and it seems to have great potential; however, it too will probably only be useful during the acute stage of infection when the virus is present.

Similar to other viruses of rats, SV has the potential to interfere with many different types of research including research in gerontology, toxicology, physiology, immunology, respiratory disease, reproduction, teratology, carcinogenesis and others (Coid and Wardman, 1971, 1972; Burek et al., 1977; Kay, 1978; Castleman, 1983, 1984; Carthew and Aldred, 1988; Castleman et al., 1988; McDonald, 1988; Lussier, 1988; Rao et al., 1989; Piedimonte et al., 1990; Baker, 1998).

Pneumonia Virus of Mice

Pneumonia virus of mice (PVM) is another paramyxovirus, although not a parainfluenza virus, which is relatively common in mice and rats (Parker et al., 1966; Tennant et al., 1966; Gannon and Carthew, 1980; Lussier and Descoteaux, 1986; Richter, 1986; Rao et al., 1989; Gilioli et al., 1996). Antibodies to PVM have also been detected in hamsters, gerbils, guinea pigs, rabbits, mongooses and perhaps even monkeys and humans (Pearson and Eaton, 1940; Eaton and Van Herick, 1944; Horsfall and Curnen, 1946; Tennant et al., 1966; Pringle and Eglin, 1986). In addition, guinea pigs have been experimentally infected with PVM, but neither clinical signs nor lesions could be attributed to PVM (Griffith et al., 1997).

PVM is usually considered to be a relatively innocuous virus in rodents since it usually does not cause disease nor lesions in natural infections (Gannon and Carthew, 1980; Baker, 1998). However, natural disease and lesions do occur in some cases. In particular, athymic nude mice seem to be especially susceptible to PVM which can result in a wasting type syndrome, dyspnea, cyanosis, a necrotizing and hemorrhagic pneumonia and death (Richter et al., 1988; Weir et al., 1988). Similar lesions, along with desquamation and hyperplasia of the bronchial epithelium, have been reported in natural infections involving **euthymic mice**; however, clinical signs and deaths were not observed (Carthew and Sparrow, 1980b). Experimentally infected rats reportedly develop interstitial pneumonia, but clinical signs were not observed (Eaton and Van Herick, 1944; Vogtsberger et al., 1982). **Vasculitis** may also be present in areas of pneumonia in experimentally infected mice and rats.

PVM is probably transmitted by direct animal-to-animal contact (Pearson and Eaton, 1940). The virus is tropic for the bronchial and alveolar epithelium of mice (Carthew and Sparrow, 1980b).

PVM reportedly does not cause clinical disease nor lesions in natural infections in rats; therefore, it is usually detected in rats with serology (HAI, ELISA and IFA) during routine monitoring (ACLAD, 1991). Although virus isolation can be used to detect PVM in tissues, it can be time consuming, whereas immunohistochemistry (e.g. immunoperoxidase) can also be used and is faster (Carthew and Sparrow, 1980b; Weir et al., 1988; ACLAD, 1991).

Reports of PVM interfering with research involving rats are rare. For example, Rao et al. (1989) reported that PVM and Sendai were associated with significant decreases in the body weights of rats in carcinogenicity studies. In contrast, there have been slightly more reports of PVM interfering with research involving mice (Horsfall and Curnen, 1946; Tennant et al., 1966; Richter, 1986). PVM has the potential to have devastating effects on research using athymic nude mice since they are particularly prone to develop fatal disease (Richter et al., 1988; Weir et al., 1988). Although similar fatal infections have yet to be reported in athymic rats, PVM might have the same effect with research involving them.

Infectious Diarrhea of Infant Rats Virus

Vonderfecht and his colleagues (1984) were the first to identify a virus which caused diarrhea in suckling rats. The virus was morphologically identical to typical rotaviruses, but it was antigenically different from other rotaviruses. They gave this virus the name of *Infectious diarrhea of infant rats virus* because it apparently only caused diarrhea in infant rats. Subsequent to their discovery, the IDIR virus was assigned to the group B rotavirus group which contains similar atypical rotaviruses that infect and cause similar disease in humans, calves and pigs (Mebus et al., 1978; Vonderfecht et al., 1988; Chasey et al., 1989; Eiden et al., 1991). The prevalence of IDIR virus in rats is not known since rats are not routinely tested for this virus.

Diarrhea was the only clinical sign described in the original report of the natural outbreak with IDIR virus (Vonderfecht et al., 1984; Huber et al., 1989). However, in experimental infections not only was diarrhea described, but also erythema, cracking and bleeding of the perianal skin along with anorexia, dehydration and rapid weight loss (Vonderfecht et al., 1984; Salim et al., 1995). The animals may also be stunted and have dry flaky skin during the latter stages of the infection. The infection is self-limiting, with the rats rapidly returning to normal.

The mode of transmission is not known, but probably involves the fecal-oral route of infection.

Rats older than 14 days of age are apparently resistant to infections, but the exact reason for this age-associated resistance is not known (Vonderfecht et al., 1984). The virus is tropic for the small intestinal villous epithelium, particularly on the luminal one-third to one-fourth of the villi (Vonderfecht et al., 1984; Huber et al., 1989). IDIR virus seems to have more of an affinity for the middle and distal small intestines and less affinity for the proximal small intestines and even less for the colon. The virus causes loss of small intestinal villous enterocytes which are quickly replaced with immature cuboidal epithelium. These changes lead to a reduction in the absorption of water and sodium which results in diarrhea (Salim et al., 1995). The diarrhea continues until the villi are again lined by mature columnar epithelium.

Gross lesions which may be observed in suckling rats include perianal fecal staining, hyperemia, cracking and hemorrhage. The intestinal contents are watery and gaseous and may also contain mucus and poorly formed fecal pellets (Vonderfecht et al., 1984). The rats' stomachs contain curdled milk.

Microscopic lesions are restricted to the small intestine and are characterized by villous atrophy, villous epithelial necrosis, villous epithelial syncytial cell formation and mucosal flattening (Vonderfecht et al., 1984; Huber et al., 1989; Salim et al., 1995). As expected, these lesions are most prominent in the distal small intestine. Small, eosinophilic intracytoplasmic inclusion bodies may be observed in the syncytial cells. Little if any inflammation is present in the intestine; however, there maybe compensatory hyperplasia of the small intestinal crypt epithelium.

Good timing and correct sampling are critical for establishing the diagnosis (Vonderfecht et al., 1988; Huber et al., 1989; Salim et al., 1995). The chance of making a diagnosis is greatly enhanced if samples for histopathology or other tests (e.g. immunofluorescent staining of tissues) are collected from the distal small intestine during the first 24 hours of the infection. During this time the characteristic syncytial cells and sometimes eosinophilic intracytoplasmic inclusion bodies may be observed with histopathology. IDIR viral antigens are also more abundant during this time period and are rapidly eliminated after that time. Other laboratory tests are being investigated to detect group B rotaviruses in feces and intestinal specimens, but they may not be commercially available (Vonderfecht et al., 1985, 1988; ACLAD, 1991). A combined reverse transcriptase reaction–PCR assay seems to have potential as a diagnostic tool for the detection of IDIR virus in fecal samples (Eiden et al., 1991).

This virus has the potential to interfere with any research utilizing suckling rats, as evidenced by the concerns of the researcher who submitted the original rats which were experiencing diarrhea (Huber et al., 1989).

Bacterial and Mycoplasmal Diseases

Murine Respiratory Mycoplasmosis

Mycoplasma pulmonis is the etiology of murine respiratory mycoplasmosis (MRM). *M. pulmonis* causes natural disease in rats and mice; however, it also has been cultured from hamsters and guinea pigs (Tully, 1986).

The infection in young rats is usually clinically silent. In older rats, nonspecific clinical signs such as snuffling, sneezing, rattling, **moist rales, dyspnea, hyperpnea,** head shaking, chromodacryorrhea, face and ear rubbing, ruffled hair coat, twirling when suspended by the tail, head tilts, weight loss and decreased breeding efficiency may be observed (Lane-Petter et al., 1970; Lindsey et al., 1971; Jersey et al., 1973; Broderson et al., 1976; Fox, 1977; Cassell et al., 1979, 1981a; Harkness and Ridgeway, 1980; Cassell, 1982; Schunk et al., 1995).

M. pulmonis is transmitted both horizontally (airborne and possibly sexually) and vertically (Jersey et al., 1973; Cassell et al., 1979, 1981a; Cassell, 1982; Lindsey et al., 1985; Cassell et al., 1986). The infection progresses slowly and may eventually result in respiratory and/or genital disease.

The principal portal of entry is the respiratory tract, beginning in the nasal cavity with probable progressive colonization of the middle ears, larynx, trachea and inconsistently the lungs (Cassell et al., 1973, 1979; Lindsey et al., 1985). The exact means by which it reaches the genital tract is not clear. It has been speculated that the organism may reach the genital tract from the oropharynx during the rat's coprophagic activities or via the blood from the respiratory tract (Cassell, 1982).

The disease outcome depends on a complex interaction of host factors, environmental factors and *M. pulmonis* factors. Host factors include the rat strain, age and microbial status. For example, LEW and CFE rats appear to be more susceptible than F-344, CFHB and CFY rats to the disease-producing potential of *M. pulmonis*, and the lesions in the respiratory and genital tracts tend to be more severe in LEW rats (Lane-Petter et al., 1970; Cassell, 1982; Davis and Cassell, 1982). Older rats tend to have more severe disease than suckling rats, probably because of the declining immune function, the slow progression of the disease, and lung involvement in older rats (Jersey et al., 1973; Cassell et al., 1981a; Lindsey et al., 1985). Intercurrent infections with Sendai virus, rat coronaviruses, opportunistic bacteria and possibly cilia-associated respiratory (CAR) bacillus can also significantly influence the disease outcome (MacKenzie et al., 1981; Lindsey et al., 1985; Schoeb and Lindsey, 1985, 1987; Schoeb et al., 1985; Schunk et al., 1995). High environmental ammonia levels and other irritating gases can also exacerbate the disease (Lane-Petter et al., 1970; Cassell et al., 1973, 1981a; Broderson et al., 1976; Schoeb et al., 1982; Lindsey et al., 1985; Pinson et al., 1988). Such increases in environmental irritating gases may result from faulty ventilation systems, overcrowding and infrequent bedding changes. Similarly, exposure to some toxic chemicals (e.g. hexamethylphosphoramide) can also exacerbate the disease (Cassell et al., 1973; Overcash et al., 1976). Some nutritional deficiencies (e.g. vitamins A and E) may predispose rats to infection with *M. pulmonis* (Tvedten et al., 1973). Apparently, most strains of *M. pulmonis* are capable of causing upper respiratory tract lesions; however, not all are capable of causing significant pulmonary lesions (Lindsey et al., 1971; Cassell et al., 1973). In addition, the inoculation dose of *M. pulmonis* also influences the disease outcome, especially in mice (Cassell et al., 1973, 1981a).

As was alluded to above, the pathologic expression of the disease can vary considerably because of a number of factors; therefore, the gross and microscopic lesions can also vary or not be present at all. Rats of all ages may have evidence of acute (suppurative) to chronic rhinitis, otitis media, otitis interna and laryngotracheitis (Lane-Petter et al., 1970; Lindsey et al., 1971, 1985; Broderson et al., 1976; Cassell et al., 1981a; Davis and Cassell, 1982; Schoeb et al., 1985; Schoeb and Lindsey, 1987). In addition, there may be pseudoglandular epithelial hyperplasia and/or squamous metaplasia in the nasal and tracheal

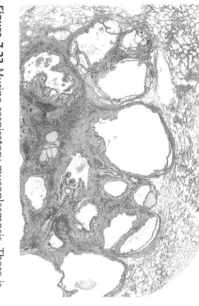

Figure 7.23 Murine respiratory mycoplasmosis. There is severe bronchiectasis and inflammation in the lung. Hematoxylin and eosin. × 2.4.

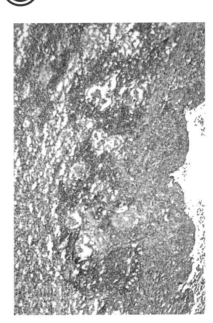

Figure 7.24 Murine respiratory mycoplasmosis. There is moderate hyperplasia and dysplasia of the bronchiolar epithelium along with moderate inflammation and luminal exudate. Hematoxylin and eosin. × 24.

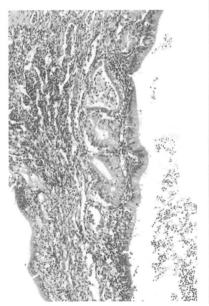

Figure 7.25 Murine respiratory mycoplasmosis. This is a higher magnification of Figure 7.23 showing a few peribronchiolar pseudoglands. Hematoxylin and eosin. × 24.

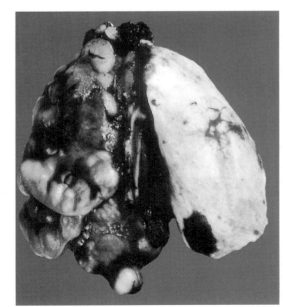

Figure 7.26 Murine respiratory mycoplasmosis. One lobe of the lung from an adult rat is dark and has multiple, raised, opaque blebs (bronchiectasis) on its surface.

mucosa, as well as a reduction in the number of cilia which normally lines different parts of the airways (Lindsey *et al.*, 1971, 1985; Davis and Cassell, 1982; Schoeb and Lindsey, 1987). In contrast, lesions in the lower respiratory tract are most common in rats beginning at 4 weeks old and may include one or more of the following lesions: hyperplasia of the bronchial-associated lymphoid tissue, bronchiectasis (Figure 7.23), bronchiolectasis, suppurative bronchopneumonia, suppurative bronchiolitis, epithelial hyperplasia with associated submucosal mononuclear cell infiltrates in the upper and lower air passages (Figure 7.25), peribronchial and perivascular mononuclear cell infiltrates, nonsuppurative to suppurative alveolitis, atelectasis and peribronchial pseudoglands (Figure 7.25) (Lindsey *et al.*, 1971, 1985; Cassell *et al.*, 1973; Jersey *et al.*, 1973; Broderson *et al.*, 1976; Davis and Cassell, 1982; Schoeb and Lindsey, 1985, 1987; Schoeb *et al.*, 1985). In addition, abscess-like structures, apparently arising from

airways, and squamous metaplasia of the bronchial epithelium may be observed. Grossly, the lungs of adult rats may have a cobblestone appearance (Figure 7.26), due to the bronchiectasis and/or abscess-like structures, or there may only be dark red, purple, brown, or gray depressed foci with or without yellow areas (Lane-Petter *et al.*, 1970; Lindsey *et al.*, 1971; Davis and Cassell, 1982; Schoeb and Lindsey, 1985). Mucopurulent exudate may be observed in the upper respiratory tract and the tympanic bullae.

Lesions outside the respiratory tract are less common and are more likely to be observed microscopically. In the female genital tract there may be **salpingitis**, perioophoritis, endometritis, **pyometra**, partially resorbed fetuses, vaginitis and cervicitis (Lane-Petter *et al.*, 1970; Cassell *et al.*, 1979, 1981a,b;

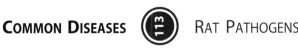

Cassell, 1982; Lindsey *et al.*, 1985). In addition, there also may be epithelial hyperplasia in the oviducts with associated submucosal mononuclear cells. Chronic inflammation of the epididymis, vas deferens and urethra may be observed in male rats. Arthritis has been reported with some *M. pulmonis* infections in rats (Cassell *et al.*, 1986).

The diagnosis can be made with a variety of tests and a combination of methods is recommended, because no one test alone is entirely perfect (Lindsey *et al.*, 1971, 1985; Cassell *et al.*, 1979, 1986; Davidson *et al.*, 1981, 1982; Schoeb and Lindsey, 1985). Microbiologic cultures of the respiratory tract, particularly the upper respiratory tract (e.g. the nasopharyngeal duct), is effective. Serology (IFA and ELISA), IFA or immunohistochemical staining of tissues, and electron microscopy may also be helpful. It is not recommended that pathology alone be used to make a diagnosis because lesions may be either absent or minimal, and when present, similar lesions can be caused by other bacteria (e.g. CAR bacillus) and viruses (e.g. Sendai virus and coronaviruses) (Lindsey *et al.*, 1985; Matsushita and Joshima, 1989; Weir *et al.*, 1990).

M. pulmonis can interfere with many different types of research, including that in the fields of immunology, respiratory disease, tissue culture, gerontology, toxicology, carcinogenesis, nutrition, behavior, pathophysiology and reproduction (Lindsey *et al.*, 1971; Tvedten *et al.*, 1973; Overcash *et al.*, 1976; Cassell *et al.*, 1979, 1981a; Naot *et al.*, 1979; Barile, 1981; Davis *et al.*, 1982; Naot, 1982; Schoeb *et al.*, 1985; Aguila *et al.*, 1988; McDonald, 1988).

Pseudotuberculosis

Corynebacterium kutscheri is the cause of pseudotuberculosis, a naturally occurring disease in mice and rats (Giddens *et al.*, 1968; Weisbroth and Scher, 1968; McEwen and Percy, 1985; Fox *et al.*, 1987). *C. kutscheri* has been cultured from hamsters which had neither clinical signs nor lesions (Amao *et al.*, 1991). Vallee *et al.* (1969), as cited by Weisbroth (1979), also isolated *C. kutscheri* from guinea pigs.

In the rat, transmission is supposedly via the fecal-oral route (Baker, 1998). Direct and indirect contact is reported to be the mode of exposure in mice (Shechmeister and Adler, 1953). Both modes of transmission are probably operative in both the rat and the mouse.

C. kutscheri apparently resides quietly in the upper and lower digestive tract, submaxillary lymph nodes,

and the upper respiratory tract of rats and mice (Amao *et al.*, 1995a,b). These latent infections may be precipitated by a number of stressors including shipping, overcrowding, nutritional deficiencies (e.g. pantothenic acid), immunosuppressive drugs (e.g. corticosteroids), irradiation, experimental manipulations, and concurrent infections (Antopol, 1950; Wolff, 1950; LeMaistre and Tompsett, 1952; Shechmeister and Adler, 1953; Seronde, 1954; Zucker and Zucker, 1954; Seronde *et al.*, 1955, 1956; Giddens *et al.*, 1968; Fujiwara, 1980; McEwen and Percy, 1985). In addition, one of the authors observed an epizootic which was associated with high environmental temperatures and elevated ammonia levels in an animal room with a defective ventilation system (Gaillard, 1998, unpublished observation). High ammonia levels may have also been responsible for an epizootic reported by Giddens *et al.* (1968). Apparently some strains of mice do not require stress or experimental manipulations for the disease to occur (Weisbroth and Scher, 1968).

The bacteria are spread throughout the body via the blood and septic emboli become lodged in organs with extensive capillary networks (e.g. lung, kidney and liver) or those which filter blood (e.g. kidney, choroid plexus and synovial membrane) (Weisbroth and Scher, 1968). This accounts for the distribution of most lesions in the host. Although virtually any organ can develop lesions, the lung is the most frequently involved organ in the rat, whereas the kidney and liver are the most common organs in mice (Seronde, 1954; Giddens *et al.*, 1968; Weisbroth and Scher, 1968).

Clinical signs, when present, are nonspecific and may include porphyrin and mucopurulent ocular and nasal discharge, respiratory rales, dyspnea, hyperpnea, hunched posture, lethargy, emaciation, weight loss, subcutaneous nodules, swollen joints and lameness (Zucker and Zucker, 1954; Giddens *et al.*, 1968; Nelson, 1973; Fox *et al.*, 1987).

External gross lesions may include subcutaneous abscesses, preputial gland abscesses and suppurative arthritis (Giddens *et al.*, 1968). Internal gross lesions may include necrosis and/or abscesses in the lung (Figures 7.27 and 7.28), liver, kidney, brain and other tissues (Giddens *et al.*, 1968; McEwen and Percy, 1985; Fox *et al.*, 1987). In addition, there may also be hepatic necrosis, and fibrinous or fibrous pleuritis, and fibrinous pericarditis (LeMaistre and Tompsett, 1952; Zucker and Zucker, 1954; Seronde *et al.*, 1956; Giddens *et al.*, 1968; McEwen and Percy, 1985; Fox *et al.*, 1987).

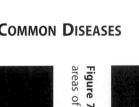

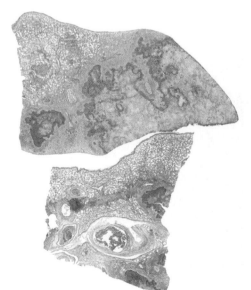

Figure 7.27 Pseudotuberculosis. Note the irregular pale areas of acute caseous necrosis in the lung of a rat.

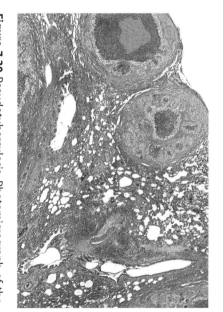

Figure 7.28 Pseudotuberculosis. There are multiple pale abscesses on the dorsal aspect of the lung.

Figure 7.29 Pseudotuberculosis. Subgross photograph of the lung in Figure 7.27. Note the large, irregular areas of caseous necrosis. Hematoxylin and eosin.

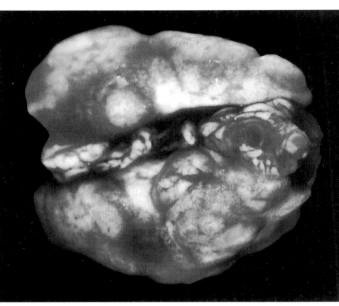

Figure 7.30 Pseudotuberculosis. Photomicrograph of the lung in Figure 7.28. There are multiple abscesses in the pulmonary parenchyma. Note that the airways near the center and the right of the photomicrograph are normal. Hematoxylin and eosin. × 4.

The microscopic lesions are related to the gross lesions (LeMaistre and Tompsett, 1952; Seronde, 1954; Giddens *et al.*, 1968; McEwen and Percy, 1985; Fox *et al.*, 1987). In the lungs there may be either irregular foci of caseous necrosis surrounded by mixed inflammatory cells (Figure 7.29) or there may be abscesses (Figure 7.30). The lesions in the lungs are primarily found in the interstitium; however, in some instances abscesses can erode through the airways and parietal pleura resulting in the seepage of septic exudate and ultimately pleuritis. In contrast to some reports in the literature, multinucleated giant cells may be present at the margins of the lesions (Figure 7.31). Necrosis and/or abscesses may be also present in the liver, kidney, subcutaneous tissues (Figure 7.32), brain (Figure 7.33), and other sites. Clusters of pleomorphic Gram-positive rods can be observed in the lesions. These bacterial colonies typically have either a Chinese letter (Figure 7.34) or bottle brush configuration.

Pathology, with the help of a Gram stain, is very helpful in making a diagnosis when lesions are present. However, the major problem is identifying animals which are latently infected with *C. kutscheri.*

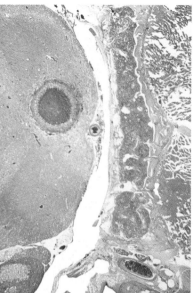

Figure 7.31 Pseudotuberculosis. Photomicrograph of the lung in Figures 7.27 and 7.29. Note the multinucleated giant cells at the margin of the area of caseous necrosis. Hematoxylin and eosin. × 60.

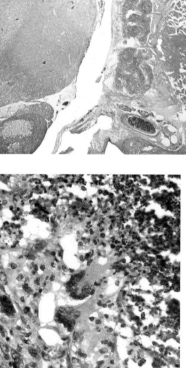

Figure 7.32 Pseudotuberculosis. Subgross photograph of the muzzle from the same rat in Figure 7.28. Note the abscesses in the subcutaneous tissues. Hematoxylin and eosin.

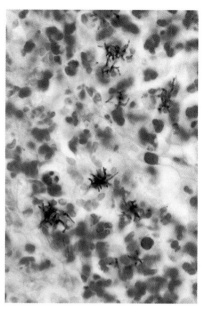

Figure 7.33 Pseudotuberculosis. Photomicrograph of an abscess in the brain of the same rat in Figure 7.32. Hematoxylin and eosin. × 15.

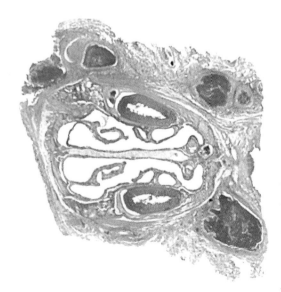

Figure 7.34 Pseudotuberculosis. Several clusters of Gram-positive bacilli arranged in a Chinese letter configuration. Gram stain. × 240

(Antopol 1950; Antopol *et al.*, 1951; LeMaistre and Tompsett, 1952; Seronde, 1954; Zucker and Zucker, 1954; Baker, 1998).

Amao *et al.* (1995b) recommended culturing the oral cavities of rats, using furazolidone–nalidixic acid–colimycin (FNC) agar to detect **latent infections** with *C. kutscheri*. Additional sites along the upper and lower digestive tract also had a very high isolation rate, but the oral cavity was the best site. Serological tests (e.g. ELISA) as well as DNA–DNA hybridization techniques on tissue touch blots may also be helpful if available (Saltzgaber-Muller and Stone, 1986; Fox *et al.*, 1987; Boot *et al.*, 1995). Subcutaneous injections with cortisone can also be used to detect latent infections by precipitating the disease (Fauve *et al.*, 1964).

C. kutscheri has the potential to interfere with virtually any type of research which causes stress, immunosuppression, nutritional deficiencies, etc.

Streptococcal Infections

At least several bacteria of the genus *Streptococcus* can cause clinical disease in rats. All of the streptococci of concern in rats are Gram-positive cocci, and are catalase-negative, nonfermentative, and generally nonmotile (Ruoff, 1995). The name *Streptococcus* is derived from the tendency of many members of the genus to form chains, visible on wet mounts of cultured colonies or in histologic section. Streptococci are differentiated on their ability to hemolyse erythrocytes in blood agar. **Beta hemolysis** refers to a clear, colorless zone of red cell lysis surrounding the bacterial colonies. This contrasts with **alpha hemolysis**, an often greenish to brownish indistinct zone of partially lysed erythrocytes, as well as with **gamma hemolysis**, the term used when no hemolysis is observed. Of primary interest in the rat is *S. pneumoniae*, which is alpha-hemolytic. There is also lesser interest for various members of the beta-hemolytic group, and for *Enterococcus* spp., which are not truly streptococci.

Pneumonia caused by *S. pneumoniae* has previously been referred to as streptococcosis, but this term should be avoided, as it is inherently nonspecific. *S. pneumoniae* may be said to have more notoriety than true impact, and it has been recently considered to be of low significance in laboratory animals (National Research Council, 1991). Humans are the natural host for *S. pneumoniae* (Austrian, 1998), with both adults and children frequently colonized. Transmission is primarily via aerosol; fomites may play a less important role. Infection in rats is usually asymptomatic although disease has, albeit infrequently, been reported. Asymptomatic rats harbor the infection in the nasopharynx. Numerous serotypes of *S. pneumoniae* exist; disease is predominantly associated with infection by more pathogenic serotypes, especially 2, 3, 8, 16 and 19 (Fallon *et al.*, 1988).

Grossly, disease begins with suppurative inflammation in the upper respiratory tract, then spreads to the lung. In the lung, multifocal areas of bronchopneumonia (Figure 7.35) expand and may coalesce (Kohn and Barthold, 1984), and may be accompanied by fibrinopurulent pleuritis (Figure 7.36).

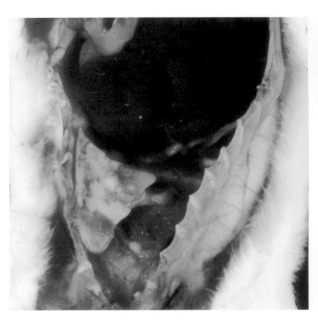

Figure 7.35 *Streptococcus pneumoniae* bronchopneumonia. Note the ventral consolidation in the lung lobe.

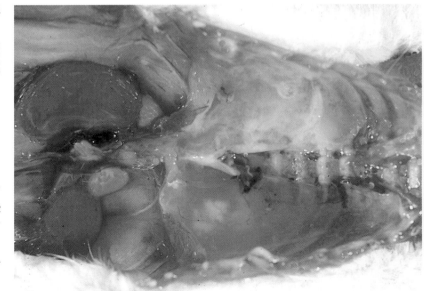

Figure 7.36 *Streptococcus pneumoniae* fibrinopurulent pleuritis. The lungs have been removed and there is exudate on the parietal pleura.

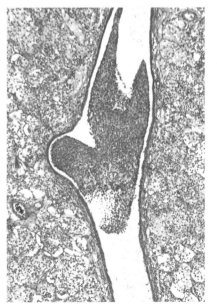

Figure 7.37 *Streptococcus pneumoniae* fibrinopurulent bronchopneumonia. Hematoxylin and eosin. × 15.

Histologically, the bronchopneumonia is characterized by edema, fibrinopurulent inflammation (Figure 7.37) and necrosis of the pulmonary parenchyma, often with fibrinopurulent pleuritis. Affected rats may become **bacteremic**, and develop fibrinopurulent inflammation of other serous surfaces (peritoneum, synovium, etc.) and other tissues. Colonies of laboratory rats are screened for *S. pneumoniae* infection by nasopharyngeal culture onto with a carpet of Gram-positive cocci (Figure 7.38). Disease is clearly associated with some strains of enterococci and not with others. The factors determining the pathogenicity, however, have not been elucidated, but may involve the ability of the pathogenic isolates to adhere to the microvillous surface.

Control of *Streptococcus* spp. and *Enterococcus* spp. is problematic. The organisms are virtually ubiquitous, including being present in a high percentage of the human population (Weisbroth, 1982; Facklam and Sahm, 1995). Some *Enterococcus* spp. are even considered **autochthonous flora** of the rat (Savage, 1971). Clearly, the bacteria can be excluded by aseptic microisolator technique or by use of isolators (Pleasants, 1974), yet the low incidence of disease may not warrant the additional time, money and other resources such housing techniques would require.

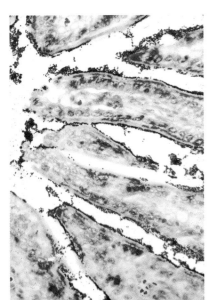

Figure 7.38 Enterococcal (streptococcal) enteropathy in a suckling rat. Gram-positive cocci form a thick blue layer on the surface of the small intestine's villi. Gram stain. × 180.

blood agar (Kohn and Barthold, 1984). However, *S. pneumoniae* must be differentiated from other alpha-hemolytic streptococci. This is most often performed by the **optochin inhibition test** which measures the sensitivity of the test isolate to optochin disks; most *S. pneumoniae* strains are inhibited to a greater degree than other alpha-hemolytic streptococci. Isolates displaying intermediate degrees of inhibition should be tested for bile solubility for confirmation; *S. pneumoniae* colonies are bile soluble (Ruoff, 1995). However, due to the occurrence of nonpathogenic isolates (Fallon *et al.*, 1988), isolation of *S. pneumoniae* from rats, even if a respiratory problem is present, does not necessarily provide a diagnosis, nor does isolation of *S. pneumoniae* from asymptomatic rats necessarily indicate a colony health threat.

Beta-hemolytic streptococci are also present in many rats, with disease only a rare occurrence. Beta-hemolytic streptococci are divided into groups based on Lancefield antigens, with Lancefield groups B and G most commonly isolated from rats. On rare occasions, they may be isolated from abscesses, but exclusion from most colonies is neither practical nor necessary.

So-called 'streptococcal enteropathy' is actually due to nonhemolytic Lancefield group D enterococci, including *Enterococcus hirae*, *E. faecium-durans-2*, and *E. fecalis-2* (Barthold, 1997). Enterococci are differentiated from streptococci by biochemical tests, as well as by 16S rRNA sequencing (Facklam and Sahm, 1995). Streptococcal enteropathy is a disease of suckling rats, and does not affect post-weaning animals. Affected litters develop diarrhea or soft stool, with bright yellow, pasty feces. Microscopically, the villi in the small intestine are covered

Cilia-associated Respiratory Bacillus

Often referred to as CAR bacillus, cilia-associated respiratory bacillus is not taxonomically classified in the genus *Bacillus*. Rather, it has recently been tentatively placed in a group of bacteria known as 'gliding bacteria' based on the fact that they are motile, but without visible means for such motility, and thus may be related to *Flavobacterium* or *Flexispira*, based on 16S ribosomal RNA sequencing (Cundiff *et al.*, 1995). At this point, however, final identification is still pending.

Amongst the common laboratory animals CAR bacillus has been identified in rats, mice, and rabbits (van Zwieten *et al.*, 1980; MacKenzie *et al.*, 1981; Waggie *et al.*, 1987; Griffith *et al.*, 1988). In rats, infection is usually asymptomatic although nonspecific clinical signs, such as weight loss and dyspnea, may be observed.

Transmission is probably primarily via direct contact with infected animals. Bedding does not transmit the infection well (Cundiff *et al.*, 1995), so the role of fomites in natural transmission of CAR bacillus is probably insignificant (Matsushita *et al.*, 1989). Airborne exposure is not an important means of transmission (Itoh *et al.*, 1987).

Gross lesions in uncomplicated CAR bacillus infections may not always be present, although translucent gray cystic lesions may be visible on the pleural surface (Figure 7.39) (Itoh *et al.*, 1987). If there is coinfection with *Mycoplasma pulmonis* or other

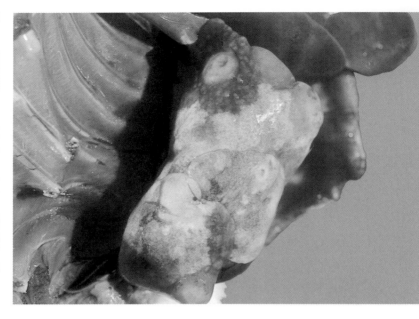

Figure 7.39 Cilia-associated respiratory (CAR) bacillus infection in a rat. The lung has multiple red areas of consolidation and a few gray, translucent, cystic areas on the pleural surface.

pathogens, the resulting lesions resemble those of chronic respiratory disease (CRD) (MacKenzie et al., 1981). Although *Mycoplasma pulmonis* is accepted as the cause of chronic respiratory disease (Jersey et al., 1973), some think that CAR bacillus may contribute to the lesions of CRD.

Histopathologically, hyperplastic peribronchial lymphoid tissue and peribronchiolar mononuclear cell cuffs are observed in the lungs (Itoh et al., 1987; Matsushita and Joshima, 1989). Additionally, there may be bronchiectasis and considerable amounts of mucopurulent exudate in the airways and alveolar spaces (Figure 7.40). A thin basophilic layer may be observed on the surface of the respiratory epithelium of airways in hematoxylin and eosin stained sections (Figure 7.41), giving the impression that the cilia are more basophilic than normal, but this is not specific and should not be used as a definitive diagnostic feature. With a Warthin-Starry or Grocott's methenamine silver stain, filamentous bacilli are readily observed among cilia of respiratory epithelium from the nasal cavity to the bronchioles

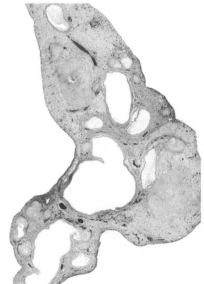

Figure 7.40 CAR bacillus infection in a rat. There is severe bronchiectasis and intense inflammation and mucus in the interstitium. Hematoxylin and eosin. × 1.5

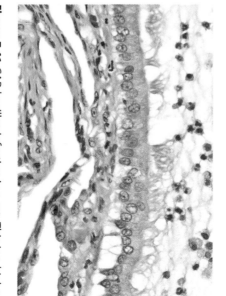

Figure 7.41 CAR bacillus infection in a rat. This is a higher magnification of Figure 7.40. Note the pale basophilic structures on the luminal surface of the bronchial epithelial cells. Additionally, there are moderate numbers of neutrophils in the lumen. Hematoxylin and eosin. × 95.

(Figure 7.42). The upper respiratory tract is involved earlier than the lower tract during the course of the infection, and both sites should be included in histologic examinations of the disease. With secondary bacterial infections, there may also be a suppurative bronchopneumonia.

CAR bacillus infection should be distinguished from murine respiratory mycoplasmosis, other bacterial pneumonias (i.e. *Streptococcus pneumoniae*, *Corynebacterium kutscheri*, etc.) and viral pneumonias. Diagnosis of CAR bacillus infection should also raise the suspicion of coinfection with the other pathogens that often accompany CAR bacillus infections (van Zwieten et al., 1980; MacKenzie et al., 1981).

Colony screening is usually performed by serologic techniques, such as ELISA or IFA (Matsushita et al., 1987; Lukas et al., 1987; Shoji et al., 1988). As false positive reactions can occur (Hook et al., 1998), any

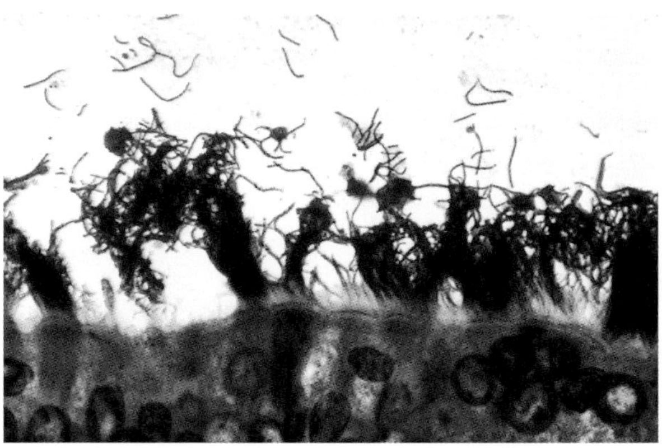

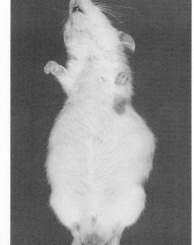

Figure 7.42 CAR bacillus infection in a rat. Darkly stained bacteria are readily visible in the normally pale layer of cilia on the surface of the bronchial epithelium. Bacilli are also present in the lumen. Warthin–Starry Silver. × 240

Figure 7.43 Tyzzer's disease. A 3–4-week-old Wistar rat has a distended abdomen due to megaloileitis associated with Tyzzer's disease.

positive results should be confirmed by a Steiner stain of tracheal mucosal scrapings or histopathology with use of special stains, as discussed previously. Interestingly, infection is not readily transmitted by soiled bedding (Cundiff *et al.*, 1995), so many sentinel programs may fail to detect this organism. Infection is lifelong, and the organisms are readily retrievable by tracheal lavage or scraping (Medina *et al.*, 1998). Therefore, CAR bacillus can also be detected by PCR (Cundiff *et al.*, 1994), which may serve as an important confirmatory test should serologic screening be positive.

The interference of CAR bacillus with research is unknown. Interference with ciliary function has been suspected but not measured. Effects of CAR bacillus on other respiratory functions and on the immune response have also been postulated but not documented in the scientific literature.

Tyzzer's Disease

Tyzzer's disease, first discovered in Japanese waltzing mice (Tyzzer, 1917), is caused by *Clostridium piliforme* (Duncan *et al.*, 1993), formerly known as *Bacillus piliformis*. The host range is extremely broad (Kohn and Barthold, 1984), including numerous rodent species, rabbits, carnivores, horses, and both nonhuman and human (Skelton *et al.*, 1995) primates.

C. piliforme infections are most often clinically silent (Motzel and Riley, 1992; Hansen *et al.*, 1992a). Overt disease in rats, as in other species, is most likely to be observed in young, recently weaned animals. In these, the clinical signs are nonspecific (anorexia, lethargy, emaciation, ruffled fur and diarrhea with or

without mucus and blood), but may also include acute death without clinical signs. In the rat, in particular, a distended abdomen (Figure 7.43) has been observed in weanlings with Tyzzer's disease (Hansen *et al.*, 1992b).

C. piliforme is transmitted horizontally in rats via the fecal–oral route by spores, which are highly resistant to desiccation and some disinfectants (Ganaway, 1980; Hansen *et al.*, 1992b). The vegetative form, however, survives only inside cells.

After a rat ingests *C. piliforme* spores, the spores produce the vegetative form, which is actively phagocytosed by mucosal epithelial cells covering the gut-associated lymphoid tissue or Peyer's patches in the jejunum, ileum and cecum (Franklin *et al.*, 1993; Riley and Franklin, 1997). The vegetative form escapes from the phagosome and multiplies in the epithelial cells and possibly the reticuloendothelial cells in Peyer's patches. The vegetative form reaches the liver, probably via the portal circulation. It then infects and multiplies in the hepatocytes, following which it may enter the bloodstream or lymphatics to colonize the myocardium. It may also possibly enter the biliary epithelium to multiply and be shed into the bile to reinfect the intestine and liver (autoinfection). Alternatively, the infection may be cleared (Motzel and Riley, 1992).

A number of factors influence the infection and disease outcome, especially age; recently weaned rats are more susceptible to overt disease. Immune function also is important (Livingston *et al.*, 1996), and immunosuppression from stress or immunosuppression by treatment with cyclophosphamide or corticosteroids may precipitate a latent infection (Boivin *et al.*, 1990).

Bacterial factors also play an important role in the pathogenesis of Tyzzer's disease. Pathogenicity has

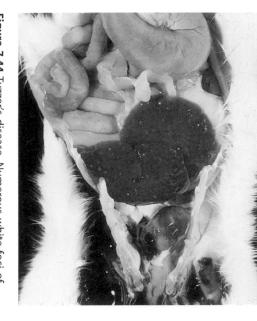

Figure 7.44 Tyzzer's disease. Numerous white foci of necrosis and inflammation are scattered in the liver of this 3–4-week-old Wistar rat.

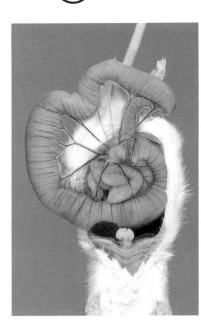

Figure 7.45 Tyzzer's disease. This is the same 3–4-week-old Wistar rat depicted in Figure 7.43. The megaloileitis is due to *Clostridium piliforme*.

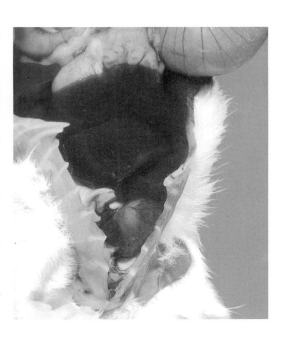

Figure 7.46 Tyzzer's disease. A distinct white area of necrosis and inflammation is present in the heart of this 3–4-week-old Wistar rat.

been associated with production of a high-molecular weight, cytotoxic protein (Riley *et al.*, 1992). In addition, some degree of species-specificity has been demonstrated for *C. piliforme* isolates, such that a rat isolate may not readily infect other host species, and vice versa (Motzel and Riley, 1992; Franklin *et al.*, 1994).

Grossly, Tyzzer's disease may cause perianal fecal staining, but the most characteristic lesions are internal (Tyzzer, 1917; Duncan *et al.*, 1993). Multiple, pinpoint or larger, pale foci of necrosis are often visible on the surface of and within the liver (Figure 7.44). Megaloileitis (Figure 7.45), a greatly dilated, flaccid and hyperemic small intestine (ileum) may be present (Hansen *et al.*, 1992a). Hyperemia, edema, hemorrhage and possibly ulceration may affect any part of the intestine, especially the terminal ileum, cecum and colon. Probably as a consequence of intestinal involvement, mesenteric lymph nodes may be enlarged, hyperemic and edematous. In the heart, pale, circumscribed, sometimes raised foci may be present on the surface. Myocardial necrosis and inflammation due to Tyzzer's disease may also appear as pale linear streaks or circumscribed raised areas on the heart (Figure 7.46), especially near the apex.

Histopathologically, characteristic lesions (Duncan *et al.*, 1993) may be observed in the liver, ileum, cecum, colon, and less frequently the heart (Kohn and Barthold, 1984). In the intestinal tract there is often necrotizing enteritis, typhlitis and colitis, which may be accompanied by edema, blunted and fused villi, crypt epithelial hyperplasia, ulceration and hemorrhage, with cellular debris in crypts and lymphatics. In the liver, coagulative necrosis (Figure 7.47) is a frequent finding, and is often accompanied by a moderate leukocytic infiltrate (neutrophils, mononuclear cells, macrophages and, rarely, multinucleated giant cells) at the periphery of the lesions. Hemorrhage may accompany acute lesions, and mineralization may be visible with time as a consequence of the necrosis. In the heart, myocardial degeneration and necrosis occurs in a minority of cases, often associated with a mixed leukocytic infiltrate and dystrophic calcification.

Histopathology is diagnostic if the characteristic bacilli are observed (Tyzzer, 1917; Kohn and Barthold, 1984; Duncan *et al.*, 1993). The vegetative form of the organism is a filamentous bacillus, 8.0–20.0 × 0.3–0.5 μm. One or usually more bacilli are present in cells in either a jumbled array (pickup stick) or parallel arrangement, as dictated by the shape of the cell. Occasionally, the vegetative form

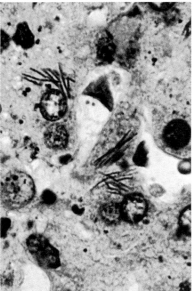

Figure 7.47 Tyzzer's disease. Foci of hepatic necrosis and inflammation. Hematoxylin and eosin. × 15

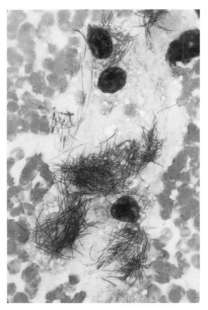

Figure 7.48 Tyzzer's disease. Numerous basophilic organisms lie in a jumbled array within the cytoplasm of a hepatocyte at the periphery of a focus of necrosis. Hematoxylin and eosin. × 295.

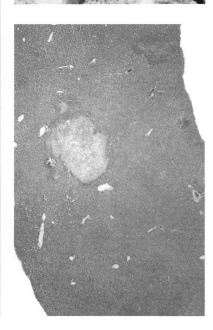

Figure 7.49 Tyzzer's disease. Numerous argyrophilic organisms lie in a jumbled array within the cytoplasm of hepatocytes. Warthin–Starry silver. × 295.

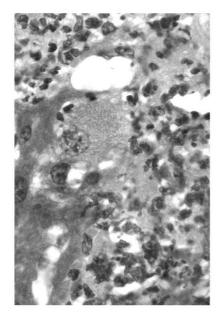

Figure 7.50 Tyzzer's disease. A Giemsa-stained impression smear from liver lesions demonstrates numerous intracellular and extracellular bacilli. × 740.

may be visible in hepatocytes in tissue sections stained with hematoxylin and eosin (Figure 7.48), but usually special stains are necessary, including Warthin–Starry silver (best), Giemsa and methylene blue stains. The organism is Gram-negative, but stains very poorly with Gram stains. In the liver, the organisms are most often observed in surviving hepatocytes at the periphery or within lesions (Figure 7.49), but may also be in hepatocytes not associated with a lesion. In the intestine, normal gut flora within mucosal crypts and superimposed upon the mucosal epithelial cells may complicate evaluation. Organisms may also be observed in myocytes of the heart when there is cardiac involvement. Less frequently, they may be seen in myocytes of the tunica muscularis of the intestine.

Differential diagnoses for necrotizing hepatitis in the rat should include other bacterial septicemias, such as *Corynebacterium kutscheri*, as well as infection with *Rat virus*. Diagnosis of clinical disease depends on demonstration of the organism in tissue. Tissue

smears may facilitate rapid diagnosis (Figure 7.50); Giemsa-stained smears of suspicious liver lesions are especially useful (Percy and Barthold, 1993b).

Colony screening for latent infections is problematic. Serologic screening is rapid and technically simple (Motzel *et al.*, 1991), but subject to false positives, yielding results which can be difficult to put into context. Disease provocation tests to exacerbate latent infections are widely used, and are recommended as a follow-up test when serologic positive results are obtained. However, there is some doubt as to the efficacy of these tests which rely on immunosuppression, usually with cyclophosphamide (Boivin *et al.*, 1990) and less frequently with corticosteroids, followed by histopathologic evaluation. The doubt arises since animals may clear the *C. piliforme* infection and, therefore, would no longer be susceptible to activation of 'latent' infection (Motzel and Riley, 1992). Alternatively, sentinel animals can be placed on soiled bedding, but this may require sentinels to be of the same species (to

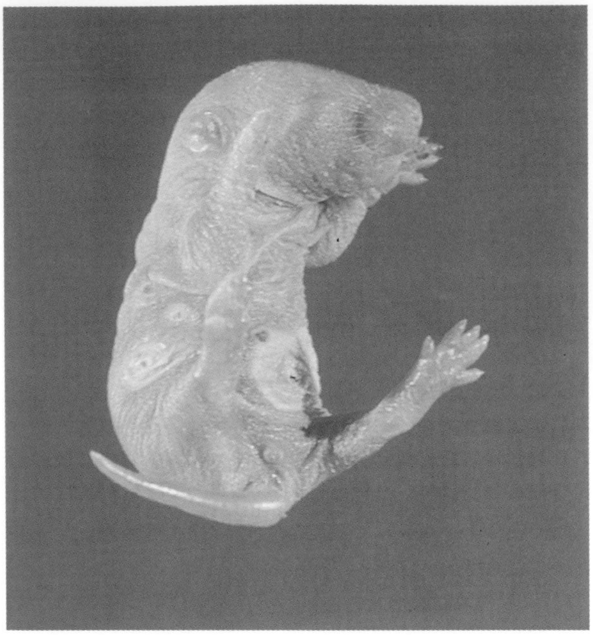

Figure 7.51 Staphylococcal dermatitis in a neonatal rat. Culture of vesicles on the skin yielded heavy growth of *S. aureus* in pure culture.

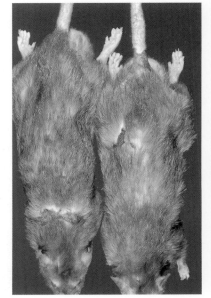

Figure 7.52 Staphylococcal dermatitis. Multiple ulcerated skin lesions on the shoulders, back and base of the tail may have originated from bite wounds in these group-housed Brown-Norway rats.

Staphylococcosis

Despite the attention given to more exotic organisms, one of the most widespread and mundane of bacteria, *Staphylococcus aureus*, may cause some of the most frequently observed lesions in laboratory rats (National Research Council, 1991). *S. aureus* is present as a commensal in laboratory rodents, as well as most other mammals, including humans. In fact, it is probably accurate to say that *S. aureus* is always present unless strictly excluded.

In any given rat population, most will be asymptomatic carriers. Occasionally, an ulcerative dermatitis (Figure 7.51) will be observed in one or more adults or, rarely, a vesicular or ulcerative condition in young animals (Clifford, 1998, unpublished observation).

S. aureus is a Gram-positive, coagulase-positive coccus (Schleifer, 1986). The name is derived from Greek, *staphyle*, meaning like a cluster of grapes. It is readily cultured from the nasopharynx, skin, bedding

avoid species-specificity causing false negatives), as not even gerbils are susceptible to all strains of *C. piliforme* (Motzel and Riley, 1992).

Research effects of *C. piliforme* have primarily been ascribed to the morbidity and mortality, although recent effects on coagulation and leukokines (Van Andel *et al.*, 1996) have also been reported.

and surfaces onto blood agar, where it produces yellow-gold colonies.

Transmission is horizontal. Caretakers may serve as reservoirs for *S. aureus* and may spread it directly or by fomites (Blackmore and Francis, 1970). The organism can also multiply in dirty bedding or other materials.

S. aureus normally inhabits the skin and mucous membranes (National Research Council, 1991), and results in disease only when there is a break in the integrity of these structures from trauma or foreign bodies. It can also penetrate the oral mucosa at the gingival-tooth margin, resulting in periodontal abscesses. Some *S. aureus* strains produce an exfoliative toxin which may predispose the skin of neonatal rats to gentle rubbing, therefore, possibly providing a portal of entry for this opportunist. It is also one of the most common organisms isolated from preputial glands, although less frequently in rats than in mice. Involvement of deeper tissues or hematogenous spread is rare in immunocompetent rats.

Gross lesions generally are those of an ulcerative dermatitis, although subcutaneous abscess may also, rarely, be observed (National Research Council, 1991). Lesions are typically intensely pruritic, and are most frequent on the dorsolateral surface of the anterior thorax, head and neck (Figures 7.52 and 7.53).

Histopathologically (Carlton and Hunt, 1978), ulcerative dermatitis is a chronic suppurative condition, usually with numerous prominent dense colonies of large Gram-positive cocci embedded in serum exudate and occasionally in the dermis. Clusters of Gram-positive cocci in the dermis or other tissues may be surrounded by an eosinophilic amphophilic dense ring or corona, referred to as Splendore–Hoeppli material.

of conjunctivitis, **metritis** and mastitis (Percy and Barthold, 1993b). Histologically, lesions are characterized by necrotizing, suppurative inflammation.

Control of the agent may not be necessary in immunocompetent animals due to the rarity of *P. pneumotropica*-induced disease. However, treatment with enrofloxacin has been described (Goelz *et al.*, 1997). Rederivation by either cesarean section or embryo transfer will also eliminate the agent (National Research Council, 1991). Antibiotic treatment of infected dams prior to cesarean section is recommended by at least one major rodent vendor (Clifford, 1998, unpublished observation), since *P. pneumotropica* can be present in the uterus. The probability of successful elimination of *P. pneumotropica* by cesarean section can be further increased by culturing all uteri after the pups have been removed, and eliminating any offspring from a culture-positive uterus. Offspring should also be held in strict isolation (i.e. not mixed in with a breeding colony) until repeatedly cultured negative for *P. pneumotropica*. *P. pneumotropica* is not transmitted to a significant degree by fomites, does not persist or multiply in the environment, and only rarely colonizes humans. Therefore, once a colony is free of the agent there is relatively little risk of reinfection except through introduction or incursion of infected animals.

Streptobacillus moniliformis

A cause of 'rat-bite fever', *Streptobacillus moniliformis* is primarily of historic interest. Although this zoonotic agent is virtually nonexistent in modern laboratory animals, it nonetheless bears brief mention due to the potential consequences of infection (Wullenweber, 1995). The agent is a Gram-negative pleomorphic bacillus, which will grow nonhemolytically on sheep blood agar, although trypticase soy agar enriched with 20% horse serum is preferred (Weisbroth, 1982; Savage, 1984).

S. moniliformis is commensal in wild rats, inhabiting the nasopharynx, middle ear and respiratory tract. It is also present in blood and urine of infected rats, and is transmitted to humans by bite wounds, aerosols and fomites (Will, 1994). The organism is nonpathogenic in rats. Clinical signs in humans follow a 3–10 day incubation period, and include fever, vomiting, **arthralgia** and rash. Disease is treated with antibiotics, and mortality is usually low. Colonies of laboratory rats are monitored by culture of blood and nasopharyngeal swabs for *S. moniliformis*, and any colony in which the organism is

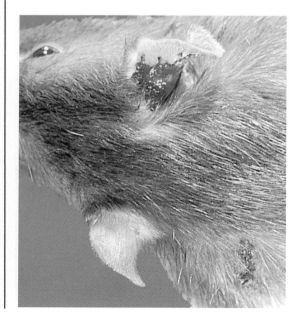

Figure 7.53 Staphylococcal dermatitis. The ulcerated skin lesion on the ear of this Long-Evans rat may have originated as a self-inflicted wound. The rat was negative for mites.

The list of differential diagnoses to be considered should include other bacterial infections, especially *Corynebacterium kutscheri*, as well as higher bacteria (*Actinomyces* spp., *Actinobacillus* spp., *Nocardia* spp.) and fungi. Chemical injury, such as inadequate rinsing of sterilants from gloves or forceps can also result in ulcerative skin lesions. Trauma from handling, sharp edges in cages and from fighting should also be considered as primary causes of ulcerative skin lesions.

Diagnosis is made by bacterial culture or by identification of characteristic organisms in ulcerative and/or suppurative lesions.

Pasteurellosis

Pasteurella pneumotropica is a Gram-negative coccobacillus. It grows aerobically on sheep blood agar without producing hemolysis, producing smooth, gray translucent colonies (Carter, 1984). It has been isolated from numerous mammalian species, including humans, and is generally considered to be of low significance in immunocompetent rats (National Research Council, 1991).

P. pneumotropica has a high prevalence in positive colonies, and is most often isolated from the nasopharynx, cecum, vagina, uterus and conjunctiva during routine monitoring (National Research Council, 1991). The vast majority of animals are asymptomatic, with only rare instances

Parasitic Diseases

Oxyuriasis

Three species of oxyurid nematodes (pinworms), *Syphacia muris*, *S. obvelata*, and *Aspiculuris tetraptera*, occur in the laboratory rat. Their continued occurrence, despite the dramatic progress in the last decades in eliminating and excluding viral and bacterial pathogens, is due both to the persistence of the eggs in the environment and to the low degree of attention paid to these parasites.

Syphacia muris is the most common oxyurid of the rat (National Research Council, 1991; Owen, 1992). *Syphacia obvelata* is more frequently found in mice, hamsters and gerbils, but is also occasionally found in the rat, especially when housed in the same room as mice with the parasite.

Syphacia spp. have a direct life cycle, requiring 11–15 days for completion (Flynn, 1973b). Transmission is horizontal via ingestion of eggs. Eggs, which remain viable at room conditions for weeks to months, are deposited by the female in the colon and around the anus, and become infective in approximately 6 hours. They are ingested during self-cleaning behavior, and hatch in the small intestine. The larvae then mature in the cecum in 10–11 days. The morphology of adults of both species is similar,

although *S. muris* is slightly smaller and the male has a longer tail, measured as a proportion of body width (Flynn, 1973b). Eggs vary more markedly between the species, with *S. muris* (Figure 7.54) being 72–82 × 25–36 μm, compared to 118–153 × 33–55 μm for *S. obvelata*. In addition, the eggs of *S. obvelata* (Figure 7.55) are almost completely flat along one side, whereas those of *S. muris* are only slightly flattened on one side.

Aspiculuris tetraptera is also transmitted horizontally by ingestion of eggs which are extremely persistent in the environment (Flynn, 1973b). The direct life cycle is longer than *Syphacia*, requiring 23–25 days. Also unlike *Syphacia*, *Aspiculuris* eggs are passed in the feces, and are not deposited around the anus. They become infective in 6–7 days. After ingestion they hatch in the colon where the larvae also mature. Adult *A. tetraptera* are readily recognized by the four alae present at the anterior end of the body (Figure 7.56). The bilaterally symmetrical eggs (Figure 7.57) are smaller than those of *Syphacia obvelata*; however, they are approximately the same size as *S. muris*, measuring 89–93 × 36–42 μm.

Gross lesions of **oxyuriasis** are very rare (Flynn, 1973b). Rectal prolapse, constipation and intussusception have been reported in mice infested with *S. obvelata*, but these findings were not experimentally reproduced. The authors also did not exclude other potential causes of rectal prolapse in mice which have since been discovered (Percy and Barthold, 1993a; Ward et al., 1996), such as *Citrobacter rodentium* or *Helicobacter hepaticus*. Histologic lesions of oxyuriasis have not been reported.

Diagnosis of oxyuriasis is most practically accomplished by direct examination of macerated

confirmed should immediately be terminated. As wild rats are the reservoir for *S. moniliformis*, its detection in a laboratory rat colony would indicate exposure to infected wild rats.

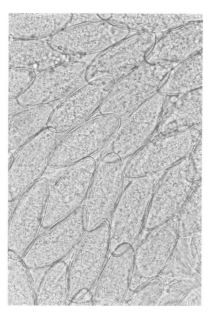

Figure 7.54 *Syphacia muris* eggs inside the uterus of an adult parasite. × 295

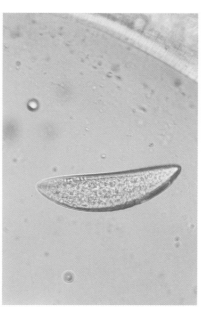

Figure 7.55 *Syphacia obvelata* egg. Compared to the eggs in Figure 7.54, this egg is larger and more markedly flattened along one side. × 295.

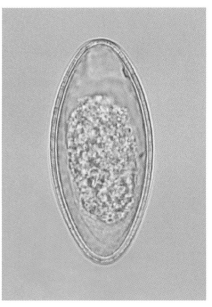

Figure 7.57 *Aspiculuris tetraptera* egg. The egg is symmetrical, and approximately the same size as the egg of *Syphacia muris*.

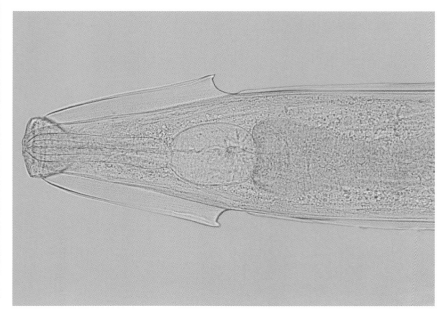

Figure 7.56 Adult *Aspiculuris tetraptera*. Lateral alae are visible along the sides of the parasite. × 295.

Numerous research effects of oxyuriasis have been described. In rats, oxyuriasis has been reported to interfere with adjuvant arthritis (Pearson and Taylor, 1975), growth rate (Wagner, 1988), and intestinal electrolyte transport (Lubcke *et al.*, 1992). In mice, oxyuriasis has been reported to alter exploratory behavior (McNair and Timmons, 1977) and to increase antibody production to other antigens (Sato *et al.*, 1995).

cecum and colon under low magnification with a stereomicroscope. Although not quite as sensitive as complete direct examination of the large bowel, it is significantly less time consuming. Examination for eggs must be tailored to the suspected infesting species of nematode. As dictated by the method of egg transmission, the perianal tape test is effective only for *Syphacia* spp., and fecal flotation is only effective for *A. tetraptera*. Screening for oxyurid eggs is significantly less sensitive than direct examination of the bowel for the adult helminths (West *et al.*, 1992; Klement *et al.*, 1996).

Oxyuriasis can be eliminated in individual rats with Ivermectin (Hasslinger and Wiethe, 1987; Huerkamp, 1993; Klement *et al.*, 1996). However, the source of the original infestation should be identified, and the premises should be thoroughly disinfected so as to prevent reinfestation. Ivermectin is not effective against eggs, which can persist for long periods in the environment. Oxyuriasis can also be eliminated by rederivation. It is readily excluded by proper adherence to modern practices of barrier room technology (Hasslinger and Wiethe, 1987).

Acariasis

Radfordia ensifera is the only ectoparasite of rats that one is likely to encounter in a laboratory animal environment, although it should be distinguished from other acarids, such as *Myobia musculi*, which could possibly be harbored briefly on the rat's pelage. *R. ensifera*, like *R. affinis*, which is more commonly found in mice, has two empodial claws on the second pair of legs (Figures 7.58 and 7.59), whereas *Myobia* only has one (Flynn, 1973a). In *R. ensifera* the empodial claws are unequal in length, whereas in *R. affinis* they are equal. In the author's experience, this difference in length is subtle.

The infestation is transmitted by eggs, which can persist in the environment for long periods. The eggs hatch in 7–8 days, and females can begin to lay eggs after another 16 days. Infestation can result in pruritus, self-excoriation and secondary bacterial infections. In mice, **acariasis** has also been associated with increased mitotic activity in the skin, immunologic alterations and amyloidosis (Weisbroth, 1982).

Acariasis is most practically diagnosed by direct examination of the animals with a dissecting scope

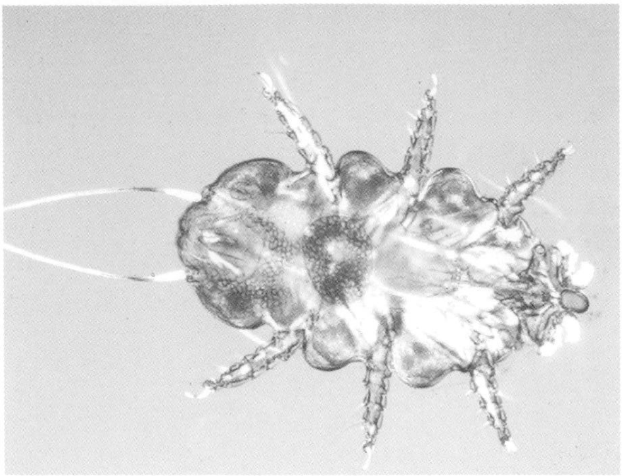

Pneumocystosis

Pneumocystosis, caused by *Pneumocystis carinii*, has long been recognized as a disease of immunodeficiency in a multitude of mammalian host species (Franklin and Riley, 1993). Molecular biology techniques have determined that *P. carinii* is a fungus (Stringer, 1993; Keely *et al.*, 1994), and have also demonstrated considerable genetic variation between the *P. carinii* strains infecting different host species (Cushion *et al.*, 1993). For example, *P. carinii* strains infecting humans and rats are so widely divergent that they are not considered to be cross-infective.

In rats, clinical signs are observed only with congenital immunodeficiency (Furuta *et al.*, 1993) or prolonged impairment of host defenses, including administration of immunosuppressive agents (Sukura *et al.*, 1991; Armstrong *et al.*, 1991; Oz and Hughes, 1996), such as cyclophosphamide and corticosteroids. Infection is persistent and progressive; therefore, clinical signs are more likely to be observed in animals older than six months of age. In immunodeficient animals, emaciation, dyspnea and cyanosis may be observed (Furuta *et al.*, 1993).

P. carinii spores are widespread in the environment, and infection is transmitted via inhalation of these spores (Chandler *et al.*, 1979). Trophozoites attach primarily to type I alveolar epithelial cells, and to a lesser extent type II alveolar epithelial cells (Yoneda and Walzer, 1980). Infection results in pulmonary insufficiency through damage to type I alveolar epithelial cells, damage to alveolar capillaries and filling of alveoli with a frothy material. This material is composed of disintegrating parasites, antigen–antibody complexes, fibrin and other serum proteins. Infection interferes with research utilizing immunodeficient and immunosuppressed animals primarily through the morbidity it causes.

Gross lesions are absent in **occult infections**. In clinical infections, lungs often fail to collapse when the thorax is opened, and may have gray-brown foci suggestive of interstitial pneumonia (Figure 7.60). The affected animals are often emaciated and occasionally cyanotic.

Histopathologic examination of hematoxylin and eosin stained sections from affected rats reveals a frothy to honeycombed, eosinophilic material with small, faint, basophilic granules (trophozoite nuclei) in alveolar spaces and the lumina of the airways (Figures 7.61 and 7.62) (Chandler *et al.*, 1979; Lanken *et al.*, 1980). In some occult infections, only meager amounts of the honeycombed material

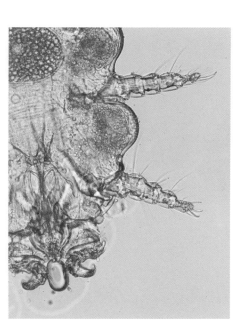

Figure 7.58 Female *Radfordia* sp. Use of polarized light helps in assessment of the two claws on the second pair of legs, since the more sclerotized body parts are anisotropic, as is the internal striated musculature. The first pair of legs, located near the mouth parts, is short and compressed for grasping hairs. × 74.

Figure 7.59 Female *Radfordia* sp. The second pair of legs has two claws. × 295.

(Flynn, 1973a). As an alternative, dead rats or their pelts can also be placed in a sealed clear glass or plastic container and refrigerated overnight, then examined against a black background.

Control of acariasis is similar to that for other parasitic metazoa. As with oxyuriasis, acariasis can be eliminated in individual rats with Ivermectin (West *et al.*, 1992). However, the source of the original infestation should be identified, and the premises should be thoroughly disinfected so as to prevent reinfestation. Ivermectin is not effective against eggs, which can persist for long periods in the environment. Infestation can also be eliminated by rederivation, and is readily excluded by proper adherence to modern practices of barrier room technology (Weisbroth, 1982).

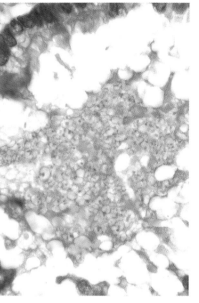

Figure 7.62 *Pneumocystis carinii* pneumonia in an athymic nude rat. This is a higher magnification of Figure 7.61. At this magnification the trophozoite nuclei (pale basophilic coccoid bodies) can be visualized. Hematoxylin and eosin. × 180.

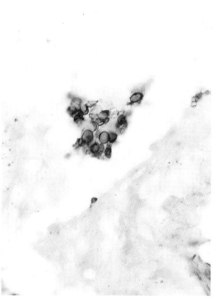

Figure 7.63 *Pneumocystis carinii* pneumonia in an athymic nude rat. There are numerous dark staining mature *P. carinii* cysts. Grocott's methenamine silver. × 180.

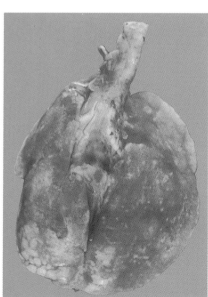

Figure 7.60 *Pneumocystis carinii* pneumonia in an athymic nude rat. The posterior portion of both lung lobes is pale and consolidated.

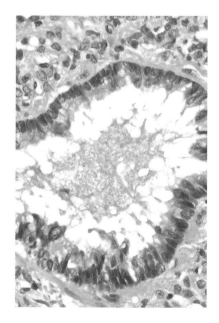

Figure 7.61 *Pneumocystis carinii* pneumonia in an athymic nude rat. There is a modest amount of a frothy eosinophilic material in the lumen of a bronchiole. Pale basophilic coccoid bodies (trophozoite nuclei) are barely visible in the frothy material. Hematoxylin and eosin. × 95.

may be observed attached to alveolar septa. An interstitial pneumonia may or may not be observed in association with the infection. Methenamine silver stains (Kusnitz *et al.*, 1994) reveal round, oval and folded cysts (Figure 7.63), although these may be few in number, and should not be confused with artifactual staining of host cells. Immunohistochemical stains are sometimes employed as an adjunct for definitive identification.

Diagnosis of pneumocystosis is most often based on histopathologic examination of appropriately stained sections. Molecular biologic techniques employing the polymerase chain reaction have been developed in recent years, and are useful in both immunocompetent and immunodeficient animals (Kitada *et al.*, 1991; Lu *et al.*, 1995).

Immunosuppression, followed by histologic techniques, is sometimes used to screen immunocompetent rats for latent infection (Sukura *et al.*, 1991; Oz and Hughes, 1996). Serologic screening of immunocompetent rat populations is also possible, but is not widely employed.

Acknowledgments

The authors wish to acknowledge and thank Ann Chavis and Carrie Barfield who provided invaluable service in transcribing this manuscript, Patricia Mirley for her persistence in the library, and Beth Gaul, Maureen Puccini and David Sabio for their help in the preparation of the illustrations.

References

ACLAD (American Committee on Laboratory Animal Disease) (1991) *Lab. Anim. Sci.* **41**, 199–225.

Aguila, H.N., Wayne, C.L., Lu, Y.S. and Pakes, S.P. (1988) *Lab. Anim. Sci.* **38**, 138–142.

Amao, H., Akimoto, T., Takahashi, K.W., Nakagawa, M. and Saito, M. (1991) *Lab. Anim. Sci.* **41**, 265–268.

Amao, H., Komukai, Y., Sugiyama, M., Takahashi, K.W., Sawada, T. and Saito, M. (1995a) *Lab. Anim. Sci.* **45**, 6–10.

Amao, H., Komukai, Y., Akimoto, T. *et al.* (1995b) *Lab. Anim. Sci.* **45**, 11–14.

Antopol, W. (1950) *Proc. Soc. Exp. Biol. Med.* **73**, 262–265.

Antopol, W., Glaubach, S. and Quittner, H. (1951) *Rheumatism* **7**, 187–196.

Armstrong, M.Y., Smith, A.L. and Richards, F.F. (1991) *J. Protozool.* **38**, 136S–138S.

Austrian, R. (1998) In: Gorbach, S.L., Bartlett, J.G. and Blacklow, N.R. (eds) *Infectious Diseases*, 2nd edn, pp. 1719–1723. Philadelphia: W.B. Saunders.

Baker, D.G. (1998) *Clin. Microbiol. Rev.* **11**, 231–266.

Ball-Goodrich, L.J., Leland, S.E., Johnson, E.A., Paturzo, F.X. and Jacoby, R.O. (1998) *J. Virol.* **72**, 3289–3299.

Barile, M.F. (1981) *Isr. J. Med. Sci.* **17**, 555–562.

Baringer, J.R. and Nathanson, N. (1972) *Lab. Invest.* **27**, 514–522.

Barthold, S.W. (1997) In: Jones, T.C., Popp, J.A. and Mohr, U. (eds) *Digestive System*, pp. 416–418. Berlin: Springer-Verlag.

Barthold, S.W., de Souza, M.S. and Smith, A.L. (1990) *Lab. Anim. Sci.* **40**, 481–485.

Besselsen, D.G., Besch-Williford, C.L., Pintel, D.J., Franklin, C.L., Hook, R.R. and Riley, L.K. (1995) *J. Clin. Microbiol.* **33**, 1699–1703.

Bhatt, P.N. and Jacoby, R.O. (1977) *Arch. Virol.* **54**, 345–352.

Bhatt, P.N. and Jacoby, R.O. (1985) *Lab. Anim. Sci.* **35**, 129–134.

Bhatt, R.N., Jacoby, R.O. and Jonas, A.M. (1977) *Infect. Immun.* **18**, 823–827.

Bihun, C.G.D. and Percy, D.H. (1995) *Vet. Pathol.* **32**, 1–10.

Blackmore, D.K. and Francis, R.A. (1970) *J. Comp. Pathol.* **80**, 645–651.

Boivin, G.P., Wagner, J.E. and Besch-Williford, C.L. (1990) *Lab. Anim. Sci.* **40**, 545 (abstract).

Boot, R., Thuis, H., Bakker, R. and Veenema, J.L. (1995) *Lab. Anim.* **29**, 294–299.

Broderson, J.R., Lindsey, J.R. and Crawford, J.E. (1976) *Am. J. Pathol.* **85**, 115–130.

Burek, J.D., Zurcher, C., Van Nunen, M.C.J. and Hollander, C.F. (1977) *Lab. Anim. Sci.* **27**, 963–971.

Carlton, W.W. and Hunt, R.D. (1978). In: Benirschke,

K., Garner, F.M. and Jones, T.C. (eds) *Pathology of Laboratory Animals*, Vol. 2, pp. 1368–1480. New York: Springer-Verlag.

Carter, G.R. (1984) In: Krieg, N.R. and Holt, J.G. (eds) *Bergey's Manual of Systematic Bacteriology*, Vol. 1, pp. 552–557. Baltimore: William & Wilkins.

Carthew, P. and Aldred, P. (1988) *Lab. Anim.* **22**, 92–97.

Carthew, P. and Sparrow, S. (1980a) *Res. Vet. Sci.* **29**, 289–292.

Carthew, P. and Sparrow, S. (1980b) *J. Pathol.* **130**, 153–158.

Cassell, G.H. (1982) *Rev. Infect. Dis.* **4** (Suppl.), S18–S34.

Cassell, G.H., Lindsey, J.R., Overcash, R.G. and Baker, H.J. (1973) *Ann. N.Y. Acad. Sci.* **225**, 395–412.

Cassell, G.H., Wilborn, W.H., Silvers, S.H. and Minion, F.C. (1981b) *Isr. J. Med. Sci.* **17**, 593–598.

Cassell, G.H., Lindsey, J.R., Baker, H.J. and Davis, J.K. (1979) In: Baker, H.J., Lindsey, J.R. and Weisbroth, S.H. (eds) *The Laboratory Rat*, Vol.1, pp. 243–269. New York: Academic Press.

Cassell, G.H., Lindsey, J.R. and Davis, J.K. (1981a) *Isr. J. Med. Sci.* **17**, 548–554.

Castleman, W.L., Sorkness, R.L., Lemanske, R.F., Grasee G. and Suyemoto, M.M. (1988) *Lab. Invest.* **59**, 387–396.

Chandler, F.W., Frenkel, J.K. and Campbel, W.G. (1979) *Am. J. Pathol.* **571**–574.

Chasey, D., Higgins, R.J., Jeffrey, M. and Banks J. (1989) *J. Comp. Pathol.* **100**, 217–222.

Coid, C.R. and Wardman, G. (1971) *J. Reprod. Fertil.* **24**, 39–43.

Coid, C.R. and Wardman, G. (1972) *Med. Microbiol. Immunol.* **157**, 181–185.

Cole, G.A., Nathanson, N. and Rivet, H. (1970) *Am. J. Epidemiol.* **91**, 339–350.

Coleman, G.L., Jacoby, R.O., Bhatt, P.N., Smith, A.L. and Jonas, A.M. (1983) *Vet. Pathol.* **20**, 49–56.

Compton, S.R. and Vivas-Gonzalez, B. (1998) *Contemp. Topics* **37**, 91 (abstract).

Compton, S.R., Gaertner, D.J. and Smith, A.L. (1998) *Contemp. Topics* **37**, 91 (abstract).

Cundiff, D.D., Besch-Williford, C.L., Hook, R.R., Franklin, C.L. and Riley, L.K. (1994) *J. Clin. Microbiol.* **32**, 1930–1934.

Cundiff, D.D., Besch-Williford, C.L., Hook, R.R., Franklin, C.L. and Riley, L.K. (1995a) *Lab. Anim. Sci.* **45**, 22–26.

Cundiff, D.D, Riley, L.K, Franklin, C.L., Hook, R.R. and Besch-Williford, C.L. (1995b) *Lab. Anim. Sci.* **45**, 219–221.

Cushion, M.T, Kasellis, M., Stringer, S.L. and Stringer, J.R. (1993) *Infect. Immun.* **61**, 4801–4813.

Davidson, M.K., Lindsey, J.R., Brown, M.B., Schoeb, T.R. and Cassell, G.H. (1981) *J. Clin. Microbiol.* **14**, 646–655.

Davidson, M.K., Lindsey, J.R, Brown, M.B. and Schoeb, T.R. (1982) *Rev. Infect. Dis.* **4**(Suppl.), S272 (abstract).

Davis, J.K. and Cassell, G.H. (1982) *Vet. Pathol.* **19**, 280–293.

Davis, J.K., Thorp, R.B, Maddox, P.A., Brown, M.B. and Cassell, G.H. (1982) *Infect. Immun.* **36**, 720–729.

Duncan, A.J., Carman, R.J., Olson, G.J. and Wilson, K.H. (1993) *Int. J. System. Bacteriol.* **43**, 314–318.

Eaton, M.D. and Van Herick, W. (1944) *Proc. Soc. Exp. Biol. Med.* **57**, 89–92.

Eiden, J.J., Wilde, J., Firoozmand, F. and Yolken, R. (1991) *J. Clin. Microbiol.* **29**, 539–543.

ElDadah, A.H., Nathanson, N., Smith, K.O., Squire, R.A., Santos, G.W. and Melby, E.C. (1967) *Science* **156**, 392–394.

Facklam, R.R. and Sahm, D.F. (1995) In: Murray, P.R., Baron, E.J., Pfaller, M.A., Tenover, F.C. and Yolken, R.H. (eds), *Manual of Clinical Microbiology,* 6th edn. pp. 308–314. Washington DC: ASM Press.

Fallon, M.T., Reinhard, M.K., Gray, B.M., Davis, T.W. and Lindsey, J.R. (1988) *Lab. Anim. Sci.* **38**, 129–132.

Fauve, R.M., Pierce-Chase, C.H. and Dubos, R. (1964) *J. Exp. Med.* **120**, 283–304.

Flynn, R.J. (1973a) In: *Parasites of Laboratory Animals,* pp. 425–492. Ames: Iowa State University Press.

Flynn, R.J. (1973b) In: *Parasites of Laboratory Animals,* pp. 203–320. Ames: Iowa State University Press.

Fox, J.G. (1977) *J. Environ. Pathol. Toxicol.* **1**, 199–226.

Fox, J.G., Niemi, S.M., Ackerman, J. and Murphy, J.C. (1987) *Lab. Anim. Sci.* **37**, 72–75.

Franklin, C.L. and Riley, L.K. (1993) Charles River Laboratories Reference Paper 110.

Franklin, C.L., Kinden, D.A., Stogsdill, P.L. and Riley, L.K. (1993) *Infect. Immun.* **61**, 876–883.

Franklin, C.L., Motzel, S.L., Besch-Williford, C.I., Hook, R.R. and Riley, L.K. (1994) *Lab. Anim. Sci.* **44**, 568–572.

Fujiwara, K. (1980) *Lab. Anim. Sci.* **30**, 298–303.

Furuta, T., Fujita, M, Machii, K., Kobayashi, K., Kojima, S. and Ueda K. (1993) *Lab. Anim. Sci.* **43**, 551–556.

Gaertner, D.J., Jacoby, R.O., Smith, A.L., Ardito, R.B. and Paturzo, F.X. (1989) *Arch. Virol.* **105**, 259–268.

Gaertner, D.J., Jacoby, R.O, Paturzo, F.X., Johnson, E.A., Brandsma, J.L. and Smith, A.L. (1991) *Arch. Virol.* **118**, 1–9.

Gaertner, D.J., Jacoby, R.O., Johnson, E.A., Paturzo, F.X., Smith, A.L. and Brandsma, J.L. (1993) *Virus Res.* **28**, 1–18.

Gaertner, D.J., Smith, A.L. and Jacoby, R.O. (1996) *Virus Res.* **44**, 67–78.

Ganaway, J.R. (1980) *Lab. Anim. Sci.* **30**, 192–196.

Gannon, J. and Carthew, P. (1980) *Lab. Anim.* **14**, 309–311.

Giddens, W.E., Keahey, K.K, Carter, G.R. and Whitehair, C.K. (1968) *Pathol. Vet.* **5**, 227–237.

Giddens, W.E., Van Hoosier, G.L. and Garlinghouse, L.E. (1987) *Lab. Anim. Sci.* **37**, 442–447.

Gilioli, R., Sakurada, J.K., Andrade, L.A.G., Kraft, V., Meyer, B. and Rangel, H.A. (1996) *Lab. Anim. Sci.* **46**, 582–584.

Goelz, M.F., Thigpen, J.E., Mahler, J. *et al.* (1997) *Lab. Anim. Sci.* **46**, 280–285.

Griffith, J.W., White, W.J., Danneman, P.J. and Lang, C.M. (1988) *Vet. Pathol.* **25**, 72–76.

Griffith, J.W., Brasky, K.M. and Lang, C.M. (1997) *Lab. Anim.* **31**, 52–57.

Hajjar, A.M., DiGiacomo, R.F., Carpenter, J.K., Bingel, S.A. and Moazed, T.C. (1991) *Lab. Anim. Sci.* **41**, 22–25.

Hansen, A.K., Dagnaes-Hansen, F. and Mollegaard-Hansen, K.E. (1992a) *Lab. Anim. Sci.* **42**, 449–453.

Hansen, A.K., Skovgaard-Jensen, H.J., Thomsen, P., Svendsen, O., Dagnaes-Hansen, F. and Mollegaard-Hansen, K.E. (1992b) *Lab. Anim. Sci.* **42**, 444–448.

Harkness, J.E. and Ridgeway, M.D. (1980) *Lab. Anim. Sci.* **30**, 841–844.

Hawthorne, J.D., Lorenz, D and Albrecht, P. (1982) *Infect. Immun.* **37**, 1037–1041.

Hook, R.R., Franklin, C.L., Riley, L.K., Livingston, B.A. and Besch-Williford, C.L. (1998) *Lab. Anim. Sci.* **48**, 234–239.

Horsfall, F.L. and Curnen, E.C. (1946) *J. Exp. Med.* **83**, 43–64.

Huber, A.C., Yolken, R.H., Mader, L.C., Strandberg, J.D. and Vonderfecht, S.L. (1989) *Vet. Pathol.* **26**, 376–385.

Huerkamp, M.J. (1993) *Lab. Anim. Sci.* **43**, 86–90.

Ishida, N. and Homma, M. (1978) *Adv. Virus Res.* **23**, 349–383.

Itoh, T., Kohyama, K., Takakura, A., Takenouchi, T. and Kagiyama, N. (1987) *Exp. Anim.* **36**, 387–393.

Jacoby, R.O., Bhatt, P.N. and Jonas, A.M. (1979) In: Baker, H.J., Lindsey, J.R. and Weisbroth, S.H. (eds) *The Laboratory Rat,* Vol. I, pp. 271–306. New York: Academic Press.

Jacoby, R.O., Bhatt, P.N., Gaertner, D.J., Smith, A.L., and Johnson, E.A. (1987) *Arch. Virol.* **95**, 251–270.

Jacoby, R.O., Gaertner, D.J., Bhatt, P.N., Paturzo, F.X. and Smith, A.L. (1988) *Lab. Anim. Sci.* **38**, 11–14.

Jacoby, R.O., Johnson, E.A., Paturzo, F.X., Gaertner, D.J., Brandsma, J.L. and Smith, A.L. (1991) *Lab. Anim. Sci.* **117**, 193 205.

Jacoby, R.O., Ball-Goodrich, L.J., Besselsen, D.G., McKisic, M.D., Riley, L.K. and Smith, A.L. (1996) *Lab. Anim. Sci.* **46**, 370–380.

Jersey, G.C., Whitehair, C.K. and Carter, G.R. (1973) *J. Am. Vet. Med. Assoc.* **163**, 599–604.

Kay, M.M.B. (1978) *Proc. Soc. Exp. Biol. Med.* **158**, 326–331.

Keely, S., Pai, H.J., Baughman, R. *et al.* (1994) *J. Eukaryotic Microbiol.* **41**, 94S.

Kilham, L. (1961) *Proc. Soc. Exp. Biol. Med.* **106**, 825–829.

Kilham, L. and Ferm V.H. (1964) *Proc. Soc. Exp. Biol. Med.* **117**, 874–879.

Kilham, L. and Margolis, G. (1965) *Science* **148**, 244–246.

Kilham, L. and Margolis, G. (1966) *Am. J. Pathol.* **49**, 457–475.

Kilham, L. and Margolis, G. (1969) *Teratology* **2**, 111–124.

Kilham, L. and Margolis, G. (1974) *J. Infect. Dis.* **129**, 737–740.

Kilham, L. and Oliver, L.J. (1959) *Virology* **7**, 428–437.

Kitada, K., Oka, S., Kimura, S. *et al.* (1991) *J. Clin. Microbiol.* **29**, 1985–1990.

Klement, P., Augustine, J.M., Delaney, K.H., Klement, G. and Weitz, J.I. (1996) *Lab. Anim. Sci.* **46**, 286–290.

Kohn, D.F. and Barthold, S.W. (1984) In: Fox, J.G., Cohen, B.J. and Loew, F.M. (eds) *Laboratory Animal Medicine*, pp. 91–122. San Diego: Academic Press.

Kusnitz, A.L., Bray, M.V. and Smith, A.L. (1994) *J. Histotechnol.* **17**, 349–351.

Lai, Y., Jacoby, R.O., Bhatt, P.N. and Jonas, A.M. (1976) *Invest. Ophthalmol.* **15**, 538–541.

Lane-Petter, W., Olds, R.J., Hacking, M.R. and Lane-Petter, M.E. (1970) *J. Hygiene (Cambridge)* **68**, 655–662.

Lanken, P.N., Minda, M., Pietra, G.G. and Fishman, A.P. (1980) *Am. J. Pathol.* **99**, 561–588.

La Regina, M., Woods, L., Klender, P., Gaertner, D.J. and Paturzo, F.X. (1992) *Lab. Anim. Sci.* **42**, 344–346.

LeMaistre, C. and Tompsett, R. (1952) *J. Exp. Med.* **95**, 393–408.

Liang, S.-C., Schoeb, T.R., Davis, J.K., Simecka, J.W., Cassell, G.H. and Lindsey, J.R. (1995) *Vet. Pathol.* **32**, 661–667.

Lindsey, J.R., Baker, H.J., Overcash, R.G., Cassell, G.H. and Hunt, C.E. (1971) *Am. J. Pathol.* **64**, 675–718.

Lindsey, J.R., Davidson, M.K., Schoeb, T.R. and Cassell, G.H. (1985) *Lab. Anim. Sci.* **35**, 597–607.

Lipton, H., Nathanson, N. and Hodous, J. (1973) *Am. J. Epidemiol.* **96**, 443–446.

Livingston, R.S., Franklin, C.L., Besch-Williford, C.L., Hook, R.R. and Riley, L.K. (1996) *Lab. Anim. Sci.* **46**, 21–25.

Lu, J.-J., Chen, C.-H., Bartlett, M.S., Smith, J.W. and Lee, C.-H. (1995) *J. Clin. Microbiol.* **33**, 2785–2788.

Lubcke, R., Hutcheson, F.A.R. and Barbezat, G.O. (1992) *Dig. Dis. Sci.* **37**, 60–64.

Lukas, V., Ruehl, W.W. and Hamm, T.E. (1987) *Lab. Anim. Sci.* **37**, 553.

Lussier, G. (1988) *Vet. Res. Commun.* **12**, 199–217.

Lussier, G. and Descoteaux, J.P. (1986) *Lab. Anim. Sci.* **36**, 145–148.

Machii, K., Otsuka, Y., Iwai, H. and Ueda, K. (1989) *Lab. Anim. Sci.* **39**, 334–337.

MacKenzie, W.F., Magill, L.S. and Hulse, M. (1981) *Vet. Pathol.* **18**, 836–839.

Macy, J.D., Weir, E.C. and Barthold, S.W. (1996) *Lab. Anim. Sci.* **46**, 129–132.

Margolis, G. and Kilham, L. (1970) *Lab. Invest.* **22**, 478–488.

Margolis, G., Kilham, L. and Ruffolo, P.R. (1968) *Exp. Mol. Pathol.* **8**, 1–20.

Margolis, G. and Kilham, L. (1972) *Exp. Mol. Pathol.* **16**, 326–340.

Maru, M. and Sato, K. (1982) *Arch. Virol.* **73**, 33–43.

Matsushita, S. and Joshima, H. (1989) *Lab. Anim.* **23**, 89–95.

Matsushita, S., Kashima, M. and Joshima, H. (1987) *Lab. Anim.* **21**, 356–359.

Matsushita, S., Joshima, H., Matsumoto, T. and Fukutsu, K. (1989) *Lab. Anim.* **23**, 96–102.

McDonald, D.M. (1988) *Am. Rev. Resp. Dis.* **137**, 1432–1440.

McEwen, S.A. and Percy, D.H. (1985) *Lab. Anim. Sci.* **35**, 485–487.

McNair, D.M. and Timmons, E.H. (1977) *Lab. Anim. Sci.* **27**, 38–42.

Mebus, C.A., Rhodes, M.B., and Underdahl, N.R. (1978) *Am. J. Vet. Res.* **39**, 1223–1228.

Medina, L.V., Chladny, J., Fortman, J.D., Artwohl, J.E., Bunte, R.M. and Bennett, B.T. (1998) *Lab. Anim. Sci.* **46**, 113–115.

Morzel, S.L. and Riley, L.K. (1992) *Lab. Anim. Sci.* **42**, 439–443.

Morzel, S.L., Meyer, J.K. and Riley, L.K. (1991) *Lab. Anim. Sci.* **41**, 26–30.

Naot, Y. (1982) *Rev. Infect. Dis.* **4** (Suppl.), S205–S209.

Naot, Y., Merchav, S., Ben-David, E. and Ginsburg, H. (1979) *Immunology* **36**, 399–406.

Nathanson, N., Cole, G.A., Santos, G.W., Squire, R.A. and Smith, K.O. (1970) *Am. J. Epidemiol.* **91**, 328–338.

National Research Council (1991a) In: *Infections Diseases of Mice and Rats*, pp. 33–84. Washington DC: National Academy Press.

National Research Council (1991b) In: *Infections Diseases of Mice and Rats*, pp. 164–197. Washington DC: National Academy Press.

National Research Council (1991c) In: *Infections Diseases of Mice and Rats*, pp. 85–163. Washington DC: National Academy Press.

Nelson, J.B. (1973) *Lab. Anim. Sci.* **23**, 370–372.

Novotny, J.F. and Hetrick, F.M. (1970) *Infect. Immun.* **2**, 298–303.

Overcash, R.G., Lindsey, J.R., Cassell, G.H. and Baker, H.J. (1976) *Am. J. Pathol.* **82**, 171–189.

Owen, D.G. (1992) In: *Parasites of Laboratory Animals*, pp. 39–116. London: Royal Society of Medicine Services.

Oz, H.S. and Hughes, W.T. (1996) *Lab. Anim. Sci.* **46**, 109–110.

Parker, J.C. and Reynolds, R.K. (1968) *Am. J. Epidemiol.* **88**, 112–125.

Parker, J.C., Tennant, R.W. and Ward, T.G. (1966) *Natl Cancer Inst. Monograph* **20**, 25–36.

Parker, J.C., Cross, S.S. and Rowe, W.P. (1970) *Arch. Ges. Virusforsch.* **31**, 293–302.

Pearson, H.E. and Eaton, M.D. (1940) *Proc. Soc. Exp. Biol. Med.* **57**, 677–679.

Pearson, D.J. and Taylor, G. (1975) *Immunology* **29**, 391–396.

Percy, D.H. and Barthold, S.W. (1993a) In: *Pathology of Laboratory Rodents and Rabbits*, pp. 70–114 Ames: Iowa State University Press.

Percy, D.H. and Barthold, S.W. (1993b) In: *Pathology of Laboratory Rodents and Rabbits*, pp. 3–69. Ames: Iowa State University Press.

Percy, D.H. and Palmer, D.J. (1997) *Lab. Anim. Sci.* **47**, 132–137.

Percy, D.H. and Williams, K.L. (1990) *Lab. Anim. Sci.* **40**, 603–607.

Percy, D.H. and Wojcinski, Z.W. (1986) *Lab. Anim. Sci.* **36**, 665–666.

Percy, D.H., Hanna, P.E., Paturzo, F. and Bhatt, P.N. (1984) *Lab. Anim. Sci.* **34**, 255–260.

Percy, D.H., Lynch, J.A. and Descoteaux, J.P. (1986) *Vet. Pathol.* **23**, 42–49.

Percy, D.H., Wojcinski, Z.W and Schunk, M.K. (1989) *Vet. Pathol.* **26**, 238–245.

Piedimonte, G., Nadel, J.A., Umeno, E. and McDonald, D.M. (1990) *J. Appl. Physiol.* **68**, 754–760.

Pinson, D.M., Schoeb, T.R., Lin, S.L. and Lindsey, J.R. (1988) *Lab. Anim. Sci.* **38**, 143–147.

Pleasants, J.R. (1974) In: Melby, E.C. and Altman, N.H. (eds) *Handbook of Laboratory Animal Science*, pp. 119–174. Cleveland: CRC Press.

Pringle, C.R. and Eglin, R.P. (1986) *J. Gen. Virol.* **67**, 975–982.

Profeta, M.L., Lief, F.S. and Plotkin, S.A. (1969) *Am. J. Epidemiol.* **89**, 316–324.

Rao, G.N., Haseman, J.K. and Edmondson, J. (1989) *Lab. Anim. Sci.* **39**, 389–393.

Richter, C.B. (1986) In: Bhatt, P.N., Jacoby, R.O., Morse, H.C. and New, A.E., (eds) *Viral and Mycoplasmal Infections of Laboratory Rodents*, pp. 137–192. New York: Academic Press.

Richter, C.B., Thigpen, J.E., Richter, C.S. and Mackenzie, J.M. (1988) *Lab. Anim. Sci.* **38**, 255–261.

Riley, L.K. and Franklin, C.L. (1997) In: Jones, T.C., Popp, J.A. and Mohr, U. (eds) *Digestive System*, 2nd edn, pp. 201–209. Berlin: Springer-Verlag.

Riley, L.K., Caffrey, C.J., Musille, V.S. and Meyer, J.K. (1992) *J. Med. Microbiol.* **37**, 77–80.

Robey, R.E., Woodman, D.R. and Hetrick, F.M. (1968) *Am. J. Epidemiol.* **88**, 139–143.

Rogers, A.E. (1979) In: Baker, H.J., Lindsey, J.R. and Weisbroth, S.H. (eds) *The Laboratory Rat*, Vol. I, pp. 123–152. New York: Academic Press.

Rottinghaus, A.A., Gibson, S.V. and Wagner, J.E. (1986) *Lab. Anim. Sci.* **36**, 496–498.

Ruffolo, P.R., Margolis, G. and Kilham, L. (1966) *Am. J. Pathol.* **49**, 795–824.

Ruoff, K.L. (1995) In: Murray, P.R., Baron, E.J., Pfaller, M.A., Tenover, F.C. and Yolken, R.H. (eds) *Manual of Clinical Microbiology*, pp. 299–307. Washington DC: ASM Press.

Salim, A.F., Phillips, A.D., Walker-Smith, J.A. and Farthing, M.J.G. (1995) *Gut* **36**, 231–238.

Saltzgaber-Muller, J. and Stone, B.A. (1986) *J. Clin. Microbiol.* **24**, 759–763.

Sato, Y., Ooi, H.K., Nonaka, N., Oku, Y. and Kamiya, M. (1995) *J. Parasitol.* **81**, 559–562.

Savage, D.C. (1971) In: National Research Council (eds) *Defining the Laboratory Animal. IV Symposium, International Committee on Laboratory Animals*, pp. 60–73. Washington DC: National Academy of Sciences.

Savage, N. (1984) In: Krieg, I.N.R. and Holt, J.G. (eds) *Bergey's Manual of Systematic Bacteriology*, Vol. I, pp. 598–600. Baltimore: Williams & Wilkins.

Schleifer, K.H. (1986) In: Sneath, P.H.A., Mair, N.S., Sharpe, M.E. and Holt, J.G. (eds) *Bergey's Manual of Systematic Bacteriology*, Vol. 2, pp. 999–1103. Baltimore: Williams & Wilkins.

Schoeb, T.R. and Lindsey, J.R. (1985) In: Jones, T.C., Mohr, U. and Hunt, R.D. (eds) *Respiratory System*, pp. 213–217. New York: Springer-Verlag.

Schoeb, T.R., Kervin, K.C. and Lindsey, J.R. (1985) *Vet. Pathol.* **22**, 272–282.

Schoeb, T.R. and Lindsey, J.R. (1987) *Vet. Pathol.* **24**, 392–399.

Schoeb, T.R., Davidson, M.K. and Lindsey, J.R. (1982) *Infect. Immun.* **38**, 212–217.

Schunk, M.K., Percy, D.H. and Rosendal, S. (1995) *Can. J. Vet. Res.* **59**, 60–66.

Seronde, J. (1954) *Proc. Soc. Exp. Biol. Med.* **85**, 521–524.

Seronde, J., Zucker, L.M. and Zucker, T.F. (1955) *J. Infect. Dis.* **97**, 35–38.

Seronde, J., Zucker, T.F. and Zucker, L.M. (1956) *J. Nutr.* **59**, 287–298.

Shechmeister, I.L. and Adler, F.L. (1953) *J. Infect. Dis.* **92**, 228–239.

Shoji, Y., Itoh, T. and Kagiyama, N. (1988) *Exp. Anim.* **37**, 67–72.

Singh, S.B. and Lang, C.M. (1984) *Lab. Anim.* **18**, 364–370.

Skelton, H., Smith, K., Hilyard, E. *et al.* (1995) *J. Invest. Dermatol.* **104**, 687.

Stringer, J.R. (1993) *Infect. Agents Dis.* **2**, 109–117.

Sukura, A., Soveri, T. and Lindberg, L.-A. (1991) *J. Clin. Microbiol.* **29**, 2331–2332.

Taylor, K. and Copley, C.G. (1994a) *Lab. Anim.* **28**, 26–30.

Taylor, K. and Copley, C.G. (1994b) *Lab. Anim.* **28**, 31–34.

Tennant, R.W., Parker, J.C. and Ward, T.G. (1966) *Natl Cancer Inst. Monograph* **20**, 93–104.

Thigpen, J.E. and Ross, P.W. (1983) *Lab. Anim. Sci.* **33**, 446–450.

Toolan, H.W. (1960) *Science* **131**, 1446–1448.

Toolan, H.W. (1961) *Bull. NY Acad. Med.* **37**, 305–310.

Toolan, H.W. (1966) *Nature* **209**, 833–834.

Toolan, H.W., Dalldorf, G., Barclay, M., Chandra, S. and Moore, A.E. (1960) *Proc. Natl Acad. Sci. USA* **46**, 1256–1258.

Toolan, W., Buttle, G.A.H. and Kay, H.E.M. (1962) *Proc. Am. Assoc. Cancer Res.* **3**, 368.

Tully, J.G. (1986) In: Bhatt, P.N., Jacoby, R.O., Morse, H.C. and New, A.E. (eds) *Viral and Mycoplasmal Infections of Laboratory Rodents*, pp. 63–85. New York: Academic Press.

Tvedten, H.W., Whitehair, C.K. and Langham, R.F. (1973) *J. Am. Vet. Med. Assoc.* **163**, 605–612.

Tyzzer, E.E. (1917) *J. Med. Res.* **37**, 307–338.

Ueno, Y., Sugiyama, F. and Yagami, K. (1996) *Lab. Anim.* **30**, 114–119.

Ueno, Y., Sugiyama, F., Sugiyama, Y., Ohsawa, K., Sato, H. and Yagami, K. (1997) *J. Vet. Med. Sci.* **59**, 265–269.

Vallee, A., Guillon, J.C. and Cayeux, R. (1969) *Bull. Acad. Vet. France* **42**, 797–800.

Van Andel, R.A., Franklin, C.L., Besch-Williford, C.L., Hook, R.R. and Riley, L.K. (1996) *Contemp. Topics* **35**, 67 (abstract).

van Zwieten, M.J., Solleveld, H.A., Lindsey, J.R., de Groot, F.G., Zurcher, C. and Hollander, C.F. (1980) *Lab. Anim. Sci.* **30**, 215–221.

Vogtsberger, L.M., Stronberg, P.C. and Rice, J.M. (1982) *Lab. Anim. Sci.* **32**, 419.

Vonderfecht, S.L., Huber, A.C., Eiden, J., Mader, L.C. and Yolken, R.H. (1984) *J. Virol.* **52**, 94–98.

Vonderfecht, S.L., Eiden, J.J., Miskuff, R.L. and Yolken, R.H. (1985) *J. Clin. Microbiol.* **22**, 726–730.

Vonderfecht, S.L., Eiden, J.J., Miskuff, R.L. and Yolken, R.H. (1988) *J. Clin. Microbiol.* **26**, 216–221.

Waggie, K.S., Spencer, T.H. and Allen, A.M. (1987) *Lab. Anim. Sci.* **37**, 533.

Wagner, M. (1988) *Lab. Anim. Sci.* **38**, 476–478.

Ward, J.M., Lock, A., Collins, M.J., Gonda, M.A. and Reynolds, C.W. (1984) *Lab. Anim.* **18**, 84–89.

Ward, J.M., Anver, M.R., Haines, D.C. *et al.* (1996) *Lab. Anim. Sci.* **46**, 15–20.

Weir, E.C., Brownstein, D.G., Smith, A.L. and Johnson, E.A. (1988) *Lab. Anim. Sci.* **38**, 133–137.

Weir, E.C., Jacoby, R.O., Paturzo, F.X., Johnson, E.A. and Ardito, R.B. (1990) *Lab. Anim. Sci.* **40**, 138–143.

Weisbroth, S.H. (1979) In: Baker, H.J., Lindsey, J.R. and Weisbroth, S.H. (eds) *The Laboratory Rat*, Vol. I, pp. 193–241. New York: Academic Press.

Weisbroth, S.H. and Peress, N. (1977) *Lab. Anim. Sci.* **27**, 466–473.

Weisbroth, S.H. and Scher, S. (1968) *Lab. Anim. Care* **18**, 451–458.

West, W.L., Schofield, J.C. and Bennett, B.T. (1992) *Contemp. Topics Lab. Anim. Sci.* **31**, 7–10.

Will, L.A. (1994) In: Beran, G.W. (ed) *Handbook of Zoonoses Section A: Bacterial, Rickettsial, Chlamydial and Mycotic*, 2nd edn, pp. 231–242. Boca Raton: CRC Press.

Wojcinski, Z.W. and Percy, D.H. (1986) *Vet. Pathol.* **23**, 278–286.

Wolff, H.L. (1950) *Antonie Van Leeuwenhoek* **16**, 105–110.

Wullenweber, M. (1995) *Lab. Anim.* **29**, 1–15.

Yagami, K., Goto, Y., Ishida, J., Ueno, Y., Kajiwara, N. and Sugiyama, F. (1995) *Lab. Anim. Sci.* **45**, 326–328.

Yang, F., Paturzo, F.X., and Jacoby, R.O. (1995) *Lab. Anim. Sci.* **45**, 140–144.

Yoneda, K. and Walzer, P.D. (1980) *Infect. Immun.* **29**, 692–703.

Zucker, T.F. and Zucker, L.M. (1954) *Proc. Soc. Exp. Biol. Med.* **85**, 517–521.

Zurcher, C., Burek, J.D., Van Nunen, M.C.J. and Meihuizen, S.P. (1977) *Lab. Anim. Sci.* **27**, 955–962.

CHAPTER 8

Control of SPF Conditions: FELASA Standards

Ivo Kunstyr
Medizinische Hochschule Hannover, Hannover, Germany

Werner Nicklas
Deutsches Krebsforschungszentrum, Heidelberg, Germany

Introduction

Only experimental animals of a good microbiological quality will give any kind of guarantee of an experiment undisturbed by health hazards. It is for this reason that so-called **'SPF' (or specific pathogen free)** animals are used for animal experiments. Here we focus on 'SPF' rats, although experimental rats of conventional and possibly even **germ-free** hygienic status are also used in research and testing.

Most infectious agents can severely influence experimental results. Therefore the detection and subsequent elimination of infectious agents is essential if improved and more reliable results from animal experiments are to be obtained. At the same time, the use of such animals reduces the number of animals needed and therefore makes an important contribution to animal welfare.

Definition of 'SPF'

The term 'SPF' means that the absence of individually listed microorganisms has been demonstrated for a population by regular monitoring of a sufficient number of animals at appropriate ages by appropriate and accepted methods. 'SPF' animals originate from germ-free animals. These are usually associated with a defined microflora and subsequently lose their **gnotobiotic** status by contact with environmental and human microorganisms. Such animals are bred and housed under conditions that prevent the introduction of unwanted microorganisms, i.e. organisms that have the potential to induce disease in animals (or humans) or which are known to influence the physiological properties of their host and thus the outcome of experiments (Table 8.1). 'SPF' animals are morphologically and

Table 8.1 Possible consequences of infectious agents for experimental animals

- Outbreak of clinically apparent infections, eventually with deadly outcome
- Hazardous for personnel if the agent is zoonotic
- Reduction of the lifespan
- Increase in interindividual variation
- Impact on physiological parameters (immunology, haematology, histomorphology, enzymology, clinical chemistry)
- Modulation of oncogenesis (induction of tumours, reduction of the incidence of tumours, enhancement or suppression of chemical or viral carcinogenesis, altered growth rate of transplantable tumours)

Table 8.2 Potential research complications due to infectious agents in absence of clinical signs

- Changed behaviour
- Suppressed increase in body weight (lower growth rate)
- Reduced life expectancy (changed tumour rate)
- Contamination of samples and tissue specimens (cells, transplantable tumours, sera, monoclonal antibodies)
- Reduced breeding efficacy

physiologically 'normal', well suited for modelling the situation of a human population.

It has to be stressed that most infections in experimental rodents are subclinical. The absence of clinical manifestations therefore has very limited diagnostic value. However, modifications of research results due to natural infections often occur in the absence of clinical disease. Such modifications may be devastating for experiments because they often remain undetected (Table 8.2).

The types of interference of an agent with experimental results may be diverse. As an example, a detailed list of the potential influences of *Kilham rat virus* (KRV), a frequently occurring rat pathogen, on research results is given in Table 8.3 (see also Mossmann *et al.*, 1998). More information about the considerable effects on research due to infectious agents can be found in various review articles (Bhatt *et al.*, 1986; Lussier, 1988; National Research Council, 1991; Hansen, 1994; Mossmann *et al.*, 1998; Baker, 1998; Nicklas *et al.*, 1999).

Most infectious diseases are multifactorial. An infectious agent alone or in insufficient quantities is usually not able to elicit the disease. Support by other factors is necessary. Some factors that can lead to an overt disease are listed in Table 8.4.

The potential clinical consequences of an infection with two of the most frequent bacterial 'intruders' into 'SPF' animal units, *Staphylococcus aureus* and so-called *Pasteurella pneumotropica*, are shown in Figures 8.1 and 8.2.

Requirements for Housing 'SPF' Animals

Certain requirements are necessary to maintain the desired hygienic quality. Physical barriers together with appropriate operating methods aim at preventing contamination with pathogens and penetration by wild rodents. As a consequence, barrier units are not easily accessible for personnel, which is sometimes considered a disadvantage by experimenters. Finally, monitoring programmes help to detect and control potential sources of contamination and may therefore be of crucial importance for the management of a facility housing animals of a good microbiological quality.

Table 8.3 Examples of interference with research: *Kilham rat virus* (KRV)

Immunology
Infection of T and B lymphocytes and suppression of various lymphocyte functions
Stimulation of autoreactive T lymphocytes specific for pancreatic antigens
Altered susceptibility to autoimmune diabetes in rats
Altered cytotoxic lymphocyte activity
Depression of lymphocyte viability and various T cell functions
Stimulation of interferon production

Microbiology
Supports secondary colonization with other microorganisms
Influence on the prevalence of *Yersinia*-induced arthritis in rats
Persistent infection of cell lines

Physiology
Inhibition of lipid formation in rat kidney cells *in vitro*
Increased leukocyte adhesion in the aortic epithelium
Congenital malformation
Death and resorption of fetuses

Oncology
Suppression of leukaemia induction by *Moloney virus*
Contamination of leukaemias or leukaemia virus preparations
Contamination of tumours

Table 8.4 Some factors supporting the infectious agent and leading to an overt disease

- Experimental burden (the experiment itself)
- Physical, social, nutritional stress (environmental influences)
- Emergence of a second (or more) infectious agent (interaction of microorganisms)
- Introduction of a genetically more susceptible animal strain (genetic susceptibility)

Keeping rodents free of pathogens is a much more complex problem in research facilities than in breeding units. It is necessary that all potential sources of infections are considered and evaluated. They have been discussed in more detail by Nicklas (1993).

Risk Factors

Unwanted microorganisms may be introduced into a barrier unit by various routes and materials. The most important sources of infections are infected animals of the same or closely related species (e.g. mice). In addition, biological materials (e.g. cell lines, sera, monoclonal antibodies, transplantable tumours, isolated organs, virus strains or parasites after animal-to-animal passages) may be contaminated (Collins and Parker, 1972; Nicklas *et al.*, 1993a). The contaminating agents may survive for years or decades when contaminated samples are stored frozen or freeze-dried. Therefore, such materials must be included in regular health monitoring programmes to avoid transmission of unwanted

Table 8.5 Rat antibody production test (RAP test) procedure

a) *Specimen:* concentrated and diluted 1:10. In the case of tumour cells repeated freezing and thawing is recommended to destroy tumour cells and avoid tumour growth

b) *Animals:* Virus-antibody-free young rats
per dilution:	4 rats
controls:	2 rats

c) *Inoculation:* 0.5 mL i.p. and 0.05 mL i.n.

d) *Serology*
   28 days post inoculation: bleeding of animals for serology

Abbreviations: i.p., intraperitoneally; i.n., intranasally.

microorganisms. Monitoring is usually done by the rat antibody production test (RAP test). This test is based on the immune response to rat viruses which is stimulated in pathogen- and antibody-free animals if the material injected is contaminated. A short protocol is given in Table 8.5; for more details see Nicklas *et al.* (1993a). The **polymerase chain reaction** (PCR) can also be used to demonstrate the presence or absence of microorganisms in such materials but is more expensive and time consuming to perform.

All additional materials that have been in contact with infected animals may be contaminated and may act as potential **vectors**. However, many of them (e.g. cages, feeders, bottles, etc.) can easily be decontaminated by hygienic procedures or appropriate disinfection.

Another important factor is human contact. Although the risk of transmitting rat pathogens by humans is very low if all personnel (caretakers, technicians, researchers) are properly educated and motivated, in practice pathogens are often transmitted as a consequence of a lack of discipline or thoughtlessness.

Health Monitoring Programme

Aim

The main purpose of health monitoring is to detect or prevent infections which might influence physiological characteristics of animals or their health. Appropriate health monitoring helps to avoid

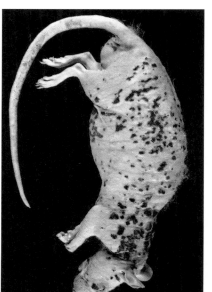

Figure 8.1 Possible consequence of introducing unwanted microorganisms into an animal colony. Multiple scratch wounds due to intradermal abscesses caused by *Staphylococcus aureus* in an *rnu/rnu* rat.

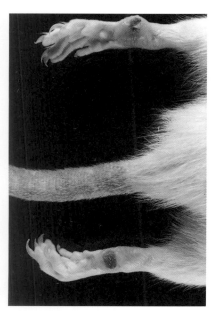

Figure 8.2 Possible consequence of introducing unwanted microorganisms into an animal colony. Pododermatitis in an older rat due to infection by *Pasteurella pneumotropica.*

imprecise results and allows all the experiments necessary to be carried out with a minimum number of animals. In contrast to troubleshooting, which means an *ad hoc* search and identification of unknown causes of abnormalities in an experiment, health monitoring describes a scheduled programme for monitoring the microbiological status of an animal population. The health monitoring programme aims at determining the microbiological status of a population before and during an experiment through regular and repeated examination and monitoring for previously defined, known infectious agents. Another aim of health monitoring is prevention of the introduction of unwanted organisms.

As the major risk factor, the animal remains the main target of the monitoring laboratory. We must emphasize that all diseased or dead animals should be examined in addition to regular and scheduled monitoring of clinically healthy animals. They are a valuable source of information about the hygienic status of the colony.

The Federation of the European Laboratory Animal Science Associations (FELASA) publish recommendations dealing with health monitoring of either breeding colonies or experimental units (Kraft *et al.*, 1994; Rehbinder *et al.*, 1996). In experimental units in particular, the monitoring programme will differ between institutions or between different units of the same facility in its dependence on (a) research objectives, (b) physical conditions and the layout of the animal house, (c) husbandry methods, (d) sources of animals, (e) staff quantity and qualification, (f) diagnostic laboratory support, (g) finances. An overview on monitoring of experimental rodent colonies has been given by Nicklas (1996).

Sentinels

In most experimental units, animals of appropriate ages will not always be available for random sampling to monitor the microbiological status. Furthermore, diverse special experimental animals – transgenic, **immunodeficient**, pretreated – which are only available in small quantities, have been used increasingly during recent years. The use of **sentinel animals** is therefore advisable. Sentinels are animals from a breeding colony of known hygienic status (negative for all known pathogens) which aid in the evaluation of the microbiological status of the colony. They must be housed in the population to be monitored for a sufficiently long time (minimum of

4–6 weeks) in order to develop detectable antibody titres or parasitic stages. Sentinels should be kept in such a way that they receive maximum exposure to potential infections (on bottom shelves of different racks within an animal room, open cages, use of 'dirty bedding') (National Research Council, 1991).

Number and Age of Animals to be Monitored

A sufficient number of animals has to be monitored to obtain relevant information on a given population. Clearly, infections with an attack rate of 50% or more (*Sendai virus*, *Rat coronavirus/sialodacryoadenitis virus*, RCV/SDAV) require far fewer animals to detect their presence than infections with low attack rates.

It has been recommended by the ILAR Committee on Long-term Holding of Laboratory Rodents (1976) that at least eight randomly sampled animals should be monitored, which is (theoretically) sufficient to detect an infection with a 95% probability if at least 30% of a population is infected. The formula which can be used to calculate the number of animals for an estimated prevalence rate is given in Table 8.6.

In breeding units these animals should be at least 10 weeks old, which ensures that they have reached immunological maturity and had sufficient time to develop detectable antibody titres or parasitic stages (e.g. worm eggs). For experimental units, the time animals have been housed in the unit to be monitored may be more important than their age. As already mentioned for the sentinel animals, they should have been housed in the respective population for a minimum of 4–6 weeks before serological monitoring is conducted.

According to the FELASA recommendations two additional weanlings should be monitored because they may be better suited for the detection of specific parasites or bacterial pathogens than older animals.

Frequency of Monitoring

Monitoring must be performed on a regular basis to detect unwanted microorganisms in good time. The recommended frequency is every 12 weeks. Most commercial breeders test more frequently (e.g. every 6 weeks). In most multipurpose experimental units animals are regularly bought and introduced

Table 8.6 Calculation of the number of animals to be monitored

Assumption
1) both sexes are infected at the same rate
2) population size > 100 animals
3) random sampling

$$\frac{\log 0.05}{\log N} = \text{no. of animals}$$

N = percentage noninfected
0.05 = 95% confidence limit

No. of animals required to detect an infection

Suspected prevalence rate (%)	Confidence limit		
	95%	99%	99.9%
1	299	459	688
2	149	228	324
3	99	152	227
5	59	90	135
10	29	44	66
20	14	21	31
30	9	13	20
40	6	9	14
50	5	7	10

Example: Nine animals should be monitored to have at least one positive animal if the suspected prevalence rate of an infection is 30% (confidence level: 95%).

into a facility. It may, in such cases, be reasonable to test with a higher frequency (e.g. 3–5 animals every 4–6 weeks instead of 10 every three months) as this will result in the earlier detection of an infection (Kunstyr, 1992).

Agents

For each facility or even for every single unit within a facility, the agents that are acceptable must be defined. Besides FELASA (Kraft et al, 1994), various other organizations (Kunstyr, 1988; National Research Council, 1991; Waggie et al, 1994) have published similar lists of microorganisms which should be monitored for in routine programmes. The list will usually be restricted to organisms that pose a threat to animals (or humans) or organisms which are known to affect experiments and that can be eliminated. However,

infections in immunodeficient animals frequently result in increased mortality due to reduced or lack of resistance to weakly pathogenic or even saprophytic microorganisms. It may therefore be necessary to include organisms with low pathogenicity in a monitoring protocol for immunodeficient animals.

On the other hand, some pathogens of laboratory rats have disappeared during domestication or **gnotobiotic** derivation (e.g. *Francisella tularensis*, *Leptospira* sp., *Rickettsia* sp., *Spirillum minus*) and are less likely to infect laboratory animals housed behind barriers. Some parasites (e.g. most **cestodes**) need an intermediate host not found in barrier units. Monitoring for these agents may therefore be less urgent or even unnecessary and may be performed less frequently. FELASA recommends testing once a year for such agents, i.e. agents of lower priority (Kraft et al, 1994). Some of the most important bacteria, fungi and parasites for which rats should be monitored are given in Table 8.7.

Table 8.7 Some of the most common bacteria, fungi and parasites infecting laboratory rats

1) Bacteria	2) Mycoplasmas
Actinobacillus sp.	Mycoplasma pulmonis
Bordetella bronchiseptica	Mycoplasma arthriditis
CAR bacillus	
Clostridium piliforme	3) Fungi
Corynebacterium kutscheri	Microsporum sp.
Haemophilus sp.	Trichophyton sp.
Helicobacter sp.	Yeasts
Klebsiella pneumoniae	Pneumocystis carinii
Klebsiella oxytoca	
Listeria monocytogenes/ivanovii	4) Parasites (all parasites)
Pasteurella multocida	Aspiculuris tetraptera
Pasteurella pneumotropica	Syphacia muris
Other Pasteurellaceae	Trichosomoides crassicauda
Pseudomonas aeruginosa	Hymenolepis sp.
Salmonella sp.	Spironucleus muris
Staphylococcus aureus	Coccidia
Streptobacillus moniliformis	Giardia sp.
Streptococcus pneumoniae	Trichomonads
β-Haemolytic streptococci	Amoebae
Yersinia pseudotuberculosis	Demodex sp.
	Notoedres sp.
Others if associated with lesions or	Polyplax spinulosa
clinical signs	
Streptobacillus moniliformis	Radfordia ensifera
	and others

Methods

In general, the examination methods are: (a) necropsy – following after sacrifice, (b) serology, (c) bacteriology and (d) parasitology. Most of these methods are described in special publications (Feldman and Seely, 1988; Kunstyr, 1992; Owen, 1992; Kraft *et al.*, 1994) and in various textbooks. Reliable results are only obtained if appropriate and sufficiently sensitive methods are used for health monitoring. It is therefore evident that the methods must be adapted to the actual 'state of art', i.e. to introduce new proven methods as they become available.

Microscopic methods such as stereomicroscopy are commonly used for monitoring for ectoparasite sites. Adhesive tape, flotation or direct microscopy of wet mounts taken from the intestinal tract are used for detection of endoparasites.

A number of new organisms have emerged during recent years and are not included in existing lists. A number of Pasteurellaceae that have not yet been definitely classified seem to infect rats, in addition to the only known species, *Pasteurella pneumotropica* (Nicklas *et al.*, 1993b). Several *Helicobacter* species have been isolated recently from rats, such as *H. muridarum* (Lee *et al.*, 1992), *H. hepaticus* (Fox *et al.*, 1994; Riley *et al.*, 1996), *H. bilis* (Fox *et al.*, 1995; Riley *et al.*, 1996), *H. trogontum* (Mendes *et al.*, 1996). A rat parvovirus has also been detected (Ueno *et al.*, 1995, 1997; Jacoby *et al.*, 1996) in addition to those parvoviruses already known (*Kilham rat virus, Toolan's H-1 virus*). Other organisms, such as *Clostridium piliforme*, have been renamed recently (Duncan *et al.*, 1993), which leads to some confusion in those scientists who are not sufficiently familiar with health monitoring of laboratory rats.

Table 8.8 Acceptable serological methods to test for common rat pathogens

	Acceptable methods
Viruses	
RCV/SDAV	IIF, ELISA
KRV	HI, ELISA, IIF
H-1	HI, ELISA, IIF
PVM	ELISA, IIF, HI
Reo 3	ELISA, IIF
Sendai	ELISA, IIF, HI
TMEV (GD VII)	ELISA, IIF, HI
Mouse adenovirus	ELISA, IIF
LCMV	ELISA, IIF
Hantaan virus	ELISA, IIF
Bacteria	
Mycoplasma pulmonis	ELISA, IIF
Mycoplasma arthritidis	ELISA,
Clostridium piliforme	ELISA, IIF
CAR bacillus	ELISA, IIF
Unexpected results should be confirmed by alternative methods (serology, virus isolation).	

Abbreviations: IIF, indirect immunofluorescence assay; HI, haemagglutination inhibition assay; ELISA, enzyme-linked immunosorbent assay.

Monitoring for bacteria is usually done by culture methods. However, serology or PCR may in some cases be superior or the only reliable approaches (e.g. for *Streptobacillus moniliformis*, *Clostridium piliforme* or *Mycoplasma pulmonis*) (van Kuppeveld et al., 1993; Goto and Itoh, 1994).

Monitoring for viral infections is primarily done by serological methods. PCR, as an example of a new method, might be applicable in the case of acute infections (clinical disease) or for agents causing persistent infections (e.g. parvoviruses under specific conditions; Gaertner et al., 1995; Besselsen et al., 1995). However, the lack of macroscopical changes during necropsy or lack of histopathological changes are still commonly used as the sole basis for declaring a population negative for a specific organism. This must be considered insufficient and unacceptable.

Serological methods must be selected properly as they may differ in their sensitivity and specificity (Smith, 1986; Lussier, 1991). Unexpected serological results should always be confirmed by an independent method or, preferably, by virus isolation or

antigen detection in order to avoid false-positive results. Some acceptable serological methods for the most common viral and some bacterial pathogens are given in Table 8.8.

Health Report

A health status report is usually requested and necessary when animals are shipped from breeders or between scientific institutions. It must contain sufficient data to provide reliable information on the quality of a population. Usually, each animal facility or breeder has its own style of report sheets which are sometimes difficult to read and to interpret. The FELASA (Kraft et al., 1994; Rehbinder et al., 1996) recommends using a uniform health report for breeding and for experimental colonies. Some additional information might be reasonable (e.g. housing conditions, treatment) and should be included. Table 8.9 gives a checklist of the basic information that should be included in a health status report.

Table 8.9 Information which should be included in a health report when animals are shipped to external colonies

- Exact location (designation) of the colony
- Housing conditions (conventional, barrier, isolator)
- Name(s) of laboratory/ies involved in monitoring
- Date of restocking/rederivation of the colony
- Date of last monitoring
- No. of animals monitored since date of restocking or during the last 12 months
- Methods used (clinical signs, microscopy, microbiological culture, serology)
- Name(s) of pathogens detected in the colony
- Name(s) of pathogens not detected in the colony
- Treatment, vaccination, etc.

Detailed results of the last monitoring should be added.

References

Baker, D.G. (1998) *Clin. Microbiol. Rev.* **11**, 231–266.

Besselsen, D.G., Besch-Williford, C.L., Pintel, D.J., Frankin, C.L., Hook, R.R. and Riley, L.K. (1995) *J Clin. Microbiol.* **33**, 1699–1703.

Bhatt, P.N., Jacoby, R.O., Morse, H.C. and New, A. (eds) (1986) *Viral and Mycoplasma Infections of Laboratory Rodents: Effects on Biomedical Research.* New York: Academic Press.

Collins, M.J. and Parker, J.C. (1972) *J. Natl Cancer Inst.* **49**, 1139–1143.

Duncan, A.J., Carmen R.J., Olsen, G.J. and Wilson K.H. (1993) *Int. J. Syst. Bacteriol.* **43**, 314–318.

Feldman, D.B. and Seely, J.C. (1988) *Necropsy Guide: Rodents and the Rabbit.* Boca Raton, FL: CRC Press.

Fox, J.G., Dewhirst, F.E., Tully, J.G. *et al.* (1994) *J. Clin. Microbiol.* **32**, 1238–1245.

Fox, J.G., Yan, L., Dewhirst, F.E. *et al.* (1995) *J. Clin. Microbiol.* **33**, 445–454.

Gaertner, D.J., Jacoby, R.O., Paturzo, F.X. and Smith, A.L. (1995) *Lab. Anim. Sci.* **45**, 249–253.

Goto, K. and Itoh, T. (1994) *Jikken Dobutsu* **43**, 389–394.

Hansen, A.K. (1994) In: Svendsen, P. and Hau, J. (eds) *Handbook of Laboratory Animal Science*, Vol. 1, pp. 125–153. Boca Raton, FL: CRC Press.

ILAR Committee on Long-term Holding of Laboratory Rodents (1976) Long-term holding of laboratory rodents. *ILAR News* **XIX** (4), L1–L25.

Jacoby, R.O., Ball-Goodrich, L.J., Besselsen, D.G., McKisic, M.D., Riley, L.K. and Smith, A.L. (1996) *Lab. Anim. Sci.* **46**, 370–380.

Kraft, V., Deeny, A.A., Blanchet, H.M. *et al.* (1994) *Lab. Anim.* **28**, 1–12.

Kunstyr, I. (ed.) (1988) *List of Pathogens for Specification in SPF Laboratory Animals.* Society for Laboratory Animal Science Publication No. 2, Biberach.

Kunstyr, I. (ed.) (1992) *Diagnostic Microbiology for Laboratory Animals*, GV-SOLAS Vol. 11. Stuttgart: Gustav Fischer.

Lee, A., Phillips, M.W., O'Rourke, J.L. *et al.* (1992) *Int. J. Syst. Bacteriol.* **42**, 27–36.

Lussier, G. (1988) *Vét. Res. Contrib.* **12**, 199–217.

Lussier, G. (ed.) (1991) *Lab. Anim Sci.* **41**, 199–225.

Mendes, E.N., Queirez, D.M.M., Dewhirst, F.E., Paster, B.J., Moura, S.B. and Fox, J.G. (1996) *Int. J. Syst. Bacteriol.* **46**, 916–921.

Mossmann, H., Nicklas, W. and Hedrich, H.J. (1998) In: Kaufmann, S.H.E. and Kabelitz, D. (eds) *Methods in Microbiology*, Vol. 25, *Immunology of Infection*, pp. 109–188. San Diego, CA: Academic Press.

National Research Council, Committee on Infectious Diseases of Mice and Rats (1991) *Infectious Diseases of Mice and Rats.* Washington DC: National Academy Press.

Nicklas, W. (1993) *Scand. J. Lab. Anim. Sci.* **20**, 53–60.

Nicklas, W. (1996) *Scand. J. Lab. Anim. Sci.* **23**, 69–75.

Nicklas, W., Homberger, F.R., Illgen-Wilcke, B. *et al.* (1999) *Lab. Anim.* **33**, Supps. 1, S1: 39–51: 87.

Nicklas, W., Kraft, V. and Meyer, B. (1993a) *Lab. Anim. Sci.* **43**, 296–300.

Nicklas, W., Staut, M. and Benner, A. (1993b) *Zentralbl. Bakt.* **279**, 114–124.

Owen, D.G. (1992) *Parasites of Laboratory Animals*, Laboratory Animal Handbooks No. 12. London: Laboratory Animals.

Rehbinder, C., Baneux, P., Forbes, D. *et al.* (1996) *Lab. Anim.* **30**, 193–208.

Riley, L.K., Franklin, C.L., Hook, R.R. and Besch-Williford, C. (1996) *J. Clin. Microbiol.* **34**, 942–946.

Smith, A.L. (1986) In: Bhatt, P.N. *et al.* (eds) *Viral and*

Mycoplasmal Infections of Laboratory Rodents, pp. 731–749. Orlando, FL: Academic Press.

Ueno, Y., Sugiyama, F. and Yagami, K. (1995) *Lab. Anim.* **30**, 14–19.

Ueno, Y., Sugiyama, F., Sugiyama Y, Ohsama, Y., Sato, H. and Yagami, K. (1997) *J. Vet. Med. Sci.* **59**, 265–269.

van Kuppeveld, F.J.M., Melchers, W.J.G., Willemse,

H.F.M., Kissing, J., Galama, J.M.D. and van der Logt, J.T.M. (1993) *J. Clin. Microbiol.* **31**, 524–527.

Waggie, K., Kagiyama, N., Allen, A.M. and Nomura, T. (eds) (1994) *Manual of Microbiologic Monitoring of Laboratory Animals*, 2nd edn. U.S. Department of Human Health and Human Services, NIH Publication No. 94-2498.

PART 4

Reproduction and Breeding

Contents

CHAPTER 9

Physiology of Reproduction

Kei-ichiro Maeda
Graduate School of Bioagricultural Sciences, Nagoya University,
Nagoya 484–8601, Japan

Satoshi Ohkura
Primate Research Institute, Kyoto University,
Aichi 484–8506, Japan

Hiroko Tsukamura
Graduate School of Bioagricultural Sciences, Nagoya University,
Nagoya 464–8601, Japan

Introduction

The rat is one of the most popular experimental animals for studying reproductive physiology. One of the advantages of using rats rather than other animals, such as sheep and monkeys, in which the physiology of reproduction has been intensively investigated, is that they have much shorter reproductive cycles compared with larger animals. Stages such as puberty, the estrous cycle, pregnancy and lactation are all much shorter. In addition, rats display various types of estrous cycle, such as estrous cycle with luteal phase or spontaneous ovulation, when they receive certain stimuli. This is another advantage of using the rat as a model for other mammals in experiments in reproduction. This chapter reviews the characteristics of reproduction in the rat.

Sexual Differentiation

Sexual Differentiation of Reproductive Organs

As in other mammalian species, the **default sex** in the rat is the female. The *SRY* gene on the Y chromosome is a testis-determining gene in humans and mice (George and Wilson, 1994), but there have been few reports on the role of the testis-determining gene in rats. The gonadal ridge has developed by day 13 when the ridge contains primordial germ cells in both sexes (Hebel and Stromberg, 1986). Primordial germ cells derived from outside the embryo proper migrate and reach the genital ridge (tissue covering the ventral area of the primitive kidney, called mesonephros). The tissue becomes oogonia in the female or prospermatogonia in the male, and then finally forms the ovary or testis (Huckins and Clermont, 1968).

It has been well established that gonadotropin-releasing hormone (GnRH) neurons derive from the embryonic olfactory placode and migrate caudally to the hypothalamus in various animal species, including birds and mammals. In rats, GnRH neurons appear in the olfactory placode on day 13.5 of pregnancy and go on to migrate caudally to the septum/preoptic area by day 17 of pregnancy (Jennes, 1989; Daikoku-Ishido et al., 1990). The fetal hypothalamus contains radioimmunoassayable GnRH by gestational day 15 in the rat. Luteinizing hormone (LH) and follicle-stimulating hormone (FSH) can first be detected in the fetal pituitary around gestational days 15–19. The LH receptor content in the testis starts to increase from around gestational day 15.5 and reaches its maximum around the time of birth. The number of interstitial cells and testosterone content increases coincidentally with the rise in LH receptors in the testis. The fetal rise in testosterone secretion is quite important for the induction of sexual differentiation of the brain as described below.

The müllerian duct starts to degenerate in the male fetus and the wolffian duct degenerates in the female on day 17 of gestation (Hebel and Stromberg, 1986). The degeneration of the müllerian duct in the male is induced by the antimüllerian hormone, which is a 145 kDa dimeric protein (Picard and Josso, 1984; Picard et al., 1986; Haqq et al., 1992). In the male rat, immunoreactive antimüllerian hormone protein and mRNA are first detected in the immature Sertoli cells when sex cords begin to differentiate at day 13–14 of gestation (Tran et al., 1987; Hirobe et al., 1992). The immunoreactivity of the antimüllerian hormone in the Sertoli cells peaks between days 15 and 17, then decreases and is not detectable 9 days after birth. Testosterone formation coincides with the spermatogenic cord and fetal Leidig cell differentiation in the male rat (George and Wilson, 1994). Testosterone and its reduced metabolite, 5α-dihydrotestosterone, have separate roles in the muscularization of the reproductive organ (Wilson and Lasnitzki, 1971; Schultz and Wilson, 1974; George and Wilson, 1994). In the male rat, testosterone is responsible for the **virilization** of the wolffian duct. On the other hand, 5α-dihydrotestosterone is responsible for the virilization of the anlage of the prostate and external genitalia; 5α-reductase activity is high in these organs during the development of the wolffian duct. The female urogenital tract, however, develops from the müllerian duct in the absence of gonads.

The sex of the neonatal rats can be determined by visual observation, comparing the distance between the external genitalia and anus immediately after birth. The distance is larger in the male than the female. It is sometimes difficult to identify the sex immediately after birth but comparison of this distance in all the pups in a litter make sex identification easier. The difference in the distance becomes much bigger as the pups grow up and is more obvious after their hair starts to grow because the external genitalia and anus are separated by hair in the male but not in the female.

Sexual Differentiation of the Brain

The sexual differentiation of the brain has been well established in the rat, because the critical period continues into the neonatal period in this species. The critical period for sexual differentiation of the brain is 7–9 days after birth: administration of testosterone to a female neonate by this time inhibits the proestrous LH surge and **lordosis** behavior in adulthood, indicating defeminization of the brain (Davis et al., 1995; Diaz et al., 1995). Androgenized females exhibit persistent estrus with many matured follicles in their ovaries primarily because of the absence of the LH surge and then ovulation. Defeminization of the brain is induced by estrogen, which is produced from testosterone locally by the brain aromatase, since defeminization of the brain is also induced by neonatal estrogen treatment but not by dihydrotestosterone (DHT), which is nonaromatizable testosterone. Aromatase has been found in various areas of the male rat brain (Shinoda, 1994). Localization of estrogen receptors and aromatase correlate well (Kawata, 1995; Hayashi, S. et al., 1997). The fetus is protected from maternal estrogen by an elaborate system as described later.

Sexual dimorphic nuclei (SDN) were first identified in the preoptic area in the rat brain (Nelson, 1995). Then, they were found in various other areas of the brain (Figure 9.1), including the olfactory bulb, preoptic/septal regions, hypothalamus, limbic system including the amygdala (Arai, 1981; Segovia

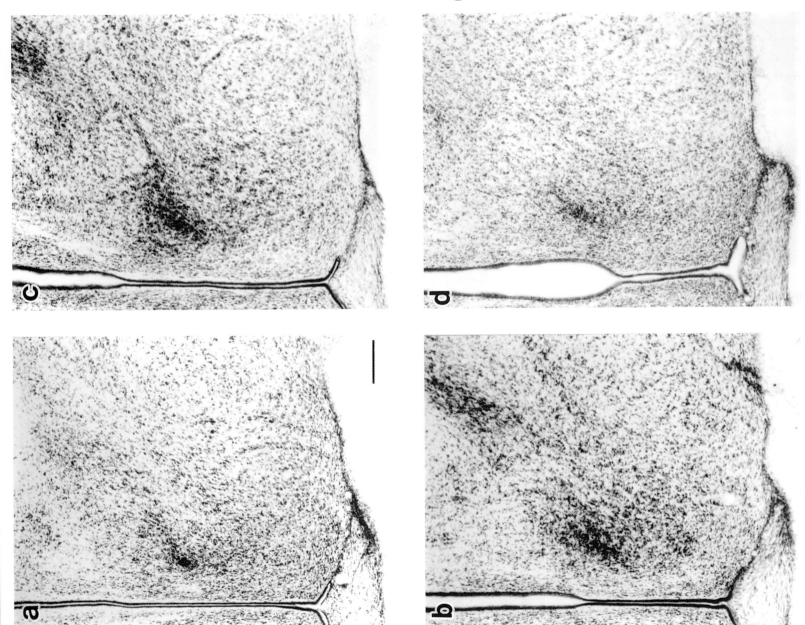

Figure 9.1. Sexual dimorphic nucleus (SDN) in the preoptic area (POA) in 10-day-old female (a) and male (b) rats. The medial preoptic nucleus (MPN) is one of the SDNs in the brain and its size is determined by the perinatal hormonal condition. The MPN is larger in the male rat (b) than in the female (a). Testosterone propionate injections into the female neonate for 9 days after birth (c) make the nucleus larger than that of the control female. The size decreases in the castrated male rat immediately after birth compared with the control male (d). Scale bar = 100 μm. Courtesy of Drs M. Yokosuka and S. Hayashi of the Tokyo Metropolitan Institute of Neurosciences.

and Guillamon, 1993) with different sizes and synaptic organization between the genders. Aromatase activity and androgen receptors in various brain regions during adulthood are also sexually differentiated by neonatal steroid treatment, with higher activity in the male than the female (Roselli and Klosterman, 1998). Recent studies indicate that maternal progesterone plays an important role in brain sexual differentiation, because a numerous number of progesterone receptors are found in the neonatal male rat but not in the female (Wagner et al., 1998).

Mechanisms Protecting Sexual Differentiation from Maternal Estrogen

The fetus is considered to be protected from the vast amount of maternal estrogen secreted from the ovary by a fetus-specific estrogen-binding protein, α-fetoprotein, which is synthesized by the perinatal rat liver in both sexes (MacLusky and Naftolin, 1981; Toran-Allerand, 1984). The protein binds to estrogen but not to androgen, so that androgen secreted from fetal testis enters the brain freely. On the other hand, the maternal estrogen is trapped by the α-fetoprotein in the fetal blood and does not act on the perinatal tissues. However, some artificial estrogenic substances, such as diethylstilbesterol (DES), do not bind well to α-fetoprotein, so they may affect the morphological development or sexual differentiation of the brain and then change the physiology and behavior in adulthood.

Puberty

Puberty in the Male

The development of the reproductive organs in males was extensively investigated by Suzuki in the early 1950s using Wistar strain animals (Suzuki, 1952, 1954a,b; Sakuma, 1997). Sperm first appear in the testis at day 20–30 after birth and 100% of animals contain testicular sperm at day 70. In the tail of the epididymis, some males contain sperm at around day 40 and almost all animals do so by day 90. The relative weights of the testis and epididymis reach their peak value at around day 70. Testicular weight is around 1% at 50 days after birth, the time of puberty.

The rapid increase in testicular weight during the peripubertal period is suggested as being due to an increase in the number of follicle-stimulating hormone (FSH) receptors in the Sertoli cells (Ojeda and Urbanski, 1994). Both FSH and testosterone stimulate FSH receptor number. The number of androgen receptors in the Sertoli cells markedly increases from postnatal day 10–20 to 35–60 after birth, during which puberty occurs, suggesting that androgen plays an important role in puberty in the male.

Descent of the testes occurs at around day 30–60. The penis of the male rat looks similar to the clitoris of the female and the glans of the penis is difficult to expose by 30 days after birth. The shape of the penis shows the 'V type' at this stage (Figure 9.2) (Suzuki, 1954b). The 'W type' of the penis is a transient type from V to U type. The W or U type of the penis first appears at around day 20–30 and 100% of the animals show these types at around day 70 after birth. The relative weight of the sexual accessories (total weight of the coagulating and prostate glands and seminal vesicle) starts to increase at around day 70 when testis and penis developments reach their peak (Figure 9.3).

The hypothalamic levels of GnRH continue to increase during postnatal development and even during adulthood (Ojeda and Urbanski, 1994). There are considerable discrepancies in previous reports on LH secretion during postnatal development, probably because LH is secreted in a pulsatile manner. On the other hand, puberty in the male rat has been reported to be associated with an increase in FSH secretion. Serum FSH concentration reaches its maximum level at around 30–40 days of age.

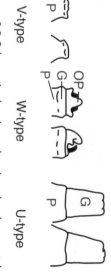

Figure 9.2 Schematic drawings showing developmental changes in the penis in prepubertal male rats. The V type of penis changes to the U type, which is the mature state. The W type is a transient type, which first appears at 20–30 days after birth. P, praeputium; OP, os priapi; G, glans penis. Adapted from Suzuki (1954b).

Puberty in the Female

Puberty in the female rat is associated with the vaginal opening and first proestrus. Vaginal opening

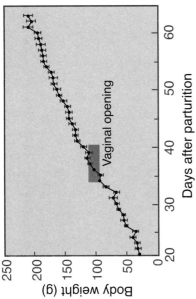

Figure 9.4 Change in body weight related to vaginal opening in the female rat. Vaginal opening occurs around 33–42 days of age (horizontal shaded bar) with the body weight more than 100 g.

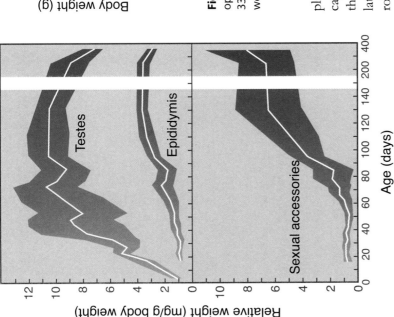

Figure 9.3 Changes in the relative weight of the testes, epididymis and sexual accessories (total weight of the coagulating and prostate glands and seminal vesicle) after birth. Solid lines and shaded area show the means and standard deviations. Adapted from Suzuki (1954a).

usually occurs around 33–42 days after birth with the body weight just above 100 g (Figure 9.4). In the female rat, the first nucleated cells in the vaginal smear are usually observed after vaginal opening with a body weight of approximately 120 g at around 35–40 days after birth. The animal starts to show regular estrous cycles about one week after the vaginal opening. It seems that the timings of the vaginal opening and first proestrus are much more dependent on body weight than the time after birth. There is a big difference in growth rates between the pups in a litter. Pups with rapid growth have an earlier vaginal opening and first proestrus than those with slow growth.

The secretion of gonadotropin, especially FSH, increases immediately after birth, reaching its maximum by day 12, and then gradually decreases (Ojeda and Urbanski, 1994). GnRH contents in the hypothalamus continuously increase from the time of birth until puberty. LH profiles during postnatal development are not so evident as FSH, but the moderately elevated LH levels are interrupted by sporadic surge-like release.

Ovariectomy in infant female rats elevates the plasma LH level but estrogen treatment is not capable of reducing the hormone level because of the high level of α-fetoprotein present in the circulation. Aromatizable androgens seem to play a major role in the feedback regulation of gonadotropin secretion before the α-fetoprotein level shows a marked decrease between days 12 and 28 of age (Ojeda and Urbanski, 1994). After 20 days of age, the proestrous estrogen level is sufficient to induce an LH surge. The magnitude of the estrogen-induced surge increases by days 30–32 of age. The estrogen-induced surge at this period is very similar to that in the first estrus, suggesting that the positive feedback system matures during this period.

Neuroendocrine Mechanism Governing Puberty

The physiological mechanism of puberty in the rat has been intensively investigated. The 'gonadostat theory' has been proposed in order to explain the physiological mechanism underlying puberty, because prepubertal gonadectomy induces a rise in the gonadotropin secretion in both genders (Ramirez and McCann, 1963, 1965). The hypothesis proposes that the sensitivity of the GnRH-releasing system to estrogen feedback action is high before puberty, so that the basal level of estrogen strongly suppresses GnRH/LH secretion. Sensitivity decreases toward puberty and then GnRH/LH release increases around puberty.

Other investigators disagree with this hypothesis, since the sensitivity to estrogen feedback action changes after the first proestrous surge. They put more emphasis on the mechanism in the brain itself than the feedback action of ovarian steroids. Ojeda and Urbanski (1994) have reviewed in detail the central mechanism governing the onset of puberty in the rat.

Spermatogenesis and Testicular Functions

Spermatozoa

The process of spermatozoa production in the testes is called spermatogenesis. Spermatozoa in rodents are longer than those of the other mammalian species, including humans and common domestic animals (Setchell, 1984), and are approximately 150–200 mm long in the rat. The rat sperm head is a hook-shaped, as in other rodents (Eddy and O'Brien, 1994) (Figure 9.5).

Spermatogenesis

A considerable body of knowledge has been built up about spermatogenesis in the rat (Russell et al., 1990; de Kretser and Kerr, 1994; Sharpe, 1994). Primodial germ cells that have ceased to migrate are surrounded by Sertoli cells and a prominent basement membrane in the seminiferous tubules in the male sex cord. The male gonocytes remain inactive until just before puberty, which is around 50 days after birth. At that stage they start to divide and become spermatogonia; they then continue to divide until the animal loses its ability to produce spermatozoa.

The spermatogonia are roughly classified into three types: A, intermediate and B types (Figure 9.5) (Clermont, 1962; Sharpe, 1994). Type A spermatogonia are further subdivided into type A0 (also called stem cells) and types A1–A4. Type A0 spermatogonia remain on the basement membrane of the seminiferous tubules and have the ability to divide into two daughter cells, one of which becomes A1 spermatogonia, which continue further in the process of spermatogenesis, while the other remains as a stem cell. In the rat, A1 spermatogonia then divide six mitotic divisions, and they subsequently become **preleptotene** spermatocytes. The spermatocytes are then in the meiotic phase, during which they develop through **leptotene, zygotene** and **pachytene** to become a secondary spermatocyte in the adluminal component of the Sertoli cell in the seminiferous tubule. During this meiotic phase, each spermatocyte becomes one of four haploid spermatids, which then enter the acrosomal phase, during which the acrosome develops. Nuclear condensation and elongation takes place next, followed by the phase of cytoplasmic elimination and release.

In the rat, 14 stages of the spermatogenic cycle are recognized in the seminiferous tubule (Figure 9.6). The tubule has a segmental arrangement, and each cross-section of the tubule shows a homogeneous stage involving four or five generations of germ cells in synchrony (Figure 9.5) (Perey et al., 1961; Sharpe, 1994). The seminiferous tubule in the rat is well characterized by this segmental structure, while that in the human and other common domestic animals usually shows a mosaic pattern of several stages. In the rat, it takes 12 days to complete one cycle consisting of these 14 stages. A spermatogonium in the rat needs four cycles to finally form spermatozoa, so that 48 days are required to complete the whole spermatogenic step.

Hormonal Control of Spermatogenesis

The hormonal control of spermatogenesis has been reviewed in detail by Sharpe (1994). Spermatogenesis is initiated at the time of puberty because of an increased secretion of gonadotropins (FSH and LH) from the anterior pituitary. FSH was thought to be an essential hormone for the induction of spermatogenesis and to stimulate directly the seminiferous tubule, because complete spermatogenesis in hypophysectomized rats is restored by FSH treatment in combination with either LH or testosterone. On the other hand, the effect on spermatogenesis of LH, sometimes called the interstitial cell stimulating hormone (ICSH) in the male because of its androgenic action on Leydig cells in the interstitium, is considered to be mediated by androgen, at least in the rat. In this context, LH secretion also stimulates testosterone synthesis in Leydig cells in the testis.

FSH action on spermatogenesis is probably mediated by the Sertoli cells, since peptide hormones cannot directly reach the spermatocytes

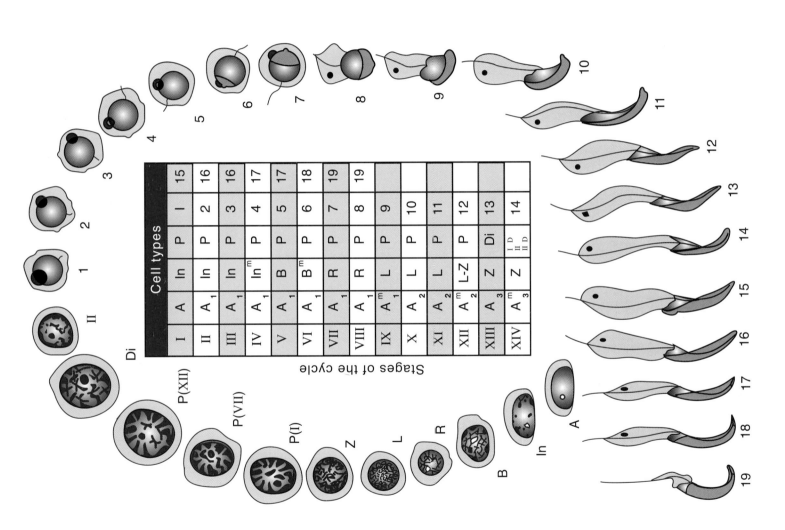

Cell types				Stages of the cycle
A	In	P	15	I
A$_1$	In	P	16	II
A$_1$	In	P	16	III
A$_1$	In^m	P	17	IV
A$_1$	B	P	17	V
A$_1$	B^m	P	18	VI
A$_1$	R	P	19	VII
A$_1$	R	P	19	VIII
A$^m_1$	L	P	9	IX
A$_2$	L	P	10	X
A$_2$	L	P	11	XI
A$^m_2$	L-Z	P	12	XII
A$_3$	Z	Di	13	XIII
A$^m_3$	Z	$^{I\ D}_{II\ D}$	14	XIV

Figure 9.5 Stage of the cell cycle in rat spermatogenesis, starting clockwise from the lower left. A, type A spermatogonium; In, intermediate type spermatogonium; B, type B spermatogonium; R, resting primary spermatocyte; L, leptotene spermatocyte; Z, zygotene spermatocyte; P(I), P(VII), P(XII), early, mid and late pachytene spermatocytes. The Roman numerals indicate the stage of the cycle at which they are found; Di, diplotene; II, secondary spermatocyte; 1–19, steps of spermiogenesis. The table in the center gives the vellular composition of the stages of the cycles of the seminiferous epithelium (I–XIV). The superscript m indicates the occurrence of mitosis. Adapted from Clermont with slight modification (1962).

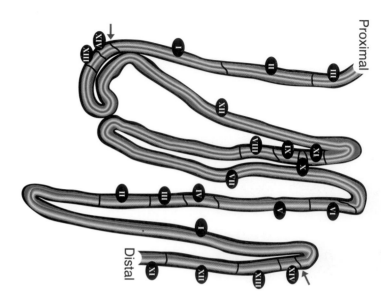

Figure 9.6 The rat seminiferous cycle distributed along the tubule. Two arrows indicate the limits of the seminiferous wave, the borderlines between segments XIV and I. Adapted from Perey et al. (1961).

and spermatids across the blood–testis barrier, which is formed during the 16–19th days post partum (de Kretser and Kerr, 1994). In contrast, testosterone can easily cross the blood–testis barrier by diffusion (and probably also by some transporting system). It has been reported that the testosterone level in the interstitial fluid (more than 50 ng/mL) in the adult rat is much higher than that in the testicular (around 30 ng/mL) or peripheral venous fluid (less than 10 ng/mL), suggesting a paracrine or autocrine action of testosterone on spermatogenesis in the testes (Sharpe, 1994). The existence of androgen receptors in germ cells is still controversial, while the receptors are found in Leydig cells, peritubular cells, Sertoli cells, and the muscular layer of most arteries in the rat testis. It is, therefore, suggested that the testosterone action on spermatogenesis is probably mediated by the latter. One of the roles for Sertoli cells is the production of androgen-binding protein, which is stimulated by FSH and testosterone. It has also been suggested that some unknown factor(s) secreted from Sertoli cells, in response to FSH and testosterone stimulation, might be involved in spermatogenesis.

Hormonal Profiles in the Male Rat

LH secretion shows a pulsatile fluctuation in both male and female rats. The steroid feedback system in the male, however, is much simpler than that in the female, because the male has only the negative feedback action of testosterone on the hypothalamo-pituitary axis. In the intact adult male, the mean plasma LH concentration is around 0.5 ng/mL in terms of NIDDK-rLH-RP-2 (rat LH standard preparation provided by the National Hormone and Pituitary Program), which is much lower than that in the adult female. LH pulses are hardly detected in intact males, because of the strong negative feedback effect of testosterone.

LH pulses are often more frequent in castrated males (around 7 pulses/3 hours, concentrations ranging from 2 to 5 ng/mL) than in ovariectomized females (around 5 pulses/3 hours, concentrations ranging from 1 to 4 ng/mL); this makes it quite difficult to get good pulses in the castrated male rat. Plasma testosterone concentrations in intact males are roughly 2–3 ng/mL.

Inhibin is secreted from the Sertoli cell and plays a major role in the inhibition of FSH secretion in the male rat (Gnessi et al., 1997). Bioactive inhibin secretion may begin in the perinatal period, although some inhibin immunoreactivities are found in the fetal testis during late gestation (Noguchi et al., 1997).

Estrous Cycle

Identification of the Estrous Cycle

The female rat shows 4- or 5-day estrous cycles. A cycle consists of proestrus, estrus and diestrus (Figure 9.7). A 4-day cycle has a 2-day diestrus (diestrus 1 and 2) and a 5-day cycle has a 3-day diestrus (diestrus 1, 2 and 3). Diestrus 1 is often called metestrus. Even within a strain, the length of the estrous cycle sometimes varies from one individual to another.

Vaginal smears are widely used to identify the phase of the estrous cycle. Observation of the cell population in the vaginal smear is the most popular and reliable method for identifying the different phases, because the populations of the different

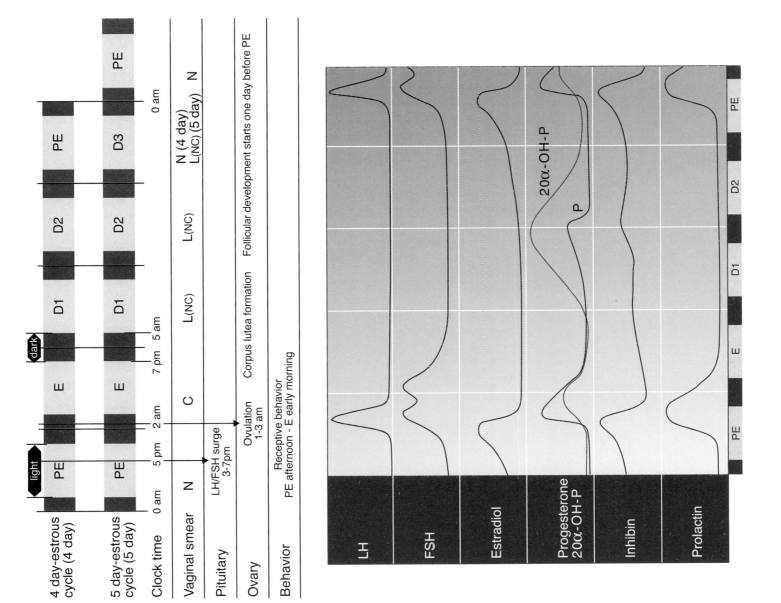

Figure 9.7 Physiological and behavioral events and hormonal profiles during the rat estrous cycle. The upper panel shows the 4- or 5-day rat estrous cycle. The middle panel shows cell populations in the vaginal smear and physiological and behavioral events during the cycle. The lower panel depicts the hormonal profiles of the 4-day estrous cycle in the circulating blood, except for 20α-OH-P in the ovarian venous blood. Upper panel: PE, proestrus; E, estrus; D1, diestrus 1; D2, diestrus 2; D3, diestrus 3. Middle panel: N, nucleated cell; C, cornified cell; L, leukocyte; N, C, L, minor cell populations in the vaginal smear. Lower panel: LH, luteinizing hormone; FSH, follicle-stimulating hormone; 20α-OH-P, 20α-dihydroxyprogesterone.

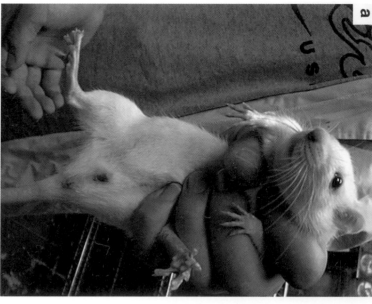

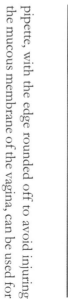

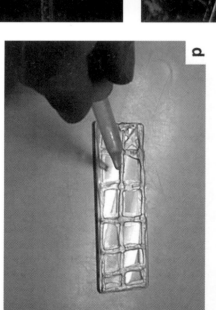

Figure 9.8 The method of taking vaginal smears in the rat. The rat is held properly (a) and the vagina is flushed with water using a pipette (b). The water, containing vaginal epithelial cells, is put on to a slide (c and d). Photograph by Dr F. Maekawa of Nagoya University.

cell types are controlled by circulating estrogen. Estrogen causes a proliferation of vaginal epithelial cells in the proestrus and lack of this steroid results in a reduction in their numbers.

It is easy to obtain vaginal samples when the rat is held properly (Figure 9.8a,b). A small glass or plastic pipette, with the edge rounded off to avoid injuring the mucous membrane of the vagina, can be used for sampling. A small amount of distilled water or even tapwater is put into the vagina and the cells are sucked up into the pipette. Use of saline is not recommended as crystals may appear on the slide as it dries out. The suspended cells are put onto a slide which has 10–12 small compartments separated by nail polish or felt pen with a mark in the first compartment to indicate the first one (Figure 9.8c,d). As a result, smears can be taken from 9–11 rats on just one slide. The cells are then examined under a microscope (usually with × 100). The slides can be reused for repeated routine checking of vaginal smears. If long-term storage is needed, the smear can be stained with 1–2% methylene blue for several minutes and dried.

Nucleated cells are the major population in the smear at proestrus (Figure 9.9a). When the smear is taken in the late afternoon of proestrus, some of the nucleated cells have already developed into cornified

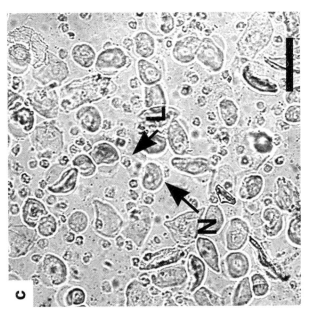

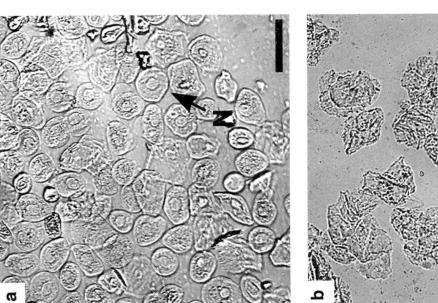

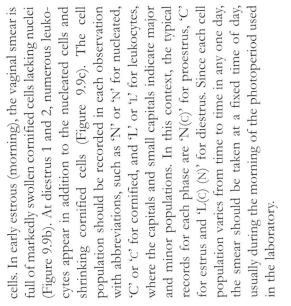

Figure 9.9 Photomicrograph of typical vaginal smears taken from rats at proestrus (a), estrus (b) and diestrus 1 (c). N, C and L indicate nucleated cells, cornified cells and leukocytes. Scale bar = 50 µm. Photograph by Dr F. Maekawa of Nagoya University.

Hormonal Profiles During Estrous Cycle

As in other mammalian species, ovarian activity during the estrous cycle is regulated by gonadotropins secreted by the anterior pituitary in the female rat. Plasma LH profiles show a pulsatile fluctuation. The frequency of LH pulses varies from phase to phase in the estrous cycle. As in other mammalian species, the frequency is highest in the proestrus and lowest in the estrus in the female rat (Gallo, 1981a,b). Using a push–pull perfusion technique, each LH pulse has been found to correspond to a GnRH pulse in the mediobasal hypothalamus or anterior pituitary (Dluzen and Ramirez, 1986; Levine and Duffy, 1988; Levine and Powell, 1989; Levine *et al.*, 1991). **Multiple unit activity (MUA)** recorded from the mediobasal hypothalamus is one of the parameters indicating the hypothalamic activity related to GnRH/LH release. The MUA volleys in the mediobasal hypothalamus are well correlated with LH pulses in the rat (Kimura *et al.*, 1991). The significance of the pulsatile pattern of GnRH/gonadotropins in the control of the gonadal activities was first demonstrated by Knobil in the monkey (Knobil, 1980). This pulsatile mode is also important in the rat, because continuous exposure of the animal to GnRH or its agonists results in

cells. In early estrous (morning), the vaginal smear is full of markedly swollen cornified cells lacking nuclei (Figure 9.9b). At diestrus 1 and 2, numerous leukocytes appear in addition to the nucleated cells and shrinking cornified cells (Figure 9.9c). The cell population should be recorded in each observation with abbreviations, such as 'N' or 'n' for nucleated, 'C' or 'c' for cornified, and 'L' or 'l' for leukocytes, where the capitals and small capitals indicate major and minor populations. In this context, the typical records for each phase are 'N(c)' for proestrus, 'C' for estrus and 'L(C) (N)' for diestrus. Since each cell population varies from time to time in any one day, the smear should be taken at a fixed time of day, usually during the morning of the photoperiod used in the laboratory.

suppressed gonadal activity (Rippel et al., 1973). In this regard, a constant-release device for GnRH agonists could be used to suppress gonadotropin release and hence gonadal functions in both genders (Sudo et al., 1991).

The level of estrogen increases together with follicular development in early proestrous (Figure 9.10) (Smith et al., 1975). The surge of estradiol-17β begins in the morning of proestrus, terminating in the late afternoon. The progesterone peak follows the estrogen peak just around the LH surge. In the rat, the timings of gonadotropin surges are fixed in terms of the LD cycle. For instance, the peak of LH surge occurs at 17:00 h under an LD cycle of 12L:12D with the lights turned on at 6:00 h (Smith et al., 1975). Plasma LH concentrations start to increase at 14:00–15:00 h, reach their peak (20–40 ng rLH-RP-2/mL) and return to the basal level during the night (Figure 9.10). The peak also occurs at 17:00 h in our lighting schedule, which is 14L:10D with lights-on at 5:00 h, returning to the basal level by 20:00 h (Figure 9.11). Periovulatory FSH secretion has dual peaks, with the first surge occurring around 17:00 h and the secondary surge at around the late dark phase. The secondary surge is considered to be associated with an abrupt decrease in inhibin after ovulation (Ackland et al., 1990; Haisenleder et al., 1990; Watanabe et al., 1990). Thus, FSH secretion is more dependent on inhibin action than on GnRH during the estrous cycle in the female rat (Figure 9.7) (Arai et al., 1996).

The term 'critical period' was first used by Sawyer (1969) to indicate the period until which pentobarbital injection blocks ovulation and after which the treatment has no effect on it. This concept is now accepted as the period related to the initiation of the GnRH surge. The levels of GnRH in portal blood have been reported by several groups. There is a rise in the GnRH level starting around 14:00 h in the afternoon (de Greef et al., 1987). The injection of pentobarbital before the rise in GnRH blocks the surge by inhibiting the excitation of the GnRH-releasing system, resulting in the blockade of the subsequent LH rise and ovulation.

In the rat, the functional corpus luteum does not last long after ovulation. Eto et al. (1962) first reported, by direct measurement of ovarian steroid in ovarian venous blood, that progesterone is converted to a inactive progesterone, 20α-dihydroprogesterone by 20α-hydroxysteroid dehydrogenase (Figure 9.7) (Hashimoto et al., 1968). As a result, cycling rats show a high level of plasma 20α-dihydroprogesterone, which is also secreted from the regressed corpora lutea for the previous 3–4 cycles. The corpus luteum becomes functional through prolactin action during pregnancy or pseudopregnancy as described later (Takahashi, 1984).

Follicular Development and Ovulation

Oogonia transform to oocytes following mitotic division and the oocytes then undergo meiosis, but this latter meiotic process is not complete by the first LH surge. The oocyte is arrested in the diplotene stage of the first meiotic division which lasts until ovulation. Meiotic germ cells are first found on days 16.5–17.5 of gestation in the rat (Hirshfield, 1991).

The details of the follicular development in mammalian species are reviewed elsewhere (Hirshfield, 1991; Fortune, 1994). According to Hirshfield's classification of follicular development using granurosa cell generation (Hirshfield, 1991), follicle development in rats is divided into 10 phases. Growth of a **primordial follicle** to the 8th generation takes more than 50 days. It takes another 2.5 days to reach the 9th generation, during which the **antrum** begins to form. In the rat, the recruitment of follicles to the ovulatory cohort and most **atresia** occur around the antrum formation when the follicles are around 0.2–0.4 mm in diameter. The follicles reach this stage under basal gonadotropin secretion without much follicular loss. Follicular recruitment is considered to be associated with FSH secretion. In the rat, the secondary FSH surge at estrus may be responsible for the recruitment of the next cohort of ovulatory follicles (Figures 9.7 and 9.10). The final follicular maturation occurs during the final 3 days before the LH surge. In the 4–5-day rat estrous cycle, the diameter of the follicle is 0.4–0.5 mm at diestrus 1 and 0.8–1.0 mm at proestrus.

Under 14L:10D lighting conditions with lights-off at 19:00 h, rats ovulate at around 12:00–2:00 h during the night of estrus and make multiple copulations from the proestrous evening to the estrous morning (Figure 9.7). The first meiotic process begins around ovulation after a prolonged period of arrested development at the diplotene stage. There is no doubt that resumption of the meiotic changes of oocytes in the Graafian follicle is triggered by the LH surge.

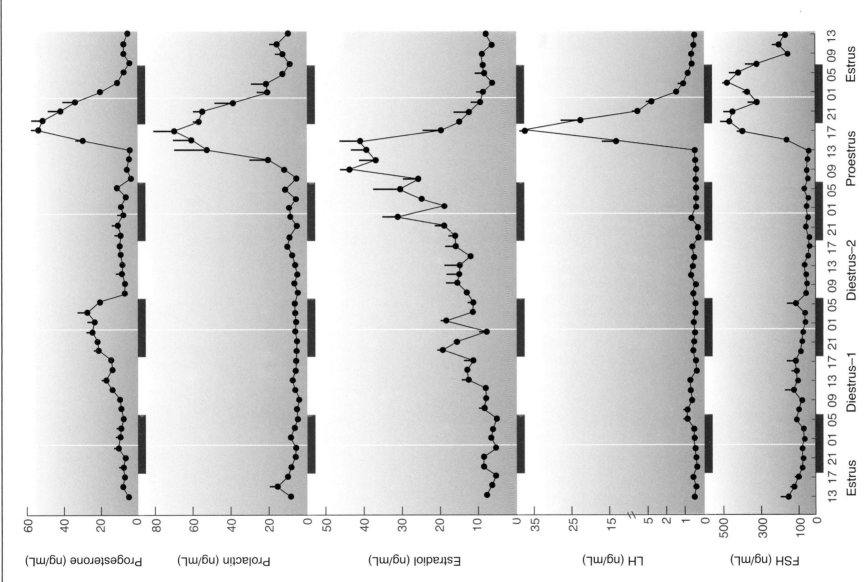

Figure 9.10 Hormonal profiles throughout the 4-day estrous cycle in the female rat. The horizontal red bars and white vertical lines indicate the dark period (18:00–6:00) and midnight. Values are means ± SEM. LH, luteinizing hormone; FSH, follicle-stimulating hormone. Adapted from Smith *et al.* (1975).

Negative and Positive Feedback Actions of Estrogen

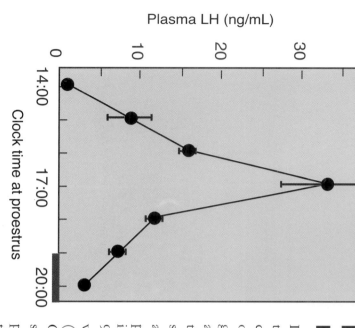

LH has two modes of secretion: one is the basal or tonic mode, called the pulse, and the other is the cyclic mode, known as the surge. When a rat is ovariectomized, plasma LH concentrations start to gradually increase and reach a plateau by 2 weeks after surgery (Maeda *et al.*, 1989), due to removal of the negative feedback effect of estrogen. The absence of this negative feedback action seems to affect both the amplitude and frequency of LH pulses. The plasma LH concentration after ovariectomy shows a typical pulsatile pattern (Figure 9.12, left panel). When the ovariectomized rats were immediately implanted with a Silastic implant (1.5 mm i.d.; 0.3 mm o.d.; 2.5 cm in length, Dow Corning, MI, USA) containing estradiol-17β dissolved in peanut oil at 20 mg/mL to produce physiological plasma levels of estrogen at diestrus, the amplitudes of LH pulses were suppressed to a level of 1–2 ng/mL (Figure 9.12, right panel) (Cagampang *et al.*, 1991).

The timing of the proestrous LH surge is fixed at late afternoon under a usual 12L:12D or 14L:10D photoperiod (Figures 9.10 and 9.11). When an

Figure 9.11 The preovulatory LH surge in the rat. The peak of the surge is fixed at around 17:00 h under lighting conditions of 14L:10D with the lights off at 19.00 h. Blood samples were taken every hour from 14.00 to 20.00 h. The shaded bar indicates the dark period. Values are means ± SEM.

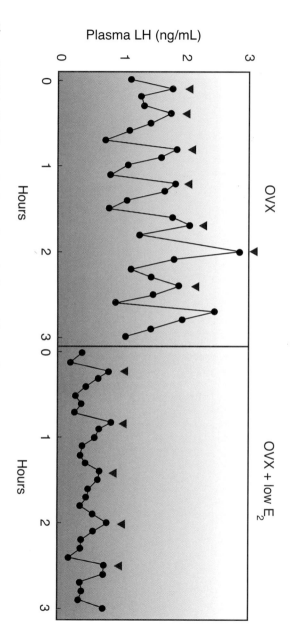

Figure 9.12 Pulsatile LH secretion in ovariectomized rats with or without estrogen treatment to produce the basal blood level needed for the negative feedback action. The animal was ovariectomized for 2 weeks (left panel), or ovariectomized and immediately implanted with a subcutaneous estrogen implant (right panel). Arrowheads above the dots indicate LH pulse peaks identified with the PULSAR computer program (Merriam and Wachter, 1982). The PULSAR is one of the most popular computer programs for detecting pulses at various intervals and baseline levels. OVX, ovariectomized; E₂, estradiol-17β.

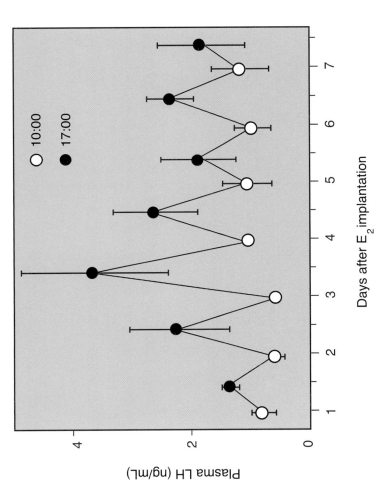

Figure 9.13 Daily LH surges induced by a local estradiol-17β (E₂) implant into the preoptic area (POA) in the ovariectomized rat. Blood samples were taken at 10:00 h (open circle) and 17:00 h (closed circle) for 7 days after implantation. The E₂ implant in the POA has the same effect on LH secretion as the subcutaneous implant, suggesting that the POA is one of the feedback sites of estrogen in female rats. Values are means ± SEM.

ovariectomized rat bears an estrogen implant to keep the plasma estradiol concentration at a proestrous level (>100 pg/mL), the daily LH surges occur at a fixed time of the day (Figure 9.13) (Legan and FJ, 1975; Chazal *et al.*, 1977; Tsukamura *et al.*, 1988).

The daily surges can be induced by a Silastic implant (1.0 mm i.d., 1.5 mm o.d., 2 cm in length, Dow Corning) containing crystalline estradiol-17β. The preovulatory progesterone surge plays a role in enhancing the LH surge, because progesterone injection in the morning is known to amplify the level of the LH surge (Kalra, 1993).

Ovarian steroids have been thought to act on specific feedback sites in the brain. One of the positive feedback sites is the preoptic area, since a microimplant containing estrogen put into the preoptic area induces an LH surge (Figure 9.13) (Goodman, 1978). The arcuate nucleus in the mediobasal hypothalamus has been reported to be one of the negative (Akema *et al.*, 1984) and positive (Naftolin *et al.*, 1996) feedback sites for estrogen. The neural mechanism mediating these positive and negative feedback effects of steroids has not yet been fully elucidated (Kalra, 1993).

Pseudopregnancy

When the females receive cervical stimulation by a vasectomized male or mechanical stimulation with a glass rod, the corpora lutea are released from their quiescent state and become functional in terms of progesterone secretion. The status, called pseudopregnancy, lasts 12–14 days, being shorter than normal pregnancy. The luteal function is maintained by an increased prolactin secretion after cervical stimulation. Cervical stimulation induces two daily surges of prolactin called the diurnal and nocturnal surges (Smith *et al.*, 1975), occurring at around 17:00–19:00 h and 03:00–07:00 h, respectively. The prolactin surges transform the corpora lutea into an active state by inhibiting the activity of 20α-hydroxysteroid dehydrogenase which converts progesterone to 20α-dihydroprogesterone (Takahashi, 1984). Interestingly, increased progesterone secretion from the active corpora lutea ensures the daily prolactin surges throughout pseudopregnancy, because prolactin surges attenuate in the late phase of pseudopregnancy around day 10–14 in ovariectomized animals but not in progesterone-implanted ovariectomized rats (Freeman, 1994).

Pseudopregnancy could be a good model for the investigation of the mechanism regulating the lifespan of the corpora luteum or luteolysis (Takahashi, 1984), because the lifespan of the corpora luteum in the pseudopregnant rat is very similar to that in other mammalian species, such as monkeys and ewes, having a 14-day luteal phase in the estrous or menstrual cycle. The endocrine mechanism underlying luteolysis is still under debate, but a series of experiments indicates that immune cells, such as splenic macrophages, are involved in the regulation of luteal functions during pseudopregnancy (Takahashi et al., 1989; Matsuyama et al., 1990, 1992; Matsuyama and Takahashi, 1995).

Environmental Regulation of the Activity of the Gonadal Axis

Photoperiod

In the rat, photoperiod has a strong influence on the activity of the hypothalamopituitary-gonadal axis and thence the estrous cycle because the neuroendocrine system is tightly coupled to the circadian clock. The time of the GnRH/LH surge is tightly linked to the circadian system. As described above, the timing of the LH surge is fixed in the late afternoon if the female has high levels of circulating estrogen (Legan and FJ, 1975; Chazal et al., 1977). In this context, a female rat has LH surges every 4 days when it has mature follicles, so there is a high level of estrogen at this time.

When placed under constant light conditions for more than 2 weeks, female rats become acyclic, and the LH surge and consequent ovulation are inhibited (Takahashi and Suzuki, 1969). As a result, the rats show persistent estrus as long as they are kept in constant light, because matured follicles are present in the ovaries and keep secreting estrogens. Under constant light conditions, the rat ovulates in response to copulation. Mechanical stimulus given to the uterine cervix by a glass rod also induces a GnRH/LH surge and then ovulation. In this context, persistently estrous rats under constant light behave as if they were reflex ovulators, like rabbits and cats (Takahashi, 1984). When female rats are kept in constant darkness, they show normal estrous cycles (Schwartz and McCormack, 1972), probably because the timing of the LH surges is controlled by the circadian clock located in the suprachiasmatic nucleus. Lesion of the suprachiasmatic nucleus results in the loss of this LH surge (Nunez and Stephan, 1977; Kawakami et al., 1980).

The female rat is equipped with neuroendocrine mechanisms controlling various options of the estrous cycle: estrous cycle with or without the luteal phase, and reflex ovulation as described above. The rat can, therefore, serve as a good experimental model for the physiological study of other types of reproductive cycles.

Nutrition

Nutrition is another key factor in the regulation of gonadal activity (Kalra and Kalra, 1996; Wade, 1996; Foster et al., 1998; Maeda et al., 1998). If the rat is subjected to 48-hour fasting, starting at the day of estrus, pulsatile LH secretion is profoundly suppressed as well as the next proestrous LH surge, resulting in the blockade of ovulation. The fasting-induced suppression of LH release is mediated by corticotropin-releasing hormone (CRH) as well as other types of stress (Figure 9.14a). The suppression of LH pulses is estrogen-dependent and the neuroendocrine mechanism is described in detail elsewhere (Maeda et al., 1996; Maeda and Tsukamura, 1996, 1997).

Stress

Stress strongly suppresses the activity of the hypothalamopituitary-gonadal axis in the rat (Rivier and Rivest, 1991). Here, electrical foot shock and immobilization or restraint are commonly used to study the effect of stress on gonadal activity (Rivier et al., 1986). When the rat is immobilized, LH pulses are immediately suppressed in the absence or presence of estrogen (Figure 9.14b). Another report showed that immobilization stress suppresses LH secretion in ovariectomized rats but stimulates the secretion in estrogen-treated rats (Higuchi et al., 1986). The effect of estrogen on acute stress-induced LH suppression is still controversial.

Lactation

The suckling stimulus profoundly suppresses LH secretion in the rat (Maeda et al., 1989). This will be described later in the section on lactation.

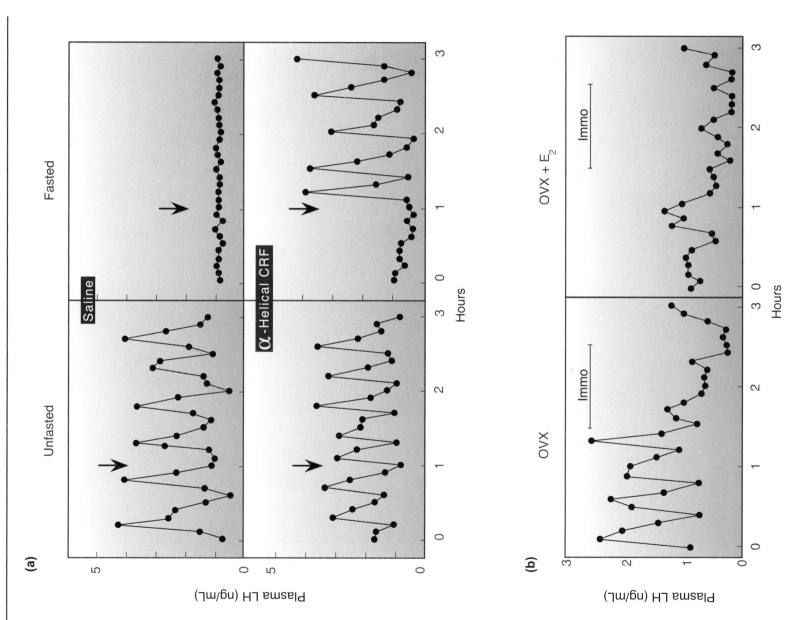

Figure 9.14 Suppression of LH secretion by 48-hour fasting (a) and immobilization stress (b) in female rats. Blood samples were taken every 6 min for 3 hours. (a) Estrogen-implanted ovariectomized rats were subjected to 48-hour fasting (right panels), or fed *ad libitum* (left panels). LH pulses are strongly suppressed by fasting. This suppression is estrogen-dependent, because 48-hour fasting has no effect on LH secretion in the ovariectomized rat (Cagampang *et al.*, 1991). Intracerebroventricular injection of a CRH antagonist (arrows in the lower panel), α-helical CRF, restored suppressed LH pulses after 48-hour fasting (right lower panel), suggesting that the inhibitory effect of fasting on LH secretion is mediated by the brain CRH system. (b) Immobilization stress (indicated by the horizontal bars) immediately suppresses LH secretion in the presence (right panel) or absence (left panel) of E_2.

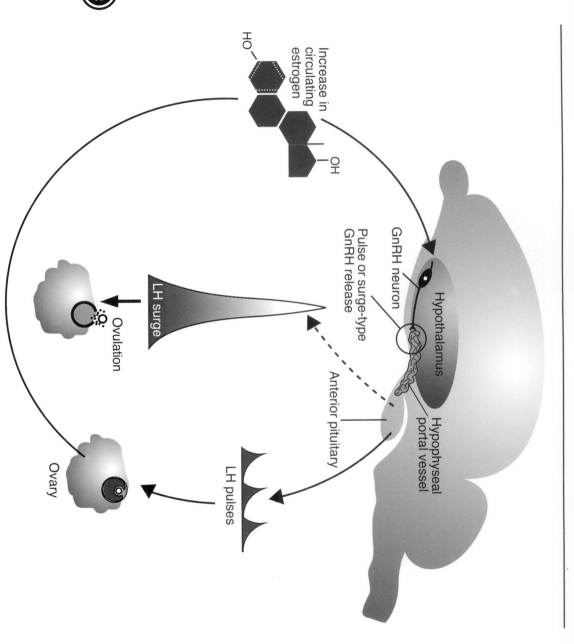

Figure 9.15 Diagram of the hypothalamo-pituitary-gonadal axis in the rat. Pulsatile GnRH release stimulates the pulse-type LH release from the anterior pituitary. The LH pulse stimulates follicular development and steroidogenesis in the ovary. The increased level of estrogen secreted from matured follicles stimulates a GnRH surge in the proestrous afternoon, and then an LH surge in the late afternoon. The LH surge causes ovulation during the dark phase. Black lines indicate GnRH/LH pulses related to the follicular development. Red lines indicate the events relating to the GnRH and LH surges and ovulation. See text for details.

Neuroendocrine Mechanisms Regulating Gonadal Activity in the Female Rat

Figure 9.15 summarizes the activity of the hypothalamopituitary-gonadal axis in the female rat. Two major GnRH neuronal systems have been found in the rat brain: one is the terminal nerve system and the other the preoptic system. The latter plays a key role in the regulation of reproductive activity in the rat; the function of the former has not been elucidated (Schwanzel-Fukuda, 1997). The midbrain

GnRH neuronal system, which is chicken GnRH II immunoreactive, has been identified in several animal species but not yet in the rat brain (Parhar, 1997).

The preoptic GnRH neurons serve as a major source supplying GnRH to the anterior pituitary in order to stimulate gonadotropin secretion. The cell bodies are scattered around the septal/preoptic region in the rat without forming a clear cell group. The GnRH fibers run from the base of the brain to project onto the external layer of the median eminence (Kawano, 1981).

GnRH is released in a pulsatile manner from the nerve terminals in the median eminence into the hypophyseal portal vessels. The pulsatile GnRH release causes a pulsatile LH and FSH release, resulting in follicular development, maturation and steroidogenesis in the ovary. The basal level of estrogen secreted from the follicles exerts a negative feedback action on GnRH/LH secretion at the hypothalamic and pituitary level. When the follicles reach their final maturation, the high level of circulating estrogen secreted from the matured follicles acts on the pituitary or hypothalamus to induce a GnRH/LH surge.

Environmental cues such as nutrition, stress or suckling stimulus (see the section on Lactation) control gonadal function through modulation of the pulse mode but not the surge mode of LH release, because the periovulatory level of estrogen is still capable of inducing an LH surge in the animals during lactation (Tsukamura *et al.*, 1988) or fasting (unpublished observation) when the pulse is suppressed at a low level.

The brain mechanism generating the GnRH surge or pulse has been intensively investigated but has not yet been elucidated (Maeda *et al.*, 1995; Nishihara *et al.*, 1997).

Pregnancy and Parturition

Making a Rat Pregnant

For mating, a proestrous rat is transferred to the cage of male rats and left overnight. The vaginal plug should be checked the next morning to ensure that successful copulation has occurred (Figure 9.16a). If the animals are kept in a cage with a mesh floor during mating, then the plug underneath the floor is easy to check. The vaginal smear can also be checked the following morning. The smear usually contains plenty of sperm if copulation has been successful (Figure 9.16b). The cell composition is different to that of the estrous phase when copulation is successful: there are many leukocytes and few cornified cells (Figure 9.16b).

Implantation

The preovulatory estrogen surge causes a proliferation of epithelial cells prior to implantation during

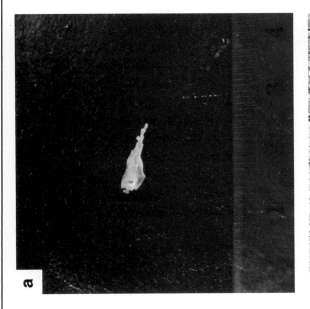

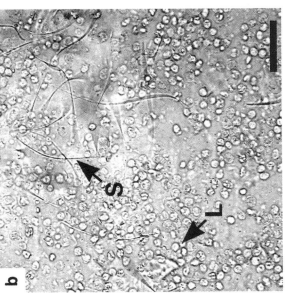

Figure 9.16 (a) A vaginal plug obtained in the morning following mating. A female rat at proestrus was mated with a male overnight. (b) A photomicrograph of the vaginal smear obtained on the following morning. Many spermatozoa (S) are present in the smear with a number of leukocytes (L). The population of the cells is different from the estrous smear, because mating induces daily prolactin surges which form functional corpora lutea and then stimulate progesterone secretion. Scale bar = 50 μm. Photograph by Dr F. Maekawa of Nagoya University.

the first few days of pregnancy. Then progesterone secreted from the newly formed corpus luteum not only stimulates stromal cell proliferation but also ensures survival of the embryo. The hatched blastocyst becomes attached to the uterine epithelium on day 5 of pregnancy. Decidualization of stromal cells at the site of implantation has already started by this time. Maternal estrogen plays an essential role in the induction of implantation in the rat (Dey and Johnson, 1986), because the rat embryo does not appear to produce estrogen, unlike other animal species, such as the pig, hamster and rabbit, whose blastocyst produces enough estrogen for implantation.

The increase in permeability of the uterine stromal capillaries and the transformation of stroma cells to decidual cells is restricted to the implantation site. This suggests that a signal(s) triggering the local changes could be provided by the embryo. Prostaglandins have been suggested as a candidate for the embryonic signal inducing these changes in the rat (Parr et al., 1988).

Growth factors have been considered to play an important role in cell–cell recognition between the embryo and the uterus at the implantation site. Epidermal growth factor (EGF) receptors and transforming growth factor α, a member of the EGF family, have been found to increase in the embryo and uterus after implantation in the rat (Chakraborty et al., 1988; Tamada et al., 1997).

The Placenta

Structure of the rat placenta

The lower panel of Figure 9.17 shows a pregnant uterus containing conceptus. The uterus is relaxed and semitransparent with dark red placentae. The rat has a discoidal placenta and the physical interaction between fetal and maternal tissues is confined to a roughly circular area (Figure 9.17, top panels) (Kaufmann and Burton, 1994). Microscopically, the rat shows hemochorial placentation, in which the invasion of the maternal tissue by the trophoblast results in disappearance of the maternal vessels (Enders, 1965), so that the trophoblast comes into direct contact with the maternal blood.

The rat has two placental structures: the choriovitelline placenta and the chorioallantoic placenta (Sores et al., 1998). The choriovitelline placenta,

Pregnancy

In the pregnant rat, progesterone is mainly produced by the ovary, but production is supplemented by the placenta in the second half of gestation (Gibori et al., 1988). The copulatory stimulus induces daily prolactin surges during the early phase of pregnancy as described for pseudopregnancy (Smith et al., 1975). In the first half of pregnancy, prolactin secreted from the pituitary is the major luteotropic hormone; hypophysectomy by day 12–13 terminates the pregnancy whereas after day 13 it does not have any effect (Heap and Flint, 1984).

The placental lactogens function as a main luteotropic hormone to ensure progesterone secretion from the corpus luteum in the second half of gestation as described in detail below (Orgen and Talamantes, 1988). The ovary continues to produce estrogen throughout pregnancy to activate the corpus luteum. Estrogen is indispensable for the maintenance of the corpus luteum by stimulating the vascularization or steroidogenesis (Gibori et al., 1988). The aromatizable androgen is supplied mainly by the theca interna cells of the follicle and interstitial cells of the ovarian stroma in the first half of the pregnancy. In the second half of pregnancy, androgens are supplied by the placenta. They are converted to estradiol in the granulosa cells for the stimulation of the luteal functions.

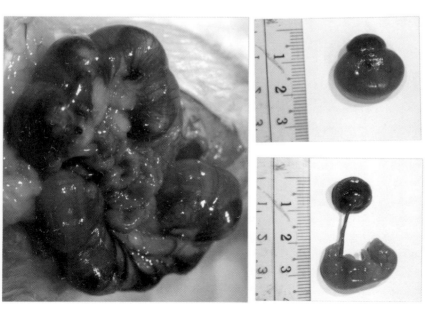

Figure 9.17 The uterus of a pregnant female rat on day 19 of pregnancy (lower panel). A 19-day-old rat fetus with (upper left panel) or without (upper right panel) fetal membranes.

The placenta as an endocrine organ

The placenta plays a key role in regulating various physiological functions during pregnancy. The major polypeptides secreted from the placenta are the placental lactogens (Soares *et al.*, 1991; Sores *et al.*, 1998). Two major molecular species have been identified and cloned in the rat: placental lactogen I and II (PL-I and II). PL-I expression is initiated immediately after implantation in the mural trophoblast giant cells of the blastocyst. The expression later extends to the choriovitelline and chorioallantoic placentae. The plasma PL-I concentration increases at the mid-phase of gestation with a maximum around day 11–12 of gestation (Orgen and Talamantes, 1988). The plasma concentration of PL-II starts to increase at mid-gestation and reaches its maximum at the end of the gestation. The placental lactogens contribute to the development of the mammary glands and to stimulation of progesterone synthesis in the corpora lutea during pregnancy. Recent studies have demonstrated that placental lactogens stimulate insulin secretion and the proliferation of maternal B cells in the pancreatic islets during the latter half of pregnancy in the rat (Brelje *et al.*, 1993; Kawai and Kishi, 1997).

Unlike the human placenta, which serves as a major source of progesterone and estrogen during pregnancy, the rat placenta does not secrete estrogen and secretes an insufficient amount of progesterone to maintain pregnancy (Gibori *et al.*, 1988). Several lines of evidence suggest that the rat placenta synthesizes androgen and that biosynthesis is limited to the fetal trophoblastic cells. On the other hand, the decidual cells have no capacity to synthesize androgen. The placenta starts to secrete androgen from day 11 of gestation onwards. In the second half of gestation, androgen secreted from the placenta is converted to estradiol by the aromatase in the corpus luteum to stimulate luteal function. In contrast, aromatizable androgen originates from the ovaries until mid-pregnancy. Estradiol converted by the corpus luteum has a local action in the activation of the corpus luteum by increasing progesterone secretion or vascularizing the luteal cells.

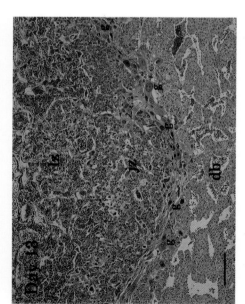

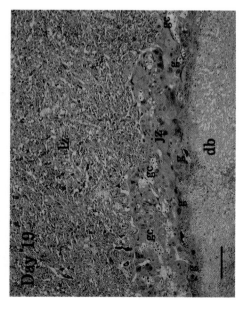

Figure 9.18 Photomicrographs of rat placentas on day 13 (upper) and 19 (lower) of gestation (hematoxylin-eosin stain). jz, junctional zone; lz, labyrinth zone; db, decidua basalis; g, trophoblast giant cell; gc, glycogen cell. Scale bars = 20 μm. Courtesy of Drs M. Kawai and K. Kishi of the Shionogi Pharmaceutical Inc.

consisting of trophoblast cells adherent to the basement membrane, is associated with the decidua capsularis. This placenta degenerates and disappears by day 14 of gestation. The chorioallantoic placenta, which is localized in the mesometrial region of the uterus, develops before the degeneration of the choriovitelline placenta. It consists of two prominent zones, called the junctional and labyrinth zones (Figure 9.18). The junctional zone, consisting of trophoblast cells and maternal vascular channels, lies adjacent to the decidua basalis. The labyrinth zone consists of trophoblast cells, maternal vascular channels and fetal vessels and is located adjacent to the embryo. A number of differentiated trophoblast cells are observed in the junctional and labyrinth zones (Sores *et al.*, 1998).

Parturition

Parturition mostly occurs during the daytime on day 21–22 of pregnancy. Under our lighting condition of 14L:10D (lights-on at 5:00), 37% of the animals give birth during the daytime on day 21, 20% of the animals during the night on day 21–22 and 42% of the animals during daytime on day 22. There are two peaks of parturition: one is 13:00–15:00 h on day 21 and the other is 9:00–11:00 h on day 22. The litter size is 12–18 in the Wistar-Imamichi strain of rat and sometimes more than 20. The litter size varies from strain to strain.

It is well known that fetal glucocorticoid secretion triggers the initiation of parturition in sheep and goats, but it is difficult to define the role of each fetus in labor in **polytocous** species. The role of fetal glucocorticoids in initiating parturition in the rat is still unclear: classical experiments have shown that removal of the fetuses allowed delivery of the placentae (Thorburn and Challis, 1979). Ovarian estradiol secretion increases during the final 24–48 hours before delivery and the increase could be involved in parturition (Thorburn and Challis, 1979). One action of estrogen could be to stimulate the synthesis and release of prostaglandins. Prostaglandin production by the uterine endometrium has been found to reach its maximum level on day 22 of gestation. This increase in synthesis is probably related to the contractile activity of the uterus during parturition. Pituitary oxytocin secretion is known to rise during parturition and this rise is closely associated with uterine contraction (Higuchi et al., 1986). The oxytocin secretion from the posterior pituitary is stimulated by a neuroendocrine reflex called the **Ferguson reflex,** in which the distension of the cervix by the descending fetus triggers a series of neuroendocrine responses. On the other hand, oxytocin is also synthesized in the uterine endometrium epithelium during parturition. The locally synthesized peptide is also involved in the contractile activity of the uterus during labor acting as a paracrine or autocrine mediator (Zigg et al., 1995). Uterine oxytocin synthesis, but not the hypothalamic (see the section on Milk ejection and Chapter 20 Endocrinology for details), is stimulated by estrogen, suggesting that estrogen is one of the factors bringing about the dramatic increase in uterine oxytocin synthesis at the final stage of gestation. There is a positive feedback loop between oxytocin and prostaglandin, because oxytocin stimulates prostaglandin release and prostaglandin increases uterine oxytocin receptors.

Relaxin plays an important role in the growth and softening of the cervix throughout the second half of pregnancy and parturition. Treatment of pregnant rats with antirelaxin serum prolongs the duration of

litter delivery and the fetuses and placentae are retained *in utero* (Sherwood et al., 1993). Relaxin is produced and secreted by the corpus luteum during the second half of pregnancy. Plasma relaxin concentrations start to increase around day 10 of pregnancy and reach a peak just before parturition. The peptide increases the growth and extensibility of the rat cervix as well as the pubic symphysis (Samuel et al., 1996) by reducing collagen concentrations along with the dispersion and random orientation of collagen fiber bundles. Relaxin may also be involved in reducing uterine contractility during the second half of pregnancy in rats. Brain relaxin has been reported to determine the time of birth (Summerlee et al., 1998) and is involved in oxytocin secretion (Heine et al., 1997).

Postpartum Ovulation

The LH surge and subsequent postpartum ovulation occurs within 24 hours after parturition (Hoffman and Schwartz, 1965). Follicular development and maturation occur in the late phase of pregnancy in the rat. The corpus luteum made by the postpartum ovulation is maintained by a high level of prolactin secretion which is stimulated by suckling. The corpus luteum is active in secretion of progesterone throughout the lactating period as described later. The postpartum LH surge is considered to be induced by the expansion of the vaginal cervix associated with parturition, because when the pups are taken out by cesarian incision, the postpartum LH surge and subsequent ovulation do not occur (Fox and Smith, 1984).

Embryo and Fetus

Early Development of the Embryo

Rat embryology has been described in detail by Hebel and Stromberg (1986). Follicles grow rapidly during proestrus and ovulation occurs in response to the LH surge. The first maturation division occurs shortly before ovulation, resulting in the formation of the first polar body. The second maturation division, which has already started before ovulation, is completed within an hour after the entrance of the

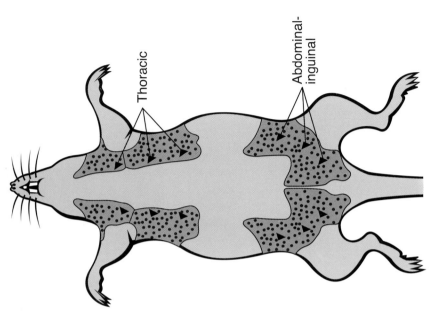

Figure 9.19 Schematic drawing of the rat mammary gland. The female rat has six pairs of mammary glands: three pairs in the thoracic region, three in the abdominal-inguinal region. Adapted from Mochizuki et al. (1968).

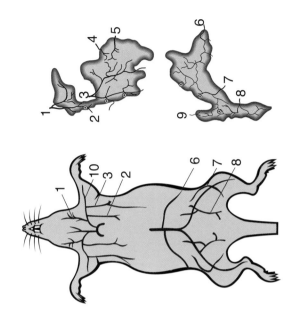

Figure 9.20 The blood supply to the mammary gland in the rat. 1, superficial cervical artery; 2, internal thoracic artery; 3, external thoracic artery; 4, branch of subscapular artery; 5, branch of intercostal artery; 6, iliolumbar artery; 7, superficial epigastric artery; 8, external pudic artery; 9, branch of cranial epigastric artery; 10, axillary artery. From Mochizuki et al. (1968).

sperm cell. The average diameter of the unfertilized ova of the rat is approximately 80 mm and that of the polar bodies is in the range of 8–13 μm. The diameter of the egg cell with the zona pellucida has been reported to be around 108 μm.

Within 3 hours after ovulation, 90% of the ova are penetrated by sperm cells. Within 10 min to 2 hours after the entry of the first sperm, zona reaction occurs. After sperm penetration, metaphase of the second maturation division of the ovum progresses and the second polar body formation is finished within 1 hour after the sperm entrance. The first cleavage of the ovum to form a two-cell embryo is finished by 25 hours after sperm penetration. At the end of the two-cell stage, the ova have reached the distal third of the oviduct. The four-cell stage is usually found between 40 and 70 hours after mating and has already arrived at the distal end of the oviduct. Eight-cell stages can be found from 65 to 90 hours and the blastocyst stage between 80 and 110 hours after mating. Hatching of blastocysts starts at about 110 hours after mating (day 4 of gestation).

Having completed hatching, the blastocysts become attached to the uterine epithelial depression on the antimesometrial side, with their inner cell mass oriented mesometrially by the end of day 5. The decidual reaction starts before the blastocysts attach to the uterine surface. The blastocyst increases in size during day 6. Then, it rapidly differentiates and proliferates to form the ectoplacental cone from the trophoblast and the ectodermal node and entoderm from the embryonal cell mass during day 7 (see section on Implantation for more details).

Lactation

The Mammary Gland

The female rat has six pairs of mammary glands: three pairs in the thoracic, three in the abdominal-inguinal region (Figure 9.19). A nipple is present on each mammary gland, giving six pairs in total. Each gland receives an abundant blood supply in order to get the enormous amount of energy and material needed for milk production (Figure 9.20). Two different types of tissue are present in the mammary gland: the parenchyma and stroma (Cowie, 1984). The parenchyma consists of a layer of epithelial

(a)

Mammary gland

(b)

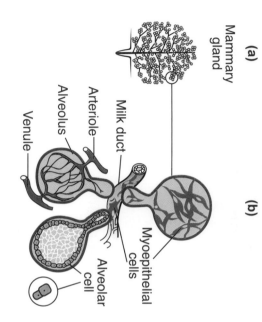

Milk duct
Arteriole
Alveolus
Venule
Myoepithelial cells
Alveolar cell

Figure 9.21 Structure of the rat mammary gland. (a) A rat mammary gland duct system. Alveoli cluster at the end of the duct system. Each alveolus opens into a small duct which then joins up with the others. These ducts eventually form one main duct, and open at the nipple. (b) An alveolus consisting of blood vessels, myoepithelial cells and alveolar cells. Adapted from Nagasawa et al. (1983).

cells, called alveolar cells. Each alveolus opens into a small duct and then these ducts join each other. These ducts in the rat eventually form one main duct, and open at the nipple (Figure 9.21). The milk is stored in the above-mentioned duct system in the lactating rat until the milk is ejected.

Development of the Mammary Gland

The pattern of fetal mammary development in the rat is similar to that in the mouse (Imagawa et al., 1994). In rodents, fetal mammary growth occurs during the last few days of gestation. In the female rat, the primary mammary cord, which originally derived from the ectoderm, remains attached to the epidermis and the distal end penetrates into the dermis, and then forms mammary ducts. In the male fetus, the primary cord loses its attachment to the epidermis by the action of androgen, and so no nipples are formed.

The duct shows little growth in females until just before the onset of reproductive cycles. When the animal starts to have regular ovarian cycles, the mammary gland begins to show active growth. In the rat, which has no relevant functional luteal phase, the ducts rapidly grow and branch at the follicular phase and their DNA production increases by the time of

ovulation. However, duct growth becomes quiescent after ovulation and DNA synthesis decreases.

Development of the mammary glands and milk secretion is induced by some hormones, such as estrogen, progesterone, prolactin, growth hormone (GH) and glucocorticoids (Cowie, 1984). The minimal hormonal requirements for mammary growth have been studied in ovariectomized, adrenalectomized and hypophysectomized rats. In the female rat, estrogen, GH and adrenal steroids are required for duct growth. In addition, prolactin and progesterone are needed for lobulo-alveolar growth. Prolactin and adrenal steroids are also required for milk secretion. Placental hormones, i.e. placental lactogens, are also involved in the development of the mammary gland during pregnancy as described below.

Initiation and Maintenance of Milk Production

Hormonal control of the induction of lactose synthesis, an indicator of lactogenesis, in the rat has been well studied by Yokoyama and his co-workers (Yokoyama and Ota, 1978). They showed that ovariectomy and placentectomy in pregnant rats induces lactose synthesis in the mammary gland during late pregnancy, suggesting that withdrawal of the effect of progesterone triggers the initiation of milk synthesis in these glands. Progesterone has been shown to inhibit prolactin binding to its receptors in the gland (Tucker, 1994). It has also been suggested that prolactin and glucocorticoids play indispensable roles in the initiation of lactation in the rat. The plasma corticosterone levels show circadian rhythmicity; a nocturnal increase during early and mid-pregnancy. However, a marked increase in the plasma concentration of corticosterone takes place even in the morning during the last few days of pregnancy (Yokoyama and Ota, 1978). The placental hormones also play an important role in the development of the mammary gland during pregnancy and in the initiation of synthesis of milk production (Tucker, 1994). Placental lactogens, the plasma levels of which increase biphasically during early (PL-I) and late pregnancy (PL-II), act through PRL receptors to maintain the function of the mammary gland, because the mammary glands develop and secrete milk even after the removal of the anterior pituitary at mid- or late gestation in the rat.

pups (Tucker, 1994). The suckling stimulus also stimulates secretion of GH and ACTH (resulting in the increase in plasma corticosterone levels). Therefore, it is easy to understand that removal of the pups from their mothers will terminate milk production.

Milk Ejection

Milk ejection occurs when the pups suckle the teat. When the milk is ejected from the teat, the rat pup shows typical behavior called the 'stretching reaction': they stretch all their legs as long as they are taking milk. As the pups attaching to their mother's nipples do not necessarily suckle, the stretching reaction can be used as a good indicator for milk ejection. The stomach milk, which can be easily detected by visual observation of a pup, is also a good marker for indicating whether milk is being ejected and a pup is taking milk. The suckled mother rat usually shows an EEG pattern of **slow-wave sleep** (Lincoln et al., 1980). It is well known that, in the lactating rat, milk ejection is regulated by a neuroendocrine loop called the 'milk ejection reflex', in which oxytocin plays a central role (Lincoln, 1984). When pups suckle the teat, the suckling stimulus is conveyed by the sensory nerve through the spinal cord and reaches the hypothalamus. The magnocellular oxytocinergic neurons in the hypothalamic nuclei show a pulsatile firing pattern with good synchronization in order to release oxytocin from their nerve terminals projecting into the posterior pituitary. The oxytocin released from the posterior pituitary into the general circulation reaches the mammary gland and causes milk ejection by stimulating contraction of the myoepithelial cells investing the alveoli of the mammary gland (Figure 9.21b).

Oxytocin is released into the general circulation in a pulsatile manner during continuous suckling (Higuchi et al., 1985, 1986; Lincoln et al., 1985). An intermittent increase in intramammary pressure follows each rise in plasma oxytocin concentration. This periodic oxytocin release is based on the periodic excitation of oxytocinergic neurons in the paraventricular and supraoptic nuclei of the hypothalamus. The firing of the neurosecretory neurons in these two nuclei are synchronized with each other to induce pulsatile oxytocin release from the posterior pituitary.

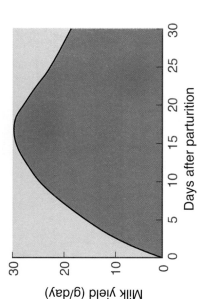

Figure 9.22 The milk yield in prolonged lactation. The yield is estimated by the gain and loss of the weight of pups that receive 30-min timed suckling every day. The pups were replaced by the younger ones every 10 days throughout lactation, so that the lactation was prolonged beyond the physiological lactational period.

Rat milk composition is as follows (% w/v): fat, 10.3; casein, 6.4; whey protein, 2.0; lactose, 2.6; minerals, 1.3 (Nagasawa et al., 1983). The values vary from report to report, probably due to differences in the sampling method.

Figure 9.22 depicts a schematic drawing of the rat milk yield. The yield is estimated by the gain and loss of the weight of pups that had 30-minute timed suckling every day. The pups were replaced by younger ones every 10 days throughout lactation, so that lactation was prolonged beyond the physiological lactational period. The yield increases immediately after parturition and reaches its peak at around day 17 of lactation and then gradually decreases, even if the mother receives a suckling stimulus of a similar strength. Russell (1980) has also estimated the daily milk yield by pup weight gain taking the pup weight loss into account. The daily milk yield per mammary gland sucked is around 1 g on day 1 postpartum, gradually increases, and reaches its maximum (around 2–2.5 g) by day 10. Along with the increase in the daily milk yield, the litter weight gain gradually increases from the day of birth, and reaches its plateau by day 10–15. The litter weight gain shows an abrupt increase from day 15 to the end of lactation at around day 20. The pattern of food consumption of the mother is very similar to the litter weight gain (Figure 9.23) (Ota and Yokoyama, 1967).

The suckling stimulus is essential for the maintenance of lactation; plasma prolactin concentrations remain at a high level in the rats with their pups, but they decrease within hours after the removal of the

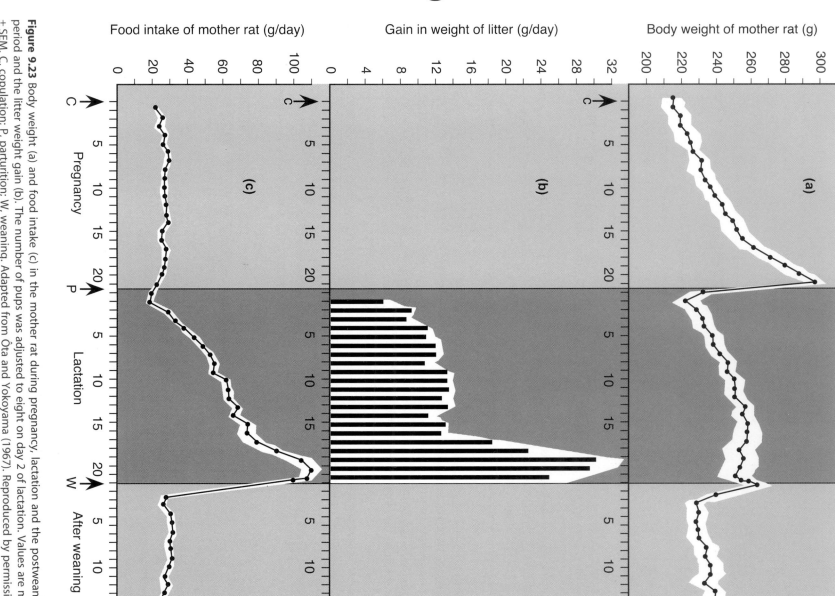

Figure 9.23 Body weight (a) and food intake (c) in the mother rat during pregnancy, lactation and the postweaning period and the litter weight gain (b). The number of pups was adjusted to eight on day 2 of lactation. Values are means ± SEM. C, copulation; P, parturition; W, weaning. Adapted from Ôta and Yokoyama (1967). Reproduced by permission of the Society for Endocrinology.

Gonadal Functions During Lactation

As in other mammalian species, ovulation in the rat will not occur as long as vigorous suckling stimulus is given to the mother. Follicular development is inhibited because of the low level of gonadotropin secretion. When fertilization is successful after postpartum ovulation, the implantation of the blastocyst located in the uterus of a lactating mother is also blocked. This ensures that the lactating mother does not become pregnant while she expends an enormous amount of energy on milk production.

Gonadal activity during lactation in rodents, including rats, is characterized by the presence of lactational corpora lutea. In the rat, the lactational corpora lutea are formed after postpartum ovulation and progesterone secretion is maintained by the high level of prolactin secretion which is stimulated by suckling until the end of lactation (Smith, 1978). Prolactin keeps stimulating the progesterone secretion from the corpora lutea by suppressing the activity of 20α-hydroxysteroid dehydrogenase, which converts progesterone to 20α-hydroxyprogesterone, as is seen in the pseudopregnant rat. In this regard, a high level of plasma progesterone concentration is maintained as long as the suckling stimulus stimulates prolactin secretion during this lactational period. The physiological importance of progesterone secreted from the lactational corpora lutea in the maintenance of lactation is not known. Ovariectomy in lactating mothers does not disturb maternal activities, including milk production and maternal behavior. It may ensure the suppression of gonadotropin secretion throughout lactation in cooperation with the suckling stimulus itself.

When fertilization is successful after postpartum ovulation, the embryo at the blastocyst stage stays in the uterus until the end of lactation. This is called delayed implantation. Implantation is delayed as long as lactation lasts, because gonadotropin secretion is suppressed by the suckling stimulus as well as progesterone secretion from lactational corpora lutea, resulting in the lack of estrogen secretion from ovarian follicles. As described above, the suckling stimulus profoundly suppresses gonadotropin secretion, so that follicular development and estrogen synthesis are inhibited during lactation. In this context, administration of estrogen induces the implantation of the embryo even during lactation so

long as the uterus is primed with progesterone secreted from lactational corpus luteum.

LH secretion is profoundly suppressed during lactation to avoid pregnancy during lactation (Maeda et al., 1989). As mentioned above, high levels of progesterone secreted from the lactational corpora lutea partly participate in the suppression of gonadotropin secretion (Smith, 1978). The suckling stimulus itself plays a major role in suppressing gonadotropin secretion during early and mid-lactation, because ovariectomized lactating rats show very low levels of plasma LH concentrations (Maeda et al., 1987, 1989). This suppression has been shown to be mainly due to the neuronal circuit originating from the suckling stimulus itself rather than humoral factors such as prolactin secretion. This is due to the fact that LH secretion is suppressed in early to mid-lactation even in ovariectomized mothers whose blood prolactin levels are pharmacologically suppressed and that neuronal disconnection of the hypothalamus, namely hypothalamic deafferentation, reverses suppression of LH secretion in lactating mothers without affecting prolactin levels (Tsukamura et al., 1990, 1991, 1992, 1993).

Reproductive Behavior

Female Sexual Behavior

Beach (1976) has proposed a classification of female sexuality using three criteria: (1) attractivity, (2) proceptivity, and (3) receptivity. In this classification, proceptivity and receptivity overlap conceptually as well as practically. A proceptive female rat initiates copulation by showing a lordosis posture, which also indicates her receptivity. Sex steroid hormones, especially estrogens, are responsible for all of these components of sexual behavior. Most information about the neuroendocrine mechanism mediating female sexual behavior has come from studies on lordosis (Sakuma, 1997).

Lordosis behavior

Lordosis behavior, one of the typical receptive behaviors, is characterized by a dorsiflexion of the vertebral column (Figure 9.24) (Pfaff, 1980).

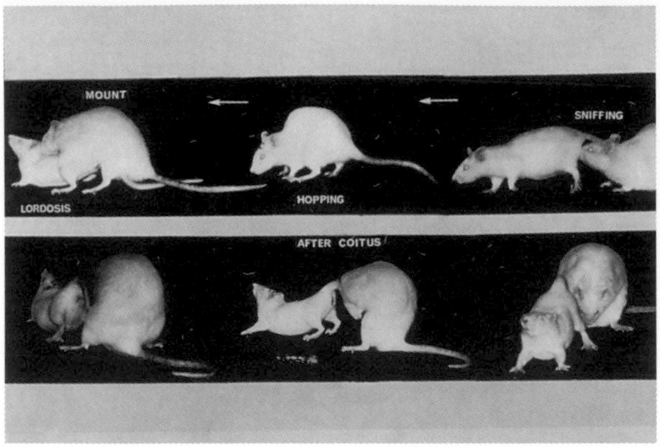

Figure 9.24 Sequence of the mating behavior in male and female rats (see text for details). Courtesy of Dr K. Yamanouchi of Waseda University.

Male Sexual Behavior

Testosterone is necessary for the mating behavior in male rats. A castrated male will not show any sexual behavior when he is kept with a female. The effect of castration on such behavior is reversed by testosterone treatment (Meisel and Sachs, 1994). The brain is the primary target for testosterone, and local implants of testosterone into various brain regions restore sexual behavior in castrated animals. The preoptic area, including the rostral hypothalamic area, is the main site of testosterone action; the posterior hypothalamus is a secondary site of action. Estrogen implants in the above-mentioned areas are as effective as testosterone. In contrast, dihydrotestosterone is not as effective as testosterone in restoring sexual behavior, suggesting that the latter may be converted to estrogen by aromatase in the brain, thus inducing male sexual behavior. Lesion of the sexual dimorphic nucleus in the preoptic area also causes a reduction in such behavior (Arendash and Gorski, 1983).

In rodents, olfactory cues play an important role in the induction of male sexual behavior (Nelson, 1995). Pheromonal information received by the vomeronasal organ is conveyed to the accessory olfactory bulb. The information is then transmitted to the medial amygdala. As described above, the preoptic area contains steroid receptors for the reception of hormonal information. The preoptic area and medial amygdala, which have a dense connection, are the key components for the regulation of male sexual behavior in rats.

Ultrasonic Vocalization During Reproductive Behavior

Adult rats have two main types of call: one at around 50 kHz and the other at approximately 22 kHz (Barfield and Thomas, 1986). Both males and females produce the 50-kHz call during copulatory behavior. The vocalization at 50 kHz in both genders is known to facilitate mating interactions. The 22-kHz call is observed in males during the postejaculatory refractory period when they exhibit a sleep-like EEG pattern.

The male 50-kHz vocalization increases in the presence of an estrous female, probably in response to olfactory stimuli. Treatment of the female partner with estrogen and/or progesterone increases the

Somatosensory pressure stimulation of the skin of the flank perineum region in the female elicits the lordosis reflex, allowing the male to insert his penis. The lordosis reflex is widely used for investigating the physiological mechanisms regulating female sexual behavior and their sexual differentiation. Ovarian steroids, such as estrogen and progesterone, are necessary for the manifestation of the reflex. Estrogen alone is sufficient for the induction of the lordosis reflex while progesterone complements the expression of proceptive behavior.

The neural mechanism mediating the lordosis reflex has been intensively investigated (Sakuma, 1997). Several brain nuclei are implicated. These are the ventromedial nucleus of the hypothalamus (VMH), preoptic area, midbrain central gray (MCG), medullary reticular formation, etc., most of which have estrogen receptors (Kawata, 1995). The VMH is one of the critical regions for the induction of lordosis by extending axons into the MCG which also receives a dense projection of GnRH neurons. In this regard, the rise in circulating estrogens during the proestrous morning activates the neural circuit for lordosis by acting on the estrogen receptors in those brain nuclei. GnRH neurons projecting into the MCG have a facilitatory role in the induction of the behavior. Interestingly, the male rat is also equipped with the neural mechanism for lordosis behavior. Yamanouchi and colleagues have discovered that the male rat, however, has two major inhibitory mechanisms: one is located in the septal region and the other in the dorsal raphe nucleus (Yamanouchi, 1997). Neonatal rises in testosterone secretion are responsible for activating these inhibitory mechanisms, resulting in lifelong suppression of lordosis behavior in the male rat.

rate of ultrasonic vocalization. The female 50-kHz vocalization observed during copulation may be associated with their steroidal condition; ovariectomized animals rarely vocalize in the presence of a male. The role of female vocalization is considered to serve as her solicitation activity and to enhance her attractiveness; devocalized females receive fewer intromissions from males.

Observation and Quantification of Rat Sexual Behavior

In order to observe sexual behavior in rats, a male rat that has already been trained to mate with normal females several times is placed in a test cage under a red dim light, e.g. a 60 × 50 × 40 cm plastic cage with bedding at the bottom to facilitate activity. After several minutes, a steroid-induced estrous female is introduced. The usual way to induce estrous behavior in female rats is to combine the injection of estradiol benzoate (10 mg) or Silastic estradiol-17β implantation for 3 days with a 0.5-mg progesterone injection on the morning of the behavioral test (Yamanouchi, 1997).

The usual sequence of events is shown in Figure 9.24. The male starts an investigation and genital sniffing if he realizes that the female is in estrus (Kondo and Yamanouchi, 1992). If the estrus is strong, she shows several kinds of soliciting behavior such as hopping and ear-wiggling. The male then shows mounting behavior with a pelvic thrust. The male rat has three distinguishable components of such activity, such as mounting without intromission, intromission (sometimes with a backward jump) and ejaculation, after which the male suddenly quits frequent pelvic thrusts and leaves the female. The female shows the lordosis behavior in response to the male mounting her.

In order to quantify this lordosis behavior, the **lordosis quotient** (LQ), i.e. the ratio of lordosis responses to 10 mounts × 100, is calculated. LQ shows a value close to 100 in females treated with estrogen and progesterone. Male sexual behavior is quantified by various parameters, such as frequencies and latencies of mounting, intromission and ejaculation (Kondo and Yamanouchi, 1992). The postejaculatory refractory period, the time between an ejaculation and the onset of the next copulation, could also be used as a parameter (Nelson, 1995).

Maternal Behavior

The presentation of foster pups is often used as an experimental paradigm to examine parental behavior in rats (Nelson, 1995). Such studies can be used to investigate how quickly the adult females (or sometimes males) start to behave in a parental manner, if they are shown the foster pups. Castrated or intact males either ignore or attack the foster pups during the first day together. Adult females which are either not pregnant or pseudopregnant act in the same way. Females in late pregnancy initiate maternal behavior immediately after the presentation of foster pups. When the pups are presented to a nulliparous female for 1–2 hours each day, she shows a maternal behavior after 5–6 days. This phenomenon is called sensitization. Sensitized rats behave just like a rat that has given birth.

The mechanism for the initiation of maternal behavior is still unknown. It is thought that a blood-borne factor could be involved in the induction of such behavior in rats, because full maternal behavior was observed in a nulliparous female within 24 hours after exchanging her blood with that of a mother rat nursing pups (Terkel and Rosenblatt, 1968). Estrogen, progesterone and prolactin have been considered as candidates for the humoral factors involved. Oxytocin may also be one of the factors, because intracerebroventicular injection of this peptide has been reported to induce maternal behavior in estrogen-primed ovariectomized rats (Pedersen et al., 1982). The neural and endocrinological regulation of the behavior is reviewed in detail by Numan (1994).

Acknowledgments

We wish to thank Drs A. Yokoyama, K. Yamanouchi, S. Hayashi, M. Yokosuka, M. Kawai, K. Kishi, F. Maekawa and S. Tsukahara for their great help in writing this manuscript and Ms. Niwa for her secretarial assistance.

References

Ackland, J.F., D'Agostino, J., Ringstrom, S.J., Hostetler, J.P., Mann, B.G. and Schwartz, N.B. (1990) *Biol. Reprod.* **43**, 347–352.

Akema, T., Tadokoro, Y. and Kimura, F. (1984) *Neuroendocrinology* **39**, 517–523.

Arai, K., Watanabe, G., Taya, K. and Sasamoto, S. (1996) *Biol. Reprod.* **55**, 127–133.

Arai, Y. (1981) *Trends Neurosci.* 291–293.

Arendash, G.W. and Gorski, R.A. (1983) *Brain Res. Bull.* **10**, 147–154.

Barfield, R.J. and Thomas, D.A. (1986) *Annals NY Acad. Sci.* **474**, 33–43.

Beach, F.A. (1976) *Horm. Behav.* **7**, 105–138.

Breje, T.C., Scharp, D.W., Lacy, P.E. *et al.* (1993) *Endocrinology* **132**, 879–887.

Cagampang, F.R.A., Maeda, K-I., Tsukamura, H., Ohkura, S. and Ota, K. (1991) *J. Endocrinol.* **129**, 321–328.

Chakraborty, C., Tawfik, O.W. and Dey, S.K. (1988) *Biochem. Biophys. Res. Commun.* **153**, 564–569.

Chazal, G., Faudon, M., Gogan, F., Hery, M., Kordon, C. and Laplante, E. (1977) *J. Endocrinol.* **75**, 251–260.

Clermont, Y. (1962) *Am. J. Anat.* **111**, 111–129.

Cowie, A.T. (1984) In: Short, R.V. and Austin, C.R. (eds) *Hormonal Control of Reproduction, Reproduction in Mammals*, Vol. 3, pp. 195–231. Cambridge: Cambridge University Press.

Daikoku-Ishido, H., Okamura, Y., Yanaihara, N. and Daikoku, S. (1990) *Dev. Biol.* **140**, 374–387.

Davis, E.C., Shryne, J.E. and Gorski, R.A. (1995) *Neuroendocrinology* **62**, 579–585.

de Greef, W.J., de Koning, J., Tijssen, A.M.I. and Karels, B. (1987) *J. Endocrinol.* **112**, 351–359.

de Kretser, D.M. and Kerr, J.B. (1994) In: Knobil, E. and Neill, D.J. (eds) *The Physiology of Reproduction*, 2nd edn, pp. 1177–1290. New York: Raven Press.

Dey, S.K. and Johnson, D.C. (1986) *Annals NY Acad. Sci.* **476**, 49–62.

Diaz, D.R., Fleming, D.E. and Rhees, R.W. (1995) *Dev. Brain Res.* **86**, 227–232.

Dluzen, D.E. and Ramirez, V.D. (1986) *Endocrinology* **118**, 1110–1113.

Eddy, E.M. and O'Brien, D.A. (1994) In: Knobil, E. and Neill, D.J. (eds) *The Physiology of Reproduction*, 2nd edn, pp. 29–77. New York: Raven Press.

Enders, A. (1965) *Am. J. Anat.* **116**, 29–68.

Eto, T., Matsuda, H., Suzuki, Y. and Hosi, T. (1962) *Jpn. J. Anim. Reprod.* **8**, 34–40.

Fortune, J.E. (1994) *Biol. Reprod.* **50**, 225–232.

Foster, D.L., Nagatani, S., Bucholtz, D.B., Tsukamura, H., Tanaka, T. and Maeda, K-I. (1999) In: Hansel, W. and McCann, S. (eds) *Nutrition and Reproduction*. Baton Rouge: LSU Press (in press).

Fox, S.R. and Smith, M.S. (1984) *Biol. Reprod.* **31**, 619–626.

Freeman, M.E. (1994) In: Knobil, E. and Neill, J.D. (eds) *The Physiology of Reproduction*, 2nd edn, pp. 613–658. New York: Raven Press.

Gallo, R.V. (1981a) *Biol. Reprod.* **24**, 100–104.

Gallo, R.V. (1981b) *Biol. Reprod.* **24**, 771–777.

George, F.W. and Wilson, J.D. (1994) In: Knobil, E. and Neill, J.D. (eds) *The Physiology of Reproduction*, 2nd edn, pp. 3–28. New York: Raven Press.

Gibori, G., Khan, I., Warshaw, M.L. *et al.* (1988) *Recent Prog. Horm. Res.* **44**, 377–429.

Gnessi, L., Fabbri, A. and Spera, G. (1997) *Endocr. Rev.* **18**, 541–609.

Goodman, R.L. (1978) *Endocrinology* **102**, 151–159.

Haisenleder, D.J., Ortolano, G.A., Jolly, D. *et al.* (1990) *Life Sci.* **47**, 1769–1773.

Haqg, C., Lee, H.M., Tizard, R. *et al.* (1992) *Genomics* **12**, 665–669.

Hashimoto, I., Hendricks, D.M., Anderson, L.L. and Melampy, R.M. (1968) *Endocrinology* **82**, 333–341.

Hayashi, S., Yokosuka, M. and Orikasa, C. (1997) In: Maeda, K-I., Tsukamura, H. and Yokoyama, A. (eds) *Neural Control of Reproduction: Physiology and Behavior*, pp. 135–152, Tokyo/Basel, Japan Scientific Societies Press/Karger.

Heap, R.B. and Flint, A.P.F. (1984) In: Short, R.V. and Austin, C.R. (eds) *Hormonal Control of Reproduction in Mammals*, Vol. 3, pp. 153–194. Cambridge: Cambridge University Press.

Hebel, R. and Stromberg, M.W. (1986) *Anatomy and Embryology of the Laboratory Rat*. Worthsee: BioMed Verlag.

Heine, P.A, Di, S., Ross, L.R., Anderson, L.L. and C.D., J. (1997) *Neuroendocrinology* **66**, 38–46.

Higuchi, T., Honda, K., Fukuoka, T., Negoro, H. and Wakabayashi, K. (1985) *J. Endocrinol.* **105**, 339–346.

Higuchi, T., Honda, K. and Negoro, H. (1986) *J. Endocrinol.* **110**, 245–250.

Higuchi, T., Tadokoro, Y., Honda, K. and Negoro, H. (1986) *J. Endocrinol.* **110**, 251–256.

Hirobe, S., He, W.-W., Lee, M.M. and Donahoe, P.K. (1992) *Endocrinology* **131**, 854–862.

Hirshfield, A.N. (1991) *Int. Rev. Cytol.* **124**, 43–101.

Hoffman, J.C. and Schwartz, N.B. (1965) *Endocrinology* **76**, 620–625.

Huckins, C. and Clermont, Y. (1968) *Arch. Anat. Histol. Embryol.* **51**, 341–354.

Imagawa, W., Yang, J., Guzman, R. and Nandi, S. (1994) In: Knobil, E. and Neill, D.J. (eds) *The Physiology of Reproduction*, 2nd edn, pp. 1033–1063. New York: Raven Press.

Jennes, L. (1989) *Brain Res.* **482**, 97–108.

Kalra, S.P. (1993) *Endocr. Rev.* **14**, 507–538.

Kalra, S.P. and Kalra, P.S. (1996) *Front. Neuroendocrinol.* **17**, 371–401.

Kaufmann, P. and Burton, G. (1994) In: Knobil, E. and Neill, J.D. (eds) *The Physiology of Reproduction*, 2nd edn, pp. 441–484. New York: Raven Press.

Kawai, M. and Kishi, K. (1997) *J. Reprod. Fertil.* **109**, 145–152.

Kawakami, M., Arita, J. and Yoshioka, E. (1980) *Endocrinology* **106**, 1087–1092.

Kawano, H.D.S. (1981) *Neuroendocrinology* **32**, 179–186.

Kawata, M. (1995) *Neurosci. Res.* **24**, 1–46.

Kimura, F., Nishihara, M., Hiruma, H. and Funabashi, T. (1991) *Neuroendocrinol* **53**, 97–102.

Knobil, E. (1980) *Recent Prog. Horm. Res.* **36**, 53–88.

Kondo, Y. and Yamanouchi, K. (1992) *J. Hum. Sci.* **5**, 2–16.

Legan, S.J. and F.J., K. (1975) *Endocrinology* **96**, 57–62.

Levine, J. E. and Duffy, M. T. (1988) *Endocrinology* **122**, 2211–2221.

Levine, J.E. and Powell, K.D. (1989) *Methods Enzymol.* **168**, 166–181.

Levine, J.E., Bauer-Dantoin, A.C., Besecke, L.M. *et al.* (1991) *Recent Prog. Horm. Res.* **47**, 97–153.

Lincoln, D.W. (1984) In: Austin, C.R. and Short, R.V. (eds) *Hormonal Control of Reproduction, Reproduction in Mammals*, Vol. 3, pp. 21–51. Cambridge: Cambridge University Press.

Lincoln, D.W., Hentzen, K., Hin, T., van der Schoot, P., Clarke, G. and Summerlee, A.J. (1980) *Exp. Brain Res.* **38**, 151–162.

Lincoln, D.W., Fraser, H.M., Lincoln, G.A., Martin, G.B. and McNeilly, A.S. (1985) *Recent Prog. Horm. Res.* **41**, 369–419.

MacLusky, N.J. and Naftolin, F. (1981) *Science* **211**, 1294–1302.

Maeda, K., Tsukamura, H. and Yokoyama, A. (1987) *Endocrinol. J.* **34**, 709–716.

Maeda, K.-I. and Tsukamura, H. (1996) *Acta Neurobiol. Exp.* **56**, 787–796.

Maeda, K.-I. and Tsukamura, H. (1997) In: Maeda, K.-I. Tsukamura, H. and Yokoyama, A. (eds) *Neural Control of Reproduction: Physiology and Behavior*, pp. 71–84. Tokyo/Basel: Japan Scientific Societies Press/Karger.

Maeda, K.-I., Tsukamura, H., Uchida, E., Ohkura, N., Ohkura, S. and Yokoyama, A. (1989) *J. Endocrinol.* **121**, 277–283.

Maeda, K.-I., Tsukamura, H., Ohkura, S. and Yokoyama, A. (1995) *Neurosci. Biobehav. Rev.* **19**, 427–437.

Maeda, K.-I., Nagatani, S., Estacio, M.A. and Tsukamura, H. (1996) *Cell. Mol. Neurobiol.* **16**, 311–324.

Maeda, K.-I., Cagampang, F.R.A., Nagatani, S. *et al.* (1998) In: Miyamoto, H. and Manabe, N. (eds) *Reproductive Biology Update: Novel Tools for Assessment of Reproductive Toxicity*, pp. 271–279. Kyoto: Shoukadoh Booksellers Co.

Matsuyama, S. and Takahashi, M. (1995) *Endocr. J.* **42**, 203–217.

Matsuyama, S., Shiota, K. and Takahashi, M. (1990) *Endocrinology* **127**, 1561–1567.

Matsuyama, S., Shiota, K., Tachi, C., Nishihara, M. and Takahashi, M. (1992) *Endocrinol. Jpn.* **39**, 51–57.

Meisel, R.L. and Sachs, B.D. (1994) In: Knobil, E. and Neill, J.D. (eds) *The Physiology of Reproduction*, 2nd edn, pp. 3–105. New York: Raven Press.

Merriam, G.R. and Wachter, K.W. (1982) *Am. J. Physiol.* **243**, E310–318.

Mochizuki, K., Fujioka, T. and Kitoh, J. (1968) In: Hoshi, T. and Naito, M. (eds) *Hinyun, Lactation* [in Japanese], pp. 1–36. Tokyo: Japan Scientific Societies Press.

Naftolin, F., Mor, G., Horvath, T.L. *et al.* (1996) *Endocrinology* **137**, 5576–5580.

Nagasawa, H., Fujiwara, K., Maejima, K., Matsushita, H., Yamada, J. and Yokoyama, A. (1983) *Jikken Dobutsu Handbook, Handbook of Experimental Animals* [in Japanese]. Tokyo: Yokendo.

Nelson, R.I. (1995) *An Introduction to Behavioral Endocrinology.* Massachusetts: Sinauer Associates.

Nishihara, M., Yoo, M.-J. and Takahashi, M. (1997) In: Maeda, K-I., Tsukamura, H. and Yokoyama, A. (eds) *Neural Control of Reproduction: Physiology and Behavior*, pp. 31–55. Tokyo/Basel: Japan Scientific Societies Press/Karger.

Noguchi, J., Hikono, H., Sato, S. *et al.* (1997) *J. Endocrinol.* **155**, 27–34.

Numan, M. (1994) In: Knobil, E. and Neill, J.D. (eds) *The Physiology of Reproduction*, 2nd edn, pp. 363–409. New York: Raven Press.

Orgen, L. and Talamantes, F. (1988) *Int. Rev. Cytol.* **112**, 1–65.

Ota, K. and Yokoyama, A. (1967) *J. Endocrinol.* **38**, 252–261.

Ojeda, S.R. and Urbanski, H.F. (1994) In: Knobil, E. and Neill, J.D. (eds) *The Physiology of Reproduction*, 2nd edn, pp. 363–409. New York: Raven Press.

Nunez, A.A. and Stephan, F.K. (1977) *Behav. Biol.* **20**, 224–234.

Parhar, I. (1997) In: Parhar, I. and Sakuma Y. (eds) *GnRH Neurons: Gene to Behavior*, pp. 99–122. Tokyo: Brain Shuppan.

Parr, M.B., Parr, E.L., Munaretto, K., Clark, M.R. and Dey, S.K. (1988) *Biol. Reprod.* **38**, 333–343.

Pedersen, C.A., Ascher, J.A., Monroe, Y.L. and Prange, A.J. (1982) *Science* **216**, 648–649.

Percy, B., Clermont, Y. and Leblond, C.P. (1961) *Am. J. Anat.* **108**, 47–77.

Pfaff, D.W. (1980) *Estrogens and Brain Function.* New York: Springer.

Picard, J.Y. and Josso, N. (1984) *Mol. Cell. Endocrinol.* **34**, 23–29.

Picard, J.Y., Benarous, R., Guerrier, D., Josso, N. and Kahn, A. (1986) *Proc. Natl Acad. Sci. USA* **83**, 5464–5468.

Ramirez, V.D. and McCann, S.M. (1963) *Endocrinology* **72**, 452–464.

Ramirez, V.D. and McCann, S.M. (1965) *Endocrinology* **76**, 412–417.

Rippel, R.H., Johnson, E.S., White, W.F., Fujino, M., Yamazaki, I. and Nakayama, R. (1973) *Endocrinology* **93**, 1449–1452.

Rivier, C. and Rivest, S. (1991) *Biol. Reprod.* **45**, 523–532.

Rivier, C., Rivier, J. and Vale, W. (1986) *Science* **231**, 607–609.

Roselli, C.E. and Klosterman, S.A. (1998) *Endocrinology* **139**, 3193–3201.

Russell, J.A. (1980) *J. Physiol.* **303**, 403–415.

Russell, L.D., Ettlin, R.A., Hikim, A.P.S. and Clegg, E.D. (1990) *Histological and Histpathological Evaluation of the Testis.* Clearwater: Cache River Press.

Sakuma, Y. (1997) In: Maeda, K.-I., Tsukamura, H. and Yokoyama, A. (eds) *Neural Control of Reproduction: Physiology and Behavior*, pp. 155–164. Tokyo/Basel: Japan Scientific Societies Press/Karger.

Samuel, C.S., Butkus, A., Coghlan, J.P. and JF., B. (1996) *Endocrinology* **137**, 3884–3890.

Sawyer, C.H. (1969) In: Haymaker, W., Anderson, E. and Nauta, W.J.H. (eds) *The Hypothalamus*, pp. 389–430. Springfield: Thomas.

Schultz, F.M. and Wilson, J.D. (1974) *Endocrinology* **94**, 979–986.

Schwanzel-Fukuda, M. (1997) In: Parhar, I. and Sakuma, Y. (eds) *GnRH Neurons: Gene to Behavior*, pp. 221–242. Tokyo: Brain Shuppan.

Schwartz, N.B. and McCormack, C.E. (1972) *Annu. Rev. Physiol.* **34**, 425–472.

Segovia, S. and Guillamon, A. (1993) *Brain Res. Rev.* **18**, 51–74.

Setchell, B.P. (1984) In: Austin, C.R. and Short, R.V. (eds) *Germ Cells and Fertilization. Reproduction in Mammals,* Vol. 1, pp. 63–101. Cambridge: Cambridge University Press.

Sharpe, R.M. (1994) In: Knobil, E. and Neill, D.J. (eds) *The Physiology of Reproduction*, 2nd edn, pp. 1363–1434. New York: Raven Press.

Sherwood, O.D., Downing, S.J., Guico-Lamm, M.L., Hwang, J.-J., O'Day-Bowman, M.B. and Fields, P.A. (1993) *Oxford Rev. Reprod. Biol.* **15**, 143–189.

Shinoda, K. (1994) *Endocr. J.* **41**, 115–138.

Smith, M.S. (1978) *Biol. Reprod.* **19**, 77–83.

Smith, M.S., Freeman, M.E. and Neill, J.D. (1975) *Endocrinology* **96**, 219–226.

Soares, M.J., Faria, T.N., Roby, K.F. and Deb, S. (1991) *Endocr. Rev.* **12**, 402–423.

Sores, M.J., Muller, H., Orwing, K.E., Peters, T.J. and Dai, G. (1998) *Biol. Reprod.* **58**, 273–284.

Sudo, K., Shiota, K., Nasaki, T. and Fujita, T. (1991) *Endocrinol. Jpn.* **38**, 39–45.

Summerlee, A.J., Ramsey, D.G. and Poterski, R.S. (1998) *Endocrinology* **139**, 479–484.

Suzuki, Y. (1954a) *Jpn. J. Vet. Sci.* **16**, 1–12.

Suzuki, Y. (1954b) *Jpn. J. Vet. Sci.* **16**, 87–100.

Suzuki, Z. (1952) *Jpn. J. Vet. Sci.* **14**, 115–126.

Takahashi, M. (1984) In: Ochiai, K., Arai, Y., Shioda, T. and Takahashi, M. (eds) *Endocrine Correlates of Reproduction*, pp. 307–315. Tokyo/Berlin: Japan Scientific Societies Press/Springer-Verlag.

Takahashi, M. and Suzuki, Y. (1969) *Endocrinol. Jpn.* **16**, 87–102.

Takahashi, M., Kasuga, F., Saito, S. et al. (1989) *Prog. Clin. Biol. Res.* **294**, 101–115.

Tamada, H., Sakamoto, M., Sakaguchi, H., Inaba, T. and Sawada, T. (1997) *Life Sci.* **60**, 1515–1522.

Terkel, J. and Rosenblatt, J.S. (1968) *J. Comp. Physiol. Psychol.* **3**, 479–482.

Thorburn, G.D. and Challis, R.G. (1979) *Physiol. Rev.* **59**, 863–918.

Toran-Allerand, C.D. (1984) *Prog. Brain Res.* **61**, 63–98.

Tran, D., Picard, J.Y., Campargue, J. and Josso, N. (1987) *J. Histochem. Cytochem.* **35**, 733–743.

Tsukamura, H., Maeda, K.-I., and Yokoyama, A. (1988) *J. Endocrinol.* **118**, 311–316.

Tsukamura, H., Maeda, K.-I., Ohkura, S. and Yokoyama, A. (1990) *J. Neuroendocrinol.* **2**, 59–63.

Tsukamura, H., Maeda, K.-I., Ohkura, S., Uchida, E. and Yokoyama, A. (1991) *Jpn. J. Anim. Reprod.* **37**, 59–63.

Tsukamura, H., Ohkura, S. and Maeda, K.-I. (1992) *J. Reprod. Dev.* **38**, 159–164.

Tsukamura, H., Ohkura, S., Coen, C.W. and Maeda, K.-I. (1993) *J. Endocrinol.* **137**, 291–297.

Tucker, H.A. (1994) In: Knobil, E. and Neill, D.J. (eds) *The Physiology of Reproduction*, 2nd edn, pp. 1065–1098. New York: Raven Press.

Wade, G.N. (1996) *Am. J. Physiol.* **270**, E1–E19.

Wagner, C.K., Nakayama, A.Y. and De Vries, G.J. (1998) *Endocrinology* **139**, 3658–3661.

Watanabe, G., Taya, K. and Sasamoto, S. (1990) *J. Endocrinol.* **126**, 151–157.

Wilson, J.D. and Lasnitzki, I. (1971) *Endocrinology* **89**, 659–668.

Yamanouchi, K. (1997) In: Maeda, K.-I., Tsukamura, H. and Yokoyama, A. (eds) *Neural Control of Reproduction: Physiology and Behavior*, pp. 219–235. Tokyo/Basel: Japan Scientific Societies Press/Karger.

Yokoyama, A. and Ota, K. (1978) In: Yokoyama, A., Mizuno, H. and Nagasawa, H. (eds) *Physiology of Mammary Glands*, pp. 266–284. Tokyo/Baltimore: Japan Scientific Societies Press/University Park Press.

Zigg, H.H., Rozen, F., Chu, K. et al. (1995). *Recent Prog. Horm. Res.* **50**, 255–273.

CHAPTER 10

Breeding and Assisted Reproduction Techniques

Frank Zimmermann
Transgene Laboratory and Animal Facility, Center for Molecular Biology,
University Heidelberg, Germany

Jüergen Weiss
Transgene Laboratory and Animal Facility, Center for Molecular Biology,
University Heidelberg, Germany

Kurt Reifenberg
Laboratory Animal Research Unit,
University Uem, Germany

Introduction

Like that of other mammalian species, the diploid rat genome is made up of 6000 million base pairs of DNA. Those regions of DNA that control discrete hereditary characteristics, usually corresponding to single proteins, are defined as genes.

The characteristic DNA sequence of genes may exhibit variations with potential impact on function. These alternative forms of genes are referred to as **alleles.** Genes occupy characteristic chromosomal regions, known as **genetic loci.**

In contrast to the **autosomes,** which exist as pairs of morphologically identical partners, the mammalian X and Y chromosomes exhibit significant morphological differences. The vast majority of genes located on the X and Y **heterosomes** lack a counterpart on the heterosomal partner, whereas few genes are shared by both chromosomes. The latter loci map to a small heterosomal region, the pseudoautosomal region. This name was well chosen, since with regard to this region heterosomes are equivalent to autosomes. In male mammals most heterosomally linked genes exist in a single allele. Only those few heterosomal genes which map to the small pseudoautosomal region exist in two alleles.

A diploid organism harbouring two identical alleles of a gene of interest, is referred to as **homozygous**. If the two alleles are distinct, the organism is **heterozygous**. The special situation of male mammals, where most heterosomally linked genes exist in a single allele, is called hemizygosity. With the emergence of transgene technology the definition of hemizygosity has had to be expanded. As described in detail in Chapter 29, pronuclear microinjection of **linearized DNA** can lead to integration of transgenic DNA sequences at a random chromosomal site of the host genome, giving rise to a new (trans)gene locus. Transgenic animals may harbour the acquired locus on one autosome but not on the partner autosome. Since the latter situation is similar to that found with regard to most heterosomal genes of male mammals, it has also been referred to as hemizygosity.

In diploid organisms, transfer of genetic information from one generation to another involves a reduction of the diploid parental genome to the intermediate haploid genome found in gametes. The special cell cycle accomplishing this genome reduction is called meiosis. During **meiosis** the two parental alleles of each heterozygous locus will be distributed randomly in different germ cells. Thus, 50% of gametes will carry one allele and 50% the other allele. This rule of inheritance was first postulated by Gregor Mendel and is referred to as the 'law of segregation'. Mendel also found that the segregation of two distinct genes is independent from one another and referred to this as the 'law of independent assortment'. As we now know, the second law of Mendel only holds true for genes which are located on distinct chromosomes. For 'linked' genes positioned on the same chromosome, the rules of inheritance are more complicated. In these cases allelic recombinations during meiosis. Whereas all autosomal partner chromosomes as well as the two X

Inbred Strains

By definition, a strain is designated as **inbred** when it has been mated brother × sister (brother–sister inbreeding, BSI) for 20 or more consecutive generations (Festing and Staats, 1973). Parent × offspring

chromosomes of female mammals recombine frequently, the situation is different with respect to the X and Y chromosome of male mammals. Since the meiotic recombination repertoire of these chromosomes is restricted to the small pseudoautosomal region, recombination occurs extremely rarely, if at all.

Nomenclature for Crossing Laboratory Animals

A specific nomenclature system has been established in order to characterize crosses between laboratory animals which carry a standardized genome. The system considers the genotype of a single gene or a group of genes of the two mating partners. To simplify matters, the system will be discussed for a single imaginary gene, characterized by the allelic repertoire A and a.

To perform an incross, homozygous animals of the genotype A/A or a/a have to be mated among one another. The **incrosses** $A/A \times A/A$ or $a/a \times a/a$ will produce offspring with the parental genotype A/A or a/a, respectively. Incrosses are used to propagate inbred strains of animals.

An **intercross** is obtained by mating heterozygous A/a animals with each other. The intercross $A/a \times A/a$ will generate animals of the genotypes A/A, A/a, and a/a at a ratio of 1:2:1, respectively.

Mating of a homozygous A/A or a/a animal with a heterozygous A/a partner is referred to as backcrossing. The backcrosses $A/A \times A/a$ or $a/a \times A/a$ will generate animals of the genotypes A/A and A/a or a/a and A/a, respectively. A series of consecutive backcrosses has to be performed to transfer individual genes or groups of linked genes of interest from undesired donor strains to desired inbred recipient strains.

Finally, matings between the homozygotes A/A and a/a are defined as **outcrosses**. The outcross $A/A \times a/a$ will result in heterozygous A/a animals and will also serve to generate hybrids.

matings may substitute for BSI, if the mating in each case is to the younger of the two parents. During BSI, the chance of individual genetic loci becoming homozygous, which is referred to as the coefficient of inbreeding F_t, is increasing continuously. For a given generation t, F_t is calculated according to the equation (Falconer, 1989):

$$F_t = 0.25 \, (1 + 2F_{t-1} + F_{t-2})$$

For strains that have been brother–sister inbred for 20, 40 and 60 generations F_t attains values of 0.986 335, 0.999 803 and 0.999 997, respectively. For some purposes it is more favourable to indicate the increment of F_t per generation, referred to as ΔF. This value is calculated according to the equation:

$$\Delta F = (F_t - F_{t-1}) \, / \, (1 - F_{t-1})$$

For the first four generations of BSI ΔF is equal to 0.250, 0.167, 0.200, and 0.188, but it approaches a constant value of 0.191 in later generations. The inbreeding coefficient indicates the chance of homozygosity of a randomly drawn genetic locus. However, since blocks of linked genes rather than individual genes are transmitted from one generation to the next, the proportion of the whole genome which will be fixed after a series of full-sib matings will be less than that calculated by the inbreeding coefficient.

The number of loci fixed in the genome of inbred animals not only depends on the number of BSI generations performed but also on the genome length and to a lesser extent on the chromosome number (Stam, 1980). For a species with a genome size of 2500 cM and a haploid chromosome number of 20, Fisher (1965) has estimated that it would take 60 generations of consecutive BSI to obtain animals with a 99% fixation of their genomes. This value most probably also holds true for inbred strains of rats, since this species has a similar genome size (estimated to be 2250 cM in the Rat Genome Database [http://ratmap.gen.gu.se/]) and the haploid rat genome is organized into 21 chromosomes. Hence, even after 60 generations of consecutive BSI inbred rats may carry a considerable number of heterozygous loci. This is referred to as residual heterozygosity. To maintain a pressure in favour of fixation of residual heterozygous loci, inbred strains are not only generated but also propagated by continuous brother × sister mating. However, if selective forces favour heterozygous genotypes, heterozygosity may persist in spite of the pressure of inbreeding due to a reduced viability or fertility of homozygotes (Hayman and Mather, 1953).

Breeding colonies of inbred strains are structured into **nucleus colonies** (NC), **pedigreed expansion colonies** (PEC) and **multiplication colonies** (MC) (Hedrich, 1990a). The NC is a self-perpetuating system which serves to maintain the inbred strain and thus is kept by strict brother × sister mating. It consists of just 10–30 breeding pairs and all animals originate from one common ancestral breeding pair. Two to three sublines are set up from the offspring of the common ancestor and allowed to diverge for 3–7 generations. The diverging sublines are carefully monitored for performance and selected genetic data. If sufficient data on each of the sublines are available, one line is selected to propagate the inbred strain further, whereas the others are removed from the NC. Between 10 and 15 rats per week can be expected from an NC. If more animals are needed, a PEC has to be set up. The breeding animals of the PEC originate from the NC exclusively. In the same way as the NC, the PEC is maintained by brother × sister mating. Since PECs primarily serve to generate breeders for MCs, the size depends on the size of the MCs to be supplied. MCs are not maintained by brother × sister mating but breeders are mated at random. MCs serve to generate sufficient numbers of animals for experimental research.

Genetic Variability of Inbred Strains

It is essential for all researchers using inbred animals to realize that the gene pool of an inbred strain, once established, is not totally stable but can be altered by three factors: residual heterozygosity, mutation and genetic contamination.

Residual heterozygosity

Even a highly inbred strain which has been **full-sib mated** for 60 or more generations may still carry a considerable number of heterozygous loci. During further propagation of the strain by brother × sister mating these loci may become fixed. Such fixation of formerly heterozygous loci represents one factor, which leads to alterations in the gene pool of an inbred strain.

Mutation

Since the exact mutation rate of particular rat genes has not yet been determined, the impact of spontaneous mutations on the gene pool of an inbred strain of rats can only be roughly estimated. The average mutation rate of eukaryotic organisms per gamete and per locus (designated as n) has been estimated to be 10^{-5} (Ohno, 1972). However, this value does not take account of the fact that mutation rates depend on genetic locus, sex and age (for review see Crow, 1997). Since in a full-sib mated inbred strain each generation is founded by two animals, each autosomal gene is represented by only four alleles. Therefore, in an inbred strain the rate of mutation occurrence at a particular locus is $4 \times n$. The chance of fixation of mutations strongly depends on whether selective forces are acting in favour or against the mutated allele. If the influence of selection is ignored, new mutations will have a one in four chance of becoming fixed in the gene pool of inbred strains. Hence, the rate of allelic substitution per generation of brother–sister inbreeding is equal to the mutation rate n (Falconer, 1989). Since the mammalian genome consists of approximately 10^5 genes, it can be postulated that a new mutation is being fixed in the gene pool of inbred rats in every generation of inbreeding. The extent to which this value reflects the actual mutation rate of rat genes is uncertain. For mice, Bailey (1977) has estimated that in every third generation one mutation is being fixed.

Genetic contamination

Genetic contamination of an inbred strain results from inadvertent introduction of foreign genes by outcrossing. In contrast to the above-mentioned mechanisms of fixation of formerly heterozygous loci and acquisition of mutations, genetic contamination is avoidable, at least in principle. However, the high frequency of genetic contaminations of inbred strains described in the past clearly demonstrates that there are no measures that can safely prevent accidental outcrossing entirely. The risk of genetic contamination is extremely high in facilities maintaining many inbred strains with identical coat colours in close proximity. Persons supervising the breeding of inbred rats are obliged to establish all measures necessary to minimize the risk of genetic contamination. This implies the safe identification of breeding animals and the training of animal caretakers. For animal facilities maintaining a broad variety of inbred variants and supplying a multitude of research groups it should be obligatory to establish genetic monitoring systems to control the authenticity of their strains. The monograph edited by Hedrich (1990b) deals with such genetic monitoring programmes, although it does not consider the use of **microsatellite marker** polymorphisms to control the gene pool of inbred strains. Today, inbred strains of rats can easily be cryopreserved in the form of frozen preimplantation embryos. This technique allows gene pools of inbred strains to be 'backed up' and enables authentic strains to be rederived in the event of genetic contamination.

In summary, changes in the gene pool of an inbred strain are unavoidable due to the fixation of residual heterozygous loci and due to the acquisition of mutations. Furthermore, the status of inbred strains is threatened by the risk of genetic contamination. Taking these factors into account, unequivocal rules have been established as to when an inbred strain has to be divided into new substrains (Festing and Staats, 1973). These rules should be followed strictly by everybody supervising the breeding of inbred strains.

Co-isogenic Strains

Inbred rats carry a highly standardized genome and thus represent ideal carriers for mutations or transgenes. Mutations of rodent genes either occur spontaneously or following treatment with mutagenic substances (Russell et al., 1979) or through exposure to ionizing radiation (Green and Roderick, 1966). Transgenes are directly introduced into inbred rats by pronuclear microinjection of appropriate DNA constructs. A **co-isogenic strain system** is generated if an inbred founder animal transmits an acquired mutation or transgene to the next generation. Each co-isogenic strain system is comprised of the original inbred strain in the nonmutated or non-transgenic form and the co-isogenic partner strain which harbours the mutated allele or the transgenic DNA sequences. The strain system thus shares an identical genetic background but differs with respect to a particular genetic locus. This feature renders co-isogenic strain systems ideal models for analysis of phenotypes induced by mutations or transgenes. Co-isogenic strains, once established, are mostly propagated by brother × sister mating.

Congenic Strains

Congenic strains are generated by transferring a specific genetic locus from an undesired donor strain to a desired recipient inbred strain. The specific

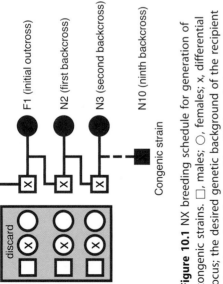

Donor strain

Recipient inbred strain

F1 (initial outcross)

N2 (first backcross)

N3 (second backcross)

N10 (ninth backcross)

Congenic strain

discard

Figure 10.1 NX breeding schedule for generation of congenic strains. □, males; ○, females; x, differential locus; the desired genetic background of the recipient inbred strain is indicated by filled symbols.

genetic locus is referred to as the differential locus and may harbour a particular allele of interest or a linked group of interesting genes such as the **major histocompatibility complex.** The function of the donor strain is to provide the differential locus. Hence, the donor strain must not necessarily be inbred and it is of no relevance whether this strain is homozygous or heterozygous for the gene of interest. In contrast, the recipient strain provides the new genetic background for the differential region and must be inbred. Transfer of the differential locus to the recipient strain is achieved by breeding measures, the basic concept of which has been developed by George Snell (1978).

Today, in almost all cases the NX breeding schedule is applied for generating congenic strains (Flaherty, 1981).

As shown in Figure 10.1, this schedule is composed of two mating steps. First, an outcross between donor and recipient strain serves to introduce the differential locus into the gene pool of the recipient strain. This initial outcross not only results in the transfer of the desired differential locus but is inevitably associated with the introduction of abundant undesired donor strain alleles. Secondly, multiple backcrosses to the recipient strain are performed in order to replace the contaminating donor strain alleles by recipient strain genes. In each backcross generation heterozygous or hemizygous carriers of the differential locus are selected from noncarrier animals. Selected animals are mated with members of the recipient inbred strain to generate the consecutive backcross. The first outcross generation should be designated as generation 1 (F1), the first

backcross generation as 2 (N2), the second backcross generation as 3 (N3), etc. By definition (Greenhouse et al., 1990), 10 crosses (counting the initial outcross as number 1) to the recipient inbred strain have to be performed in order to consider the resulting variant as congenic. If the transferred gene is dominant, established congenic strains can be maintained by further backcrossing to the recipient strain. Alternatively the congenic strain may be propagated by brother × sister mating.

Although the NX breeding system leads to extensive replacement of unwanted donor strain alleles by desired recipient strain genes, it should be noted that congenic strains still harbour considerable residual genetic contamination of donor strain origin. In this context it is important to mention that replacement of donor strain alleles with chromosomal linkage to the differential locus by recipient strain alleles strictly depends on chromosomal recombination, whereas meiotic recombination is not necessary for the replacement of unlinked donor alleles. Therefore, attempts to estimate the rate of residual contamination of congenic variants by donor strain alleles have to determine whether or not there is linkage to the differential locus. If we assume all genes of the donor and recipient strain to be polymorphic, the animals resulting from the initial outcross will carry genomes consisting of heterozygous loci exclusively. In those parts of the genome which have no linkage to the differential locus each step of the backcrossing schedule will reduce the proportion of heterozygous loci by 50%. Hence, with regard to these loci the fraction of heterozygosity can be calculated as 0.5^{n-1} for a given backcrossing generation n. According to this equation, congenic animals crossed to the recipient inbred strain for 10 generations ($n = 10$) will harbour 0.20% of heterozygous loci in those parts of their genomes not linked to the differential region. This value is generally regarded as acceptable. However, the contamination rate of congenic strains by donor strain alleles is more critical with regard to the chromosome which carries the differential locus. This chromosome will, together with the differential region, acquire a chromosomal segment of the donor strain of considerable size. The size Ln (in centimorgans) of this segment can be estimated according to the equation (Flaherty, 1981)

$$Ln = 200 \times (1 - 2^{-n}) / n \; cM$$

for a given number n of crosses to the recipient inbred strain. For all values of n greater than 5 this equation can be simplified to (Bartlett and Haldane, 1935):

$$L_n = 200/n$$

Both equations are based on the assumption that the differential locus is not located at the chromosomal end. Using these equations the size of the donor chromosomal segment flanking the differential locus can be estimated to 20 cM or 10 cM in congenic strains crossed to the recipient inbred strain for 10 or 20 generations, respectively. Since the size of the rat genome has been estimated to approximately 2250 cM these values are equivalent to approximately 1.0% and 0.5% of the genome of congenic rats, respectively.

The above-mentioned calculations demonstrate that newly established congenic strains harbour a considerable amount of residual genetic contamination by donor strain alleles. If congenic strains are further maintained by backcrossing this contamination will further decrease. However, in many cases congenic strains are propagated by brother × sister mating which will lead to fixation of heterozygous loci. Since donor and recipient strain alleles of heterozygous loci have an equal chance of fixation, 50% of such loci will be fixed with donor strain alleles. These regions of donor strain origin will be scattered throughout the genome of full-sib-mated congenic animals and are referred to as passenger loci. Importantly, in congenic strains maintained by full-sib mating all contaminating alleles located in the donor chromosomal fragment flanking the differential locus are being fixed. It should therefore be noted that congenic strains, maintained by full-sib mating, are not the same as co-isogenic strains. A co-isogenic strain only differs from the partner strain with respect to a particular genetic locus. Hence, phenotypic differences observed in co-isogenic strain systems can safely be attributed to this locus. In contrast, a full-sib-mated congenic strain differs from the recipient inbred strain with regard to passenger loci and to a multitude of donor strain alleles included in the donor chromosomal segment flanking the differential locus. Therefore, phenotypic differences observed in congenic strain systems may be induced by the differential allele, but can also be caused by residual contamination by donor strain alleles.

In the NX breeding system only heterozygous (or hemizygous) carriers of the differential locus are used for further backcrossing to the recipient inbred strain. Prior to the availability of molecular genetic tools, heterozygous carriers could be identified only if the allele was dominant and thus expressed phenotypically. Today the use of molecular biological methods will also allow recessive alleles in heterozygous carriers to be identified. In those rare cases where the differential locus is recessive and cannot be identified in heterozygotes by means of DNA analysis, a modified breeding schedule is applied for generating congenic strains. In this breeding system, which is referred to as the **M system** (Flaherty, 1981), a series of alternate intercrosses and backcrosses are performed. The former are intended to generate homozygous carriers of the differential allele which can be discriminated from heterozygous and noncarrier littermates by phenotype and the latter serve to further replace donor strain alleles by recipient strain genes.

Another factor to be considered during the establishment of congenic strains is the special situation of sex chromosomes. If the differential locus is located on an autosome, introduction of both heterosomes of the recipient inbred strain must be ensured by appropriately selecting the sex of breeding partners used for outcrossing and backcrossing. Whereas male rats of the recipient inbred strain are mated with donor strain females in the initial outcross, females of the recipient strain are paired with male carriers of the differential locus in all following backcrosses. This sex combination guarantees on the one hand that the Y chromosome of the recipient strain is introduced into the congenic strain during the initial outcross and that it is preserved during all following backcross generations. On the other hand, the choice of male carrier rats of the differential locus for backcrossing to the recipient inbred strain ensures that the congenic strain possesses a nonrecombined X chromosome of recipient strain origin. If the differential locus to be transferred to a new congenic strain is located on the X heterosome, backcrossing has to be performed by mating female carrier rats of the differential locus to males of the recipient inbred strain. This enables meiotic recombinations between the donor and recipient strain X chromosome. If the breeding schedule for autosomally linked differential loci is applied to transfer X chromosomally linked alleles, the resulting animals harbour the entire donor strain X chromosome. Such strains are termed **consomic**. The establishment of a consomic strain cannot be avoided if a Y chromosomally linked differential locus has to be transferred to a new recipient strain.

'Speed Congenic' Strains

'Traditional congenic' strains are produced by crossing animals carrying the differential locus to a recipient inbred strain for at least 10 consecutive generations. Since the generation time of rats is about three months, it will take about 3 years to generate such a congenic strain. This considerable time factor resulted in consideration as to how congenic strains could be created in a considerably shorter time by using additional selection criteria. The rationale behind this idea was to not only select for transmission of the desired donor-derived differential region but also to select against the transmission of unwanted donor genes. For this additional selection the establishment of an adequate number of genetic polymorphisms between the donor and recipient strain was required. Furthermore, the polymorphisms should be chosen so as to allow their rapid and economic determination. With the detection of microsatellite markers (Miesfeld *et al.*, 1981; Hamada *et al.*, 1982) a genomic element was identified that fulfilled all of these criteria. Microsatellites – also known as simple sequence repeats – consist of tandem repeats of basic DNA motifs composed of 2–4 single base pairs. Microsatellites are found frequently in all mammalian genomes and exhibit an extreme intraspecific polymorphism, characterized by the number of repetitions of the underlying motif. Importantly, microsatellite polymorphisms can easily be detected by polymerase chain reaction (PCR)-based amplification using primers homologous to the specific DNA sequences flanking the locus. Variations in the length of the PCR products, referred to as simple sequence length polymorphisms, can easily be evaluated by electrophoresis.

Microsatellites have provided the genetic tool necessary for accelerated generation of congenic strains. As shown by computer simulations (Weil *et al.*, 1997; Markel *et al.*, 1997), the inclusion of microsatellite-based selective breeding strategies should allow the generation of congenic strains of rodents in significantly fewer generations than is possible with random backcrossing. Lander and Schork (1994) have introduced the term '**speed congenics**' to describe congenic strains developed using such methods. The generation of 'speed congenic' strains of mice is already practised today (Serreze *et al.*, 1996). In contrast, 'speed congenic' rat strains are not produced routinely yet. This should be the case, however, as soon as adequate numbers of microsatellite markers have been characterized for this species. Recently, James and Lindpaintner (1997) have published a variety of internet addresses, where detailed information about rat microsatellites is available.

Segregating Inbred Strains

Once established, co-isogenic and congenic strains are often propagated by brother × sister mating. Sometimes homozygosity of the gene of interest of such strains will interfere with strain viability or fertility. In these cases the strain is full-sib mated with this gene forced to the heterozygous state. Heterozygosity can be forced by either backcrossing or by intercrossing. In the former case heterozygous and homozygous carriers of the gene of interest are mated with each other and in the latter case heterozygous carriers are crossed. An example of segregating inbred strains are congenic rat strains carrying the recessive *rnu* (Rowett nude) allele, which induces a severe immunodeficiency. Since *rnu/rnu* females have difficulties in raising their young, these strains are maintained by mating homozygous *rnu/rnu* males with heterozygous *rnu/+* females.

Hybrids

Hybrid rats are generated by outcrossing members of two distinct inbred strains. They therefore carry a haploid chromosome set from each parental strain. Since the X and the Y chromosome in male hybrids will originate exclusively from the maternal and paternal strain, respectively, it is essential for a hybrid generation to discriminate which inbred strain has been used as the paternal or maternal progenitor. The specific genome of F1 hybrids can only be generated by crossing the parental inbred strains. Thus, for hybrid production these strains have to be maintained permanently. If F1 hybrids are intercrossed, random segregation and independent assortment of heterozygous loci will lead to F2 animals which are genetically distinct.

Inbred animals and hybrids share the feature of genetic uniformity. However, in contrast to the high degree of homozygosity of inbred genomes, hybrids exhibit a high degree of heterozygosity. For a variety of characters and species, inbred animals have been shown to demonstrate more variation due to environmental factors than noninbred animals (Livesay, 1930; Hyde, 1973). In such experiments the method of choice to obtain genetic uniformity without increased environmental variation is the use of hybrids. Another reason why hybrids are attractive experimental animals is their higher viability and enhanced fertility as compared with inbred animals,

Recombinant Inbred Strains

The breeding schedule for the generation of **recombinant inbred (RI) strains** starts with an outcross between two well-established inbred strains, which are referred to as **progenitor strains**. The resulting F1 hybrids are intercrossed to generate a large number of F2 animals. At this stage, pairs of F2 animals are chosen at random to serve as founders for new inbred strains of rats. Hence, the offspring from each F2 pair has to be maintained separately from all other offspring and two of these animals are chosen randomly to perform the first generation of full-sib mating. Twenty consecutive generations of strict brother–sister inbreeding have to be performed with the descendants of each F2 pair to consider the resulting strains as **RI strains**. The breeding schedule mentioned will generate a broad panel of new RI strains for a particular combination of progenitor strains. Different RI strains established with the same progenitor strains are considered as members of the same RI set.

Each strain of a particular RI set will harbour multiple recombined chromosomes, made up of fragments from each progenitor strain. Importantly, every strain of the set will carry a unique pattern of chromosomal recombinations, which is stably inherited upon further strain propagation by inbreeding. Donald Bailey had the foresight to realize the importance of recombinant inbred strains for genetic analysis (Bailey, 1971, 1981). The most important use

of RI strains is to determine map positions and linkage. For mapping of a newly cloned gene, the progenitor strains of existing sets of RI strains have to be checked for polymorphism of the gene of interest. Once alternative alleles have been distinguished for the progenitors of a set, all RI strains of this set are typed. In principle, 50% of the strains of a set should carry one and 50% the other allele. The results of this analysis is referred to as the **strain distribution pattern (SDP)** of the specific locus. The SDP of a single locus is not informative. However, the more SDPs that are available for a set of RI strains, the higher the chances for a new gene to be mapped by comparing its SDP with that of other genes. Appropriate computer programs for such analyses are available (Manly, 1993).

If SDPs of two defined loci are compared for linkage analysis, the result is usually presented in terms of concordance or discordance. Two distinct genetic loci of interest are considered to be concordant within a particular RI strain, if this strain exclusively carries alleles from one progenitor strain. If a particular RI strain harbours alleles from both progenitors, the loci are designated as discordant. For a pair of unlinked loci 50% of RI strains of a given set should show concordance and 50% should exhibit discordance. On the other hand, for two closely linked loci about 100% of RI strains of a certain set will exhibit concordance and virtually no strains will show discordance. For loci which are less closely linked, levels of concordance and discordance will lie between the described extremes. The terms N and i denote the total number of RI strains typed for discordance and the number of discordant strains observed, respectively. The fraction $R = i/N$ gives the level of discordance observed in one or multiple sets of RI strains. Importantly, the level of discordance observed in RI sets for two particular loci reflects the mean estimate of the loci's map distance. Based on a mathematical approach by Haldane and Waddington (1931), the probability of recombination of two linked loci r, which represents a direct measure of the map distance of these loci, can be calculated according to the equation

$$r = R / (4 - 6R)$$

This equation allows the direct estimation of the distance of two genetic loci of interest (in centimorgans/100) from the fraction R of discordance observed in one or multiple RI sets. For further reading, the excellent book by Silver (1995) is recommended.

Outbred Stocks

The basic concept of outbred stocks is to preserve a broad genetic variety and thus to more closely mimick the genetic situation of human populations. Outbred animals are usually used to evaluate pharmacological actions of drugs and to investigate the toxicological potential of chemicals. Outbred stocks may also serve as initial populations in selection experiments. Furthermore, transgenic strains are frequently established by using outbred rats as embryo donors.

During breeding of outbred stocks three important points have to be respected. First, outbred stocks once established have to be maintained as closed populations, into which no new animals should be introduced. Secondly, loss of alleles from the initial outbred gene pool should be reduced to a minimal level. Thirdly, formation of stock sublines with significant differences in gene frequencies should be prevented. The extent to which loss of alleles or subline formation can be avoided is determined by various parameters (Rapp, 1972), including population size, sequence of generations, choice of animals for breeding and breeding systems.

Population size

The primary factor influencing the decrease of average heterozygosity associated with outbreeding is the effective population size, which is defined as the total number of those breeding animals supplying offspring to the next stock generation. Using computer simulations Eggenberger (1973) has proposed that an effective population size of 400 animals is required to reduce the loss of alleles from the gene pool of an outbred stock to a negligible level. It should be noted that loss of alleles from outbred gene pools, once it has occurred, cannot be reversed by breeding measures. Furthermore, rederivation of outbred stocks by embryo transfer is usually associated with bottleneck effects of population size and thus may lead to an additional increase of average stock homozygosity.

Sequence of generations

Since the loss of alleles from gene pools of outbred stocks depends on meiotic events, breeding pairs should be exchanged as rarely as possible. This measure will slow down the process of decreasing average heterozygosity.

Choice of animals for breeding

Artificial selection for specific phenotypes should be strictly avoided for breeding of outbred stocks (Eggenberger, 1973). If strong selective forces are acting, particular alleles may be fixed in the gene pools of outbred populations within few generations. This rule should also be followed with respect to breeding and growth performance. An increase of these parameters, although very attractive for economic reasons, should not be the objective of a standardized outbreeding population.

Breeding systems

A variety of breeding systems have been developed to maintain a high degree of average heterozygosity within a population. Random breeding is characterized by the rule that any animal has an equal chance of mating with any other animal in the population (Falconer, 1989). However, since this does not exclude the mating of close relatives, random breeding cannot be recommended for minimizing loss of average heterozygosity from a population's gene pool. Other breeding systems are based on maximum avoidance of inbreeding by mating least-related animals (Wright, 1921). These systems depend on knowledge of kinship of mating animals and thus require a pedigree of the colony. Such pedigree-based breeding systems have a low initial rate of decrease of average heterozygosity. However, in later generations rotation breeding systems were found to be superior to pedigree-based breeding schedules for minimizing loss of heterozygosity.

In the **circular mating rotation breeding system** (Kimura and Crow, 1963) the population is subdivided into an equal number of female and male breeding animals, which are allocated odd and even numbers, respectively. The total number of breeding animals is kept constant in all following generations. The circular mating system provides rules of how breeding animals of a new generation are generated by mating particular breeders of the last generation. In Table 10.1 these rules are depicted for $n = 4$, $n = 6$ and $n = 8$ breeding animals. The table presents pairs of numbers of breeding animals. The first and second number of a particular pair indicate the father and the mother of the new breeding animal, respectively. For example, circular mating is performed with 8 animals ($n = 8$), the female breeder no. 1 [1(f)] of a new generation is created by mating the male breeder no. 8 of the last generation with the female breeder no. 1 of the last generation.

Table 10.1 Circular mating (Kimura and Crow, 1963) for n = 4, n = 6 and n = 8 breeding animals

n	F	Breeding animals							
		1(f)	2(m)	3(f)	4(m)	5(f)	6(m)	7(f)	8(m)
4	1	4/1	2/1	2/3	4/3				
	2≅1								
6	1	6/1	2/1	2/3	4/3	4/5	6/5		
	2≅1								
8	1	8/1	2/1	2/3	4/3	4/5	6/5	6/7	8/7
	2≅1								

F, generation; f, female; m, male; 2≅1, equivalent to.

Table 10.2 Circular pair mating (Kimura and Crow, 1963) for n = 3, n = 4, n = 5, n = 6, n = 7 and n = 8 breeding pairs

n	F	Breeding pairs							
		1	2	3	4	5	6	7	8
3	1	3/1	1/2	2/3					
	2≅1								
4	1	4/1	1/2	2/3	3/4				
	2≅1								
5	1	5/1	1/2	2/3	3/4	4/5			
	2≅1								
6	1	6/1	1/2	2/3	3/4	4/5	5/6		
	2≅1								
7	1	7/1	1/2	2/3	3/4	4/5	5/6	6/7	
	2≅1								
8	1	8/1	1/2	2/3	3/4	4/5	5/6	6/7	7/8
	2≅1								

F, generation; ≅, equivalent to.

As can be seen from Table 10.1 the circular mating system requires that each breeder has to be mated twice. Since this effort cannot be justified in an economically managed breeding facility, circular mating is hardly ever used for the propagation of outbred stocks. The **circular pair mating system** (Kimura and Crow, 1963) overcomes this disadvantage. This breeding system uses permanently mated breeding pairs. The cages of the breeding pairs are numbered and the total number of pairs (cages) is kept constant for the subsequent generations. For providing breeding animals to a particular cage n of the next generation a female offspring of cage n and a male offspring of cage $n-1$ of the last generation are mated. In Table 10.2, the circular pair mating system is shown for $n = 3$, $n = 4$, $n = 5$, $n = 6$, $n = 7$ and $n = 8$ breeding pairs, respectively. The table consists of pairs of cage numbers. The first and second number of a particular pair specifies from which cage (breeding pair) of generation F_{n-1} the male and female partner has to be chosen for establishing a new breeding pair in generation F_n, respectively.

Although the circular pair mating system is easily managed, it is rarely used for maintaining outbred populations. **Rotation breeding systems**

Table 10.3 Systematic breeder rotation (Poiley, 1960) for m = 3, m = 4, m = 5, m = 6, m = 7 and m = 8 blocks

m	F	Blocks							
		1	2	3	4	5	6	7	8
3	1	3/2	1/3	2/1					
	2≅1								
4	1	3/4	4/1	1/2	2/3				
	2≅1								
5	1	5/4	1/5	2/1	3/2	4/3			
	2≅1								
6	1	3/6	6/1	5/2	1/3	2/4	4/5		
	2≅1								
7	1	2/6	3/7	6/1	7/2	4/3	5/4	1/5	
	2≅1								
8	1	6/7	1/8	7/1	8/2	2/3	3/4	4/5	5/6
	2≅1								

F, generation; ≅, equivalent to.

Table 10.4 Mating system by Robertson (Falconer, 1967) for m = 4 and m = 8 blocks

m	F	Blocks							
		1	2	3	4	5	6	7	8
4	1	1/2	3/4	2/1	4/3				
	2≅1								
8	1	1/2	3/4	5/6	7/8	2/1	4/3	6/5	8/7
	2≅1								

F, generation; ≅, equivalent to.

commonly used for propagating outbred stocks include the **systematic breeder rotation** by Poiley (1960), the mating system by Robertson (Falconer, 1967), the **cyclical system** by Falconer (1967) and the **Han-rotation system** (Rapp, 1972). These four systems are characterized by subdivision of the outbred population into a number of equally large blocks. Whereas in the other three systems the number of blocks can be chosen freely, the system by Robertson only allows the choice of 4 or 8 or 16 or 32 etc. blocks. The total number of blocks is kept constant for all generations. A single block is composed of an equal number of male and female breeders, such as a single breeding pair or – usually – a multitude of breeding pairs. It is important for

providing breeders to the next generation, that the offspring from each block are kept separately from the offspring of the other blocks. During transition from one generation to the next, rotation system-specific rules have to be followed as to how new breeders for a particular breeding block are recruited from the offspring of the last generation. In Tables 10.3, 10.5 and 10.6 the systematic breeder rotation by Poiley, the cyclical system by Falconer and the Han-rotation system are presented for m = 3, m = 4, m = 5, m = 6, m = 7 and m = 8 blocks, respectively. Table 10.4 shows the mating system by Robertson for m = 4 and m = 8 blocks. These tables consist of pairs of block numbers. The first and second number of a particular pair specifies from

Table 10.5 Cyclical system by Falconer (1967) for m = 3, m = 4, m = 5, m = 6, m = 7 and m = 8

m	F	Blocks							
		1	2	3	4	5	6	7	8
3	1	1/2	2/3	3/1					
	2	1/3	2/1	3/2					
	3≅1								
4	1	1/2	2/3	3/4	4/1				
	2	1/3	2/4	3/1	4/2				
	3	1/4	2/1	3/2	4/3				
	4≅1								
5	1	1/2	2/3	3/4	4/5	5/1			
	2	1/3	2/4	3/5	4/1	5/2			
	3	1/4	2/5	3/1	4/2	5/3			
	4	1/5	2/1	3/2	4/3	5/4			
	5≅1								
6	1	1/2	2/3	3/4	4/5	5/6	6/1		
	2	1/3	2/4	3/5	4/6	5/1	6/2		
	3	1/4	2/5	3/6	4/1	5/2	6/3		
	4	1/5	2/6	3/1	4/2	5/3	6/4		
	5	1/6	2/1	3/2	4/3	5/4	6/5		
	6≅1								
7	1	1/2	2/3	3/4	4/5	5/6	6/7	7/1	
	2	1/3	2/4	3/5	4/6	5/7	6/1	7/2	
	3	1/4	2/5	3/6	4/7	5/1	6/2	7/3	
	4	1/5	2/6	3/7	4/1	5/2	6/3	7/4	
	5	1/6	2/7	3/1	4/2	5/3	6/4	7/5	
	6	1/7	2/1	3/2	4/3	5/4	6/5	7/6	
	7≅1								
8	1	1/2	2/3	3/4	4/5	5/6	6/7	7/8	8/1
	2	1/3	2/4	3/5	4/6	5/7	6/8	7/1	8/2
	3	1/4	2/5	3/6	4/7	5/8	6/1	7/2	8/3
	4	1/5	2/6	3/7	4/8	5/1	6/2	7/3	8/4
	5	1/6	2/7	3/8	4/1	5/2	6/3	7/4	8/5
	6	1/7	2/8	3/1	4/2	5/3	6/4	7/5	8/6
	7	1/8	2/1	3/2	4/3	5/4	6/5	7/6	8/7
	8≅1								

F, generation; ≅, equivalent to.

Table 10.6 Han-rotation system (Rapp, 1972) for m = 3, m = 4, m = 5, m = 6, m = 7 and m = 8 blocks

m	F	Blocks 1	2	3	4	5	6	7	8
3	1	3/1	1/2	2/3					
	2	2/1	3/2	1/3					
	3≅1								
4	1	4/1	1/2	2/3	3/4				
	2	3/1	4/2	1/3	2/4				
	3≅1								
5	1	5/1	1/2	2/3	3/4	4/5			
	2	4/1	5/2	1/3	2/4	3/5			
	3	2/1	3/2	4/3	5/4	1/5			
	4	3/1	4/2	5/3	1/4	2/5			
	5≅1								
6	1	6/1	1/2	2/3	3/4	4/5	5/6		
	2	5/1	6/2	1/3	2/4	3/5	4/6		
	3	3/1	4/2	5/3	6/4	1/5	2/6		
	4≅1								
7	1	7/1	1/2	2/3	3/4	4/5	5/6	6/7	
	2	6/1	7/2	1/3	2/4	3/5	4/6	5/7	
	3	4/1	5/2	6/3	7/4	1/5	2/6	3/7	
	4≅1								
8	1	8/1	1/2	2/3	3/4	4/5	5/6	6/7	7/8
	2	7/1	8/2	1/3	2/4	3/5	4/6	5/7	6/8
	3	5/1	6/2	7/3	8/4	1/5	2/6	3/7	4/8
	4≅1								

F, generation; ≅, equivalent to.

which blocks of generation F_{n-1} male and female breeders have to be recruited for establishment of new breeding blocks in generation F_n, respectively.

As shown by Eggenberger (1973) the systematic breeder rotation by Poiley, the mating system by Robertson, the cyclical system by Falconer and the Han-rotation system are equally well suited for the preservation of a high level of average heterozygosity of outbred stocks. However, the breeder rotation by Poiley cannot be recommended, since it will lead to subline formation.

Embryo Transfer

General

Modern laboratory animal facilities usually possess knowledge about embryo transfer techniques. This important technology allows new strains to be introduced into animal facilities in the form of preimplantation embryos and thereby minimizes the risk of concomitant contamination with specific pathogens. In addition, the efficient transfer of embryos allows the establishment of further assisted reproduction techniques, such as cryopreservation of preimplantation embryos and *in vitro* fertilization (IVF). Furthermore, efficient transgene technology is based on transfer of DNA-microinjected embryos to recipient females.

In order to obtain embryos of rats either naturally cycling females or females with an ovulation induced by hormonal treatment (**superovulation**) are mated with fertile males. Application of ovulation-inducing hormones should be carefully matched with the illumination cycle of the laboratory animal facility. All information about timing of superovulation provided in this chapter refers to light and dark periods of 12 hours each. Ovulation of female rats, irrespective of whether hormone-induced or naturally occurring, will take place approximately at the midpoint of the dark cycle. Females mated with males during this dark period will most probably tolerate copulation. Only those females which have copulated are used for embryo recovery. The developmental stage of the isolated embryos depends on the time point of embryo recovery. The first, second, etc. light periods following ovulation and copulation are referred to as day 0.5, 1.5, etc. of pregnancy, respectively. Generally, the development of preimplantation embryos of rats is slightly delayed in comparison to that of mice (Sullivan and Ouhibi, 1995). However, this developmental difference is negligible until day 1.5 of pregnancy. Hence, equivalent to the murine situation, rat embryos of the one- and two-cell stage can be obtained at days 0.5 and 1.5 of pregnancy, respectively. Rat embryos from the one-cell to the morula stage are isolated from the oviducts of donor females and rat blastocysts are derived from the uteri.

Specific manipulations are usually performed with rat embryos of certain developmental stages. For generation of transgenic rats embryos of the one-cell stage, designated as zygotes, are microinjected with appropriate DNA constructs. Although it is also possible to cryopreserve rat embryos of other developmental stages with high efficiency, we prefer to use embryos of the two-cell stage for freezing. For embryo transfers performed for reasons of hygiene we also recommend the use of embryos of the two-cell stage.

Once manipulated *in vitro*, rat embryos, should be transferred to the reproductive tract of suitable recipient females immediately. If the embryos are subjected to additional culture periods, it should be noted that they will easily develop to the two-cell stage *in vitro*. However, culture beyond the two-cell stage is problematic, because rat embryos show a complete developmental blockage at the two-cell or four-cell stage *in vitro* (Mayer and Fritz, 1974). In principle, embryo transfers to pregnant recipients are also possible, but the transferred embryos and the recipient's own embryos would have to compete for maternal resources. It is recommended, therefore, to use pseudopregnant rats as recipients. Although pseudopregnancy in rat females can be induced by mechanical stimulation (DeFeo, 1966; Yang, 1968), pseudopregnant recipients are usually generated by providing a natural copulation stimulus by mating with vasectomized males. The first, second, etc. light periods following the night of sterile copulation are referred to as days 0.5, 1.5, etc. of pseudopregnancy. Rat embryos from the one-cell to the morula stage have to be transferred into the oviducts of females at day 0.5 of pseudopregnancy and rat blastocysts are transferred into the uteri of recipients at day 3.5 of pseudopregnancy. Embryos transferred into oviducts of rats must be protected by an intact zona pellucida, whereas this structure is not necessary for blastocysts transferred into the uterus.

Materials and Equipment

Anaesthesia

For implantation of **osmotic pumps**, female rats are subjected to short-term inhalation anaesthesia using ether. Embryo transfers and vasectomies are performed under injection anaesthesia whereby rats are injected intraperitoneally with a combination of 11.5 mg ketamine hydrochloride and 0.1 mg xylasine per 100 g body weight. In order to prevent the eyes of anaesthetized animals from drying up, a tear-substitute liquid or eye ointment must be applied.

Pipettes for embryo handling and embryo transfer

Micropipettes for embryo handling are pulled from Pasteur pipettes as described by Rafferty (1970) and micropipettes for transfer of embryos into oviducts are pulled from borosilicate glass capillaries with an inner diameter of 0.78 mm and an outer diameter of 1.0 mm (Clark Electromedical Instruments, Pangbourne, UK). For production of both kinds of pipettes the glass is softened by rotating the capillaries in a flame (small Bunsen burner or microflame) and pulled immediately after removal from the flame. Resulting micropipettes should have an internal diameter of between 150 and 200 μm. Such pipettes are scratched with a diamond pen and are then neatly broken. Pasteur pipettes for embryo handling are directly attached to a silicone tube and a mouthpiece. Pipettes for embryo transfer are shortened to a length of 8–10 cm. Each piece is inserted into a Pasteur pipette, leaving a 2–3-cm piece protruding from it, and fixed in that position with silicone. Once the silicone has hardened, the opening of these pipettes is fire-polished using a microforge (Stoelting, Chicago, USA). This measure will protect the oviduct epithelium from damage during embryo transfer.

approximately 600 μl of M16 medium. Alternatively, microdrop cultures as described by Hogan *et al.* (1994) can also be set up.

Surgical instruments

For incisions, surgical scissors and forceps are used. For oviduct dissection, oviduct flushing and embryo transfer we recommend using Dumont no. 5 forceps. Dissection of the bursa ovarica should be performed using extra fine straight scissors. For closing of the body wall resorbable suture material such as catgut is applied. Skin incisions are closed with autoclips.

Preparation of Donor Females and Embryo Recovery

Small numbers of rat embryos may be obtained by setting up natural matings. Since the oestrous cycle of rats lasts 4–5 days, only 20–25% of a random group of mature females will be in the proestrous stage at a certain time point and tolerate copulation. The copulation rate of naturally cycling females can be markedly increased by allowing only those females to mate which are in the proestrous stage, judging from the external appearance of the genitals or suggested by vaginal cytological analysis. As described by Baker (1979), rats in the proestrous stage are characterized by a slightly swollen vulva and dry vagina. As shown in Chapters 9 and 25 vaginal smears obtained from proestrous females are typically characterized by large numbers of nucleated epithelial cells.

For all experiments requiring large numbers of rat embryos, superovulation will be induced in donor females. The aims of hormone treatment of embryo donors are to synchronize the oestrous cycle and to achieve a high embryo yield. In mice superovulation can be reliably induced by application of pregnant mare serum gonadotropin (PMSG) and human chorionic gonadotropin (HCG) at an interval of 47–48 h. However, this treatment is considered to be of limited value for superovulation of rats (Whittingham, 1975; Wood and Whittingham, 1981). In our hands, however, immature rats of 31–33 days of the Crl:CD strain responded excellently to PMSG and HCG treatment. Superovulation was induced in these animals by intraperitoneal treatment with 20–30 IU PMSG and HCG each.

Media

Rat embryos can be transferred into the same media as that used for murine embryos. We recommend M2 medium for embryo recovery and handling and M16 medium for embryo culture (Hogan *et al.*, 1994) since these media can be produced easily from concentrated stocks. For *in vitro* fertilizations we use modified Whittingham's medium supplemented with 30 mg/ml bovine serum albumin (Whittingham, 1971; Fraser and Drury, 1975). We recommend a reduction in the concentration of phenol red in modified Whittingham's medium from 10 mg/100 ml as originally supplied to 5 mg/100 ml. All cultivation steps are performed in a humidified incubator at a CO_2 concentration of 5% and a temperature of 38.5°C. M16 medium and modified Whittingham's medium should be preincubated for 1 h before use.

Microscopes

For oviduct rupture and flushing and for embryo handling we recommend M8 (Leica, Bensheim, Germany). For embryo transfer we use M650 (Leica).

Tissue culture dishes

Oviducts are flushed in 60-mm plastic tissue culture dishes available from a variety of companies. For culture of rat embryos we recommend organ tissue culture dishes (60 × 15 mm with centre well; Becton Dickinson Labware, New York, USA) filled with

PMSG was applied 7.5 h after onset of the light cycle and HCG application was performed 48 h thereafter. Hormone-treated females were mated at the end of the light cycle in which HCG had been applied. In immature Crl:CD females this superovulation treatment induced average ovulation rates of 20–40.

Armstrong and Opavsky (1988) have described an alternative approach to induce superovulation in rats. Their protocol combines continuous infusion of a highly purified preparation of follicle-stimulating hormone (FSH, Folltropin®, Vetrepharm Inc., London, Ontario, Canada) by means of an osmotic pump and a single intraperitoneal HCG application. Filling of the osmotic pump (type 1003 D with a pumping rate of 1 μl per hour, Alza Corp, Palo Alto, USA) is prepared by resuspending 35 mg Folltropin® (one vial) in sterile saline. The pump is filled with 200 μl of this solution and then allowed to equilibrate in sterile saline for at least 4 h. Implantations of osmotic pumps are performed 5.5 h after onset of the light cycle. Therefore, females are anaesthetized and the cervical region is shaved and disinfected with 80% ethanol. As illustrated in Figure 10.2 a small transverse skin incision of a length of 1.0 cm is made dorsally on the neck, above the cervical region. Using a pair of closed scissors a subcutaneous canal is built from this incision in the caudal direction. The osmotic pump is pushed through this canal to the region adjacent to the lumbar spine. Alternatively, osmotic pumps may be implanted intraperitoneally. Fifty-four hours after implantation of the pump (= 0.5 h prior to the end of the second light period following implantation), females are treated intraperitoneally with 20–30 IU of HCG and are immediately mated. The protocol of Armstrong and Opavsky (1988) yields optimal results when applied to immature rats. Superovulated females may yield 60–80 oocytes regardless of the strain used. In mature females the ovulation rate will be considerably lower.

A third method for the induction of superovulation of rats has been described by Rouleau et al. (1993). The protocol combines the superovulation treatment of Armstrong and Opavsky (1988) with a previous application of des-Gly^{10} [D-Ala^{6}] LH-RH ethylamide, referred to as LH-RH. LH-RH is applied subcutaneously at a dose of 40–60 μg 5.5 h after the onset of the light period. In the second light period following LH-RH application an osmotic pump with Folltropin® is implanted as described. Fifty-four hours after pump implantation the animals are injected intraperitoneally with 20–30 IU of HCG and are immediately mated with males. The superovulation protocol of Rouleau et al. (1993) is especially suited for the superovulation of mature females of an age of 54–70 days. Depending on the strains used, it will yield 8–30 oocytes per female.

Irrespective of the way in which superovulation is induced, hormone-treated females are mated individually with fertile males. Mating frequency of fertile males should be twice per week in order to maintain plugging performance. Superovulated females are checked for signs of copulation at the beginning of the light cycle following mating. In immature rats the copulatory plug is usually easily detectable, whereas adult rats may loose the vaginal plug shortly after copulation or the plug may be located deeply within the vagina (Voipio and Nevalainen, 1998). For adult females it is recommended therefore to control for copulatory

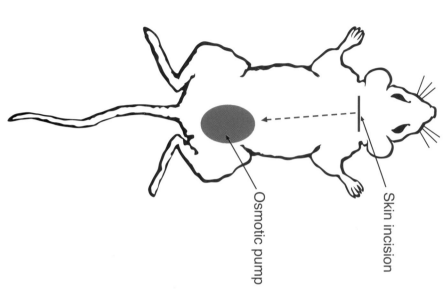

Figure 10.2 Subcutaneous implantation of osmotic pumps into female rats. A skin incision is made in the cervical region and the osmotic pump inserted into the subcutis. The final location of the pump is as shown.

3–5 min of enzyme treatment the zygotes are washed by passing through at least three drops of M2 medium and are cultured in M16 medium until DNA injection.

Embryos of the two-cell stage needed for cryo-preservation are isolated by flushing the oviducts under the microscope. A blunt-ended 30G needle is inserted into the opening of the oviduct (the infundibulum), fixed with a pair of no. 5 microforceps, and flushed with approximately 100 μL of M2 medium. Isolated two-cell-stage embryos are rinsed by passing them through at least three drops of M2 medium. For embryos that may be contaminated with a pathogenic rat virus additional rinsing steps are recommended (Rouleau *et al.*, 1993). Embryos of the two-cell stage are cultured in M16 medium until further use.

Vasectomy of Rats

Males of an outbred strain such as Crl:CD should be used for vasectomy, because such animals exhibit a high plugging performance. Vasectomy should be performed at 10 weeks of age. The rats are anaesthetized, placed on their backs, their ventral abdomen shaved and disinfected with 80% ethanol. Transverse incisions of approximately 1.5 cm are made through the skin and body wall at a point level with the knees. The testes, including their surrounding fat pads, are exteriorized. Each ductus deferens, which can easily be recognized by a blood vessel running along one side, is separated from the mesentery membrane and an approximately 5-mm piece is removed using a **thermocauter.** The body wall is closed and the skin clipped together with autoclips. Animals should be allowed to recover from surgery for 2 weeks before allowing them to mate. Vasectomized males should be mated twice per week to maintain plugging performance and may be used until they attain an age of 1 year.

Preparation of Recipient Females and Embryo Transfer

As embryo recipients, females of an outbred strain such as Crl:CD and of an age of 12–26 weeks should be used. Such females are mated with vasectomized sterile males at the end of the light period. By mating only those females that are in the proestrous cycle stage, the copulation rate can be markedly increased. At the beginning of the light period after mating, the

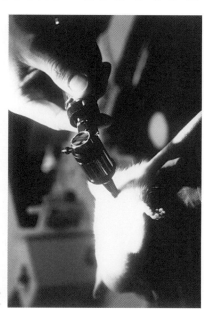

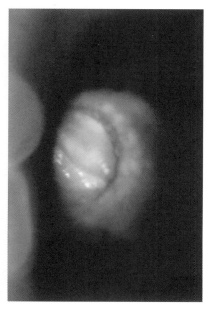

Figure 10.3 Otoscopic investigation of the rat vagina for copulatory plug. (a) Otoscope introduced into the vagina of a mature rat. (b) Copulatory plug in the depth of the vagina as observed through the otoscope.

plugs by means of **otoscopic** inspection of the vagina (Figure 10.3). For safe evaluations it may also be necessary to check for the presence of sperm in vaginal smears.

For the recovery of zygotes for pronuclear injections the copulation-positive females are sacrificed 5 hours after onset of day 0.5 of pregnancy. If two-cell-stage embryos are required, females are sacrificed at the onset of day 1.5 of pregnancy. For embryo recovery the abdominal cavity is opened and the oviducts are dissected as described by Hogan *et al.* (1994). Dissected oviducts are transferred into drops of M2 medium. For isolation of zygotes, the swollen proximal part of the oviduct, called the ampulla, is ruptured under the microscope using a 30G needle. In most cases the zygotes, surrounded by masses of cumulus cells, will spontaneously pour out of the ruptured ampulla. To remove cumulus cells zygotes are transferred into a solution of hyaluronidase (Calbiochem, Corp., La Jolla, USA) in M2 medium (5000 IU/mL). After

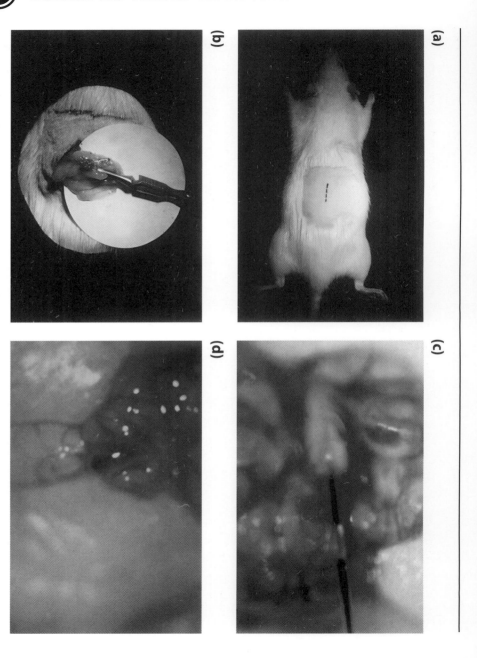

Figure 10.4 Embryo transfer to the oviduct of a pseudopregnant recipient rat. (a) Position of the skin incision used to transfer embryos into both oviducts. (b) Anaesthetized recipient female with exteriorized and serafine-fixed ovary. (c) Micropipette introduced into the infundibulum of the oviduct. (d) Ampulla of the oviduct filled with methylene blue staining solution.

vagina of the females is otoscopically checked for a copulatory plugs. In our hands 30 Crl:CD females in a random oestrous cycle stage or 10 females in the proestrous stage have to be mated to obtain two to seven copulation-positive pseudopregnant females.

Since most manipulations on rat embryos are performed with zygotes or two-cell-stage embryos, virtually all embryo transfers are to the oviducts of females at day 0.5 of pseudopregnancy. For this procedure the recipient female is anaesthetized, placed on its abdomen, and the back is shaved and disinfected with 80% ethanol. As depicted in Figure 10.4 a longitudinal skin incision 1.5 cm long is made above the lumbar spine. The subcutaneous connective tissue surrounding the incision is loosened with a pair of scissors. This incision can be used to transfer embryos to both oviducts of the recipient female. For transfer into the left oviduct a transverse incision of approximately 1.0 cm is made into the left body wall about 1.0 cm to the left of the spinal cord. The left ovary and oviduct together with the surrounding fat pad are exteriorized, placed

on a sterile filter paper and fixed by clipping a **serrefine** onto the fat pad. Since the bursa ovarica of rats is extensively vascularized, 1–3 drops of Suprarenin® (1:1000, Hoechst, Frankfurt, Germany) should be added to the bursa before dissection. The bursa is opened cautiously using extrafine straight scissors. At this stage of the surgery, the transfer micropipette is loaded with embryos. To allow visual control of the transfer procedure, small air bubbles are included in the pipette; these can be seen clearly in the oviduct. First the transfer pipette is almost entirely filled with medium to prevent suction. Then it is loaded with a small air bubble followed by a small amount of medium, then a second small air bubble followed by the embryos (in medium), and finally a third small air bubble followed by a small amount of medium. The infundibulum, which always points to the back of the animal, is prepared under the stereomicroscope. The embryo-loaded pipette is cautiously inserted into the infundibulum and fixed with forceps. By blowing into the pipette the embryos are released into the ampulla of the

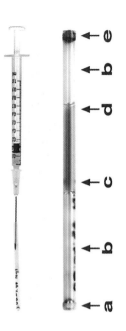

Figure 10.5 Plastic straw for cryopreservation of rat embryos. Upper part: Application of freeze medium to a Minitüb® straw with a syringe. Lower part: Filled Minitüb® straw with arrows a and e indicating the position of the metal and glass bulbs, respectively. The terminal regions of the straw are filled with air (b). Arrow c indicates the position of the embryos and arrow d shows the straw region used for seeding.

oviduct. The complete transfer of the embryos into the ampulla can be confirmed by checking for the presence of the air bubbles. After removal of the serafine and cautious redeposition of the oviduct and ovary into the abdominal cavity, the body wall is closed.

Embryos are always transferred in equal number to both oviducts of a recipient female. The total number of transferred embryos depends on the developmental stage of the embryos and the kind of manipulation performed with the embryos. For generation of transgenic rats, we transfer 30 zygotes previously microinjected with DNA per recipient female. After *in vitro* fertilization, we transfer 20 fertilized oocytes per recipient. For revitalization of cryopreserved strains we transfer 16 thawed two-cell-stage embryos per female. These numbers of transferred embryos usually result in litter sizes of 8–15 pups per recipient.

Storage of Rat Strains as Frozen Preimplantation Embryos

With the development of efficient transgene technology, the number of co-isogenic and congenic rat strains will increase dramatically within the near future. This will pose a severe space problem, which may be solved by the preservation of rat strains as frozen preimplantation embryos. Furthermore, shipment of rat strains in the form of cryopreserved embryos avoids transport stress and the escape of transgenic animals into the environment and prevents contamination of the recipient facility with rat pathogens.

Conventional Cryopreservation of Rat Two-cell-stage Embryos

A multitude of methods have been developed for cryopreservation of mammalian embryos. As also recommended by Hedrich and Reetz (1990), we prefer to use two-cell-stage embryos for cryopreservation of rat strains and to freeze such embryos

using a conventional two-step freezing protocol (Willadsen, 1977; Whittingham *et al.*, 1979). This protocol is described below.

As containers of embryos we recommend Minitüb® plastic straws (Minitüb, Tiefenbach, Germany). The freezing medium is M2 medium supplemented with 1,2-propanediol (PROH) (final concentration 1.5 M) and sucrose (final concentration 0.1 M). The addition of sucrose enhances embryo survival (Ruelicke and Autenried, 1995). Minitüb® straws are sealed on one side with a metal bulb and are then filled with 100 μL of freezing medium (Figure 10.5). After transfer of embryos into the freezing medium using a micropipette the straws are closed with a glass bulb. Filled straws are stored at 0°C until the freezing process. We prefer to freeze the embryo-loaded straws in a programmable automatic methanol cooling bath (F8C50 Cryostate, Haake, Karlsruhe, Germany). The freezing programme starts with a 5-min equilibration period at 0°C. Subsequently, the straws are cooled to −7°C at a rate of 1°C/min. This temperature is maintained for 5 min to allow for seeding. For seeding the straws are touched with large forceps precooled by immersion into liquid nitrogen. The programme continues to cool the straws down to −32°C at a rate of 0.4°C/min. Straws are maintained at this temperature for 5 min before they are plunged into liquid nitrogen.

It should be mentioned that rat embryos can also be cryopreserved by directly plunging into liquid nitrogen, a process referred to as vitrification (Takeda *et al.*, 1984; Krag *et al.*, 1985; Rall and Fahy, 1985; Biery *et al.*, 1986; Chupin and DeReviers, 1986; Williams and Johnson, 1986). Since vitrification does not depend on the availability of a cryostat, the choice of this technique for cryopreserving embryos may help to save costs. However, in our hands the survival rate of embryos frozen by vitrification was extremely susceptible to minor deviations of the freezing protocol.

Thawing of Embryos Following Two-step Freezing

A dilution medium is prepared by supplementing M2 medium with sucrose (final concentration 0.1 M). For thawing, the straws are removed from liquid nitrogen and are immediately transferred to a 37°C waterbath. The end of the Minitüb® straw with the metal bulb is cut off and the open end is connected to a silicone tube with an air-filled syringe. After removal of the glass bulb at the other end, the freezing medium (volume 100 μl) containing the embryos is transferred to a tissue culture dish. Subsequently, the embryos are subjected to a series of elution steps with each step followed by 5 min of equilibration. Three portions of 100 μl of dilution medium are pipetted on to the freezing medium at intervals of 5 min, which reduces the PROH concentration stepwise to 50.0%, 33.3% and 25.5%. After the final elution step the embryos are washed by passing through three drops of M2 medium (without sucrose) and cultured in M16 medium until transfer. In our hands, the viability of thawed embryos is in the range 90–97%.

Setting Up an Embryo Bank

The type of liquid nitrogen tank and carrier system (for uptake of freezing containers) used depends on the type of freezing containers (straws, vials). To minimize the risk of accidental embryo thawing it is strongly recommended that all storage tanks are furnished with an alarm system controlling the temperature and that sufficient numbers of embryos of the same strain are stored in two separate tanks. Each freezing run should be controlled by a temperature recording. Hedrich and Reetz (1990) recommend controlling each freezing run by freezing additional 'control' embryos concomitantly with the embryos of interest. These 'control' embryos are revitalized shortly thereafter and the percentage of morphologically intact embryos is evaluated. This vitality control is obligatory for those cases where embryos are cryopreserved by vitrification; we do not perform it regularly when embryos are frozen according

to the more reliable conventional two-step protocol described.

As transgene technology makes the rapid establishment of new rat strains feasible, the highest demand for embryo cryopreservation will concern congenic and congenic transgenic strains. Since the background strain of these variants will probably be continuously maintained by breeding, it is not essential to freeze embryos derived from full-sib matings.

Hence, for cryopreservation of co-isogenic or congenic strains, embryos can easily be obtained from multiplication colonies without strict brother × sister mating. Depending on the efficiency of cryopreservation and breeding performance we recommend freezing 200–400 embryos of each co-isogenic or congenic strain.

For cryopreservation of inbred strains strictly maintained by brother × sister mating, it is necessary to freeze embryos originating from full-sib matings of the nucleus colony. All embryos originating from a particular mating are frozen together in one batch and each batch is considered as a potential breeding nucleus. Each batch should contain at least 10 embryos to increase chances for establishment of one fertile breeding pair upon revitalization. According to Hedrich and Reetz (1990) 8–10 such batches are required to achieve a 99.9% chance that the cryopreserved inbred strain can be rederived by a full-sib mating.

In Vitro Fertilization (IVF)

The chances of establishing a transgenic lineage depends on the inheritance of a specific transgene locus from a single founder individual developed directly from a microinjected embryo. In case transgenic founder males are reluctant to mate, IVF has to be performed for the successful establishment of transgenic lineages. For IVF such a male is sacrificed and sperm are obtained from its epididymes. The sperm are incubated for capacitation and are then used to fertilize oocytes in vitro. Successfully fertilized oocytes are transferred to pseudopregnant recipients. In this context it should be noted that artificial insemination of rats is not routinely performed since the sperm suspension has to be applied by puncturing the uterus wall (Villalon et al.,

1982) and since a copulatory stimulus or an adequate signal must also be provided to the inseminated female for the establishment of pregnancy.

A modified method for IVF of rat oocytes is based on the work of Toyoda and Chang (1974). Since the embryo yield of IVF experiments depends on the number of available oocytes, we use at least three immature females per experiment. These females should be derived from a strain highly responsive to superovulation. For superovulation Folltropin® and HCG are applied as described above. The sperm donor is sacrificed 11 h after the females are treated with HCG, i.e. 1.5 h before the end of the dark period. Since sperm are extremely susceptible to low temperatures, all equipment used for IVF has to be prewarmed to 38.5°C. After opening the abdominal cavity of the male and exteriorization of the testes, the epididymes are carefully dissected and each subjected to 1 mL of preincubated modified Whittingham's medium. Using the stereomicroscope each epididymis is carefully squeezed with a no. 5 forceps, which will force the sperm out. The sperm suspension is incubated for 1.5 h to allow for capacitation. During this time oocytes are recovered from the superovulated females. The females are sacrificed and the oviducts are dissected and ruptured as described above. All oocytes obtained from a single oviduct are released into 300 μL of preincubated modified Whittingham medium. After capacitation 20–30 μL of sperm suspension is transferred to each oocyte suspension. The germ cells are incubated together for 5–6 h for fertilization. Subsequently, the fertilized oocytes are transferred to preincubated M16 medium. Successful fertilization can be confirmed by checking for the development of pronuclei. We recommend transferring fertilized oocytes immediately into recipients at day 0.5 of pseudopregnancy. Alternatively, they may be left in culture for development to the two-cell stage and then transferred to recipients.

References

Armstrong, D.T. and Opavsky, M.A. (1988) *Biol. Reprod.* **39**, 511–518.

Bailey, D.W. (1971) *Transplantation* **11**, 325–327.

Bailey, D.W. (1977) *Ciba Found. Symp.* **52**, 291–303.

Bailey, D.W. (1981) In: Foster H.L., Small, J.D. and Fox, J.G. (eds) *The Mouse in Biomedical Research*, Vol. 1, pp. 223–239. New York: Academic Press.

Baker, D.E.J. (1979) In: Baker, H.J., Lindsey J.R. and Weisbroth S.H. (eds) *The Laboratory Rat*, Vol. 1, pp. 153–168. New York: Academic Press.

Bartlett, M.S. and Haldane, J.B.S. (1935) *J. Genet.* **31**, 327–340.

Biery, K.A., Seidel, G.E. and Elsden, R.P. (1986) *Theriogenologie* **25**, 140.

Chupin, D. and DeReviers, M.M. (1986) *Theriogenologie* **26**, 157–166.

Crow, J.F. (1997) *Proc. Natl Acad. Sci. USA* **94**, 8380–8386.

DeFeo, V.J. (1966) *Endocrinology* **79**, 440–442.

Eggenberger, E. (1973) *Z. Versuchstierkd.* **15**, 297–331.

Falconer, D.S. (1967) In: Lane-Petter, W. (ed.) *UFAW Handbook on the Care and Management of Laboratory Animals*, 3rd edn, pp. 72–96. Edinburgh: Livingstone.

Falconer, D.S. (1989) *Introduction to Quantitative Genetics*. New York: Longman Scientific & Technical.

Festing, M.F. and Staats J. (1973) *Transplantation* **16**, 221–245.

Fisher, R.A. (1965) *The Theory of Inbreeding*, 2nd edn. Edinburgh: Oliver & Boyd.

Flaherty, L. (1981) In: Foster, H.L., Small, J.D. and Fox, J.G. (eds) *The Mouse in Biomedical Research*, Vol. 1, pp 215–222. New York: Academic Press.

Fraser, L.R. and Drury, L.M. (1975) *Biol. Reprod.* **13**, 513–518.

Green, E.L. and Roderick, T.H. (1966) In: Green, E.L. (ed.) *Biology of the Laboratory Mouse*, pp. 165–185. New York: McGraw-Hill.

Greenhouse, D.D., Festing, M.F., Hasan, S. and Cohen, A.L. (1990) In: Hedrich, H.J. (ed.) *Genetic Monitoring of Inbred Strains of Rats*, pp. 410–480. Stuttgart: Gustav Fischer.

Haldane, J.B.S. and Waddington, C.H. (1931) *Genetics* **16**, 357–374.

Hamada, H., Petrino, M.G. and Kakunaga, T. (1982) *Proc. Natl Acad. Sci. USA* **79**, 6465–6469.

Hayman, B.I. and Mather, K. (1953) *Heredity* **7**, 165–183.

Hedrich, H.J. (1990a) In: Hedrich, H.J. (ed.) *Genetic Monitoring of Inbred Strains of Rats*, pp. 11–22. Stuttgart: Gustav Fischer.

Hedrich, H.J. (1990b) *Genetic Monitoring of Inbred Strains of Rats*. Stuttgart: Gustav Fischer.

Hedrich, H.J. and Reetz, I.C. (1990) In: Hedrich, H.J. (ed.) *Genetic Monitoring of Inbred Strains of Rats*, pp. 274–288. Stuttgart: Gustav Fischer.

Hogan, B., Beddington, R., Costantini, F. and Lacy, E. (1994) *Manipulating the Mouse Embryo. A Laboratory Manual*. New York: Cold Spring Harbor Laboratory.

Hyde, J.S. (1973) *Behav. Genet.* **3**, 233–245.

James, M.R. and Lindpaintner, K. (1997) *Trends Genet.* **13**, 171–173.

Kimura, M. and Crow, J.F. (1963) *Genet. Res. Cambridge* **4**, 399–415.

Krag, K.T., Koehler, I.M. and Wright, R.W. (1985) *Theriogenologie* **23**, 199.

Lander, E.S. and Schork, N.J. (1994) *Science* **265**, 2037–2048.

Livesay, E.A. (1930) *Genetics* **15**, 17–54.

Manly, K.F. (1993) *Mamm. Genome* **4**, 303–313.

Markel, P., Shu, P., Ebeling, C. *et al.* (1997) *Nature Genet.* **17**, 280–284.

Mayer, J.F. and Fritz, H.I. (1974) *J. Reprod. Fertil.* **9**, 99–102.

Miesfeld, R., Krystal, M. and Arnheim, N. (1981) *Nucleic Acids Res.* **9**, 5931–5947.

Ohno, S. (1972) *Dev. Biol.* **27**, 131–136.

Poiley, S.M. (1960) *Proc. Anim. Care Panel* **10**, 159–166.

Rafferty, Jr, K.A. (1970) *Methods in Experimental Embryology of the Mouse*. Baltimore: Johns Hopkins Press.

Rall, W.F. and Fahy, G.M. (1985) *Nature* **313**, 573–575.

Rapp, K.G. (1972) *Z. Versuchstierkd.* **14**, 133–142.

Rouleau, A.M.J., Kovacs, P.R., Kunz, H.W. and Armstrong, D.T. (1993) *Lab. Anim. Sci.* **43**, 611–615.

Ruelicke, T. and Autenried, P. (1995) *Lab. Anim.* **29**, 320–326.

Russell, W.L., Kelly, P.R., Hunsicker, P.R., Bangham, J.W., Maddux, S.C. and Phipps, E.L. (1979) *Proc. Natl Acad. Sci. USA* **76**, 5918–5922.

Serreze, D.V., Chapman, H.D., Varnum, D.S. *et al. J. Exp. Med.* **184**, 2049–2053.

Silver, L.M. (1995) *Mouse Genetics*. New York: Oxford University Press.

Snell, G.D. (1978) In: Morse, H.C. (ed.) *Origins of Inbred Mice*, pp. 1–31. New York: Academic Press.

Stam, P. (1980) *Genet. Res.* **35**, 131–155.

Sullivan, N. and Ouhibi, N. (1995) In: Monastersky, G.M. and Robl, J.M. (eds) *Strategies in Transgenic Animal Science*, pp. 37–55. Washington DC: ASM Press.

Takeda, T., Elsden, R.P. and Seidel, G.E. (1984) *Theriogenologie* **21**, 266.

Toyoda, Y. and Chang, M.C. (1974) *J. Reprod. Fertil.* **36**, 9–22.

Villalon, M., Ortiz, M.E., Aguayo, C., Munoz, J. and Croxatto, H.B. (1982) *Biol. Reprod.* **26**, 337–341.

Voipio, H.M. and Nevalainen, T. (1998) *Scand. J. Lab. Anim. Sci.* **25**, 5–9.

Weil, M.M., Brown, B.W. and Serachitopol, D.M. (1997) *Genetics* **146**, 1061–1069.

Whittingham, D.G. (1971) *J. Reprod. Fertil. (suppl.)* **14**, 7–21.

Whittingham, D.G. (1975) *J. Reprod. Fertil.* **43**, 575–578.

Whittingham, D.G., Wood, M., Farrant, J., Lee, H. and Halsey, J.A. (1979) *J. Reprod. Fertil.* **56**, 11–21.

Willadsen, S.M. (1977) In: Elliot, K. and Whelan, J. (eds) *The Freezing of Mammalian Embryos*, pp. 175–189. Amsterdam: Elsevier.

Williams, T.J. and Johnson, S.E. (1986) *Theriogenologie* **26**, 125–133.

Wood, M.J. and Whittingham, D.G. (1981) In: Zeilmaker, G.H. (ed.) *Frozen Storage of Laboratory Animals*, pp. 119–128. Stuttgart: Gustav Fischer.

Wright, S. (1921) *Genetics* **6**: 11–178.

Yang, W.H. (1968) *Endocrinology* **82**, 423–425.

CHAPTER 11

Reproductive and Developmental Toxicology Safety Studies

Paul Barrow
Phoenix International Preclinical Services Europe (Chrysalis),
Les Oncins, L'Arbresle, France

Choice of Species and Strains

The rat is the undisputed species of choice for regulatory assessments of reproductive and developmental toxicology. This in itself is surprising when we consider that the first guidelines for the detection of **teratogenic effects** (FDA, 1966) appeared in the immediate aftermath of the thalidomide tragedy, an agent to which the rat embryo is insensitive (Neubert and Neubert, 1997), despite occasional reports to the contrary (e.g. Parkhie and

Webb, 1983). The rat offers many advantages over other laboratory species and is by far the best studied species for reproductive assessments, but it is by no means universally relevant for the testing of all substances. The selection of species and/or strains should be based on the same considerations as for general toxicology (see Chapter 1), plus other factors pertinent to reproductive assessments such as comparative embryology/physiology (e.g. hormonal differences), **pharmacokinetics** in pregnant animals, metabolic changes during pregnancy (e.g. differences in plasma binding) and the susceptibility to known developmental toxicants. The regulatory guidelines require embryotoxicity studies in one rodent and one 'nonrodent' (usually the rabbit) species.

The choice of the strain of rat to be used for the reproductive toxicology studies will depend on the individual experience of the testing laboratory and in particular the amount of historical data available. Commercial outbred strains offer the advantages of high fertility, large litter sizes, genetic stability and low spontaneous malformation incidences. Strains of low **fecundity**, such as Fischer 344, should be avoided. The Fischer 344 also differs from other strains in its postnatal period of development (Francis, 1994).

Definitions

The term reproductive toxicology will be used in this chapter to cover all adverse reproductive outcomes resulting from the exposure of the adult or developing organism (it is sometimes used elsewhere to denote only influences on the fertility of the adult). Developmental toxicology will be used to cover any adverse influences, whenever they are manifested, resulting from the exposure of the organism before reaching adult maturity.

It is unfortunate that the term teratology was misused in the first FDA guidelines (Christian and Goeke, 1997). It will be used herein to describe a congenital effect characterized by the induction of structural birth defects. This definition may be extended to include functional defects, as in 'behavioural teratology'. So called 'teratology' studies are renamed embryotoxicity studies for drugs and prenatal development studies for chemicals (see below). These investigations test for all manifestations of toxic influences on the pregnant dam or embryo in addition to structural defects arising from teratogenic mechanisms.

The term drugs will be used to designate all pharmaceutical or medicinal agents whether they are used for therapeutic or social purposes. Chemicals will be used to designate all chemical agents to which humans are likely to be exposed (e.g. pesticides, fungicides, industrial reagents, agrochemicals and food additives) except drugs.

The day of identification of mating (i.e. when a vaginal plug is found or sperm appear in a vaginal smear) is taken as day 0 of gestation. Likewise, the day of parturition is termed day 0 postpartum.

Regulatory Requirements for Reproductive Toxicology

Harmonization of Guidelines

For drugs, the regulatory agencies of Europe, the USA and Japan successfully consolidated their requirements at the first International Conference on Harmonization and the resulting guidelines have since been ratified and accepted worldwide (ICH, 1994). The remarkable success of the ICH harmonization initiative has stimulated efforts to harmonize the international regulatory requirements for other chemicals. The Environmental Protection Agency of the USA (EPA, 1997a) harmonized only with itself, by blending its guidance requirements for the control of toxic substances and pesticides. The Organization for Economic Co-operation and Development (OECD, 1996) intends to accommodate the EPA study designs in its updated guidelines, without, however, requiring the more radical EPA requirements based on unproven methodology.

There are still many notable contradictions between the requirements for drugs and chemicals. The reasons for these differences are generally more pertinent to risk assessment than to hazard identification. A single consolidated testing strategy for chemicals and drugs would reduce the risk of borderline substances, such as therapeutic food additives or medicinal cosmetics, falling into the gaps between the divergent regulations.

The latest EPA final guidelines are legally superfluous: all signatory members of the OECD are contractually obliged to apply the OECD texts. Whether or not the EPA texts can be safely ignored in favour of the OECD texts, and by whom, remains to be seen. The technical and practical differences in the various regulatory guidelines are highlighted in the relevant sections of this chapter.

Regulatory Requirements for Drugs and Chemicals

The guidelines for reproductive toxicity testing issued by the regulatory agencies are intended for the primary detection of toxic influences on reproduction. Once an effect has been detected, further experiments are usually necessary to characterize fully the nature of the response.

The strategy of regulatory testing for reproductive and developmental toxicology testing varies between drugs and chemicals. The regulatory requirements for chemicals (including industrial reagents, pesticides and food additives) include an evaluation of possible toxic influences of all phases of development and adult fertility in one or more generations. The testing strategy for drugs includes an evaluation of all of these phases except that there is no requirement to expose the developing offspring from weaning through puberty to sexual maturity. This remains true even though the ICH guidelines state that: 'The combination of studies selected should allow exposure of mature adults at all stages of development from conception to sexual maturity'.

All regulatory assessments of reproductive and developmental toxicity of drugs are now performed according to the harmonized ICH guidelines. The most common ICH testing strategy involves a three-segment study design comprising two embryotoxicity studies (one rodent and one nonrodent), a fertility study and a pre- and postnatal study. Alternatively, the embryotoxicity and fertility studies can be blended into a single protocol.

The regulatory assessment of the reproductive toxicity of chemicals is usually performed in two segments, embryotoxicity (one rodent and one nonrodent) followed by a two-generation study (OECD, 1981, 1982a, 1983a). The OECD has issued guidelines for a one-generation study design, but this study design is not sufficient for the detection of many manifestations of developmental toxicity and the guideline is likely to be revoked in the near future (OECD, 1982b, 1983b).

Regulatory Requirements for Other Specific Agents

Foods and food additives

Foods and food additives are tested for reproductive toxicity using embryotoxicity and multigeneration study designs similar to those required for chemicals. The existing FDA guidelines (1982) include routine embryotoxicity studies and a technically complex protocol for the multigeneration study design comprising three or more generations, each with two or more mating phases. Draft guidelines, which show no signs of being finalized, propose simplifying these requirements to bring them in line with those for other chemicals (FDA, 1993).

The FDA draft requirements for foods also require that an *in utero* exposure phase be added to one of the **carcinogenicity** studies in rodents, preferably the rat. The parental animals are exposed to the test substance from at least 4 weeks before mating and then throughout **gestation** and lactation of the inseminated females. One pup of each sex per litter is then selected for the main investigations which are similar to a conventional carcinogenicity study. This protocol is designed to detect hazards, such as cross-placental carcinogenesis, which may occur when the human embryo or fetus is exposed *in utero* to food additives consumed by the mother.

Products of biotechnology

Many biotechnology products are intended for use in women of childbearing potential. These include hormones, hormone releasing factors, **cytokines**, vaccines, blood components and **gene therapies**. Reproductive toxicity testing of these agents is a challenging topic of vital importance (Henck *et al.*, 1996). The products to be tested are often only bioactive in humans or primate species, so the rat may not always be an appropriate species for their safety assessment.

Recombinant human proteins can provoke antibody production in animals, resulting in the progressive neutralization of the test substance. These immune reactions may also cause pathological lesions in the test species, confounding the interpretation of the study. It may be necessary to subdivide the treatment period in the reproductive toxicity studies to ensure that different groups of rats are exposed at all stages of development to the test substance before it can be neutralized. The route and rate of administration also influence antibody production: continuous intravenous infusion may be less immunogenic than other methods of administration (Kung *et al.*, 1994). A novel solution to the problem posed by immunogenic proteins uses the 'rodent' version of the molecule, in which the immunogenic portions of the human protein have been replaced by the corresponding amino acid sequences from the rat (or more often, the mouse).

Since the majority of biopharmaceuticals have to be administered by the i.v. route, the maximum dose that can be given is often limited by the solubility of the test substance in physiological solutions; so it may not be possible to achieve the **maximum tolerated dose**. In this case, the animal studies should aim to demonstrate an adequate safety margin with respect to the proposed clinical dose (FDA, 1997) Assessments of immune function, such as antibody titres and immune complex levels, should be included in the study designs as appropriate.

Vaccines and medicinal agents for once-only or very infrequent administration

Most vaccines are not given to pregnant or lactating women, so embryotoxicity and pre- and postnatal studies are not normally required. Possible effects on the reproductive organs in the adult are adequately assessed in the general toxicology studies (provided that appropriate methods are used), so fertility studies are not usually necessary.

Embryotoxicity studies are required for those medicinal products (e.g. vaccines), dietary supplements or other prophylactic agents that are likely to be given to pregnant women. A typical example could be a vitamin supplement for use in parts of the developing world, where a medical team will travel from village to village treating the entire population, say once a year. Each woman will only be treated once during any given pregnancy, but it is not possible to predict the stage of pregnancy at which the exposure will occur. In view of the stage-specific nature of teratogenic and other embryotoxic effects, it is therefore necessary to expose the test animals throughout the entire period of **organogenesis**, even though this may result in an exaggerated total exposure with regard to the intended clinical application.

Data on possible influences on embryo—fetal development are frequently requested when a microorganism used to prepare a vaccine has been implicated in reprotoxic effects (European Agency for the Evaluation of Medicinal Products, 1997). Also, some live vaccines (e.g. rubella), although safe for nonpregnant women, may cause fetal infection. Special considerations apply to antifertility vaccines. **Adjuvants** or **exipients** used in vaccine preparation may need to be tested alone or in combination with the final product.

Gene therapy products

Gene therapy products may be comprised of **viral or nonviral vectors** containing nucleic acid, or of naked DNA. The preclinical evaluation of these products is, in principle, similar to that of other biotechnology-derived products.

Molecular biology techniques, such as the polymerase chain reaction (PCR), can be used to assess the distribution of an introduced gene. An important issue to address is the possibility of germ-line alterations (European Agency for the Evaluation of Medicinal Products, 1998). The best evidence of the absence of germ-line alterations is the lack of the introduced gene in the gonads of the treated animal. If the gene persists in these organs, PCR analysis of the gametes may be considered. Species other than the rat may be better suited for this purpose. The chances of detecting a germ-line alteration in the offspring of the treated animal is remote, in view of the small proportion of germ cells that actually receive the gene and the even lower proportion of these that will give rise to gametes that will eventually be fertilized and develop into viable young.

The distribution of a gene therapy product in the **conceptus** can be determined by PCR analysis following treatment during pregnancy.

Paediatric drugs

Medicines and drugs intended for use in children or adolescents may need additional testing in view of the gap in the ICH guidelines concerning treatment after weaning. Direct treatment of rat pups is feasible by all conventional routes except i.v. from the day of birth. Neonatal studies are best designed with each dam raising a mixture of treated and control pups. It may be necessary to continue treatment of the offspring up to sexual maturity. The duration of the treatment period should take into account the timing of secondary sexual development (i.e. hormone surges, the onset of spermatogenesis and ovulation, etc.). The postweaning period is particularly pertinent for the testing of drugs (and chemicals) with possible **androgenic** or antiandrogenic properties (Ashby and Lefevre, 1997).

Cosmetics

Animal studies are no longer specifically required for cosmetics, and may even be outlawed in Europe. This principle is rational for cosmetics entirely

Safety testing of classes of substance which have known teratogenic or reproductive toxic potential

Certain therapeutic classes of compound present an inherent risk of teratogenesis or of other reproductive effects. The consequences of the disease (e.g. epilepsy or diabetes) may be so serious that the therapeutic benefits outweigh the risk of birth defects. In these cases, the need to find nontoxic medicines is so great that, while perhaps not strictly necessary for approval purposes, it would be unethical not to test for reproductive toxicity. Any new drug intended for use as a dual therapy with a known reproductive toxicant (e.g. valproic acid) will need to be tested both alone and in the anticipated drug combination.

The Timing of Reproduction Toxicology Studies for Drugs

A male fertility study is required before the start of phase III clinical trials. No reproductive toxicology studies are necessary before the start of phase I and II trials in males on condition that the reproductive organs have been adequately assessed in the general toxicology studies.

The requirements differ between agencies when women of procreational potential are to be included in clinical trials. The embryotoxicity studies must be complete before phase I in Europe and Japan. This is not necessary in the USA provided that the women use an effective contraceptive and have given their informed consent concerning the risks of falling pregnant during the trial. The inclusion of women in clinical trials is likely to become more common in the USA because of a recent government directive. A female fertility study is required before phase I in Japan and before phase III in Europe or the USA, along with the embryotoxicity studies if not performed before. Pre- and postnatal studies are not required before the start of clinical trials.

Nonregulatory Investigative Studies

Regulatory studies are intended only to detect potential toxic influences. Additional studies are often necessary in order to elucidate the mechanisms

formulated from compounds which have already been tested individually. Whether or not the vendor should then be allowed to claim that no animals have been used in the development of the product is another question.

Difficulties may arise when the cosmetic product contains one or more novel chemicals which have never been tested, or when medicinal claims are made for the finished product. In practice, the manufacturer is held accountable for the safety of the product (EEC, 1996) and will usually elect to test any product which has real biological efficacy. It may be more appropriate to test some cosmetics according to the guidelines for chemicals, since the occupational exposure of the workers that handle the product (e.g. hairdressers) often outweighs that of the consumer.

The pharmacokinetic properties of cosmetic ingredients may determine which safety studies are necessary. The risk is greatly reduced, for instance, when the conditions of handling and use of the product do not result in systemic exposure. For this reason, reproductive toxicity studies may not be required for topically applied products which are not absorbed across the skin.

Previously untested high-production chemicals

Many existing 'high-production volume chemicals' have never been tested for reproductive toxicity. The EPA Toxic Substances Control Act inventory currently lists over 80 000 chemicals. The OECD 'reproduction/developmental toxicity screen' was proposed as a preliminary study to detect those chemicals that warrant further investigation. The Chernoff–Kavlock assay is also used for this purpose.

When are reproductive toxicology tests not required?

There is no specific need to test drugs that will only be administered to adults who are not of reproductive potential (i.e. permanently sterile men and women). Because of the need to develop medicines for use during sensitive stages of development, the regulatory agencies may request reproductive toxicology studies even for drugs that are intended to be contraindicated during pregnancy.

of any effects. The following study designs are frequently employed for this purpose.

Subdivided treatment periods for embryotoxicity studies

Several groups of females are treated over different periods, so that together they cover the entire period of organogenesis. Dosing of each group may be performed on consecutive days for a short duration, or each group may be treated at given intervals instead of every day. This type of protocol may be used to determine the period of sensitivity to a teratogenic agent, or it may replace the standard regulatory study when continuous treatment during organogenesis results in unacceptable maternal toxicity.

Peer-feeding

Reduced food consumption frequently accompanies maternal toxicity and may also result from poor palatability of the diet mixture in multigeneration studies. It is often difficult to determine whether observed developmental effects are the indirect consequence of reduced maternal food consumption or of a direct influence on the offspring. This question can be addressed in peer-feeding studies, where the quantity of food offered to a group of untreated females is adjusted to match that consumed by a treated group at the same stage of gestation and/or lactation. Reduced pup growth may be mediated by effects on maternal milk production.

Cross-fostering

Like peer-feeding, cross-fostering studies are used to distinguish between maternal- or pup-mediated effects. One group of rats is treated with the test article during late gestation and throughout lactation. A control group is not treated. On day 1 postpartum the offspring from one half of the dams in each group are exchanged to produce four subgroups: untreated dams and litters, treated dams and litters, untreated foster mothers raising pups born to treated dams and treated foster mothers raising pups born to untreated dams.

Continuous breeding protocol

The continuous breeding protocol may be used to detect influences on fertility affecting the duration of reproductive capacity, which are not necessarily manifest under the conditions of routine regulatory toxicology tests. Groups of adult male and female rodents are treated for one week before pairing. Treatment is continued during a 98-day cohabitation period. Each litter is removed from the cage and necropsied soon after birth. The last F1 litter is then allowed to survive and selected offspring are treated from weaning and mated to produce an F2 litter which is in turn terminated at weaning.

Alternative tests

Much progress has been made in the development of *in vivo* and *in vitro* techniques for the assessment of reproductive toxicology (ECETOC, 1989; Harris, 1997). At present these tests cannot replace conventional safety studies. They can, and should, be employed however to reduce the number of animals used in safety studies by screening substances, such as series of structural analogues, to identify those which are most worthy of further development. Alternative tests can also provide additional information on mechanisms of reproduction and its relevance to humans.

There are two main areas of progress where *in vitro* methods may have the potential to replace live animal studies: fertility effects and teratogenic activity. In general all *in vitro* tests suffer the same disadvantages: they are static closed systems in which maternal biotransformation and excretion are not taken into account. *In vivo* tests include studies of the development of free living nonmammalian embryos when exposed to a test agent. The species most studied are hens, frogs, brine shrimp, various fish and *Drosophila*. Another test assesses the ability of dissociated adult hydra cells to aggregate and form a complete organism. *In vitro* tests examine toxic effects on cultured cells, organs or intact embryos. The most promising *in vitro* methods have been developed to model specific stages in the reproductive process. The available methods have been reviewed by Fielder *et al.* (1997).

In vitro tests for effects on fertility

While some components of the female reproductive system, such as pituitary, hypothalamus and ovary, can be maintained *in vitro*, the main interest is in the detection and characterization of effects on male fertility. Testicular toxicity can be investigated with cultures of primary cell lines or intact seminiferous tubules. To date, no models have been developed to assess epididymal sperm maturation. Sperm function can be assessed using *in vitro* fertilization.

In vitro tests for effects on embryonic development
A great deal of effort has been expended over the last 20 years to validate rodent embryo culture techniques. So far the results have been disappointing. Whole embryo culture assesses the growth and development of isolated postimplantation rodent embryos, which can be maintained in culture for several days. Isolated embryonic rat organs, such as limb buds and midbrain, can also be evaluated in micromass cultures. Preimplantation embryos from the rat may also be cultured *in vitro*.

Routes of Administration

For drugs, the proposed human route of administration is preferred for the reproductive toxicology studies, provided that this route provides an adequate exposure to the test article with respect to humans. For chemicals, the principal route of human exposure should be used (see Chapter 2), unless the pharmacokinetic properties of the test article suggest otherwise.

Gavage administration has the advantage of allowing the administration of an exact predefined dosage to each animal and is the preferred method of oral administration for embryotoxicity studies and of drugs for all reproductive studies. Administration by admixture in the diet or by dissolution in the drinking water are the preferred methods of oral administration for the multigeneration studies with chemicals. There are marked pharmacokinetic differences between oral administration by daily gavage and admixture in the diet, which often result in divergent toxicological responses. In dietary studies the rats are fed with the treated diet continuously during the course of the study. They are most often given a fixed concentration of test article, but it is also possible to vary the concentration according to the predicted parental food consumption and body weight in order to administer a constant dose level relative to body weight. It is not usual to exceed a concentration of 5% of the test article in the diet for any toxicology study in the rat; otherwise vitamin deficiencies may result. This danger is particularly pertinent to reproductive studies (Barrow *et al.*, 1995). Maternal food consumption on average doubles during the course of gestation and lactation,

with a corresponding increase in the amount of ingested test article. The pups generally start to eat solid food during the second week postpartum, from which time they are directly exposed to the test article in the diet. Poor palatability of the treated diet or water will result in a dosage-related reduction in food or water consumption and influences on the achieved test article intake.

When the route of exposure is by inhalation, particularly with pregnant or lactating rats, nose-only exposure is preferred because of the stress associated with the restraint necessary in whole-body exposure.

Rat pups can be treated by gavage practically from birth, but this becomes impractical before weaning under the conditions of a reproductive toxicology study, when hundreds or thousands of pups have to be treated daily.

Selection of Dose Levels

The selection of correct dose levels is critical. Fortunately, prior to commencement of the reproduction studies a great deal of toxicity data in the rat are available from the general toxicity studies. This is rarely true for embryotoxicity studies in other species. The selected doses need to allow for extrapolation to humans from the results obtained. At least three dose levels are generally needed for all regulatory reproductive toxicology studies. The intervals between doses must not be too large to permit the evaluation of any dose-dependent changes, so additional dose groups may also be needed. It is often convenient to keep the dose levels constant between the subchronic general toxicity studies and the various reproductive segments, but this is not always possible in view of the different treatment durations.

All regulatory agencies now require **toxicokinetic principles** to be taken into account in the selection of dose levels. There is little point in administering more than one dose which is above the limit of absorption. The ICH guidelines for drugs (1994) suggest that dose levels should be assessed in terms of total body burden (i.e. Area Under the Curve) rather than as administered dosages. Peak plasma levels also influence developmental effects and need to be taken into account.

The emphasis in the reproductive toxicology studies is on the detection of effects on reproduction which are more prominent than other toxicological hazards. Therefore, if toxic influences which will limit the use of the test article have already been identified at a given exposure level in the general toxicity studies, there is usually no need to exceed these dose levels in the reproduction studies.

For drugs and chemicals, it is not normally necessary to exceed the limit dose of 1 g/kg/day on condition that this provides a good margin of safety with respect to the anticipated human exposure. For chemicals, the regulatory texts recommend that the high dose levels should be selected to induce some manifestations of parental or developmental toxicity without excessive suffering. Mortality should not in any case exceed 10%. The intermediate dose group should induce 'minimal' toxicity.

When the test article causes little or no toxicity at very high doses (e.g. penicillin in rats) the inclusion of just one treated group and control may be justified.

The low dose level should result in a total exposure that is comparable with or, preferably, slightly higher than the anticipated exposure in humans.

Toxicokinetics

The aim of toxicology studies is not to make the world a safer place for rats! There is no justifiable reason to perform regulatory toxicology studies in animals if the data generated are not pertinent to the detection of possible toxicological hazards in humans. Pharmacokinetic differences between species often account for marked differences in susceptibility to toxic insult and therefore need to be investigated before any results can be extrapolated to humans.

The pharmacokinetic properties of the test substance (and of any active metabolites) have a particular relevance in reproductive toxicology. Many of the physiological changes which occur during pregnancy and lactation in the rat may potentially influence the toxicokinetic and pharmacodynamic properties of the test article. These changes, with regard to the nonpregnant female include: reduced gastric secretion, increased intestinal transit time, increased plasma volume, increased extracellular fluid volume, increased body fat, decreased xenobiotic hepatic transformation, increased kidney function and differences in protein binding (Clarke, 1993).

Rats, being much smaller than humans, have a faster rate of metabolism and eliminate most potential toxicants much more rapidly, resulting in a less prolonged exposure. This difference needs to be taken into account in the selection of dose levels and dose regimes for safety testing. An opposing argument relevant to teratogenicity is that the gestation length is much shorter in the rat so a relatively short duration of exposure will cover more developmental stages in the rat than in the human. It may be impossible to reproduce the human pharmacokinetic profile in the rat using the proposed route of human exposure; in such instances other routes of administration may be more appropriate. Methods of programmable intravenous infusion have recently been developed and validated for all types of reproductive toxicology study (Barrow and Heritier, 1995, 1996; Barrow and Guyot, 1996; Barrow et al., 1996) and may be employed to better simulate the human pharmacokinetic profile in the rat when this cannot be achieved by conventional methods.

Because of their stage-dependent nature, developmental effects may be differentially dependent on peak plasma levels and the total exposure (AUC) of a given toxicant. For example, high maternal plasma levels (C_{max}) of sodium valproate at a specific stage of gestation in rodents have been shown to cause exencephaly in the developing rodent embryo, while sustained exposure to lower levels results in embryonic resorption (Nau, 1985). This type of observation has led to a dual classification of embryotoxic agents as either C_{max}- or AUC-dependent. Because of the important influence of pharmacokinetic factors, when testing a substance of unknown toxicity, it is prudent to maximize both peak and total plasma levels. For example, the highest possible plasma level of a new anticoagulant may be limited by the acute toxicity in the healthy rat when administered by i.v. bolus, the proposed method of clinical administration. In this case the only way of obtaining a superior AUC in the rat with respect to the clinical dose is to prolong the exposure using continuous i.v. infusion. In other cases, multiple dosing regimes may have to be tested in the same study in order to maximize both the C_{max} and the AUC.

The treatment regime may need to be adapted in consequence of the duration of activity (or half-life) of the test article and any active metabolites in the organism. A substance with a very long half-life will tend to accumulate in the test animal if it is administered at a greater rate than it can be metabolized or eliminated. On the other hand, a substance with a short half-life will be disactivated rapidly and may no longer be active when certain target events take place. Because of the very stage-specific responses in reproductive toxicology, the time of day when the rats are dosed may also influence the results of the study, particularly for compounds that are rapidly metabolized or eliminated. A frequent oversight of this type involves the duration of exposure to the test substance with respect to the time of copulation. In most studies, rats are dosed once per day in the morning. The rat, however, being nocturnal, tends to copulate at night. Because of the delay between dosing and copulation, the plasma or target tissue levels of the test article may have declined or been completely eliminated at the time of mating, so possible influences on mating behaviour could remain undetected.

Preliminary Studies

The results from the subchronic rat studies are often sufficient for the selection of dose levels in the reproduction studies, provided that the same routes and methods of administration are used. Otherwise, preliminary reproduction studies may be performed. A preliminary study is always advisable when the test article is to be given to lactating females in the diet because of the great increase in food consumption, and hence test article intake, that occurs when the dam has to produce enough milk to feed a litter of eight or more growing pups.

To aid in the evaluation of risk and extrapolation of the results, it is useful to know if the test substance crosses the placental barrier to reach the fetus, or if it is secreted in the milk. Biodistribution studies performed in pregnant or lactating dams are useful for this purpose. Rapid stage-dependent physiological changes during the course of gestation of lactation have to be taken into account when performing theses studies. Milk can be sampled and analysed for test article concentration (see Chapter 25).

The fact that a test article does not cross the placenta is not sufficient justification for discounting a potential embryotoxic effect. Maternal metabolic or physiological influences (caused by hypoglycaemic or antiarrhythmic agents for example) have been shown to cause teratogenic outcomes (Danielsson et al, 1989; Schardein, 1993). The same principle is true for secretion of the test article in the milk and possible effects in the suckling offspring. Maternal effects on milk production, in particular, have a marked influence on the development of the pups.

Satellite animals that will not be included in the toxicological evaluations of the experiment are generally needed for toxicokinetic investigations in the rat because of the limited volume of blood that can be sampled. It is normally considered sufficient to examine a very limited number of time points in the pregnant and lactating rat. Provided that no marked differences are found in the pregnant or lactating rat compared with the more complete toxicokinetic profile determined during the general toxicology studies, more detailed determinations are not usually justified. Satellite groups of about 5–10 rats per dose level may be included alongside the main groups of the reproductive toxicology studies for this purpose (or in the corresponding preliminary studies, where applicable). It is usually sufficient to take blood samples at the start and the end of the embryonic period and on one or two days during lactation.

For a preliminary study prior to an embryotoxicity study, it is usual to allocate about six pregnant rats per group (plus satellite animals for toxicokinetics, if required – see above) which are then submitted to the same in-life and caesarean examinations as will be employed in the main study. Detailed fixed fetal examinations are not usually necessary.

The function of preliminary studies is essentially to evaluate dose levels based on parental toxicity; they should not be used to select nondevelopmentally toxic levels, which would undermine the objectives of the main studies. For this reason, most regulatory agencies now expect the reports of all preliminary studies to be submitted as supplementary investigations. It is not strictly necessary, however, to perform preliminary studies under GLP (good laboratory practice) conditions.

In these studies the emphasis is placed on generating data which facilitate the selection of the high dose levels for the main studies, the lower dose levels are generally imposed by other criteria, including the anticipated human exposure and comparative toxicokinetics. Therefore, it is advisable to choose preliminary dose levels that are relatively high with respect to the anticipated human exposure level.

OECD reproductive toxicology screen

When a single method of administration is to be used, a simple preliminary study can be designed to cover all of the ensuing studies. The OECD reproductive toxicology screen (1995) is useful for this purpose: 10 male and 10 females are treated for 2 weeks before pairing, the females are allowed to give birth and the adults and litters are necropsied at weaning.

For embryotoxicity and pre- and postnatal studies it is possible to obtain time-mated females, avoiding the need to maintain a large breeding facility in-house. These rats are mated by the supplier and delivered to the laboratory before the start of treatment on day 6 of gestation. Ideally, they should arrive at the testing facility on day 0 of gestation, so that their body weights can be recorded on arrival and they can acclimate to the laboratory for as long as

Animal Supply and Husbandry

The criteria for the selection of an animal supplier are the same as for other types of study (see Chapter 1). Particular attention needs to be given to fertility, fecundity and the incidences of fetal abnormalities and *in utero* deaths. Within- and between-studies animals should be of comparable age, weight and parity at the start (ICH, 1994). Strains of low fecundity should not be used. The final choice of the strain of rat will probably rest with the experience of the laboratory and the amount of background data available.

Chernoff–Kavlock assay

The Chernoff–Kavlock assay was developed for the rapid screening of high numbers of chemicals for potential developmental toxicity (Chernoff and Kavlock, 1982). The original species of choice was the mouse, but as the study design has evolved over the years the rat has become the preferred species. Pregnant rodents are exposed to the test article for about 5 days during early organogenesis and allowed to give birth. The viability and growth of the pups is then monitored for 4–7 days. Embryotoxicity is manifest as a reduction in live litter size at birth in relation to the number of implantations on the uterus of the dam, or as a reduction in birth weight. If treatment-related effects on pup weight are detected during the first week postpartum, the dams and litters may be retained until weaning. The limited sensitivity of this test is commented on in Chapter 12.

Treatment of Controls

The control groups of rats are sham-treated with a placebo formulation or the vehicle used to formulate the test article for administration. When different treatment volumes are used for the various treatment groups, the control group is normally given the volume administered to the highest treated group. If the reproductive toxicity of the placebo or vehicle has not been properly evaluated beforehand, it may be necessary to treat a second control group with an innocuous control article for purposes of comparison under the conditions of the study. At least one of the control articles should allow an assessment of the method of dosing, or of the vehicle, on the pharmacokinetics or metabolism of the test article (including possible effects mediated by influences on food or water intake).

A comparative control group, treated with a well-studied compound of similar chemical, physical or therapeutic properties to the test article may be considered. For example, if the solution of a test article given by injection is nonisotonic, it might be prudent to include a control group treated with a placebo solution of comparable osmolarity in addition to a negative control given an isotonic solution.

possible before the start of treatment. It is important to verify that all of the mating records (including paternal identity) are correctly recorded by the breeder. The pregnant rats must be transported under suitable environmental conditions with an adequate supply of food and water. They should preferably be weighed before and after transport in order to assess any adverse reactions. Pregnancy rates of over 90% can be expected.

Animal husbandry requirements for rats in reproductive toxicology studies are similar to those for general toxicology or maintenance of a breeding colony (see Chapter 4). Pregnant and lactating rats have particular nutritional requirements, which have a marked influence on reproductive performance. Nutritional deficiency and hypervitaminosis are known causes of birth defects. Most commercial rodent diets are suitably formulated for use in all types of reproduction study. In case of doubt, a specific breeding diet should be used.

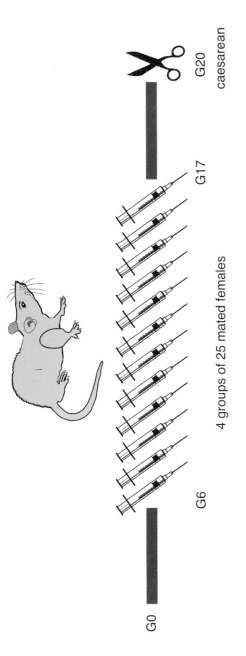

G0

G6

G17

G20

caesarean

4 groups of 25 mated females

Figure 11.1 Embryotoxicity study: basic study design. G, day of gestation.

Positive control groups are used when the available data suggest that the test article may induce reproductive effects similar to those produced by a known toxicant. Valproic acid may be used when testing a novel anticonvulsant agent, for instance, in order to demonstrate that the test system is sensitive to the types of toxic effects that are likely to result from treatment with the test article.

The animals are randomly assigned to the various treatment and control groups at the start of the study. This can be achieved using stratified allocation procedures to ensure that the mean body weights of all groups are similar at the start of the study. When allocating pregnant rats (as in embryotoxicity or pre- and postnatal studies), consideration should also be given to the distribution across the groups of the males used to inseminate the dams.

Embryotoxicity or Prenatal Development Studies

Study Design

Embryotoxicity studies are still sometimes called segment II or teratogenicity studies, as stated in the original FDA guidelines (1966).

Until recently, the assessment of embryotoxicity (which includes teratogenicity) was identical for all categories of drugs and chemicals. This harmony disappeared in 1997 as the result of a harmonization initiative undertaken by the Environmental Protection Agency of the United States, when new more stringent guidelines for prenatal development studies were issued by the Office of Prevention, Pesticides and Toxic Substances (EPA, 1997b). Similar guidelines have been prepared by the OECD (1996) and are expected to be finalized shortly.

All regulatory assessments of reproductive and developmental toxicity of drugs are now performed according to the ICH (1994) harmonized guidelines.

The ICH guidelines for this type of study (Figure 11.1) adhere in most respects to the FDA study protocol which came into being 30 years ago.

For both chemicals and drugs, the embryotoxicity study is often the first type of reproductive toxicology test performed. This strategy allows the detection of potentially embryotoxic agents before animals and resources are unnecessarily assigned to the more complex reproductive studies. Alternatively, savings in the number of animals used for the total package of studies can be made by combining the embryotoxicity assessments with the fertility studies (see below).

The ICH guidelines require treatment from implantation of the embryo until the end of the embryonic period. Palatal closure, which marks the end of the embryonic period, is normally complete in most strains of rat on day 17 of gestation (Marsden and Roche, 1997).

Technical Procedures

In-life

At least four groups of about 25 mated female rats are allocated to the study in order to provide at least 20 pregnant rats at term per group. They should ideally be 10-12 weeks old at the start of the study. Each female is treated from day 6 of gestation (i.e. soon after implantation of the embryos on the uterus) until the end of the embryonic period (day 17 – see above) for drugs or until the day before caesarean examination for chemicals (EPA, 1997b). When gavage or parenteral administration is used, the rats are normally dosed once daily, though more or less frequent dosing may be imposed by the pharmacokinetic characteristics of the test article. Where possible, the daily dose given to each rat is adjusted according to the most recent body weight. The rats are monitored for changes in clinical condition throughout the study, body weights and the amount of food consumed are recorded at intervals of 3 or 4 days. A caesarean examination is performed on day 20 or 21 of gestation (i.e. 1 or 2 days before parturition normally occurs).

Caesarean examination

The dams are euthanized by carbon dioxide inhalation and given a detailed macroscopic necropsy examination to detect any lesions in the maternal organs. The number of visible implantation sites on each horn of the uterus is recorded. Any undetected implantation sites can be stained by immersing the uterus in 10% ammonium sulfide solution for about 10 minutes; this is a regulatory requirement at least for **nongravid** females. The entire reproductive tract, including the ovaries, fallopian tubes, uterus, cervix and vagina, is removed and pinned to a dissection board. The number of corpora lutea (not to be confused with the smaller, paler Graafian follicles) in each ovary are counted. The weight of the gravid uterus may be recorded, as required for chemicals, and is occasionally useful for the elucidation of possible maternal body weight effects or for an estimation of the quantity of amniotic fluid. Alternatively, the quantity of amniotic fluid may be estimated by weighing the entire conceptuses, complete with fetus, placenta and membranes, before rupturing the amniotic sac. The uterine horns are cut open and the chorionic and amniotic sacs are broken to expose the fetuses. Any discoloration of the amniotic fluid is noted. The uterus is carefully examined for the presence of embryonic or fetal resorptions and the nature and position of each implantation is recorded. Resorptions are classified as early (embryonic) or late (fetal). For early resorptions only placental remnants are visible. For late resorptions both placental and fetal remnants can be distinguished. Each fetus is examined for gross abnormalities and is checked for breathing following gentle stimulation. Any mature fetus which fails to breathe is considered to be dead. The fetuses are removed from the uterus and separated from the placenta by cutting the umbilical cord, which is first clamped with a pair of forceps to prevent excessive blood loss. Abnormalities in the colour, size and shape of the placentae are noted. Any rats that die during the course of the study are subjected to similar necropsy procedures.

The time of day when the rats are submitted to the caesarean examination has an impact on the relative state of development of the fetus and on the recorded fetal weight, since the fetuses grow very quickly at the end of gestation. Therefore, each session of caesarean examinations should be completed as quickly as possible and the order in which the dams are euthanized should be equalized between the treatment groups.

It is also important to minimize operator bias in the recorded data. The same precautions as those taken to minimize bias in other types of toxicology study are also relevant to reproductive toxicology. For some unspecified reason, fetal examinations are singled out in the EPA guidelines as requiring 'blind' examination, where the operator is unaware of the identity of the fetus (i.e. treatment group or control) at the time of examination. Most experienced researchers would dispute that fetal examinations are any more prone to operator bias than other types of examination and argue that the dubious benefits of 'blind' examination do not warrant the additional cost and effort involved in coding the specimens and recompiling the results.

Fresh fetal examinations

The fetuses are blotted dry and then weighed individually. The placentae may also be weighed. Each fetus is carefully examined for any external abnormalities and the sex is determined by inspection of the genital tubercle. The fetuses are euthanized by subcutaneous or intraperitoneal injection of sodium pentobarbitone solution or by placing them on an

Table 11.1 Composition of fixatives for fixed-visceral examination of fetuses

Constituent	Relative volumes
Bouin's fixative	
Saturated picric acid solution	7.5
40% Formaldehyde solution	2.5
Glacial acetic acid	0.5
Harrison's fixative	
95% Ethanol	8.0
Glycerol	1.0
40% Formaldehyde solution	2.0
9% Saline	7.5

ice-cold tray for a few minutes. One half of the fetuses (i.e. every second fetus in the uterus) is preserved whole for subsequent fixed soft tissue examination. The selected fetuses are individually identified with plastic tie-on tags, or more conveniently by writing on their skin with an indelible marker pen, and then fixed in Bouin's fluid. Harrison's fixative (Table 11.1) has less noxious constituents and is a convenient alternative to Bouin's fluid; it also has the advantage of rendering the soft tissues less brittle after fixation. The remaining half of the fetuses are given a fresh internal examination prior to processing for skeletal examination. The internal examination is best performed under a dissecting microscope. The abdomen is cut open along its ventral aspect so that the presence, size and shape of all of the internal organs can be checked *in situ*. The kidneys are sectioned to examine the cortex and renal papillae. The sex is confirmed internally. Taking care not to damage the skeleton, the rib cage is cut open to expose the thoracic organs, which are also examined *in situ*. Following removal of the thymus and the pericardium, the heart and major blood vessels can be examined. The ductus arteriosis is examined and should still be patent. The atria are removed to expose the foramen ovale and the ventricles are cut open to check the integrity of the septum. After examination of the thoracic and abdominal organs the fetus is eviscerated, individually identified with a tie-on label or plastic tag and fixed in ethanol. Care is always taken to ensure that any fetuses with external abnormalities are allocated to the most appropriate type of subsequent examination.

Alternatively, if sufficient resources are available,

a detailed fresh examination of the fetuses by microdissection (Staples, 1976) performed at the time of caesarean examination may replace the more common fixed soft tissue examination (see below). This has the advantage of allowing all of the fetuses to be examined for both soft tissue and skeletal abnormalities. The high level of technical skill involved in the microdissection technique and the limited time in which it must be performed on the day of the caesarean contribute to logistical hurdles which make the *in situ* examination technique impracticable for most laboratories.

Fetal soft tissue examinations

Examination of the fixed soft tissues (also called visceral examination) may be performed by serial sectioning (Wilson, 1965) or by a combination of serial sectioning of the head and *in situ* microdissection of the thorax and abdomen (Barrow and Taylor, 1967). Both techniques give comparable results (Sterz and Lehmann, 1985). The serial sectioning technique (Figure 11.2) can be performed rapidly if one or two technicians cut sections for examination by a more experienced operator. A high level of experience is needed by the examiner, however, to be capable of identifying possible abnormalities and in particular to transform the two-dimensional image of the cut sections into a three-dimensional mental picture of the intact fetus. The microdissection technique (Figure 11.3) demands a high degree of manual dexterity and anatomical knowledge on the part of the technician, but any abnormalities are more easily visualized and described.

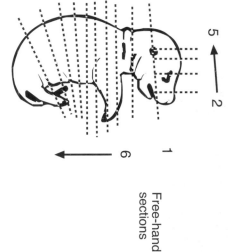

Figure 11.2 Fixed soft tissue examination of a rat fetus by serial sectioning (Wilson method).

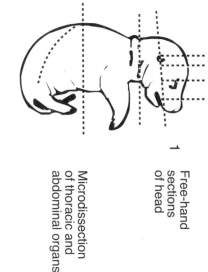

Figure 11.3 Fixed soft tissue examination of a rat fetus by microdissection (Barrow–Taylor method).

The fetuses must be thoroughly fixed before the soft tissue examination can commence. During fixation the skeleton is decalcified and softened and the soft tissues hardened, so that the organs are less easily deformed or squashed during sectioning. For both examination techniques, the head and upper neck are sectioned by hand using a razor blade into about 1-mm transverse sections. Both surfaces of the cut sections are then examined under a low-power binocular microscope so that the presence and form of all of the internal structures (e.g. eyes, ears, brain and major blood vessels) can be verified.

In the serial sectioning technique, transverse slices continue to be cut through the thorax, taking care to check the cardiac chambers and valves and to trace the major blood vessels from one cut section to the next in order to detect any cardiovascular defects. The abdominal cavity is examined in a similar manner. If certain features are not visible (e.g. retina, pituitary, pineal, thyroid, ductus arteriosus or renal pelves) it may be necessary to shave the sections or probe them with a fine wire.

In the microdissection technique, the thoracic and abdominal cavities are carefully opened under the binocular microscope so that the organs can be examined *in situ*. The heart is carefully cut and dissected in place to scrutinize its internal structures. The kidneys are sectioned to allow an examination of the renal papillae.

Whatever the method of examination used, the examined tissues are retained for archiving (often for much longer than their state of preservation would allow retrospective evaluation, because of overzealous interpretations of GLP requirements).

Dawson (1926). The specimens are dehydrated, defatted, macerated and stained with Alizarin red S. The stained specimens can be stored indefinitely in glycerol. They may be conveniently archived in heat-sealed plastic sachets. Several modifications of the technique have been developed according to different laboratory conditions. Automated processors are available. The end result is very attractive, all of the ossified parts of the skeleton are stained bright red and are strikingly visible through the other tissues which have become completely transparent (Figure 11.4). The entire ossified skeleton can now be examined, checking the presence, size and shape of every bone (Barrow, 1990).

The latest EPA guidelines for chemicals, again in disconcordance with the harmonized requirements for drugs, suggest an examination of the fetal cartilage in addition to the ossified bones. Why this is requested for rodents, but not rabbits is unclear. The cartilage can be differentially stained (Figure 11.5) using alcian blue in a modification of the Wilson technique (Whitaker and Dix, 1979). Also, if the maceration step with potassium hydroxide in the original single staining technique is carefully controlled and kept short the cartilaginous areas of the skeleton remain partially visible as light shadowy regions. With acquired experience of the cartilage staining techniques and of the interpretation of the observations made, it is likely that this evaluation

Fetal skeletal examinations

Before examination, the fetal carcasses which were preserved in ethanol following the fresh internal examination must be prepared and stained using a modification of a technique first described by will one day be regarded as indispensable for all potential toxicants, including drugs.

X-ray imaging has also been used for skeletal examination of fetuses which can then be submitted to soft tissue examination, but the technique has fallen from favour in recent years because of the expensive material investment required, the long preparation time and difficulty in obtaining reliable results.

Specific Requirements for Chemicals

The latest EPA guidelines and OECD drafts for chemicals modify the traditional study design by requiring the prolongation of the treatment period to include the fetal period. The extended duration of treatment is intended to improve the sensitivity of the test for the detection of toxic influences on fetal development, such as effects on early nephron development. There is a danger, however, that treatment during the fetal period may cause maternal toxicity or increased levels of fetal loss which could mask teratogenic effects induced during the preceding embryonic period. For this reason it is important to pay particular attention to the incidence of late resorptions following an extended treatment period.

Fertility and Postnatal Investigations

Study Designs

For drugs, the evaluation of fertility of the adult generation and the assessment of postnatal effects are most often made in separate experiments (i.e. segments I and III). For chemicals, both of these evaluations are part of the two-generation 'reproduction study'.

ICH fertility study

In this protocol a minimum of 20 male rats per group are treated for 4 weeks before pairing. Previous regulatory requirements specified a longer pre-pairing treatment period for males of 8–10 weeks, based on the length of the spermatogenic cycle in the rat. The ICH (1996) concluded, however, that a

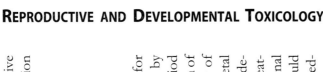

Figure 11.4 Alizarin-stained rat fetus (gestation day 20). Courtesy of the UK Fetal Pathology Terminology Group.

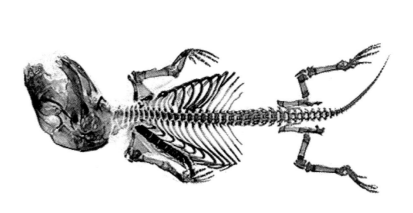

Figure 11.5 Double stained rat fetus (gestation day 20). Courtesy of the UK Fetal Pathology Terminology Group.

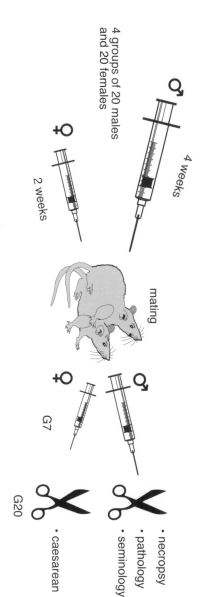

Figure 11.6 ICH fertility study: basic study design. G, day of gestation.

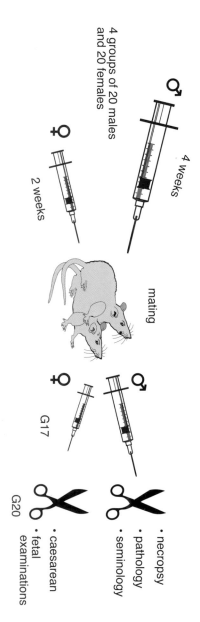

Figure 11.7 ICH combined fertility and embryotoxicity study. G, day of gestation.

shorter period of 4 weeks is sufficient to detect all known toxicants affecting spermatogenesis. This presumption is logical when the physiology of the seminiferous epithelium is considered, since any adverse influence on a particular stage of spermatogenesis would affect several generations of developing sperm. Nevertheless, it is a condition of the shortened ICH preparing treatment period that histopathological data of the reproductive organs must be available from a general toxicology study of at least 13 weeks duration.

The decision by the ICH to shorten the premating treatment period for males may have weakened the testing strategy in an unanticipated manner, however. In the past, with a premating treatment period of 8–10 weeks, most laboratories started the study with males of 4–5 weeks of age in order that they would be at an optimum age for mating two months later. These males were therefore exposed to the test substance from soon after weaning and during puberty. The investigator was therefore inadvertently testing for effects on spermatogenesis at a time when the developing test system could be expected to be particularly sensitive to toxic insult (i.e. during the postweaning androgen surges). Now, with the shorter treatment period, the males are already sexually mature when they are allocated to the study. Note that the animals of the second generation of the pre- and postnatal study are not exposed to the test article during sexual maturation.

At least 20 female rats per group are treated for 2 weeks (to cover at least two oestrous cycles) before pairing (Figure 11.6). One male and one female from the same treatment group are then paired. The females are submitted to a caesarean examination 2 weeks after insemination in order to determine their pregnancy status and evaluate litter data. The males and any noninseminated females are also necropsied at this time. This study design can be conveniently merged with the ICH embryotoxicity protocol by extending the treatment of the mated females until the end of the embryonic period and then retaining the females until day 20 of gestation, so that all of the required caesarean examinations and fetal examinations for the embryotoxicity evaluation can be performed (Figure 11.7).

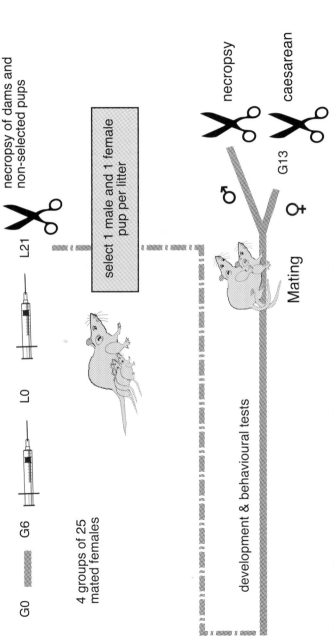

Figure 11.8 ICH pre- and postnatal study. G, day of gestation; L, day of lactation.

ICH pre- and postnatal development study

In this study mated females are treated from the start of the embryonic period, during littering and throughout lactation until weaning of the offspring (Figure 11.8). The treatment period was modified by the ICH to encompass the embryonic period in addition to the fetal and postweaning periods to be sure of detecting possible developmental effects which are induced during organogenesis, but are manifest only after birth. The group sizes and animal specifications are identical to those of the embryotoxicity study.

Multigeneration (reproduction) studies

This type of study is applicable to the testing of industrial chemicals, pesticides, fungicides and food additives. The most usual study design involves feeding a treated diet continuously to two generations of rats with one mating of each generation (Figure 11.9). Alternatively, the test article may be dissolved in the drinking water. If equivocal effects are found during the course of the study it may be necessary to extend the protocol to evaluate a third generation of rats and/or to include a second (or third) mating to produce additional litters in one or more generations.

Paternal teratogenicity

At the present time there is no convincing evidence of a paternally mediated teratogenic mechanism that can cause malformed offspring without exposure of the female. Malformations have been reported following treatment of male rabbits (Lutwack-Mann, 1964) and rats (Husain and Pellerin, 1970) with thalidomide but the results have not been reproducible. If such an undiscovered mechanism does exist, the resulting defects would not be detected in the standard ICH fertility study for drugs (where the offspring are not examined for structural changes). They would, however, be manifest in a combined ICH embryotoxicity and fertility study and in the routine reproduction (multigeneration) protocols used to test chemicals.

Male-mediated teratogenicity can occur following an occupational exposure of the male, who then carries the toxicant home on his body or clothing resulting in exposure of the pregnant women. Another mechanism involves exposure of the pregnant women via a developmental toxicant excreted in the seminal fluid. This method of exposure cannot be directly tested in the rat, which does not mate during gestation. If such an exposure is suspected, a specific embryotoxicity study has to be designed with intravaginal administration of an appropriate dose level of the test substance.

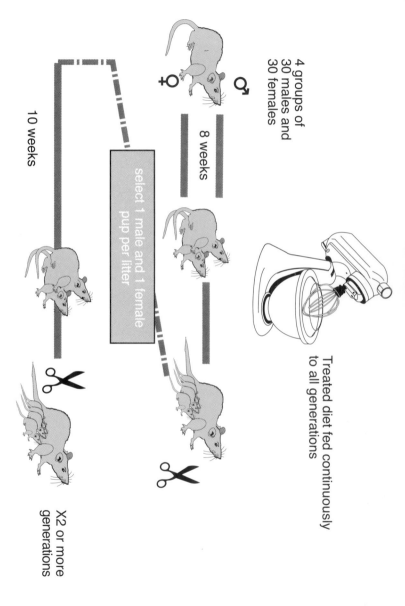

4 groups of
30 males and
30 females

♂ ♀

8 weeks

select 1 male and 1 female
pup per litter

10 weeks

Treated diet fed continuously
to all generations

X2 or more
generations

Figure 11.9 A typical reproduction (multigeneration) study for testing chemicals.

Technical Procedures

Before mating

Before mating, the rats are maintained under similar conditions to those in general toxicity studies (Chapter 4). For drugs, treatment of the males and females begins at least 4 and 2 weeks respectively before pairing. During this period, the rats are weighed and their food intake recorded at 2-weekly intervals. For chemicals, most regulatory agencies require at least 8 weeks of treatment of the males and females before pairing. During this time, the body weights and food consumption are normally recorded weekly.

An evaluation of the oestrous cycle of the females may be performed prior to pairing. This is a specific requirement of the EPA guidelines, which specify that oestrous cycles should be examined for each female daily for 3 weeks before pairing. Two weeks is otherwise normally sufficient. A small sample of cells is removed from the vaginal lumen of the female rat each morning and examined microscopically. The samples may be taken using a dry cotton swab (i.e. 'dry smearing') or by flushing the vagina with a small volume of saline (i.e. 'wet smearing').

The stage of oestrous cycle is determined and recorded (see Chapters 9 and 25). There is a danger that the procedure of vaginal smearing if not expertly performed may interfere with mating performance by provoking pseudopregancy. Evaluation of the oestrous cycles during the mating period is required by the EPA and is optional in the OECD draft. The most frequent toxic influences on the oestrous cycle include an arrested cycle (which may be the result of general poor clinical condition of the female or a direct influence of the test article on the hormonal control of the uterus), irregular cycles, or extended oestrus.

Mating and gestation

Treated rats are usually paired on the basis of one male to one female. If the aim is just to supply pregnant females for the subsequent allocation to an embryotoxicity or pre- and postnatal study, it is possible to pair two or more females with each male in order to optimize the number of females inseminated per day. The female should normally be introduced into the cage of the male, but in practice cage dominance does not appear to have a significant influence on mating performance. The animals may be left together in the same cage until insemination is detected, or they may be separated every morning and re-paired in the evening.

Each morning during the cohabitation period, the vagina of the female is inspected for the presence of an *in situ* vaginal plug. If no plug is found, a vaginal smear is taken (see Chapters 9 and 25) and examined for the presence of sperm. Once insemination has been detected, by the presence of vaginal plug or by sperm in the vaginal smear, the rats are separated and the female is placed in a littering cage. It should be possible to detect the day of copulation for all of the inseminated females. The consequences of failing to detect the day of insemination for occasional females depend on the study design. At best only the body weights and food consumption data of the female during gestation will not be collected. At worst the gestation data, the caesarean data and fetal observations will be lost. The day of identification of insemination is best termed day 0 of gestation, the use of day 1 instead leads to confusion. A mating period of 2 weeks is normally sufficient to detect any toxic influences on mating behaviour; the ICH guidelines for drugs require 3 weeks. It is possible, but not necessary, to change the mating combinations of any rats in the same treatment group which have not copulated within a given number of days. More than 90% of rats normally copulate during the first available oestrus. The precoital interval for each pair of rats is recorded; the interval is considered normal if rats mate within 4 or 5 days.

During gestation, the body weights and food consumption of the female rats are recorded at 3–4 day intervals. Depending on the study design (see above), the pregnant rats may be subjected to a caesarean examination on day 13 or 20 of gestation or allowed to give birth.

Parturition, lactation and postpartum observations

Littering

The pregnant females are placed in solid-bottomed cages with a suitable bedding material such as sawdust and a paper tissue. Starting from day 20 of gestation the females are examined two or three times per day for bleeding from the vagina, which is the first sign of the onset of parturition. The duration of gestation is recorded for each female, calculated as the number of days between the day of identification of mating and the delivery of the first pup. Any parturition difficulties (dystocia) are noted.

If necessary, any female which fails to complete parturition within 24 hours and shows a marked deterioration in clinical condition is euthanized.

The female is disturbed as little as possible during parturition, but stillborn or noticeably malformed pups are removed and examined before the mother can make a meal of them. Dosing of the female may have to be suspended until after completion of parturition. The time of completion of parturition, when there is no more bleeding from the vagina and the dam starts to clean and feed the pups, is noted. After the last pup has been delivered, or the day after completion of parturition, the pups are counted, examined, sexed and individually weighed. If necessary the pups can be individually identified by tattooing on the paws or using other acceptable methods.

Any moribund or dead pups are submitted to a necropsy examination in order to determine the cause of death (if possible) and detect any congenital anomalies.

Preweaning assessment of pup viability and development

The lactating dams and litters are examined daily for any changes in clinical condition or behaviour; any dead pups are removed from the nest and necropsied as soon as possible. Each pup is weighed at specified intervals (e.g. days 4, 7, 11, 14, 17 and 21 postpartum) until weaning. Although required by some test guidelines, the utility of individually weighing pups is open to question, since these data are almost always presented as the mean and/or total weight per litter. It may be more cost effective to weigh the whole litter together at each interval except at birth and weaning. It is now common to present pup weight data by sex, as preferred by the EPA.

Preweaning development tests are required for the testing of drugs, but not for chemicals. The pups are examined daily for a series of developmental milestones in order to evaluate their physical development. The day of occurrence of some or all of the following is noted for each pup: pinna unfolding (i.e. detachment of the outer margin of the external ears from the scalp), incisor eruption (appearance of the first tooth), hair growth and eye opening. If the pups are not individually identified the proportion of the litter is recorded until completion of the litter. Reflexes of the pups are also tested on specific days or at intervals until all pups in the litter are positive, these include surface righting reflex (the pup is placed on its back on a hard surface and must demonstrate the ability to turn over onto its feet), air righting reflex (the pup is turned into a supine position and dropped from a height of 30 cm over a padded surface and must demonstrate the ability to turn to land on its feet), pupil reflex (both pupils must constrict in response to light) and startle response to a sharp sound. The anogenital distance of the male and female pups may be measured; this parameter is a possible indicator of oestrogenic or antiandrogenic interference, as is abnormal nipple development in male and female rat pups.

Culling (or not)

Many laboratories try to make litter responses uniform by standardizing litter sizes, usually on day 4 postpartum. This is done by randomly selecting and discarding the appropriate number of excess pups from each litter to leave a predefined number of males and females (usually four or five of each sex). No attempt is made to standardize litters with less than the total required litter size. When there are insufficient numbers of pups of one sex, additional pups of the opposing sex are retained where possible to maintain the desired total litter size.

There has been much discussion recently concerning the validity of this practice, with arguments for and against its continued use (Chapin and Heck, 1997; Agnish and Keller, 1997; Palmer and Ulbrich, 1997a). At present, all of the regulatory texts state that culling is optional. The most powerful (but not often stated) argument in favour of culling is the decreased technical workload resulting from the reduced number of pups to be examined. The jury is still out but, unless its utility can be proved, culling is likely to fall from favour. For the time being, most laboratories will elect to carry on with their present practice in order to remain consistent with their historical data. Any laboratory starting from scratch or re-initializing its historical database would be best advised not to cull litters. In any case, each investigator should be prepared to justify his or her decision.

Estimation of milk production and quality

Milk is relatively easily sampled from the rat (see Chapter 25). The collected milk can then be analysed using standard clinical pathology instruments or analytical chemistry to determine its composition. It is not easy, on the other hand, to estimate the quantity of milk produced by the dam (at least not without resorting to radiochemistry). In the final analysis, the best measure of milk production is probably pup growth.

Selection of pups at weaning

At weaning (day 21 postpartum) the appropriate number of pups are randomly selected to form the subsequent generation (where required). It is usual to select one male and one female pup from each litter, though it may be necessary to select additional pups from some litters to make up the required number. The method of selection within the litter must be random, it is not appropriate to select on the basis of body weight or any other parameter. Runts should not normally be excluded from the selection, but exceptions can be justified for pups considered unlikely to survive. The selected pups are renumbered and allocated to new cages. The data records must clearly indicate the litter origin of each rat. The nonselected pups and their mothers are euthanized and given a necropsy examination.

Postweaning

There is some disagreement between toxicologists over whether rats should be individually or group housed. The consensus in Europe is that rats should be group housed whenever possible (Council of Europe, 1997). Within the context of developmental toxicology, the choice is more clear-cut, since it has been shown that socially deprived rats do not show a normal **neurobehavioural** development (Levitsky and Barnes, 1972). It is justified, therefore, to sacrifice the accuracy of food consumption recordings during the postweaning development phase in favour of a more appropriate assessment of neurological development.

The F1 rats continue to be examined daily for any mortality or changes in clinical condition. They are weighed individually at least once weekly.

The day of vaginal opening is recorded for each female. The day of **balanopreputial** skinfold cleavage is noted for each male; this milestone is a more appropriate indicator of secondary sexual development in the male than testes descent, which is very variable (ICH, 1994). The body weight on the day of occurrence of these milestones is also recorded and is useful for the evaluation of possible effects of treatment when accompanied by body weight effects.

A functional test battery of behavioural tests is performed on the young rats before mating (see Chapter 21). Until recently, these tests were only required for drugs, but the OECD now recommends functional testing for chemical agents also. There are EPA and OECD guidelines for developmental neurotoxicity studies for pesticides and industrial chemicals which include detailed behavioural testing.

Most strains of rats can be mated from about 11 weeks of age (see above).

Post-mortem

While the requirements for the assessment of adult fertility understandably figure in the various regulatory texts for reproductive toxicology, this does not mean that the seminology and histopathological examinations are only applicable to reproductive studies. The more shrewd investigator thinks of including these examinations much earlier in the safety testing programme, preferably during the subchronic toxicology studies. This strategy makes better use of each experimental animal and allows an earlier detection of potential toxic influences on fertility. If such effects are anticipated the design of the reproduction studies can then be modified accordingly.

Seminology

Sperm analysis was a requirement in the initial ICH guidelines for drugs (ICH, 1994). An amendment was later issued to make sperm analysis optional (ICH, 1996). This unprecedented reversal occurred after several purpose-commissioned studies (Takayama et al., 1995a,b; Ulbrich and Palmer, 1995) questioned whether the increased sensitivity to detect reprotoxic effects in routine safety studies warrants the increased cost and effort of seminology investigations. Nonetheless, sperm analysis persisted as a formal requirement in the final EPA (1997a) and draft OECD (1996) guidelines for chemicals. Sperm analysis involves quantitative evaluations of epididymal sperm reserves, sperm motility and morphology and spermatid counts in the testes. Recent evidence (Chapin et al., 1997) shows that at least one sperm parameter, epididymal sperm count, is predictive of fertilizing capacity in rodents (the mouse).

Sperm motility can be assessed visually, but the most accurate and cost-effective methods make use of computer-assisted sperm analysis (CASA). Several commercial systems are available (Working and Hurtt, 1987). These machines give reliable, accurate measures of sperm counts and motility. The measurements are, however, very dependent on the methods of sample preparation (Klinefelter et al., 1991). The investigator can easily be deceived by the false precision of the recorded parameters if the experimental variables are not carefully

standardized. Validation and calibration of the techniques and equipment are particularly tedious.

Methods of sperm collection by ejaculation have the advantage of allowing repeated sampling, so that several measurements can be taken for each rat (before and after the start of treatment for instance). Unfortunately, in rats these methods are too invasive for use during the course of routine safety studies (see Chapter 25), so samples can only be taken at necropsy.

Samples of sperm for motility and morphology evaluations are best obtained at necropsy from the cauda epididymis, which is isolated, sectioned and placed in an incubated physiological solution so that the sperm diffuse out of the tissue. A sample of the mixed sperm suspension is then transferred to the counting chamber for analysis. The depth of this chamber is vitally important, since the sperm must have enough space to swim unimpeded without moving in and out of the depth of focus of the microscope objective (Slott et al., 1991). Enough microscopic fields are analysed to allow the examination of at least 200 sperm cells. The machine must be calibrated in such a way that it can distinguish the sperm cells from cellular debris. CASA systems print out a long series of parameters, many more than can be adequately interpreted. Of these parameters, the following are reported to be the most predictive of fertilizing capacity of the rat: epididymal sperm content, percentage normally motile sperm, and measures of forward sperm motion such as linearity (calculated as straight line velocity divided by curvilinear velocity). Video recording of the samples, either on tape or optical disk, allows retrospective analysis of the data; but unless the machine can memorize the exact temporal and physical location on the recording of the fields analysed, there is no guarantee that repeated analysis of the video records will give consistent results. If visual assessment is used without video recording, the EPA requires analysis of all groups. When video recording is made for all groups it is acceptable in the first instance to analyse only the control and high dose data. This concession is largely superfluous since almost no effort is needed to analyse the data once the CASA recordings have been made.

Testicular spermatid counts are obtained by mincing a weighed sample of one or both testes in a physiological solution and counting the number of homogenization-resistant spermatids in the suspension. The results are expressed as number of spermatids per gram of testis and the estimated total count per testis (calculated from the relative weight of the sample).

The EPA guidelines also require an evaluation of sperm morphology. This is an option on some CASA systems. The morphological assessments made by automated systems are sometimes limited to an evaluation of the sperm head, while the mid-piece and tail also have to be examined. As primary assessment, a detailed description of every morphological abnormality is not generally necessary. Provided that there are no treatment-related changes, the data compiled can be limited to the proportion of sperm in a few simple categories (e.g. abnormalities of the head, mid-piece or tail, and normal).

Histopathology of male reproductive organs

No assessment of reproductive toxicity can be considered complete without a thorough evaluation of possible toxic influences on the testicular function. Because the rat has a large reserve capacity of sperm production, mating performance may not be the most predictive indication of testicular effects in this species.

Several regulatory texts justifiably make a reference to 'good' histopathology of the testes. The routine methods of examination following fixation in formaldehyde employed in the past result in shrinkage of the tubules and are not suitable for the detection of influences on spermatogenesis (Chapin, 1989). Fixation in Bouin's fluid followed by H/E and PAS staining is now regarded as the minimum requirement. Interpretation of potential effects is complicated by the complex three-dimensional structure of the seminiferous epithelium, involving four generations of interacting cells developing in synchronization with each other.

The duration of sperm development in the rat testis is about 53 days (Foster, 1989), during which time the cell works its way from the basal compartment towards the lumen. Because of the overlapping sperm cell populations, the seminiferous epithelium shows a 13-day longitudinal cycle. Fourteen stages of this cycle can be identified in the rat. In addition to gross lesions of the types normally detected in general toxicology studies (i.e. atrophy or tumours), the pathologist needs to check for abnormalities of the spermatogenic cycle such as retained spermatids, germ cell depletion and sloughing of spermatogenic cells into the lumen (Creasy, 1997).

Tubular staging, a quantitative evaluation of the number of cross-sections of tubules showing each of the 14 stages of the cycle, is a useful (but time-consuming) technique for the characterization of spermatogenic disruption following an acute exposure (Hess and Moore, 1993). The technique is not of value following chronic exposure, as in routine reproductive toxicology studies, where multiple successive reproductive cycles are disrupted to the extent that no point of action can be identified. The regulatory guidelines for drugs and chemicals are often incorrectly interpreted to require quantative tubular staging, which is not the case.

Examination of the intact epididymis can be accomplished by examination of a stained longitudinal section after fixation in Bouin's fixative. It should be possible to identify such lesions as sperm granulomas, leukocytic infiltration (inflammation), **aberrant cell types** in the lumen, or the absence of clear cells in the cauda epididymal epithelium (EPA, 1997a). The presence of spermatozoids and the absence of cellular debris are the best indicators of intact spermatogenesis.

Histopathology of female reproductive organs

The EPA guidelines state that the histopathological examination of the ovaries must be capable of detecting a depletion of the primordial follicle population. A quantitative evaluation of primordial follicles (e.g. Smith *et al.*, 1991) in the F1 females is required if there were any possible effects in the previous generation on the male or female germ cells or on oestrous cycles or ovary weights. Differential follicle counts are thought to be a quantifiable endpoint of ovarian injury (Bolon *et al.*, 1997). The techniques for this type of evaluation are still being refined and urgently need to be validated (EPA, 1997a). This endpoint is the only attempt in any regulatory guideline, including those for drugs, to detect possible toxic effects that could result in reduced female fertility later in life or premature menopause.

Reporting of Data from Reproductive Toxicology Studies

The presentation and analysis of data from reproductive toxicology studies is hampered by the complex nature of the parameters examined. Each dam may have up to about 20 offspring, so the number of litter-based values is not constant or predictable. Also, many reproductive parameters follow non-normal, asymmetric, skewed or dichotomous distributions which necessitate complex methods of analysis.

Presentation of Results

The final report of a regulatory toxicology study has to address several conflicting objectives. First, all of the relevant (and often irrelevant) data must be complete and accurately presented. The regulatory assessors often insist that all of the findings from the study, however trivial, are fully detailed in the report. At the same time, other assessor's claim that they don't have time to read the complete text and will probably only scan through the summary tables (Palmer and Ulbrich, 1997b). In order to meet these objectives a great deal of care needs to be taken over the preparation of the report tables, appendices and text. The report must be clear, concise and complete. Quality and quantity should not be confused. The preparation of a clear, concise, but complete report is much more demanding than that of a poorly planned voluminous document. Various computer systems can be used for the reporting of reproductive toxicology data and greatly reduce the human workload. Unfortunately, to date, computer-produced reports all too often fall into the confused voluminous category. This is because computer programs rely heavily on pre-set table formats which are relatively inflexible and difficult to adapt according to the design and results of a given study.

Basic Sampling Unit: Litter or Fetus?

When analysing litter data (fetal weight for instance) the basic sampling unit has to be defined: the litter or the fetus? A litter-based approach is strongly preferred. That is to say that the mean of the individual fetal values is first calculated for each litter and the litter means are then used for the analysis. If a fetal-based analysis is used, a single treated dam with 18 fetuses, for example, will influence the result nine times more than another treated dam with only two fetuses.

Terminology

A great deal of effort has been devoted in recent years towards the harmonization of the terms used to describe structural developmental abnormalities. Much of this work has been coordinated on an international level by the International Federation of Teratology Societies, which has published a glossary of developmental abnormalities in common laboratory animals (Wise et al., 1997). This glossary, while not perfect (especially in its annoying habit of indiscriminately mixing nouns, verbs and adjectives), is a first step towards agreeing a common language to describe morphological abnormalities encountered in reproductive toxicology studies. Regulatory toxicologists would be well advised to make full use of this glossary when describing their findings, since it is very likely to become the *de facto* standard with the regulatory authorities.

The French Teratology Association, working in conjunction with the International Federation of Teratology Societies, will shortly publish a bilingual comparative atlas of malformations in humans and animals. It is hoped that this effort will help to coordinate international efforts to consolidate the terms used to describe fetal abnormalities encountered in laboratory animals and in humans.

A group of experienced fetal pathologists from UK laboratories (R. Clark et al., personal communication) is currently engaged in the preparation of a reference manual of common observations in the fetal rat skeleton. The aim is to encourage clarity and consistency in the descriptive terminology used by fetal pathologists and also to set a standard which can be followed by academic researchers as well as those performing regulatory studies for the safety evaluation of drugs and other chemicals. It is intended that the manual will be made available in hard copy and on CD-ROM. The bulk of the publication will be presented in two main sections containing fully labelled, high quality, coloured images of normal and abnormal fetuses. A third section, providing accompanying text, will give the background and reasoning behind the recommended terminology and will also include technical aspects.

There remain, of course, many disagreements over the use of certain terms, but these arguments are mainly of trivial consequence (such as the spelling of foetus or fetus, harmonised or harmonized).

Statistical Analysis (Inferential Statistics)

Before commencing the statistical analysis, numerical data must be examined to determine which statistical tests are applicable. This can be done on a study-by-study basis, or the historical database can be analysed to evaluate the distribution of the data population with a view to selecting the most appropriate methods with the greatest degree of confidence. Even when the distribution of the historical data is known, it is still necessary to verify that the data from each study conform to the expected distribution. It is advisable to apply the most powerful statistical test possible for each data set. In practice, this means that parametric methods are applied wherever possible. A test of homogeneity of variance, or more rarely a test of normality, is usually used for this purpose. Nonhomogeneous data are mathematically transformed, where possible, to approximate to a normal distribution to allow the use of parametric methods. As a last resort nonparametric tests are used.

Some litter parameters (again, fetus and pup weights are good examples) are influenced by litter size. The pups in a litter of 18, for instance, tend to be smaller and grow more slowly than those in a litter of only two pups. One way to take this influence into account in the analysis of the data is to analyse both the mean and total weights for the litter. Analysis of covariance (Freund and Wilson, 1997) is a more powerful method for evaluating possible treatment-related effects on interrelated variables. Fetal and pup weights are also influenced by sex, so male and female weights should be analysed separately.

Incidence and observational data present a particular challenge for the statistician. For high-frequency events, such as the incidence of the more common fetal variations, the observations can be transformed into a numeric distribution by calculating the percentage of affected fetuses in each litter, but the artificial nature of the resulting pseudo-continuous distribution should be kept in mind throughout the analysis. Low- to mid-frequency events, such as the incidence of fetal malformations or the incidence of **resorptions**, cannot be analysed in the same way and require more sophisticated methods. However, routine statistical analysis of these data is not always considered worthwhile, since a treatment-related increase in malformation incidence is regarded with so much caution that biological significance is almost always reached long before statistical significance is attained. An extremely powerful method for analysis of low-frequency incidence data, permutation analysis (Crump et al., 1991), has become feasible with the recent advances in microprocessor power. This method allows the calculation of the exact probability of any combination of findings in the control and treated groups.

Electronic Reporting Methods – The Way Forward?

Toxicology reports for regulatory submission must address multiple, often conflicting, objectives. Ever increasing GLP constraints have undoubtedly brought a vast improvement in the reliability of the reported data, but the scientific quality of the reports has often suffered as a result. Numerous attestations, certificates and other 'paper chase documents' bulk out the reports and seriously detract from their legibility (Palmer and Ulbrich, 1997b).

Using modern database technology it should now be possible to reverse the trend towards ever more complicated and cumbersome reports. Intelligent electronic documents will allow the reader to individually adapt the presentation of the document to his or her needs. 'Paper chase documents' will remain invisible until requested. The reader will be able to sort and display the data at will without having to submit to a predefined presentation imposed by the author. For instance, in order to evaluate a possible relationship not envisaged by the author, the reader may want to display maternal food consumption data alongside the fetal incidence of spina bifida and the historical control data. In the future it will be possible to include much more detailed data without overloading the report. Good reporting will always be very time consuming, with or without digital methods.

A previous premature attempt to define electronic reporting standards called CANDA, on a global rather than a per study level, by the FDA (1995) has now apparently been abandoned. At the present time, many laboratories already produce reports in electronic formats in order to facilitate the transmission and distribution of documents. In most cases, however, the actual form of the electronic file is a dumb conventional-type document with no added value.

Interpretation of Results

The aim of toxicological safety testing is to provide information for use in the estimation of human health risks. The data from these studies will be used in reproductive and developmental toxicity risk assessment for the purposes of hazard identification and dose–response evaluation (Kimmel and Kimmel, 1997).

There are four manifestations of developmental toxicity: death, structural abnormalities, growth alterations and functional defects. The conditions under which such effects occur also need to be considered, particularly with respect to maternal or paternal toxicity.

Maternal toxicity is assessed by the evaluation of mortality or **morbidity**, clinical signs, body weight gain, food and water consumption, organ weights and pathological lesions. One of the first manifestations of maternal toxicity is often a reduction in food consumption; the resulting change in nutritional status of the dam may directly or indirectly influence the development of the embryos, fetus or pups. Maternal body weight gain during the second half of gestation in the rat is influenced by the rate of growth of the litter. Retarded fetal development resulting in reduced fetal growth, also impacts on maternal weight gain. Litter influences on maternal weight can be assessed by subtracting the weight of the gravid uterus – determined at necropsy – from the weight gain of the dam during gestation. This type of analysis is suggested in the latest EPA guidelines; it is less appropriate for embryotoxicity studies with drugs where the rats are not treated during the fetal period. Treatment-related effects on gestation length have an influence on the relative state of development of the pups at birth and need to be taken into account in the evaluation of pup growth and postnatal development.

When evaluating embryotoxic agents, it is unusual to find malformations in the absence of growth retardation and embryo lethality (thalidomide being a notable exception). The incidence of these events usually varies in frequency depending on the dose level. Likewise, malformations rarely occur without an associated increase in the incidence of less serious structural alterations. In the past there has been a tendency to concentrate on the more dramatic, but rare, manifestations of developmental toxicity, such as malformations. It is now accepted that it is essential to also evaluate the more subtle morphological modifications, which usually give a more sensitive indication of developmental toxicity. The entire spectrum of effects needs to be consolidated in the report. It is not sufficient to consider each element in isolation, otherwise important clues may be missed.

To facilitate the visual assessment of the data,

it is usual to sort fetal abnormalities according to their severity. Structural defects which are rare in the control population and are thought to be life threatening or of major physiological consequence are classed as malformations. Minor defects which are relatively rare in the control population and/or are not considered to be of major physiological consequence are classed as anomalies. Other minor abnormalities or alternative forms which are common in the control population and are of no known physiological consequence are classed as variations. Palmer, who first proposed such a classification, now claims that its overzealous use is detrimental to the detection of developmental effects because of a failure to consolidate the evaluation of the fragmented data (Palmer and Ulbrich, 1997b).

The conclusion of the study includes a statement concerning the reproductive toxicity caused by the test substance, the degree of any maternal or paternal toxicity, and the dose level(s) at which each type of toxicity was observed.

Historical Control Data

Historical (or background) control data are used to verify that the results obtained in the concurrent control group(s) are representative for the strain; they become essential for the interpretation of the study when equivocal results are found. It is therefore preferable to evaluate the quantity and quality of historical data available before initiating a study. Data generated in-house are more valuable than results obtained under different experimental conditions. Failing this, relevant data may be obtained from other sources, such as animal suppliers, contract research organizations and independent associations (e.g. MARTA, 1997).

All laboratories, therefore, need to maintain a database of control results. The data should be compiled by species, strain, period and study. The database should be constructed to allow sorting of the data by criteria (such as route of administration, type of vehicle, etc.) and to detect and monitor background fluctuations. It is convenient to tabulate the data by year and by study. The EPA (1997b) states that the historical incidence of fetal abnormalities should be compiled by fetus and by litter. Electronic reporting should soon provide the tools for making better use of historical data in reports.

References

Agnish, N.D. and Keller, K.A. (1997) *Appl. Toxicol.* **38**, 2–6

Ashby, J. and Lefevre, P.A. (1997) *Regul. Toxicol. Pharmacol.* **26**, 330–337.

Barrow, M.V. and Taylor, W.J. (1967) *J. Morphol.* **127**, 291–306.

Barrow, P. (1990) *Technical Procedures in Reproduction Toxicology: Laboratory Animals Handbooks 11.* London: Royal Society of Medicine.

Barrow, P.C., Heritier, B. and Marsden, E.K.S. (1996) *Toxicol. Meth.* **6**, 139–147.

Barrow, P.C. and Guyot, J.Y. (1996) *Hum. Exp. Toxicol.* **15**, 214–218.

Barrow, P.C. and Heritier, B. (1995) *Toxicol. Meth.* **5**, 61–67.

Barrow, P.C. and Heritier, B. (1996) *Contemp. Top. Lab. Anim. Sci.* **35**, 66–69.

Barrow, P.C., Olivier, P. and Marzin, D. (1995) *Reprod. Toxicol.* **9**, 389–398.

Bolon, B., Bucci, T.J., Warbritton, A.R., Chen, J.J., Mattison, D.R. and Heindel, J.J. (1997) *Fundam. Appl. Toxicol.* **39**, 1–10.

Chapin, R.E. (1989) In: Working, P.K. (ed.) *Toxicology of the Male and Female Reproductive Systems*, pp. 1–14. New York: Hemisphere.

Chapin, R.E. and Heck, H. d'A. (1997) *Appl. Toxicol.* **38**, 1 [culling].

Chapin, R.E., Sloane, R.A. and Haserman, J.K. (1997) *Fundam. Appl. Toxicol.* **38**, 129–142.

Chernoff, N. and Kavlock, R.J. (1982) *J. Toxicol. Environ. Health* **10**, 541.

Christian, M.S. and Goeke, J.E. (1997) In: Hood, R.D. (ed.) *Handbook of Developmental Toxicology*, pp. 529–595. Boca Raton: CRC Press.

Clarke, D.O. (1993) Pharmacokinetic studies in developmental toxicology: practical considerations and approaches. *Toxicol. Meth.* **3**, 223–251.

Council of Europe (1997) Cons 123 (96) 10.

Creasy, D.M. (1997) *Toxicol. Pathol.* **25**, 119–131.

Crump, K.S., Howe, R.B. and Kodell, R.L. (1991) In: Krewski, D. and Franklin, C. (eds) *Statistics in Toxicology*, pp. 349–377. New York: Gordon & Breach.

Danielsson, B.R.G., Reiland, S., Rundqvist, E. and Danielsson, M. (1989) *Teratology* **40**, 351–358.

Dawson, A.B. (1926) *Stain Tech.* **1**, 123–124.

ECETOC (1989) Monograph No. 12. Alternative approaches for the assessment of reproductive toxicity. European Chemical Industry and Toxicology Centre, Brussels.

EEC (1996) Directive 93/95 Sixth amendment to Cosmetic Directive.

EPA (US Environmental Protection Agency) (1997a) *Fed. Reg.* 43820–43864.

EPA (1997b) *Fed. Reg.* 40, 799, 9370.

European Agency for the Evaluation of Medicinal Products (1997) Note for guidance on pre-clinical pharmacological and toxicological testing of vaccines, draft 9. Available on-line: http://www.eudra.org/emea.html.

European Agency for the Evaluation of Medicinal Products (1998) Annex to note for guidance on gene therapy product quality aspects in the production of vectors and genetically modified somatic cells. Available on-line: http://www.eudra.org/emea.html.

Fielder, R.J., Atterwill, C.K., Anderson, D. *et al.* (1997) *Hum. Exp. Toxicol.* **16**, S1–S40.

FDA (1966) Guidelines for reproduction studies for the evaluation of drugs for human use, National Technical Information Service, Springfield, VA.

FDA (Food and Drug Administration) (1982) Toxicological principles for the safety assessment of direct food additives and color additives in food, National Technical Information Service, Springfield, VA.

FDA (1993) *Redbook II – Draft*, pp. 123–137. Washington DC: Center for Food Safety and Applied Nutrition.

FDA (1995) *Fed. Reg.* **59**, 48745–48752.

FDA (1997) *Fed. Reg.* **62**, 61515–61519. Available on-line http://www.cber.gov.

Foster, P.M. (1989) In: Working, P.K. (ed.) *Toxicology of the Male and Female Reproductive Systems*, pp. 1–14. New York: Hemisphere.

Francis, E.Z. (1994) In: Kimmel, C.A. and Buelke-Sam, J. (eds) *Developmental Toxicology*, 2nd edn, pp. 403–428. New York: Raven.

Freund, R.J. and Wilson W.J. (1997) In: *Statistical Methods*, revised edn, pp. 520–528. San Diego: Academic Press.

Harris, C. (1997) In: Hood, R.D. (ed.) *Handbook of Developmental Toxicology*, pp. 465–510. Boca Raton: CRC Press.

Henck, J.W., Hilbish, K.G. Serabian, M.A. *et al.* (1996) *Teratology* **53**, 185–195.

Hess, R.A. and Moore, B.J. (1993) In: Chapin, R.E. and Heindel, J.J. (eds) *Methods in Toxicology*, Vol. 3, Pt A, pp. 86–94. San Diego: Academic Press.

Husain, S.M. and Pellerin M. (1970) *CMAJ* **18**, 163–164.

ICH (1994) In: D'Arcy, P.F. and Harron, D.W.G. (eds) *Proceedings of the Second International Conference on Harmonization, Orlando*, pp. 557–578. Belfast: Queen's University.

ICH (1996) Tripartite guideline on detection of toxicity to reproduction for medicinal products: addendum. *Fed. Reg.* **61**, 15359–15361.

Kimmel, C.A. and Kimmel, G.L. (1997) In: Hood, R.D. (ed.) *Handbook of Developmental Toxicology*, pp. 667–693. Boca Raton: CRC Press.

Klinefelter, G.R., Grey, L.E. and Suarez, J.D. (1991) *Reprod. Toxicol.* **5**, 39–44.

Kung, A.H.C., Kong, K.N., Achilles, K.A., Mohler, V.I. and White, M.L. (1994) *J. Am. Coll. Toxicol.* **13**, 64–75.

Levitsky D. and Barnes R.H. (1972) *Science* **176**, 68–71.

Lutwak-Mann, C. (1964) *BMJ* **1**, 1090–1091.

Marsden, E.K.S. and Roche, F. (1997) *Teratology* **6**, 393.

MARTA (Middle Atlantic Reproduction and Teratology Association) (1997) In: Hood, R.D. (ed.) *Handbook of Developmental Toxicology*, pp. 713–733. Boca Raton: CRC Press.

Nau, H. (1985) *Toxicol. Appl. Pharmacol.* **80**, 243–250.

Neubert, R. and Neubert, D. (1997) In: Kavlock, R.J. and Daston, G.P. (eds) *Drug Toxicity in Embryonic Development*, pp. 41–105. Berlin: Springer.

OECD (1981) Teratogenicity, OECD guideline for testing chemicals 414.

OECD (1982a) Two-generation reproduction toxicity study. OECD guideline for testing chemicals 416, 1.

OECD (1982b) One-generation reproduction toxicity study. OECD guideline for testing chemicals 415, 1.

OECD (1983a) First addendum to OECD guideline for testing chemicals 416, 1.

OECD (1983b) First addendum to OECD guideline for testing chemicals 415, 1.

OECD (1995) Reproduction/developmental toxicity screening test. OECD guideline for testing chemicals 421.

OECD (1996) Draft guidelines available on-line: http://www.oecd.org/ehs/test/testlist.htm.

O'Flaherty, E.J. and Clarke, D.O. (1994) In: Kimmel, C.A. and Buelke-Sam, J. (eds) *Developmental Toxicology*, 2nd edn, pp. 215–244. New York: Raven.

Palmer, A.K. and Ulbrich, B.C. (1997a) *J. Appl. Toxicol.* **38**, 7–22.

Palmer, A.K. and Ulbrich, B.C. (1997b) In: Hood R.D.

(ed.) *Handbook of Developmental Toxicology*, pp. 227–290. Boca Raton: CRC Press.

Parkhie, M. and Webb, M. (1983) *Teratology* **27**, 327–332.

Schardein, J.L. (1993) In: Schardein, J.L. (ed.) *Chemically Induced Birth Defects*, pp. 416–435. New York: Marcel Dekker.

Slott, V.L., Suarez, J.D. and Perreault, S.D. (1991) *Reprod. Toxicol.* **5**, 449–458.

Smith, B.J., Plowchalk, D.R., Sipes, I.G. and Mattison, D.R. (1991) *Reprod. Toxicol.* **5**, 379–383.

Staples, R.E. (1976) *Environ. Health Prospect.* **18**, 95.

Sterz, H. and Lehmann, H. (1985) *Teratog. Carcinog. Mutag.* **5**, 347–354.

Takayama, S., Akaike, M., Kawashima, K., Takahashi, M. and Kurokawa, Y. (1995a) *J. Toxicol. Sci.* **20**, 173–182.

Takayama, S., Akaike, M., Kawashima, K., Takahashi, M. and Kurokawa, Y. (1995b) *J. Am. Coll. Toxicol.* **14**, 266–292.

Ulbrich, B. and Palmer, A.K. (1995) *J. Am. Coll. Toxicol.* **14**, 293–327.

Whitaker, J. and Dix, K.M. (1979) *Lab. Anim.* **13**, 309–310.

Wilson, J.G. (1965) In: Wilson, J.G. and Warkany, J. (eds) *Teratology Principles and Techniques*, pp. 262–277. Chicago: University Press.

Wise, D.L., Beck, S.L., Beltrame, D. et al. (1997) *Teratology* **55**, 249–292.

Working, P.K. and Hurtt, M.E. (1987) *J. Androl.* **8**, 330–337.

CHAPTER 12

Developmental Neurotoxicity

Wolfgang Kaufmann
BASF AG, Ludwigshafen,
Germany

Introduction

In recent years, the public and the scientific community have become increasingly alarmed about the rise in the numbers of unexplained mental disorders in human infants. Research, especially in the last two decades, has suggested that some disorders with no genetic background can be attributed to exposure to xenobiotics during the early development of the nervous system (Slikker, 1994). *In utero* and postnatal exposure to toxic agents, such as ethanol, lead or methylmercury, is known to be responsible for brain-related disorders in children. In addition, many drugs, chemical agents and pesticides have been shown to have the potential to cause developmental neurotoxicity in humans (Goldey *et al.*, 1995). Many of these experiments were conducted using the rat.

The development of the nervous system is a complex process and there are important differences between the vulnerability and reactivity of the immature brain and that of the mature brain. This chapter describes the different stages of brain development and their specific susceptibilities to toxic insults, especially focused on rats. Then, a recommended test strategy is proposed.

The Value of Experimental Animal Data

Rats and mice are the most commonly used animals in behavioral teratology (Meyer, 1998). According to Meyer (1998) the distinct advantages in using rats (or mice) are: '(1) the small size and relatively low purchase and maintenance costs; (2) ease of handling, treatment, and testing; (3) simplicity of breeding in the laboratory setting; (4) short gestation periods; (5) relatively large litter sizes, thereby providing many offspring for study; and (6) extensive background information concerning normal behavioral and neural development.' These advantages have led to the rat becoming one of the favored test animals in experimental studies designed to screen for toxin-induced injuries during brain development, covering the fetal, perinatal, postnatal and preadolescent periods. Regulatory agencies, such as the US Environmental Protection Agency (EPA) and the Organization for Economic Cooperation and Development (OECD) require the use of Wistar or Sprague-Dawley rats (not Fischer 344, as developmental timings are different) as test animals for developmental neurotoxicity (DNT) studies. Exceptions are possible (and have to be considered carefully) but ample justification has to be provided for a different selection. As the results of such studies aim to achieve a prognostic risk assessment for humans, it is important to consider the comparability of the data gained experimentally from using laboratory animals. In principle, the basic brain development is quite similar in all mammal species. Although the relative sizes of the main brain compartments (telencephalon, diencephalon, mesencephalon, metencephalon and myelencephalon) differ considerably between the different species, the development of the nervous system and the cytoarchitecture are closely related (Schlote, 1983). The gain in brain weight is a reliable criterion for this purpose.

Himwich (1973) showed in his investigations that, in general, the different developmental periods follow the same schedule. The developmental periods of the human brain may be directly related to the developmental periods of other mammal species when the periods of the 'brain growth spurt' are synchronized. This important event in brain development is quite differently positioned in relation to the time of birth. In humans, guinea pigs and dogs, the 'brain growth spurt' is almost completed before birth. In rats, it begins after birth and lasts up to the third postnatal week. These differences between rats and humans should be kept in mind, as they have important implications when planning a DNT study with rats and carrying out risk assessment for human infants. The concordance between the behavioral and structural changes in humans and rats exposed to the same developmental neurotoxicants is, in many cases, impressively high (Schardein, 1998); rat pups of alcohol-treated dams were more emotional and had significantly lower learning abilities, abolition of reflexes, microcephaly and other effects on suckling behavior (cited after Schardein, 1998). Even subtle hypoplasia of the optic nerve has been observed in Wistar rat fetuses as well as in children (Stromland and Pinazo-Duran, 1994). Animal and human data on the developmental neurotoxicity effects of alcohol correlate quite well, even with regard to subtle changes, and this correlation is also shown for other well-known developmental neurotoxicants (Stanton and Spear, 1990). This does not mean that animal rat models will always mimic the neurobehavioral effects seen in humans, and even when a model shows a comparable neuropathology it is unlikely to adequately parallel the neurobehavioral changes in humans, as shown for lead encephalopathies in rats and children (Davies et al., 1990). In addition, rats are not suitable experimental animals for testing toxicant effects on higher cognitive functions (Meyer, 1998).

In conclusion, despite the differences in species sensitivity and interindividual variability, animal data from experimental developmental neurotoxicity studies make good predictors for the risk of developmental neurotoxicity in humans, when developmental neurobehavioural and neuropathology endpoints are considered carefully (Kimmel, 1998; Schardein, 1998).

Vulnerability – Some Fundamental Differences between the Developing and the Adult Nervous Systems

Impact of the Timing of Exposure on the Neurotoxic Outcome

Adult rats treated with a certain dose of any specific neurotoxin will show a characteristic pattern of behavorial changes and topography of structural lesions throughout their adolescent life-time. Given the same test conditions, there are no principle differences, apart from those caused by the general aging process, and the timing of exposure has no relevance for the nature and extent of the observed adult neurotoxicity.

In contrast, the developing nervous system will respond to the same neurotoxic insult with a different susceptibility depending on the stage of development (Table 12.1). Timing of exposure is critical for the nature and extent of neurotoxic effects in the developing nervous system. Bayer et al. (1993) reported a series of experiments using X-irradiation in which a different neuropathology occurred, depending on exposure during certain 'critical periods'. Critical periods are the periods of neurogenesis, neuronal migration and settling, and neuronal differentiation. It is well known, and the thalidomide embryopathy (Smithells and Newman, 1992) is a prominent example, that there are vulnerable periods during prenatal development in which severe malformations can be induced (limb reduction effects after thalidomide treatment). Facial nerve paralysis, autistic disorders and developmental delays in children may be the result of the interference by thalidomide with the development of the nervous system. The susceptibility for thalidomide in humans is limited to gestational days 20–36 after conception during the period of organogenesis (embryonic stage). Developmental neurotoxicants may be toxic only during such a 'time window'. Alternatively, they may be toxic during most or all of the developmental stages of the nervous system but the nature of the lesion changes, depending on which developmental stage is affected.

The antimitotic agent methylazoxymethanol (MAM) can cause a severe microencephaly in 7- or 10-week-old rats when administered at gestational day 15. The forebrain weight is reported to be decreased by 53%, compared with the controls (Johnston and Coyle, 1979). However, a single dose administered at gestational day 17 did not cause any microencephaly (Spatz and Laquer, 1968). MAM administered to newborn mice and hamsters within 24 hours after birth produced extensive necrosis of the external granular layer of the cerebellum and caused defective maturation and ataxia and gait disturbances in surviving adult animals of that treatment group (Hirono et al., 1969). Postnatal treatment of rats with MAM produces morphological features of a congenital cerebellar

hypoplasia (Politis et al., 1980). The timing of exposure, and not the toxic potential of an agent alone, determines the neurotoxic outcome in the developing nervous system.

Some of the well-known, potent, adult neurotoxicants, e.g. hexane or acrylamide, are not selective developmental neurotoxicants and their characteristic neurotoxic changes in adult animals (distal axonopathy) were not found in the offspring of dams treated during organogensis and early postnatal life (Howd et al., 1983; Wise et al., 1995). Ethanol, in contrast, is both an adult (causing the Wernicke–Korsakoff syndrome) and a severe developmental neurotoxicant (causing the fetal alcohol syndrome), but the neurotoxic outcome is quantitatively and qualitatively different depending on the time of exposure during pregnancy or adulthood (Horvath et al., 1997; Harper and Butterworth, 1997; Nulman et al., 1998).

Significance of the Immature versus Mature Blood–Brain Barrier (BBB) on the Neurotoxic Outcome

Morphology and function of the BBB in the mature brain

The blood–brain barrier (BBB) is a specific structure of the central nervous system not found in other organs or tissues. For a long time it was believed that astrocytic endfeet were the morphological substrate of the BBB. Nowadays, at least in vertebrates, it is known that the BBB is represented by specialized endothelial cells which do not show the normal fenestrated pattern of capillaries in peripheral tissues but are continuously linked by tight junctions ('zonulae occludentes'). Those cerebral endothelial cells are further characterized by high levels of the BBB-specific enzyme γ-glutamyl transpeptidase (γ-GT).

The BBB has a protective effect for the brain as it actively isolates the brain from the blood. A pivotal function is that of the regulation of the selective transport and metabolism of substances from the blood or the brain (Aschner, 1998). Lipophilic molecules can pass freely across the BBB into the CNS, but hydrophilic solutes and macromolecules can only pass using specific carrier mechanisms, localized at the luminal or abluminal membrane of the BBB

Table 12.1 Critical (vulnerable) periods of the rat nervous system development

Stage		
1	Predifferentiation stage:	
	(1) 'All or nothing' period	GD 0 to GD 5
	(2) Neural plate formation completed	GD 0 to GD 5
2	Embryonic stage:	
	(1) Period of organogenesis	GD 5 to GD 6
	(2) Neural tube formation	GD 6 to GD 15
	(3) Three-vesicle stage	GD 6 to GD 15
	(4) Begin of neuro- and gliogenesis	GD 11
	(5) Begin of migration and settling	GD 11
	(6) Vascularization/BBB development initialized	GD 11
	(7) Neurotransmitter system development initialized	GD 11 to GD 15
	(8) Begin cholinergic synaptogenesis	GD 11?
	(9) Begin noradrenergic synaptogenesis	GD 14
	(10) Begin dopaminergic synaptogenesis	GD 14
	(11) Begin serotinergic synaptogenesis	GD 15
3	Fetal stage:	
	(1) Five-vesicle stage	GD 15 to GD 20
	(2) Controlled neuro- and gliogenesis	GD 15 to GD 20
	(3) Controlled migration and settling	GD 15 to GD 20
	(4) Enhancement of differentiation processes	GD 15 to GD 20
	(5) Accelerated vascularization and BBB development	GD 15 to GD 20
	(6) Steady increase of neurotransmitter system differentiation processes	GD 15 to GD 20
	(7) Sexual brain differentiation initialized	GD 18
4	Birth	GD 21
5	Postnatal stage (preweaning period):	
	(1) 'Brain growth spurt'	PD 0 to PD 21
	(2) Myelination gliosis (oligodendroglia cell proliferation)	PD 0 to PD 21
	(3) Rapid rate of myelination	PD 16 to PD 30
	(4) Controlled neuro- and gliogenesis from both primary and secondary germinal matrix	PD 0 to PD 21
	(5) Controlled migration and settling	PD 0 to PD 21
	(6) High rate of vascularization and BBB development	PD 0 to PD 21
	(7) High rate of differentiation processes	PD 0 to PD 21
	(8) Sexual brain differentiation completed	PD 10
	(9) Steady increase of neurotransmitter system differentiation processes	PD 0 to PD 21
	(10) Maturation of noradrenergic neurotransmitter system	PD 14
	(11) Maturation of serotinergic neurotransmitter system	PD 21
6	Weaning	PD 21
7	Preadolescent stage:	
	(1) BBB maturation completed	PD 22 to PD 60
	(2) Rapid rate of myelination terminated	PD 24
	(3) Maturation of cholinergic neurotransmitter system	PD 30
	(4) Maturation of dopaminergic neurotransmitter system	PD 30 to PD 60
		PD 35

GD = gestational day, PD = postnatal day.

Data adapted from the literature reviewed and cited in this chapter. For references see text and reference list.

(Romero *et al.*, 1996). Toxic proteins for which no active transport mechanism exists are excluded from the brain (e.g. diphtheria, tetanus and staphylococcus toxins) (Jacobs, 1980).

However, there are also CNS regions which lack a true BBB, e.g. circumventricular organs or the choroid plexus (Gross, 1992; Jacobs, 1994), and these regions have to be considered as potential sites for the accumulation of neurotoxins (Aschner, 1998).

trigeminal and spinal sensory ganglia, a part of the nervous system which is not protected by the BBB (Reuhl, 1988).

The second effect of developmental neurotoxicants (e.g. peptides and opiates) is to interfere directly with the maturation of the brain microvasculature, i.e. the development of a fully functional BBB in neonates. This may lead to a long-lasting dysfunction of the BBB, affecting later transport of peptides and opiates into the brain (Aschner, 1998).

Impact of developmental neurotoxicants on the morphological/functional development of the BBB

Endothelial cells in the developing brain grow in a close relationship to the developing CNS cells, forming capillaries which become progressively ensheathed by resident astrocytes. The BBB features of the nonfenestrated cerebral capillaries are believed to be primarily induced by trophic factors from astrocytes. A survey of data by Aschner (1998) both gives evidence and casts doubt on the inductive effects of astrocytes in BBB formation and maintenance. According to Schulze and Firth (1992), the BBB in rats is fully developed at postnatal day 24. The maturation of the BBB develops progressively from the onset of intraneural vascularization, but morphological characteristics are not fully developed until the neonatal period (Aschner, 1998).

Developmental neurotoxicants may affect the brain capillaries in two ways. First, they may be directly toxic to cerebral endothelial cells, altering the growing pattern and leading to severe edema and hemorrhage. This is the effect described for acute infantile lead encephalopathy. Acute lead encephalopathies are not a feature of lead poisoning in adults (Verity, 1997). Heavy metals in general and lead and mercury in particular are the most critical developmental and adult neurotoxicants with a different outcome of structural and functional neurotoxicity during the different stages of nervous system development and the adolescent stage. The protective function of the BBB can be seen in the effects of cadmium poisoning. In neonates, cadmium poisoning causes a characteristic broad distribution of hemorrhages in the brain, whereas in adults a highly localized hemorrhage is observed only in the

Receptor Acting Agents May Cause Permanent Changes During Brain Maturation

Similar to the induction of a lasting dysfunctional BBB, a variety of receptor-acting xenobiotics may interfere with the differentiation process of the brain during neonatal development, causing a permanent, irreversible insult instead of only a transient, reversible 'pharmacological' effect. A critical period outlined for this developmental stage is the period of the 'brain growth spurt'.

Insecticides (DDT, pyrethroids) have been shown to alter the normal development of the cholinergic neurotransmitter system, causing a permanent dysfunction (Eriksson *et al.*, 1992). Some drugs (anxiolytics, antidepressants) show effects which are essentially transient in nature but may permanently affect the growing brain. Treatment may cause an irreversible 'imprinting' of receptor densities with a lasting functional and structural change in the nervous system, e.g. a lifelong, higher sensitivity to the substances which were responsible for the developmental imprinting may be caused (IEH, 1996).

The special plasticity of the growing brain is better demonstrated when the sexual differentiation of the nervous system is considered. According to the theory of developmental host specificity, certain target tissues in the brain develop a sensitivity to the hormone appropriate to one sex or the other. This occurs during a critical perinatal period during which the brain is maximally sensitive to gonadal hormones. In rats, the critical period of sexual differentiation starts around gestational day 18 and lasts up to postnatal day 10 (Kelly, 1985; Goy and McEwen, 1980). At this stage a 'blueprint' of appropriate sexual behavior in response to hormonal stimulation is created. How does the gender identity develop? In principle, the developing nervous system of either gender is bipotential. The fetuses of both sexes are exposed to high levels of circulating estrogens in the maternal blood. Without an additional hormonal influence, a female pattern of anatomical and behavioral organization takes place, independently of the genetic status. In genotypic males, androgens are needed to express the right phenotype. Androgens are produced by the immature gonads in the developing male rat between gestational day 13 and postnatal day 10. The specialized testicular Leydig cells of male rat fetuses are normally differentiated between gestational days 16 and 18. Rats castrated after parturition ('deandrogenized' rats) in this critical period develop the behavioral characteristics of genotypic females. Androgens given during pregnancy will cause hermaphroditism in genotypic females and a blend of male and female behavior. Normally, an androgenized brain exhibits a tonic secretory pattern of luteinizing (LH) and follicle-stimulating (FSH) hormone from the anterior pituitary gland, whereas the pattern of the female brain is cyclic. The cyclical secretion of the 'gonadotropins' LH and FSH is only established in the absence of androgens during the perinatal period of sexual differentiation. Female neonatal rats exposed to a single dose of androgens on postnatal day 4 do not develop the ability to go through cyclical secretions, are unable to ovulate as adults and are infertile.

But sexual differentiation may not only be influenced by the presence or absence of androgens. Interestingly, the female hormone estrogen plays a central role in the process of masculinization, since on a cellular level testosterone is converted to estradiol by target nerve cell enzymes. It has been shown experimentally that estradiol has an 8 times higher efficacy than the same levels of testosterone (Kelly, 1985). What endogenously produced steroid hormones are able to do, a variety of steroids and endocrine active environmental agents normally not present in the body are also able to do: i.e. modulate/alter the normal sexual differentiation of the individual, when exposed during the critical maturational period. Among these, pesticides (e.g. DDT), testosterone, diethylstilbestrol and drugs (e.g. barbiturates) are compounds which have been shown experimentally to be capable of inducing brain masculinization (Kelly, 1985).

Other Factors Affecting the Developing Brain

During the brain growth spurt, when oligodendroglial cell proliferation accelerates and differentiation processes such as dendritic development and arborization take place, a corresponding capillary sprouting is observed. It is thought that the amount of vascularization represents the metabolic needs in direct correlation with the rapidly growing brain regions (Jacobson, 1978). Malnutrition at this developmental stage is seen to be especially critical. Indeed, undernourishment of rats during the interval from birth to postnatal day 14 (when the brain growth spurt in rats takes place) is the period identified for the establishment of permanent myelin deficits after rehabilitation. Earlier undernourishment or malnutrition after weaning has no lasting adverse effects.

Epidemiological studies in humans show that nutritionally rehabilitated children continue to suffer from various behavioral disorders, such as a lag in learning, speech, problem solving, eye–hand coordination, and social–personal behavior. Postnatally undernourished infants are neurologically abnormal (Wiggins, 1982).

Besides the steroids, thyroid hormones play a profound role in the regular growth of the developing brain (Stein et al., 1991). This is dramatically demonstrated in the outcome of the severe thyroid anomaly cretinism, which results in mental retardation and deafness.

The higher sensitivity of young rats compared with adults to the toxicity of many organophosphorous, acetylcholinesterase inhibiting pesticides is most probably due to the immaturity of detoxifying enzyme systems. For example, the same dose of chlorpyrifos will cause fatalities in rat pups but almost no behavioral disorders in adult rats. Chlorpyrifos is detoxified by binding to carboxylesterases and hydrolysis by A-esterases in adult rats. Both enzymes are deficient in the rat fetus or the neonate, which may explain the higher sensitivity at much lower doses than in adults (Padilla et al., 1998).

Developmental Stages and Critical (Vulnerable) Periods in the Development of the Nervous System – an Anatomical Approach

In order to plan and assess a rat study screening for possible developmental neurotoxic effects and to understand the special vulnerability of the developing nervous system it is necessary to have a basic knowledge of the natural development of the central nervous system. This section gives an overview, with special consideration of the neurotoxic outcome at the stages described.

Predifferentiation Stage

The predifferentiation stage is characterized by germ cells with no distinct morphological differentiation (Suzuki, 1980). For rats, this stage (the 'all-or-nothing' period) covers the time from conception to postconceptional day 5. Damage during this period normally has only two consequences: (1) all the cells are killed and no embryo is formed (severe damage) or (2) there are enough surviving cells to compensate for the insult and a normal embryo is formed (minimal damage).

Embryonic Stage

The embryonic stage is characterized by the mobilization and organization of cell and tissue groups to form individual organ systems (Suzuki, 1980). The periods of organogenesis are different from one mammalian species to another. In rats, organogenesis proceeds from gestational day (GD) 6 to 15, in humans from GD 20 to 55, in monkeys from GD 20 to 45, and in mice from GD 7 to 16 (Schardein, 1998; Slikker, 1994).

Development of the neural tube

Nerve and glial cells of the nervous system derive from a specialized region of the ectoderm called the neural plate (Martin, 1985). The neural plate indents and forms the neural groove from which the lateral lips close to create the neural tube. In rats, the neural tube is formed around gestational day 11.

Damage during that early period results in either anencephaly (closure of the neural tube fails at rostral levels) or spina bifida (the caudal portion of the neural tube fails to close). The neural tube itself has a central fluid-filled lumen which gives rise to the ventricular system of the central nervous system.

Start of neurogenesis

The epithelial cells lining the neural tube are called the neuroepithelium. The neuroepithelium is the source of all neurons and glial cells of the central nervous system. The nerve cells of the peripheral nervous system (dorsal root ganglion cells, postganglionic neurons of the autonomic nervous system) originate from the neural crest, a population of cells whose cell bodies lie outside the neural tube.

There is growing evidence that the neuroepithelium contains a 'Bauplan' (blueprint) of the whole central nervous system (Bayer and Altman, 1995).

The precursors of nerve cells, the neuroblasts, divide repeatedly but do not proliferate uniformly along the length of the neural tube: the neuroepithelium appears to be a 'spatiotemporal mosaic' where neuroblasts seem to be committed to generate specific neuron populations according to strict timetables.

In a strictly time-dependent sequence, programmed cell proliferation occurs at specific sites in the neuroepithelium which gives rise to the occurrence of the three primary brain vesicles, the rostral prosencephalon (primitive forebrain), the mesencephalon (primitive midbrain) and the caudal rhombencephalon (primitive hindbrain). This is known as the three-vesicle stage (Figure 12.1). More programmed cell proliferation leads to an enormous expansion of the primary brain vesicles with a further subdivision.

Fetal Stage

This stage is characterized by a significant increase in brain size and also by enhanced cellular proliferation and differentiation.

The prosencephalon divides into (from rostrally to caudally) the telencephalon with the cerebral

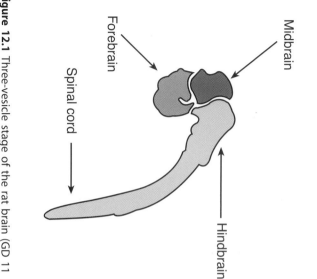

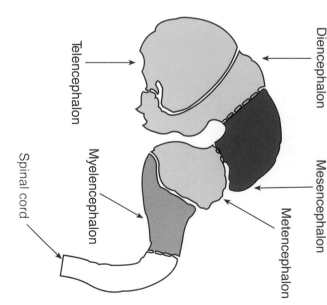

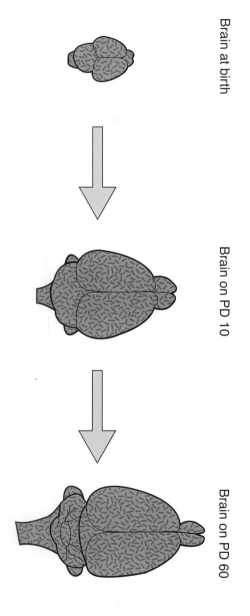

Three-vesicle stage

Forebrain

Midbrain

Hindbrain

Spinal cord

Figure 12.1 Three-vesicle stage of the rat brain (GD 11 to GD 15).

Early five-vesicle stage

Diencephalon

Mesencephalon

Telencephalon

Metencephalon

Myelencephalon

Spinal cord

Figure 12.2 Five-vesicle stage of the rat brain (GD 15 to GD 20).

cortex and basal ganglia and the diencephalon with the thalamus and hypothalamus. The mesencephalon remains undivided, with the tectum and the tegmentum. The rhombencephalon divides into the metencephalon with the cerebellum and pons and myelencephalon with the medulla oblongata. This is known as the five-vesicle stage (Figure 12.2).

In the caudal part of the neural tube programmed cell proliferation forms the spinal cord which contains the sensory and motor neurons and many interneurons (second-order neurons).

Peri- and Postnatal Stage

The postnatal stage is characterized by an extensive growth of the brain (brain growth spurt). In rats, neuronal cell populations are produced up to postnatal day 21 (at weaning); in the rat cerebrum, around half of all the cell population is produced in the postnatal period (Krinke and Eisenbrandt, 1994). Figure 12.3 shows the postnatal size development of the rat brain between birth and PD 60.

Brain at birth

Brain on PD 10

Brain on PD 60

Figure 12.3 Postnatal size development of the rat brain to PD 60.

Although CNS cellular proliferation and differentiation continues after birth in many species (important examples are the cerebellum, olfactory bulb and hippocampus), other processes gain increasing significance. These may be referred to as the 'maturation of neuronal circuitry' (Bayer and Altman, 1995). Postnatal processes that have to be considered when assessing potential developmental neurotoxins are:

- Axonogenesis
- Dendritic arborization
- Synaptogenesis
- Rapid development of all major neurotransmitter systems
- Developmental ('apoptotic') cell death
- Trimming (selective elimination of unimportant synapses, while preserving the most advantageous ones)
- Myelination (initiated by a marked proliferation of oligodendroglial cells = 'myelination gliosis').

The number of different processes during the remarkable growth of the postnatal brain may also demonstrate the importance of that period for the overall assessment of developmental neurotoxicity.

Neurobehavioral and neuropathological examinations for developmental neurotoxicity studies designed to meet the requirements of regulatory agency guidelines (e.g. EPA, OECD) are carried out within or at the end of this period of nervous system development.

Developmental Stages and Critical (Vulnerable) Periods of the Development of the Nervous System – a Cellular Approach

During the stages of CNS development (embryonic, fetal, peri- and postnatal stages) described above, the developing brain cells may be altered differently depending on their cellular stage of development. Three stages can be defined:

(1) Neurogenesis and gliogenesis
(2) Migration and settling (neuronal migration to predetermined locations)
(3) Differentiation (synchronized neuronal aggregation to certain structures with predefined oriented axons and dendrites).

Damage occurring during these three periods of brain development may show a variety of consequences.

Neurogenesis and Gliogenesis

The neuron does not stand alone; the glia–neuronal association represents the functional unit of the nervous system. This means that a neuron-centric definition of the nervous system is inadequate. The complexity of these interactions provides numerous possibilities for interference with neurotoxic chemicals (LoPachin and Aschner, 1993). For that reason development and interference with development are viewed separately for the two cell populations, i.e. the neurons and the glial cells.

Impact during neuronal cell proliferation ('neurogenesis')

There is one important principle to be recognized: the loss of precursor neurons will be not compensated! The surviving precursor neurons produce only the programmed number of neurons during a programmed time window (Bayer and Altman, 1995; Bayer et al., 1993). Should a massive injury causing an entire loss of a certain neuronal population, this would have further consequences for cell migration, settlement and differentiation of neuronal populations which have already been produced or will be produced after the injury. Antimitotic agents (e.g. methylazoxymethanol or methylmercury) are known to kill a large number of precursor neurons in the germinal matrix. The consequence of the cell loss is a hypoplasia of neuronal cell populations.

The qualitative, morphological diagnosis of the presence of a 'hypoplasia' in the developing brain may be difficult. A loss of neurons reduces the overall volume of the neuronal population but does not change the density of the structure (which would be the case in the adult brain); this means that reduced cell numbers are primarily observed as changes in the size of structures (Rodier, 1990; Rodier and Gramann, 1979). This is in concordance with the observation in human infants with mental retardation, where the brain may be small but with no abnormal cytoarchitecture patterns (Suzuki, 1980). ENU (ethylnitrosourea)-injection in rats at gestation day 14 or 15 causes a thin cerebral cortex and a reduction of cortical neurons to about 41% of the controls. Despite the thinness of the cortex, the six cortical neuronal layers were well retained (Halls and Das, 1978).

Size reduction without an obvious, histomorphological recognizable change in the normal cytoarchitecture led Rodier and Gramann (1979) to suggest the use of 'simple morphometry' as a valuable tool for evaluating cell loss in the developing brain. Gliosis, the classical neuromorphological marker for injury-induced neuronal eliminations in the adult CNS, is not a regular feature in injury (neurotoxin)-induced cell death during the developmental stage of neurogenesis/cell proliferation.

The anticonvulsant valproic acid, a developmental neurotoxin which causes mental retardation in humans, also interferes with neuronal cell production. It is a good example for such agents with an extremely time-dependent effect. Exposure in rats on gestation day 12 will cause a loss of motor neurons in the nucleus abducens. Exposure on gestation day 13 will cause a diminution of the oculomotor nucleus. The nucleus abducens stays unaffected, because all the cells were produced before day 13 (IEH, 1996).

Another example is provided by the neuroteratogen methylazoxymethanol (MAM). When delivered on day 14 of rat gestation – that is when growth hormone-releasing neurons (located in the arcuate nucleus) are formed – a retarded postnatal growth rate of the treated offspring was noted (Fischer et al., 1971). When the treatment day was changed from 14 to 16, i.e. when the somatotropin release-inhibiting factor neurons located in the anterior periventricular region are formed (a factor which inhibits growth hormone release), the MAM-exposed neonates were not smaller, but significantly larger than controls (Johnston and Coyle, 1979). In cases of postnatal administration of MAM in newborn mice, rats and hamsters, a hypoplastic cerebellum (Hirono et al., 1969) is induced (through extensive degenerative changes in the external germinal/granular layer).

The two examples given above show that each population of neurons in the CNS is generated according to a precise time schedule. Bayer and Altman (1995) postulated that chronology of neuron production is a prerequisite for the proper anatomical and functional development of the CNS.

It is important to bear in mind that cell production in the developing CNS occurs at specific times in specific regions, and when testing for developmental neurotoxic effects it is a precondition that the adequate tissue is examined for the exposure time selected.

Impact during developmental glia cell production ('gliogenesis')

Astrocytic cells belong to a dynamic class of brain cells with important and diverse functions. They are estimated to include as much as 20–25% or even 50% of the total volume in some brain areas and are far beyond the classical reduction to playing only a supportive role for forming and maintaining the structure of the CNS tissue. According to the concept of astrocytic heterogeneity, astrocytes from different brain regions may show different biochemical properties and may respond in different ways to injuries. In principle, the major diverse functions of mature astrocytes may be summarized in two categories: (1) the maintenance of the neural microenvironment (regulation of pH, ion concentration and osmolarity) and (2) immunocompetence (antigen presentation), phagocytosis and repair function (Montgomery, 1994). Guidance and support of neuronal migration during brain development (Rakic, 1971) belong to another category of function as this process is carried out by immature astrocytes being in a transient stage of differentiation for a defined time period. These 'immature' astrocytes are known as 'radial glia cells'.

Early in development, glia cells and neurons establish a highly dynamic reciprocal relationship which influences subsequent nervous tissue growth, morphology and behavior (LoPachin and Aschner, 1993). There are 'primary' and 'secondary' radial glia cell populations. Primary radial glia differentiate from the neuroectoderm, secondary radial glia from the secondary germinal matrix (e.g. external granular layer in the cerebellar cortex). At the end of neuronal migration the astrocytes differentiate and lose their radial structure, except in three regions. The radial scaffold persists in the mature brain in the cerebellar cortex as Bergmann glia, as Müller cells in the retina, and as tanycytes in the hypothalamus (Berry and Butt, 1997).

Interference of several neuroteratogens (X-irradiation, cytotoxic drugs, ethanol) with the developing brain induces ectopias (heterotopias). One of the presumed mechanisms not discussed in detail before is that via the effect on radial glia cells. Zhang *et al.* (1995) identified several abnormalities of radial glia which are interpreted to be the cause of periventricular neuronal heterotopias observed after exposure to methylazoxymethanol (MAM).

Morphological techniques used to reveal radial glia are Golgi staining, immunostaining and electron microscopy (Zhang *et al.*, 1995). The most useful technique for demonstrating structural abnormalities of early radial glia cells (up to GD 19) was the oldest of these three, Golgi staining, which allows viewing of the radial glia in their entirety, with sufficient resolution to determine accurately structural changes at high optical magnification. Immunohistochemistry is not sufficiently specific for early radial glia detection and electron microscopy is much too focused on parts of the radial glia cell only. However, in principle, immature astrocytes ('primary radial glia') have been shown to contain vimentin and glial fibrillary acidic protein (Levitt and Rakic, 1980; Bignami *et al.*, 1982). Differentiating astrocytes lose their vimentin reactivity and express GFAP more extensively (Montgomery, 1994; Berry and Butt, 1997).

There are many other effects on glia cells in developmental neurotoxicity processes. For example, neonatal exposure to organic tin leads to a decrease in the glial fibrillary acidic protein (GFAP) in Long-Evans rat pups (O'Callaghan and Miller, 1988). In the fetal human brain, a diffuse white matter gemistocytic astrocytosis (prominent in the cerebrum and cerebellum) was described after methylmercury poisoning *in utero*. The gemistocytic astrocytes contained mercury grains in their cytoplasm (Choi *et al.*, 1978). Astrogliosis is recognized as 'reactive' gliosis during neurodegenerative events in mature brains of adults. GFAP is an excellent indirect marker for evaluating a neurodegenerative change in the brain. Astrogliosis and gemistocytic astrocytes are morphological substrates for the repair function of the astroglia cell population and an indirect marker for neuronal damage. This ability seems to be limited to mature astrocytes. Radial glia cells ('immature' astrocytes) may be induced by developmental neurotoxicants to differentiate into mature astrocytes too early, with loss of their characteristic radial scaffold. Gressens *et al.* (1992) report an ethanol-induced disturbance of gliogenesis which

leads to a premature transformation of the radial glia into mature astrocytes during neuronal migration resulting in almost complete absence of a normal, vertical, neuronal columnization in the cortex cerebri. The increased number (hyperplasia, astrocytosis) or (hypertrophy, astrogliosis) of mature astroglial cells is nowadays quite easily recognized by applying antibodies against GFAP. Nevertheless, negative or weak results from GFAP immunohistochemistry/GFAP assays on the developing, immature brain should be considered critically. They do not exclude developmental neurotoxicity.

Migration and Settling of Neurons

Once a presumptive neuron turns off cell division in its germinal matrix (as a rule the neuroepithelium) it migrates to its predetermined location in the brain parenchyma and settles. Most neurons are postmitotically fixed from the beginning of migration. Not all neurons lose their ability to divide. In the cerebellum, neuroblasts of the neuroepithelium migrate to form a second germinal layer, the external granular layer which produces billions of granular cells and interneurons of the cerebellar cortex. The cerebellar cortex is a good site to demonstrate one important pattern of neuronal migration: neuronal migration is characterized by an astrocyte-guided translocation of nerve cells from their primary or secondary germinal layers to their adult locations (Rakic, 1971). In the cerebellar cortex, migration of granular cells occurs along radial glia fibers which develop from GFAP-positive cells in the external granular layer (Sievers *et al.*, 1994). The physical contact between glia cells and migrating neurons is mediated by adhesion molecules. These cell-cell contacts have been considered recently as a putative site of neurotoxicant action (LoPachin and Aschner, 1993; Reuhl *et al.*, 1994).

However, Bayer and Altman (1995) found increasing evidence that migrating neurons also follow complex trajectories unrelated to the presence of a radial glia fiber network.

Impact on migration and settling of neurons

Damage to the process of migration and settling may lead to aberrant neuronal migration and settlement in wrong locations. Neuronal cell clusters in wrong locations are called 'ectopia' (syn: heterotopia).

Up to now it was not known what kind of interference by a toxic agent might give rise to misplaced neurons. Is it the actual process of migration, including the effect on radial glia cells as described above? Do the toxicants disturb the territory which has to be passed by the migrating neurons? Or do they injure the amoeboid moving abilities of the neuronal cell in migration?

Although the mechanisms are still unclear, ectopias were described as malformations in the brain a long time ago. Methylmercury and X-irradiation exposure have been shown to interfere with migrating neurons. Ectopic cells are described in reports of prenatal methylmercury poisoning in Japan (fetal minamata disease) and Iraq (Matsumoto et al., 1975; Choi et al., 1978). Clusters of misplaced neurons (supposed Purkinje cells) were found in the white matter of the cerebellum. X-irradiation on gestation day 13 or 14 produced subcortical ectopias in rats (Hicks et al., 1959).

Bayer et al. (1993) assumed that the granular cell ectopias in the cerebellar cortex after X-irradiation were caused by the effect of X-irradiation during migration, killing many precursor cells in the external granular layer. This would result in a break in the normal steady stream of new granular cells settling in their proper locations ('outside-in organization'). Consequently, many mossy fibers (axons that normally contact granule cell dendrites in the granule layer) do not find their normal complement of granule cell targets and grow upwards into the molecular layer. There, they arrest the downward migration of the granule cells produced by the surviving precursors. However, this seems to be only one possible mechanism for the development of ectopias.

Major ectopias seem to require high doses of neuroteratogens and indicate a massive disturbance of development. They often occur in conjunction with cell loss. Once ectopia has been produced by abnormal migration, it becomes a permanent anatomical feature of the brain (Bayer et al., 1993). Small ectopias are less reliable as a morphological marker for early injury during brain development as there are also reports of a 'spontaneous' occurrence or a disappearance of ectopic cells over time in the brain (Schmechel and Rakic, 1979). However, in working out a possible neurodevelopmental toxic effect, the small ectopias detected should be assessed quantitatively as they are also observed in normal tissue.

The schizophrenia phenomenon

A neurodevelopmental toxic impact on migration and settling is nowadays believed to induce the human pathological phenomenon of schizophrenia. Throughout most of this century schizophrenia was seen as the result of a psychopathological process which occurs in young adult life a short time before the diagnosis is made. For around two decades, the neurodevelopmental hypothesis has been increasingly favored, in which schizophrenia is seen as a neurodevelopmental encephalopathy (Weinberger, 1995a). This conclusion is based on the observation that nonprogressive morphological deviations have been found in neuroimaging studies using computed tomography (CT) and magnetic resonance imaging (MRI). Compared with controls, and taking into account the physiological variability of ventricular size, schizophrenic patients often exhibit a ventricular enlargement. This implies that the brain tissue volume is reduced in schizophrenia. MRI studies confirmed this assumption. The most consistent finding was a 5–10% reduction of the overall brain and cortical gray matter volume (Andreasen et al., 1994).

Surprisingly for many researchers, in most cross-sectional studies of ventricular and brain volume assessment, correlations with duration of the illness were not found. These results indicated that a progressive, neurodegenerative model does not fit the anatomical data in most cases of schizophrenia (Jaskiw et al., 1994).

Necropsy studies, using appropriate controls, reliable diagnostic methods and objective morphometric techniques, confirmed ventricular enlargement. Light microscopy of cortical areas showed volumetric changes and slight reductions in neuronal cell counts and density. Reduced neuronal density, however, was not as consistent as was reduced cortical thickness. The most consistent histomorphological observation has been the absence of 'gliosis.' Most adult-onset brain injuries and neurodegenerative disorders are characteristically accompanied by astrogliosis. Gliosis is not found in many neuropathological events occurring early in development.

The most important evidence for the neurodevelopmental hypothesis of schizophrenia came from histomorphological studies of the cortical cytoarchitecture. Examination of Nissl-stained sections of the entorhinal cortex showed attenuated cellularity in superficial layers I and II, incomplete clustering of neurons into glomerular structures in layer II, and the presence of such neuronal clusters in deeper layers ('ectopic cells') where they are not normally found (Arnold *et al.*, 1991). In the prefrontal and cingulate cortices, small neurons were analogously reduced in number, while larger neurons in deeper layers were overabundant (Benes *et al.*, 1991). All these studies describe a similar defect in the cortical organization: the laminar distribution of cortical neurons is displaced inwards. A defect in the 'inside-out' organization of cortical layers suggests a defect in the normal processes of neuronal migration during this developmental stage (second trimester of human pregnancy). These results provide a central piece to the jigsaw puzzle and correlate well with the findings from neuroimaging and from necropsy data. If cellular relations are maldeveloped through migratory deficits, it is understandable that neuronal connectivity and circuitry are also likely to be anomalous and will lead to behavioral abnormalities (Falkai and Bogerts, 1995; Weinberger, 1995a,b).

Suzuki (1980), this emphasizes the usefulness of the Golgi preparation in the investigation of developmental disorders of the brain. Rodier (1990) agreed that descriptions of changes in dendritic extent and connectivity from Golgi-impregnated tissue can be highly informative, but pointed out that they require sophisticated and very time-consuming quantitative methods, which may be a severe disadvantage for routine studies. The discovery of synapse-associated molecules provided an immunocytochemical alternative for studying a toxic impact on synapses (Kinney *et al.*, 1993; Kinney and Armstrong, 1997).

Several nonmorphologic approaches to the evaluation of synaptogenesis are described by O'Callaghan and Miller (1988).

Impact on the development of neurotransmitter systems ('neurochemical synaptogenesis') in rats

During the neonatal 'brain growth spurt', a rapid development of all of the major neurotransmitter systems is observed. These systems include the major monoaminergic neurotransmitters, such as norepinephrine, dopamine, histamine and serotonin, and the excitatory and inhibitory amino acids, such as glutamate and GABA, respectively, which are particularly implicated in the fast transmission of information in neural networks (e.g. in the cortex) (IEH, 1996).

The process of noradrenergic synaptogenesis is observed as early as GD 14 in rats (locus coeruleus) and reaches adult values in density and distribution at PD 14 (neocortex). Mesencephalic dopaminergic nuclei are shown to give rise to fiber projections at GD 14 (diencephalon), achieve adult topology at PD 12 (neocortex) and adult densities at PD 35. Sprouting of serotin-ergic raphe nuclei axons begins at GD 15 (pons), and adult levels of terminal field densities are noted at PD 21 (cortex, hippocampus, septal regions, brainstem) (Broening and Slikker, 1998).

Another neurotransmitter system that is highly important in developmental neurotoxicity is the cholinergic system. Its major role in neurotransmission is less direct and more a modulatory one, influencing the excitatory and inhibitory actions of other neurotransmitters (Jett, 1998). Cholinergic neurons (interneurons or projection neurons) are found all over the brain in association with other

Maturation of Neuronal Circuits

Damage due to neurodevelopmental toxicants may have a variety of consequences dependent on the maturational process involved. An overview of maturational processes and some known impacts during these developmental periods is given below.

Axonogenesis, dendritic arborization and synaptogenesis in general

The development of interneuronal connections and the connectivity between neuronal aggregations follows a predetermined pattern but is also dependent on and influenced by several intrinsic and environmental factors. Strabismus, for example, must be corrected as early as possible to avoid permanent deficits in vision, because normal stimulation is necessary for the normal development of connections (IEH, 1996).

Defective dendritic development and the abnormal configuration or absence of dendritic spines have been observed after X-irradiation ('dysplasia' according to Bayer *et al.*, 1993), malnutrition (Salas *et al.*, 1974) and an endogenous disorder, hypothyroidism (Earys, 1955). Many of these changes were only recognized using a Golgi impregnation of the tissue which depicts spines and axonal boutons. For neurotransmitter systems. The disperse and diffuse character of distribution differs clearly from the more localized nature of other neurotransmitter systems. The development of the cholinergic system occurs at a relatively late stage in rat neonates (demonstrated immunocytochemically by a gradual increase in the number of muscarinic (MAChR) and nicotinic (NAChR) acetylcholine receptors; Buwalda, 1995). It is not fully mature before postnatal day 30. Acetylcholine and acetylcholinesterase levels show a steady increase from the embryonic through the postnatal period to adulthood (Jett, 1998).

The cholinergic systems are associated with the development of behavioral inhibitory systems, e.g. to reduce high levels of motor output and promote attentional and associative processes (IEH, 1996).

Milestones of behavioral development are partly correlated with the development of neurotransmitter systems (e.g. increasing locomotor activities of pups) or newly produced neuropeptides, e.g. cortico-trophin-releasing factor is known to be active during separation of the rat pup from its mother.

Damage may have various consequences. Drugs of abuse, like methamphetamine, are detected neuro-toxicants for adults and neonates. Methamphetamine administration results in clear disparities between neurotoxic outcomes in adult rats and developing rats. In adult rats there is evidence that methamphetamine injures the monoaminergic terminals. This leads to permanent deficits in dopamine. Astrogliosis and argyrophilia is observed in the corresponding dopaminergic and serotoninergic nuclei, addressing secondary neuronal damage (Pu et al., 1994). In developing rats, neither long-term reductions in dopamine, nor astrogliosis or argyrophilia are found in corresponding nuclei (Pu and Vorhees, 1993). The neurotoxicity outcome is different but not less dramatic with regard to persistance. Neonates exposed to methamphetamine during a specific period from PD 10 to PD 20 develop learning and memory deficits when tested as adults (Vorhees et al., 1994 a,b), which are absent or rarely seen when treated with methamphetamine as adult rats (Broening and Slikker, 1998). Drug challenge methods (pharmacological challenge with known agonists or antagonists) may be extremely useful in developmental neurotoxicity assessment of monoaminergic neurotransmitter systems. They can unmask functional deficits or detect an altered sensitivity of the offspring to the same toxicant which was prenatally given to the dam (Meyer, 1998).

A variety of chemicals investigated have been shown to affect the cholinergic system, e.g. DDT and pyrethroid insecticides. Their basic mechanism of action is interference with the sodium channels of the nerve membrane, leading to prolonged depolarization and induction of repetitive activity, enhancing neurotransmitter release (Narahashi, 1985). The MAChR receptor density in the cerebral cortex was increased through neonatal treatment. Neonatal exposure also led to permanent changes in the adult cholinergic system in mice which had reached four months of age. In the same brain region (the cerebral cortex) where an increase in MAChR receptor density was observed neonatally, a decrease was noted at four months (Eriksson et al., 1992). This could be correlated with behavioral disturbances as there was an absence of or delayed habituation to a novel environment in the adult mice. In contrast to behavioral disturbances observed 24 hours after adult exposure to a type I pyrethroid (bioallethrin), which nearly disappeared after two months, neonatally exposed animals showed permanent deficits. Interestingly, adult behavior was only altered when neonatal exposure was induced during a short period of neonatal development (PD 10–14) (Ahlbom et al., 1995; Eriksson, 1997).

These recent investigations point out the vulnerability of the neonatal brain cholinergic system to the influence of pesticides capable of affecting the nerve membrane sodium channel at doses that apparently have no permanent effect when administered to the adult animal (Eriksson, 1997; Desaiah, 1998). Further neurotoxic impact on the development of the cholinergic system is attributed to acetylcholinesterase-inhibiting agents, e.g. carbamate and organophosphate pesticides, polychlorinated biphenyls (PCBs), nicotine, lead and mercury (Jett, 1998).

The assessment of receptor densities and distribution in the developing nervous system requires biochemical and immunohistochemical techniques. Quantitation may be required.

Developmental cell death (controlled, programmed cell destruction by apoptosis)

The elimination of excess neurons (i.e. all neurons which are not selected to be target neurons during differentiation) is a basic principle of the differentiating nervous system. As the main mechanism for the initiation of developmental apoptotic cell death, a growth factor deprivation was recognized and clearly demonstrated in the dorsal root ganglion of rats. Around gestational day 14–16 almost half of the dorsal root ganglia show apoptotic cell death (Chu Wang and Oppenheim, 1978). Neuronal maintenance or death seem to be dependent on the synthesis and release of nerve growth factors by the peripheral targets and regular synaptic uptake and retrograde axonal transport (Deckwerth and Johnson, 1993). Up to now, no toxic agents have been linked to inhibition of this active cell death, but it seems likely that there is a connection, considering the role of apoptosis and toxic agents in adults.

The significance of this process may be highlighted by the human brain abnormality called autism, in which the limbic system may show an excess of neurons (Baumann and Kemper, 1985). Rodier *et al.* (1996) and Rodier (1998) found clear evidence that autism is an organic disorder which can be induced by some teratogens. Research on autism is handicapped by the lack of appropriate animal models.

Disturbances in the developmental, programmed cell death process can be recognized by histomorphological screening of the brain showing the presence of an abnormally high number of neuronal cells when compared with homologous control sections.

An overview of experimental approaches to the detection of apoptotic cells in the developing, immature brain is given by Shield and Mirkes (1998).

Trimming

Like in the process of programmed developmental cell death, the synapses that are not needed are selectively eliminated during the maturation of the neuronal network. Weak or unimportant synapses are eliminated and the most advantageous ones are preserved (IEH, 1996). It is supposed that some action of lead on the brain of young children occurs by disturbing this mechanism (Goldstein, 1992).

Myelination

The postnatal brain growth spurt is believed to result primarily from two processes: the so-called myelination gliosis (oligodendroglial cell proliferation period) and the rapid rate of myelination. At birth there are no oligodendrocytes, but by postnatal day 5 approximately 10% of all glial cells in the optic nerve of rats are oligodendrocytes. With myelination gliosis the relative number of oligodendrocytes increases dramatically, reaching a level of 50% of all optic glial cells by PD 20 and finally comprising up to 60% in the adult rat (PD 57) (Vaughn and Peters, 1971).

In rats, the proliferation phase of oligodendroglial cells is completed approximately 3 weeks after birth (at weaning, PD 21). Beginning around PD 10, myelination is highly accelerated between PD 16 and PD 30 (period of the rapid rate of myelination), with a maximum at PD 20. After day 30 a low level of myelination appears to be maintained throughout life (Miller, 1992). In the brain, the cerebellum is one of the first and the cerebrum is one of the last regions to begin myelination (Yakovlev and Lacours, 1967; Norton and Poduslo, 1973). In principle, a caudal–rostral progression of myelination is observed.

Copper deficiency (Dipaolo *et al.*, 1974), malnutrition or undernourishment (Krigman and Hogan, 1976; Wiggins, 1982; Diaz-Cintra *et al.*, 1990) and chronic lead intoxication in suckling rats (Krigman *et al.*, 1974) or young children (Pentschew, 1965) are well-known examples of conditions which affect myelination.

Alteration of the process of active myelination results in hypomyelination. One important mechanistic pathway was discussed by Wiggins (1982): after postnatal undernourishment, hypomyelination probably results from the failure of oligodendroglia to mature and to initiate myelin formation, as only a slight reduction in total cell numbers and brain size was observed.

Recently, Duffard *et al.* (1996) described CNS myelin deficits in suckling rats exposed to 2,4-dichlorophenoxyacetic acid (2,4-D), a widely used phenoxyherbicide. Significant myelin deficits were only observed when the exposure time occurred in the period of rapid myelination (PD 16 to PD 30). No significant changes occurred in pups of dams exposed from PD 9 to PD 15 only. No information was given as to whether the effect on myelination was a transient or permanent change. However, undernourishment during the interval from PD 0 to PD 14 caused a lasting deficit in the myelin concentrations of the cerebral cortex, cerebellum and other brain areas. Undernourishment confined to the actual period of rapid myelin synthesis (PD 14 to PD 30) caused no lasting deficit after rehabilitation (Wiggins, 1982).

Hypomyelination in the neonatal brain can be revealed using various histomorphological techniques. (1) The cresyl violet stain is a classical stain for demonstrating myelinating glial cells (characteristics: strong basophilic cytoplasm at a paranuclear, unilateral position, according to Schlote, 1983). (2) The Klüver Barrera technique is a well-known myelin stain which stains complex lipids not affected by solvent extraction (during paraffin processing). The gold chloride stain does not work on frozen sections where the free lipids have been extracted by alcohol. (3) The histochemical stain for myelin on frozen sections according to Schmued (1990) stains other lipid components and seems to be more sensitive than the Klüver Barrera stain.

Immunohistochemistry with polyclonal antibodies to myelin basic protein (MBP) was used by Carratu et al. (1996) to evaluate hypomyelinating disorders after intrauterine exposure to carbon monoxide.

It is also well known that adult glio- or myelinopathic agents may act as developmental neurotoxicants (Krinke and Eisenbrandt, 1994) and disturb either myelination gliosis or the myelination process itself. Examples are 6-aminonicotinamide (Aikawa and Suzuki, 1988), triethyltin (Cook et al., 1984) and hexachlorphene (Nieminen and Bjondahl, 1973). Brzoska and Adhami (1975) report Schwann cell swellings in the sciatic nerve after 6-aminonicotinamide treatment of newborn rats. This indicates that the peripheral nervous system has also to be considered when assessing developmental neurotoxicity.

Developmental Neurotoxicity Studies in Rats

This section focuses on recommendations and requirements of the final EPA DNT study guidelines of August 1998 and some considerations of the first draft of OECD DNT study guidelines.

The Actual Regulatory View for the Conduct of DNT Studies

Since the first US EPA DNT guideline was finalized in 1991 (OPPTS Developmental Neurotoxicity Testing Guideline, §83-6), only a limited number of DNT studies have been conducted. Recently, Makris et al. (1998) reviewed a total of 12 DNT studies that have been evaluated by OPPTS in support of the registration and/or use of pesticides and toxic substances; among them are carbamates, organophosphates and solvents. Since August 1998, a slightly revised version (OPPTS 870.6300) is available (EPA, 1998).

Up to now, OPPTS has required DNT studies on the basis of the chemical database (weight-of-evidence) as a second tier toxicity study. Triggers for the conduct of DNT studies are summarized by Levine and Butcher (1990) as CNS teratogens, psychoactive drugs and chemicals, adult neurotoxicants, hormonally active agents, peptides and amino acids, and structurally related agents.

The US Food Quality Protection Act (FQPA) and the Safe Drinking Water Act Amendments of 1996 focused on children as a susceptible population and required much more extensive evaluation of risks to children, as neurotoxicity data following pesticide exposures during pre- and postnatal development were often lacking (Fenner-Crisp, 1998). In the meantime, an EPA toxicology working group was established which recommended the inclusion of a developmental neurotoxicity study in the minimum core toxicology data set for all chemical food-use pesticides (EPA X10 Task Force Draft, Toxicology working group, 1998). Two main reasons seem to be behind this recommendation: (1) there is insufficient scientific information to predict the developmental neurotoxicity of agents neurotoxic to adults and (2) it is important to test whether an agent that shows no CNS malformations or is not an adult neurotoxicant is nevertheless neurotoxic to the developing nervous system.

Ulbrich and Palmer (1996) published a review of pharmaceuticals which were submitted for regulatory purposes to the German agencies. Eighty-five drugs showed behavioral effects in developmental neurotoxicity tests; these drugs included a wide variety of therapeutic classes, many of which were not suspected as causing any effect on the nervous system (seven of them were antibiotics). They concluded that it was necessary to conduct developmental neurotoxicity studies for all substances to which the developing human brain might be exposed. Similarly, only about 65% of known developmental neurotoxicants were detected in a developmental toxicity screen, the Chernoff-Kavlock assay (see Chapter 11) which uses prenatal exposure and birth weight, growth, fetal viability and neonatal survival as endpoints. The authors concluded, that this screen is not reliable enough to serve as a developmental neurotoxicity screen to identify a potential developmental neurotoxicity (Goldey et al., 1995). This conclusion is not surprising when considering the 2 major limitations inherent to this

Table 12.2 Observation in an open arena ('open field observation') according to OPPTS 870.6300

1 Automatic functions: Lacrimation, salivation, piloerection, exophthalmus, pupillary function, palpebral closure, urination and defecation

2 Convulsions, tremors, abnormal movements

3 Posture and gait abnormalities

4 Unusual or abnormal behaviors, excessive or repetitive actions, emaciation, dehydration, hypo- or hypertonia, altered fur appearance, red or crusty deposits (around eyes, nose, mouth)

The table lists the parameters that should be assessed and recorded in 40 dams (2 times during gestational and lactational period each) and 80 offspring (on PD 4, PD 11, at weaning, PD 35, PD 45, PD 60).

screening test: exposure limited to only part of the period of nervous system development and absence of any functional tests.

The Developmental Neurotoxicity Study as Recommended by the EPA

The purpose of the DNT study in rats is to develop data on the potential functional and morphological hazards to the nervous system which may arise in the offspring from exposure to the mother during two periods: pregnancy and lactation. The study may be conducted as a standalone or combined study (with the F1 generation in developmental toxicity studies). As a rule, Wistar or Sprague-Dawley rat strains are preferred. The Fischer 344 rat strain should not be used.

One control and three dosage groups are required as a minimum. As the route of exposure, oral administration (diet or gavage) is recommended. But it is important to take the most relevant human exposure route into consideration when planning the study.

Comparable to developmental toxicology studies in general, at least 20 litters should be included for each dose group. Under practical considerations, at least 25 females should be cohabitated. First, conception may be unsuccessful in single cases and second, the litter size needed for further testing procedures is not reached in all cases. So, for the first step a minimum of 100 females and males are needed.

The litter size required is at least 8 pups (4 males and 4 females, or at least a relation of 5 to 3 or 3 to 5)

per litter. The adjustment of litters by random selection of pups occurs at PD 4. In total, 640 pups (320 males and females each) are required for further testing.

The dosing period will last from GD 6 to PD 10 (early lactation period), except parturition. The dosing period is a matter of controversy (are all critical periods covered?). The first draft of the OECD DNT study guidelines recommends a dosing during pregnancy and throughout lactation from GD 0 (conception) to PD 21 (weaning). In the case of the danger of a treatment-related preimplantation loss, the beginning of treatment at GD 6 is recommended. Early developmental changes during pregnancy and lactation may give cause to end treatment at PD 10.

In DNT studies only the dams are dosed. This led to considerations about the effective dose reaching the developing brain of the fetus or the suckling pup. Such (pharmacokinetic) data are of high value for a risk assessment but are rarely available. This is clearly an area requiring further research.

In principle, the dosing procedure may be adapted to the most relevant exposure route for human infants: if a direct exposure of infants is anticipated, the suckling rats should also be directly exposed (recommended in the first draft of the OECD 426 DNT study guidelines, 1998).

The body weight of all dams has to be measured at least weekly, on the day of delivery and at PD 11 and PD 21 (at weaning). Ten dams per group should be observed clinically in an open arena in more detail ('open field observation'), twice during the gestational period and twice during the lactational period. Parameters to be investigated are summarized in Table 12.2. Signs of all kinds of toxicity should be noted. These data must be taken into account in

Table 12.3 Proposal for an assignment of pups to different subsets

Subset I	Interim sacrifice group. Brain weight measurements on PD 11. Ten male and 10 female pups per group are selected for further brain neuropathology and morphometry
Subset II	Open field observation
Subset III	Motor activity
Subset IV	Auditory startle test
Subset V	Learning and memory test (on PD 21)
Subset VI	Learning and memory test (on PD 60 ± 2)
Subset VII	Brain weight measurements on PD 60 ± 2
Subset VIII	In situ perfusion fixation of 10 male and 10 female pups per group, neuropathology of brain and peripheral nervous system, and brain morphometry on PD 60 ± 2

One subset consists of 80 pups (10 males and 10 females per group: 1 male or 1 female out of 20 litters). Under practical considerations, the subset for the Auditory startle test may be also used for neuropathology at termination. Furthermore, our experience with weight measurements of immersion or perfusion fixed brains is signaling that they detect weight changes in the same sensitive way native (unfixed) brains do. So far, there is no necessity for an additional subset for the brain weight measurements only.

interpreting the effects on offspring in order to answer questions relating to whether the noted effects are direct or indirect. Are the effects on the developing nervous system found in the offspring caused by a general, maternal toxicity of the substance? Developmental effects, especially altered behavior, may occur as a consequence of maternal toxicity during gestation and/or lactation rather than being a direct effect on the offspring (Francis, 1992).

A broad spectrum of endpoints should be evaluated in the offspring. For that purpose, subsets of 80 pups (10 males and 10 females per group) are formed after culling (PD 4) on the basis of a random selection. One subset will be humanely killed on PD 11 and brain weights measured. All these pups (10 males and 10 females per group) are recommended for further neuropathology and morphometry of the brain. With further subsets, motor activity testing (on PD 13, 17, 21, 60 ± 2), auditory startle response (on PD 21 and PD 60 ± 2), and learning and memory testing (on PD 21 and PD 60 ± 2) is carried out. An open field observation must be done using a set of parameters identical to that used with the dams; 80 pups should be tested on six different observation days (Table 12.2). Developmental landmarks, such as body weight, vaginal opening and preputial separation, must be recorded for all live pups. At study termination, 80 of the offspring are sacrificed for brain weight measurements, and an additional group of 80 animals are perfusion fixed (an *in vivo* fixation method which guarantees an especially high quality of tissue fixation for further neuropathology). Table 12.3 gives an example of what an assignment of pups to different subsets may look like.

In the OECD-426 DNT study a similar approach is taken. Instead of the PD 11 histopathology, pups have to be sacrificed on PD 22. Furthermore, less emphasis is put on the motor activity testing (limited to PD 22, 35 and 60) while, in addition to the investigations in the OPPTS test guidelines, development of behavioral functions (behavioral ontogeny) and an additional test of learning and memory around PD 35 are suggested. The OECD approach more closely resembles the approach taken in child neurology where delays in development of specific functions are used to control ongoing therapy and/or to predict functional deficits at adulthood. In addition, exposure to the test substance is provided over a larger part of the brain and nervous system development.

Beside testing for potential functional effects, data for potential morphological changes to the nervous system have to be determined (EPA, 1998). As described above, brain weight measurements are carried out with one subset at PD 11 (end of dosing period) and another one at termination of the study. At both time points, neuropathological and morphometric examinations are required. Immersion fixation of brain and nervous system tissue is sufficient for PD 11 pups, whereas perfusion fixation is required for PD 60 young adult animals. In both cases an appropiate fixative (as a rule an aldehyde fixative) should be used. The guideline does not give any further guidance, but formaldehyde solution should be sufficient for most routine cases and may be recommended for the cases where immunohistochemistry is scheduled (as many immunohistochemical stains do not work on glutaraldehyde-fixed tissues). Glutaraldehyde or a fixative according to Karnovsky (fixative containing a certain percentage of glutaraldehyde) should be considered when electron microscopic examinations are scheduled.

All major brain regions should be investigated (e.g. olfactory bulbs, cerebral cortex, hippocampus, basal ganglia, thalamus, hypothalamus, midbrain with tectum, tegmentum, cerebral peduncles, the brainstem and the cerebellum). A trimming proposal which includes the major brain regions is given in Figure 12.4.

The whole nervous system of all animals assigned for neuropathology at termination of the study should be examined, according to the extent recommended for adult animals (EPA, 1998a). In addition to what is required for PD 11 pups, the spinal cord and possible target sites in the peripheral nervous system should be investigated (e.g. spinal root ganglia and peripheral nerves). Neuromorphological analysis of different brain regions should identify types of neuropathological alterations caused by the test substance and should assess their severity. Indications of developmental insults to the brain are of particular importance. For example, any of the following should be recorded:

- Deviations of normal size and shape of cerebral hemispheres or the normal pattern of foliation of the cerebellum
- Evidence of hydrocephalus
- Abnormal proliferations
- Neurohistologically: Hypoplasia? Heterotypias? Hypomyelination? Increased apoptotic cell death? Alterations in transient developmental structures (e.g. external germinal matrix of the cerebellum)? Abnormal differentiation?

Besides a qualitative and semiquantitative morphological analysis of the nervous system, the EPA

guideline requires a 'simple' morphometric analysis which may allow the assessment of deviations in the normal rate of growth of different, 'major' brain layers. Representative measurements of major layers in the brain are required at least for the neocortex, hippocampus and the cerebellum. The only reference given by the guidelines is Rodier and Gramann (1979). K. Jensen (personal communication) recommends the following procedure for morphometry:

- Prepare homologous sections which are preconditions for comparable measurements.
- Two sections will cover the minimum of major brain layers. One coronal section (Sherwood and Timiras, 1970, p. 50 (PD 10 pups) or p. 110 (PD 21 pups)) will give measurements of the neocortex (perpendicular to a tangent of the pial surface where the neocortex exhibits its greatest thickness), corpus callosum (at the midline) and hippocampus (greatest dorso-ventral extent). One sagittal section (Sherwood and Timiras, 1970, p. 70 (PD 10 pups) or p. 134 (PD 21 pups)) will give measurement of the cerebellum (width of selected folia (e.g. the pyramis) perpendicular to its long axis at the midpoint between its tips and base).

Since it first came up as a guideline requirement in 1991, the value of time-consuming morphometric (stereologic) measurements in a first-step analysis for the evaluation of a potential of developmental neurotoxicity has been a matter of controversy. Alternative proposals are that morphometry should only be carried out if brain weight changes are noted or that regional brain weight measurements should be used instead. In general, brain weight changes seem to be a sensitive indicator for developmental neurotoxicity (Walker et al., 1989).

The use of morphometry only if brain weight changes are noted (K. Jensen, personal communication) is in accordance with recommendations in the newest draft of an OECD 426 DNT study guideline (OECD, 1998). Morphometric analysis is only taken into consideration as one of possibilites for a further characterization of brain weight or neuropathological changes.

Regional brain weight measurements (Figure 12.5) might also give additional information concerning the rate of growth, but is not a requirement of any guideline. Nevertheless, it should be considered as a less time-consuming alternative to morphometric measurements when conducting a DNT study.

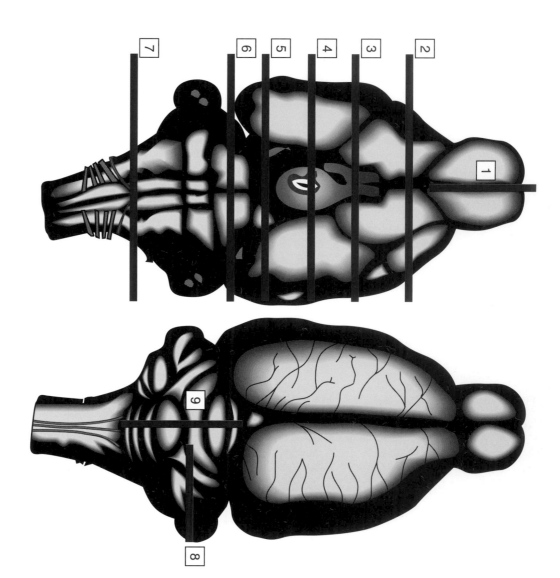

Figure 12.4 Trimming proposal for the brain of PD 11, PD 22 and PD 60 (± 2) young rats. Ventral view of the brain (left).

1 The olfactory bulbs are dissected midsagittally and both halfs are embedded with the cut surface down into the cassette.

2 Half-way between the ventral base of the olfactory bulbs and the optic chiasm/mamillary body.

3 Anterior to the mamillary body through the optic chiasm.*

4 Through the infundibulum.

5 Posterior to the mamillary body.

6 Through the pons.*

7 Through the posterior medulla oblongata, directly behind the caudal end of the cerebellar cortex. Dorsal view of the brain (right).

8 Through the midcerebellum.

9 The midsagittal section of the cerebellar cortex is embedded the cut surface down into the cassette.

The cerebellar cortex will be removed from the rest of the brain. It is cut into two halfs (midsagittal section) from which one will be used to prepare a cross-section (midcerebellum), the other one to prepare a midsagittal section.

All cross-sections are embedded the anterior surface down into the cassettes.

*under practical considerations, we do without level 3 and 6 in the PD 11 brains.

Regional brain weight measurements

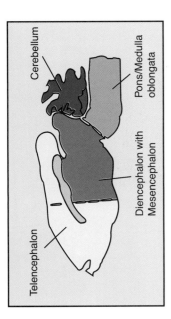

Figure 12.5 Regional brain weight measurements.

The brain is carefully removed, blotted, chilled and weighed in total in a first step. According to Glowinski and Iversen (1966), the following dissection may be performed on an ice-cooled glass plate in a second step:

The rhombencephalon is separated by a transverse section from the rest of the brain and dissected into cerebellum and medulla oblongata/pons.

(2) The second transverse section is made at the level of the chiasma opticum which delimits the anterior part of the hypothalamus and passes through the anterior commissure.

(3) The cortex cerebri is peeled off the posterior part and added to the anterior section.

Immediately after dissection the weight measurement of the brain regions is carried out as follows:

- Telencephalon (anterior part of the prosencephalon with added cortex cerebri of the posterior part)
- Diencephalon (posterior part of the prosencephalon) together with the mesencephalon (midbrain)
- Pons/medulla oblongata (rhombencephalon)
- Cerebellum (rhombencephalon).

The decision as to which approach is most appropriate should be done on a 'weight-of-evidence' basis for each substance under consideration for DNT testing.

References

Ahlbom, J., Fredriksson, A. and Eriksson, P. (1995) *Brain Res.* **677**, 13–19.

Aikawa, H., and Suzuki, K. (1988) In: Jones, T.C., Mohr, U. and Hunt, R.D. (eds) *Monographs on Pathology of Laboratory Animals, Nervous System*, pp. 53–57. Berlin: Springer-Verlag.

Andreasen, N.C., Flashman, L., Flaum, M. *et al.* (1994) *JAMA* **272**, 1763–1769.

Arnold, S.E., Hyman, B.T., Van Hoesen, G.W. and Damasio, A.R. (1991) *Arch. Gen. Psychiatry* **48**, 625–632.

Aschner, M. (1998) In: Slikker, Jr., W. and Chang, L.W. (eds) *Handbook of Developmental Neurotoxicology*, pp. 339–351. San Diego: Academic Press.

Bauman, M.L. and Kemper, T.L. (1985) *Neurology* **35**, 866–874.

Bayer, S.A. and Altman, J. (1995) In: Paxinos, G. (ed.) *The Rat Nervous System*, pp. 1079–1098. San Diego: Academic Press.

Bayer, S.A., Altman, J., Russo, R.J. and Zhang, X. (1993) *Neurotoxicology* **14**, 83–144.

Benes, F.M., McSparran, J., Bird, E.D., San Giovanni, J.P. and Vincent, S. (1991) Deficits in small interneurons in prefrontal and cingulate cortices of schizophrenic and schizoaffective patients. *Arch. Gen. Phych.* **48**, 996–1001.

Berry, M. and Butt, A.M. (1997) In: Graham, D.I. and Lantos, P.L. (eds), *Greenfield's Neuropathology*, pp. 63–83. London: Arnold.

Bignami, A., Raju, T. and Dahl, D. (1982) *Dev. Biol.* **91**, 286–295.

Broening, H.W. and Slikker, Jr, W. (1998) In: Slikker, W. Jr and Chang, L.W. (eds) *Handbook of Developmental Neurotoxicology*, pp. 245–256. San Diego: Academic Press.

Brzoska, H.R. and Adhami, H. (1975) *Acta Neuropathol. (Berlin)* **33**, 59–66.

Buwalda, B. (1995) *Dev. Brain Res.* **84**, 185–191.

Carratu, M.R., Cagiano, R., De Salvia, M.A., Trabace, L. and Cuomo, V. (1995) Developmental Neurotoxicity of Carbon Monoxide. *Arch. Toxicol.* Suppl. 17, 295–301.

Choi, B.H., Lapham, L.W., Amin-Zaki, L. and Saleem, T. (1978) *J. Neuropathol. Exp. Neurol.* **37**, 719–733.

Chu Wang, I.W. and Oppenheim, R.W. (1978) *J. Comp. Neurol.* **177**, 33–58.

Cook, L., Jacobs, K.S. and Reiter, L.W. (1984) *Toxicol. Appl. Pharmacol.* **72**, 75–81.

Davies, J.M., Otto, D.A., Weil, D.E. and Grant, L.D. (1990) *Neurotoxicol. Teratol.* **12**, 215–229.

Deckwerth, T.L. and Johnson, E.M. (1993) *Ann. NY Acad. Sci.* **679**, 121–131.

Desaiah, D. (1998) In: Slikker, Jr, W. and Chang, L.W. (eds) *Handbook of Developmental Neurotoxicology*, pp. 559–565. San Diego: Academic Press.

Diaz-Cintra, S., Cintra, L., Ortega, A., Kemoer, T. and Morgane, P.J. (1990) *J. Comp. Neurol.* **292**, 117–126.

Diapaolo, R.V., Kanfer, J.K. and Newberne, P.M. (1974) *J. Neuropathol. Exp. Neurol.* **33**, 226.

Duffard, R., Garcia, G., Rosso, S. et al. (1996) Neurotoxicol. Teratol. 18, 691–696.

Earys, J.T. (1955) Acta Anat. 25, 160.

EPA (US Environmental Protection Agency) (1998a) Health Effects Test Guidelines OPPTS 870.6200 Neurotoxicity Screening Battery. http://www.epa. gov/epahome/research.htm

EPA (US Environmental Protection Agency) (1998b) Health Effects Test Guidelines OPPTS 870.6300 Developmental Neurotoxicity Study. http://www.epa. gov/epahome/research.htm

EPA X10 Task Force Draft, Toxicology working group guidelines. Abstracts. 16th International Neurotoxicology Conference, Little Rock, AK, USA.

Eriksson, P. (1997) Neurotoxicology 18, 719–726.

Eriksson, P., Ahlbom, J. and Fredriksson, A. (1992) Brain Res. 582, 277–281.

Falkai, P. and Bogerts, B. (1995) In: Hirsch, S.R., and Weinberger, D.R. (eds) Schizophrenia, pp. 275–292. Oxford: Blackwell Science.

Fenner-Crisp, P. (1998) New legislation, regulations and guidelines. Abstracts. 16th International Neurotoxicology Conference, Little Rock, AK, USA. Pesticides and susceptible populations – who is at risk and when?

Fischer, M.H., Welker, C. and Waisman, H.A. (1971) Teratology 5, 223–232.

Francis, E. (1992) Neurotoxicology 13, 77–84.

Glowinski, J. and Iversen, L.L. (1966) J. Neurochem. 13, 655–669.

Goldey, E.S., Tilson, H.A. and Crofton, K.M. (1995) Neurotoxicol. Teratol. 17, 313–332.

Goldstein, G.W. (1992) Neurologic concepts of lead poisoning in children. Pediatric Annals. 21 (6) 384–388.

Goy, R.W. and McEwen, B.S. (1980) Sexual Differentiation of the Brain. Cambridge, MA: MIT Press.

Gressens, P., Lammens, M., Picard, J.J. and Evrard, P. (1992) Alcohol Alcoholism 27, 219–226.

Gross, P.M. (1992) Prog. Brain Res. 91, 219–234.

Halls, B.H. and Das, G.D. (1978) J. Neurol. Sci. 39, 111.

Harper, C. and Butterworth, R. (1997) Graham, D.I. and Lantos, P.L. (eds) Greenfield's Neuropathology, pp. 603–626. London: Arnold.

Hicks, S.P., D'Amato, C.A. and Lowe, M.J. (1959) J. Comp. Neurol. 113, 435–469.

Himwich, W.A. (1973) In: Ford, D.H. (ed.) Neurobiological Aspects of Maturation and Aging Progress in Brain Research, Vol. 40, p. 13. Amsterdam: Elsevier Scientific.

Hirono, I., Shibuya, C. and Hayashi, K. (1969) Proc. Soc. Exp. Biol. Med. 131, 593–598.

Horvath, E., Scheithauer, B.W., Kovacs, K. and Lloyd, R.V. (1997). In: Graham, D.I. and Lantos, P.L. (eds), Greenfield's Neuropathology, pp. 1047–1048. London: Arnold.

Howd, R.A., Rebert, C.S., Dickinson, J. and Pryor, G.T. (1983) Neurobehav. Toxicol. Teratol. 5, 63–68.

IEH (Institute of Environment and Health) (1996) Developmental Neurotoxicology in the Neonate. Leicester: Medical Research Council.

Jacobs, J.M. (1980) Vascular permeability and neural injury. In: Spencer, P.S. and Schaumburg, H.H. (eds), Experimental and Clinical Neurotoxicology, pp. 102–117. Baltimore, London: Williams & Wilkins.

Jacobs, J.M. (1994) Blood–brain and blood–nerve barriers and their relationships. In: Chang, L.W. (ed.), Principles of Neurotoxicology, pp. 35–68. New York: Marcel Dekker, Inc.

Jacobson, M. (1978) Histogenesis and morphogenesis of the central nervous system. In: Jacobson, M. (ed.), Developmental Neurobiology, pp. 57–114. New York: Plenum Press.

Jaskiw, G.E., Juliano, D.M., Goldberg, T.E., Hertzman, M., Urow-Hamell, E. and Weinberger, D.R. (1994) Schizophr. Res. 14, 23–28.

Jett, D.A. (1998) In: Slikker, Jr, W. and Chang, L.W. (eds) Handbook of Developmental Neurotoxicology, pp. 257–274.

Johnston, M.V. and Coyle, J.T. (1979) Brain Res. 170, 135–155.

Kelly, D.D. (1985) Sexual differentiation of the nervous system. In: Kandel, E.A. and Schwartz, J.H. (eds), Principles of Neural Science, pp. 771–783. New York, Amsterdam, Oxford: Elsevier.

Kimmel, C.A. (1998) In: Slikker, Jr, W. and Chang, L.W. (eds) Developmental Neurotoxicology, pp. 675–685. San Diego: Academic Press.

Kinney, H.C. and Armstrong, D.D. (1997) In: Graham, D.I. and Lantos, P.L. (eds), Greenfield's Neuropathology, pp. 535–599. London: Arnold.

Kinney, H.C., Rava, L.A. and Benowitz, L.I. (1993) J. Neuropathol. Exp. Neurol. 52, 39–54.

Krigman, M.R. and Hogan, E.L. (1976) Brain Res. 107, 139.

Krigman, M.R., Druse, M.J., Traylor, T.D., Wilson, M.H., Newell, L.R. and Hogan, E.L. (1974) J. Neuropathol. Exp. Neurol. 33, 58.

Krinke, G.J. and Eisenbrandt, D.L. (1994) In: Mohr, U., Dungworth, D.L. and Capen, C.C. (eds) Pathobiology of the Aging Rat, pp 3–9. Washington DC: ILSI Press.

Levine, T.E. and Butcher, R.E. (1990) Workshop on the qualitative and quantitative comparability of human and animal developmental neurotoxicity, work group IV report: Triggers for developmental neurotoxicity testing. Neurotox. Teratol., 12, 281–284.

Levitt, P. and Rakic, P. (1980) J. Comp. Neurol. 193, 815–840.

LoPachin, R.M. and Aschner, M. (1993) Toxicol. Appl. Pharmacol. 118, 141–158.

Makris, S., Raffaele, K., Sette, W. and Seed, J. (1998) A retrospective analysis of twelve developmental neurotoxicity studies submitted to the USEPA Office of Prevention, Pesticides, and Toxic Substances (OPPTS). Presented to the Science Advisory Panel, 8–9 December 1998.

Martin, J.H. (1985) Development as a guide to the regional anatomy of the brain. In: Kandel, E.A. and Schwartz, J.H. (eds), *Principles of Neural Science*, pp. 244–258. New York, Amsterdam, Oxford: Elsevier.

Matsumoto, H., Koya, G. and Takeuchi, T. (1975) *J. Neuropathol. Exp. Neurol.* **34**, 563–574.

Meyer, J. (1998) In: Slikker, Jr, W. and Chang, L.W. (eds) *Handbook of Developmental Neurotoxicology*, pp. 403–426. San Diego: Academic Press.

Miller, S.L. (1992) In: Boulton, A., Baker, G. and Butterworth, R.) (eds) *Neuromethods*, Vol. 21, *Animal Models of Neurological Disease*, pp. 205–273. Clifton, NJ: The Humana Press.

Montgomery, D.L. (1994) *Vet. Pathol.* **31**, 145–167.

Narahashi, T. (1985) *Neurotoxicology* **6**, 3–22.

Nieminen, L. and Bjondahl, K. (1973) *Food Cosmet. Toxicol.* **11**, 635–639.

Norton, W.T. and Poduslo, S.E. (1973) *J. Neurochem.* **21**, 759–773.

Nulman, I., O'Hayon, B., Gladstone, J. and Koren, G. (1998) In: Slikker, Jr, W. and Chang, L.W. (eds) *Handbook of Developmental Neurotoxicology*, pp. 567–586. San Diego: Academic Press.

O'Callaghan, J.P. and Miller, D.B. (1988) *J. Pharmacol. Exp. Ther.* **244**, 368–378.

OECD (1998) Proposal for a new guideline 426: Developmental neurotoxicity study. http:www.oecd.org/ehs/test/health.htm

Padilla, S., Lassiter, T.L., Hunter, D. *et al.* (1998) Abstracts. 16th International Neurotoxicology Conference, Little Rock, AK, USA.

Pentschew, A. (1965) *Acta Neuropathol.* **5**, 133.

Politis, M.J., Schaumburg, H.H. and Spencer, P.S. (1980) In: Spencer, P.S. and Schaumburg, H.H. (eds) *Experimental and Clinical Neurotoxicology*, pp. 613–630. Baltimore: Williams & Wilkins.

Pu, C. and Vorhees, C.V. (1993) *Dev. Brain Res.* **72**, 325–328.

Pu, C., Fisher, J.E., Cappon, G.D. and Vorhees, G.V. (1994) *Brain Res.* **649**, 217–224.

Rakic P. (1971) Guidance of neurons migrating to the fetal monkey neocortex. *Brain Res.* **33**, 471–476.

Reuhl, K.R. (1988) In: Jones, T.C., Mohr, U. and Hunt, R.D. (eds) *Monographs on Pathology of Laboratory Animals, Nervous System*, pp. 104–107. Berlin: Springer-Verlag.

Reuhl, K.R., Lagunowich, L.A. and Brown, D.L. (1994) *Neurotoxicology* **15**, 133–146.

Rodier, P.M. (1990) *Toxicol. Pathol.* **18**, 89–95.

Rodier, P.M. (1998) In: Slikker, Jr, W. and Chang, L.W. (eds) *Handbook of Developmental Neurotoxicology*, pp. 661–672. San Diego: Academic Press.

Rodier, P.M. and Gramann, W.J. (1979) *Neurobehav. Toxicol.* **1**, 129–135.

Rodier, P.M., Ingram, J.L., Tinsdale, B, Nelson, S. and Romano, J. (1996) *J. Comp. Neurol.* **370**, 247–261.

Romero, I.A., Abbott, N.J. and Bradbury, M.W.B. (1996)

In: Chang, L.W. (ed.) *Toxicology of Metals*, pp. 561–585. Boca Raton: CRC Press.

Salas, M., Diaz, S. and Nieto, A. (1974) *Brain Res.* **73**, 139.

Schardein, J.L. (1998) In: Slikker, Jr, W. and Chang, L.W. (eds) *Handbook of Developmental Neurotoxicology*, pp. 687–708. San Diego: Academic Press.

Schlote, W. (1983) In: Doerr, W. and Seifert, G. (eds) *Spezielle pathologische Anatomie. Pathologie des Nervensystems II*, pp. 2–172. Berlin: Springer-Verlag.

Schmechel, D.E. and Rakic, P. (1979) *Anat. Embryol.* **156**, 115–152.

Schmued, L.C. (1990) *J. Histochem. Cytochem.* **38**, 717–720.

Schulze, C. and Firth, J.A. (1992) *Dev. Brain Res.* **69**, 85–95.

Sherwood, N.M. and Timiras, P.S. (1970) *A Stereotaxic Atlas of the Developing Rat Brain*. Los Angeles: University of California Press.

Shield, M.A. and Mirkes, P.E. (1998) In: Slikker, Jr, W. and Chang, L.W. (eds) *Handbook of Developmental Neurotoxicology*, pp. 159–188. San Diego: Academic Press.

Sievers, J., Pehlemann, F.W. and Gude, S. (1994) *J. Neurocytol.* **23**, 97–115.

Slikker, W. (1994) *Neurotoxicology* **15**, 11–16.

Smithells, R.W. and Newman, C.G.H. (1992) *J. Med. Genet.* **29**, 716–723.

Spatz, M. and Laqueur, G.L. (1968) *Proc. Soc. Exp. Biol. Med.* **129**, 705–710.

Stanton, M.E. and Spear, L.P. (1990) *Neurotoxicol. Teratol.* **12**, 261–267.

Stein, S.A., Adams, P.M., Shanklin, D.R., Mihailoff, G.A. and Palnitkar, M.B. (1991) Thyroid hormone control of brain and motor development: Molecular, neuroanatomical, and behavioral studies. *Advances Exp. Med. Biol.* **229**, 47–105.

Stromland, K. and Pinazo-Duran, M.D. (1994) *Teratology* **50**, 100–111.

Suzuki, K. (1980) In: Spencer, P.S. and Schaumburg, H.H. (eds) *Experimental and Clinical Neurotoxicology*, pp. 48–61. Baltimore: Williams & Wilkins.

Ulbrich, B. and Palmer, A.K. (1996) Neurobehavioral aspects of developmental toxicity testing. *Environ. Health Perspect.* 104/SUPPL **2**, 407–412.

Vaughn, J.E. and Peters, A. (1971) In: Pease, D.C. (ed.) *Cellular Aspects of Growth and Differentiation*, pp. 103–140. Los Angeles: University of California Press.

Verity, M.A. (1997) In: Graham, D.I. and Lantos, P.L. (eds) *Greenfield's Neuropathology*, pp. 755–811. London: Arnold.

Vorhees, C.V., Ahrens, K.G., Acuff-Smith, K.D., Schilling, M.A. and Fisher, J.E. (1994a) *Psychopharmacology* **114**, 392–401.

Vorhees, C.V., Ahrens, K.G., Acuff-Smith, K.D., Schilling, M.A. and Fisher, J.E. (1994b) *Psychopharmacology* **114**, 401–408.

Walker, R.F., Guerriero, F.J., Toscano, T.V. and Weidemann, C.A. (1989) *Neurotoxicol. Teratol.* **11**, 251–255.

Weinberger, D.R. (1995a) *Lancet* **346**, 552–557.

Weinberger, D.R. (1995b) In: Hirsch, S.R. and Weinberger, D.R. (eds) *Schizophrenia*, pp. 293–323. Oxford: Blackwell Science.

Wiggins, R.C. (1982) *Brain Res. Rev.* **4**, 151–175.

Wise, L.D., Gordon, L.R., Soper, K.A., Duchai, D.M. and Morrissey, R.E. (1995) *Neurotoxicol. Teratol.* **17**, 189–198.

Yakovlev, P.I. and Lacours, A.R. (1967) In: Minikowski, A. (ed.) *Regional Development of the Brain in Early Life*, pp. 3–70. Oxford: Blackwell.

Zhang, L.L., Collier, P.A. and Ashwell, K.W.S. (1995) *Neurotoxicol. Teratol.* **17**, 297–311.

PART 5

Anatomy

Contents

CHAPTER 13

Gross Anatomy

Vladimír Komárek
Agricultural University, Prague, Czech Republic

Introduction

Although this book does not aim to provide a comprehensive description of rat anatomy, this chapter presents illustrations of areas likely to be of practical importance to those working with laboratory rats. These areas include body surface, body regions, muscles, and dissection of the neck, thorax and abdomen with pelvic cavity.

For further anatomical details, readers are referred to Chapter 15 and the excellent works of Green (1963), Hebel and Stromberg (1986) and Popesko et al. (1990).

The terminology used here is based on the international veterinary anatomical nomenclature published by Schaller et al. (1992). In the figure captions, XY denotes male and XX female.

Acknowledgement

With her kind consent, some of the figures presented in this chapter were drawn following the concept of Professor Dr Viera Rajtova (Popesko et al., 1990).

References

Green, E.C. (1963) *Anatomy of the Rat.* New York: Hafner Publishing.

Hebel, R. and Stromberg, M.W. (1986) *Anatomy and Embryology of the Laboratory Rat.* Wörthsee: BioMed Verlag.

Popesko, P., Rajtova, V. and Horak, J. (1990) *Atlas anatomie malych laboratornych zvierat*, Vol. 2. Bratislava: Priroda. (English version published by Wolfe Publishing Ltd, London, 1992.)

Schaller, O., Constantinescu, G.M., Habel, R.E., Sack, W.O., Simoens, P. and de Vos, N.R. (1992) *Illustrated Veterinary Anatomical Nomenclature.* Stuttgart: Enke Verlag.

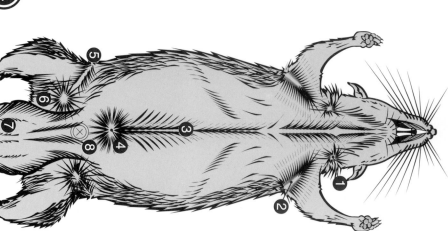

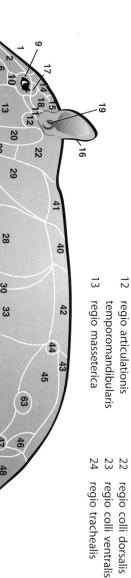

(a)

Figure 13.1 The hair coat, ventral view (XY). The rat hair is arranged to form whirls and streams (vortices et flumina pilorum).

1 at the level of arm joints there are divergent whirls (vortices pilorum divergentes)

2 in the axillary region there is divergent stream (flumen pilorum divergens axillaris)

3 in the ventromedial area there is a convergent stream (flumen pilorum convergens trunci).

4 in the umbilical area there is convergent umbilical whirl (vortex pilorum convergens umbilicalis)

5 the inner surface of the thigh is separated from the caudal abdomen (inguinal region) by divergent inguinal stream (flumen pilorum divergens inguinalis)

6 at the caudal end of the above stream there is a whirl (vortex pilorum divergens inguinalis)

7 the ventral surface of scrotum is hairless (planum depilatum)

8 preputium, penis

Figures 13.2a, b, (XY) and **c** (XX): The regions of rat body

Regions of the body (regiones corporis).

Regions of the face (regiones faciei)

1 regio dorsalis nasi
2 regio lateralis nasi
3 regio naris et apex nasi
4 regio oralis
5 regio mentalis
6 regio buccalis
7 regio mandibularis
8 regio intermandibularis
9 regio orbitalis
10 regio infraorbitalis
11 regio zygomatica
12 regio articulationis temporomandibularis
13 regio masseterica

Regions of the skull (regiones cranii)

14 regio frontalis
15 regio parietalis
16 regio occipitalis
17 regio supraorbitalis
18 regio temporalis
19 regio auricularis et auricula

Regions of the neck (regiones colli)

20 regio parotides
21 regio subhyoidea et laryngea
22 regio colli dorsalis
23 regio colli ventralis
24 regio trachealis

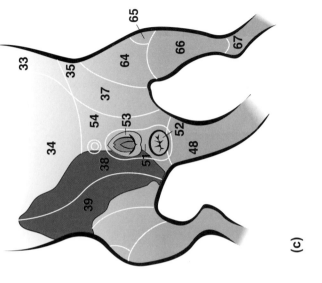

(c)

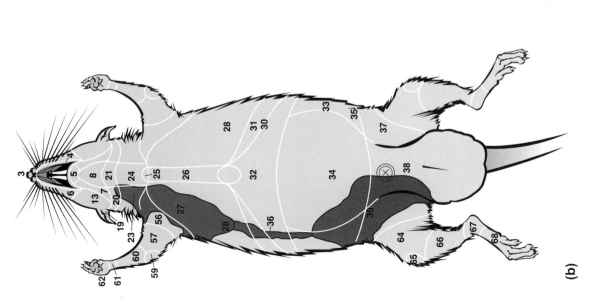

(b)

Figures 13.2a, b, c (*continued*)

Regions of the breast (regiones pectoris)
25 regio presternalis
26 regio sternalis
27 regio mammaria thoracica
28 regio costalis
29 regio scapularis
30 arcus costalis
Cranial abdominal regions (regiones abdominis craniales)
31 regio hypochondriaca
32 regio xiphoidea
Median abdominal regions (regiones abdominis mediae)
33 regio abdominis lateralis
34 regio umbilicalis
35 regio plicae genus
36 regio mammaria abdominalis
Caudal abdominal regions (regiones abdominis caudales)
37 regio inguinalls
38 regio pubica (scroti et preputialis in XY)
39 regio mammaria inguinalis

Dorsal regions (regiones dorsi)
40 regio vertebralis thoracis
41 regio interscapularis
42 regio lumbalis
Pelvic regions (regiones pelvis)
43 regio sacralis
44 regio tuberis coxae
45 regio glutea
46 regio clunis
47 regio tuberis ischiadici
48 regio radicis caudae
49 regio corporis caudae
50 regio apicis caudae
51 regio perinealis
52 regio analis
53 regio vulvae (XX)
54 regio clitoridis (XX)
Regions of the thoracic extremity (regiones membri thoracici)
55 regio articulationis humeri
56 regio axillaris
57 regio brachii
58 regio tricipitalis
59 regio cubiti
60 regio antebrachii (cranialis, lateralis, caudalis, medialis)
61 regio carpi (cranialis, lateralis, caudalis, medialis)
62 regio manus (metacarpi et digiti, dorsalis, lateralis, volaris/palmaris, medialis)
Regions of the pelvic extremity (regiones membri pelvini)
63 regio articulationis coxae
64 regio femoris (cranialis, lateralis, caudalis, medialis)
65 regio genus
66 regio cruris (cranialis, lateralis, caudalis, medialis)
67 regio tarsi (cranialis, lateralis, caudalis, medialis)
68 regio pedis (metatarsi et digiti, dorsalis, lateralis, plantaris, medialis)

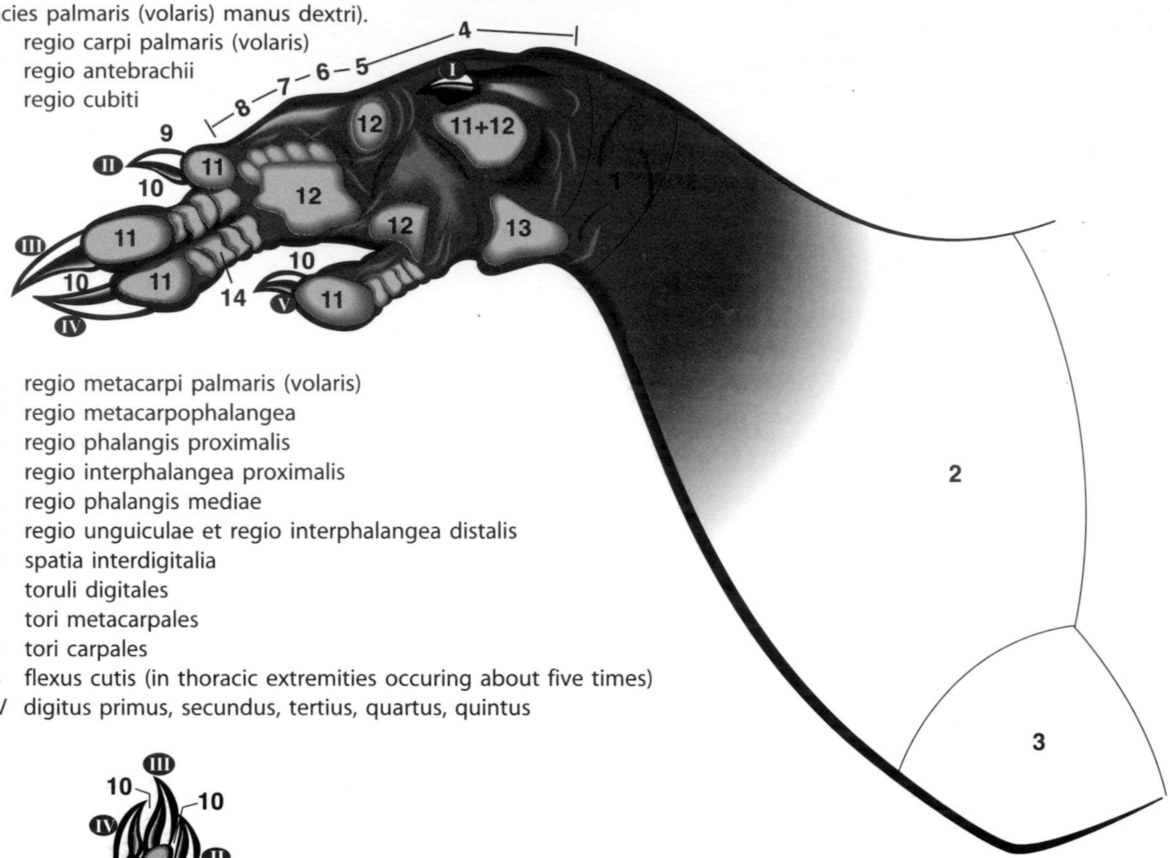

Figure 13.3 Palmar (volar) surface of the right frontal paw (facies palmaris (volaris) manus dextri).

1 regio carpi palmaris (volaris)
2 regio antebrachii
3 regio cubiti
4 regio metacarpi palmaris (volaris)
5 regio metacarpophalangea
6 regio phalangis proximalis
7 regio interphalangea proximalis
8 regio phalangis mediae
9 regio unguiculae et regio interphalangea distalis
10 spatia interdigitalia
11 toruli digitales
12 tori metacarpales
13 tori carpales
14 flexus cutis (in thoracic extremities occuring about five times)
I–V digitus primus, secundus, tertius, quartus, quintus

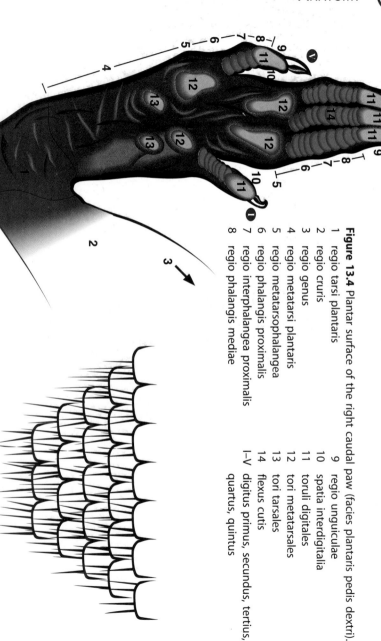

Figure 13.4 Plantar surface of the right caudal paw (facies plantaris pedis dextri).

1 regio tarsi plantaris
2 regio cruris
3 regio genus
4 regio metatarsi plantaris
5 regio metatarsophalangea
6 regio phalangis proximalis
7 regio interphalangea proximalis
8 regio phalangis mediae
9 regio unguiculae
10 spatia interdigitalia
11 toruli digitales
12 tori metatarsales
13 tori tarsales
14 flexus cutis
I–V digitus primus, secundus, tertius, quartus, quintus

Figure 13.5 Scales on the tail. The tail is covered by square scales, underneath which grow two to six straight hairs, extending over the next row of scales.

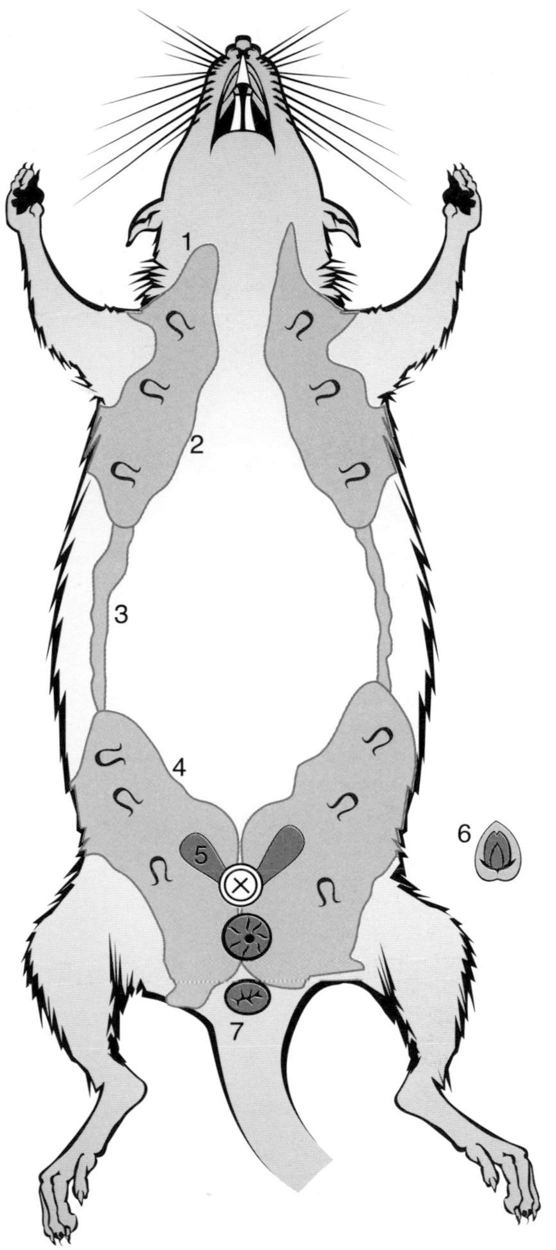

Figure 13.6 The mammary gland (XX). The mammary tissue is distributed bilaterally, reaching from the neck to the anus. In males the nipples do not develop well.

1 cervical mammary gland, devoid of nipples
2 thoracic mammary gland usually has three pairs of nipples; it does not cover the sternum, but fills the axillary region, surrounds partly the basis of forelimbs and extends towards the costal region
3 abdominal mammary gland has only little, irregularly developed tissue
4 inguinal mammary gland usually has three pairs of nipples and is located in the inguinal region, partly surrounding the basis of hindlimbs
5 clitoral preputium is equipped with a paired clitoral gland. In female rats the urethra opens at the clitoris so that there is no vaginal vestibulum
6 vaginal entrence (vulva) has small labia
7 anus

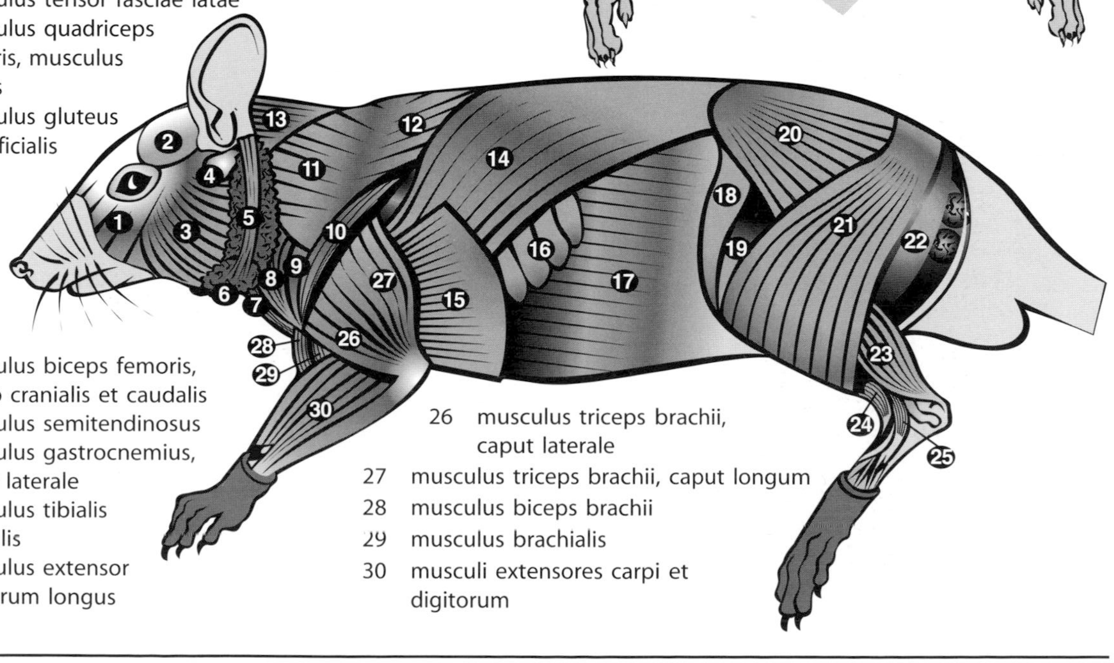

Figure 13.7 The superficial muscles. **(See also Colour Plate 1.)**

1 musculi faciales
2 musculus temporalis
3 musculus masseter
4 glandula lacrimalis extraorbitalis
5 glandula parotidea with the ventral auricular muscle
6 glandula mandibularis
7 musculus sternocephalicus, pars mastoidea
8 musculus brachiocephalicus, pars occipitalis
9 musculus deltoideus, pars acromialis
10 musculus deltoideus, pars scapularis
11 musculus trapezius, pars cervicalis
12 musculus trapezius, pars thoracica
13 musculus cervicoauricularis
14 musculus latissimus dorsi
15 musculus cutaneus trunci
16 musculus serratus ventralis thoraci
17 musculus obliquus externus abdominis
18 musculus tensor fasciae latae
19 musculus quadriceps femoris, musculus rectus
20 musculus gluteus superficialis

21 musculus biceps femoris, portio cranialis et caudalis
22 musculus semitendinosus
23 musculus gastrocnemius, caput laterale
24 musculus tibialis cranialis
25 musculus extensor digitorum longus

26 musculus triceps brachii, caput laterale
27 musculus triceps brachii, caput longum
28 musculus biceps brachii
29 musculus brachialis
30 musculi extensores carpi et digitorum

Figure 13.8 The deep muscles, forelimb removed. **(See also Colour Plate 2.)**

1 glandula parotidea
2 glandula and lymphonodus mandibularis
3 lymphonodus retropharyngeus
4 lymphonodus cervicalis profundus
5 vena jugularis
6 plexus brachialis
7 arteria et vena subclavia
8 musculus sternocephalicus, pars mastoidea
9 musculus brachiocephalicus, pars occipitalis
10 clavicula
11 musculi pectorales
12 musculus rectus thoracis et abdominis
13 musculus rhomboideus capitis
14 musculus rhomboideus cervicis
15 musculus splenius
16 musculus longissimus capitis et atlantis
17 corpus adiposum nuchae (multivesiculare s. plurivacuolare s. hiberneticum)
18 musculus longissimus cervicis
19 musculus longissimus thoracis
20 musculus longissimus lumborum
21 musculus serratus ventralis (cervicis et thoracis)
22 musculus serratus dorsalis cranialis
23 musculus serratus dorsalis caudalis
24 musculus iliocostalis
25 musculi intercostales externi
26 musculus obliquus externus abdominis
27 musculus obliquus internus abdominis
28 musculus gluteus medius
29 musculus quadriceps femoris
30 musculus biceps femoris
31 musculus semimembranosus et semitendinosus
32 musculus tibialis cranialis
33 musculus triceps surae

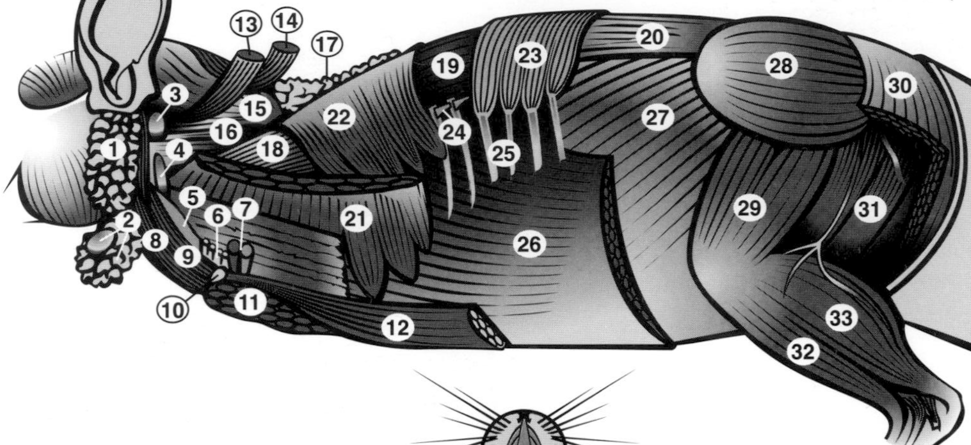

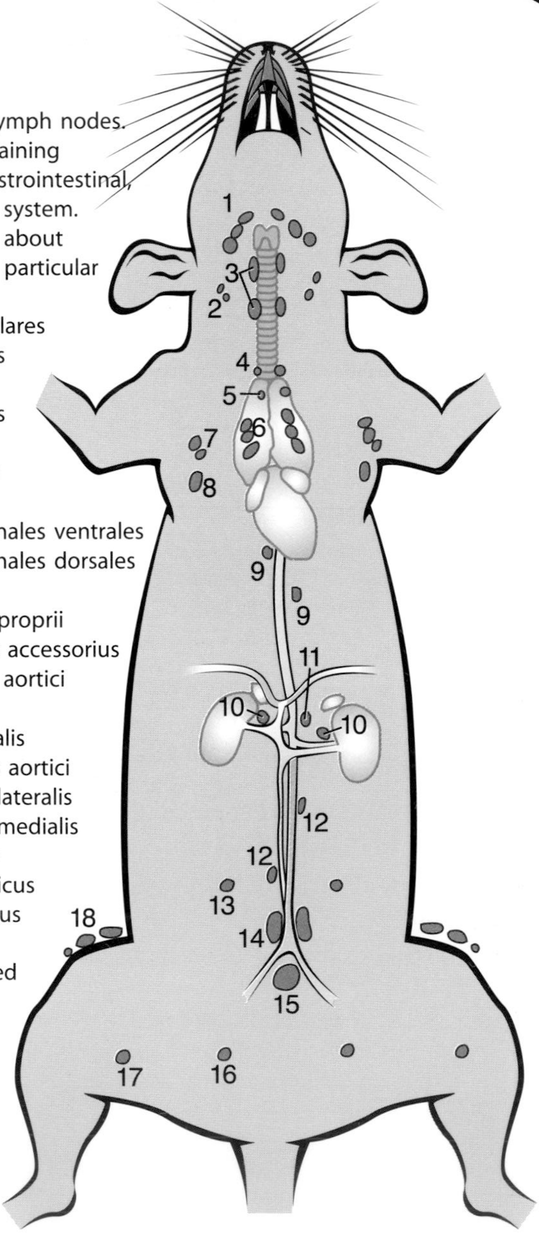

Figure 13.9 Locations of lymph nodes. Does not include those draining specific viscera such as gastrointestinal, respiratory and urogenital system. See Chapter 28 for details about the lymph nodes draining particular body areas.

1 lymphonodi mandibulares
2 lymphonodi cervicales superficiales
3 lymphonodi cervicales profundi
4 lymphonodi sternales craniales
5 lymphonodi mediastinales ventrales
6 lymphonodi mediastinales dorsales (et thymus)
7 lymphonodi axillares proprii
8 lymphonodus axillaris accessorius
9 lymphonodi thoracici aortici
10 lymphonodi renales
11 lymphonodus cisternalis
12 lymphonodi lumbales aortici
13 lymphonodus iliacus lateralis
14 lymphonodus iliacus medialis
15 lymphonodus sacralis
16 lymphonodus ischiadicus
17 lymphonodus popliteus
18 lymphonodi subiliaci

The trachea is accompanied by truncus trachealis and the (abdominal) aorta by truncus lumbalis, which joins with truncus intestinalis, producing cisterna chyli, from which truncus thoracicus leads towards the heart.

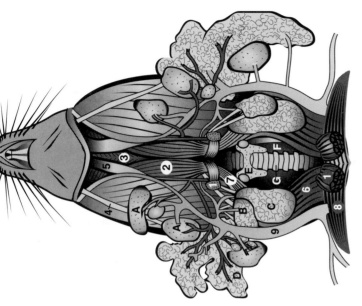

Figure 13.12 Organs of the ventral neck, ventral view, deep layer (organa colli ventralis, norma ventralis, stratum profundum). **(See also Colour Plate 4.)**

A lymphonodi mandibulares
B glandula sublingualis
C glandula mandibularis (submandibularis)
D glandula parotis et lymphonodus cervicalis superficialis
E glandula thyreoidea et parathyreoidea
F esophagus
G trachea
1 musculus sternohyoideus et sternothyreoideus (resectus)
2 musculus digastricus, venter rostralis
3 musculus mylohyoideus
4 musculus masseter et ductus parotideus
5 mandibula
6 musculus sternomastoideus
7 musculus omohyoideus
8 musculus pectoralis major
9 vena jugularis externa

6 glandula mandibularis et ductus glandulae mandibularis (also called submandibular)
7 musculus masseter et ductus parotideus
8 venter rostralis musculi digastrici
9 musculus sternomastoideus
10 musculus sternohyoideus
11 musculus pectoralis major
12 vena jugularis externa dextra

Figure 13.10 Ventral view of the head.

1 labium maxillare pars externa
2 labium maxillare pars interna
3 palatum durum
4 glandulae mentales

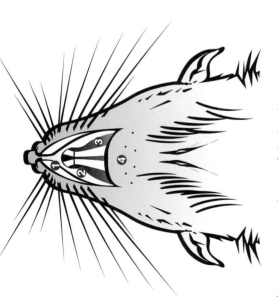

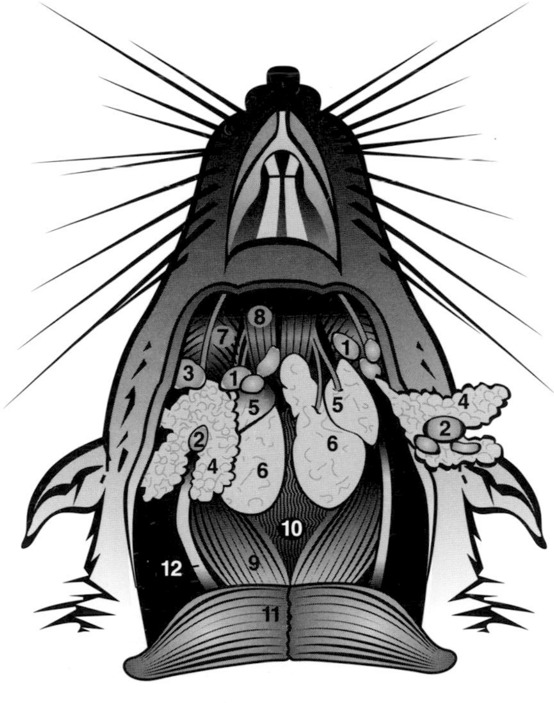

Figure 13.11 Subcutaneous organs of the ventral neck, ventral view (organa subcutanea colli ventralis, norma ventralis). **(See also Colour Plate 3.)**

1 lymphonodi mandibulares and deep underneath, close to the atlas lymphonodi retropharyngei
2 lymphonodi cervicales superficiales
3 glandula lacrimalis extraorbitalis
4 glandula parotis
5 glandula sublingualis major et ductus glandulae sublingualis and deep underneath glandula thyreoidea et parathyreoidea. Caudally to them lymphonodi cervicales craniales

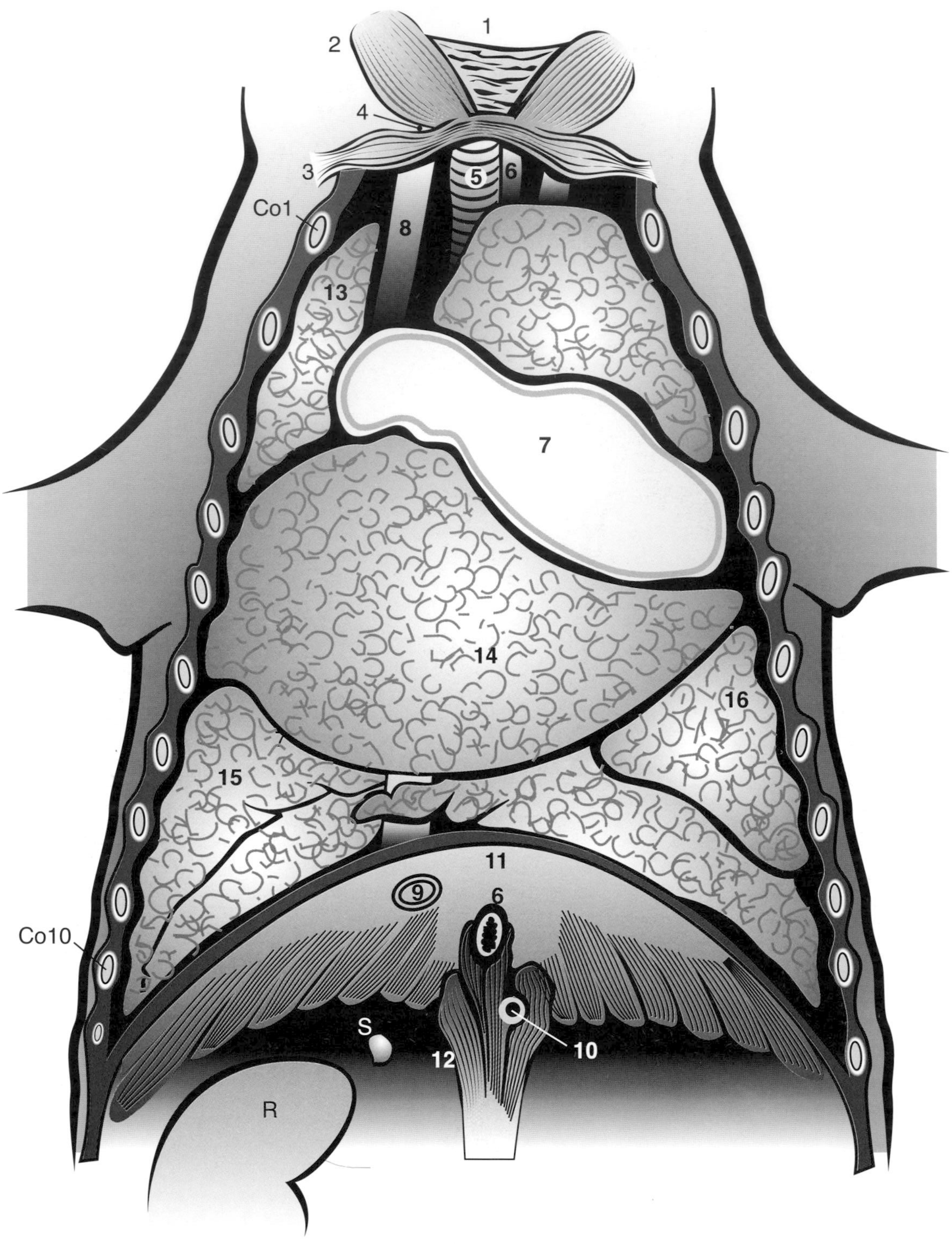

Figure 13.13 Ventral view at the thorax, after removal of the sternum and portions of the ribs.

1　platysma colli
2　musculus sternomastoideus
3　musculus pectoralis transversus
4　clavicula grown into musculus cleidobrachialis
5　trachea
6　esophagus et hiatus esophageus
7　open pericardium, adhering to the thoracic wall
8　vena cava cranialis dextra
9　vena cava caudalis et foramen venae cavae caudalis
10　hiatus aorticus

11　diaphragma, centrum tendineum
12　pars lumbalis diaphragmae
13　lobus cranialis pulmonis dextri
14　lobus accessorius pulmonis dextri
15　lobus caudalis pulmonis dextri
16　pulmo sinister (pars caudalis)
Co 1　costa prima
Co 10　costa decima (other ribs are out of the section level)
R　ren dexter
S　glandula adrenalis dextra

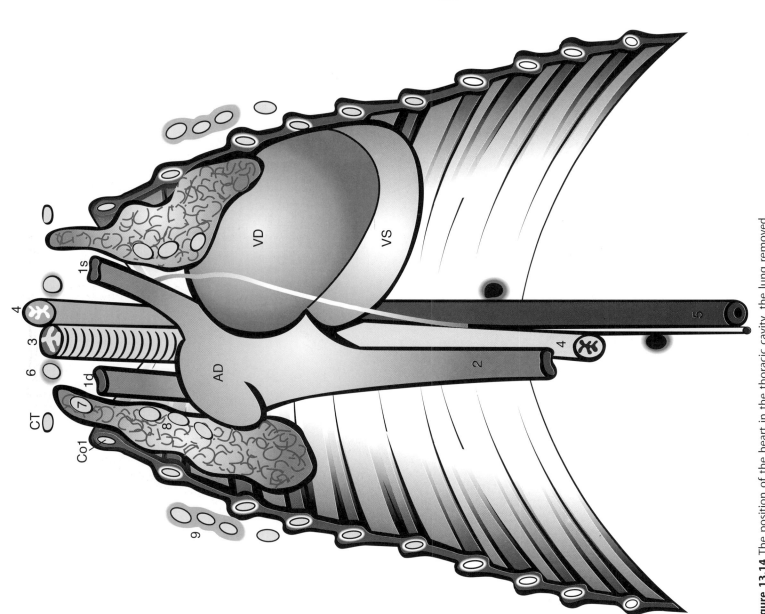

Figure 13.14 The position of the heart in the thoracic cavity, the lung removed.

Co 1 costa prima
CT   clavicula
1 d,s vena cava cranialis dextra et sinistra
2   vena cava caudalis
3   trachea
4   esophagus
5   aorta descendens et ductus thoracicus (leading to
      vena cava sinistra), lymphonodi aortici, usually small
6   lymphonodi sternales craniales

7   lymphonodi mediastinales ventrales
8   thymus et lymphonodi mediastinales dorsales (the
      thymus and the lymph nodes are displaced laterally,
      to uncover the heart basis over which they are
      normally located)
9   lymphonodi axillares proprii et accessorii
AD   atrium dextrum
VD   ventriculus dexter
VS   ventriculus sinister

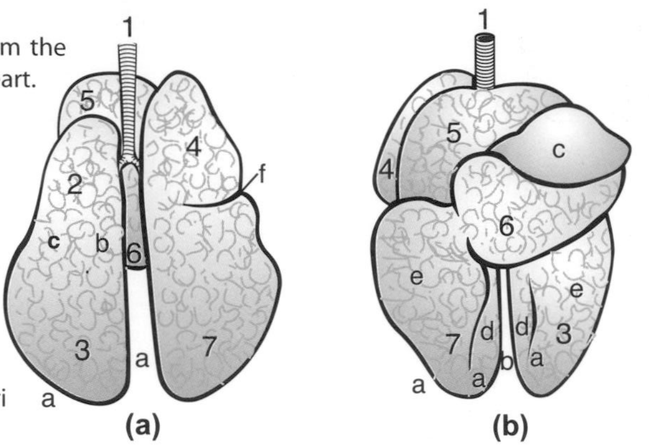

Figure 13.15 The lungs removed from the thoracic cavity, together with the heart.

A norma dorsalis
B norma ventralis
C cor
1 trachea
2 pulmo sinister (pars cranialis)
3 pulmo sinister (pars caudalis)
4 lobus cranialis pulmonis dextri
5 lobus medius (cardiacus) pulmonis dextri
6 lobus accessorius pulmonis dextri ('postcaval lobe', lobus azygos)
7 lobus caudalis pulmonis dextri
a margo acutus
b margo dorsalis (obtusus)
c facies costalis

d facies medialis
e facies diaphragmatica
f fissura interlobaris

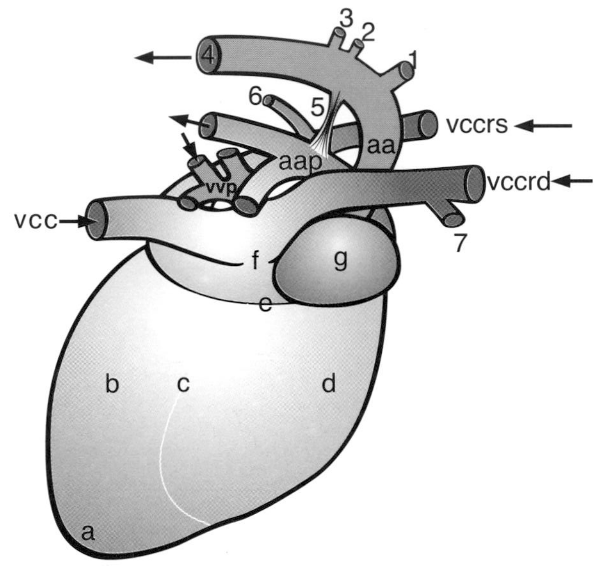

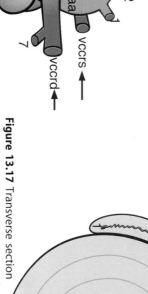

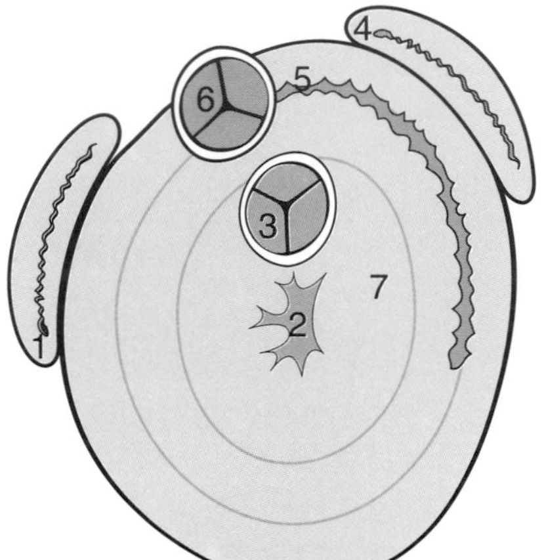

Figure 13.16 The heart, from the right side (cor, adspectus dexter).

a   apex cordis
aa   arcus aortae
aap   arteriae pulmonales
b   ventriculus sinister
c   sulcus interventricularis subsinuosus
d   ventriculus dexter
e   sulcus coronarius
f   sinus venarum cavarum et atrium dextrum
g   auricula dextra
vcc   vena cava caudalis
vccrd vena cava cranialis dextra
vccrs vena cava cranialis sinistra
vvp   venae pulmonales
1   truncus brachiocephalicus
2   arteria carotis communis sinistra
3   arteria subclavia sinistra
4   aorta thoracica
5   ligamentum arteriosum (Botalli)
6   vena azygos sinistra
7   vena subclavia dextra

Figure 13.17 Transverse section through the heart at the level of exits of large vessels.

1 cavum auriculae sinistrae
2 cavum ventriculi sinistri
3 ostium et valva aortae
4 cavum auriculae dextrae

5 cavum ventriculi dextri
6 ostium et valva trunci pulmonalis
7 septum interventriculare

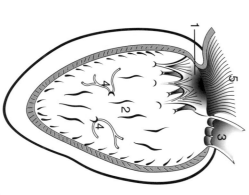

Figure 13.18 The heart, right ventricle opened (cor, ventriculus dexter apertus).

1 valva atrioventricularis dextra (tricuspidalis), ostium atrioventriculare dextrum shimmering through
2 septum interventriculare
3 ostium et valva trunci pulmonalis
4 trabeculae septomarginales
5 outer wall of the right ventricle, detached and deflected

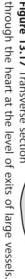

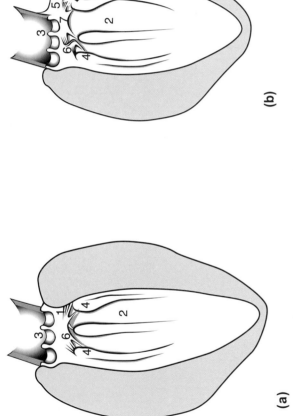

(a)

(b)

Figure 13.19a,b The heart, left ventricle cut open (cor, ventriculus sinister resectus).

1 valva atrioventricularis sinistra (bicuspidalis)
2 septum interventriculare
3 ostium et valva aortae
4 musculi papillares
5 ostium atrioventriculare sinistrum
6 cuspis parietalis
7 cuspis septalis

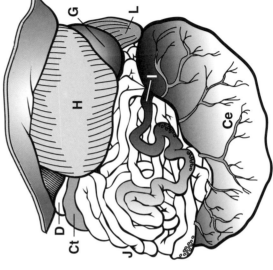

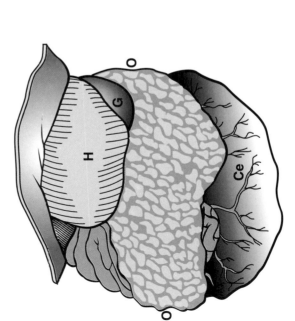

Figure 13.20 Ventral view of the abdominal cavity, superficial layer. Organs and tissues seen after opening the abdominal cavity.

Ce intestinum cecum
G gaster (ventriculus, stomach)
H hepar (liver)
O saccus omenti majoris (in well-nourished individuals exhibiting prominent adipose tissue located along the lymphatic vessels)

Figure 13.21 Ventral view of the abdominal cavity after removal of the omentum.

Ce cecum
Ct colon transversum
D duodenum
G gaster
H hepar
I ileum
J jejunum
L lien

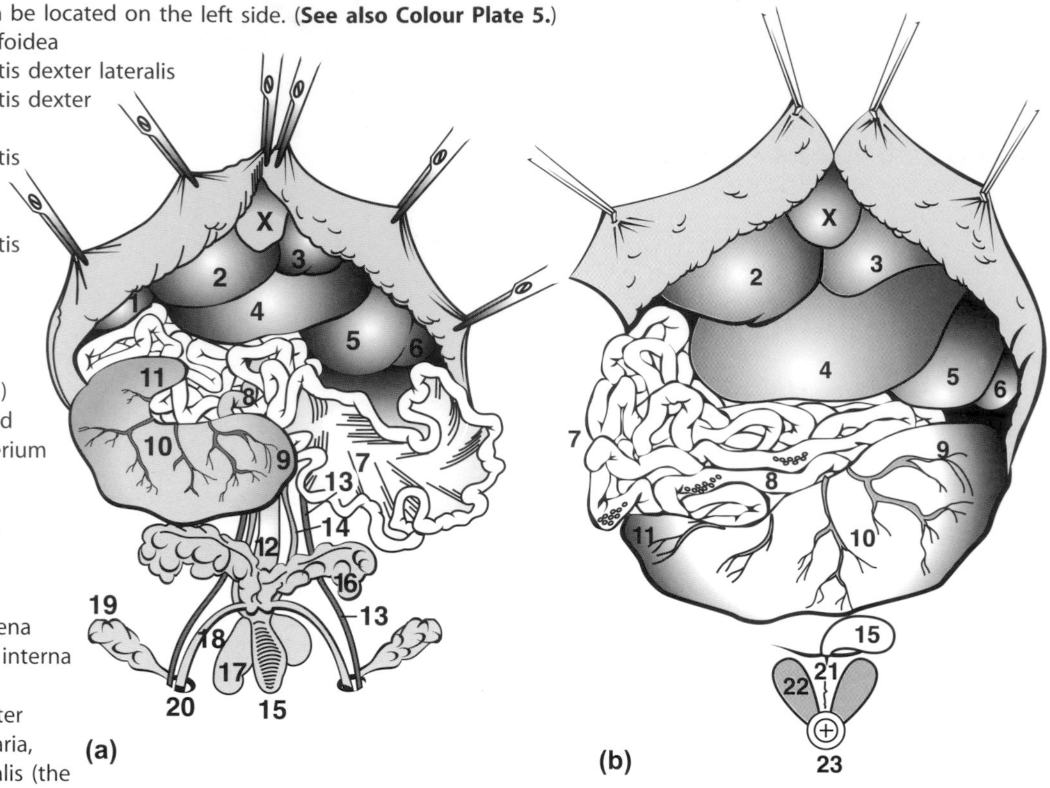

Figure 13.22a,b Ventral view of the abdominal cavity (XY), cecum in right (a) or central (b) position. In some instances the cecum can even be located on the left side. (**See also Colour Plate 5.**)

X   cartilago xifoidea
1   lobus hepatis dexter lateralis
2   lobus hepatis dexter medialis
3   lobus hepatis sinister medialis
4   lobus hepatis sinister lateralis
5   fundus ventriculi
6   lien (spleen)
7   jejunum and its mesenterium
8   ileum
9   basis ceci
10 corpus ceci
11 apex ceci
12 rectum
13 arteria et vena spermatica interna sinistra
14 ureter sinister
15 vesica urinaria, facies dorsalis (the urinary bladder is turned over caudally)
16 glandula vesicularis sinistra

(a)
17 prostata ventralis, lobus dexter
18 ductus deferens dexter
19 paniculus adiposus

(b)
20 canalis inguinalis dexter
21 symphysis pelvis
22 glandula preputialis
23 preputium

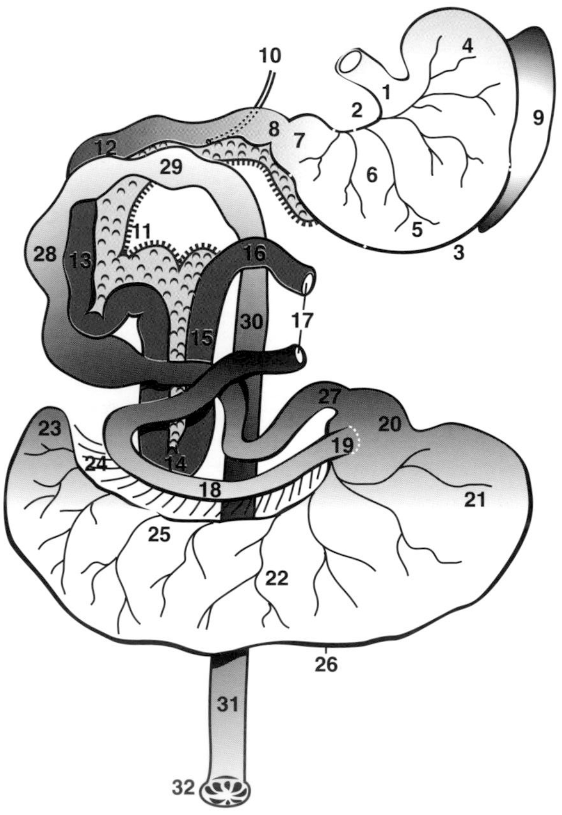

Figure 13.23 Ventral view of the gastrointestinal tract after removal of the jejunum.

1   esophagus et ostium cardiacum
2   curvatura ventriculi minor
3   curvatura ventriculi major
4   saccus cecus (proventriculus)
5   fundus ventriculi
6   corpus ventriculi
7   pars pylorica ventriculi
8   ostium pyloricum
9   lien (spleen)
10 ductus hepatoentericus (choledochus)
11 pancreas
12 flexura duodeni cranialis
13 pars descendens (duodeni)
14 flexura duodeni caudalis
15 pars ascendens (duodeni)
16 flexura duodenojejunalis
17 jejunum
18 ileum
19 ostium ileocecale
20 excavatio ceci
21 basis ceci
22 corpus ceci
23 apex ceci
24 ligamentum ileocecale
25 curvatura ceci minor
26 curvatura ceci major
27 ostium cecocolicum
28 colon ascendens (with fluid contents)
29 colon transversum (with solid contents)
30 colon descendens
31 rectum
32 anus

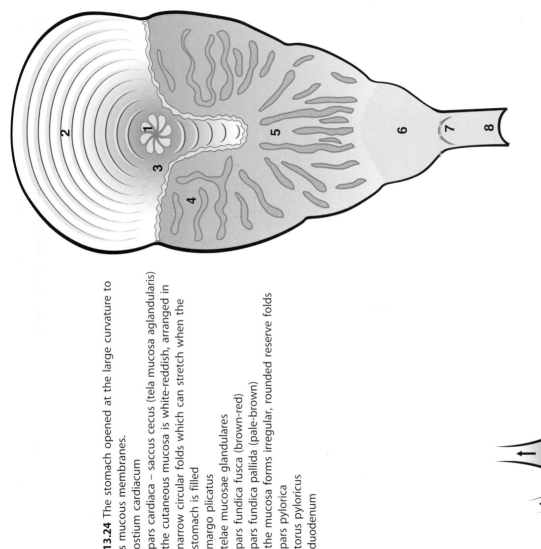

Figure 13.24 The stomach opened at the large curvature to show its mucous membranes.

1   ostium cardiacum
2   pars cardiaca – saccus cecus (tela mucosa aglandularis) the cutaneous mucosa is white-reddish, arranged in narrow circular folds which can stretch when the stomach is filled
3   margo plicatus
4,5,6 telae mucosae glandulares
4   pars fundica fusca (brown-red)
5   pars fundica pallida (pale-brown)
4,5   the mucosa forms irregular, rounded reserve folds
6   pars pylorica
7   torus pyloricus
8   duodenum

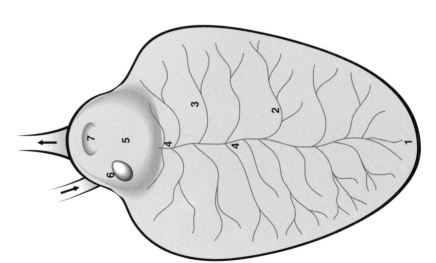

Figure 13.25 The cecum opened at the large curvature to show the mucous membrane.

1   apex ceci
2   corpus ceci
3   basis ceci
4   blood vessels, seen underneath the mucosa, arrive from the small curvature
5   excavatio ceci
6   ostium ileocecale
7   ostium cecocolicum

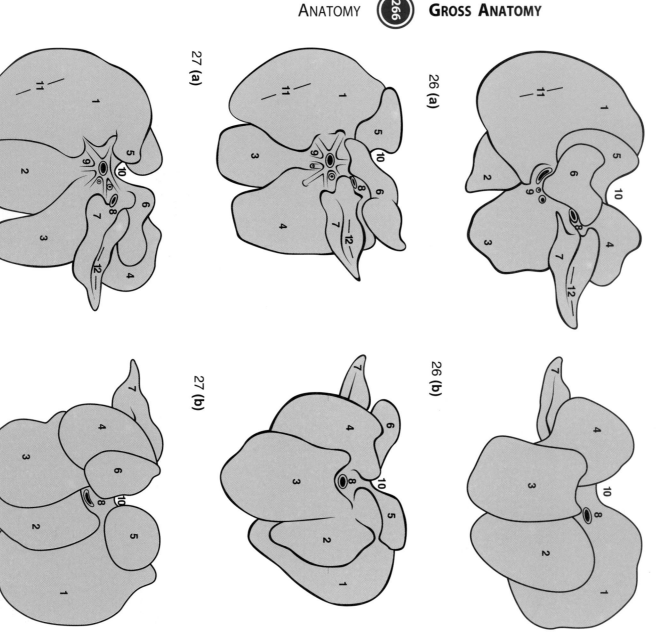

Figures 13.26–13.29 The liver. (a) Facies visceralis; (b) facies diaphragmatica. The rat does not possess a gall bladder so that the liver is connected to the duodenum by ductus choledochus (enterohepaticus). This series of figures demonstrates the great individual variation of hepatic lobulation in rats. Lobus quadratus is not described in rats.

1 lobus lateralis sinister
2 lobus medialis sinister
3 lobus medialis dexter
4 lobus lateralis dexter
5 processus papillaris pars preventricularis (lobus caudatus)
6 processus papillaris pars retroventricularis (lobus caudatus)
7 processus caudatus (lobus caudatus)

8 vena cava caudalis growths into the liver collecting venae hepaticae
9 at the porta hepatis, arteria hepatica and vena portae enter, and ductus hepatoentericus (hepaticus communis, choledochus) exits the liver
10 margo dorsalis with sulcus esophagicus (impressio esophagica)
11 on the facies visceralis lobi lateralis sinistri there is impressio gastrica
12 on the processus caudatus there is impressio renalis

26 (a)

26 (b)

27 (a)

27 (b)

28 (a)

28 (b)

Figures 13.26–29 (continued)

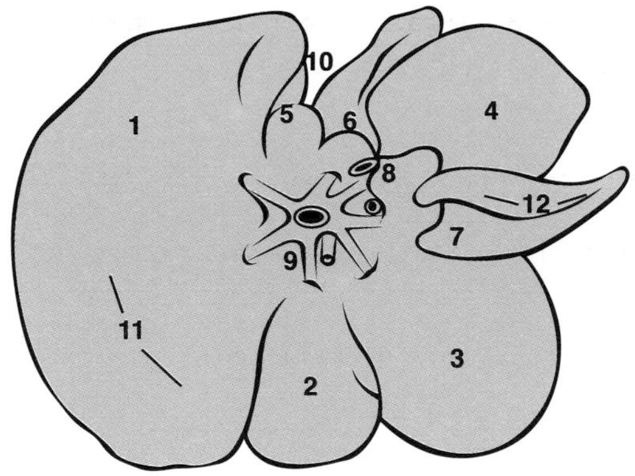

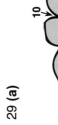

29 (a)

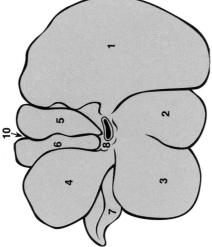

29 (b)

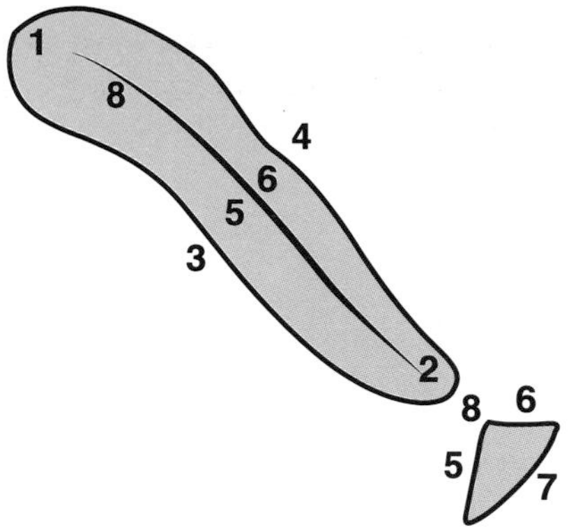

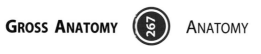

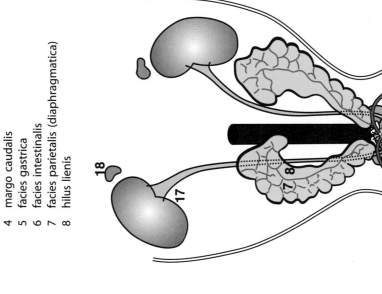

Figure 13.30 The spleen (lien) – visceral surface and transverse section (facies visceralis et sectio transversa lienis).

1 extremitas dorsalis
2 extremitas ventralis
3 margo cranialis
4 margo caudalis
5 facies gastrica
6 facies intestinalis
7 facies parietalis (diaphragmatica)
8 hilus lienis

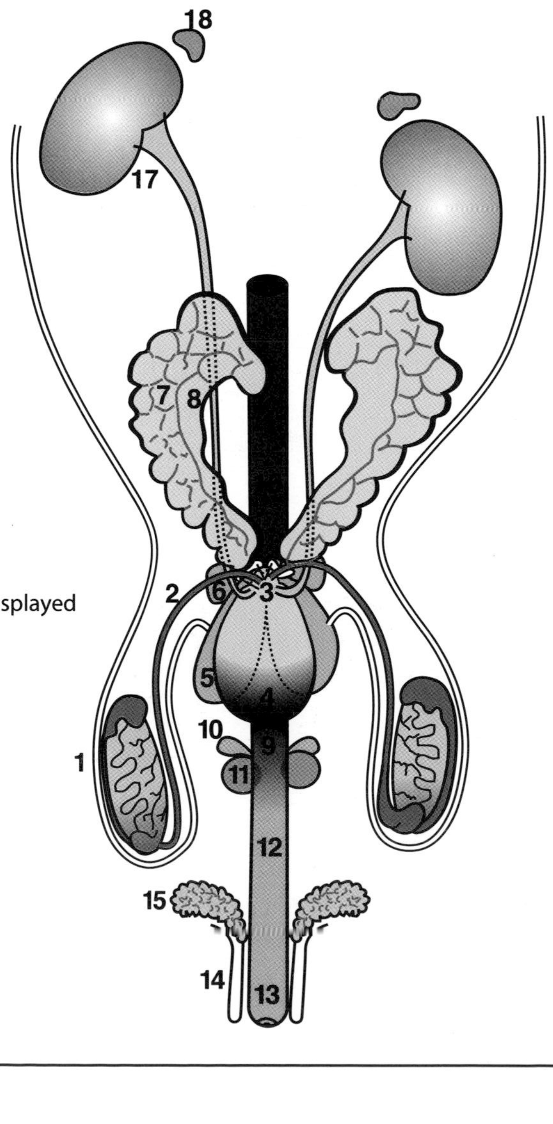

Figure 13.31 Ventral view of the male urogenital tract.

1 testis dexter in scroti
2 ductus deferens dexter
3 glandula ductus deferentis
4 vesica urinaria is turned over, so that the facies dorsalis is displayed
5 prostata ventralis
6 prostata dorsolateralis
7 glandula vesicularis
8 glandula coagulationis
9 musculus urethralis
10 glandula bulbourethralis
11 musculus bulbocavernosus
12 corpus penis
13 glans penis
14 preputium
15 glandula preputialis
16 rectum
17 ren dexter et ureter dexter
18 glandula suprarenalis dextra

Plate 13.32 Ventral view of the main blood vessels of the abdominal and pelvic cavity (XY). **(See also Colour Plate 6.)**

1 aorta abdominalis
2 arteriae phrenicae caudales (inferiores)
3 arteria suprarenalis cranialis (superior)
4 arteria celiaca
5 arteria et vena renalis
6 arteria et vena suprarenalis caudalis (inferior)
7 arteria mesenterica cranialis (superior)
8 arteria et vena testicularis have rami epididymales et ramus testicularis where the vein forms around the artery plexus pampiniformis (8')
9 arteria et vena iliolumbalis
10 arteria mesenterica caudalis
11 arteria et vena iliaca communis
12 arteria et vena iliaca interna
13 arteria et vena ductus deferentis
14 vena cava caudalis
15 venae caudalis
A hiatus aorticus
B foramen venae cavae caudalis
C glandula suprarenalis (adrenalis) sinistra
D ren sinister
E ureter sinister
F vesica urinaria
G ductus deferens sinister
H urethra

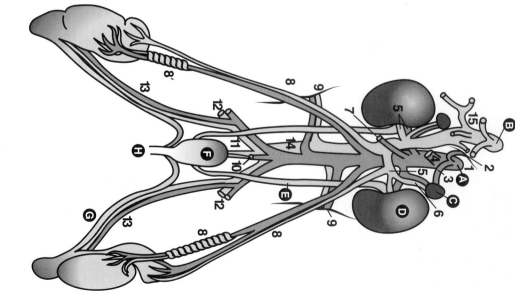

Figure 13.33 Location of the male genital organs viewed from the left.

1 testis dexter in scroti
2 ductus deferens dexter
3 glandula ductus deferentis
4 vesica urinaria
5 prostata ventralis
6 prostata dorsolateralis
7 glandula vesicularis
8 glandula coagulationis
9 musculus urethralis
10 glandula bulbourethralis
11 musculus bulbocavernosus
12 corpus penis
13 glans penis
14 preputium
15 glandula preputialis
16 rectum
S1 os sacrum

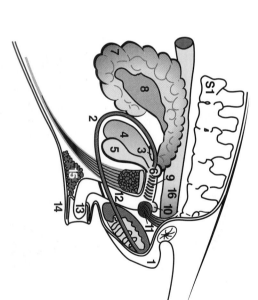

Figure 13.34 Testis in scrotum, dorsal view (testis in scroti, aspectus dorsalis).

1 testis dexter
2 caput epididymidis
3 corpus epididymidis
4 cauda epididymidis removed from the scrotum to demonstrate its relatively large size, obviously related to high fertility of rodents
5 ductus deferens dexter
6 funiculus spermaticus, arteria, vena et nervus spermaticus internus, et musculus cremaster internus
7 paniculus adiposus which maintains the widths of canalis inguinalis (8) and enables easy translocation of the testicle between the abdominal cavity and scrotum
8 canalis inguinalis
9 ligamentum testis proprium
10 mesorchium
11 septum scroti

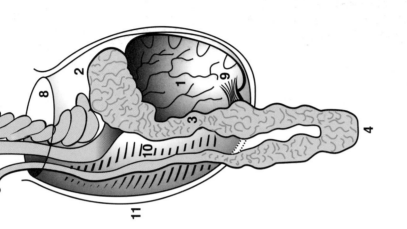

Figure 13.35 Glans nudus penis et crura penis ischiadica.

1 processus urethrae et orifitium urethrae externum
2 pars libera penis
3 lamina interna preputii
4 anulus preputialis
5 lamina externa preputii
6 cutis resecta
7 glandulae preputiales
8 corpus penis
9 crura penis attached to arcus ischiadicus (radix penis)
10 urethra entering the penis from the pelvic cavity

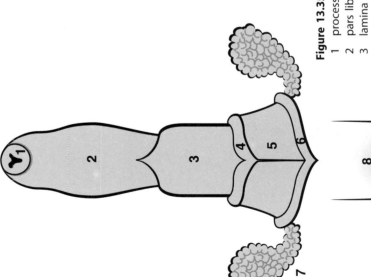

Figure 13.36 Ventral view of the main blood vessels of the abdominal and pelvic cavity (XX). **(See also Colour Plate 7.)**

1 aorta abdominalis
2 arteriae phrenicae caudales (inferiores)
3 arteria suprarenalis cranialis (superior)
4 arteria coeliaca
5 arteria et vena renalis
6 arteria et vena suprarenalis caudalis (inferior)
7 arteria et vena ovarica have ramus ovaricus, ramus tubarius et ramus uterinus
8 arteria et vena iliolumbalis
9 arteria et vena iliolumbalis
10 arteria mesentrica caudalis
11 arteria et vena iliaca communis
A hiatus aorticus
C glandula suprarenalis sinistra
D ren sinister
E ureter sinister
I ovarium sinistrum
J uterus

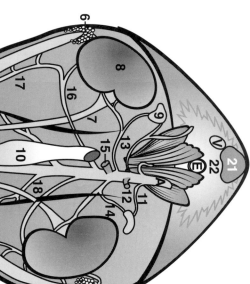

Figure 13.37 Ventral view of the abdominal cavity of a nonpregnant female. The gastrointestinal tract is removed and the veins are not depicted. **(See also Colour Plate 8.)**

1 rectum et anus
2 vesica urinaria, facies dorsalis – turned over, so that it covers introitus vaginae et clitoris
3 vagina
4 cervix uteri
5 uterus dexter
6 ovarium dextrum
7 ureter dexter
8 ren dexter
9 glandula suprarenalis (adrenalis) dextra
10 colon descendens
11 arteria suprarenalis cranialis sinistra
12 arteria celiaca
13 arteria renalis dextra
14 arteria suprarenalis caudalis sinistra
15 arteria mesenterica caudalis
16 arteria ovarica dextra
17 ramus uterinus dexter
18 arteria circumflexa ilium profunda
19 arteria mesenterica caudalis
20 arteria iliaca communis sinistra
21 cartilago xiphoidea
22 diaphragma
A aorta abdominalis
E hiatus esophagicus
V foramen venae cavae caudalis

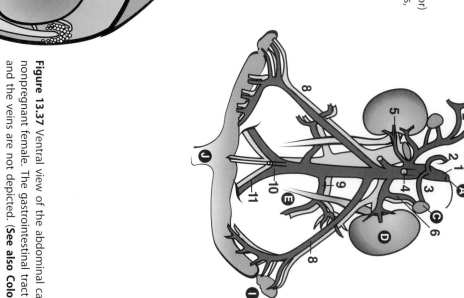

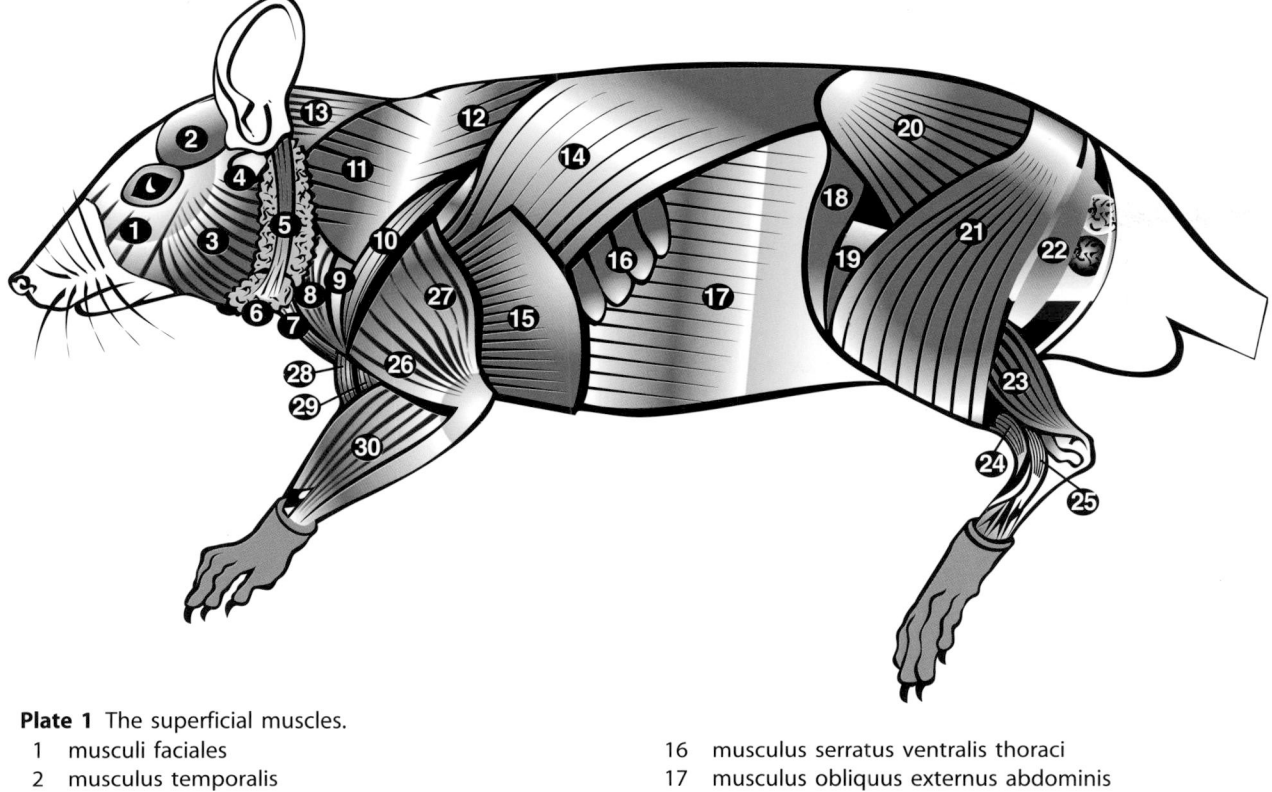

Plate 1 The superficial muscles.

1 musculi faciales
2 musculus temporalis
3 musculus masseter
4 glandula lacrimalis extraorbitalis
5 glandula parotidea with the ventral auricular muscle
6 glandula mandibularis
7 musculus sternocephalicus, pars mastoidea
8 musculus brachiocephalicus, pars occipitalis
9 musculus deltoideus, pars acromialis
10 musculus deltoideus, pars scapularis
11 musculus trapezius, pars cervicalis
12 musculus trapezius, pars thoracica
13 musculus cervicoauricularis
14 musculus latissimus dorsi
15 musculus cutaneus trunci

16 musculus serratus ventralis thoraci
17 musculus obliquus externus abdominis
18 musculus tensor fasciae latae
19 musculus quadriceps femoris, musculus rectus
20 musculus gluteus superficialis
21 musculus biceps femoris, portio cranialis et caudalis
22 musculus semitendinosus
23 musculus gastrocnemius, caput laterale
24 musculus tibialis cranialis
25 musculus extensor digitorum longus
26 musculus triceps brachii, caput laterale
27 musculus triceps brachii, caput longum
28 musculus biceps brachii
29 musculus brachialis
30 musculi extensores carpi et digitorum

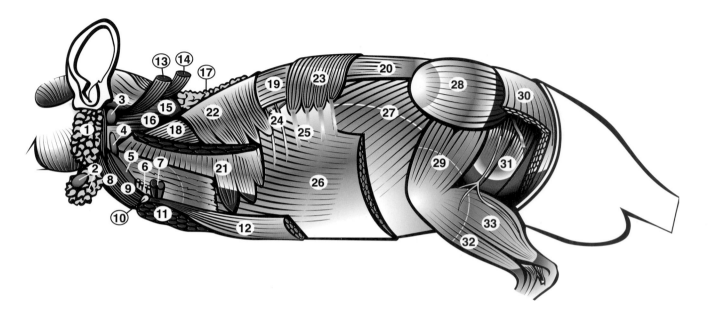

Plate 2 The deep muscles, forelimb removed.

1 glandula parotidea
2 glandula and lymphonodus mandibularis
3 lymphonodus retropharyngeus
4 lymphonodus cervicalis profundus
5 vena jugularis
6 plexus brachialis
7 arteria et vena subclavia
8 musculus sternocephalicus, pars mastoidea
9 musculus brachiocephalicus, pars occipitalis
10 clavicula
11 musculi pectorales
12 musculus rectus thoracis et abdominis
13 musculus rhomboideus capitis
14 musculus rhomboideus cervicis
15 musculus splenius
16 musculus longissimus capitis et atlantis
17 corpus adiposum nuchae (multivesiculare s. plurivacuolare s. hiberneticum)

18 musculus longissimus cervicis
19 musculus longissimus thoracis
20 musculus longissimus lumborum
21 musculus serratus ventralis (cervicis et thoracis)
22 musculus serratus dorsalis cranialis
23 musculus serratus dorsalis caudalis
24 musculus iliocostalis
25 musculi intercostales externi
26 musculus obliquus externus abdominis
27 musculus obliquus internus abdominis
28 musculus gluteus medius
29 musculus quadriceps femoris
30 musculus biceps femoris
31 musculus semimembranosus et semitendinosus
32 musculus tibialis cranialis
33 musculus triceps surae

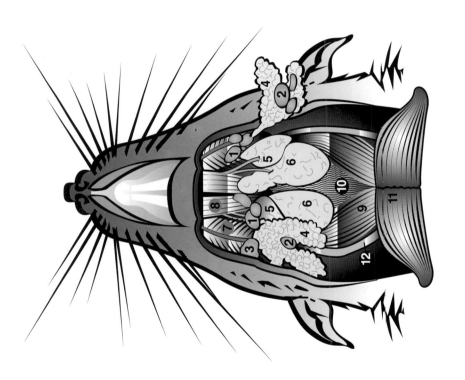

Plate 3 Subcutaneous organs of the ventral neck, ventral view (organa subcutanea colli ventralis, norma ventralis).

1 lymphonodi mandibulares and deep underneath, close to the atlas lymphonodi retropharyngei
2 lymphonodi cervicales superficiales
3 glandula lacrimalis extraorbitalis
4 glandula parotis
5 glandula sublingualis major et ductus glandulae sublingualis and deep underneath glandula thyreoidea et parathyreoidea. Caudally to them lymphonodi cervicales craniales
6 glandula mandibularis et ductus glandulae mandibularis (also called submandibular)
7 musculus masseter et ductus parotideus
8 venter rostralis musculi digastrici
9 musculus sternomastoideus
10 musculus sternohyoideus
11 musculus pectoralis major
12 vena jugularis externa dextra

Plate 4 Organs of the ventral neck, ventral view, deep layer (organa colli ventralis, norma ventralis, stratum profundum).

A lymphonodi mandibulares

B glandula sublingualis

C glandula mandibularis (submandibularis)

D glandula parotis et lymphonodus cervicalis superficialis

E glandula thyreoidea et parathyreoidea

F esophagus

G trachea

1 musculus sternohyoideus et sternothyreoideus (resectus)

2 musculus digastricus, venter rostralis

3 musculus mylohyoideus

4 musculus masseter et ductus parotideus

5 mandibula

6 musculus sternomastoideus

7 musculus omohyoideus

8 musculus pectoralis major

9 vena jugularis externa

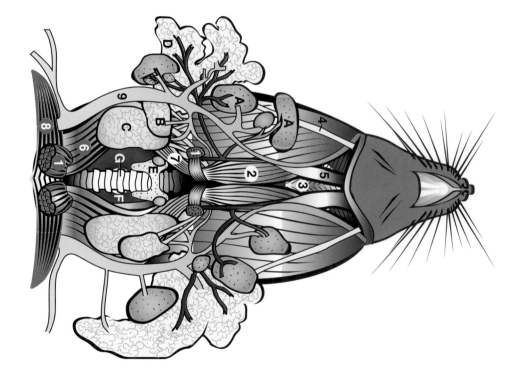

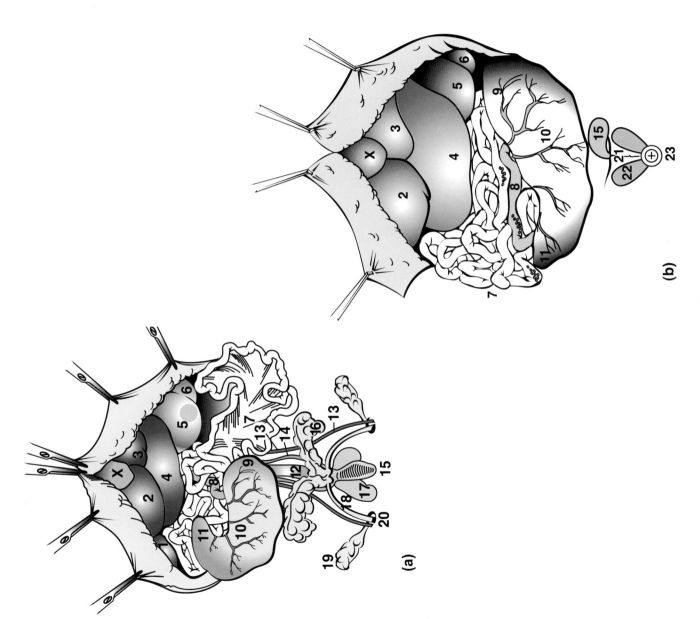

Plate 5 Ventral view of the abdominal cavity (XY), cecum in right (a) or central (b) position. In some instances the cecum can even be located on the left side.

X cartilago xifoidea
1 lobus hepatis dexter lateralis
2 lobus hepatis dexter medialis
3 lobus hepatis sinister medialis
4 lobus hepatis sinister lateralis
5 fundus ventriculi
6 lien (spleen)
7 jejunum and its mesenterium
8 ileum
9 basis ceci
10 corpus ceci
11 apex ceci
12 rectum

13 arteria et vena spermatica interna sinistra
14 ureter sinister
15 vesica urinaria, facies dorsalis (the urinary bladder is
     turned over caudally)
16 glandula vesicularis sinistra
17 prostata ventralis, lobus dexter
18 ductus deferens dexter
19 paniculus adiposus
20 canalis inguinalis dexter
21 symphysis pelvis
22 glandula preputialis
23 preputium

Plate 6 Ventral view of the main blood vessels of the abdominal and pelvic cavity (XY).

1   aorta abdominalis
2   arteriae phrenicae caudales (inferiores)
3   arteria suprarenalis cranialis (superior)
4   arteria celiaca
5   arteria et vena renalis
6   arteria et vena suprarenalis caudalis (inferior)
7   arteria mesenterica cranialis (superior)
8   arteria et vena testicularis have rami epididymales
    et ramus testicularis where the vein forms around
    the artery plexus pampiniformis (8')
9   arteria et vena iliolumbalis
10 arteria mesentrica caudalis
11 arteria et vena iliaca communis

12 arteria et vena iliaca interna
13 arteria et vena ductus deferentis
14 vena cava caudalis
15 venae hepaticae
A   hiatus aorticus
B   foramen venae cavae caudalis
C   glandula suprarenalis (adrenalis) sinistra
D   ren sinister
E   ureter sinister
F   vesica urinaria
G   ductus deferens sinister
H   urethra

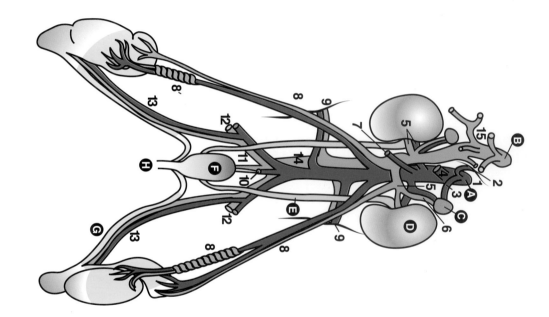

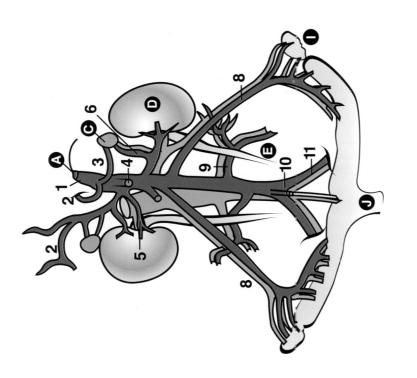

Plate 7 Ventral view of the main blood vessels of the abdominal and pelvic cavity (XX).

1 aorta abdominalis
2 arteriae phrenicae caudales (inferiores)
3 arteria suprarenalis cranialis (superior)
4 arteria coeliaca
5 arteria et vena renalis
6 arteria et vena suprarenalis caudalis (inferior)
8 arteria et vena ovarica have ramus ovaricus, ramus tubarius et ramus uterinus
9 arteria et vena iliolumbalis

10 arteria mesentrica caudalis
11 arteria et vena iliaca communis
A hiatus aorticus
C glandula suprarenalis sinistra
D ren sinister
E ureter sinister
I ovarium sinistrum
J uterus

Plate 8 Ventral view of the abdominal cavity of a nonpregnant female. The gastrointestinal tract is removed and the veins are not depicted.

1 rectum et anus
2 vesica urinaria, facies dorsalis – turned over, so that it covers introitus vaginae et clitoris
3 vagina
4 cervix uteri
5 uterus dexter
6 ovarium dextrum
7 ureter dexter
8 ren dexter
9 glandula suprarenalis (adrenalis) dextra
10 colon descendens
11 arteria suprarenalis cranialis sinistra
12 arteria celiaca

13 arteria renalis dextra
14 arteria suprarenalis caudalis sinistra
15 arteria mesenterica caudalis
16 arteria ovarica dextra
17 ramus uterinus dexter
18 arteria circumflexa ilium profunda
19 arteria mesenterica caudalis
20 arteria iliaca communis sinistra
21 cartilago xiphoidea
22 diaphragma
A aorta abdominalis
E hiatus esophagicus
V foramen venae cavae caudalis

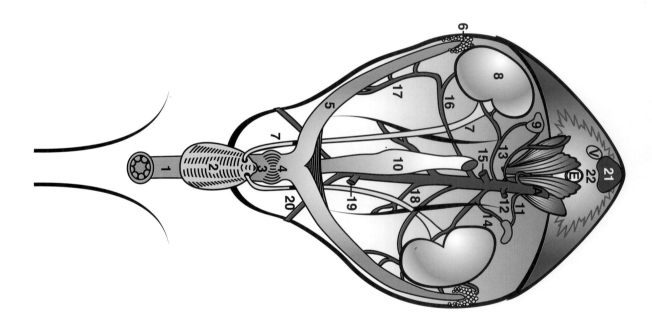

Figure 13.38 Vagina simplex, dorsal median section, dorsal view (vagina simplex, sectio mediana dorsalis, adspectus dorsalis).

1 introitus vaginae
2 corpus vaginae
3 portio vaginalis cervicis
4 canales cervicis uterorum et portio prevaginalis cervicis
5 uterus duplex
S uterus sinister
D uterus dexter

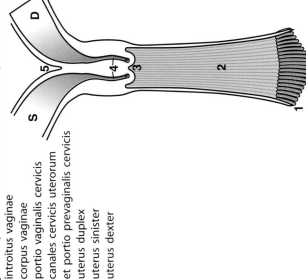

Figure 13.39 Position of the pregnant uterus, day 11 of pregnancy, view from the left.

L6 vertebra lumbalis VI
S os sacrum
1 anus
2 introitus vaginae
3 clitoris et ostium urethrae externum
4 glandulae clitoridis
5 symphysis pelvis et m. gracilis
6 rectum
7 vagina
8 cervix uteri
9 uterus sinister with embryos
10 ren sinister et ovarium cum oviducti
11 ureter sinister
12 vesica urinaria
13 urethra feminina et musculus urethralis

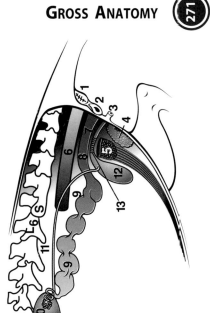

Figure 13.40 Shape of the abdomen of pregnant female, day 19 of pregnancy, ventral view with indication of the extent of the mammary gland. At this stage, the abdomen is the most voluminous part of the body. The abdominal cavity is mostly filled by the pregnant uterus, whereas the other organs, such as the intestines, stomach, spleen and liver are squeezed into the diaphragm. The gastrointestinal tract has little content. The body length of the animal used for this preparation is indicated, (0/21cm) as are the section levels of the following Figures 13.41–13.48 (41–48). These transverse sections are presented as caudal views.

A anus
B pudendum femininum
C clitoris et ostium urethrae externum

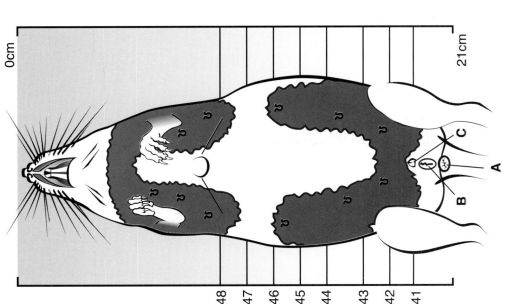

Figure 13.41 Transverse section at the level of the first caudal vertebrae (scale = 1 cm).

A rectum
B vagina
C urethra
D fascia et tela pelvis
1 muscles of the tail
2 musculus biceps femoris
3,4 musculi semitendinosus et semimembranosus
5 caudal muscles of the leg (extensors of the tarsus and flexors of the toes)
6 dorsal muscles of the leg (extensors of the toes and flexors of the tarsus)
7 muscle of the clitoris
8 ossa cruris (tibia and fibula grown together)

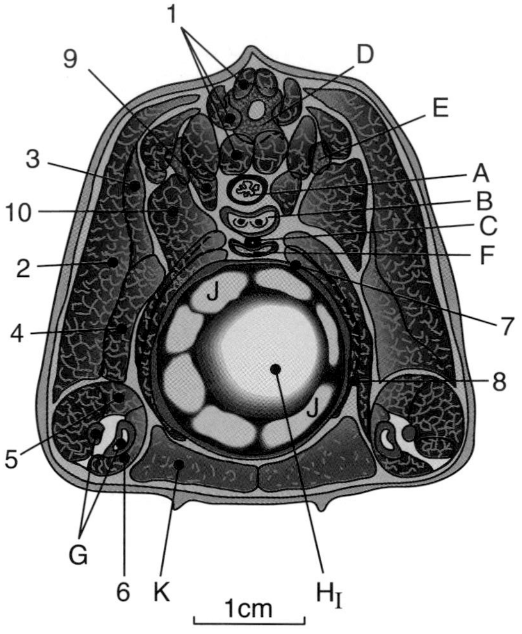

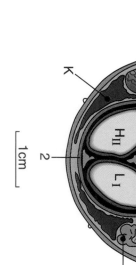

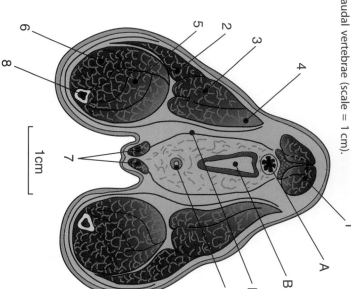

Figure 13.42 Transverse section at the level of the pelvis caudally to the acetabulum (scale = 1 cm).

A rectum
B cranial end of the vagina with opening of the left and right uterus (portio vaginalis cervicis – ostia uteri sinistri et dextri externa)
C urethra
D os sacrum
E os ischii
F symphysis pelvis
G ossa cruris
H_I uterus sinister (fetus I)

J paniculi adiposi
K mamma
1 dorsal, lateral and ventral muscles of the tail
2 musculus biceps femoris
3,4 musculi semitendinosus et semimembranosus
5 caudal muscles of the leg
6 dorsal muscles of the leg
7 abdominal wall
8 musculus gracilis
9 musculi obturatorii
10 musculus adductor

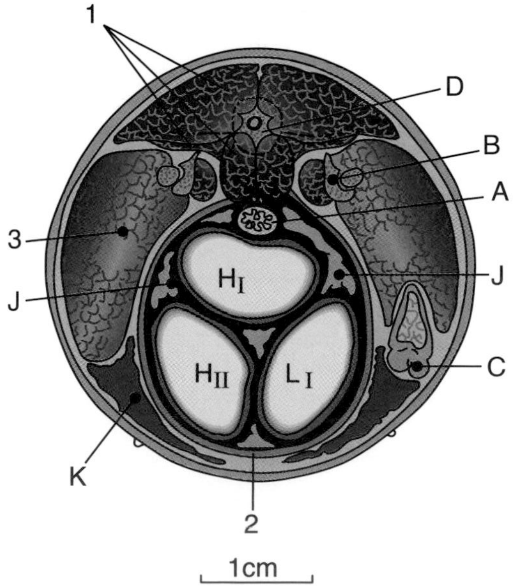

Figure 13.43 Transverse section at the level of acetabulum (scale = 1 cm).

A colon descendens
B articulatio coxae
C femur (epiphysis distalis)
D os sacrum
H_I uterus sinister (fetus I)
H_II uterus sinister (fetus II)
J paniculi adiposi
K mamma
L_I uterus dexter (fetus I)
1 dorsal, lateral and ventral muscles of the tail
2 abdominal wall
3 musculus quadriceps femoris

Figure 13.44 Transverse section 6 cm cranial to anus (scale = 1 cm).

A   colon descendens, above it are aorta abdominalis et vena cava caudalis
B   vertebra lumbalis surrounded by the long muscles of the vertebral column
D   abdominal wall
H   uterus sinister (fetus I, II, III)
J   paniculi adiposi
K   mamma
L   uterus dexter (fetus I)
M   placenta discoidea (disciformis)
S   intestinum

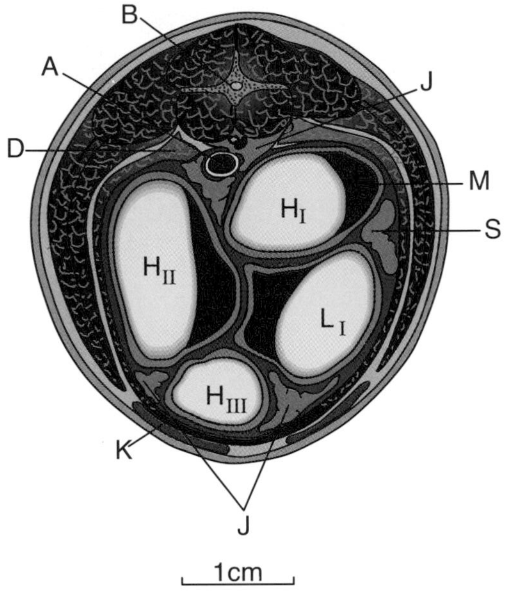

Figure 13.45 Transverse section 7.5 cm cranial to anus (scale = 1 cm).

A   colon descendens et flexura coli, above it are aorta abdominalis et vena cava caudalis
B   vertebra lumbalis
D   abdominal wall
H   uterus sinister (fetus III, IV, V)
J   paniculi adiposi
K   mamma
L   uterus dexter (fetus II, IV, V, VI)
M   placenta discoidea
S   intestinum tenue

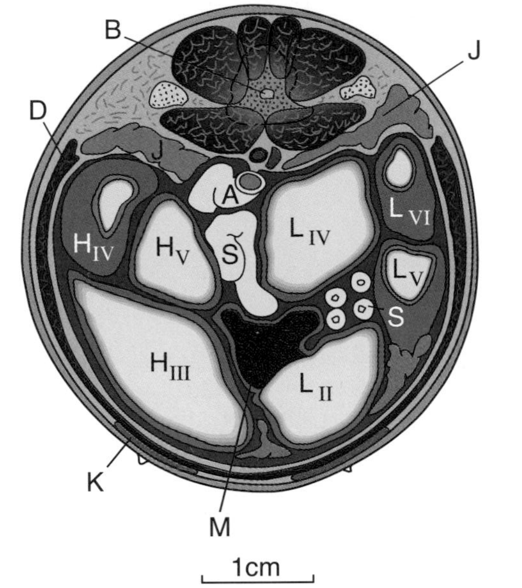

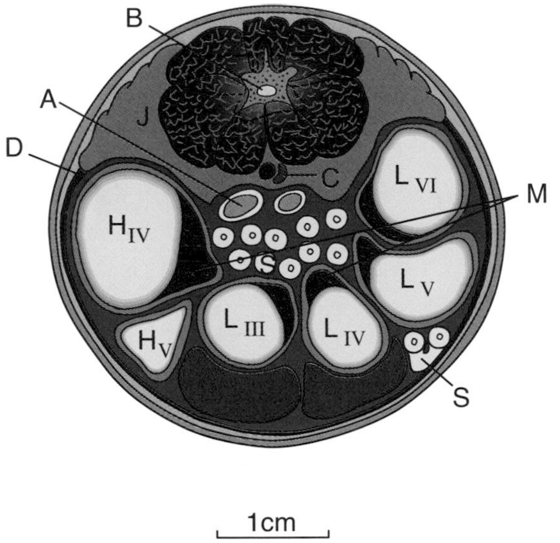

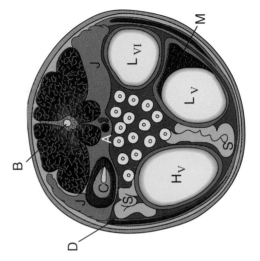

Figure 13.46 Transverse section 9 cm cranial to anus (scale = 1 cm).

A   colon transversum
B   vertebra lumbalis surrounded by the long muscles of the vertebral column
C   aorta descendens et vena cava caudalis
D   abdominal wall
H   uterus sinister (fetus IV, V)
J   paniculi adiposi
L   uterus dexter (fetus III, IV, V, VI)
M   placenta discoidea
S   intestinum tenue

Figure 13.47 Transverse section 10 cm cranial to anus, at the level of the left kidney (scale = 1 cm).

A   aorta descendens (abdominalis) et vena cava caudalis
B   vertebra lumbalis surrounded by the long muscles of the vertebral column
C   ren sinister
D   abdominal wall
H   uterus sinister (fetus V)
J   paniculi adiposi
L   uterus dexter (fetus V et VI)
M   placenta discoidea
S   intestinum tenue

Figure 13.48 Transverse section 11.3 cm cranial to anus, at the level of the right kidney (scale = 1 cm).

A aorta descendens (abdominalis) et vena cava caudalis

B first lumbar vertebra surrounded by the long muscles of the vertebral column

C abdominal wall

D ren dexter

E cecum

F colon transversum

G hepar

J paniculi adiposi

K mamma

L uterus dexter (fetus VI)

N gaster

O diaphragma

|___1cm___|

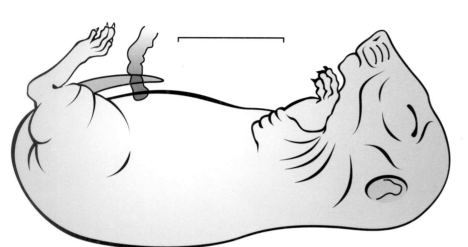

Figure 13.49 Uterus, day 20 of pregnancy, ventral view after opening the abdomen in the midline (scale = 5 cm).

A cartilago xiphoidea

B lobi hepatici

C intestinum tenue

D intestinum cecum, detached and removed

E paniculus adiposus

UD uterus dexter (contains 5 fetuses, 1 XX and 4 XY)

US uterus sinister (contains 8 fetuses, 4 XX and 4 XY)

The arrows are directed towards the head of each fetus; the heads are mostly, but not always directed to the vagina.

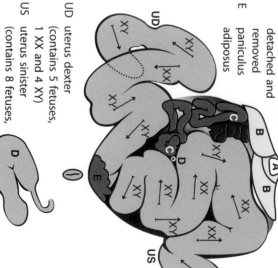

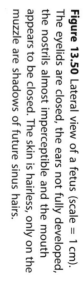

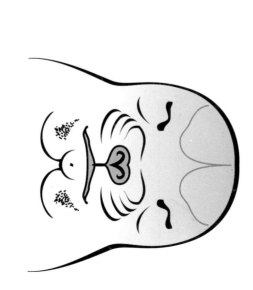

Figure 13.50 Lateral view of a fetus (scale = 1 cm). The eyelids are closed, the ears not fully developed, the nostrils almost imperceptible and the mouth appears to be closed. The skin is hairless, only on the muzzle are shadows of future sinus hairs.

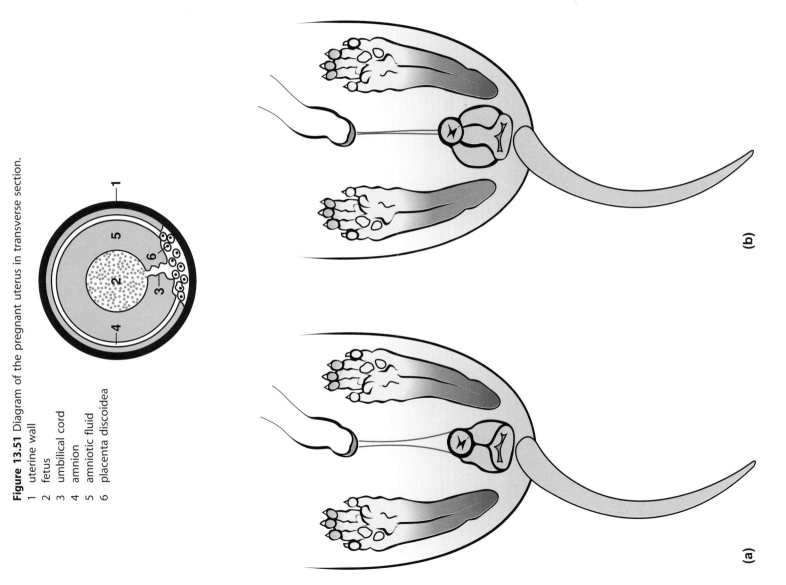

Figure 13.51 Diagram of the pregnant uterus in transverse section.

1 uterine wall
2 fetus
3 umbilical cord
4 amnion
5 amniotic fluid
6 placenta discoidea

Figure 13.52a,b Sexual differentiation. In males (a) the distance between the anus and preputium is shorter (about 2 mm) than in females (b) (about 3 mm). Moreover, in females the labia and the introitus vaginae are indicated.

(a)

(b)

CHAPTER 14

Imaging

Peter R Allegrini
Novartis Pharma AG, Basel, Switzerland

Introduction

For the images in this chapter magnetic resonance imaging (MRI) was performed on a 4.7-Tesla 30-cm-bore Spectrospin DBX (Bruker, Karlsruhe, Germany) equipped with a 20-cm actively shielded gradient system (max. 100 mT/m; rise time < 250 µs). The animal's body was positioned either with the head in a 35-mm resonator or the entire animal in a 72-mm birdcage resonator.

Longitudinal whole-body images were acquired in three parts, i.e. lower abdomen, abdomen and chest, with a T_2 weighted multislice SE sequence. The imaging parameters were as follows: slices with a thickness of 2.5 mm, field of view (FOV) 100 mm, echo time, 55 ms, repetition time 1.660 ms. The total measuring time was 3×29 minutes. The data

matrix of 512×256 pixel was zero-filled to 512^2 pixel before Fourier transformation, resulting in the in-plane spatial resolution of $195 \,\mu m \times 195 \,\mu m^2$.

For transverse and longitudinal head images one imaging cycle was applied, respectively, in which T_2-weighted slices of the brain were taken using a multislice spin echo sequence. The imaging parameters were as follows: slice thickness 1.2 mm, FOV 35 mm, repetition time 2.150 ms and 1.330 ms respectively, echo time 55 ms. The data matrix of 512×256 pixel was zero-filled to 512^2 pixel before Fourier transformation, resulting in the in-plane spatial resolution of $78 \,\mu m \times 78 \,\mu m^2$. The total measuring time was 73 and 45 minutes, respectively.

MR images were displayed with the image analysis software Analyze® (CNSoftware, Southwater, UK) on a Silicon Graphics 02 computer for presentation.

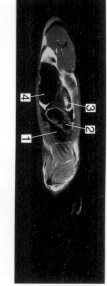

Figure 14.1 Longitudinal view of the body.
1 liver
2 stomach
3 left kidney
4 cecum

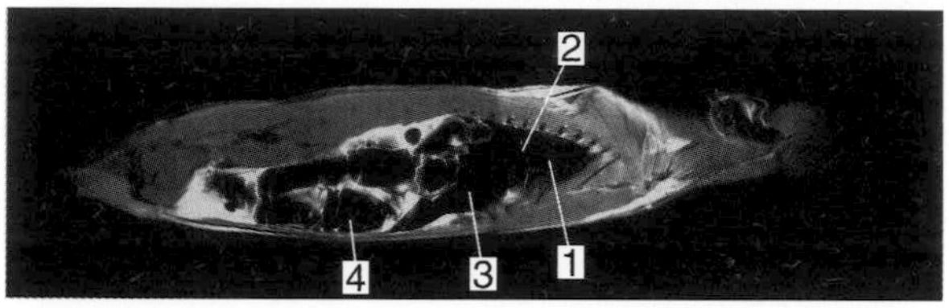

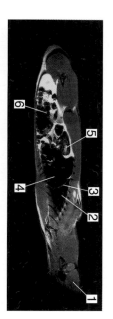

Figure 14.2 Longitudinal view of the body.
1 lung
2 diaphragm
3 liver
4 cecum

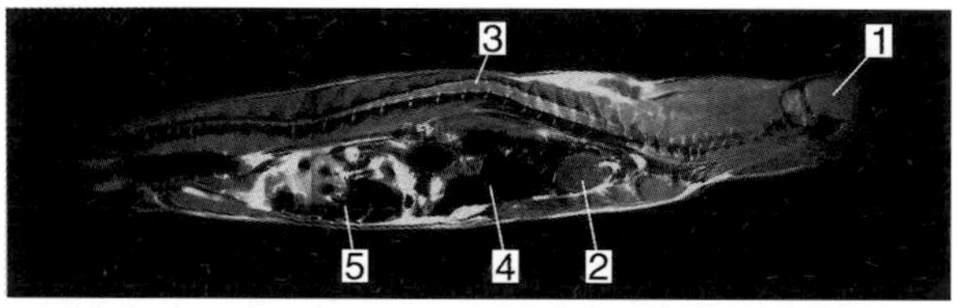

Figure 14.3 Longitudinal view of the body.
1 brain
2 heart
3 spinal cord
4 liver
5 liver

Figure 14.4 Longitudinal view of the body.
1 brain
2 lung
3 diaphragm
4 liver
5 right kidney
6 intestinal tract

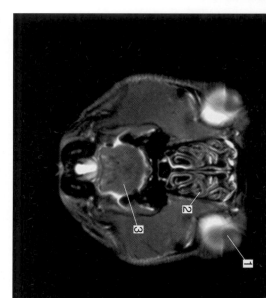

Figure 14.5 Transverse view of the head.
1 eye
2 nasal cavity
3 tongue

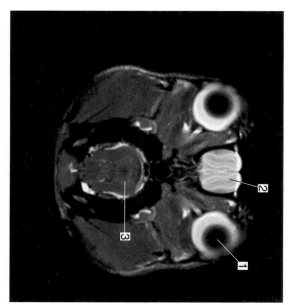

Figure 14.6 Transverse view of the head.
1 eye
2 bulbus olfactorius
3 tongue

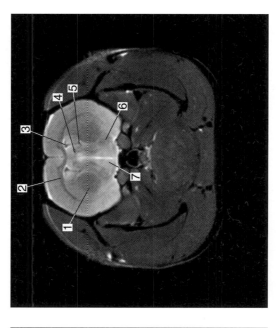

Figure 14.7 Transverse view of the head.

1 optic nerve   3 frontal cerberal
2 fissura rhinalis   hemisphere

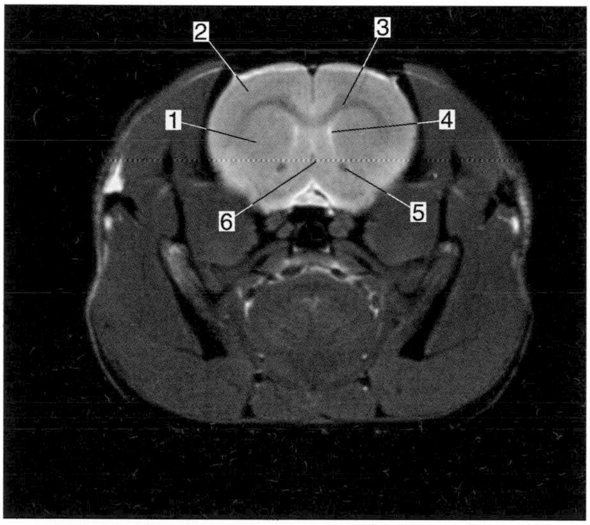

Figure 14.8 Transverse view of the head.

1 basal ganglia   4 lateral cerebral
  (caudatoputamen)   ventricle
2 frontal cortex   5 commissura anterior
3 corpus callosum   6 area parolfactoria

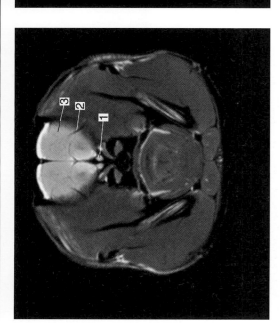

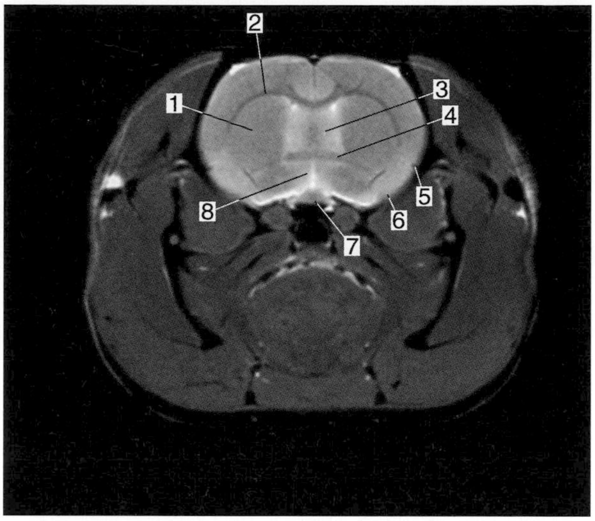

Figure 14.9 Transverse view of the head.

1 basal ganglia   5 fissura rhinalis
  (caudatoputamen)   6 cortex piriformis
2 corpus callosum   7 chiasma opticum
3 septum   8 area preoptica
4 commissura anterior

Figure 14.10 Transverse view of the head.

1 basal ganglia   4 septum
  (caudatoputamen)   5 stria medullaris thalami
2 corpus callosum   6 fasciculus medialis
3 lateral cerebral   telencephali
  ventricle   7 anterior hypothalamus

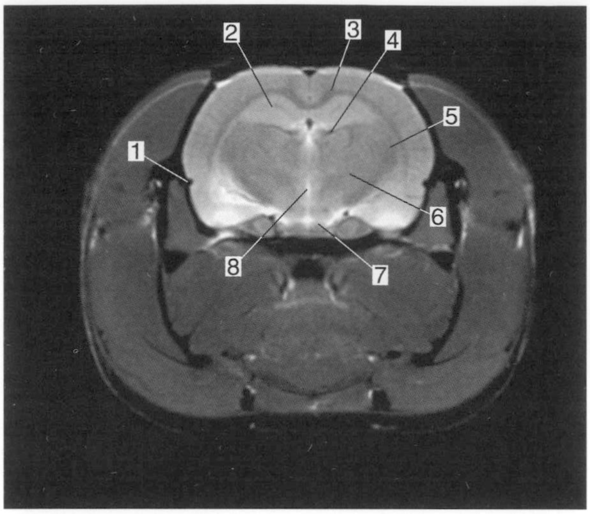

Figure 14.11 Transverse view of the head.

1	fissura rhinalis	5	thalamus
2	dorsal hippocampus	6	lemniscus medialis
3	corpus callosum	7	hypothalamus
4	stria medullaris thalami	8	3rd cerebral ventricle

Figure 14.13 Transverse view of the head.

1	fissura rhinalis	6	corpus geniculatum mediale
2	tegmentum mesencephali	7	pedunculus cerebri
3	hippocampus	8	nucleus interpeduncularis
4	colliculus superior	9	pituitary gland
5	substantia grisea centralis	10	trigeminal root

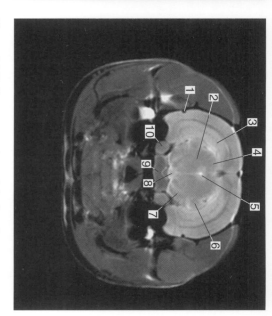

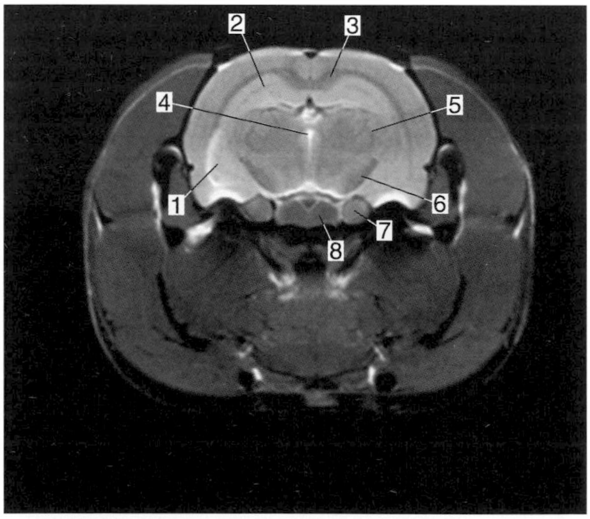

Figure 14.12 Transverse view of the head.

1	ventral hippocampus	5	thalamus
2	dorsal hippocampus	6	pedunculus cerebri
3	corpus callosum	7	trigeminal nerve
4	3rd cerebral ventricle	8	pituitary gland

Figure 14.14 Transverse view of the head.

1	raphe	6	formatio reticularis
2	fissura rhinalis	7	pedunculus cerebellaris
3	colliculus inferior		medius and trigeminal root
4	colliculus superior	8	pons and tractus corticospinalis
5	aqueductus cerebri		

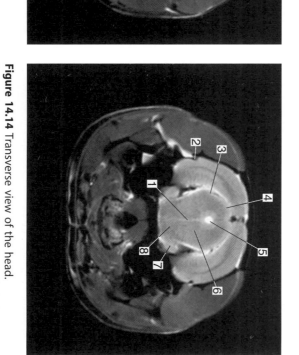

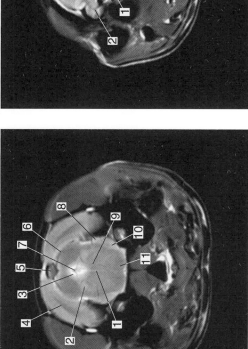

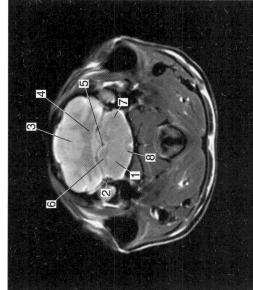

Figure 14.15 Transverse view of the head.

1 raphe
2 pedunculus cerebellaris superior
3 substantia grisea centralis
4 occipital cortex
5 pineal body
6 colliculus inferior
7 aqueductus cerebri
8 pedunculus cerebellaris medius
9 formatio reticularis
10 spinal trigeminal root
11 tractus corticospinalis

Figure 14.17 Transverse view of the head.

1 reticular nuclei
2 paraflocculus
3 deep cerebellar nuclei
4 cerebellar cortex
5 4th cerebral ventricle
6 spinal trigeminal tract and nucleus
7 corticospinal tract

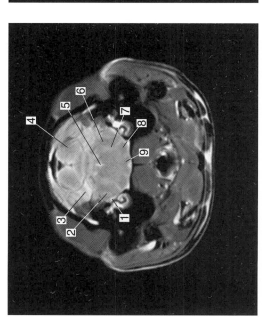

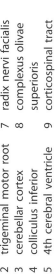

Figure 14.16 Transverse view of the head.

1 spinal trigeminal root
2 trigeminal motor root
3 cerebellar cortex
4 colliculus inferior
5 4th cerebral ventricle
6 trigeminal motor nucleus
7 radix nervi facialis
8 complexus olivae superioris
9 corticospinal tract

Figure 14.18 Transverse view of the head.

1 reticular nuclei
2 spinocerebellar tract
3 cerebellar cortex
4 deep cerebellar nuclei
5 4th cerebral ventricle
6 vestibular nuclei
7 spinal trigeminal tract and nucleus
8 corticospinal tract

Figure 14.19 Transverse view of the head.

1 raphe
2 cerebellar cortex
3 4th cerebral ventricle
4 cuneate nucleus and fascicle
5 spinal trigeminal root and nucleus
6 corticospinal tract

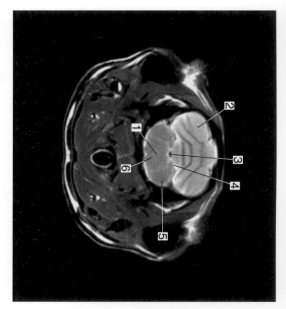

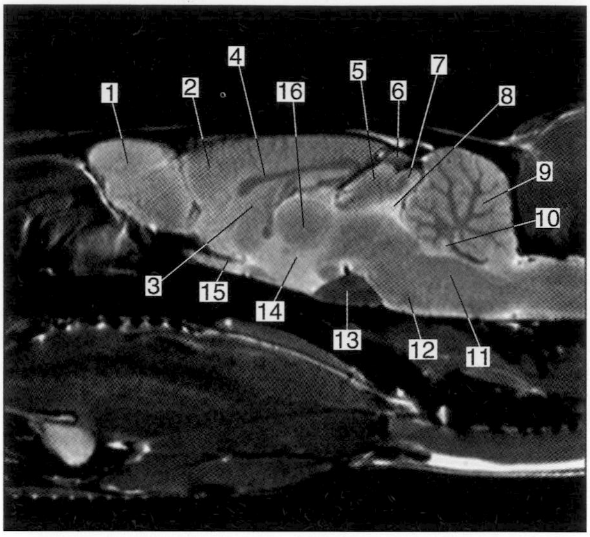

Figure 14.20 Mid-longitudinal view of the head.

1 bulbus olfactorius
2 cerebral cortex
3 septum
4 corpus callosum
5 colliculus anterior
6 pineal body
7 colliculus posterior
8 aqueduct
9 cerebellum
10 4th cerebral ventricle
11 medulla oblongata
12 pons
13 pituitary gland
14 3rd cerebral ventricle
15 optic nerve
16 thalamus

CHAPTER 15

Synopsis of the Organ Anatomy

Vladimír Komárek
Agricultural University, Prague, Czech Republic

Christian Gembardt
BASF AG, Ludwigshafen, Germany

Anneliese Krinke
PATHEV, Frenkendorf, Switzerland

Talaat A Mahrous
Novartis Crop Protection AG, Stein, Switzerland

Philippe Schaetti
Novartis Crop Protection AG, Stein, Switzerland

Introduction

This synopsis provides concise descriptions of particular organs arranged in alphabetical order. The descriptions are focused on features characteristic for the rat. They are based mostly on the data presented by Olds and Olds (1979), Hebel and Stromberg (1986), Boorman et al. (1990a), Mohr et al. (1992, 1994), and supplemented by selected references and personal observations. For the description of bilateral organs the word 'paired' is consistently used. Bilaterally symmetrical organs, however, such as the brain, nasal cavity, etc., are not considered as 'paired'. Morphological features relevant for organ function are also addressed in great detail in the physiology chapters of this book. The anatomical nomenclature used for description of lobes and portions of the organs such as the liver, lung, pancreas etc. differs from author to author. This synopsis includes synonyms and compares organ subdivisions in order to facilitate the understanding of other texts. We suggest that the terms selected by the International Veterinary Anatomical Nomenclature should be used, although this nomenclature was not established for rodents (Schaller, 1992).

In addition to the morphological characteristics of young, healthy individuals, some characteristic spontaneous changes and changes related to aging are described as well. The spontaneous and aging changes cannot always be discriminated, since a variety of changes known to occur increasingly with age can be encountered in adolescent or young adult individuals (Dixon et al., 1995). Artefactual postmortem changes (autolysis) were described by Seaman (1987). Proliferative and neoplastic lesions, albeit commonly related to advanced age, have been exempted. There are a number of excellent publications dealing with rat hyperplasia and neoplasia (Greaves and Faccini, 1984; Boorman et al., 1990a; Stinson et al., 1990; Turusov and Mohr, 1990; Bannasch and Gössner, 1994, 1997; Mohr 1997). The incidences of spontaneous neoplasms for different rat strains have been published: for the Fischer rat by Boorman et al. (1990a) and Stinson et al. (1990); for the Sprague-Dawley by Chandra et al. (1992) and McMartin et al. (1992); and for the Wistar by Bomhard (1992), Bomhard and Rinke (1994), Walsh and Poteracki (1994), and Poteracki and Walsh (1998). Furthermore, there is a computerized information system providing internationally approved diagnostic criteria, illustrations, references and incidence data. This system, called RENI, was developed at the Fraunhofer Institute of Toxicology and Aerosol research in Hannover, Germany, in cooperation with RITA – Registry of Industrial Toxicology Animal-data (Morawietz et al., 1992). The RENI Web Site is at: http://www.ita.fhg.de/reni.

All the photographs in Figures 15.1–15.87 show hematoxylin and eosin-stained paraffin sections, except where noted otherwise.

Adrenal Gland (Glandula Suprarenalis, Glandula Adrenalis) (Figure 15.1)

The paired adrenal glands lie within the retroperitoneal fat tissue cranially to the kidneys. According to Hebel and Stromberg (1986), there is a shape difference between the right (bean-like) and left (ovoid) one, and there is a sexual difference in the size of the organ: the relative weight of both cortex and medulla is higher in females than in males. The organ is covered by a connective tissue capsule and consists of two parts: cortex and medulla. In the center of the medulla lies the central vein. The medulla is totally covered by the cortex, but around the central vein which runs to the hilus, medullary cells can be scattered. The cortex consists of an outer zona glomerulosa, an intermediate zona fasciculata and an inner zona reticularis. Their denomination indicates the pattern of their cell arrangement. Their size changes with age and varies individually, but the zona fasciculata is generally the widest zone. The arterial supply is provided by capsular vessels which run into the arterial plexus in the zona glomerulosa, or penetrate the medulla. The medulla is composed of polyhedral (secretory) cells, among which different nerve cells and fibers are occasionally encountered. Adrenal medullary cells are often referred to as chromaffin cells since the oxidation of their catecholamine-containing secretory granules by chromate solutions results in red-brown coloration (Hamlin and Banas, 1990).

In the aged rats the following, spontaneously occurring changes can be seen (Tischler and Coupland, 1994; Yarrington and Johnston, 1994): thickening of the capsule due to proliferation of collagen, accumulation of lipid droplets in the cortical cells which may vary depending on strain and possibly sex, but which generally declines after 600 days in the Wistar rat. There is also formation of dilated blood-filled sinuses and cysts lined by endothelium occasionally containing thrombi (commonly found in females), occurrence of focal changes in the adrenal cortex which can show tinctorial differences or hypertrophy of the cortical cells, accumulation of lipogenic pigment (lipofuscin, ceroid), and diffuse or nodular hyperplasia of the medulla.

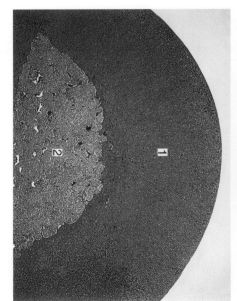

Figure 15.1 Adrenal gland.
1 cortex   2 medulla

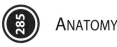

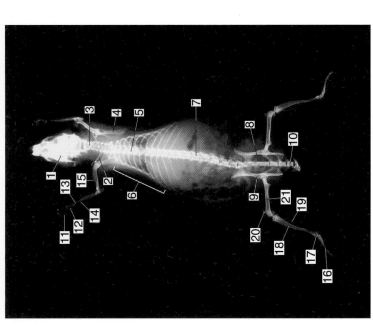

Figure 15.3b Skeleton.

1	cranium	11	metacarpus
2	clavicula	12	carpus
3	vertebrae cervicales	13	radius
4	scapula	14	ulna
5	vertebrae thoracicae	15	humerus
6	costae	16	metatarsus
7	columna vertebralis	17	tarsus
8	vertebrae sacrales (os sacrum)	18	tibia
9	pelvis	19	fibula
10	vertebrae caudales (coccygeae)	20	patella
		21	femur

Bone (Os) (Figures 15.3 and 15.4)

The structure of rat bones is similar to that of other mammalian species. A notable exception is that the cartilaginous growth plates (physes) of long bones are not totally resorbed in the rat. The physis is divided into zones which, from the epiphyseal side to the metaphyseal side, are termed resting, proliferative, hypertrophic and mineralizing. The zone of ossification in the proximal metaphysis (primary spongiosa) is the site where cartilage is resorbed and replaced by osteoid (Leininger and Riley, 1990).

Usually, histological evaluation of rat bone tissue is done on the femur together with the knee joint, sternum and vertebrae. Occasionally, fibrous osteo-dystrophy occurs and is associated with renal disease and secondary hyperparathyroidism; these changes taken together form the osteo-renal syndrome.

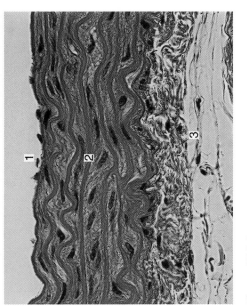

Figure 15.2 Aorta.

1 lumen, lined by   2 media, with wavy elastic fibers
intima   3 adventitia

Aorta (Figure 15.2)

The aorta is the largest artery in the body. Originating in the heart, its ascending portion, still in the pericardium, gives rise to the right and left coronary arteries. After penetrating the pericardium, the aorta forms an aortic arch giving rise to the following branches: innominate artery (arteria anonyma or truncus brachiocephalicus, branching further into the right subclavian and right common carotid arteries), the left common carotid and the left subclavian artery. It then turns downwards as the descending portion. The wall is composed of three layers: the intima with an endothelial lining, the thick media formed predominantly by elastic fibers with muscle fibers, and the adventitia.

Mural mineralization associated with osteo-renal syndrome is occasionally found spontaneously (Lewis, 1992).

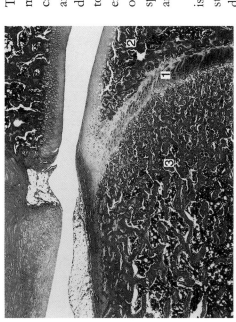

Figure 15.3a Bone.

1 growth plate   2 epiphysis   3 metaphysis

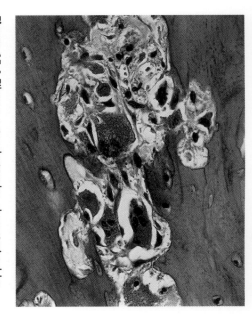

Figure 15.4 Fibrous osteodystrophy, characterized by formation of 'resorption tunnels' with (multinucleated) osteoclasts removing the bone tissue.

Whereas fibrous osteodystrophy results in destruction of bone, another spontaneous change, myelofibrosis, results in the replacement of the bone marrow by fibrous tissue and this process progresses to hyperostosis – formation of additional new bone.

Bone Marrow (Medulla Ossium)

(Figures 15.5–15.7)

The bone marrow consists of a highly vascular, loose connective tissue stroma and the hematopoietic cells. The stroma supporting the vessels and hematopoietic cells consists of adventitial reticular cells, adipocytes, macrophages and reticulin fibers. In rats, the sternum, femur and humerus are frequently used for the assessment of bone marrow. In decalcified, hematoxylin and eosin-stained paraffin sections an estimate of general hematopoietic activity (cellularity) and myeloid/erythroid ratio can be made. The erythroid elements are rather small with round, dense, deeply basophilic nuclei. The myeloid (granulocytic) elements have large, bean-shaped nuclei that are less basophilic and more vesicular than the erythroid cells. Megakaryocytes are easily recognized by their large size and multilobulated nuclei (MacKenzie and Eustis, 1990).

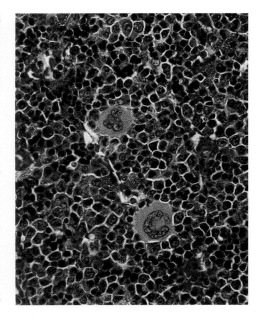

Figure 15.5 Bone marrow. Two large megakaryocytes with multilobulated nuclei, erythroid elements with deeply basophilic nuclei, myeloid elements with larger, bean-shaped vesicular nuclei; occasional mast cells have blue cytoplasmic granules, mature erythrocytes are red.

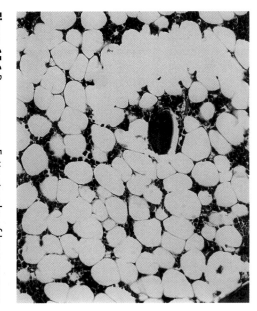

Figure 15.6 Bone marrow. Fatty atrophy of bone marrow is characterized by the presence of large adipose cells (round clear structures) replacing the hematopoietic tissue.

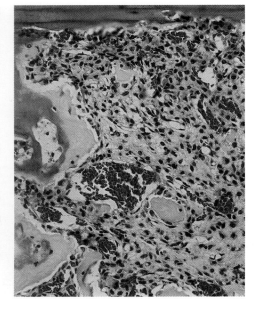

Figure 15.7 Bone marrow. This bone is affected by myelofibrosis, characterized by loss and replacement of the bone marrow by fibrovascular tissue.

Cline and Maronpot (1985) described variations in the histological distribution of rat bone marrow cells with respect to age and anatomical site. A characteristic change seen in aging is that of fatty atrophy.

Brain (Cerebrum, Encephalon)

(Figures 15.8–15.10)

The rat brain is lissencephalic, i.e. the cerebral cortex is devoid of gyri (convolutions). Unlike other species, the basal ganglia are not subdivided by the capsula interna and they form a structure called caudatoputamen. In the basal cortex (tuberculum olfactorium) there are groups of small neurons (insulae Calleja) which, because of their striking lymphocyte-like appearance, are frequently mistaken for inflammatory infiltrates or for developmental anomalies. Views on how the rat brain can be subdivided into anatomical portions are somewhat controversial as sometimes (in chemical safety test guidelines) the imprecise term 'center of cerebrum' is used. The preferential subdivision is: forebrain (cerebral cortex, hippocampus and olfactory bulbs), the upper brainstem (basal ganglia, septum, epithalamus, thalamus and hypothalamus), and the midbrain, cerebellum with pons, and medulla oblongata.

A list of atlases and books dealing with the rat central nervous system anatomy is presented in Chapter 27. The brain tissue consists of functional cells (nerve cells, neurons) and the supporting cells (macroglia and microglia). The macroglia are oligodendrocytes, which are the central myelin-forming cells, and astrocytes which occur in both the gray and the white matter. Rat astrocytes react positively for the GFAP (glial fibrillary acidic protein) immunohistochemical reaction, but only when they are producing cytoskeleton, e.g. the so-called reactive astrocytes. Positive staining is increasingly encountered in the aging brain, especially in areas compressed due to an increased intracranial pressure, e.g. due to the presence of tumors. The brain grows continuously, as is indicated by the increasing brain weight during the first 24 months of life. Therefore, there is no brain atrophy with advancing age, at least during this period. Spontaneous age-related findings are: neuroaxonal dystrophy in the gracile nucleus, multifocal degeneration of nerve fibers, vascular changes associated with hemorrhage, necrosis and ischemic changes, demyelination, and

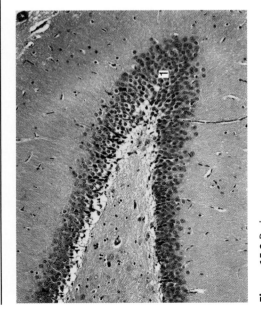

Figure 15.8 Brain.
1 neuronal cell layer of the hippocampal fascia dentata; the inner margin of this layer shows artificial edema characteristic of imperfect fixation.

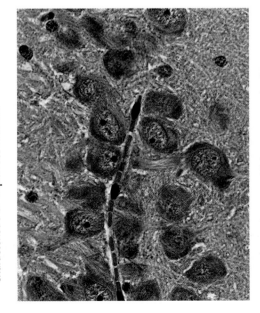

Figure 15.9 Brain. Pyramidal neurons in the hippocampus have large, pale nuclei and basophilic cytoplasm.

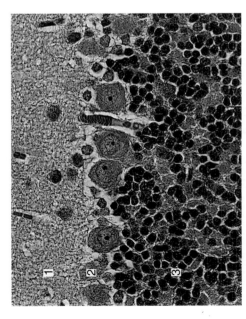

Figure 15.10 Brain. Layers of the cerebellar cortex
1 molecular layer
2 Purkinje cell layer, with pericellular artificial
   edema characteristic of imperfect fixation
3 granular cell layer

sporadic multifocal spongiform encephalopathy (Krinke and Eisenbrandt, 1994).

Bulbourethral Gland (Glandula Bulbourethralis)

The paired bulbourethral glands are the male accessory genital glands. They lie laterally to the rectum between the ischiocavernosus and bulbocavernosus muscles. The excretory ducts open into the urethral bulb. The gland is formed by wide, highly branched tubules containing a single cell layer of mucous and seromucous cells. The cells are high, pyramid-shaped and contain secretory granules. The whole organ is covered by striated muscle.

Cecum

See intestine.

Clitorial Gland ('Female Preputial Gland') (Glandula Clitoridis)

'Female preputial gland' (paired) — *see preputial gland, urethra.*

Colon

See intestine.

Ductus Deferens (Vas Deferens)

The paired ductus deferens emerges from the medial aspect of the epididymal tail. It runs along the medial side of the testis, enters the abdominal cavity, attaches to the contralateral duct, penetrates the dorsolateral lobe of the prostate and opens dorsally into the urethra, commonly with the excretory ducts of seminal vesicles into so-called ampullae, where the openings are located in the seminal collicle. The terminal part of ductus deferens is equipped with the gland of the ductus deferens. The wall is formed by ciliated columnar epithelial lining, thick circular and longitudinal smooth muscle layer, and adventitia.

Duodenum

See intestine.

Ear (Auris)

The paired ears are composed of three parts, the external ear, the middle ear and the inner ear. The external ear (auris externa) is formed by concha auriculae (the pinna) and the external auditory canal. It is supported by elastic auricular cartilage. The middle ear (auris media) consists of the tympanic cavity with the tympanic membrane and the Eustachian tube. The tympanic membrane is covered by simple squamous epithelium. Besides the squamous epithelium, the middle ear cavity contains an arrangement of ciliated cells interspersed with secretory cells. The Eustachian tube is nearly horizontal and contains a large number of goblet cells but few mucous glands (Hebel and Stromberg, 1986). Within the tympanic cavity lie the auditory ossicles malleus, incus and stapes. The inner ear (auris interna) consists of the labyrinth (organ of equilibrium) and the cochlea (the organ of audition). In the cochlea there is the organ of Corti with sensory hair cells which are arranged into a single inner row and three outer rows. The hair cells are innervated by spiral ganglion cells.

With advancing age numerous hair cells, as well as ganglion cells, degenerate and disappear. The observed normal hair cell population in Sprague-Dawley rats is approximately 960 inner and 3740 outer hair cells. In aged animals the ganglion cells can accumulate lipofuscin pigment (Feldman, 1994). A spontaneous change occasionally occurring in the pinna is auricular chondropathy.

Epididymis (Figures 15.11 and 15.12)

The paired epididymides consist of the head (caput), attached to the cranial pole of the testis, the body (isthmus) located medially and the tail (cauda) located at the caudal pole of the testis. The organ is formed by several ductuli efferentes in the head which open into the ductus epididymidis, continuing as the vas deferens. The ducts are lined by ciliated epithelium. The ductus deferens emerges from the tail and passes through the prostate to open into the urethra.

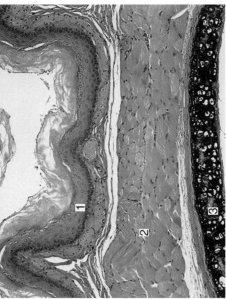

Figure 15.13 Esophagus.
1   stratified sqamous
    epithelium
2   striated muscle layers
3   tracheal cartilage

Eye (Oculus) (Figures 15.14–15.16)

The paired rat eyeballs are nearly spherical. With advancing age they grow independently of the body weight, until 400 days of life. The thickness of cornea and sclera doubles between days 21 and 400 (Leopold and Calcins, 1951).

The rat cornea is composed of corneal epithelium (generally five layers thick), corneal stroma (lamina propria) consisting of collagen fibers, Descemet's membrane and endothelium. The Bowman's membrane is missing.

The rat conjunctival epithelium is, in contrast to other species, squamous rather than polyhedral or

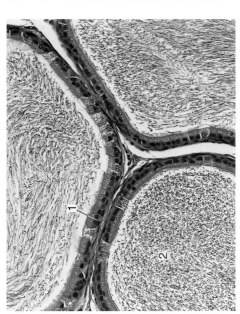

Figure 15.11 Epididymis. Caput.
1   ciliated epithelium
2   spermatozoa in the lumen

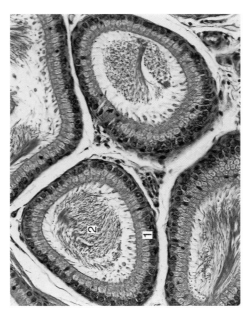

Figure 15.12 Epididymis. Cauda.
1   ciliated epithelium
2   spermatozoa in the lumen

Esophagus (Figure 15.13)

The esophagus is located dorsally to the trachea, slightly to the left of the medial level. The wall is composed of a stratified squamous epithelial layer, the submucosa, which is free of glands, and two coats of striated muscular layers, with different arrangement of muscle fibers: the outer coat consists of an outer longitudinal and inner circular layer, whereas the inner coat is oriented longitudinally only.

Estrous Cycle

For comparison of changes in the vagina as described in the vaginal smears or the histological preparations *see vagina*; for uterine histology *see uterus*.

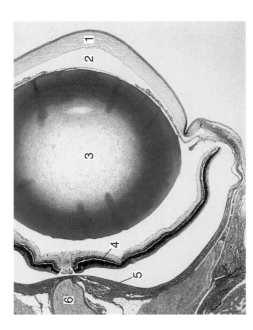

Figure 15.14 Eye.
1   cornea
2   anterior chamber
3   lens
4   retina
5   sclera (with choroid)
6   optic nerve

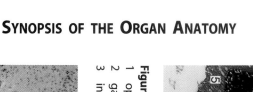

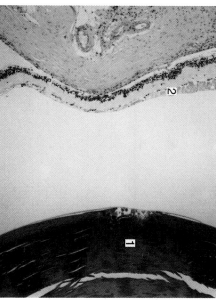

Figure 15.15 Eye. Central fundus.

1 optic papilla
2 ganglionic cell layer
3 inner granular cell layer
4 outer granular cell layer
5 photoreceptor (outer segment) layer

Figure 15.16 Eye.

1 early formation of cataract in posterior subcapsular area, breakdown of lens fibers to fragments
2 retinal atrophy, loss of photoreceptor layer and outer granular cell layer, and thinning of inner granular cell layer

(Johansson, 1987). In albino rats the choroid is devoid of pigment and consists mostly of two layers of thin-walled vessels.

The ciliary body is relatively small. The ciliary muscle consists of single fibers or small fiber bundles; there is little or no accommodation. The pupilla is circular.

The rat retina shows a relatively thick outer nuclear layer, this being common to nocturnal animals (Leopold and Calcins, 1951). Most of the receptor cells are rods. According to some authors, sparse, randomly distributed cones are present. The area centralis or the horizontal streak are missing.

In albino rats the pigment epithelium is devoid of pigment. It has a low mitotic rate and remains *in situ* for life. Its phagocytic mechanism is not restricted to removal of the outer photoreceptor discs, since the pigment epithelium can phagocytize carbon particles, latex beads or chloroquine, for example (Feeney, 1973).

The rat lens is relatively large and, like the whole eye, nearly spherical. It doubles in size between days 21 and 850 (Leopold and Calcins, 1951). The lens capsule, which at the embryonic stage is thinner anteriorly, becomes thicker with age, so that by 600 days, the anterior capsule is 7.5 times thicker than the posterior one (Parmigiani and McAvoy, 1989). The lens epithelium, which at 21 days is nearly columnar, becomes cuboidal at 400 days. In the embryonic stage, the lens is supplied with nutrients through the temporary vascular network formed by the tunica vasculosa lentis and vasa hyaloidea propria. There are often hyaloid remnants with some hemorrhage. The vitreous body is covered by an approximately 100-μm-thick cortical area formed by extracellular matrix (collagen fibers, proteins and proteoglycans) and cellular components called hyalocytes. The majority of these cells are considered to be resting macrophages. The most external structure is formed by the hyaloid membrane (Salu et al., 1985).

Spontaneous corneal dystrophy, associated with general basement membrane changes, can occur even in young rats (Bruner et al., 1992). Characteristic changes occurring with advanced age are cataract formation and retinal atrophy.

columnar. The goblet cells are aggregated into clusters. There are no lymphoid follicles (Setzer et al., 1987).

Like the human eye, the sclera is thickest next to the optic nerve and thinnest posteriorly to the anterior muscle ring. It consists of collagen fibers with sparse elastic ones. The rat eye has the least developed lamina cribrosa within the mammalian species. It is formed by only 1–2 layers of sparse connective tissue. Therefore, the rat eye could be a good model for studying glaucomatous eyes, where a possible influence of the lamina cribrosa can be excluded

Harderian Gland (Figures 15.17 and 15.18)

The paired Harderian glands lie deep within the orbit and encircle the bulbus oculi and the optic nerve

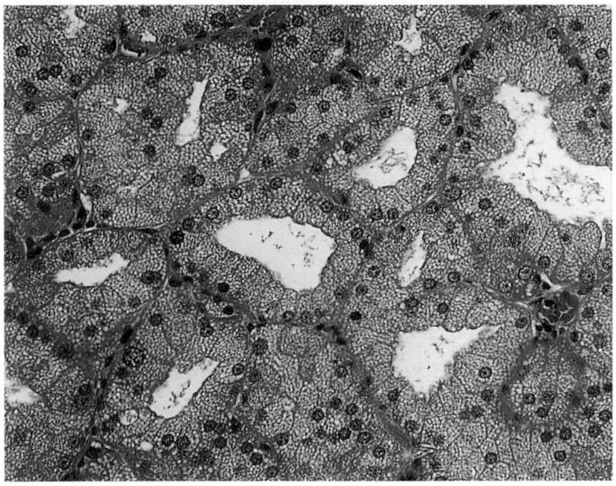

Figure 15.17 Harderian gland. Acinar cells have clear, finely vacuolated cytoplasm.

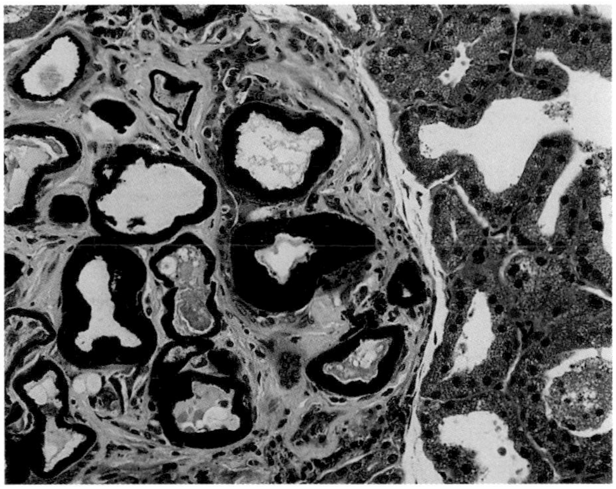

Figure 15.18 Harderian gland. Porphyrin granuloma consisting of porphyrin accretions surrounded by multinucleated giant cells and fibrous tissue.

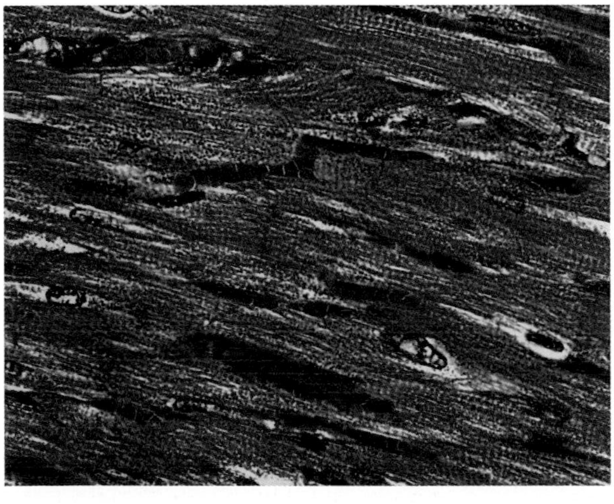

Figure 15.19 Heart. Cross-striated myocardial fibers.

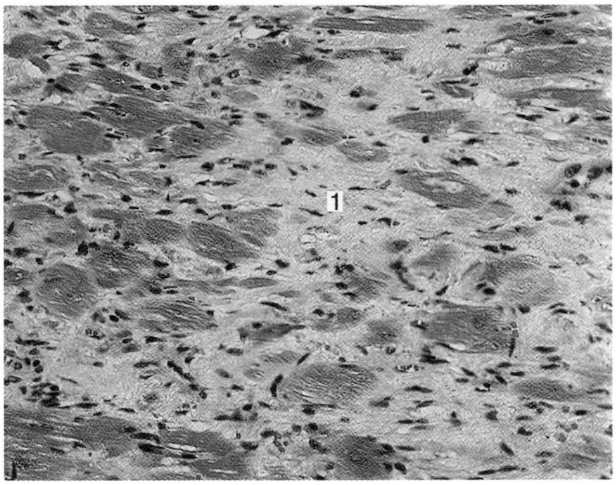

Figure 15.20 Heart. Myocardial fibrosis: the myocardial fibers are lost and replaced by fibrous tissue.
1 fibrous tissue

from the medial, superior and inferior sides. The gland exhibits a tubuloalveolar organization devoid of an intraglandular duct system. A single duct opens in the inner canthus of the eye. The secretory cells are columnar with an eosinophilic cytoplasm that contains many clear, lipid-containing, secretory vacuoles. The secretory cells are surrounded by a network of myoepithelial cells.

With advancing age, intraluminal porphyrin accumulates predominantly at the periphery of the gland. This is associated with atrophy of the secretory cells and a granulomatous inflammatory reaction, which is followed by proliferation of the interstitial connective tissue resulting in sclerosis of the gland (Krinke, 1991).

Heart (Cor) (Figures 15.19 and 15.20)

The heart is located in the thoracic cavity, nearly in the central axis, with the heart apex pointing to the left. It is a hollow muscular organ covered by a delicate, transparent pericardium. A septum divides the organ into a left and a right half. Each half is in turn divided into a ventricle and a less muscular atrium. The left ventricle is also more muscular than the right one. Between the ventricles and the atria there is a groove – the sulcus coronarius – which carries the coronary vessels. The blood supply for the heart is provided by these coronary vessels and also by blood vessels running along the lateral walls of the ventricles and not in the longitudinal sulci as in other species. Therefore, in the rat the longitudinal sulci which mark the boundary between the left

Figure 15.21 Intestine. Duodenum (small intestine).
1 the tips of the villi are post-mortally digested by intraintestinal enzymatic activity
2 tunica muscularis

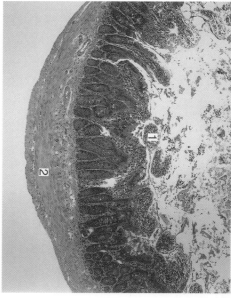

Figure 15.24 Intestine. Cecum (large intestine).

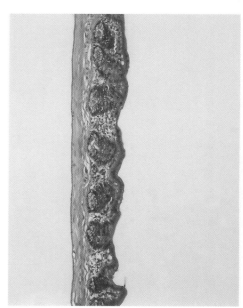

and right ventricles are not very prominent. The heart wall consists of three layers: the endocardium, myocardium and epicardium. As in other species, the myocardial fibers are striated and have centrally located nuclei.

Characteristic aging changes include myocardial fibrosis, initially associated with inflammatory cell infiltration, occurring mainly in the males (Lewis, 1992).

Ileum

See intestine.

Intestine (Intestinum)

(Figures 15.21–15.26)

Small intestine (intestinum tenue)

The small intestine ranges in total length from 107 cm in five-month-old to 122 cm in aged (F-344) rats (Elwell and McConnell, 1990). It consists of three parts: the duodenum, the jejunum and the ileum.

The duodenum runs towards the right kidney (duodenum descendens), continues towards the midline (flexura duodeni caudalis) and then turns cranially (duodenum ascendens). It contains the duodenal papilla, an elevated area where the hepatic duct (ductus hepatoentericus) opens out. The jejunum forms the longest part of the intestine; it consists of garland-like loops filling the right ventral part of the abdomen. The ileum is connected with the base of the cecum, near to the beginning of the colon.

Figure 15.22 Intestine. Jejunum (small intestine).

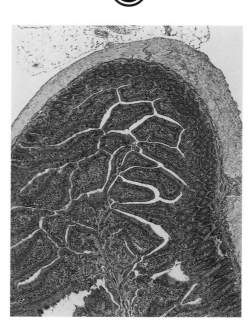

Figure 15.23 Intestine. Ileum (small intestine).
1 Peyer's patch

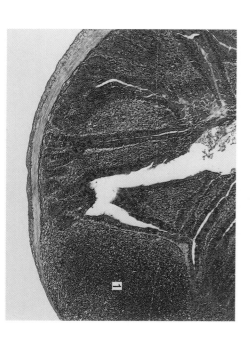

muscle (outer longitudinal and inner circular layers) and the serous membrane (serosa = adventitia exposed to the abdominal cavity). The mucous membrane forms crypts and, in the small intestine, villi, these being longest in the duodenum. The submucosa contains loose connective tissue with blood and lymphatic vessels and is separated from the lamina propria of the mucosa by a thin circular smooth muscle, the lamina muscularis mucosae. The mucosa and submucosa of the colon and rectum form prominent folds. Lymphatic tissue (GALT) is distributed throughout the whole intestine as foci of varying size. The small intestine is richer in lymphatic tissue than the large one. The biggest aggregations of lymphatic foci are the Peyer's patches. They are predominantly located at the antimesenteric border of distal ileum. The epithelial lining of the mucosa consists of columnar epithelial cells with microvilli on the luminal surface, of the mucous (goblet) cells. Among the specialized cell types of the intestine are the M cells (lymphoepithelial cells) in the mucosa overlying Peyer's patches, the Paneth's cells with brightly eosinophilic cytoplasmic granules, located at the base of the crypts in the small intestine, and the enteroendocrine cells. The submucosa of the initial 6–8 mm of the duodenum contains tubular Brunner's glands. At the end of the rectum there is a short zone of stratified squamous epithelium with circumanal (modified sebaceous) glands (Elwell and McConnell, 1990).

Morphometric data on the villus and crypt size in the small intestine were published by Altmann (1975). Whiteley *et al.* (1996) investigated the influence of diet and colonic microflora on colonic mucosal growth: they report a marked individual variability with respect to the thickness of the tunica mucosa and tunica muscularis.

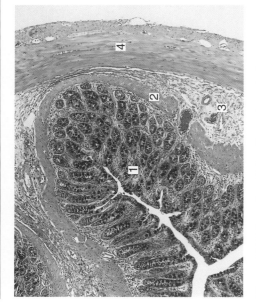

Figure 15.25 Intestine. Colon (large intestine).

1 tunica mucosa	3 submucosa
2 lamina muscularis mucosae	4 tunica muscularis

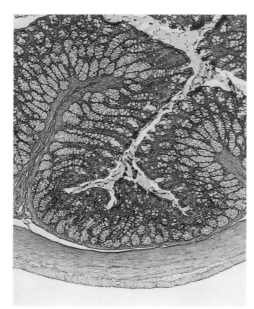

Figure 15.26 Intestine. Rectum (large intestine).

Large intestine (intestinum crassum)

The total length of the colon and rectum in F-344 rats is approximately 15 cm (Elwell and McConnell, 1990). It consists of three parts: the cecum, the colon and the rectum.

The cecum is located in the right part of the abdominal cavity, but may show considerable positional variation (Green, 1963; Hebel and Stromberg, 1986). It consists of the base (basis), the body (corpus) and the apical part (apex). The colon initially ascends (colon ascendens) rostrally from the cecum and then behind the right kidney it turns in a transverse direction (colon transversum), finally going over into the caudally directed colon descendens and rectum. The rectum runs along the midline and terminates in the anus.

The intestinal wall is formed from three layers: the mucous membrane with submucosa, the smooth

Jejunum

See intestine.

Joint (Articulatio) (Figure 15.27)

The structure of rat joints is essentially the same as in other mammalian species. They are generally composed of a joint capsule, ligaments and articular cartilage covering the ends of the bones. A synovial membrane covers the inner aspect of the joint capsule, ligaments and tendon sheaths, but not the

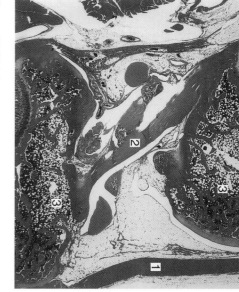

Figure 15.27 Joint.
1 capsule
2 ligaments
3 epiphyses (ends of bones)

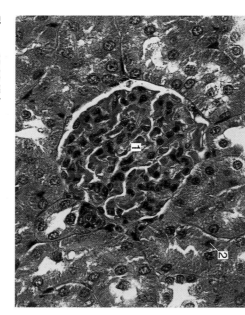

Figure 15.28 Kidney.
1 glomerulus
2 cortical tubules

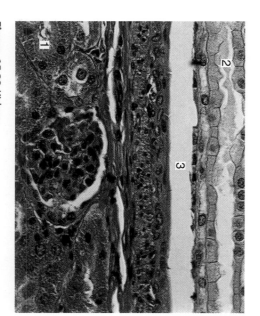

Figure 15.29 Kidney.
1 cortex
2 papilla
3 pelvis

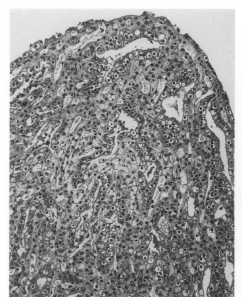

Figure 15.30 Kidney. Papilla.

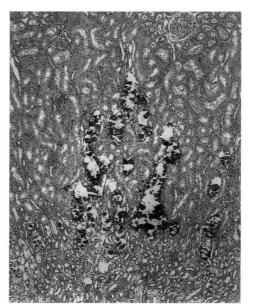

Figure 15.31 Kidney. Nephrocalcinosis: mineralization at the corticomedullary junction.

articular cartilage or menisci. Menisci, which are semilunar cartilages within the joint space, undergo partial ossification in the rat (Leininger and Riley, 1990).

The knee joint is frequently used to represent the rat joint tissue. Of particular interest is the articular cartilage, which, since it is devoid of innervation or a vascular system, is considered a biologically privileged tissue with respect to the effects of xenobiotics. The aged mammalian articular cartilage is prone to erosive and degenerative lesions (Gough et al., 1992).

Kidney (Ren) (Figures 15.28–15.32)

The paired kidneys are located retroperitoneally in the dorsal abdominal cavity, the left kidney shifted slightly caudally. The rat kidney is unipapillate. The whole organ is covered by a fibrous capsule and

and divides into interlobar arteries which branch further into arcuate arteries following the pattern seen in other mammalian species (Montgomery and Seely, 1990).

The male rat is prone to hyaline droplet formation in proximal tubular cells. These droplets are secondary lysosomes involved in metabolism of α_2-microglobulin (Read, 1991). Nephrocalcinosis (mineralization in the corticomedullary junction) occurs frequently, especially in females (nearly 100%). In both sexes the age-related changes comprise tubular atrophy, tubular basophilic proliferation and chronic progressive nephropathy.

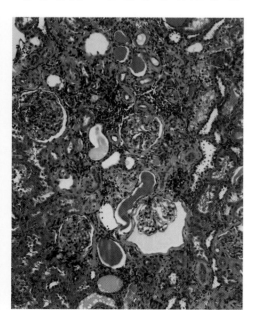

Figure 15.32 Kidney. Chronic progressive nephropathy, characterized by thickening of the basement membrane, formation of tubular hyaline casts, and interstitial lymphocytic infiltration.

embedded in adipose tissue (capsula adiposa). Each kidney is composed of a cortex, a medulla with papilla, and the renal pelvis. The cortex contains glomeruli and convoluted proximal and distal tubules, forming the so-called cortical labyrinth. The proximal tubular cells have a brush border composed of microvilli, which is positive for the periodic acid Schiff (PAS) stain. The glomeruli are located within the Bowman's capsule lined by epithelium, which is initially squamous but with age it is transformed into a columnar structure (Hebel and Stromberg, 1986). The juxtaglomerular apparatus consists of the macula densa (the specialized termination of the distal tubule), the renin-producing (modified smooth muscle) cells of the afferent arteriole, and the extraglomerular mesangial cells. The medulla is subdivided into an outer and an inner zone: the inner zone forms the papilla. The outer zone can be further subdivided into an inner and an outer stripe. The outer stripe of the outer zone extends into the cortex, forming so-called medullary rays. The medulla is composed of proximal, intermediate, distal and collecting tubules. The thin intermediate tubules are found in the inner medullary stripe and the papilla. The collecting tubules run into papillary ducts lined by simple cuboidal to columnar epithelium. The papillary ducts form the papilla and open into the renal pelvis. The renal pelvis has a parenchymal portion lined by simple cuboidal epithelium, and a nonparenchymal surface, which is lined by transitional epithelium of 3–4 layers. The pelvis opens into the ureter. The kidney is supplied by the renal artery which enters the organ at the hilus

Lacrimal Gland (Glandula Lacrimalis) (Figure 15.33)

The rat has two pairs of lacrimal glands: superior (extraorbital, exorbital) and inferior (infraorbital). Usually, the exorbital glands are collected for examination. This gland is a flattened, disc-like structure located just below the ear, rostrodorsally to the parotid gland. Its main duct arises at the anterior border of the gland, runs forward, and is joined by the duct of the infraorbital gland just before reaching the lateral corner of the dorsal and ventral conjunctival sacs. These glands are associated with the outer canthus of the eye. The lacrimal gland is serous and tubuloacinar, with many intraglandular excretory ducts.

With advanced age (from about 300 days), nuclear pleomorphism (irregular size and shape), intranuclear pseudoinclusions, lymphocytic infiltration and

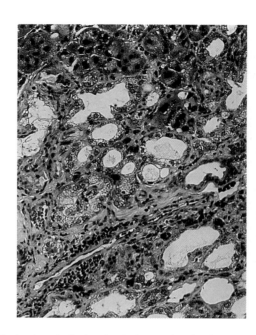

Figure 15.33 Lacrimal gland. The gland shows 'Harderinization' (metaplasia to Harderian gland-like acini), and lymphocytic infiltration.

occurrence of Harderian alveoli appear spontaneously, especially in male animals (Krinke *et al.*, 1994).

Large Intestine (Intestinum Crassum)

See intestine.

Larynx

The entrance of the larynx is bordered ventrally by the epiglottis. In the laryngeal vestibule, a distinct medial laryngeal recess is located ventrally (ventral laryngeal diverticulum, ventral pouch). The wall of the larynx is composed of three layers. The inner one is formed by epithelial lining, which on the anterior and upper posterior surface of the epiglottis, the upper half of the laryngeal surface, a portion of the ventricular folds and the vocal cords is nonkeratinized, stratified squamous epithelium. The remainder of the larynx is mostly lined by pseudostratified ciliated columnar epithelium and nonciliated columnar epithelium. In the ventral portion of the larynx the cells have inconspicuous microvilli and no cilia (Boorman *et al.*, 1990b). There is a site located cranially to the laryngeal recess with underlying seromucinous glands, which is recognized as a preferred site for histopathological evaluation in inhalation studies (Sagartz *et al.*, 1992). The central layer contains cartilage, muscle and vocal cords. The outer layer is formed by loose connective tissue. Histologic methods and interspecies variations in the laryngeal histology were described by Renne *et al.* (1992, 1993).

Germann *et al.* (1995) demonstrated in aging F-344 rats spontaneous formation of inflammatory and degenerative changes in the oropharyngeal and laryngotracheal cavity.

Leydig Cells

See testis.

Liver (Hepar) (Figures 15.34–15.40)

The liver is subdivided into lobes. This subdivision is differently interpreted by various authors (Table 15.1). Moreover, there is a great individual

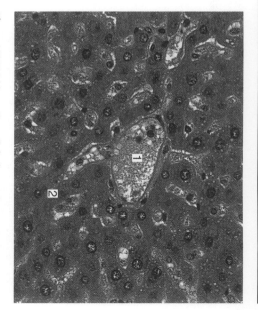

Figure 15.34 Liver. Centrilobular region.
1 central vein 2 hepatocytes

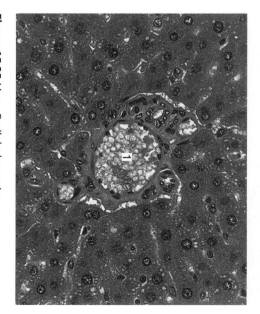

Figure 15.35 Liver. Perilobular region.
1 branches of portal vein, hepatic artery and bile ducts

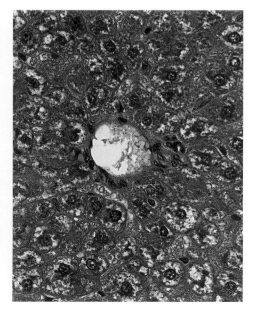

Figure 15.36 Liver. Glycogen. In H/E stain following formalin fixation the glycogen is washed out from the hepatocytes, leaving irregular clear spaces in their cytoplasm.

Table 15.1 Four different interpretations of liver lobes

Authors	Left lobes	Middle lobes	Right lobes
Green (1963)	Large left lobe	Median or cystic lobe, a small caudate lobe, which fits around the esophagus	Right lobe, partially subdivided into anterior and posterior lobes
Hebel and Stromberg (1986)	Left lobe, subdivided into greater lateral and smaller medial lobes	Intermediate lobe, subdivided into a caudate process and two papillary processes, the pars infraportalis and the pars supraportalis	Right lobe, small, not subdivided
Popesko et al. (1990)	Left lateral and left medial lobes	Caudate lobe, subdivided in processus caudatus and processus papillaris, which in turn is subdivided into pars preventricularis and pars retroventricularis	Right lateral and right medial lobes
Eustis et al. (1990a)	Left lobe	Median lobe, subdivided into right and left sublobes, and the caudate lobe (process) subdivided into cranial and caudal sublobes	Right lateral lobe, subdivided into cranial and caudal sublobes

variability. Generally, the lobes are: left, middle and right. The overview in Table 15.1 probably reflects differences in description as well as the real individual differences in the liver shape.

The rostral surface of the liver contacts the diaphragm (diaphragmatic surface), the caudal surface the viscera (visceral surface) such as stomach, spleen, duodenum, jejunum, colon and the right kidney. The

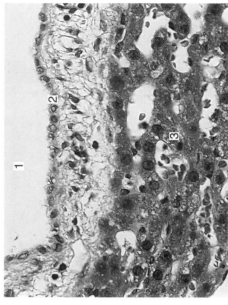

Figure 15.38 Liver. Biliary cyst.
1 lumen of the cyst
2 cuboidal epithelial lining
3 hepatic parenchyma

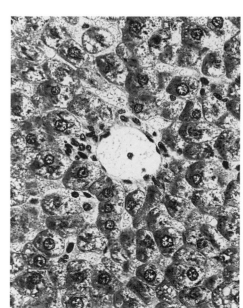

Figure 15.37 Liver. Glycogen. In special stain for glycogen (Best carmin) the red staining glycogen is artificially shifted towards the cell membranes, indicating the direction of fixative penetration during immersion

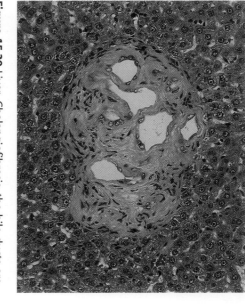

Figure 15.39 Liver. Cholangiofibrosis: the bile ducts are enclosed by fibrous tissue.

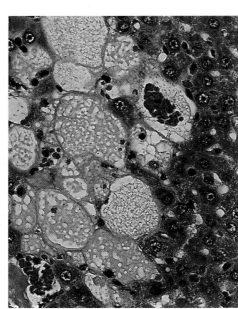

Figure 15.40 Liver. Spongiosis hepatis: formation of spongy areas without any cellular lining.

unit of the liver, referred to as an acinus, is centered around the portal vein and branches of the hepatic artery, i.e. around the lobular periphery (Rappaport et al., 1954).

Among the nonparenchymal cells, the following types have been identified: bile duct, endothelial, Kupffer, and fat-storing (Ito) cells. Kupffer cells have microvilli at the surface and are located preferentially in the periportal regions. They are highly phagocytic cells. The endothelial cells have pores and fenestrations. The liver weight, mitotic activity, glycogen and lipid contents can vary due to circadian rhythm.

Common age-associated changes in the liver are the presence of lipofuscin pigment in the hepatocytes, hemosiderin pigment in the hepatocytes and Kupffer cells, variations in the size of the nuclei and increase in the volume and variations in ploidy of the hepatocytes, and formation of intranuclear pseudoinclusion bodies (Irisarri and Hollander, 1994). Furthermore, aging is frequently associated with cholangiofibrosis and occasional formation of biliary cysts, especially in females. A rather rare spontaneous change is spongiosis hepatis. Parker and Gibson (1995) described necrotic and inflammatory liver lesions produced by wrapping the torso in a percutaneous toxicity study.

Lung (Pulmo) (Figures 15.41 and 15.42)

The right lung consists of cranial (anterior, apical), middle (cardiac), caudal (posterior, diaphragmatic, phrenic) and a subdivided accessory lobe. The synonyms used for accessory lobe are 'median lobe',

hepatoenteric duct originates from the connection of bile ducts in the portal area. It runs among the pancreatic lobules towards the duodenum, and receives several (2–8) pancreatic ducts. The liver has no gall bladder. The liver is covered by a delicate connective tissue capsule. The liver tissue consists of parenchymal (hepatocytes) and nonparenchymal cells. The rather uniform hepatocytes are organized in trabeculae with blood sinusoids on one and bile canaliculi on the other side of each cell. Between the hepatocytes and the wall of blood sinusoids there is the space of Disse. The liver parenchyma is divided through a small amount of interstitial tissue into hexagonal lobules which are identical with the morphologic hepatic units. In the middle of each lobule (centrilobular region) lies a central vein, while the periphery is surrounded by branches of the hepatic artery, portal vein and the bile ducts. The functional

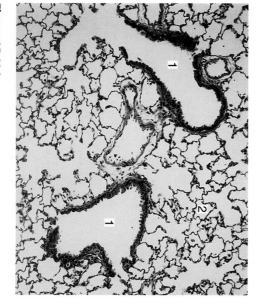

Figure 15.41 Lung.
1 terminal bronchioles 2 alveoli

Lymph Nodes (Lymphonodi, Nodi Lymphatici)

(Figures 15.43–15.46)

The lymph nodes are connected with the lymphatic system and distributed through the whole body. Regional distribution of lymph nodes is partly depicted in Chapter 13 and their draining areas are commented on in Chapter 28. Lymphatic tissue incorporated in selected organ systems is commonly known as NALT (nose-associated lymphatic tissue), BALT (bronchial-associated lymphatic tissue) in the lung and GALT (gut-associated lymphatic tissue) in the intestine. The lymph nodes are separate lymphatic organs. Each lymph node is covered by a connective tissue capsule which can penetrate into

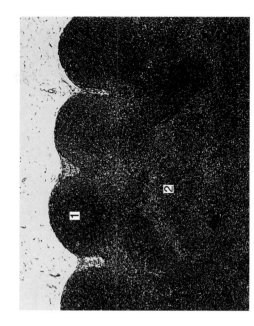

Figure 15.43 Lymph node.
1 cortex   2 paracortex

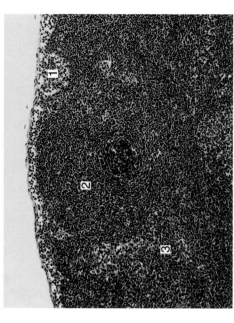

Figure 15.44 Lymph node.
1 marginal sinus   3 paracortex
2 lymphatic follicle (cortex)

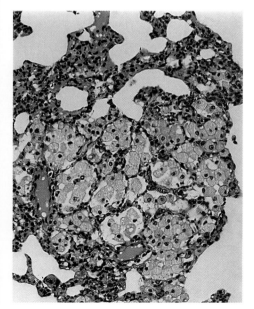

Figure 15.42 Lung. Intra-alveolar foam cells.

'azygous lobe' or 'postcaval lobe'. The smaller left lung is not separated into lobes. The whole organ is organized as a tubuloalveolar gland. The bronchus entering each lobe gives rise to secondary bronchi from which the bronchioles originate. The pulmonary acinus consists of a branching system of alveolar ducts ending in alveolar sacs. The epithelium of intrapulmonary bronchi and bronchioles is simple and includes the ciliated cells and nonciliated secretory cells (goblet cells, serous cells, Clara cells). There are also neurosecretory cells, basal cells and intermediate cells. The alveolar epithelium consists of type I (flat) and type II (cuboidal) pneumocytes. Alveolar brush cells which are provided with short microvilli are referred to as type III pneumocytes. There are interstitial septae rich in elastic and collagen fibers. Within the septae run numerous blood and lymph vessels. Some of the larger pulmonary arteries (mainly so-called right-angle branches of the axial arteries supplying each lobe) have an oblique muscle layer external to the external elastic lamina and additional to the circular muscle layer. The wall of these arteries appears unusually thick relative to their small lumen and this can be misinterpreted as hypertrophy of the media. In the rat lung the veins have an internal subendothelial layer of smooth muscle and an external layer of striated cardiac muscle similar to that in the heart (Boorman and Eustis, 1990). The lung is covered by the pleura formed by connective tissue together with elastic and muscle fibers, covered by a serous membrane with a single layer of tesselated epithelium.

A characteristic spontaneous change seen in the rat lung is the accumulation of intra-alveolar foam cells (alveolar histiocytosis, alveolar lipidosis).

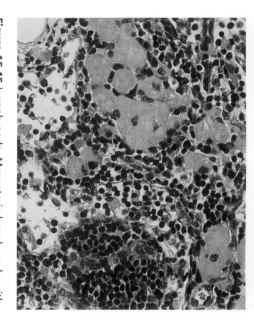

Figure 15.45 Lymph node. Mesenteric lymph node with 'phagocytic cells' characterized by abundant pink cytoplasm.

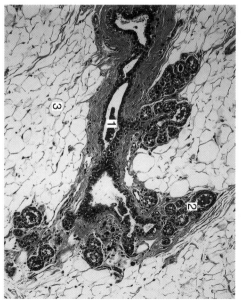

Figure 15.46 Lymph node. Axillary lymph node affected by chronic reactive hyperplasia manifested by the presence of numerous plasma cells.

the organ, forming short septae. The nodes consist of numerous endothelial sinuses and reticular tissue, forming a meshwork filled with lymphatic cells. The organ is divided into cortex with paracortex and medulla. The cortex is densely filled with lymphocytes arranged in follicles, mainly composed of B-cells. The paracortex is the lymphatic tissue between the follicles and the medulla and is composed mainly of T cells. The periphery of the paracortex has the highest concentration of 'high endothelial venules'. The medulla forms medullary cords and spreads from the center of the organ to the concave side and the hilus. Under the capsule there is a subcapsular sinus which is connected to paratrabecular and medullary sinuses. The lymph enters through vasa afferentia which penetrate the capsule and exits through the vas efferens in the hilus.

Characteristic changes occurring in the lymph nodes of aging rats are chronic reactive hyperplasia in the axillary lymph node, and occurrence of large 'phagocytic cells' in the mesenteric lymph node. Occasionally, aging rat mesenteric lymph nodes exhibit angiomatous proliferation considered by some authors as vascular tumors (Losco and Harleman, 1992).

Mammary Gland (Glandula Lactifera, Mamma)

(Figures 15.47–15.49)

In the female rat there are usually six pairs of mammary glands with nipples, located symmetrically on both sides of the body. Three of them on each side in the thoracic region, and three on each side in the

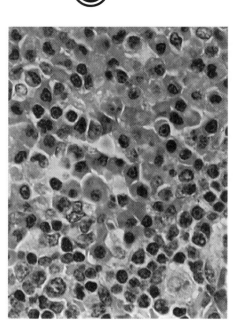

Figure 15.47 Mammary gland.
1 lactiferous duct 2 secretory alveoli 3 adipose tissue

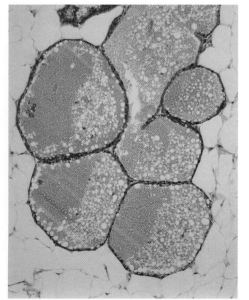

Figure 15.48 Mammary gland. Secretory activity with accumulation of milk in the lumen of distended alveoli.

types of epithelium: stratified squamous epithelium in the vestibulum and partially in the ventral meatus; respiratory epithelium in dorsal and medial meatus and partially in the ventral meatus, and in the nasopharyngeal duct; olfactory epithelium in the ethmoturbinates and in the caudal part of the dorsal meatus. The respiratory epithelium contains ciliated cells, goblet cells, cuboidal cells, nonciliated columnar cells and brush cells. There is a subset of the respiratory epithelium formed by transitional epithelium. The olfactory epithelium is a uniform pseudostratified columnar structure composed of bipolar neurons, sustentacular cells and basal cells (Boorman et al., 1990a). It is of yellow or orange color, which intensifies with age. In the propria of the nasal wall there are serous and mucous glands (Hebel and Stromberg, 1986).

Monticello et al. (1990) developed a simplified method for quantification of cell proliferation in nasal epithelia by relating the number of labeled cells to unit length of epithelial basement membrane. Comparative aspects of nasal airway anatomy were described by Harkema (1991). Mery et al. (1994) produced nasal diagrams which can be used as a tool for recording the distribution of nasal lesions. In his review of formaldehyde carcinogenesis, Morgan (1997) presented a number of anatomical and functional features of the rat nasal airways. Cytokeratin expression patterns in the rat respiratory tract, including the nose, larynx, trachea and lung, were described by Schlage et al. (1998).

Optic Nerve (Nervus Opticus)

The paired optic nerves of the normal rat consist of 100 000–140 000 nerve fibers with maximum diameter about 2 μm. About 90% of the fibers cross in the optic chiasma to reach the contralateral side of the brain. There are no distinct connective tissue septae (Lessell and Kuwabara, 1974).

Oral Cavity (Cavum Oris)

The upper lip is cleaved by a deep, hairless groove called philthrum, which forms a ventral continuation of the 'Nasenspiegel' phinarium. The dorsal wall of the oral cavity is formed by the hard palate, equipped with prominent palatal ridges, and the soft palate containing a thick layer of mucous glands. The tongue is grooved by the median sulcus in the rostral third. At the transition from the middle to the caudal third, there is a distinct dorsal prominence.

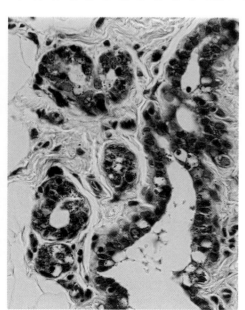

Figure 15.49 Mammary gland. Deposition of brownish pigment (probably lipofuscin) in the acinar cells.

inguinal region. Between the thoracic and inguinal mammary glands, there is a narrow segment without nipples. The nomenclature of the six mammary gland pairs is controversial, for example, Boorman et al. (1990c) describe cervical, cranial thoracic, caudal thoracic, abdominal, cranial inguinal and caudal inguinal, or, alternatively, left first, right first, left second, right second, etc., which sounds practical but applies individually, since the number of mammary glands can vary. During lactation the mammary glands and nipples increase considerably in size, reaching from the parotid glands cranially to the anal region caudally. The mammary gland is a compound tubuloalveolar gland consisting of branched ducts and terminal secretory alveoli arranged in lobules. Each gland has a main lactiferous duct forming the nipple sinus which opens into the nipple canal. The cuboidal to columnar secretory cells are surrounded by myoepithelial cells. Distal tips of the developing gland form 'buds' containing several layers of undifferentiated 'cap' cells (Boorman et al., 1990c). The male animals have small amounts of mammary glandular tissue, but no well-developed nipples.

The aging mammary gland can exhibit dilatation of ducts, secretory activity, or deposition of pigment.

Nasal Cavity (Cavum Nasi)

The nasal cavity is subdivided by the dorsal middle and ventral turbinates (conchae) into dorsal, middle and ventral meatus. The meatus are incompletely separated from the common meatus in vestibulum nasi. In the posterior nasal cavity there is a labyrinth of the ethmoturbinates composed of ecto- and endoturbinates. The lining is formed by three

Ovary (Ovarium) (Figures 15.50 and 15.51)

The paired ovaries are located caudally to the kidneys. They are surrounded by ovarian bursa and connected to the uterine horns by the convoluted oviducts. The ovary is covered by simple cuboidal or columnar epithelium, which at the hilus merges into simple squamous epithelium of the ovarian bursa. The major part of the ovary is formed by the parenchymatous zone containing follicles, clusters of polygonal interstitial cells, and loose central vascular zone. Close to the hilus numerous elastic and smooth muscle fibers occur. Hebel and Stromberg (1986) described the average size of follicles and oocytes as shown in Table 15.2.

The primordial follicle consists of an egg enclosed by a single layer of cells. For quantitative evaluation, the eggs with no surrounding granulosa cells are included in this category. In growing follicles the egg is surrounded by multiple cell layers but formation of a cavity is not evident. Graafian follicles means 'folliculi ovarici vesiculosi'; some authors use the term 'antral follicles' which describes the presence of a cavity within the follicle.

The presence of a regular number of oocytes and follicles is considered an indicator of intact fertility. Therefore, quantitative evaluation may be needed. Standard follicle-counting procedures were originally developed for mice and it is reported that they can be readily employed in rats (Plowchalk et al., 1993; Heindel, 1998). Tissue processing requirements (Bolon et al., 1997) for both species are identical, but in the rat each ovary yields approximately 600

6-μm-thick serial sections. For the conventional method, morphological criteria (Pedersen and Peters, 1968; Hirshfield and Midgley, 1978) are used to differentiate three major follicle classes (small, growing, antral) in every tenth section (i.e. a nonrandom 10% sample). However, preliminary data demonstrate that, as with mice, the analysis may be abbreviated either by (1) acquiring total counts in lieu of differential follicle counts (Bolon, unpublished data) or by (2) reducing the number of sections sampled (e.g. 5% or 1%; Bucci et al., 1997). Additional work will be necessary to validate these simplified counting schemes for regulatory use.

Table 15.2 Sizes of follicles and oocytes according to Hebel and Stromberg (1986)

Type	Size (μm)
Follicles	
Primordial	25–30
Growing	30–400
Graafian	650–700
Oocytes	
Primordial	18–20
Growing	40–60
Graafian	80–90
Corpora lutea	
Periodicum	about 700
Graviditatis	about 1100

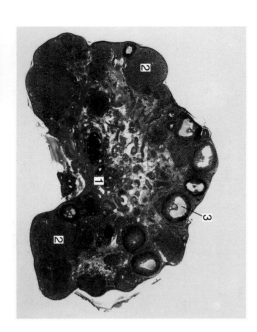

Figure 15.50 Ovary.
1 hilus
2 corpora lutea (yellow bodies)
3 Graafian follicle

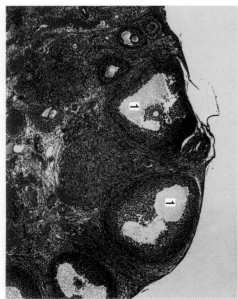

Figure 15.51 Ovary.
1 Graafian follicles

Ovulation occurs during estrus. Simultaneously, the next generation of primary follicles starts to grow and this growth is continuously maintained through the following cycle stages until the next estrus.

In the aging rats there is often accumulation of ceroid pigment, and the whole organ may become atrophic.

Oviduct (Tuba Uterina, Tuba Fallopii) (Figure 15.52)

The paired oviducts begin with the infundibulum, projecting into the ovarian bursa. Then they continue forming multiple garland-like loops and finally enter the uterine horns. The oviduct can be subdivided into four segments: the preampulla, the ampulla which has a larger lumen, the isthmus which is narrow, and the junctura of the uterus (Del Vecchio, 1992). The wall of all segments consists of tunica mucosa, with partly ciliated epithelium, smooth muscular tunica muscularis and tunica adventitia.

Pancreas (Figures 15.53–15.55)

The pancreas consists of the body, the right lobe and the left lobe. The body and the right lobe are located in the mesoduodenum and the beginning of the mesojejunum. The left lobe stretches along the dorsal aspect of the stomach towards the intestinal surface of the spleen (in the dorsal part of the greater omentum). Eustis et al. (1990b) quote subdividing of

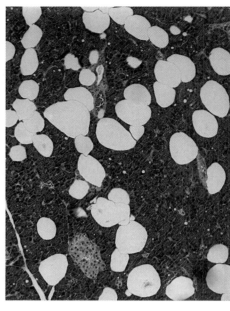

Figure 15.54 Pancreas. Acinar atrophy of the exocrine pancreas: the acinar cells are replaced by pale cells resembling the ductal or insular cells.

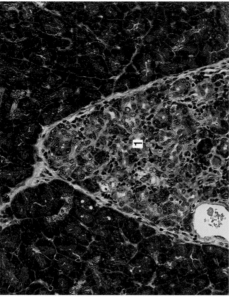

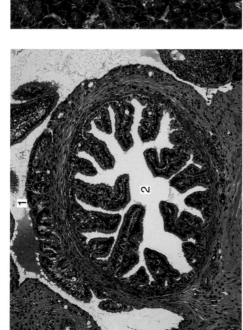

Figure 15.52 Oviduct.
1 infundibulum (within the ovarian bursa)
2 lumen of the oviduct

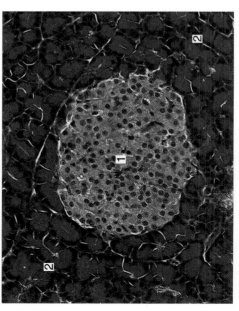

Figure 15.55 Pancreas. Fatty atrophy of the exocrine pancreas: the acinar cells are replaced by adipose cells (clear round spaces).

Figure 15.53 Pancreas.
1 pancreatic islet (endocrine pancreas)
2 exocrine pancreas, acinar cells

Table 15.3 Comparison of subdivisions of the pancreas suggested by different authors

Author	Left	Middle	Right
Hebel and Stromberg (1986)	Left lobe	Body	Right lobe
Eustis et al (1990b)	Tail	Body	Head (and neck?)
Richard et al. (1964), quoted by Eustis et al. (1990b)	Terminal part of the splenic segment	Gastric and splenic segments	Parabiliary and duodenal segments

the pancreas according to the location of ducts and vessels into: parabiliary segment, duodenal segment, small gastric segment and splenic segment. However, they also use subdivisions based on human anatomy: the head (corresponding to the parabiliary and duodenal segments) is located in the mesoduodenum, the body (gastric and splenic segments) extends from the head into the dorsal sheet of the greater omentum adjacent to the stomach, and the tail (terminal part of the splenic segment) extends into the gastrosplenic ligament and ends near the hilus of the spleen. Table 15.3 compares these subdivisions; the borders of particular regions are not clearly defined.

The exocrine pancreas is a compound acinar gland, consisting of acini connected to excretory ducts. The acinar secretory cells contain zymogen granules. Numerous excretory ducts join to form at least two, sometimes 5–8 main ducts which open into the hepatoenteric duct.

Characteristic spontaneous changes are acinar atrophy and fatty atrophy. Occasionally, accessory spleen is encountered in the rat pancreas.

Pancreatic Islets (Insulae Pancreaticae)

The endocrine pancreatic islets are irregularly distributed in the exocrine pancreas. They are more frequent and greater in diameter in the head (right lobe) than in other pancreatic regions. The islets consist of several types of cells. Alpha cells, which secrete glucagon, occur at the islet periphery, and insulin-producing beta cells are located in the center of the islet. The beta cells represent 80% of the total islet cell population (Stromberg and Capen, 1994). The other cell types are somatostatin-producing delta cells, pancreatic polypeptide-producing PP cells, and substance P-producing enterochromaffin cells (Riley

et al., 1990). The islets are separated from the exocrine pancreas by a fine connective tissue sheath.

Age-related changes were examined by Dillberger (1994). They were more common in males than females and started at 3.5 months of age. They consisted of B-cell hyperplasia giving rise to enlarged islets, then fibrosis, separating the islets into smaller cell groups. At a very advanced age the islets are rather small.

Parathyroid Gland (Glandula Parathyroidea)

(Figure 15.56)

The paired parathyroid glands are located anterolaterally to each lobe of the thyroid gland. Accessory parathyroid glands can be often seen. The parenchyma consists mainly of 'chief cells', usually characterized by large prominent nuclei. The cells are arranged into irregular, anastomosing cords. Total volume of parathyroid tissue is twice as great in females as in males of equal age (Hebel and Stromberg, 1986).

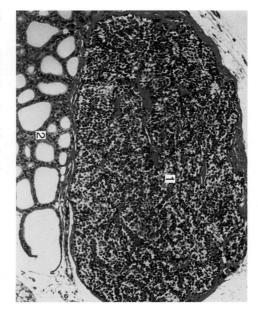

Figure 15.56 Parathyroid gland.
1 parathyroid gland
2 thyroid gland

Penis

The penis is attached by the crura to the ischiadic arch. It consists of the body and the apical glans and contains cartilaginous and bony os penis (os priapi), corpus cavernosum penis, and the distal part of the urethra.

Peripheral Nerve (Figures 15.57–15.59)

As in other species, the peripheral nerves consist of unmyelinated and myelinated nerve fibers and connective tissue sheets. The sciatic nerve (nervus

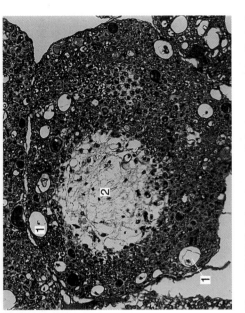

Figure 15.59 Peripheral nerve. Spinal nerve root affected by segmental demyelination.
1 swollen myelin sheaths
2 focal lipid accumulation, probably originating from damaged myelin

ischiadicus) is frequently taken for examination of rat peripheral nerve tissue, because it is the largest nerve containing the longest nerve fibers. The sensory fibers of the rat sciatic nerve originate in the dorsal root ganglia L3 to L6, but L4 and L5 are most important and contribute nearly 98–99% of all sensory fibers (Swett et al., 1991).

Peripheral nerves of aging rats undergo spontaneous degeneration and demyelination of nerve fibers. The demyelination is most prominent in lumbosacral spinal nerve roots (Krinke, 1988).

Pineal Body (Glandula Pinealis, Epiphysis)

The pineal body lies under the skull between the cerebral hemispheres and the cerebellum. It is covered by a thin capsule formed mostly by reticular fibers, which penetrate the organ causing a follicular appearance of the parenchyma. The whole organ is covered by pia mater. The vascular supply is formed by a dense capillary network.

Pituitary Gland (Glandula Pituitaria, Hypophysis)

(Figures 15.60–15.62)

The gland is located ventrally to the diencephalon, caudal to the optic chiasma. It consists of the adenohypophysis and the neurohypophysis. The adenohypophysis, in turn, consists of the pars distalis,

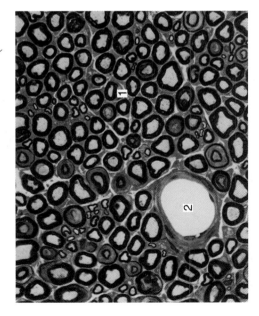

Figure 15.57 Peripheral nerve. Transverse section, epoxy resin, toluidine blue.
1 the nerve contains large and small myelinated nerve fibers in which the pale axons are surrounded by dark myelin sheaths
2 blood vessel, empty and distended owing to perfusion fixation

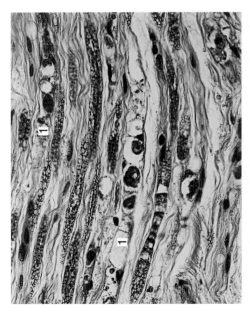

Figure 15.58 Peripheral nerve. Degeneration of nerve fibers.
1 degenerating nerve fibers, breaking down to ovoidal fragments

Table 15.4 Cell types in the pituitary gland

Azan or HE stains	Cell type	Location[b]	Hormone
Basophils	LH cells Luteotropes	Pars distalis	Luteinizing hormone (LH), (inter-stitial cell stimulating hormone)
Basophils	TSH cells Thyreotropes	Pars distalis	Thyroid-stimulating hormone (TSH) (thyrotropin)
Basophils or chromophobes	ACTH cells Corticotropes	Pars distalis, pars intermedia	Adrenocorticotropic hormone (ACTH)
Basophils	FSH cells Gonadotropes	Pars distalis	Follicle-stimulating hormone (FSH)
Acidophils	GH cells Gonadotropes	Pars distalis	Growth hormone (GH) (Somatotropin, STH)
Acidophils	PRL cells Mammotropes	Pars distalis	Prolactin (PRL) (lactogenic hor-mone, mammotropic hormone, luteotropic hormone)
Chromophobes	MSH cells Melanotropes	Pars intermedia, pars distalis	Melanocyte-stimulating hormone (MSH) (melanotrophins)
Hypothalamic neurons	'Neurosecretory cells'	Paraventricular and supraoptic nuclei, with endings in neurohypophysis	Vasopressin Antidiuretic hormone (ADH) Oxytocin

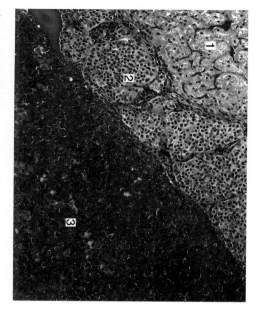

Figure 15.60 Pituitary gland.
1 neurohypophysis
2 pars intermedia (adenohypophysis)
3 pars distalis (adenohypophysis)

pars tuberalis and pars intermedia. Between the pars distalis and pars intermedia there is a horizontal hypophyseal cleft lined by one layer of epithelial cells. The whole organ is covered by dura mater. Microscopically (especially with azan staining) the adenohypophysis is seen to contain different cellular elements: (1) Acidophils occur mostly in clusters and contain red intracellular granules. (2) Basophils are distributed individually and their granules stain blue. (3) Chromophobes are the largest ovoid-shaped cells with dark blue granules.

The proportion of the different cellular types changes continuously depending on demands for specific hormones (Aoki *et al.*, 1993). Using immunohistochemistry, the cell types can be characterized more precisely. Table 15.4, modified from MacKenzie and Boorman (1990), compares the cell types, their location and function.

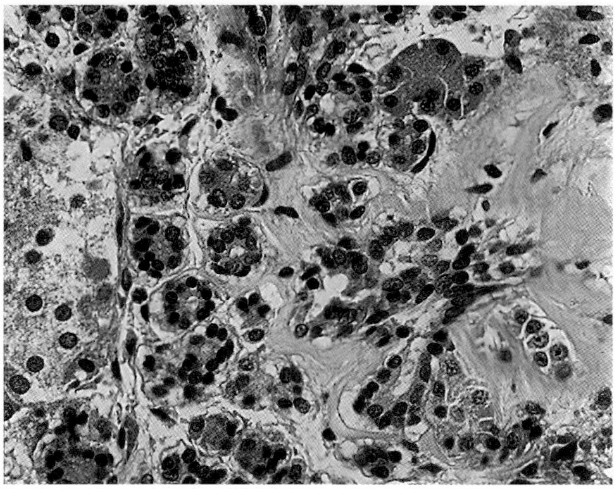

this gland is denominated the clitorial gland or female preputial gland. The whole organ is covered by a connective tissue capsule which spreads into the parenchyma forming septae. The acinar cells contain prominent cytoplasmic eosinophilic granules. The excretory ducts are lined by stratified squamous epithelium and are frequently dilated.

Prostate Gland (Glandula Prostatica) (Figure 15.63)

The bilaterally symmetrical prostate consists of three lobes: dorsocranial (called coagulation gland), ventral and dorsolateral. The dorsocranial lobes (coagulation gland) are attached to the seminal vesicles. The ventral lobes are located along the ventrolateral surface of the urinary bladder. The dorsolateral lobes surround the proximal end of the urethra. All three lobes open into the urethra, near to the seminal collicle. This tubuloalveolar gland consists of alveoli (acini) lined by epithelium and surrounded by smooth muscle. The type of epithelium can vary depending on location within the organ and physiological stage; from tall pseudo-stratified to cuboidal and low cuboidal epithelium (Hebel and Stromberg, 1986).

A characteristic spontaneous aging change is in-flammation, especially of the chronic purulent type.

Rectum

See intestine.

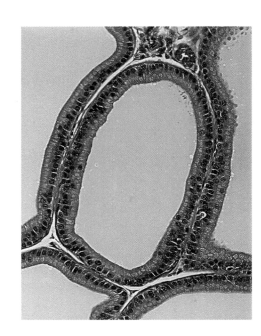

Figure 15.63 Prostate gland. The alveoli are lined by tall columnar epithelium (characteristic for ventral lobes).

Figure 15.61 Pituitary gland. Aberrant craniopharyngeal structures in the form of serous glandular acini.

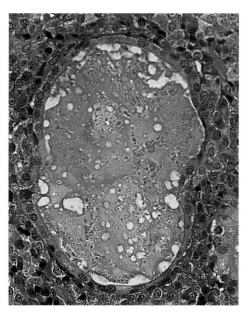

Figure 15.62 Pituitary gland. Developmental cyst in the pars distalis, partly lined by ciliated epithelium.

The well-developed vascular supply of the whole organ is formed by wide sinusoids and capillaries. The sexual difference in the volume and the weight of the organ (larger in females) is mainly due to the bigger adenohypophysis of the females.

The rat pituitary gland occasionally shows developmental cysts and sometimes a malformation known as 'craniopharyngeal structures' (Schaetti et al., 1995).

Preputial Gland (Glandula Preputialis)

The paired preputial glands are modified sebaceous glands, located in the subcutaneous adipose tissue lateral to the penis. The gland opens at the border of the parietal preputial layer and the skin. In females,

Salivary Glands (Glandulae Salivales)

(Figures 15.64 and 15.65)

There are so-called lesser and greater salivary glands. The lesser glands are represented by the minor sublingual, the buccal, the palatine and the lingual glands. The paired greater salivary glands are the parotis, (sub)mandibular (submaxillary) and greater sublingual.

The glands are composed of acinar cells and numerous ducts. The parotis consists of 3–4 distinct serous lobes, attached to the base of the auricle and rostrally is in contact with extraorbital lacrimal gland. The submandibular gland has serous and mucous acinar cells. The greater sublingual gland is tightly attached to the submandibular gland, is darker in color and mucous. The submandibular salivary gland shows sexual dimorphism of ducts: their diameter is larger in males.

The aging gland can show foci of atrophy.

Seminal Vesicle (Glandula Vesicularis) (Figure 15.66)

The paired seminal vesicles, which occur in males, lie dorsolaterally to the urinary bladder. Their ventromedial side is attached to the dorsocranial lobes of the prostate gland (coagulating glands). Both seminal vesicles unite in the middle and open into the ampulla of the urethra, joining with the ductus deferens in seminal colliculus. The seminal vesicle has a wall composed of smooth muscle and tall columnar epithelium.

Skeletal Muscle (Figures 15.67 and 15.68)

Skeletal muscle consists of cross-striated extrafusal and intrafusal muscle fibers, connective tissue, blood vessels and nerve fibers.

Age-related changes in skeletal muscle fibers are fiber atrophy, fiber splitting, increased accumulation of lipofuscin, and fiber loss and fibrosis.

Skin (Cutis, Derma, Integumentum Commune)

(Figures 15.69 and 15.70)

The skin covers the whole body. It is composed of epidermis, dermis (corium) and subcutis

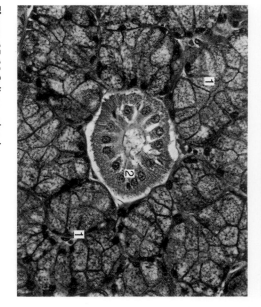

Figure 15.64 Salivary gland.
1 mucous acini   2 intralobular duct

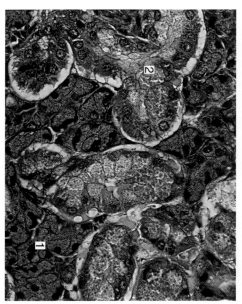

Figure 15.65 Salivary gland.
1 serous acini
2 so-called 'convoluted' ducts (submandibular gland)

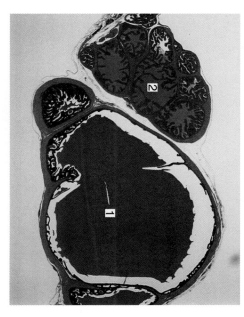

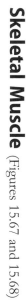

Figure 15.66 Seminal vesicle.
1 seminal vesicle
2 dorsocranial lobe of the prostate (coagulating gland)

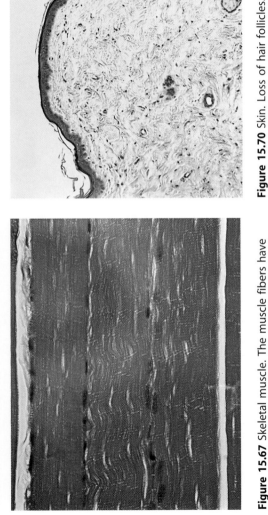

Figure 15.70 Skin. Loss of hair follicles.

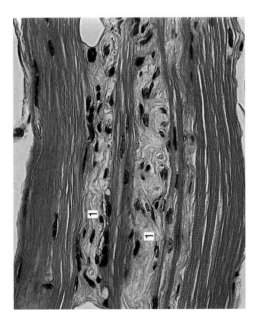

Figure 15.67 Skeletal muscle. The muscle fibers have cross-striation and nuclei located at the periphery.

Figure 15.68 Skeletal muscle. Some striated muscle fibers are lost and replaced by interstitial fibrosis.
1   fibrous tissue

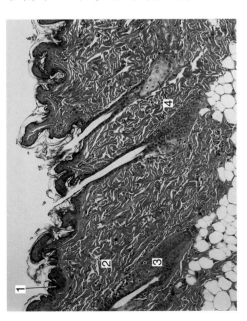

Figure 15.69 Skin.
1   epidermis
2   dermis

3   hair follicle
4   sebaceous glands

(hypodermis). The epidermis is of epithelial origin and contains four layers: stratum basale, spinosum, granulosum and corneum. The rat epidermis is relatively thin because it is densely covered by hair. The dermis is formed by connective tissue with collagen and elastic fibers and, especially in young animals, is highly cellular. The dermis is divided into stratum papillare and stratum reticulare, which contains coarser collagen fibers. The subcutis is formed by loose connective tissue with moderate amounts of fat tissue. The latter depends on the nutritional condition and it is predominantly white fat. In the rat, brown fat is located between the scapulae, in the ventral neck and in the axillary and inguinal regions. The hair coat of the rat is formed by guard hairs and underhairs. The hair follicles are arranged in groups, usually with a central follicle of a guard hair in the middle and follicles of the underhair around it. These groups are in turn arranged in rows parallel to the long axis of the body. On the upper and lower lip, nose, chin, above the eyelid, near the ear and on the caudal side of the thoracic limbs there are sinus (tactile) hairs. They are important for orientation of the animal. The sinus hair follicles are well supplied with blood vessels and nerves. Around the hair follicles there are sebaceous glands. In the rat, the sweat glands are located only in the skin of the foot pads (Hebel and Stromberg, 1986).

Spontaneous changes occurring with aging are loss of hair, reflected by atrophy and loss of hair follicles.

Small Intestine (Intestinum Tenue)

See intestine.

Spinal Cord (Medulla Spinalis)

(Figure 15.71)

A particular feature of the rat spinal cord is the presence of corticospinal (pyramidal) fibers in the deep portion of the dorsal spinal columns. Otherwise, the rat spinal cord is organized similarly to other mammalian species. It consists of 8 cervical, 13 thoracic, 6 lumbar and 4 sacral segments.

Spleen (Lien) (Figure 15.72)

The greatest lymphoreticular organ of the body is located in the left dorsal part of the abdominal cavity. Dorsally, it contacts the liver, then extends between the stomach and the left kidney to the abdominal wall in the ventrocaudal direction. It lies between two layers of omentum and is covered by a connective tissue capsule containing a few muscle fibers. The capsule spreads into the spleen parenchyma, forming trabeculae. The parenchyma consists of white and red pulp. The white pulp is organized into periarteriolar lymphoid sheets (PALS, representing mainly T cells) and lymphatic follicles, which become prominent in a response to stimulation. The periphery of white pulp is formed by a less densely cellular marginal zone. The red pulp consists of reticular tissue and venous sinuses.

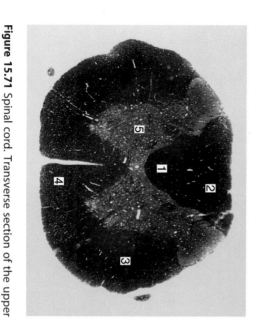

Figure 15.71 Spinal cord. Transverse section of the upper cervical cord, epoxy resin, toluidine blue.
1 corticospinal (motor) fibers in the deep portion of dorsal columns
2 sensory fibers in the
3 lateral columns
4 ventral columns
5 gray matter
superficial portion of the dorsal columns

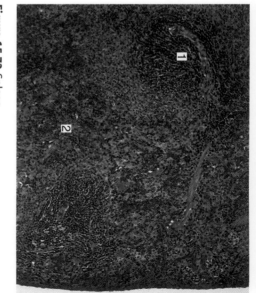

Figure 15.72 Spleen.
1 white pulp, arranged into inner PALS (periarteriolar lyphoid sheaths) and outer marginal zone
2 red pulp

Stomach (Gaster, Ventriculus)

(Figures 15.73–15.75)

The stomach is located transversally in the left cranial part of the abdominal cavity. Most of the parietal surface and part of the visceral surface are covered by the liver. The esophagus enters at the middle of the lesser curvature. The stomach is subdivided into nonglandular (forestomach, pars cardiaca, saccus cecus) and glandular (pars fundica et pars pylorica) portions. The forestomach is equipped with a cutaneous (stratified squamous epithelium) mucous

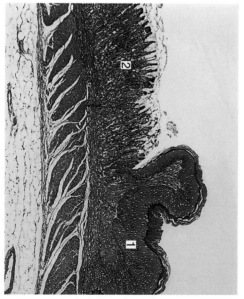

Figure 15.73 Stomach. Transition of nonglandular and glandular stomach, called margo plicatus.
1 nonglandular stomach (forestomach)
2 glandular stomach

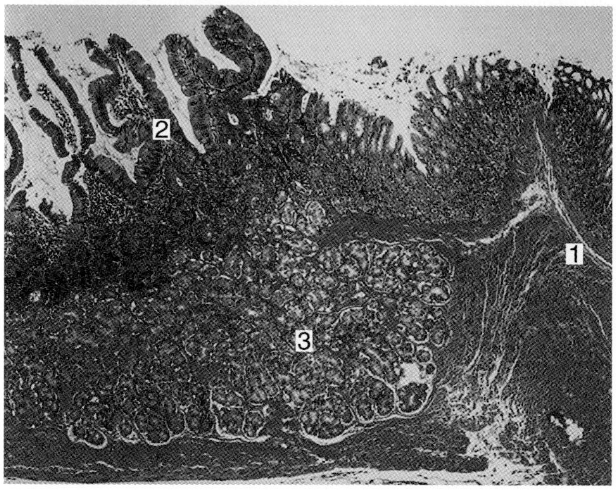

membrane, the glandular stomach has a glandular mucous membrane forming fundic (gastric) glands. The cutaneous mucous membrane is separated from the glandular mucous membrane by a line of transition (limiting ridge, margo plicatus). The cell types of the glandular mucosa include: simple columnar cells, forming so-called gastric pits, chief (zymogen/peptic), parietal (oxyntic, producing hydrochloric acid), mucous, and enteroendocrine cells: G (producing gastrin), ECL (enterochromaffin-like, producing histamine and other peptides), A (producing glucagon), and D (producing somatostatin). The parietal cells do not occur in the pyloric area, which contains short, coiled mucous glands (Brown and Hardisty, 1990). The tunica muscularis is composed of inner oblique, middle circular and outer longitudinal smooth muscle layers.

Tuch *et al.* (1992) compared the frequency of enterochromaffin-like cells in various rat strains. The methodology of morphometric evaluation of enterochromaffin-like cells in the gastric mucosa was described by White *et al.* (1998).

In aging rats, the gastric glands are frequently dilated.

Testis (Testis, Orchis)

(Figures 15.76–15.78)

The paired testes, normally located in the scrotum, can be easily withdrawn into the abdominal cavity through the open inguinal canal. The organ is

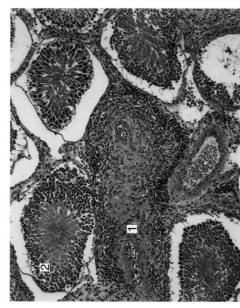

Figure 15.77 Testis.
1 polyarteritis characterized by fibrinoid necrosis, massive thickening and inflammatory cell infiltration of the vessel wall
2 seminiferous tubules are preserved

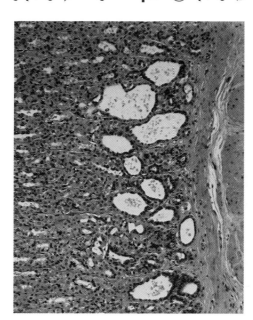

Figure 15.75 Stomach. Dilatation of gastric glands in the glandular stomach.

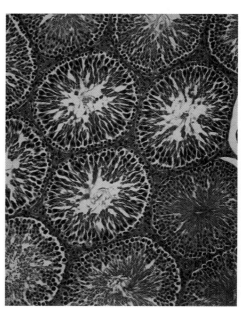

Figure 15.76 Testis. Transverse section showing seminiferous tubules and interstitial cells.

Figure 15.74 Stomach. Transition from pylorus to duodenum.
1 pylorus   2 duodenum   3 Brunner's glands

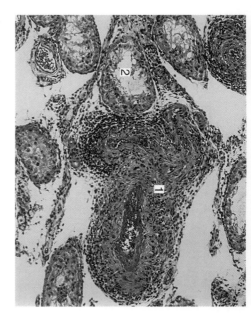

Figure 15.78 Testis.

1 polyarteritis   2 tubular atrophy

covered by thick tunica albuginea and thin tunica vaginalis which also covers the inner surface of the scrotum. There are about 20 seminiferous tubules in the adult rat testis. They form convoluted loops that are connected at both ends to the rete testis (Russel, 1992). The seminiferous tubules contain germ cells arranged in discrete layers: spermatogonia, spermatocytes, and one or two layers of spermatids. The Sertoli cells reach from the basal lamina to the tubular lumen. The rete testis conducts the sperm from the seminiferous tubules to the epididymis. The endocrine Leydig cells are located among the tubules, together with other peritubular cells, interstitial macrophages and interstitial vasculature. The methodology of spermatogenic staging (determination of the stages of spermatogenic cycle) was described by Russel et al. (1990) and reviewed by Creasy (1997). Details are described in Chapter 9 of this book dealing with the physiology of reproduction. The quality of histological preparations enabling high resolution is of critical importance. In the view of some authors, formalin fixation is only acceptable when combined with plastic embedding (Chapin et al., 1984; Creasy, 1997), while others argue that the essential details can be easily identified in formalin-fixed, paraffin-embedded tissue (Harleman and Nolte, 1997).

Spontaneous changes occurring in aging rats include tubular atrophy and occasionally polyarteritis. Impaction of spermatozoa with dystrophic calcification may occur spontaneously as well. Lee et al. (1993) described spontaneous changes such as tubular degeneration and spermatid retention occurring in young male rats at the age of 10–12 weeks. Tubular atrophy is usually associated with hyperplasia of Leydig cells (Takahashi et al., 1992).

Thymus (Figures 15.79 and 15.80)

The thymus, consisting of two lobes, lies partly in the cervical area and mostly in the thoracic cavity behind the sternum. It nearly reaches the larynx cranially and the heart caudally. It is covered by a connective tissue capsule. The parenchyma is divided into distinct lobules by septae. The organ is composed of cortex and medulla. The medulla is rich in epithelial cells, forming Hassall's bodies, which, however, are not as characteristically shaped as in other species. The cortex is densely filled with lymphocytes (essentially differentiating T cells).

The thymus retains its size until the maturation of the organism; thereafter it regresses and becomes atrophic.

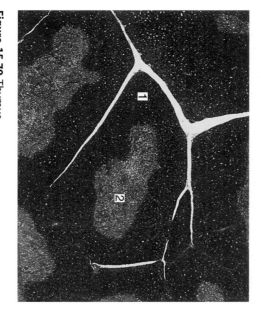

Figure 15.79 Thymus.

1 cortex   2 medulla

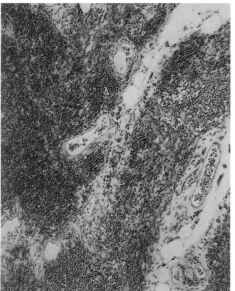

Figure 15.80 Thymus. Atrophy manifested by loss of lymphatic tissue; the regular lobular structure is effaced.

Thyroid Gland (Glandula Thyroidea)

(Figures 15.81–15.83)

The thyroid gland lies ventrolaterally and on either side of the trachea just below the larynx. It spreads over the fourth and fifth tracheal ring. It consists of two lobes connected by an isthmus. There is controversy as to whether the gland is to be considered as a paired, or unpaired, bilaterally symmetrical organ. The organ is covered by a capsule consisting predominantly of collagenous fibers. The parenchyma consists of follicles of different sizes. The follicles contain colloid, the amount and staining

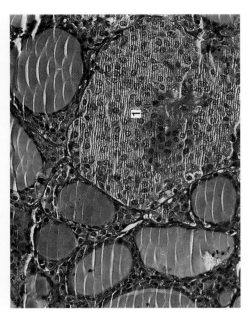

properties of which, as well as the shape of the follicular epithelium, depend on the physiologial stage. The follicular cells are columnar when active, flattened when inactive. Active follicles have a decreased amount of colloid. Between the follicles there are parafollicular or C cells. They are distributed over the whole organ, but occur more frequently in the center of each lobe. The pathophysiology of thyroid gland in rat and other species was reviewed by Capen (1997).

Occasionally, aberrant thymic tissue or developmental cysts are found in the rat thyroid gland. The number of thyroid C cells in the rat increases with age (Delverdier et al., 1990).

Figure 15.83 Thyroid gland.
1 a group of proliferated parafollicular C cells

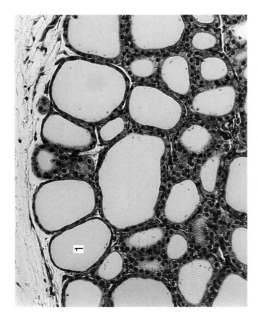

Figure 15.81 Thyroid gland.
1 the flattened epithelial cell lining of the peripheral follicles indicates low degree of activity

Tongue (Lingua)

See oral cavity.

Tooth (Dens)

The rat has 16 teeth, the formula being I 1/1 C 0/0 PM 0/0 M 3/3, i.e. an incisor and three molars on each side of the jaws. The gap between incisors and molars is called the diastema. The skin folds behind the incisors can close the mouth, preventing the swallowing of indigestible material (Olds and Olds, 1979). The anatomy and pathology of rat incisors was reviewed by Kuijpers et al. (1996).

Spontaneous changes occur mainly in the incisors and include traumatic, necrotic, inflammatory and proliferative lesions commonly known as dental dysplasia (Losco, 1995).

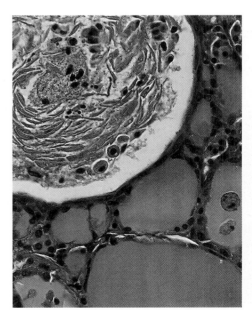

Figure 15.82 Thyroid gland. Cavity lined by squamous epithelium and filled with desquamated cells; though considered developmental cysts, such structures can become more frequent in aged animals.

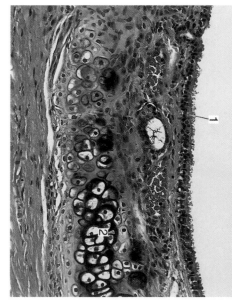

Figure 15.84 Trachea.
1 epithelial cell lining 2 cartilage

Trachea (Figure 15.84)

The trachea connects the larynx to the left and right principal bronchi, and is located ventrally to the esophagus in the cervical area. The trachea is formed by about 24 C-shaped cartilages, with smooth muscles joining the ends. The epithelial lining is pseudostratified, in the proximal part mainly nonciliated, (basal, goblet, Clara, neurosecretory cells), while distally, towards the bifurcation there is an increased number of ciliated cells. In the proximal part the submucosa contains seromucous glands (Boorman et al., 1990b).

The cartilages calcify in adult and older animals (Hebel and Stromberg, 1986).

Urinary Bladder (Vesica Urinaria) (Figure 15.85)

The bladder is located in the dorsocaudal area of the abdominal cavity. The lumen is lined by a transitional epithelial layer, the urothelium, which normally is three cells thick (representing the basal, intermediate and superficial cell layers). In the empty or contracted bladder the epithelial cells are pushed together, giving the appearance of more than three cell layers (Jokinen, 1990). The rat urothelium shows low cell turnover (Kunze and Gassner, 1986). The wall is further formed by submucosa, three smooth muscle layers, and adventitia. The thickest muscle layer is the middle one, consisting predominantly of circular or oblique fibers. Cohen et al. (1996) observed that extensive handling of rats can result in mild (urothelial) hyperplasia.

transitional epithelium and equipped with urethral glands, mainly in the pelvic part and urethral bulb. The submucosa consists of fibrous and cavernous vascular tissue. The proximal urethra usually contains an eosinophilic mass known as the 'urethral plug' (Kunstyr et al., 1982; Jokinen, 1990).

In the female, the urethra (feminina) opens independently of the vagina and ventrally to it. The external urethral orifice lies dorsally to the clitoris in a common cone-shaped skin protrusion, which also receives the openings of the paired clitoral gland ('female preputial gland').

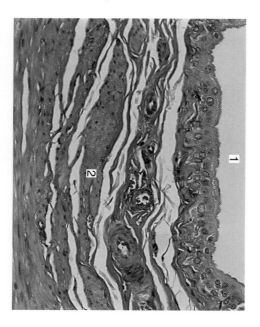

Figure 15.85 Urinary bladder.
1 lumen lined by urothelium (transitional epithelium)
2 muscular wall

Ureter

The paired ureters connect the kidneys to the urinary bladder. The ureteral wall consists of transitional epithelium, muscularis and adventitia.

Urethra

In the male, the urethra (masculina) is made up of the pelvic part, the urethral bulb (receiving the ducts of bulbourethral glands) and the penile part ending at glans penis. The initial part of the pelvic urethra forms the ampulla, containing the seminal collicle with openings of the ductus deferens and the seminal vesicles. Excretory ducts of the prostate gland enter the urethra lateral and posterior to the ducts of the other glands. The wall of the urethra is lined by

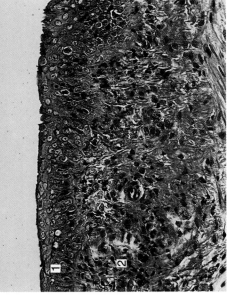

Figure 15.86 Uterus.
1 lumen lined by endometrium; the high columnar epithelium is characteristic of diestrus
2 uterine glands
3 endometrial stroma

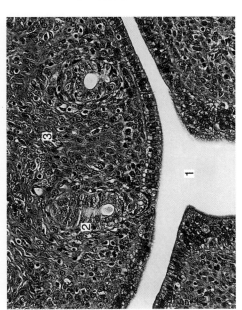

Figure 15.87 Vagina. The appearance corresponds to features of diestrus.
1 stratified squamous epithelium
2 submucosa with leukocytic infiltration

Uterus (Figure 15.86)

The rat uterus is uterus duplex (subseptus). Usually, it is considered as a single, bilaterally symmetrical rather than a paired organ. The lumina of the uterine horns are completely separate and open into the vaginal lumen as a paired external orifice (portio vaginalis uteri). The uterine horns lie in the dorsal abdominal cavity, the uterine body and vagina lie between the dorsally located rectum and ventrally located urinary bladder. The wall is composed of mucosa (endometrium), two smooth muscle layers (myometrium), and adventitia. The single row of the columnar epithelial lining of the mucosa forms uterine glands projecting into the endometrial propria (stroma). During the estrous cycle the uterus undergoes the following changes (Hebel and Stromberg, 1986):

- Proestrus: the lumen is distended with fluid so that the epithelial cells are cuboidal rather than columnar, the stroma and myometrium show an extensive infiltration with leukocytes.
- Estrus: the endometrium is hyperemic, the lumen maximally distended, the leukocytic infiltration persists.
- Metestrus: the liquid content diminishes, the low cuboidal epithelium shows vacuolar degeneration, leukocytic infiltration of the stroma and myometrium is decreased.
- Diestrus: the epithelium is regenerated, high columnar; the leukocytic infiltration is reduced to a minimum.

The age-related uterine changes are: an increase in connective tissue (collagen) in the endometrium, the glands are quiescent, widely scattered without mitotic activity, leukocytes are absent. Occasionally, endometrial cysts and (glandular) cystic hyperplasia occur in aged females (Brown and Leininger, 1992).

Vagina (Figure 15.87)

The vagina opens to the outside separately from the urethra, just below the anus. In the young females the vagina is closed by a membrane, or plug, until the beginning of puberty. It opens at about 72 days and ovulation begins at about 77 days (Green, 1963). Hebel and Stromberg (1986) describe this membrane as transverse epithelial septum which begins to degenerate at about 20–35 days, so that the continuous lumen opens at about 40–80 days. The vagina is lined by stratified squamous epithelium, exhibiting characteristic changes during the estrous cycle. Table 15.5 compares the cycle stages and findings of exfoliative cytology and histology.

A detailed description of the exfoliative cytology and histology of the vagina during the stages of estrous cycle was published by Yuan and Carlson (1987).

Zymbal's Gland

The paired Zymbal's glands are auditory sebaceous glands. The gland consists of acinar sebaceous cells and excretory ducts lined by stratified squamous epithelium. It opens into the external ear canal.

Table 15.5 Cycle stages and exfoliative cytology and histology findings of the rat vagina

Smear		Histology
Weiss et al. (Chapter 25)	Maeda et al. (Chapter 9)	Hebel and Stromberg (1986)
Proestrus Predominantly nucleated epithelial cells, few cornified epithelial cells, few leukocytes	**Proestrus 'N'** Predominantly nucleated cells, some cornified cells in the late afternoon of proestrus	**Proestrus** Vaginal epithelium is thick (8–12 layers), cornified epithelium begins to develop, superficial layers show mucous change
Estrus Almost exclusively epithelial cells, most of them cornified with pyknotic nuclei	**Estrus 'C'** Abundant cornified cells, characterized by swollen shape and loss of nuclei	**Estrus** The vaginal epithelium is formed by 6–10 layers, of which 3–5 superficial layers are cornified
Metestrus Predominantly leukocytes and cornified epithelial cells	**Diestrus 1 'L'** Numerous leukocytes in addition to nucleated cells and shrinking cornified cells	**Metestrus** The cornified cell layers become detached and partly fill the vaginal lumen
Diestrus Predominantly leukocytes, few epithelial cells and mucus	**Diestrus 2** (4-day cycle) **Diestrus 3** (5-day cycle) Similar to diestrus 1	**Diestrus** The epithelium is thin, but the number of cell layers increases again up to 10; there are numerous leukocytes

References

Altmann, G.G. (1975) *Am. J. Anat.* **143**, 219–240.

Aoki, A., Yoseph, S., Pasolli, H.A. and Torres, A.I. (1993) *Exp. Toxic. Pathol.* **45**, 39–40.

Bannasch, P. and Gössner, W. (1994) *Pathology of Neoplasia and Preneoplasia in Rodents.* Stuttgart: Schattauer.

Bannasch, P. and Gössner, W. (1997) *Pathology of Neoplasia and Preneoplasia in Rodents,* Vol. 2. Stuttgart: Schattauer.

Bolon, B., Bucci, T.J., Warbritton, A.R., Chen, J.J., Mattison, D.R. and Heindel J.J. (1997) *Fundam. Appl. Toxicol.* **39**, 1–10.

Bomhard, E. (1992) *Exp. Toxicol. Pathol.* **44**, 381–392.

Bomhard, E. and Rinke, M. (1994) *Exp. Toxic. Pathol.* **46**, 17–29.

Boorman, G.A. and Eustis, S.L. (1990) In: Boorman, G.A., Eustis, S.L., Elwell, M.R., Montgomery Jr, Ch.A. and MacKenzie, W.F. (eds) *Pathology of the Fischer Rat,* pp. 339–368. San Diego: Academic Press.

Boorman, G.A., Eustis, S.L., Elwell, M.R., Montgomery

Jr, Ch.A. and MacKenzie, W.F. (eds) (1990a) *Pathology of the Fischer Rat.* San Diego: Academic Press.

Boorman, G.A., Morgan, K.T. and Uriah, L.C. (1990b) In: Boorman, G.A., Eustis, S.L., Elwell, M.R., Montgomery Jr, Ch.A. and MacKenzie, W.F. (eds) *Pathology of the Fischer Rat,* pp. 315–337. San Diego: Academic Press.

Boorman, G.A., Wilson, J.Th., van Zwieten, M.J. and Eustis, S.L. (1990c) In: Boorman, G.A., Eustis, S.L., Elwell, M.R., Montgomery Jr, Ch.A. and MacKenzie, W.F. (eds) *Pathology of the Fischer Rat,* pp. 295–314. San Diego: Academic Press.

Brown, H.R. and Hardisty, J.F. (1990) In: Boorman, G.A., Eustis, S.L., Elwell, M.R., Montgomery Jr, Ch.A. and MacKenzie, W.F. (eds) *Pathology of the Fischer Rat,* pp. 9–30. San Diego: Academic Press.

Brown H.R. and Leininger, J.R. (1992) In: Mohr, U., Dungworth, D.L. and Capen, C.C. (eds) *Pathobiology of the Aging Rat,* pp. 377–388. Washington DC: ILSI Press.

Bruner, R.H., Keller, W.F., Stitzel, K.A. *et al.* (1992) *Toxicol. Pathol.* **20**, 357–366.

Hebel, R. and Stromberg, M.W. (1986) *Anatomy and Embryology of the Laboratory Rat*. Woerthsee: BioMed Verlag.

Heindel, J.J. (1998) In: Daston, G. and Kimmel, C. (eds) *An Evaluation and Interpretation of Reproductive Endpoints for Human Health Risk Assessment*, pp. 57–74. Washington DC: ILSI Press.

Hirshfield, A.N. and Midgley, A.R. Jr. (1978) Morphometric analysis of follicular development in the rat. *Biol. Reprod.* **19**, 597–605.

Irisarri, E. and Hollander, C.F. (1994) In: Mohr, U., Dungworth, D.L. and Capen, C.C. (eds) *Pathology of the Aging Rat*, pp. 341–350. Washington DC: ILSI Press.

Johansson, J.O. (1987) *Acta Anat.* **128**, 55–62.

Jokinen, M.P. (1990). In: Boorman, G.A., Eustis, S.L., Elwell, M.R., Montgomery Ch.A., Jr. and MacKenzie, W.F. (eds) *Pathology of the Fischer Rat*, pp. 109–126. San Diego, CA: Academic Press.

Krinke, A.I., Schaetti, Ph. and Krinke, G.J. (1994) In: Mohr, U., Dungworth, D.L. and Capen, C.C. (eds) *Pathobiology of the Aging Rat*, pp. 109–119. Washington DC: ILSI Press.

Krinke, G.J. (1988) In: Jones, T.C., Mohr, U. and Hunt, R.D. (eds) *ILSI Monographs on the Pathology of Laboratory Animals, Nervous System*, pp. 203–208. Berlin: Springer Verlag.

Krinke, G. (1991) In: Jones, T.C., Mohr, U. and Hunt, R.D. (eds) *ILSI Monographs on the Pathology of Laboratory Animals, Special Sense*, pp. 203–208. Berlin: Springer Verlag.

Krinke, G.J. and Eisenbrandt, D.L. (1994) In: Mohr, U., Dungworth, D.L. and Capen, C.C. (eds) *Pathobiology of the Aging Rat*, pp. 3–19. Washington DC: ILSI Press.

Kuijpers, M.H.M., Van de Kooiju, A.J. and Slootweg, P.J. (1996) *Toxicol. Pathol.* **24**, 346–360.

Kunstyr, I., Küpper, W., Weisser, H., Naumann, S. and Messow, C. (1982) *Lab. Anim.* **16**, 151–155.

Kunze, E. and Gassner, G. (1986) *J. Cancer Clin. Oncol.* **112**, 11–18.

Lee, K.P., Frame, S.R., Sykes, G.P. and Valentine, R. (1993) *Toxicol. Pathol.* **21**, 292–302.

Leininger, J.R. and Riley, M.G.I. (1990) In: Boorman, G.A., Eustis, S.L., Elwell, M.R., Montgomery Ch.A., Jr. and MacKenzie, W.F. (eds) *Pathology of the Fischer Rat*, pp. 209–226. San Diego, CA: Academic Press.

Leopold, J.H. and Calcins, L. (1951) *Am. J. Ophthalmol.* **34**, 1735–1741.

Lessell, S. and Kuwabara, T. (1974) *Invest. Ophthal.* **13**, 748–756.

Lewis, D.J. (1992) In: Mohr, U., Dungworth, D.L. and Capen, C.C. (eds) *Pathobiology of the Aging Rat*, pp. 301–309. Washington DC: ILSI Press.

Losco, P.E. (1995) *Toxicol. Pathol.* **23**, 677–688.

Losco, P. and Harleman, H. (1992) In: Mohr, U., Dungworth, D.L. and Capen, C.C. (eds) *Pathobiology*

Bucci, T.J., Bolon, B., Warbritton, A.R., Chen, J.J. and Heindel, J.J. (1997) *Repra. Toxicol.* **11**, 689–696.

Capen, Ch.C. (1997) *Toxicol. Pathol.* **25**, 39–48.

Chandra, M., Riley, M.G.I. and Johnson, D.E. (1992) Spontaneous neoplasms in aged Sprague-Dawley rats. *Arch. Toxicol.* **66**, 496–502.

Chapin, R.E., Ross, M.D. and Lamb, J.C. (1984) *Toxicol. Pathol.* **12**, 221–227.

Cline, J.M. and Maronpot, R.R. (1985) Variations in the histologic distribution of rat bone marrow cells with respect to age and anatomic site. *Toxicol. Pathol.* **13**, 349–355.

Cohen, S.M., Cano, M., Anderson, T. and Garland, E.M. (1996) *Toxicol. Pathol.* **24**, 251–257.

Creasy, D.M. (1997) *Toxicol. Pathol.* **25**, 119–131.

Del Vecchio, F.R. (1992) In: Mohr, U., Dungworth, D.L. and Capen, C.C. (eds) *Pathobiology of the Aging Rat*, pp. 331–336. Washington DC: ILSI Press.

Delverdier, M., Cabanie, P., Roome, N., Enjalbert, F., Plaisancie, P. and van Haverbeke, G. (1990) *Acta Anat.* **138**, 182–184.

Dillberger, J.E. (1994) *Toxicol. Pathol.* **22**, 48–55.

Dixon, D., Heider, K. and Elwell, M.R. (1995) *Toxicol. Pathol.* **23**, 338–348.

Elwell, M.R. and McConnell, E.E. (1990) In: Boorman, G.A., Eustis, S.L., Elwell, M.R., Montgomery Jr, Ch. A. and MacKenzie, W.F. (ede) *Pathology of the Fischer Rat*, pp. 43–62. San Diego, CA: Academic Press.

Eustis, S.L., Boorman, G.A., Harada, T. and Popp, J.A. (1990a) In: Boorman, G.A., Eustis, S.L., Elwell, M.R., Montgomery Jr, Ch.A. and MacKenzie, W.F. (eds) *Pathology of the Fischer Rat*, pp. 71–94. San Diego: Academic Press.

Eustis, S.L., Boorman, G.A. and Hayashi, Y. (1990b) In: Boorman, G.A., Eustis, S.L., Elwell, M.R., Montgomery, P.G., Ockert, D. and Tuch, K. (1995) *Toxicol. Pathol.* **23**, 349–355.

Feeney, L. (1973) *Invest. Ophthalmol.* **12**, 635–638.

Feldman, M.I. (1994) In: Mohr, U., Dungworth, D.L. and Capen, C.C. (eds.) *Pathobiology of the Aging Rat*, pp. 121–147. Washington DC: ILSI Press.

Germann, P.G., Ockert, D. and Tuch, K. (1995) *Toxicol. Pathol.* **23**, 349–355.

Gough, A.W., Kasali, O.B., Sigler, R.E. and Baragi, V. (1992) *Toxicol. Pathol.* **20**, 436–449.

Green, E.Ch. (1963) *Anatomy of the Rat*. New York: Hafner Publishing.

Greaves, P. and Faccini, J.M. (1984) *Rat Histopathology*. Amsterdam: Elsevier.

Hamlin II, M.H. and Banas, D.A. (1990) In: Boorman, G.A., Eustis, S.L., Elwell, M.R., Montgomery Ch.A., Jr. and MacKenzie, W.F. (eds) *Pathology of the Fischer Rat*, pp. 501–518. San Diego, CA: Academic Press.

Harkema, J.R. (1991) *Toxicol. Pathol.* **19**, 321–336.

Harleman, J.H. and Nolte, T. (1997) *Toxicol. Pathol.* **25**, 414–417.

of the Aging Rat, pp. 49–73. Washington DC: ILSI Press.

MacKenzie, W.F. and Boorman, G.A. (1990) In: Boorman, G.A., Eustis, S.L., Elwell, M.R., Montgomery Ch.A., Jr. and MacKenzie, W.F. (eds) Pathology of the Fischer Rat, pp. 485–500. San Diego, CA: Academic Press.

MacKenzie, W.F. and Eustis, S.L. (1990) In: Boorman, G.A., Eustis, S.L., Elwell, M.R., Montgomery Ch.A., Jr. and MacKenzie, W.F. (eds) Pathology of the Fischer Rat, pp. 395–404. San Diego, CA: Academic Press.

McMartin, D.N., Sahota, P.S., Gunson, D.E., Han Hsu, H. and Spaet, R.H. (1992) Toxicol. Pathol. 20, 212–225.

Mery, S., Gross, E.A., Joyner, D.R., Godo, M. and Morgan, K.T. (1994) Toxicol. Pathol. 22, 353–372.

Mohr, U. (ed) (1997) International Classification of Rodent Tumours, Part I: The Rat. IARC Scientific Publications No. 122, Lyon, 1997.

Mohr, U., Dungworth, D.L. and Capen, C.C. (eds) (1992) Pathobiology of the Aging Rat, Vol. 1, Blood and Lymphoid System, Respiratory System, Urinary System, Cardiovascular System, Reproductive System. Washington DC: ILSI Press.

Mohr, U., Dungworth, D.L. and Capen, C.C. (eds) (1994) Pathobiology of the Aging Rat, Vol. 2, Nervous System and Special Sense Organs, Endocrine System, Digestive System, Integumentary System and Mammary Gland, Musculoskeletal System and Soft Tissue, General Aspects. Washington DC: ILSI Press.

Monticello, T.M., Morgan, K.T. and Hurtt, M.E. (1990) Toxicol. Pathol. 18, 24–31.

Morawietz, G., Rittinghausen, S. and Mohr, U. (1992) Exp. Toxic. Pathol. 44, 301–309.

Morgan, K.T. (1997) Toxicol. Pathol. 25, 291–307.

Olds, R. and Olds, J. (1979) A Colour Atlas of the Rat – Dissection Guide. London: Wolfe Medical Publications.

Parker, G.A. and Gibson, W.B. (1995) Toxicol. Pathol. 23, 507–512.

Parmigiani, C.M. and McAvoy, J.W. (1989) Curr. Eye Res. 8, 1271–1277.

Pedersen, T. and Peters, H. (1968) J. Reprod. Fertil. 17, 555–557.

Plowchalk, D.R., Smith, B.J. and Mattison, D.R. (1993) In: Heindel, J.J. and Chapin, R.E. (eds) Methods in Toxicology, Vol. 3, Part B, Female Reproductive Toxicology, pp. 57–68. San Diego: Academic Press.

Popesko, P., Rajtova, V. and Horak, J. (1990) Atlas anatomie malých laboratórnych zvierat, Vol. 2. Bratislava: Príroda. (English version published by Wolfe Publishing Ltd., London, 1992.)

Poteracti, J. and Walsh, K.M. (1998) Toxicol Sciences 45, 1–8.

Rappaport, A.M., Borowy, Z.J., Lougheed, W.M. and Lotto, W.N. (1954) Anat. Rec. 119, 11–34.

Read, N.G. (1991) Histochem. J. 23, 436–443.

Renne, R.A., Gideon, K.M., Miller, R.A., Mellick, P.W. and Grumbein, S.L. (1992) Toxicol. Pathol. 20, 44–51.

Renne, R.A., Sagartz, J.W. and Burger, G.T. (1993) Toxicol. Pathol. 21, 542–546.

Riley, M.G.I., Boorman, G.A. and Hayashi, Y. (1990) In: Boorman, G.A., Eustis, S.L., Elwell, M.R., Montgomery Ch.A., Jr. and MacKenzie, W.F. (eds) Pathology of the Fischer Rat, pp. 545–556, San Diego, CA: Academic Press.

Russel, L.D. (1992) In: Mohr, U., Dungworth, D.L. and Capen, C.C. (eds) Pathobiology of the Aging Rat, pp. 395–405, Washington DC: ILSI Press.

Russel, L.D., Ettlin, R.A., Sinha Hikim, A.P. and Clegg, E.D. (1990) Histological and Histopathological Evaluation of the Testis. Cache River Press, Clearwater, FL, 34–620.

Sagartz, J.W., Madarasz, A.J., Forsell, M.A., Burger, G.T., Ayres, P.H. and Coggins, C.R.E. (1992) Toxicol. Pathol. 20, 118–121.

Salu, P., Claeskens, W., De Wilde, A., Hijmans, W. and Wisse, E. (1985) Ophthal. Res. 17, 125–130.

Seaman, W.J. (1987) Postmortem change in the rat: a histologic characterization. Iowa State University Press, Ames, 420 pp.

Schaetti, Ph., Argentino-Storino, A., Heinrichs, M., Mirea, D., Popp, A. and Karbe, E. (1995) Exp. Toxic. Pathol. 47, 129–137.

Schaller, O. (ed) (1992) Illustrated Veterinary Anatomical Nomenclature. Stuttgart: Ferdinand Enke Verlag.

Schlage, W.K., Bülles, H., Friedrichs, D., Kuhn, M. and Teredesai, A. (1998) Toxicol. Pathol. 26, 324–343.

Setzer, P.Y., Nichols, B.A. and Dawson, C.R. (1987) Invest. Ophthalmol. Vis. Sci. 27, 531–537.

Stinson, S.F., Schuller, H.M. and Reznik, G.K. (1990) Atlas of Tumor Pathology of the Fischer Rat. Boca Raton: CRC Press.

Stromberg, P.C. and Capen, C.C. (1994) In: Mohr, U., Dungworth, D.L. and Capen, C.C. (eds) Pathobiology of the Aging Rat, pp. 193–198. Washington DC: ILSI Press.

Swett, J.E., Torigoe, Y., Elie, V.R., Bourass, Ch. M. and Miller, P.G. (1991) Exp. Neurol. 114, 82–103.

Takahashi, M., Shinoda, K. and Hayashi, Y. (1992) In: Mohr, U., Dungworth, D.L. and Capen, C.C. (eds) Pathobiology of the Aging Rat, pp. 407–411. Washington DC: ILSI Press.

Tischler, A.S. and Coupland, R.E. (1994) In: Mohr, U., Dungworth, D.L. and Capen, C.C. (eds) Pathobiology of the Aging Rat, pp. 245–268. Washington DC: ILSI Press.

Tuch, K., Ockert, D., Hauschke, D. and Christ, B. (1992) Pathol. Res. Pract. 188, 672–675.

Turusov, V. and Mohr, U. (eds) (1990) Pathology of Tumors in Laboratory Animals, Vol. 1, Tumours of the Rat. IARC Scientific Publications No. 99, Lyon.

Walsh, K.M. and Poteracki, J. (1994) *Fundam. Appl. Toxicol.* **22**, 65–72.

White, S.L., Smith, W.C., Fisher, L.F., Galtin, C.L., Hanasono, G.K. and Jordan, W.H. (1998) *Toxicol. Pathol.* **26**, 403–410.

Whiteley, L.O., Purdon, M.P., Ridder, G.M. and Bertram, T.A. (1996) *Toxicol. Pathol.* **24**, 305–314.

Yarrington, J.T. and Johnston, J.O. (1994) In: Mohr, U., Dungworth, D.L. and Capen, C.C. (eds) *Pathobiology of the Aging Rat*, pp. 227–244. Washington DC: ILSI Press.

Yuan, Y.D. and Carlson, R.G. (1987) In: Jones T.C., Mohr U., Hunt R.D. (eds) *ILSI Monographs on the Pathology of Laboratory Animals, Genital System*, pp. 161–168. Berlin: Springer Verlag.

PART 6

Physiology

Contents

CHAPTER 16

Respiration

Holger Schulz
GSF – National Research Center for Environment and Health,
Institute for Inhalation Biology, Munich, Germany

Hartwig Muhle
Fraunhofer Institute, Hannover, Germany

Introduction

In the present context, respiration includes all processes involved in the transport of respiratory gases between the environment and the body tissues. The respiratory system, which is the subject of this chapter, provides for the first steps – the uptake of oxygen – and for the final steps – the clearance of carbon dioxide. The system must continuously meet the body's metabolic demands, even in face of other potentially competing tasks, e.g. **phonation**, olfaction, or acid–base regulation. This requires special structural features and a high degree of adaptability of the respiratory organs. Measurement techniques and the physiological ranges of the parameters of respiratory mechanics, pulmonary ventilation and alveolar capillary gas exchange are introduced here. An overview of physiological values is provided in Table 16.1. Respiratory parameters are given in traditional units because SI units are still not common in respiratory physiology and were not applied in most of the studies cited. The conversion factors are also given (Cotes, 1975; Quanjer et al., 1993). Because rats are often used in inhalation studies on the health effects of particulate matter, an overview on particle deposition and clearance in the lung is added. Finally, information on airway reactivity and on rat models of airway hyperresponsiveness is provided, since airway hyperresponsiveness is a major feature of many lung diseases.

Structural Features

Based on anatomical and physiological characteristics, the respiratory system is divided into two regions: the conducting or nonrespiratory airways distributing the inhaled air (nose, pharynx, larynx,

Table 16.1 Overview on selected lung function parameters

Parameter	Mean	Range
Body weight (g)	270	220–300
TLC $(cm^3)^a$	11	8.2–12.2
TLC/BW $(cm^3/kg)^a$	42	36–54
VC $(cm^3)^a$	9.5	5.5–11.0
FRC $(cm^3)^a$	3.0	2.1–4.6
RV $(cm^3)^a$	1.5	1.0–2.7
C_L $(cm^3/cm\ H_2O)^a$	0.6	0.3–0.9
R_L $(cmH_2O/cm^3 \cdot s)^a$	0.3	0.1–0.55
V_T (cm^3)	1.7	1.2–2.5
f (breaths/min)	110	100–140
V $(cm^3/min/kg)$	575	460–900
V_T $(cm^3)^a$	1.6	1.1–2.5
f (breaths/min)^a	85	30–130
O_2 uptake cm^3 STPD O_2/min/kg)^a	18	12.0–21.5

^{a}Measurements performed in anesthetized animals.

BW, body weight; TLC, total lung capacity; VC, vital capacity; FRC, functional residual capacity; RV, residual volume; C_L, lung compliance; R_L, pulmonary resistance; V_T, tidal volume; f, respiratory rate; V, minute ventilation.

Conversion factors are: 1 cmH_2O = 0.0981 kPa; 1 torr = 1 mmHg = 0.1333 kPa; 1 cm^3/min = 0.045 mmol/min; 1 $cm^3/min/$ torr = 0.335 mmol/min/kPa.

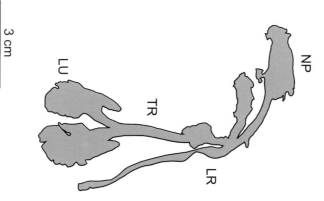

Figure 16.1 Schematic drawing of a silicon rubber cast of the respiratory system of an adult Fisher-344 rat. NP, nasopharynx; LR, larynx; TR, trachea; LU, lung. Adapted from Patra et al. (1987).

3 cm

trachea, bronchi, and nonalveolized bronchioles) and the gas-exchanging alveolized airways of the lung (respiratory bronchioles, alveolar ducts and alveolar air sacs) (Figure 16.1). Due to the close apposition of the epiglottis to the soft palate the rat is an obligate nose breather. The major nasal passages, the dorsal, middle and ventral meatus, are incompletely separated from the common meatus by the **nasal turbinates** (nasoturbinates, maxilloturbinates, **ethmoturbinates**) (Negus, 1958; Proctor and Chang, 1983; Hebel and Stromberg, 1986; Patra, 1986; Patra et al., 1986, 1987). The nasal cavity has a total volume of about 0.25 cm^3 and a surface area of approximately 13 cm^2 (Gross et al., 1982). The nasal vestibulum is lined by stratified squamous epithelium. The olfactory epithelium is located on the ethmoturbinates, constituting approximately 50% of the total surface area, while the remaining regions are lined by respiratory epithelium (Gross et al., 1982; George et al., 1986, 1993). Both respiratory and olfactory epithelium are covered with a layer of sticky mucus which provides for a defense of the lower airways against inhaled particles and gases (Morgan *et al.*, 1984; Harkema, 1990). In particular, the complex geometry of the maxillary turbinates in the anterior nasal airways contributes to an efficient filtration and absorption of airborne pollutants (Morgan *et al.*, 1991, 1993).

The pharynx, a musculomembranous tube of approximately 2.2 cm in length, connects the nasal and the laryngeal airways during breathing. While the nasopharynx is lined with respiratory epithelium, the oro- and laryngopharynx bear a nonkeratinized squamous epithelium. Among all laboratory animals, rats have the smallest bend in the nasopharynx (15°; Schreider and Raabe, 1981).

The larynx is framed by cartilage and bound by ligaments and muscles. The rostral part of the laryngeal airway lumen is lined by stratified squamous epithelium, while ciliated pseudostratified epithelium is found caudally to the vocal cords and extending into the trachea. In between, a transitional zone with nonciliated cuboidal epithelium is found in rats (Smith, 1977). The larynx is about 0.4 cm in length, its narrowest cross-sectional area being not more than 0.02 cm^2 (Schreider and Raabe, 1981). Hence, it provides a major resistive element to airflow and produces some degree of turbulence. This may lead to significant deposition of inhaled particles not only in the larynx but also in the trachea.

The trachea, approximately 3.3 cm in length and 0.3 cm by 0.15 cm in cross-sectional area, connects the extra- to the intrathoracic airways. The latter comprise a system of repeatedly branching airways, starting with the principal or main bronchi, followed by lobar, segmental and subsegmental bronchi, and bronchioles. The most distal nonrespiratory airways are defined as terminal bronchioles. They connect to the acini, i.e. to the principal unit of alveolized airways. In rats there is one short segment of respiratory bronchiole with only a few, widely scattered intramural alveoli, followed by several generations of alveolar ducts and finally ending in the alveolar sacs.

In contrast to humans, the tracheobronchial system of rats shows a monopodial branching pattern with daughter branches of unequal diameter at each bifurcation. An anatomical path length model of the rat lung estimated the cumulative volume of the conducting airways (trachea to terminal bronchioles) to be 1.2 cm^3 (Yeh *et al.*, 1979; Yeh and Harkema, 1993). Each of about 2500 terminal bronchioles is reached after an average of 15 bifurcations, but, as an indication of the wide biological variability, the number of divisions may range between 7 and 32.

Each of the terminal bronchioles has a length of 0.035 cm and a diameter of 0.02 cm. As the diameter of each individual airway decreases at successive bifurcations, their resistance should increase towards the lung periphery. However, since the summed cross-sectional area of all airways increases by more than a factor of 30, a major pressure drop occurs in the larger bronchi, and flow velocity falls rapidly along the airway tree. Hence, the significance of gas transport by convection decreases with increasing generation number while gas transport by diffusion gains more and more importance. Morphometrically, this is supported by the fact that a respired gas molecule has to travel a path of 5.1 cm within the conducting airways, while the distance within the acinus is only 0.15 cm. For the exchange of oxygen and carbon dioxide, the rat lung provides a surface area of approximately 5000 cm^2. Gas exchange takes place in 3×10^7 alveoli with diameters ranging between 50 μm and 80 μm. The alveoli are surrounded by a dense capillary meshwork. Air and blood are separated by a tissue sheet of <0.5 μm, which is approximately 1/50 of the thickness of a sheet of airmail paper (Tenny and Remmers, 1963; Johanson and Pierce, 1973; Gehr *et al.*, 1981, 1993; Hayatdavoudi *et al.*, 1981; Mercer and Crapo, 1987; Rodriguez *et al.*, 1987; Meyrick, 1990; Mercer *et al.*, 1991; Mercer and Crapo, 1993; Weibel, 1993; Valerius, 1996).

The trachea is stiffened by about 24 cartilaginous C-shaped rings to prevent dynamic airway collapse during forceful breathing. A muscular membrane makes up the dorsal tracheal wall. The bronchi have a roughly circular cross-section and are stiffened by irregular plates of hyaline cartilage separated by spirally arranged bundles of smooth muscles. Trachea and main bronchi are lined by ciliated pseudostratified epithelium mainly composed of the following cellular constituents: basal cells (13%), ciliated cells (40%), and serous cells (40%). The mucus covering the epithelium is primarily secreted by serous cells, since submucosal glands are absent in rats and mucus goblet cells are rare. Terminal bronchioles are lined by cuboidal epithelium composed of **Clara cells** ($>50\%$) and ciliated cells ($<50\%$). Ninety-six per cent of the alveolar surface is covered by type I cells, the remainder by type II cells responsible for the replacement of type I cells and for surfactant secretion. However, the number of the smaller type II cells exceeds that of type I cells by 50% (0.12×10^9/lung; Jeffrey and Reid, 1975; Plopper *et al.*, 1980, 1983; Crapo *et al.*, 1983; Hyde *et al.*, 1990; George *et al.*, 1993).

Respiratory Mechanics

Lung Volumes

Measured values of lung volumes are listed in Table 16.2 for different rat strains. The magnitude of each volume depends on the mechanical properties of the lung and chest wall tissues and on the transpulmonary pressure P_L, i.e. the pressure gradient between airway opening and pleural space. Total lung capacity (TLC), which is the lung volume at maximum inspiration, is usually determined at a P_L of 25–30 cmH$_2$O in anesthetized animals. TLC and body weight (BW) were found to correlate closely (TLC = BW $\times$ 0.0368 + 4.573 $\pm$ 1.67, r = 0.93; Sahebjami and Vassallo, 1979; Takezawa et al., 1980). At residual volume (RV), corresponding to a maximal expiration in awake animals, P_L is usually chosen to be -10 cmH$_2$O or lower. Since recoil pressure of the chest wall is extremely low in rats, airway closure appears to be the primary mechanism for setting RV. The total gas volume expelled from TLC to RV is the vital capacity (VC).

Lung volume at the end of a spontaneous expiration is called the **functional residual capacity (FRC)**. In rodents, FRC has to be distinguished from relaxation volume (V_r), which is the gas volume in the lung when the respiratory muscles are completely relaxed. V_r is set by the static balance between lung and chest wall elastic recoil forces. P_L at V_r corresponds to the pressure within the pleural space and is small (1–2 cmH$_2$O) in rodents. In case of fast breathing and/or high inspiratory muscle activity, FRC may exceed V_r considerably (Lai and Hildebrandt, 1978; Gillespie, 1983). FRC measurements performed by body plethysmography and by dilution technique were found to be similar (ratio 0.98 $\pm$ 0.02 ($\pm$ SE); Palacek, 1969), but those determined from saline displacement in excised lungs were slightly smaller (Lai and Hildebrandt, 1978). Body position and the depth of anesthesia have profound effects on the FRC (Lamm et al., 1982; Loscutoff et al., 1985); but additional effects related to muscle relaxants were not observed (Lai and Hildebrandt, 1978). Intra-animal and intracohort reproducibility of lung volume measurements performed at daily or weekly intervals was judged acceptable (Palacek, 1969; Wright et al., 1997), but

interindividual and interobserver variability as reflected in the standard deviations provided in Table 16.2 is large, even for a given strain. Some of this variability is related to biological differences, such as gender, age or body weight, but it also results from differences in measurement conditions, as partly outlined above. Alterations in lung volumes due to lung diseases are typically accompanied by a shift in the pressure volume curve (see below). Fibrotic lesions decrease lung volumes while degenerative or emphysematous lesions are reflected by increased volumes. Increased volumes are also observed in obstructive diseases, due to trapped air pockets within the lung.

Compliance

Compliance is defined as the change in lung volume per unit of pressure change. Quasi-static mechanical properties of the respiratory system are usually estimated from pressure–volume (PV) relationships during a slow inflation of the lung to TLC and subsequent deflation to RV. Typically, compliance is determined from the linear portion of the PV deflation curve near end-expiratory volume, but other analytical approaches have been introduced (Lai and Diamond, 1986). Pressure–volume curves of lung, chest wall and total respiratory system from rats are shown in Figure 16.2. Transpulmonary pressure (P_L),

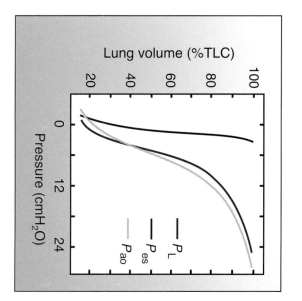

Figure 16.2 Deflation pressure–volume curves of lung (P_L), chest wall (P_{es}) and total respiratory system (P_{ao}) from anesthetized Sprague–Dawley rats. Adapted from Lai and Hildebrandt (1978).

Table 16.2 Selected lung function parameters of different rat strains

	Fisher 344				Spague-Dawley			Wistar	
	Diamond and O'Donnell (1977) Mean $\pm$ SD	Likens and Mauderly (1982) Mean $\pm$ SD	Mauderly (1982) Mean $\pm$ SD	Stevens et al. (1988) Mean $\pm$ SE	Lai et al. (1978) Mean $\pm$ SE	Loscutoff et al. (1985) Mean $\pm$ SE	Wright et al. (1997) Mean $\pm$ SD	Dormans et al. (1989) Mean $\pm$ SD	Yokoyama (1983) Mean $\pm$ SD
Body weight (g)	233 $\pm$ 32	–	222	297 $\pm$ 3	307 $\pm$ 10	450 $\pm$ 11	447 $\pm$ 30	299 $\pm$ 13	338 $\pm$ 27
Age (months)	–	3	3	4	Adult	4	–	2	2–2.8
Number	32	15	10/10	24	15	27	10	8	27
Anesthesia	Urethan	Halothan	Halothan	Pento	Pento	Urethan	Diazepam + Innovar Vet	Post-mortem (pento)	Urethane
Position	Left lat. dec.	Prone	Prone	–	Prone	Prone	–	Supine	Prone
Sex	Female	Male	Male/Female	Male	Male	Male	–	Male	Male
TLC (cm^3)	8.2 $\pm$ 1.0	13.00 $\pm$ 1.4	11.9 $\pm$ 1.7	11.19 $\pm$ 0.14	12.23 $\pm$ 0.55	17.6 $\pm$ 0.35	21.9[a]	11.78 $\pm$ 1.81	11.3 $\pm$ 1.4
TLC/BW (cm^3/kg)	36[a]	–	54[a]	38[a]	40[a]	39[a]	49[a]	40[a]	33[a]
VC (cm^3)	5.5 $\pm$ 0.9	10.7[a]	11.0 $\pm$ 1.8	10.22 $\pm$ 0.12	11.0[a]	15.8 $\pm$ 0.31	16.7 $\pm$ 2.1	–	8.4 $\pm$ 1.7
FRC (cm^3)	4.6 $\pm$ 0.6	3.75 $\pm$ 0.51	2.1 $\pm$ 0.3	2.11 $\pm$ 0.03	2.51 $\pm$ 0.20	3.9 $\pm$ 0.12	6.7 $\pm$ 0.3	3.72 $\pm$ 0.55	3.9 $\pm$ 0.8
RV (cm^3)	2.7 $\pm$ 0.8	2.31 $\pm$ 0.45	1.0 $\pm$ 0.3	0.98 $\pm$ 0.04	1.26 $\pm$ 0.13	1.9 $\pm$ 0.08	5.2 $\pm$ 0.7	–	2.9 $\pm$ 1.0
C_L (cm^3/cmH$_2$O)	0.34 $\pm$ 0.17	0.85 $\pm$ 0.17	0.59 $\pm$ 0.25	0.68 $\pm$ 0.01	0.90 $\pm$ 0.06	1.80 $\pm$ 0.07	0.92 $\pm$ 0.18	–	0.61 $\pm$ 0.16
C_{spL} (cmH$_2$O^{-1})	0.041[a]	0.065[a]	0.050[a]	0.061[a]	0.074[a]	0.10[a]	0.042[a]	–	0.054[a]
D_{Lco} (cm^3/min/torr)	–	–	0.182 $\pm$ 0.055	0.172 $\pm$ 0.005	–	0.27 $\pm$ 0.016	–	–	–

[a] Calculated values.

Pento, pentobarbital sodium; left lat. dec., left lateral decubitus position, animal lying on its left side; prone position, animal lying on its belly; supine position, animal lying on its back; BW, body weight; TLC, total lung capacity; VC, vital capacity; FRC, functional residual capacity; RV, residual volume; C_L, lung compliance; C_{spL}, specific lung compliance; D_{Lco}, diffusing capacity for carbon monoxide.

Conversion factors are: 1 cmH$_2$O = 0.0981 kPa; 1 torr = 1 mmHg = 0.1333 kPa; 1 cm^3/min = 0.045 mmol/min; 1 cm^3/min/torr = 0.335 mmol/min/kPa.

intrapleural pressure (usually approximated by esophageal pressure P_{es}), and airway opening pressure (P_{ao}) correspond to the recoil pressures of lung, chest wall and total respiratory system, respectively. The PV curve of the chest wall is much steeper in rats than in humans, with an esophageal pressure difference of only 5 cmH2O between maximum in- and expiration as compared to a 50 cmH2O difference in humans. This indicates that the structures surrounding the lung, such as the rib cage with the intercostal muscles and the diaphragm-abdomen complex, are much more compliant in rats. Reported values of chest wall compliance (C_{CW}) range between 0.73 ± 0.13 cm³/cmH2O and 2.09 ± 0.46 cm³/cmH2O (Diamond and O'Donnell, 1977; Nattie, 1977; Lai and Hildebrandt, 1978).

The elastic recoil pressure of the lung is generated from two major components: the lung tissue itself and the surface layer within the alveoli. Surface tension forces contribute substantially to lung recoil (Hayatdavoudi et al., 1981) and exert their greatest influence on PV curves at lung volumes larger than 50% of TLC (Haber et al., 1983; Mead et al., 1957). The structural elements of pulmonary tissues affecting lung compliance (C_L) are quantity and organization of collagen and elastin fibers. While loss of elastic fibers results in steeper PV curves, accumulation of lung collagen restricts lung expansion and reduces the slope of the PV curve (Kuncova et al., 1972; Damon et al., 1982). Other restrictive factors are capillary distension, edema or airway smooth muscle constriction (Dandurand et al., 1993; Hauge et al., 1977; Noble et al., 1975). Determining specific lung compliance (C_{spL}) as the ratio of C_L/TLC can reduce, but not abolish, the variance observed for C_L in rats with different lung sizes (cf. Table 16.2; Sahebjami and Vassalo, 1979; Sahebjami, 1991).

Determinants of dynamic lung compliance ($C_{L,dyn}$) are the recoil forces of the lung and the frictional forces occurring in airway and lung tissues during the breathing cycle. $C_{L,dyn}$ is defined by the ratio of tidal volume to the difference in P_L at the points of flow reversal during spontaneous breathing and is about 0.3 cm³/cmH2O in rats (range 0.19–0.39 cm³/cmH2O; King, 1966; Johanson and Pierce, 1971; Likens and Mauderly, 1982; Costa et al., 1983, 1986; Sorkness et al., 1988; Lai and Diamond, 1992; Dandurand et al., 1993). $C_{L,dyn}$ was found to be independent of the respiratory rate in healthy animals, suggesting that the time constants for filling and emptying of distal lung units are short enough to permit synchronous filling and emptying, even at respiratory rates up to 320/min (Otis et al., 1956; Diamond and O'Donnell, 1977). In the case of airway diseases, $C_{L,dyn}$ is decreased even during quiet breathing (Shore et al., 1995; Long et al., 1997; Kumar et al., 1997).

Resistance

Airway resistance (R_{aw}) is defined as the ratio of bronchial resistive pressure to gas flow. The **resistive pressure** in the airways is the pressure gradient between the alveolar space and the airway opening. Depending on whether or not the animal has been tracheotomized and/or intubated, airway resistance includes the resistance of mouth and/or nose or that of the endotracheal tube. Attempts have been made to subtract the resistance of the endotracheal tube, as determined ex vivo. However, in that case entrance effects, e.g. turbulent eddies at the open end of the tube, may lead to an overestimation of tube resistance (Loring et al., 1979). A large part of the entire respiratory resistance appears to reside in the nasal airways (0.36 cmH2O/cm³·s; King, 1966; Lung, 1987). The definition of **pulmonary resistance (R_L)** is based on the pressure drop between airway opening and pleural space. R_L, therefore also takes the resistance of lung tissues into account. Tissue resistance appears to be small; Johanson and Pierce (1971) found no significant difference between R_{aw} and R_L in rats (R_{aw} 0.43 ± 0.2 cmH2O/cm³·s (±SD) vs. R_L 0.44 ± 0.16 cmH2O/cm³·s).

Values reported for R_L range between 0.11 cmH2O/cm³·s and 0.56 cmH2O/cm³·s (Palacek, 1969; Diamond and O'Donnell, 1977; Holub and Frank, 1979; Boyd et al., 1980; Costa et al., 1983, 1986; Wang et al., 1986; Sorkness et al., 1988). This variation is partly related to strain differences. In a comparative study, the lowest R_L values were observed in Brown Norway rats, intermediate values in Wistar-Furth, and the highest values in ACI rats (0.33 ± 0.03 cmH2O/cm³·s (±SE), 0.56 ± 0.04 cmH2O/cm³·s, 0.44 ± 0.04 cmH2O/cm³·s; Wang et al., 1986). The determination of specific airway resistance (R_{sp}), defined as resistance × lung volume, accounts for the effect that increasing lung volume increases airway cross-sectional areas and therefore lowers resistance. R_{sp} in rats is only about 1/5 of that found in humans, although absolute values of R_L are higher in rats than in humans. Various anatomical and/or functional alterations, e.g. airway smooth muscle contraction, mucus secretion, epithelial cell hyperplasia, inflammatory cell infiltration and peribronchial edema, may influence airway diameters. However, the observed effect on R_L is dependent upon the airway generation that is affected. Since the summed cross-sectional area of all peripheral airways is large, changes in airway diameter have to be profound to have a measurable impact on R_L.

Maximum Expiratory Flow Volume Curve (MEFV)

The MEFV curve describes flow as a function of lung volume during a forced expiration from TLC to RV. In anesthetized animals, forced expiratory efforts are simulated by instantly exposing the airway opening to a negative pressure (generally $-40\,cmH_2O$). Except for the initial part of the maneuver, maximum expiratory flows are 'effort' (pressure) independent, they are determined by the elastic properties of lung tissue and by the airway resistance (Mead et al., 1967; Diamond and O'Donnell, 1977; Macklem, 1978). Measured values for peak expiratory flow (PEF) range between 100 and 150 cm^3/s. Forced expiratory flows at 50% of VC ($MEF_{50\%}$) vary between 55 and 120 cm^3/s. The configuration of the MEFV curve varies between animals, but repeated measurements in an individual are highly reproducible. This makes MEFV maneuvers suitable for monitoring progression of toxicant-induced diseases in follow-up studies (Diamond and O'Donnell, 1977; Harkema et al., 1982; Likens and Mauderly, 1982; Costa et al., 1983; Zhou and Lai, 1992; Wright et al., 1997; Rubio et al., 1998). Loss of elastic recoil of lung parenchyma or bronchial instability facilitates compression of airways and reduces maximal expiratory flows. Airway narrowing due to increased smooth muscle tone, wall thickening or mucus secretion also affects MEFV curves in characteristic patterns.

Kotlikoff et al., 1984; Hantos et al., 1987a,b; Peslin et al., 1990; Lutchen et al., 1996; Bates et al., 1997; Maksym and Bates, 1997). However, the work of Oostveen and co-workers (1991, 1992) showed that impedance measurements are also applicable in trained conscious animals and therefore allow analysis of respiratory system properties under more physiological conditions than most of the other lung function parameters. For detailed information concerning the complex analysis and interpretation of impedance data, the reader is referred to the reviews by Peslin (1991), Zwart and Peslin (1991) and Zwart and Van de Woestijne (1994).

Ventilation of the Lung

Oxygen Consumption

Small animals require more oxygen per unit of body weight than do large animals (Leith, 1976; Taylor et al., 1981). The rate of O_2 uptake measured in 58 adult Sprague-Dawley rats during quiet wakefulness was $23.6 \pm 0.9\,cm^3$ STPD O_2/min/kg ($\pm 2\,SD$; Olson and Dempsey, 1978). Slightly smaller values are reported for anesthetized animals. The specific rate of O_2 uptake is about 18 cm^3 STPD O_2/min/kg (range 12.2–21.7 cm^3 STDP O_2/min/kg), while the rate of CO_2 excretion is 15 cm^3 STPD CO_2/min/kg (Turek et al., 1973, 1978; Fukuda, 1991; Barnikol et al., 1994; Ardevol et al., 1995). To meet the demands during maximal treadmill exercise, rats can increase their O_2 uptake rate to almost 100 cm^3 STPD O_2/min/kg. Maximum O_2 uptake during cold exposure (ice water bath), which was also used to elicit high rates of aerobic metabolism, is approximately 20% lower (Taylor et al., 1980; Seehermann et al., 1981; Gonzalez et al., 1988).

Impedance

The complex relationships between pressure and flow determined during the application of forced oscillations of different frequencies to the lung are used to measure impedance, resistance and reactance of the respiratory system. Most measurements have been performed in anesthetized animals during spontaneous breathing or induced apneic periods, and in some cases even ventilated, open-chested animals were used (Jackson and Watson, 1982;

Ventilation

Awake, unrestrained rats are breathing tidal volumes (V_T) of approximately 1.7 cm^3 (range 1.2–2.5 cm^3) at a rate (f) of 110 breaths/min (range 100–140/min). Accordingly, **minute ventilation** is 187 cm^3/min or 575 cm^3/min/kg (range 460–900 cm^3/min/kg). During quiet breathing dead space ventilation amounts to 37% of minute ventilation and, hence, is comparable to that observed in humans. Restraining of animals can increase V_T and f substantially and may result in minute ventilations of up to 1600 cm^3/min/kg (Lai et al., 1978; Walker et al., 1985; Olson and Dempsey, 1978; Lamm et al., 1982; Walker et al., 1985; Sorkness et al., 1988). Therefore, anesthesia is deemed necessary by most investigators for measurements of ventilation. In anesthetized rats, V_T ranges between 1.1 and 2.5 cm^3, with a mean of 1.6 cm^3; values for f range between 30 and 130 breaths/min, with a mean of 85 breaths/min (Palacek, 1969; Johanson and Pierce, 1971; Diamond and O'Donnell, 1977; Nattie, 1977; Harkema et al., 1982; Costa et al., 1983, 1986; Costa and Tepper, 1988; Lai et al., 1991; Lai and Diamond, 1992; Dandurand et al., 1993). Depending upon the kind and depth of anesthesia, ventilation may become more and more depressed, primarily due to a decreased breathing frequency (Lai et al., 1978; Lamm et al., 1982), but a V_T as low as 1.1 cm^3 at a respiratory rate of 50 has been reported (Mauderly, 1982; Wang et al., 1986). Cannulation of the trachea via a tracheostomy in anesthetized animals was found to have only little effect on spontaneous breathing (Johanson and Pierce, 1971).

Regular ventilation and gas exchange in awake adult rats result in arterial blood gas tensions of approximately 91 torr for O$_2$ and 36 torr for CO$_2$. Values reported for the O$_2$ tension range between 84 and 98 torr, those for the CO$_2$ tension between 31 and 40 torr (Benignus and Annau, 1994; Lai et al., 1978; Maskrey et al., 1992; Olson and Dempsey, 1978; Walker et al., 1985). These values are comparable to those observed in humans, while arterial pH in rats appears to be slightly higher (7.43–7.49; Lahiri, 1975).

Distribution of Ventilation

A large volume of gas remains in the lungs at end expiration. Gas transport between the atmosphere and the alveolar-capillary membrane therefore is not only dependent on alveolar ventilation but also upon intrapulmonary gas mixing. The efficiency of gas transport and mixing is determined by various factors, e.g. regional differences in airway resistance, in elastic properties of the lung, or in the pleural pressure (Piiper, 1986; Piiper and Scheid, 1987; Paiva and Engel, 1988). Established approaches to the assessment of mixing efficiency are the single-breath and multi-breath washout techniques of insoluble gases (like N$_2$, He, SF$_6$) from the lung. As a measure of ventilation inhomogeneity, the single-breath procedure provides information about the change in test gas concentration during expiration of alveolar gas (slope of phase III), while the multi-breath maneuver supplies the washout kinetics in terms of the number of breaths, the decay of end-expiratory concentrations, or by moment analysis (Holub and Frank, 1979; Costa et al., 1986; González Mangado et al., 1991; Verbank et al., 1991, 1993). Washout techniques have been applied in rats to characterize the effects of elastase-induced emphysema (González Mangado et al., 1993; Loscutoff et al., 1985; Rubio et al., 1998), induced airway obstruction (Likens and Mauderly, 1982), or air pollution (Costa et al., 1986; Stevens et al., 1988). The techniques are regarded as sensitive markers of small airway disease, but the interpretation of the results is complex and may require model analysis (Costa et al., 1986; González Mangado et al., 1993; Rubio et al., 1998).

Alveolar–Capillary Gas Transfer

The pulmonary conductance for the exchange of respiratory gases, usually referred to as pulmonary diffusing capacity (D_L), is used to assess alveolar-capillary gas transfer. D_L is determined by two resistances arranged in series, that of the alveolar-capillary membrane (D_M) and that of the erythrocytes in the pulmonary capillaries (Roughton and Forster, 1957). Formally, D_L for O$_2$ ($D_{L_{O_2}}$) is derived from the ratio of oxygen uptake to the corresponding mean O$_2$ partial pressure difference between alveolar gas and capillary blood. Measurement of $D_{L_{O_2}}$ is therefore complex, and D_L for carbon monoxide ($D_{L_{CO}}$) is a well-established surrogate index of pulmonary conductance. $D_{L_{CO}}$ in anesthetized Sprague-Dawley rats was found to correlate closely with BW ($D_{L_{CO}} = -2.6 + 0.75 \log_{10} BW$, $r^2 = 0.96$; Takezawa et al., 1980). $D_{L_{CO}}$ values measured in different rat strains vary between 0.08 and 0.29 cm^3/min/torr, with a mean of 0.17 cm^3/min/torr (cf. Table 16.2; Johanson and Pierce, 1973; Turek et al., 1973; Holub and Frank, 1979; Takezawa et al., 1980; Harkema et al., 1982; Mauderly, 1982; Loscutoff et al., 1985; Stevens et al., 1988; Zhou and Lai, 1992; Rubio et al., 1998). Even by normalization to the size of the alveolar volume, the variability of $D_{L_{CO}}$ is only slightly diminished. Variations are in part related to the different measurement conditions, but many other factors may affect measurements of $D_{L_{CO}}$ (Piiper and Scheid, 1980; Takezawa et al., 1980; A decrease in $D_{L_{CO}}$ as a functional endpoint of disease may indicate a thickening of the blood–air barrier or a loss of alveolar surface area. But diminished capillary blood volume, increased ventilation–volume inhomogeneities of the lung and/or increased mismatching of ventilation and perfusion can also reduce D_{LCO}.

Aging of the Lung

It appears that body weight and lung size of rats continue to grow throughout most of their lifespan. The increase in lung volume, as in body size, is most pronounced during the postnatal period and in early adulthood, up to four months (Table 16.3; Yokoyama, 1983; Sahebjami, 1991; Wright et al., 1997). No changes in lung resistance were observed with age (King, 1966). The pressure–volume curves are shifted progressively upward and to the left, indicating that lung compliance increases with age. But when expressing PV curves and G_L relative to maximal lung volume, age-related differences became less obvious (Sahebjami and Vassallo, 1979; Mauderly, 1982; Sahebjami, 1991). Morphometrical analyses of lung parenchyma revealed an increased volume of the interstitial matrix in aging lungs, due to collagen deposition and the appearance of larger quantities of connective tissue proteins. But these changes were not severe enough to change the alveolar-harmonic mean tissue thickness of the alveolar-capillary membrane (Pinkerton et al., 1982; Sahebjami, 1991). Findings of Sugihara and Martin (1975) suggest that there were also changes in the geometric arrangement and/or in the molecular structure of connective tissues. Despite a slight enlargement of air spaces and an increase in alveolar surface area with age, no evidence was found for emphysematous processes (Johanson and Pierce, 1973; Pinkerton et al., 1982). In view of these results, larger air space dimensions rather than destructive processes appear to be responsible for changes in lung mechanics in aging rats. The alveolar capillary gas transfer, as inferred from D_{LCO}, was found to increase with age, but D_{LCO} appears to be not affected beyond maturation when adjusted to the lung volume (cf. Table 16.3; Johanson and Pierce, 1973).

Concerning the adjustment of ventilation and blood gases during growth and age, V_T was found to increase progressively with age, while f decreased until 12 months of age, with a subsequent slight increase in the older rats (Fukuda,

1991). These changes resulted in a continous decrease of alveolar ventilation normalized for body weight, which was found to be directly proportional to the metabolic rate. While the other arterial blood gas parameters remained unchanged, O_2 tension decreased progressively beyond early adulthood.

Particle Deposition in the Respiratory System

A certain fraction of particles inhaled into the lung diverge from airflow streamlines and thereby come into contact with the wet airspace surface. This phenomenon, generally referred to as particle deposition, is related to three physical mechanisms (Agnew, 1984; Schulz et al., 1999). (1) Impaction due to particle inertia: During quiet breathing inertial displacement becomes significant for particles $>2\,\mu m$ (Table 16.4) and probably occurs in the extrathoracic and large conducting airways where flow velocities are high and rapid changes in airflow direction often take place. (2) Sedimentation due to gravitational forces: Sedimentation is supported by large particle size and longer residence times as they occur in small conducting airways and in the alveolated region of the lung. (3) Diffusion related to the Brownian motion of surrounding gas molecules: Deposition due to diffusion is relevant for very small particles within the nose and the lung periphery. Summaries of deposition data for rats and other species have been published (Menache et al., 1995; Jones 1993; Raabe et al., 1977, 1988; Schlesinger, 1985; Schulz et al., 1999). Experimental studies have been carried out to assess total, regional (Dahl and Griffith, 1983; Raabe et al. 1988; Dahlbäck and Eirefelt, 1994) or extrathoracic (Cheng et al., 1990; Gerde et al., 1991) particle deposition in the respiratory system of rats, to determine the initial deposition pattern in the lung (Brody and Roe, 1983; Pinkerton et al., 1993) and to investigate the effect of exercise (Hesseltine et al., 1986) and induced chronic bronchitis on particle deposition (Sweeney et al., 1995). Theoretical deposition models have also been applied (Halik et al., 1980; Schum and Yeh, 1980; Yu and Xu, 1986; Xu and Yu, 1987; Asgharian et al., 1989, 1995; Hofmann et al., 1989; Anjilvel and Asgharian, 1995; Koblinger and Hofmann, 1995).

Table 16.3 Selected lung function parameters for Fischer-344 rats at different ages

Strain	Stevens *et al.* (1988) Mean ± SE					Mauderly (1982) Mean ± SD	
	3 weeks	6 weeks	8 weeks	10 weeks	15 weeks	77 weeks	116 weeks
Body weight (g)	32.8 ± 1.2	132.9 ± 3.1	181.6 ± 2.8	234.4 ± 1.9	222 ± 6.1	334 ± 106	332 ± 71
Number	28	26	18	20	10/10	5/5	5/5
Anesthesia	Pento	Pento	Pento	Pento	Halothan	Halothan	Halothan
Position	-	-	-	-	Prone	Prone	Prone
Sex	Male	Male	Male	Male	Male/female	Male/female	Male/female
TLC (cm^3)	1.98 ± 0.02	5.59 ± 0.05	7.33 ± 0.09	8.63 ± 0.12	11.9 ± 1.7	13.9 ± 2.2	14.4 ± 1.9
TLC/BW (cm^3/kg)	60.4[a]	42.1[a]	40.4[a]	36.8[a]	53.6[a]	41.6[a]	43.4[a]
VC (cm^3)	1.78 ± 0.02	5.14 ± 0.04	6.66 ± 0.07	7.88 ± 0.10	11.0 ± 1.8	13.4 ± 2.3	13.4 ± 1.7
FRC (cm^3)	0.66 ± 0.01	1.12 ± 0.04	1.62 ± 0.05	1.91 ± 0.04	2.1 ± 0.3	1.7 ± 0.3	2.7 ± 0.4
RV (cm^3)	0.19 ± 0.02	0.45 ± 0.02	0.67 ± 0.04	0.76 ± 0.04	1.0 ± 0.3	0.6 ± 0.2	1.1 ± 0.5
C_L (cm^3/cmH$_2$O)	0.118 ± 0.002	0.397 ± 0.006	0.49 ± 0.010	0.58 ± 0.013	0.59 ± 0.25	0.89 ± 0.23	0.85 ± 0.21
C_{spL} (cmH$_2$O^{-1})	0.063 ± 0.001	0.071 ± 0.001	0.067 ± 0.001	0.066 ± 0.001	0.050[a]	0.064[a]	0.059[a]
D_{Lco} (cm^3/min/torr)	0.023 ± 0.001	0.113 ± 0.002	0.148 ± 0.003	0.167 ± 0.004	0.182 ± 0.055	0.205 ± 0.056	0.189 ± 0.051
D_{Lco}/TLC	0.012[a]	0.020[a]	0.020[a]	0.019[a]	0.015[a]	0.015[a]	0.013[a]

[a] Calculated values.

Pento, pentobarbital sodium; prone position, animal lying on its belly; BW, body weight; TLC, total lung capacity; VC, vital capacity, FRC, functional residual capacity; RV, residual volume; C_L, lung compliance; C_{spL}, specific lung compliance, D_{Lco}, diffusing capacity for carbon monoxide.

Conversion factors are: 1 cmH$_2$O = 0.0981 kPa; 1 torr = 1 mmHg = 0.1333 kPa; 1 cm^3/min = 0.045 mmol/min; 1 cm^3/min/torr = 0.335 mmol/min/kPa.

Table 16.4 Mean displacement of unit-density spheres in 1 second due to gravitational, inertial and diffusional transport

Diameter (µm)	Settling distance (µm)	Stopping distance (µm)	Diffusional displacement (µm)	Mass (pg)
5.0	739.9	75.7	3.30	65.45
2.0	124.0	12.1	5.34	4.19
1.0	33.34	3.02	7.84	0.524
0.5	9.54	0.76	11.85	6.545×10^{-2}
0.1	0.87	0.03	39.19	5.236×10^{-4}
0.05	0.38	0.008	72.96	6.545×10^{-5}
0.01	0.071	0.0003	343.96	4.189×10^{-6}

Temperature: 37°C; atmospheric pressure: 1013 hPa; viscosity: 1.9×10^{-5} Pas; stopping distance is given for particles with an initial velocity of 1 m/s; mass is given per particle.

Total Particle Deposition

Figure 16.3 shows typical total deposition values of rats during quiet breathing (Koblinger and Hofmann, 1995; Koblinger et al., 1995). For comparison, deposition data from humans during quiet nasal breathing are also given (Heyder et al., 1986). Minimal deposition occurs for particles in the size range of 0.1 µm to 1 µm, where particle displacement related to either of the three deposition mechanisms is lowest (cf. Table 16.4). Deposition increases with increasing as well as with decreasing particle diameter and reaches almost 80% for 0.01 µm and 100% for 5 µm particles. With increasing particle size, displacement by sedimentation and impaction increasingly rises so that total deposition is enhanced. For particles <0.1 µm, total deposition increases due to diffusional displacement. Total deposition in rats appears to be similar to that observed in healthy humans during quiet nasal breathing (Heyder et al., 1986).

Regional Particle Deposition

The fractions of particles lost within the extrathoracic, the tracheobronchiolar and the alveolated region of the respiratory system, respectively, are summarized in Figure 16.3. Extrathoracic deposition occurs primarily in the nose and is only slightly smaller than total deposition, indicating the large filtration efficiency of the nose. In particular, most of the particles larger than 0.5 µm or smaller than 0.05 µm are already caught in nasal airways. The remaining fraction is mainly deposited in the alveolar region (Figure 16.4). Particle loss in the tracheobronchiolar region is relatively low, reaching almost 15% for the smallest particles, but only 1–3% for particles >0.03 µm. About 15% of the inhaled particles <0.1 µm are caught in the alveolar region. For particles in the size range of 0.1 µm to 3 µm, alveolar deposition ranges between 5 and 10%, but it is almost zero for 5-µm particles. Overall, tracheobronchiolar deposition is similar to that observed in humans. But the filtration efficiency of rat nasal airways appears to be more effective, hence the alveolar extrathoracic deposition is higher and the alveolar deposition correspondingly lower in rats than in humans. Still, a toxicant dose delivered to the alveolar region of the rat lung by 1-µm particles will be almost four times higher than that delivered to the human alveolar surface area, if the respective minute ventilation and the alveolar surface areas are taken into account.

Particle Clearance from the Respiratory System

The efficiency and the pathways of particle clearance from the respiratory system are strongly dependent on the site of particle deposition and on the physicochemical properties of the particles. This overview will mainly focus upon the clearance of poorly soluble particles. Overall aspects of lung clearance have recently been reviewed (Bailey et al., 1989; Jones, 1993; Oberdörster, 1993; Kreyling and Scheuch, 1999). Within the nose or the larger intrathoracic airways, deposited particles are transported by mucociliary action within hours to days towards the pharynx, from where they are swallowed. However, some of the particles show no measurable clearance at all within that period (Stahl-hofen, 1987; Gore and Patrick, 1978; Kreyling et al., 1999). It has been speculated that this phenomenon contributes to the induction of immunological defense mechanisms (Gehr et al., 1996). Mucociliary clearance velocities measured in the nose of rats were 1.1–5.9 mm/min in the respiratory epithelium and 0.9 mm/min on the olfactory epithelium (Morgan et al., 1986). Mucus velocities measured in the trachea ranged between 1.9 ± 0.7 and 8.1 ± 4.0 mm/min (Berke and Roslinski, 1971; Giordano and Morrow, 1972; Patrick and Stirling, 1977; Felicetti et al., 1981). Clearance rates in the tracheobronchial tree decrease towards smaller airways, corresponding to a ciliary beat frequency of 18 Hz in the main bronchi vs. only 7 Hz in the peripheral airways of rats (Iravani, 1967).

Particles penetrating into the alveolar region of the lung are removed more slowly and retention half-times range from days to months. Alveolar clearance mechanisms can be attributed to two major pathways: particle transport and particle dissolution. The main transport mechanism in rat lungs is phagocytosis of insoluble particles by alveolar macrophages (AM) and the consecutive transport towards ciliated airways. Of minor importance is the transport of particles into the alveolar interstitium by AM, which is the major clearance mechanism in humans and large mammals. These species differences are related to morphological features of the lung, i.e. to the relative short pathway length from the alveoli to the

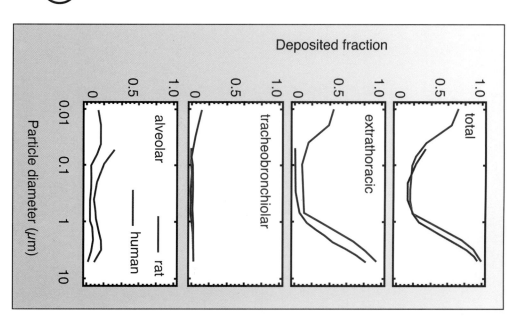

Figure 16.3 Schematic overview of total and regional particle deposition in the respiratory system for unit density spheres. Typical deposition values for adult rats and humans during quiet nasal breathing are given as a function of the inhaled particle diameter. Shown are deposition fraction curves for the extrathoracic, the tracheobronchiolar and the alveolated region of the respiratory system. Deposition data for rats are from Koblinger and Hofmann (1995, Lovelace data), those for humans are from Heyder et al. (1986).

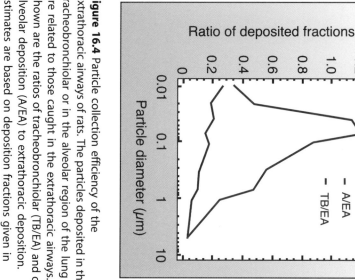

Figure 16.4 Particle collection efficiency of the extrathoracic airways of rats. The particles deposited in the tracheobronchiolar or in the alveolar region of the lung are related to those caught in the extrathoracic airways. Shown are the ratios of tracheobronchiolar (TB/EA) and of alveolar deposition (A/EA) to extrathoracic deposition. Estimates are based on deposition fractions given in Figure 16.3.

ciliated terminal bronchioles in rats (Bailey et al., 1989; Kreyling, 1990; Kreyling et al., 1991). Particles of intermediate solubility may be dissolved in phagolysosomes of AM. Particles are phagocytosed within hours after deposition (Brain, 1985), but intracellular dissolution and translocation into the blood varies according to the physicochemical properties of the material (Warheit and Hartsky, 1993; Searl, 1997) Strain-specific differences in particle clearance have been reported in rats as a result of different rates of translocation (Collier et al., 1989; Drosselmeyer et al., 1989; Patrick et al., 1989; Kreyling et al., 1993). Peripheral lung clearance was found to be impaired by chronic exposure to cigarette smoke (Finch et al., 1995) and by a general particle overload. The interpretation of clearance data therefore requires the consideration of methodological aspects, like the mode of exposure (instillation vs. inhalation) and the amount and nature of particles deposited in the lung (Oberdörster, 1995; Hesterberg et al., 1996; Oberdörster et al., 1997).

1992). Airway reactivity is assessed from the cumulative dose response curve and is quantified either by the maximum response or by the dose of substance required to double pulmonary resistance or decrease lung compliance to a certain level.

Substantial heterogeneity of responses to contractile agonists have been observed between central and peripheral airways (Munoz et al., 1989; Sakae et al., 1992). Serotonin induced little airway constriction when administered into the bronchial circulation, but acted as a strong contractile agonist when infused into the pulmonary circulation. Responses to muscarinic agonists were slightly greater in peripheral than in central airways, but were closely correlated, suggesting that both lung regions had a comparable sensitivity. Histamine elicited a biphasic response; it was a weak contractile agonist in both central and peripheral airways at low concentrations but caused progressive airway relaxation towards baseline with increasing doses.

There is evidence that genetic factors affect bronchial reactivity in rats, as strain-related differences have been reported (Joos et al., 1986; Pauwels and van der Straeten, 1986; Dandurand et al., 1993; Germonpre et al., 1995). High bronchial responsiveness was found to follow a pattern compatible with **autosomal recessive inheritance** (Pauwels et al., 1985). Intrinsic airway smooth muscle properties, regulatory mechanisms in the endogenous nitric oxide pathway, and mechanisms involving the activation of neurokinin receptors contribute to the spontaneous hyperresponsiveness observed in Fisher rats (Germonpre et al., 1995; Jia et al., 1996; Wang et al., 1997).

Different models for allergen-induced hyperresponsiveness have been established in rats. Rats were actively sensitized with ovalbumin (Dahlbäck and Eirefelt, 1984; Elwood et al., 1991; Kips et al., 1992; Wang et al., 1993; Schneider et al., 1997; dinitrophenyl-Ascaris extract (Misawa and Sugiyama, 1993) or anhydrides (Cui et al., 1997). Ovalbumin-sensitized Brown Norway rats demonstrate early and late responses (ER, LR) after inhalative allergen challenge. The ER is caused by smooth muscle contraction rather than airway wall edema (Du et al., 1992). It is mainly mediated by serotonin, while platelet-activating factor and lipoxygenase or cyclooxygenase products appear to play no role (Dandurand et al., 1994; Elwood et al., 1994). The LR is partially leukotriene (LTD$_4$) mediated and may even occur in vitro in the absence of de novo inflammatory cell recruitment (Dandurand et al., 1994). The

Airway Reactivity

Bronchial hyperresponsiveness is detected in rat models after viral infections of the respiratory tract (Knott et al., 1996) or after lung transplantation (Tavakoli and Frossard 1995). It can be induced by a choline-deficient diet (Itabashi et al., 1993) and is often observed in environmental or occupational exposures (Shore et al., 1995). Various approaches have been established to assess airway reactivity in vivo (Sakae et al., 1992; Long et al., 1997), in isolated lungs (Munoz et al., 1989; Padrid et al., 1993), or ex vivo in specimens of lung tissue by video microscopy (Wang et al., 1997) or electrical field stimulation (Aas and Fonnum, 1997). Pharmacological stimuli for the induction of airway constriction are histamine and serotonin (Munoz et al., 1989; Itabashi et al., 1993), or muscarinic agonists like acetylcholine or methacholine, which act directly on airway smooth muscles (Eidelman et al., 1991; Sakae et al., 1992; Padrid et al., 1993). Other substances like tachykinins (Munoz et al., 1989; Joos et al., 1986; Pauwels and van der Straeten, 1986) or physiological stimuli like cold air have also been used (Yoshihara et al., 1995). In living animals, contractile agents are administered either by intravenous infusion or by aerosol inhalation (Raeburn et al., densities of mast cells in the bronchial tree corre-spond closely to the sites of airway constriction, both occurring predominantly in large airways (Du et al., 1991). Allergen challenge induces a significant in-crease in eosinophils, lymphocytes and neutrophils in lung parenchyma and bronchoalveolar lavage fluid (BAL). Neutrophils appear as early as 3 hours after challenge. They peak at 24 hours in parenchyma and in BAL and decline rapidly thereafter. Marked eosinophil infiltration into lung parenchyma is ap-parent by 24 hours and peaks at 48 hours in paren-chyma and at 72 hours in BAL. Lung eosinophilia persists for at least 6 days (Elwood et al., 1991; Schneider et al., 1997). Specific inhibition of T-lymphocyte activation by cyclosporin A significantly suppresses the allergen-induced eosinophilia in BAL, but does not inhibit bronchial hyperresponsiveness (Elwood et al., 1992). Ricin, which has been shown to enhance IgE production in the rat, potentiates the inflammatory response to allergen challenge (Under-wood et al., 1995). Old animals failed to accumulate eosinophils in allergen-induced airway inflammation, probably due to age-dependent alterations in T-cell function mediated by greater amounts of interferon γ produced by lymph node cells (Yagi et al., 1997).

Exposure Methods in Regulatory Toxicology

Principles of Inhalative Exposure Systems

In conducting toxicity studies with airborne materi-als special attention should be paid to the generation and delivery of well-characterized test materials to the experimental animals. The main components of an exposure system are: (1) generation of the test atmosphere, (2) the exposure chamber, (3) monitor-ing of exposure, and (4) exposure clean-up. The principles of an inhalative exposure system are shown in Figure 16.5. After generation of the ex-posure atmosphere the output is mixed with condi-tioned air and is directed to the inhalation chamber. Exhaust fans draw the test atmosphere through the inhalation chambers. Before releasing the exposure air flow into the environment, exhaust filters remove all toxic substances from the experimental atmos-phere. An aerosol/gas sampling and measuring sys-tem supplies all of the data necessary for documentation and control. Any deviations from the set values are used to control the exposure atmosphere generator and air conditioning. Only dynamic exposure systems incorporating a flow system for the air are recommended.

The exposure chamber may be located in a sepa-rate room to which only the animal caretakers have access. The advantage of this design is that it minimizes contact of other personnel with the animals and thus lowers the risk of infection. This system is of special importance for chronic studies. The systems for the generation and control of the expo-sure atmosphere are located outside the animal room. In many cases this ideal design will be difficult to follow, e.g. for short-term inhalation studies and nose-only studies.

The principles of the exposure systems are given in the OECD Guidelines for Testing of Chemicals (OECD, 1981). For an overview of the exposure system the reader is referred to publications such as Phalen (1984) and Cheng and Moss (1995).

Aerosol Generation

The size, shape and density of particles are impor-tant parameters for deposition and retention in lungs. With regard to the deposition of aerosol there are significant species differences (Raabe et al., 1988). The rat respirable-size fraction (the fraction which reaches the lung) is considerably smaller than that for humans. The deposition of particles is governed by the aerodynamic diameter d_{ae}, which is defined by the diameter of a unit density sphere (density = 1 g/cm³) settling in air at the same velocity as the particle under consideration. For spherical particles larger than 2µm the relationship between the aerodynamic diameter, d_{ae}, and the geometric diameter, d_g, is given by

$$d_{ae} = d_g \text{ (density of the material/density of 1)}^{1/2}$$

Methods to measure the aerodynamic diameter, e.g. by cascade impactors, are described by Moss and Cheng (1995).

Aerosols can be generated by various dispersing or condensing processes. Particle generation starts from a bulk material, which is either a liquid or a powder. For the dispersion, different physical mechanisms for breaking adhesive forces are

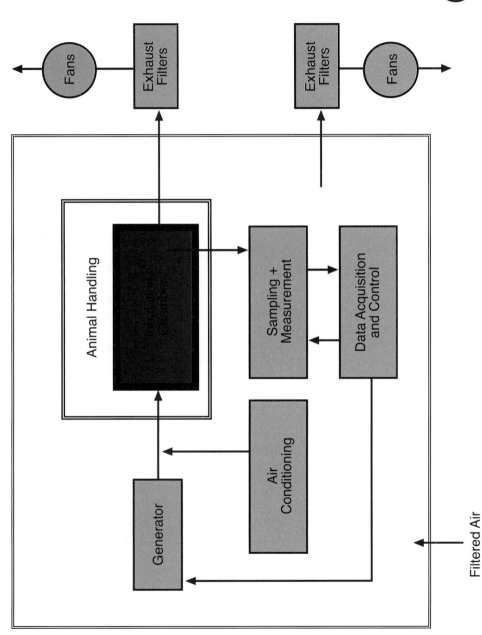

Figure 16.5 Basic elements of an inhalation exposure system. In this design two separate rooms for animal handling (including the inhalation chambers) and generation of test atmospheres are required.

employed. For example, nebulization of liquids can be achieved either by interaction with a pressurized gas or by focusing ultrasonic energy onto the surface of the liquid (Koch, 1998). Usually, a droplet spectrum with a large fraction of noninhalable coarse particles is generated. These particles have to be removed before entering the exposure chamber.

A variety of techniques are available for dispersion of dry powders. A widely used system is a rotating brush aerosol generator, where a piston filled with the dust to be dispersed is pressed against a rotating brush. The brush scrapes off material which is then dispersed by a pressurized air nozzle. Fluidized bed aerosol generators are useful for dispersion of free-flowing particles. Other powder delivery systems utilize either hoppers, screw feeders or rotating disks (Moss and Cheng, 1995). Particles may carry electrical charges after the process of aerosol generation. The deposition pattern of charged particles is different from that of neutral

particles. Therefore, aerosols are generally discharged by passing them through a cloud of bipolar air ions which can be produced with radioactive sources (e.g. krypton-85 or nickel-63).

Generation of Gaseous Test Atmospheres

The simplest method for generating a nonreactive gaseous test atmosphere is to introduce pure gas from a cylinder into the exposure system at a fixed flow rate controlled by a flowmeter. A frequently employed method for producing a vapor atmosphere is to use a constant temperature bath in which the test material is contained within a reservoir. A carrier gas is directed to flow over the surface or through the liquid at a rate controlled by a flowmeter.

Many organic gases when mixed with oxygen can produce explosive mixtures. Inflammability limits

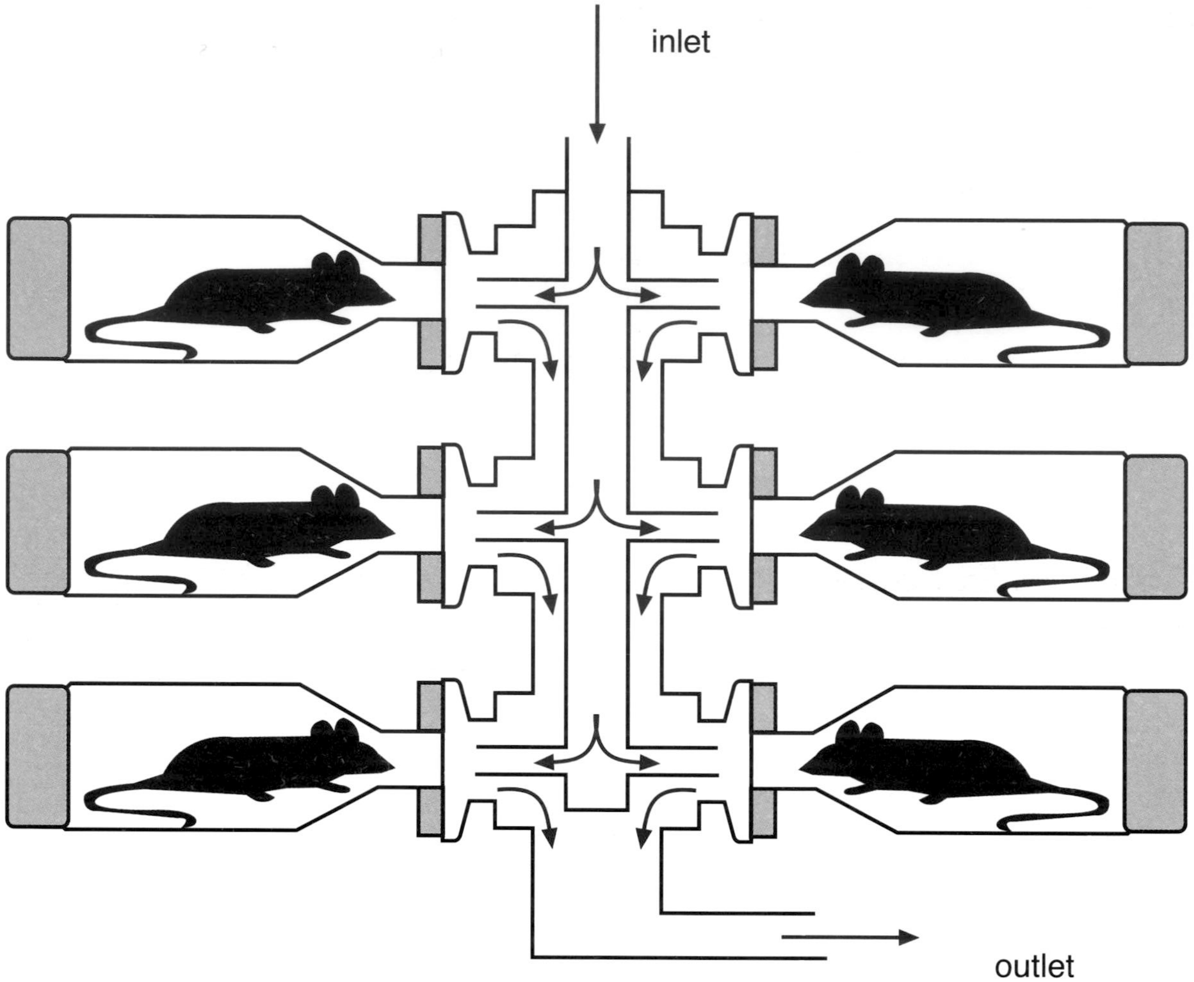

Figure 16.6 Schematic drawing of a concentric tube nose-only inhalation chamber.

inlet

outlet

must be carefully taken into account. A further problem is the reaction of gases or vapors with materials in the generator, the tubing system or the exposure chamber. For a detailed description of generation and characterization of gases and vapors the reader is referred to Wong (1995).

Exposure Systems

Rats should be tested in an exposure system which delivers a dynamic air flow of 12–15 air exchanges per hour. The oxygen content of the breathing air should be 19%. For toxic materials the maintenance of a slightly negative pressure inside the exposure chamber prevents leakage into the surrounding area.

Widely used exposure systems are: whole-body exposure, head-only and nose-only systems. Whole-body exposure systems are usually made from stainless steel and glass. The air flow rate through the chambers is either vertical or horizontal. The aerosol particles have to be homogeneously mixed with the air before entering the chamber. Whole-body exposure systems are used if enough test material is available for the generation of the exposure atmosphere. The advantages of this type of exposure system are that housing conditions are not stressful to the animals and long daily exposure durations can be applied.

The advantage of nose-only or head-only exposure systems is that only a minimum amount of the test material has to be used compared with whole-body systems. In addition, contamination of the fur, e.g. with radioactive particles, is minimized in this method. During daily exposure for up to 6 hours the animals are housed in tubes. A widely used design consists of a concentric cylinder where the freshly generated aerosol flows vertically downward (Figure 16.6). Aerosol exits by tubes are provided at different levels in a ring arrangement. The aerosol is blown directly to the breathing region of the rat sitting in a tube attached to the cylinder. The exhaled air is sucked away from the animal and flows into the outer cylinder. Detailed descriptions of exposure systems are given by Cheng and Moss (1995) and Koch (1998).

Key issues in aerosol exposure systems are the uniformity of the chamber concentration and the environmental conditions within the exposure chambers (temperature, relative humidity and air ventilation). Most systems monitor these conditions continuously and record the values automatically.

Control of Exposure Atmosphere

The concentration and the size distribution of a test aerosol should be constant during the entire length of the inhalation experiment. For the characterization of the aerosol exposure the aerosol mass concentration and size distribution have to be measured. The mass concentration can be determined gravimetrically by drawing air from the test atmosphere through a filter. The sampling flow rate and the sampling time have to be measured to determine the aerosol mass concentration. Light-scattering monitors can be used to assess real-time concentrations.

The particle size distribution of aerosols is usually measured by cascade impactors (Moss and Cheng, 1995).

Gas atmospheres can be measured by specific detection methods which usually require more widespread chemical methods. Methods for determining the gas concentration in the chambers include gas chromatography and infrared spectroscopy. Chemical analysis of trapped test materials can be used to quantify complex mixtures, where a detailed chemical analysis is necessary.

Typically, guidelines for testing of chemicals require the following to be monitored:

(1) Rate of air flow (preferably continuously).
(2) Test substance concentration. During the exposure period, the actual concentrations of the test substance should be held as constant as possible.
(3) Particle size. During the development of the generating system, particle size analysis should

be performed to establish the stability of aerosol concentrations. During exposure, analysis should be made as often as necessary to determine the consistency of the particle size distribution.
(4) Temperature and humidity (preferably continuously).

Guidelines for Regulatory Toxicology (Inhalation)

Although several mammalian species may be used in regulatory toxicology, the rat is the preferred species. The assessment of inhalation toxicity of industrial chemicals, agrochemicals or pharmaceuticals should be performed according to internationally recognized testing guidelines such as the OECD (Organization for Economic Co-operation and Development), EEC (European Economic Community), EPA (Environmental Protection Agency of the USA) Health Effects Test Guidelines for Chemicals, FIFRA (Federal Insecticide, Fungicide and Rodenticide Act of the USA) Guidelines for Agrochemicals or the regulations of the FDA (Food and Drug Administration of the USA). A recent synopsis of the US agencies for regulatory purposes can be found in publications of the Office of Prevention, Pesticides and Toxic Substances (OPPTS).

For studies which have to be accepted internationally, the OECD Guidelines are of outstanding importance. The work of the OECD related to chemical safety is carried out in the Environmental Health and Safety Division. Important documents are: *Testing and Assessment and Principles of Good Laboratory Practice and Compliance Monitoring*. Important guidelines for testing of chemicals of the OECD are *No. 403: Acute Inhalation Toxicity; No. 412: Repeated Dose Inhalation Toxicity: 28/14-Day, No. 413: Subchronic Inhalation Toxicity: 90-Day; No. 451: Carcinogenicity Studies, No. 452: Chronic Toxicity Studies, and No. 453: Combined Chronic Toxicity/Carcinogenicity Studies.*

In addition to the exposure principles mentioned above, these guidelines describe in detail the design of inhalation studies, such as the number of animals per group, housing and feeding conditions, equipment, exposure concentrations, exposure time, observation period, physical measurements, clinical examination, pathology and reporting.

References

Aas, P. and Fonnum, F. (1990) *Agents Actions Suppl.* **31**, 223–227.

Agnew, J.E. (1984) In: Clarke, S.W. and Paiva, D. (eds) *Aerosols and the Lung: Clinical and Experimental Aspects*, pp. 49–70. London: Butterworths.

Anjivil, S. and Asgharian, B. (1995) *Fundam. Appl. Toxicol.* **28**, 41–50.

Ardevol, V., Adan, C., Fernandez Lopez, J.A. *et al.* (1995) *Arch. Physiol. Biochem.* **103**, 175–186.

Asgharian, B. and Yu, C.P. (1989) *J. Aerosol Sci.* **20**, 355–366.

Asgharian, B., Wood, R. and Schlesinger, R.B. (1995) *Fundam. Appl. Toxicol.* **27**, 232–238.

Bailey, M.R., Kreyling, W.G., Andre, S. *et al.* (1989) *J. Aerosol. Sci.* **20**, 169–188.

Barnikol, W.K., Hiller, B. and Guth, S. (1994) *Biomed. Tech. Berl.* **39**, 57–62.

Bates, J.H., Schuessler, T.F., Dolman, C. and Eidelman, D.H. (1997) *J. Appl. Physiol.* **82**, 55–62.

Benignus, V. and Annau, Z. (1994) *Toxicol. Appl. Pharmacol.* **128**, 151–157.

Berke, H.L. and Roslinski, L.M. (1971) *Am. Ind. Hyg. Assoc. J.* **32**, 174–178.

Boyd, R.L., Fisher, M.J. and M.J. Jaeger (1980) *Respir. Physiol.* **40**, 181–190.

Brain, J.D. (1985) In: Fishman, A.P. and Fisher, A.B. (eds) *Handbook of Physiology*, pp. 447–471. Bethesda: American Physiological Society.

Brody, A.R. and Roe, M.W. (1983) *Am. Rev. Respir. Dis.* **128**, 724–729.

Cheng, Y.S. and Moss, O.R. (1995) In: McClellan, R.O. and Henderson, R.O. (eds) *Concepts in Inhalation Toxicology*, pp. 25–66. Washington DC: Taylor & Francis.

Cheng, Y.S., Hansen, G.K., Su, Y.F., Yeh, H.C. and Morgan, K.T. (1990) *Toxicol. Appl. Pharmacol.* **106**, 222–233.

Collier, C.G., Bailey, M.R. and Hodgson, A. (1989) *J. Aerosol Sci.* **20**, 233–247.

Costa, D.L. and Tepper, J.S. (1988) In: Gardner, D.E., Crapo, J.D. and Massaro, E.J. (eds) *Toxicology of the Lung*, pp. 147–174. New York: Raven Press.

Costa, D.L., Lehmann, J.R., Slatkin, D.N., Popenoe, E.A. and Drew, R.T. (1983) *Lung* **161**, 287–300.

Costa, D.L., Kutzman, R.S., Lehmann, J.R. and Drew, R.T. (1986) *Am. Rev. Respir. Dis.* **133**, 286–291.

Cotes, J.E. (1975) *Am. Rev. Respir. Dis.* **112**, 753–755.

Crapo, J.D., Young, S.L., Fram, E.K., Pinkerton, K.E., Barry, B.E. and Crapo, R.O. (1983) *Am. Rev. Respir. Dis.* **128**, S42–S46.

Cui, Z.H., Sjostrand, M., Pullerits, T., Andius, P., Skoogh, B.E. and Lotvall, J. (1997) *Allergy* **52**, 739–746.

Dahl, A.R. and Griffith, W.C. (1983) *J. Toxicol. Environ. Health* **12**, 371–383.

Dahlbäck, M. and Eirefelt, S. (1994) *Ann. Occup. Hyg.* **38**, Suppl. 1, 127–134.

Damon, E.G., Mauderly, J.L. and Jones, R.K. (1982) *Toxicol. Appl. Pharmacol.* **64**, 465–475.

Dandurand, R.J., Xu, L.J., Martin, J.G. and Eidelman, D.H. (1993) *J. Appl. Physiol.* **74**, 538–544.

Dandurand, R.J., Wang, C.G., Laberge, S., Martin, J.G. and Eidelman, D.H. (1994) *Am. J. Respir. Crit. Care Med.* **149**, 1499–1505.

Diamond, L. and O'Donnell, M. (1977) *J. Appl. Physiol.* **43**, 942–948.

Dormans, J.A., van Bree, L., Boere, A.J., Marra, M. and Rombout, P.J. (1989) *J. Toxicol. Environ. Health* **26**, 1–18.

Drosselmeyer, E., Müller, H.-L. and Pickering S. (1989) *J. Aerosol Sci.* **20**, 257–265.

Du, T., Sapienza, S., Eidelman, D.H., Wang, N.S. and Martin, J.G. (1991) *Am. Rev. Respir. Dis.* **143**, 132–137.

Du, T., Xu, L.J., Lei, M., Wang, N.S., Eidelman, D.H., Ghezzo, H. and Martin, J.G. (1992) *Am. Rev. Respir. Dis.* **146**, 1037–1041.

Eidelman, D.H., DiMaria, G.U., Wang, N.S., Guttmann, R.D. and Martin, J.G. (1991) *Am. Rev. Respir. Dis.* **144**, 792–796.

Elwood, W., Lötvall, J.O., Barnes, P.J. and Chung, K.F. (1991) *J. Allergy Clin. Immunol.* **88**, 951–960.

Elwood, W., Lötvall, J.O., Barnes, P.J. and Chung, K.F. (1992) *Am. Rev. Respir. Dis.* **145**, 1289–1294.

Elwood, W., Sakamoto, T., Barnes, P.J. and Chung, K.F. (1993) *J. Appl. Physiol.* **75**, 279–284.

Elwood, W., Sakamoto, T., Barnes, P.J. and Chung, K.F. (1994) *Int. Arch. Allergy Immunol.* **103**, 67–72.

Felicetti, S.A., Wolff, R.K. and Muggenburg, B.A. (1981) *J. Appl. Physiol.* **51**, 1612–1617.

Finch, G.L., Nikula, K.J., Chen, B.T., Barr, E.B., Chang, I.Y. and Hobbs, C.H. (1995) *Fundam. Appl. Toxicol.* **24**, 76–85.

Fukuda, Y. (1991) *Pflügers Arch.* **419**, 38–42.

Gehr, P., Mwangi, D.K., Ammann, A., Maloiy, G.M.O., Taylor, C.R. and Weibel, E.R. (1981) *Respir. Physiol.* **44**, 61–86.

Gehr, P., Geiser, M., Stone, K.C. and Crapo, J.D. (1993) In: Gardner, D.E., Crapo, J.D. and McClellan, R.O. (eds) *Toxicology of the Lung*, pp. 111–154. New York: Raven Press.

Gehr, P., Green, F.H.Y., Geiser, M., Im Hof, V., Lee, M.M. and Schürch, S. (1996) *J. Aerosol Med.* **9**, 163–181.

George, J.A.St., Harkema, J.R., Hyde, D.M. and Plopper, C.G. (1993) In: Gardner, D.E., Crapo, J.D. and McClellan, R.O. (eds) *Toxicology of the Lung*, pp. 81–110. New York: Raven Press.

Gerde, P., Cheng, Y.S. and Medinsky, M.A. (1991) *Fundam. Appl. Toxicol.* **16**, 330–336.

Germonpre, P.R., Joos, G.F., Everaert, E., Kips, J.C. and Pauwels, R.A. (1995) *Am. Rev. Respir. Crit. Care Med.* **152**, 1796–1804.

Gillespie, J.R. (1983) *Am. Rev. Respir. Dis.* **128**, S74–S77.

Giordano, A.M. and Morrow, P.E. (1972) *Arch. Environ. Health* **25**, 443–449.

Gonzalez, N.C., Clancy, R.L., Moue, Y. and Richalet, J.-P. (1998) *J. Appl. Physiol.* **84**, 164–168.

González Mangado, N., Peces-Barba, G., Verbank, S. and Paiva, M. (1991) *J. Appl. Physiol.* **71**, 855–862.

González Mangado, N., Peces-Barba, G., José Cabanillas, Renedo, G., Verbank, S. and Paiva, M. (1993) *Am. Rev. Respir. Dis.* **148**, 735–743.

Gore, D.J. and Patrick, G. (1978) *Phys. Med. Biol.* **23**, 730–737.

Gross, E.A., Swenberg, J.A., Fields, S. and Popp, J.A. (1982) *J. Anat.* **135**, 83–88.

Haber, P.S., Colebatch, H.J., Ng, C.K.Y. and Graves, I.A. (1983) *J. Appl. Physiol.* **54**, 837–845.

Halik, J., Lenger, V., Kliment, V. and Voboril, P. (1980) *J. Hyg. Epidemiol. Microbiol. Immunol.* **4**, 405–413.

Hantos, Z., Daroczy, B., Suki, B., and Nagy, S. (1987a) *J. Appl. Physiol.* **63**, 36–43.

Hantos, Z., Daroczy, B., Suki, B., Nagy, S. and Debreczeni, L.A. (1987b) *Acta Physiol. Hung.* **70**, 289–296.

Harkema, J.R. (1990) *Environ. Health Perspect.* **85**, 231–238.

Harkema, J.R., Mauderly, J.L. and Hahn, F.F. (1982) *Am. Rev. Respir. Dis.* **126**, 1058–1065.

Hauge, A., Bo, G. and Aarseth, P. (1977 *Acta Anesth. Scand.* **21**, 413–422.

Hayatdavoudi, G., O'Neil, J.J., Barry, B.E., Freeman, B.A. and Crapo, J.D. (1981) *J. Appl. Physiol.* **51**, 1220–1231.

Hebel, R. and Stromberg, M.W. (1986) *Anatomy and Embryology of the Laboratory Rat*, pp. 58–64. Wörthsee: BioMed Verlag.

Hesseltine, G.R., Wolff, R.D., Mauderly, J.L. and Cheng, Y.-S. (1986) *J. Appl. Toxicol.* **6**, 21–24.

Hesterberg, T.W., McConnel, E.E., Müller, W.C. *et al.* (1996) *Fundam. Appl. Toxicol.* **32**, 31–44.

Heyder, J., Gebhart, J., Rudolf, G., Schiller, C.F. and Stahlhofen, W. (1986) *J. Aerosol Sci.* **17**, 811–825.

Hofmann, W., Koblinger, L. and Martonen, T.B. (1989) *Health Phys.* **57**, Suppl. 1, 41–46.

Holub, D. and Frank, R.J. (1979) *Appl. Physiol.* **46**, 394–398.

Hyde, D.M., Plopper, C.G., George, J.A. St. and Harkema, J.R. (1990) In: Schraufnagel, D.E. (ed.) *Electron Microscopy of the Lung*, pp. 71–120. New York: Marcel Dekker.

Iravani, J (1967) *Pflügers Arch.* **297**, 221–237.

Itabashi, S., Ohrui, T., Sekizawa, K., Matsuzaki, Y. and Sasaki, H. (1993) *Respir. Physiol.* **92**, 219–225.

Jackson, A.C. and Watson, J.W. (1982) *Respir. Physiol.* **48**, 309–322.

Jeffrey, P.K. and Reid, L. (1975) *J. Anat.* **120**, 295–320.

Jia, Y., Xu, L., Turner, D.J. and Martin, J.G. (1996) *J. Appl. Physiol.* **80**, 404–410.

Johanson Jr, W.G. and Pierce, A.K. (1971) *J. Appl. Physiol.* **30**, 146–150.

Johanson Jr, W.G. and Pierce, A.K. (1973) *J. Clin. Invest.* **52**, 2921–2927.

Jones, A.D. (1993) *Ann. Occup. Hyg.* **37**, 211–226.

Joos, G., Kips, J., Pauwels, R. and van der Straeten, M. (1986) *Arch. Int. Pharmacodyn. Ther.* **280**, 176–190.

King, T.K.C. (1966) *J. Appl. Physiol.* **21**, 259–264.

Kips, J.C., Cuvelier, C.A. and Pauwels, R.A. (1992) *Am. Rev. Respir. Dis.* **145**, 1306–1310.

Knott, P.G., Henry, P.J., McWilliams, A.S., Rigby, P.J., Fernandes, L.B. and Goldie, R.G. (1996) *Br. J. Pharmacol.* **119**, 291–298.

Koblinger, L. and Hofmann, W. (1995) *J. Aerosol Med.* **8**, 21–32.

Koblinger, L., Hofmann, W., Graham, R.C. and Mercer, R.R. (1995) *J. Aerosol Med.* **8**, 7–19.

Koch, W. (1998) In: Uhlig, S. and Taylor, A.E. (eds) *Methods in Pulmonary Research*, pp. 485–507. Basel: Birkhäuser Verlag.

Kotlikoff, M.I., Jackson, A.C. and Watson, J.W. (1984) *J. Appl. Physiol.* **56**, 182–186.

Koto, H., Mak, J.C., Haddad, E.B. *et al.* (1997) *J. Clin. Invest.* **98**, 1780–1787.

Kreyling, W.G. (1990) *J. Aerosol Med.* **3**, S93–S110.

Kreyling, W.G. and Scheuch, G. (1999) In: Gehr, P. and Heyder, J. (eds) *Lung Particle Interactions*. New York: Marcel Dekker (in press).

Kreyling, W.G., André, S., Collier, C.G., Ferron, G.A., Métivier, H. and Schumann, G. (1991) *J. Aerosol Sci.* **22**, 509–535.

Kreyling, W.G., Cox, C., Ferron, G.A. and Oberdörster, G. (1993) *Exp. Lung Res.* **19**, 445–467.

Kreyling, W.G., Blanchard, J.D., Godleski, J.J. *et al.* (1999) *J. Appl. Physiol.* **87**, 269–284.

Kumar, A., Sorkness, R.L., Kaplan, M.R. and Lemanske Jr, R.F. (1997) *Am. J. Respir. Crit. Care Med.* **155**, 130–134.

Kuncova, M., Haurankova, J., Kunc, L., Holusa, R. and Palacek, F. (1972) *Arch. Environ. Health* **24**, 281–287.

Lahiri, S. (1975) *Am. J. Physiol.* **229**, 529–536.

Lai, Y.-L. and Hildebrandt, J. (1978) *J. Appl. Physiol.* **45**, 255–260.

Lai, Y.-L. and Diamond, L. (1986) *Respir. Physiol.* **66**, 147–155.

Lai, Y.-L. and Diamond, L. (1992) *J. Toxicol. Environ. Health* **35**, 63–76.

Lai, Y.-L., Tsuya, Y. and Hildebrandt, J. (1978) *J. Appl. Physiol.* **45**, 611–618.

Lai, Y.-L., Olson, J.W. and Gillespie, M.N. (1991) *J. Appl. Physiol.* **70**, 561–566.

Lamm, W.J.E., Hildebrandt, J.R., Hildebrandt, J. and Lai, Y.-L. (1982) *J. Appl. Physiol.* **53**, 1071–1079.

Leith, D.E. (1976) *Physiologist* **19**, 485–510.

Likens, S.A. and Mauderly, J.L. (1982) *J. Appl. Physiol.* **52**, 141–146.

Long, N.C., Martin, J.G., Pantano, R. and Shore, S.A. (1997) *Am. J. Respir. Crit. Care Med.* **155**, 1222–1229.

Loring, S.H., Elliot, E.A. and Drazen, J.M. (1979) *Lung* **156**, 33–34.

Loscutoff, S.M., Cannon, W.C., Buschbom, R.L., Busch, R.H. and Killand, B.W. (1985) *Environ. Res.* **36**, 170–180.

Lung, M.A. (1987) *J. Appl. Physiol.* **63**, 1339–1343.

Lutchen, K.R., Hantos, Z., Petak, F., Adamicza, A. and Suki, B. (1996) *J. Appl. Physiol.* **80**, 1841–1849.

Macklem, P.T. (1978) *Annu. Rev. Physiol.* **40**, 157–184.

Maksym, G.N. and Bates, J.H. (1997) *Ann. Biomed. Eng.* **25**, 1000–1008.

Maskrey, M., Evans, S.E., Mesch, U., Andersen, N.A. and Sherrey, J.H. (1992) *Respir. Physiol.* **90**, 47–54.

Mauderly, J.L. (1982) *Exp. Aging Res.* **8**, 31–36.

Mead, J., Whittenberger, J.L. and Radford, E.P. (1957) *J. Appl. Physiol.* **10**, 191–196.

Mead, J., Turner, J.M., Macklem, P.T. and Little, J.B. (1967) *J. Appl. Physiol.* **22**, 95–108.

Menache, M. G., Miller, F.J. and Raabe, O.G. (1995) *Ann. Occup. Hyg.* **39**, 317–328.

Mercer, R.R. and Crapo, J.D. (1987) *J. Appl. Physiol.* **63**, 749–785.

Mercer, R.R. and Crapo, J.D. (1993) In: Gardner, D.E. Crapo, J.D. and McClellan, R.O. (eds) *Toxicology of the Lung*, pp. 155–186. Raven Press, New York.

Mercer, R.R., Anjilvel, S., Miller, F.J. and Crapo, J.D. (1991) *J. Appl. Physiol.* **70**, 2193–2205.

Meyrick, B.O. (1990) In: Schraufnagel, D.E. (ed.) *Electron Microscopy of the Lung*, pp. 215–255. New York: Marcel Dekker.

Misawa, M. and Sugiyama, Y. (1993) *Arerugi* **42**, 107–114.

Morgan, K.T., Jiang, X.Z., Patterson, D.L. and Gross, E.A. (1984) *Am. Rev. Respir. Dis.* **130**, 275–281.

Morgan, K.T., Patterson, D.L. and Gross, E.A. (1986) In: Barrow, C.S. (ed.) *Toxicology of the Nasal Passages*, pp. 123–133. Washington DC: Hemisphere Publishing.

Morgan, K.T., Kimbell, J.S., Monticello, T.M., Patra, A.L. and Fleishman, A. (1991) *Toxicol. Appl. Pharmacol.* **110**, 223–240.

Morgan, K.T., Gross, E.A. and Bonnefoi, M. (1993) In: Gardner, D.E. Crapo, J.D. and McClellan, R.O. (eds) *Toxicology of the Lung*, pp. 31–53. New York: Raven Press.

Moss, O.R. and Cheng, Y.S. (1995) In: McClellan, R.O. and Henderson, R.O. (eds) *Concepts in Inhalation Toxicology*, pp. 91–128. Washington DC: Taylor & Francis.

Munoz, N.M., Chang, S.W., Murphy, T.M. *et al.* (1989) *J. Appl. Physiol.* **66**, 202–209.

Munoz, N.M., Kirchhoff, C.F., Strek, M.E., Blumenthal, R.N. and Leff, A.R. (1991) *Am. J. Physiol.* **260**, L260–267.

Nattie, E.E. (1977) *J. Appl. Physiol.* **43**, 1063–1074.

Noble, W.H., Kay, J.C. and Obdrzalek, J. (1975) *J. Appl. Physiol.* **38**, 681–687.

Negus, V.E. (1958) *The Comparative Anatomy and Physiology of the Nose and Paranasal Sinuses.* Edinburgh: Livingstone.

Oberdörster, G. (1993) *Aerosol Sci. Technol.* **18**, 279–289.

Oberdörster, G. (1995) *Regul. Toxicol. Pharmacol.* **21**, 123–135.

Oberdörster, G., Cox, C. and Gelein, R. (1997) *Exp. Lung Res.* **23**, 17–34.

Olson Jr., E.B. and Dempsey, J.A. (1978) *J. Appl. Physiol.* **44**, 763–769.

Oostveen, C.M.A. (1991) Mechanical properties of the respiratory system. A study in humans and rats by forced oscillations. Rijksuniversiteit te Utrecht.

OECD (Organization for Economic Cooperation and Development) (1981) *Guidelines for Testing of Chemicals.*

Oostveen, E., Zwart, A., Peslin, R. and Duvivier, C. (1992) *J. Appl. Physiol.* **73**, 1598–1607.

Otis, A.B., McKerrow, C.M., Bartlett, R.A. *et al.* (1956) *J. Appl. Physiol.* **8**, 427–443.

Padrid, P., Wolf, R., Munoz, N.M. *et al.* (1993) *Am. Rev. Respir. Dis.* **147**, 1514–1520.

Paiva, M. and Engel, L.A. (1988) In: Chang, H.K. and Paiva M. (eds) *Respiratory Physiology. An Analytical Approach*, pp. 245–276. New York: Marcel Dekker.

Palecek, F. (1969) *J. Appl. Physiol.* **27**, 149–156.

Patra, A.L. (1986) *J. Toxicol. Environ. Health* **17**, 163–174.

Patra, A.L., Gooya, A. and Ménache, M.G. (1986) *Anat. Rec.* **215**, 45–50.

Patra, A.L., Menache, M.G., Shaka, N.B. and Gooya, A. (1987) *Am. Ind. Hyg. Assoc. J.* **48**, 556–562.

Patrick, G. and Stirling, C. (1977) *J. Appl. Physiol.* **42**, 451–455.

Patrick, G., Batchelor, A.L. and Stirling, C. (1989) *J. Aerosol Sci.* **20**, 249–255.

Pauwels, R. and van der Straeten, M. (1986) *Arch. Int. Pharmacodyn. Ther.* **280**, Suppl. 2, 229–239.

Pauwels, R.R., van der Straeten, M., Weyne, J. and Bazin, H. (1985) *Eur. J. Respir. Dis.* **66**, 98–104.

Peslin, R. (1991) *Eur. Respir. J.* **4**, 246–247.

Peslin, R., Duvivier, C., Bekkari, H., Reichart, E. and Gallina, C. (1990) *J. Appl. Physiol.* **69**, 1080–1086.

Phalen, R.F. (1984) *Inhalation Studies: Foundations and Techniques.* Boca Raton: CRC Press.

Piiper, J. (1986) *Prax. Klin. Pneumol.* **40**, 201–204.

Piiper, J. (1987) *Keio. J. Med.* **36**, 112–115.

Piiper, J. and Scheid, P. (1980) In: West, J.B. (ed.) *Pulmonary Gas Exchange*, pp. 131–171. New York: Academic Press.

Piiper, J. and Scheid, P. (1987) In: Farhi, L.E. and Tenney, S.M. (eds) *Handbook of Physiology: The Respiratory System*, Vol. I, *Gas Exchange*, pp. 167–176. Bethesda: American Physiological Society.

Pinkerton, K.E., Barry, B.E., O'Neil, J.J., Raub, J.A., Pratt, P.C. and Crapo, J.D. (1982) *Am. J. Anat.* **164**, 155–174.

Pinkerton, K.E., Gallen, J.T., Mercer, R.R., Wong, V.C., Plopper, C.G. and Tarkington, B.K. (1993) *Microsc. Res. Tech.* **26**. 437–443.

Plopper, C.G., Mariassy, A.T. and Hill, L.H. (1980) *Exp. Lung Res.* **1**, 139–154.

Plopper, C.G., Mariassy, A.T., Willson, D.W., Alley, J.L., Nishio, S.J. and Nettesheim, P. (1983) *Exp. Lung Res.* **5**, 281–294.

Proctor, D.F. and Chang, J.C.F. (1983) In: Reznik, G. and Stinson, S. (eds) *Nasal Tumors in Animals and Man*, pp. 1–33. Boca Raton: CRC Press.

Quanjer, Ph.H., Tammeling, G.J., Cotes, J.E. *et al.* (1993) *Eur. Respir. J.* **6**, Suppl. 16, 85–100.

Raabe, O.G, Yeh, H.C., Newton, G.C., Phalen, R.F. and Velasquez, D.J. (1977) In: Walton, W.H. (ed) *Inhaled Particles IV*, pp. 3–21, New York: Pergamon.

Raabe, O.G., Al-Bayati, M.A., Teague, S.V. and Rasolt, A. (1988) *Ann. Occup. Hyg.* **32**, Suppl. 1, 53–63.

Raeburn, D., Underwood, S.L. and Villamil, M.E. (1992) *J. Pharmacol. Toxicol. Methods* **27**, 143–159.

Rodriguez, M., Bur, S., Favre, A. and Weibel, E.R. (1987) *Am. J. Anat.* **180**, 143–155.

Roughton, F.J.W. and Forster, R.E. (1957) *J. Appl. Physiol.* **11**, 290–302.

Rubio, M.L., Sánchez-cifuentes, M.V., Peces-Barba, G. *et al.* (1998) *Am. J. Respir. Crit. Care Med.* **157**, 237–245.

Sahebjami, H. (1991) *Exp. Lung Res.* **17**, 887–902.

Sahebjami, H. and Vassallo, C.I. (1979) *Respir. Physiol.* **36**, 131–142.

Sakae, R.S., Martins, M.A., Criado, P.M., Zin, W.A. and Saldiva, P.H. (1992) *J. Appl. Toxicol.* **12**, 235–238.

Schlesinger, R.B. (1985) *J. Toxicol. Environ. Health* **15**, 197–214.

Schneider, T., van Velzen, D., Moqbel, R. and Issekutz, A.C. (1997) *Am. J. Respir. Cell Mol. Biol.* **17**, 702–712.

Schreider, J. and Raabe, O. (1981) *Anat. Rec.* **200**, 195–205.

Schulz, H., Brand, P. and Heyder, J. (1999) In: Gehr, P. and Heyder, J. (eds) *Particle–Lung Interactions*. New York: Marcel Dekker (in press).

Schum, M. and Yeh, H.-S. (1980) *Bull. Math. Biol.* **42**, 1–15.

Searl, A. (1997) *Ann. Occup. Hyg.* **41**, 217–233.

Seeherman, H.J., Taylor, C.R., Maloiy, G.M.O. and Armstrong, R.B. (1981) *Respir. Physiol.* **44**, 11–23.

Shore, S., Kobzik, L., Long, N.C. *et al.* (1995) *Am. J. Respir. Crit. Care Med.* **151**, 1931–1938.

Smith, G. (1977) *Lab. Anim.* **11**, 223–228.

Sorkness, R., Blythe, S. and Lemanske, R.F. Jr. (1988) *Am. Rev. Respir. Dis.* **138**, 1152–1156.

Stahlhofen, W. (1987) In: Crapo, J.D., Smolko, E.D., Miller, F.J. and Hayes, A.W. (eds) *Extrapolation of Dosimetric Relationships of Inhaled Particles and Gases*, pp. 153–166. San Diego: Academic Press.

Stevens, M.A., Ménache, M.G., Crapo, J.D., Miller, F.J. and Graham, J.A. (1988) *J. Toxicol. Environ. Health* **23**, 229–240.

Sugihara, T. and Martin, J. (1975) *J. Clin. Invest.* **56**, 23–29.

Sweeney, T.D, Skornik, W.A., Brain, J.D., Hatch, V. and Godleski, J. (1995) *Am. J. Respir. Crit. Care Med.* **151**, 482–488.

Takezawa, J., Miller, F.J. and O'Neil, J.J. (1980) *J. Appl. Physiol.* **48**, 1052–1059.

Tavakoli, R. and Frossard, N. (1995) *Br. J. Pharmacol.* **114**, 1428–1432.

Taylor, C.R., Moloiy, G.M.O, Weibel, E.R. *et al.* (1980) *Respir. Physiol.* **44**, 25–37.

Taylor, C.R., Maloiy, G.M.O., Weibel, E.R., Langman, V.A., Kaman, J.M.Z., Seeherman, H.J. and Heglung, N.C. (1981) *Respir. Physiol.* **44**, 25–37.

Tenny, S.M. and Remmers, J.E. (1963) *Nature* **197**, 54–56.

Turek, Z., Grandtner, M., Ringnalda, B.E.M. and Kreuzer, F. (1973) *Pflügers Arch.* **340**, 11–18.

Turek, Z., Kreuzer, F. and Ringnalda, B.E.M. (1978) *Pflügers Arch.* **376**, 7–13.

Underwood, S.L., Kemeny, D.M., Lee, T.H., Raeburn, D. and Karlsson, J.A. (1995) *Immunology* **85**, 256–261.

Valerius, K.P. (1996) *J. Morphol.* **230**, 291–297.

Verbank, S., González Mangado, N., Peces-Barba, G. and Paiva, M. (1991) *J. Appl. Physiol.* **71**, 847–854.

Verbank, S., Weibel, E.R. and Paiva, M. (1993) *J. Appl. Physiol.* **71**, 847–854.

Walker, B.R., Merill Adams, E. and Voelkel, N.F. (1985) *J. Appl. Physiol.* **59**, 1955–1969.

Wang, C.G., Dimaria, G., Bates, J.H.T., Guttman, R.D. and J. Martin, J.G. (1986) *J. Appl. Physiol.* **61**, 2180–2185.

Wang, C.G., Du, T. and Martin, J.G. (1993) *Am. Rev. Respir. Dis.* **148**, 413–417.

Wang, C.G., Almirall, J.J., Dolman, C.S., Dandurand, R.J. and Eidelman, D.H. (1997) *J. Appl. Physiol.* **82**, 1445–1452.

Warheit, D.B. and Hartsky, M.A. (1993) *Microsc. Res. Tech.* **26**, 412–422.

Weibel, E.R. (1993) In: Gardner, DE., Crapo, J.D. and McClellan, R.O. (eds) *Toxicology of the Lung*, pp. 1–30. New York: Raven Press.

Wong, B.A. (1995) In: McClellan, R.O. and Henderson, R.O. (eds) *Concepts in Inhalation Toxicology*, pp. 67–90. Washington DC: Taylor & Francis.

Wright, J.L., Sun, J.-S. and S. Vedal. (1997) *Eur. Respir. J.* **10**, 1115–1119.

Xu, G.B. and Yu, C.P. (1987) *Aerosol Sci. Technol.* **7**, 117–123.

Yagi, T., Sato, A., Hayakwa, H. and Ide, K. (1997) *J. Allergy Clin. Immunol.* **99**, 38–47.

Yeh, H.-C. and Harkema, J.S. (1993) In Gardner, DE.,

Crapo, J.D. and McClellan, R.O. (eds) *Toxicology of the Lung*, pp. 55–79. New York: Raven Press.

Yeh, H.-C., Schum, F.M. and Duggan (1979) *Anat. Rec.* **195**, 482–492.

Yokoyama, E. (1983) *Comp. Biochem. Physiol.* **75A**, 77–80.

Yoshihara, S., Chan, B., Yanawaki, I., Geppetti, P., Ricciardolo, F.L., Massion, P.P. and Nadel, J.A. (1995) *Am. J. Respir. Crit. Care Med.* **151**, 1011–1017.

Zhou, K.-R. and Lai, Y.-L. (1992) *J. Appl. Physiol.* **72**, 1914–1921.

Zwart, A. and Peslin, R. (1991) *Eur. Respir. Rev.* **1**, 131–235.

Zwart, A. and Van de Woestijne, K.P. (1994) *Eur. Respir. Rev.* **4**, 114–237.

Yu, C.P. and Xu, G.B. (1986) *Aerosol Sci. Technol.* **5**, 337–347.

CHAPTER 17

Circulation

Livius V d'Uscio
Institute of Physiology, University of Zürich-Irchel, Zürich, Switzerland

Juliane Kilo
Institute of Physiology, University of Zürich-Irchel, Zürich, Switzerland

Thomas F Lüscher
Cardiology, University Hospital, Zürich, Switzerland

Max Gassmann
Institute of Physiology, University of Zürich-Irchel, Zürich, Switzerland

Anatomical Heterogeneity of Blood Vessels

Blood vessels of different anatomical origin have various functions in the circulation. Based on histologically defined criteria, the vessel wall of conduit arteries can be divided into three main layers. From the abluminal to the luminal side these consist of the outer tunica adventitia, the central tunica media and the inner tunica intima (Bloom and Fawcett, 1968).

The adventitia, the most outer layer of the vessel wall, consists of connective tissue, mainly elastin and collagen, and is important for the integration of the vessel into the surrounding tissue. The media, separated from the intima by the internal elastic lamina, has an extensive amount of elastic fibers and vascular smooth muscle cells, which are normally oriented helically around the lumen of the vessel (Bloom and Fawcett, 1968). The elastic fiber to smooth muscle cell ratio differs from vessel to vessel. Large conduit arteries such as aorta, epicardial coronary arteries, pulmonary artery or carotid artery contain a higher proportion of elastic fibers. On the other hand, **resistance arteries**, important for the regulation of peripheral vascular resistance, such as small arteries, arterioles and venules, contain more smooth muscle cells than elastic fibers. According to anatomical (location in the vascular tree) and functional (pressure drop) definitions, the resistance arteries have diameters of less than 300 µm.

Intravascular measurements show that, depending on the vascular bed, up to 50% or more of the resistance arteries appear to lie proximal to arterioles (Mulvany and Aalkjaer, 1990). In contrast to that of arteries, the media of veins, which are capacitance vessels, is thinner and very elastic. Nerve endings of mostly sympathetic origin are present at the adventitial side of the media. These structures can affect the function of the vessel wall either in an active or in a passive way (Boonen, 1992).

The intima, at the luminal side of the blood vessel wall, consists of a thin monolayer of endothelial cells forming a continuous layer covering the lumen of all blood vessels. The long axis of the endothelial cells is oriented parallel to the blood flow direction (Lüscher and Vanhoutte, 1990).

Physiology of the Blood Vessels

Role of Vascular Endothelium

The original concept of blood vessels as tubes only regulated by circulating hormones and the sympathetic nervous system has changed dramatically fairly recently. It became clear that local endothelial regulatory mechanisms as well as interactions between the cells of vessel wall and the circulating blood cells (i.e. platelets and monocytes) play an important role

Large conduit arteries gradually convert **pulsatile flow** near the heart into a more continuous flow in the more distant peripheral vessels. Small resistance arteries, however, are important for the regulation of peripheral vascular resistance and have the ability to control the lumen diameter, and thus control blood pressure (Mulvany and Aalkjaer, 1990). The physiological control mechanisms operated to maintain arterial blood pressure can be exerted through remote control or local control. Remote control is exerted by neural (mostly sympathetic nervous system) and humoral factors (such as the renin-angiotensin system, natriuretic peptides and vasopressin), while local regulation involves mechanical and metabolic factors such as carbon dioxide, pH and endothelium-derived factors (Gaskell, 1881; Judy et al., 1976; Aalkjaer, 1990; Lüscher and Vanhoutte, 1990).

(Moncada et al., 1976; Furchgott and Zawadzki, 1980). The endothelial cells, located in a strategical anatomical position, are an important source of a variety of both relaxing and constricting factors.

Endothelium-derived relaxing factors

Nitric oxide (NO)

A diffusible substance with a short half-life of a few seconds was identified as the endogenous free radical NO (Ignarro et al., 1987; Palmer et al., 1987). NO is formed from L-arginine (Figure 17.1), requiring several cofactors such as oxygen, NADPH, 5,6,7,8-tetrahydrobiopterin and Ca^{2+}/calmodulin (Moncada et al., 1991).

The formation of NO occurs via nitric oxide synthases (NOS) which can either be expressed constitutively (cNOS) or induced (iNOS). Three different isoforms of NOS have been described to date (Moncada et al., 1991).

Most of the endothelial cNOS appears to be bound to endothelial cell membrane, whereas only a small fraction is of cytosolic origin (Sessa et al., 1992). Receptor-dependent agonists (i.e. acetylcholine, bradykinin, substance P and platelet-derived products such as thrombin and adenosine diphosphate) are capable of increasing intracellular free Ca^{2+}, which in turn activates endothelial cNOS and thus endothelium-dependent relaxations in isolated rat vascular beds (Figure 17.1) (Lüscher and Vanhoutte, 1990). The endothelial L-arginine/NO pathway is further activated by shear forces exerted by the circulating blood cells, thereby causing flow-dependent vasodilation (Nadaud et al., 1996). Relaxations in response to the abluminal release of endothelium-derived NO are associated with an increase in cyclic guanosine 3',5'-monophosphate (cGMP) in vascular smooth muscle cells (Figure 17.1), which reduces intracellular Ca^{2+} and dephosphorylates myosin light chains (Rapoport et al., 1983). Soluble guanylyl cyclase, present in platelets, is activated by luminal release of endothelium-derived NO (Busse et al., 1987), and this reduces adhesion and aggregation (Radomski et al., 1992). Therefore, endothelium-derived NO causes both vasodilation and platelet deactivation and thereby represents an important **antithrombotic** feature of the endothelium. Furthermore, NO also plays a crucial role in the regulation of blood pressure (Gardiner et al., 1990). Indeed, when infused intravenously, inhibitors of NOS such as $L\text{-}N^G$-monomethyl arginine (L-NMMA) or N^G-nitro-L-arginine

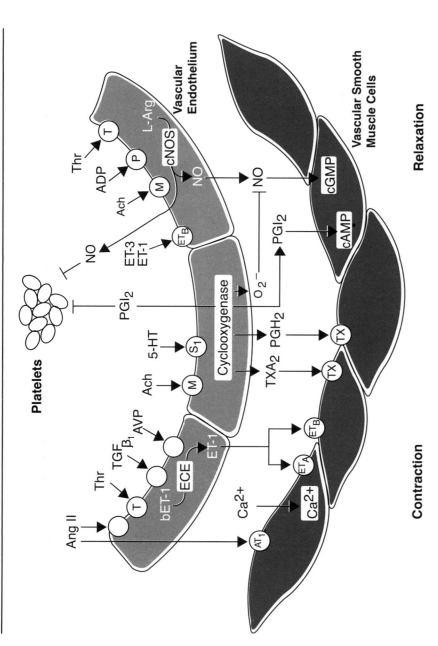

Figure 17.1 Endothelium-derived relaxing factors (right part) and endothelium-derived contracting factors (left part). Endothelial cells form nitric oxide (NO) from L-arginine via the activity of the constitutive NO synthase (cNOS). It causes increases in cyclic 3'5'-guanosine monophosphate (cGMP) in vascular smooth muscle cells and platelets, which in turn mediates relaxation and platelet inhibition, respectively. In addition, prostacyclin (PGI₂) is synthesized by endothelial cells and causes relaxation via a cyclic adenosine monophosphate (cAMP)-dependent mechanism. Stimulation of the cyclooxygenase pathway by receptor-operated agonists such as acetylcholine (Ach) and serotonin (5-HT), or physical forces, can lead to the formation of prostaglandin H₂ (PGH₂), thromboxane A₂ (TXA₂), or superoxide anions (O₂⁻), which in turn elicit direct vasoconstrictions and also inactivate NO. Furthermore, the synthesis of endothelin 1 (ET-1) is stimulated by hormones such as angiotensin II (Ang II) and arginine vasopressin (AVP), as well as coagulation factors such as thrombin (Thr) and transforming growth factor β₁ (TGFβ₁). ET-1 can activate vascular smooth muscle cell receptors (mainly ETₐ-, but also ET_B-receptors). In addition, ET-1 and ET-3 can activate ET_B-receptors in the endothelial cell membrane, which are linked to the production of NO and PGI₂. ECE, endothelin-converting enzyme; TX, thromboxane; M, muscarinerg; S, serotonin; circles, receptors.

methylester (L-NAME) induce a long-lasting increase in blood pressure and vascular resistance. This demonstrates that the vasculature is in a constant state of vasodilation due to the continuous basal release of picomolar quantities of NO by the vascular endothelium. In addition, NO is also transported after binding to hemoglobin as an S-nitrosohemoglobin complex (Jia *et al.*, 1996).

Other endothelium-derived relaxing factors

In addition to NO, prostacyclin is released by endothelial cells in response to several mediators, shear stress and hypoxia (Yang *et al.*, 1992; Chida and Voelkel, 1996). Its platelet inhibitory effects may be

probably more important than its contribution to endothelium-dependent relaxation (Moncada *et al.*, 1977).

In addition, not all endothelium-dependent relaxations are prevented by inhibitors of the L-arginine pathway. These NO-independent relaxations are even more prominent in isolated mesenteric resistance and renal arteries (Nagao *et al.*, 1992; Hwa *et al.*, 1994; Shimokawa *et al.*, 1996). Under these conditions, vascular smooth muscle cells become transiently **hyperpolarized**. A more recent study reports an identification of K⁺ as an endothelium-dependent hyperpolarizing factor (Edwards *et al.*, 1998).

Endothelium-derived contracting factors

Endothelin

Endothelin 1, a potent vasoconstrictor (Yanagisawa et al., 1988) and mitogen (Hirata et al., 1989), is the first member of the endothelin peptide family. Expression of messenger RNA and therefore release of the peptide is stimulated by vasoconstrictor hormones such as angiotensin II, epinephrine, arginine vasopressin, and also by coagulation products such as thrombin, platelet-derived transforming growth factor β_1 and cytokines (Figure 17.1) (Yanagisawa et al., 1988; Hahn et al., 1990; Dohi et al., 1992). However, endothelin is produced not only in vascular endothelial cells but also in vascular smooth muscle cells (Hahn et al., 1990) and in mesangial cells (Ikeda et al., 1995). Endothelin 1 exerts its biological effects via activation of distinct specific endothelin receptors (Arai et al., 1990; Sakurai et al., 1990). One receptor type shows high selectivity to endothelin 1 and probably represents the ET_A-receptor on vascular smooth muscle cells (Alberts et al., 1994). The other type, the ET_B-receptors, are present on endothelial cells linked to the formation of endothelium-dependent NO and prostacyclin (de Nucci et al., 1988; Takase et al., 1995). When infused intravenously, endothelin 1 produces transient vasodilatation at lower and long-lasting contractions at higher concentrations, suggesting that the vasoconstriction is far more important than vasodilation (Mortensen et al., 1990).

Cyclooxygenase-derived contracting factors

Exogenous arachidonic acid induces endothelium-dependent contractions in different isolated rat vascular beds, which are prevented by indomethacin, a cyclooxygenase inhibitor (Lüscher and Vanhoutte, 1986). Thromboxane A_2 (TXA$_2$) and the endoperoxide prostaglandin H_2 (PGH$_2$) are the most potent vasoconstrictors among the cyclooxygenase products (Figure 17.1) and are produced both in endothelial cells and in platelets. TXA$_2$ and PGH$_2$ affect not only vascular smooth muscle cells via the activation of TXA$_2$ receptors (Lang et al., 1995) but also platelets, which aggregate, and hence counteract the benefical effects of NO and prostacyclin in both cell types (Lüscher and Vanhoutte, 1990). Furthermore, prostaglandins stimulate renin secretion in vitro and in vivo (Freeman et al., 1984; Imagawa et al., 1985).

In addition, the cyclooxygenase pathway is a source of superoxide anions (O_2^-) which can evoke endothelium-dependent contractions either by the inactivation of endothelium-derived NO or by directly stimulating vascular smooth muscle cells (Figure 17.1) (Kukreja et al., 1986; Tschudi et al., 1996).

Contractile Machinery of Vascular Smooth Muscle

Contraction of vascular smooth muscle mainly results from the interaction of two contractile proteins, actin and myosin, consisting of a variety of different isoenzymes. Force development is achieved by cyclic, high-affinity cross-bridge formation of actin filaments with the larger myosin filaments (Murphy, 1994). This occurs via translocation of myosin heads that bind actin, resulting in a transaxial sliding of the filaments across each other, evoking a change in the configuration of the muscle cells. These changes are regulated from outside through a signal transduction mechanism to modify the concentrations of key intracellular second messengers (i.e. phosphoinositide), generated at the cell membrane surface passing into the intracellular space and in turn increasing intracellular free Ca^{2+} concentrations (Challiss and Gray, 1994). Three systems can be distinguished: electromechanical coupling, pharmacomechanical coupling and mechanotransduction.

Methodology

Many techniques are available to study endothelium-dependent responses and contractile responses of vascular smooth muscle of isolated conduit and small resistance arteries. The organ chambers are widely used for investigation of the responses of conduit arteries such as aorta. The rings are mounted horizontally between two stirrups in organ chambers filled with Krebs ringer bicarbonate solution (37°C, pH 7.4) aerated with 95% O$_2$/5% CO$_2$. One stirrup is connected to an anchor, and the other to a force transducer for the recording of isometric tension. Alternatively, the arteriograph system by Halpern has been developed to analyze the reactivity of small resistance arteries with an internal diameter of less than 300 μm under perfused and pressurized conditions (Halpern et al., 1984; Halpern and Kelley, 1991).

Physiology of the Heart

Morphology

As an embryological modification from a blood vessel, the heart has a structural architecture similar to a blood vessel, i.e. the endocardium is equivalent to the endothelium, the myocardium is comparable to the muscular 'media' and the pericardium is comparable to the adventitia (Bloom and Fawcett, 1968).

The circulation of the blood is maintained by the pump function of the heart. It can be divided into four chambers, i.e. left and right atrium and left and right ventricle. Left and right heart are divided by the septum, which participates in the pump function. The right heart represents the low-pressure system, receiving venous blood from peripheral organs, while the left heart is responsible for producing pressure sufficient to ensure organ perfusion. The atria are separated from the ventricles by the mitral valve (left heart) and the tricuspid valve (right heart). In order to achieve optimal flow, the ventricles are separated from the pulmonary artery by the pulmonary valve and from the aorta by the aortic valve. To fulfil its pump function, the muscle portion became predominant during evolution. Cardiac muscle cells can be divided morphologically and functionally into three different cell types: pacemaker cells, cells of the conduction system and the atrial and ventricular myocytes.

Histologically, cardiac muscle cells appear striated. This is due to the longitudinal orientation of the actin–myosin complexes that mediate contraction on the ultrastructural level. Cells of the conduction system are less striated and have indistinct boundaries (Bloom and Fawcett, 1968).

Table 17.1 Normal cardiovascular values

Parameter	Value
Heart weight (g/300 g rat)	0.95–1.19
Heart volume (mL/300 g rat)	1.2
Heart rate (beat/min)	296–388
Systolic blood pressure (mmHg)	116–145
Diastolic blood pressure (mmHg)	76–97
Pulse pressure	16–22

Adapted from Moreau et al. (1998) and Sharp and La Regina (1998). Values are from 10 rats.

can be divided into diastole and systole (Frank, 1959). In diastole, blood flows into the heart. Atrial contraction contributes to ventricular filling in addition to the passive filling. During diastole the pressure inside the ventricle remains low. After closure of the atrioventricular valves the ventricular muscle begins to contract isovolumetrically. This does not lead to shortening of the muscle fibres but only to rising intraventricular pressures. Once the ventricular pressure exceeds the aortic pressure the aortic and pulmonary valves open and ventricular ejection begins. According to the ejection of intraventricular volume, ventricular pressures drop rapidly. Closure of the aortic and pulmonary valves indicates the beginning of systole, which is followed by the phase of isovolumetric ventricular relaxation. Once ventricular pressure falls below the atrial pressure the AV valves open, permitting the ventricles to fill (Frank, 1895). The values of cardiovascular functions of normotensive rats are shown in Table 17.1.

Muscle fibre length and tension are connected in a defined relationship, so that increased ventricular volume leads to increased ventricular developed pressure. This relationship is known as the Frank–Starling mechanism (Starling, 1897).

Electrical Characteristics of the Cardiac Cell

The cell membrane is a diffusion barrier for molecules into or out of the cells which is spread differently between the cells and the extracellular matrix.

Cardiac Muscle Mechanism/ Cardiac Cycle

Isolated cardiac muscle cells can perform two different types of contraction called isotonic and isovolumetric contraction (Cooke, 1986). Both types are important for a coordinated cardiac action. The cardiac cycle, i.e. the time between two heart beats,

The extracellular environment is dominated by sodium and chloride ions, whereas intracellular fluid contains high concentrations of potassium anions. Different distribution of the various ions results in the development of a transmembrane potential, which is further enhanced by active transport mechanisms such as the Na/K pump.

The membrane of an excitable cell like a cardiac muscle cell has the ability to undergo a change in permeability according to transmembrane voltage changes. This leads to opening of ion channels in the cell membrane, permitting ions to pass across the membrane according to their concentration gradient. Since ions are charged particles, their transmembrane passage leads to voltage changes across the membrane which themselves regulate activation and inactivation of the different ion channels. The permeability to sodium, which is low at rest, increases rapidly at the beginning of the action potential and then goes down to a lower level. In contrast, potassium permeability decreases during the action potential. A short increase in permeability for chloride during the early phase of the action potential is accompanied by an increase in permeability for calcium ions which, however, remains elevated for most of the action potential. An increase in permeability for potassium finally causes repolarization (Fozzard and Gibbons, 1973).

Different cardiac cell types show different velocities of spontaneous depolarization. This is the basis for the hierarchy among the different cardiac cells which is essential for a coordinated contraction.

The connection between action potential and contraction is essentially mediated by the interaction of protein filaments that are oriented longitudinally inside the cell (Hibberd and Trentham, 1986). Thick filaments consist of myosin, thin filaments contain actin, tropomyosin and troponin. An increase in intracellular calcium during the action potential leads to increased binding of calcium to troponin C. Thus, the interaction between tropomyosin and actin is modulated, allowing myosin to bind to actin in order to induce contraction. Hydrolysis of myosin-bound ATP mediates the 'power stroke' of muscular contraction by a change in the conformation of myosin, causing thick and thin filament to slide along each other (Cooke, 1986; Thomas, 1987).

Electrocardiography

The electrocardiogram draws upon electrical variations that result from excitation expansion and not from myocardial cell contractions themselves. It provides information on heart rate, heart position, excitation formation as well as localization of heart infarcts (Pocchiari et al., 1993). The use of **telemetry** for the electrocardiogram permits evaluation of the conscious animal over a given interval (Kuwahara et al., 1994; Kramer et al., 1995; Ichimaru and Kuwaki, 1998).

Cardiac Function

The heart is an endocrine tissue and is able to produce atrial natriuretic peptides (ANPS), angiotensin II and endothelin. Normally, the major site of production, storage and release of ANP is the atrial myocytes of the heart (de Bold et al., 1981). In response to stretch of the atrial myocyte, which is the result of increased central venous pressure, ANP is released into the circulation. However, ANP is also expressed in several noncardiac tissues (i.e. vasculature and adrenal glomerulosa) (Dagnino et al., 1991). ANP is a potent vasorelaxant peptide with natriuretic and aldosterone-inhibitory properties and thus plays an important role in the regulation of blood pressure and body salt and fluid balance via autocrine or paracrine functions. In experimental models of cardiac overload ANP is expressed in overloaded ventricles (Drexler et al., 1989; Mercadier et al., 1989).

In addition to blood vessels, angiotensin-converting enzyme is present in the myocardium, especially in the microvasculature and the endocardium (Yamada et al., 1991). However, this enzyme is less active under normal conditions. The binding of angiotensin II to atrial myocyte receptors results in increased contraction. These effects are amplified by angiotensin's ability to stimulate norepinephrine release by sympathetic nerve endings, leading to positive ionotropic effects (Xiang et al., 1984).

Pathophysiology in Hypertension

Under normal physiological conditions, the **baroreceptor** reflex regulates blood pressure and heart activity. Chronic hypertension results in a resetting of the baroreceptors so that they exert less inhibition of the vasomotor centers (Gonzalez et al.,

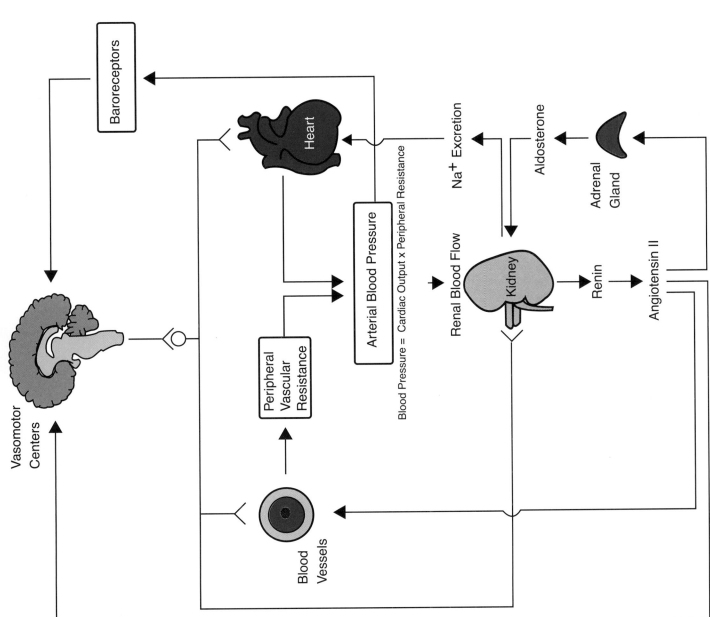

Figure 17.2 Flowchart showing the regulation of arterial blood pressure. The sympathetic nervous system plays an important role in the maintenance of cardiac output in response to increasing demand of organism both by increasing heart rate and contractility. Angiotensin II also plays an important role in cardiovascular homeostasis. Activation of the circulating renin-angiotensin system and aldosterone production is a major peripheral factor of adaptation to hemodynamic changes in cardiovascular disease and contributes to keeping arterial blood pressure normal by increasing the peripheral vascular resistance and plasma volume.

1983). As a consequence, the sympathetic activity is less inhibited, leading (1) to an increased peripheral vascular resistance needed to maintain perfusion and provide the organs with oxygen and/or (2) to an activation of the renin-angiotensin system (Figure 17.2).

In addition, these increases are considered to be related to an increase in vascular tone, via an enhanced release of endothelium-derived contract-ing factors and/or a decreased release of endo-thelium-derived relaxing factors, as well as to changes in the vascular structure of resistance ar-teries (Shepherd, 1990). To study mechanisms of blood pressure control and the pathogenesis of hypertension and to test antihypertensive drugs, different animal models of hypertension are used.

Genetic Models of Hypertension

Spontaneously hypertensive rats

Spontaneously hypertensive rats are the most widely used model for studying cardiovascular complica-tions of hypertension. They were developed by se-lective breeding from a colony of Wistar rats in which individual animals were observed to have elevated blood pressures (Okamoto and Aoki, 1963; Adams et al., 1989). Differences between spon-taneously hypertensive rats and Wistar Kyoto rats can be demonstrated in the first day postnatally, and by 3 weeks the increase in systolic blood pressure is associated with an increased wall to lumen ratio of blood vessels (Gray, 1984; Morton et al., 1990). With age, the rats develop spontaneous and long-lasting hypertension, defined as systolic blood pressure over 150 mmHg, and it becomes more severe in male than female animals. In addition, cardiac output returns to normal levels and blood vessels become hypertroph-ic (Smith and Hutchins, 1979). Thus, this genetic model of hypertension is characterized by an elevat-ed total peripheral resistance in the presence of normal cardiac output.

In spontaneously hypertensive rats less than 16 weeks old, increased baroreceptor stimulation inhi-bits sympathetic nerve activity with the same sensi-tivity as found in WKY rats. However, older spontaneously hypertensive rats appear to lose their ability to completely inhibit sympathetic nerve activity during hypertension (Judy et al., 1976; Campbell et al., 1995) (Table 17.2). The nor-mal lifespan of spontaneously hypertensive and WKY rats are 1–2 years and 2.5–3 years, respectively (Folkow and Svanborg, 1993).

Stroke-prone spontaneously hypertensive rats

Stroke-prone spontaneously hypertensive rats (SHR-SP) were derived from spontaneously hypertensive rats and have higher incidence of cerebrovascular disease. The systolic blood pressure increases up to 250 mmHg and strongly correlates with cerebral lesions (Okamoto et al., 1974). During central ische-mia, used to induce a maximal sympathetic response, the increased sympathetic nerve activity was, how-ever, significantly less than in the spontaneously hypertensive rat (Mueller and Black, 1985; Kim et al., 1992) (Table 17.2). The normal lifespan of the SHR-SP rat is 1 year and is dramatically reduced to 14 weeks of age when fed with 1% salt (Stier et al., 1989).

Dahl salt-sensitive rats

Excessive salt intake has been suggested as one of the contributing factors for the pathogenesis of Dahl salt-sensitive hypertension, in particular if associated with renal insufficiency (Dahl et al., 1962). Indeed, cross-transplantation of kidney and renal artery from a Dahl salt-sensitive into a salt-resistant rat induces hypertension in the re-cipient animal (Morgan et al., 1990). This suggests that the kidney as well as the renal artery and genetic factors contribute to the development of salt-sensitive hypertension. Supplements of 4–8% salt to the chow induces high blood pressure only in Dahl salt-sensitive rats (Table 17.2). In addition, Dahl salt-sensitive rats exposed to high salt diet suffer from glomerular sclerosis and necrosis (Jaffe et al., 1970) and a suppressed circulating renin-angiotensin system (Rapp et al., 1980).

Experimental Models of Hypertension

Deoxycorticosterone acetate salt hypertension

High blood pressure following administration of deoxycorticosterone acetate salt is a model of renin-suppressed, volume-expanded hypertension (Takeda and Bunag, 1980). Subcutaneous application of this salt occurs via either silicone rubber or os-motic minipumps (Ormsbee et al., 1973). In this rat model, blood vessels are more sensitive to norepine-phrine, vasopressin, angiotensin II and endothelin 1 (Schlegel et al., 1985; Larivière et al., 1993).

Renovascular hypertension

Renovascular hypertension (Goldblatt hyperten-sion) develops when the blood flow to the kidneys is restricted by clipping one of the renal arteries and

Table 17.2 Overview of some rat models of hypertension

Model of hypertension	Systolic blood pressure (tail-cuff (mmHg) method)	Sympathetic nerve activity	Activation of renin-angiotensin system	Vascular structure of small arteries	Vascular function	Survival
Spontaneous hypertensive rat	< 200	↑↑	⇌/↓	Hypertrophic remodeling	Impaired endothelium-dependent relaxation	12–24 months
Stroke-prone spontaneous hypertensive rat	≤ 250	⇌/↑	↑	Hypertrophic remodeling	Impaired endothelium-dependent relaxation	12 months; < 4 months after salt loading
Dahl salt-sensitive rat fed with NaCl 4%	200	↑	↓	Hypertrophic and eutrophic remodeling	Impaired endothelium-dependent relaxation	< 2–3 months after salt loading
Deoxycorticosterone acetate-salt	≤ 200	↑	↓	Hypertrophic remodeling	Impaired endothelium-dependent relaxation	
1K1C			↓	Hypertrophic remodeling		
2K1C	200–250	⇌	↑	Hypertrophic remodeling	Impaired endothelium-dependent relaxation	
NO synthase inhibition	180–230	↑	↑	Eutrophic remodeling	Impaired endothelium-dependent relaxation	

by extirpation of the other, unclipped kidney, so-called 'one-kidney, one clip' (1K1C) model (Goldblatt et al., 1934) and is associated with the inhibition of the renin-angiotensin system (Brunner et al., 1971). Peripheral vascular resistance is therefore enhanced with a small increase in cardiac output. On the other hand, the 'two-kidney, one clip' (2K1C) procedure where the unclipped kidney is left untouched, represents a pressure-overloaded, high renin model of hypertension that has been widely used in experimental studies (Okamura et al., 1986). The decrease in renal blood flow causes enhanced release of renin and thus an exaggerated activation of the renin-angiotensin-aldosterone system (Figure 17.2; Table 17.2). The result is an enhanced peripheral vascular resistance that is associated with a reduction of cardiac output (Russell et al., 1983). Interestingly, the sympathetic nervous activity seems unchanged in 2K1C hypertension (Walker et al., 1986).

Nitric oxide synthase inhibition

Because of the biological properties of endothelium-derived NO, chronic inhibition of NO synthase provides a new mechanism for the development of hypertension. Addition of N^ω-nitro-L-arginine methylester (L-NAME) to the drinking water caused marked and persistent systemic arterial hypertension in rats (over 180 mmHg) (Gardiner et al., 1992). Furthermore, high L-NAME intake results in (1) glomerular sclerosis (Baylis et al., 1992), (2) stroke (Moreau et al., 1995), (3) vascular complications (Arnal et al., 1992; Küng et al., 1995) and (4) activation of the sympathetic nervous system (Zanchi et al., 1995) and renin-angiotensin system (Takemoto et al., 1997) (Table 17.2).

Endothelium and Hypertension

Alteration of endothelial function in hypertension affecting the resistance arteries often results in increased peripheral vascular resistance. Moreover, vascular complications of the disease also occur in large and medium-sized conduit arteries. In most experimental models of hypertension, high blood pressure is associated with impaired endothelium-dependent relaxations and appears to occur as blood pressure rises and hence is a consequence rather than a cause of hypertension (Lüscher and Vanhoutte, 1990).

Nitric oxide

The mechanism of endothelial dysfunction differs in different models of hypertension. In the spontaneously hypertensive rat, the activity of constitutive NO synthase is markedly increased (Nava et al., 1995; Hayakawa and Raji, 1997), but it is inefficient probably due to an increased inactivation of NO (Tschudi et al., 1996). One possible explanation is an imbalance between the production of superoxide anions and the activity of superoxide dismutase, a superoxide anion scavenger, in the vessel wall. This effect may contribute to the impaired endothelium-dependent relaxation observed in spontaneously hypertensive rats in spite of an increased activity of the NO pathway (Dohi et al., 1990); it is more severe in male than female spontaneously hypertensive rats (Kauser and Rubanyi, 1995). Furthermore, the production of cyclooxygenase-dependent endothelium-derived contracting factors, such as PGH_2/TXA_2, is increased in the aorta (Lüscher and Vanhoutte, 1986); it offsets the effects of NO in vascular smooth muscle cells and platelets.

In isolated perfused mesenteric arteries of spontaneously, renovascular and L-NAME hypertensive rats, endothelium-dependent relaxations are also reduced (Dohi et al., 1990, 1991; Takase et al., 1996). In salt-sensitive hypertension, impaired endothelial function in isolated conduit and resistance arteries (Lüscher et al., 1987; d'Uscio et al., 1997) and reduced activity of endothelial NO synthase has been demonstrated (Hayakawa and Raji, 1997). Furthermore, endothelium-dependent hyperpolarization is reduced with aging as well as hypertension (Fujii et al., 1993). However, not all hypertensive blood vessels exhibit alterations of the L-arginine/NO pathway. Indeed, in the coronary circulation of spontaneously hypertensive rats, very little of endothelial dysfunction can be observed, with the exception of very old rats (Tschudi et al., 1991). In the WKY rat, endothelium-dependent relaxation is diminished with aging while in SHR the responses remain unchanged (Küng and Lüscher, 1995).

Endothelin

Endothelin 1 plasma levels are normal in most models of hypertension (Lüscher et al., 1992). This may be explained by the **abluminal** release of the peptide by endothelial cells (Wagner et al., 1992) and hence, plasma levels do not necessarily reflect local tissue levels of endothelin 1. In some models of hypertension, such as deoxycorticosterone acetate-salt-, angiotensin II- and salt-sensitive hypertension, tissue endothelin 1 content is increased (Larivière *et al.*, 1993; Moreau *et al.*, 1997; Barton *et al.*, 1998). In contrast, endothelin 1 production is reduced in spontaneously hypertensive rats (Larivière *et al.*, 1993). The vascular responses of the peptide are reduced in different vascular beds of experimental models of hypertension (Lüscher *et al.*, 1992) but not in the renal circulation, which is most important for long-term blood pressure regulation (Seo and Lüscher, 1995).

Vascular Structure and Hypertension

The elevated peripheral vascular resistance observed in hypertension is associated with increases in both the thickness of the media and the ratio of media to lumen diameter in small resistance arteries, but not in arterioles (Mulvany and Aalkjaer, 1990). However, the relationship between the ratio of media to lumen and arterial blood pressure does not imply any causal relationship, suggesting that pressure-independent factors such as genetic (Lee, 1987) or neurohumoral (Mulvany and Aalkjaer, 1990) may also be involved in vascular remodeling. There are two types of vascular remodeling in hypertension (Heagerty *et al.*, 1993). Resistance arteries show a narrowing of their lumen and a thickening of their media without any change in cross-sectional area of the media. Hence, this structural alteration is mainly due to a rearrangement of the same amount of vascular material around a smaller lumen, a process of so-called **inward eutrophic remodeling**. This development probably represents an adaptive mechanism necessary to compensate for the increased wall tension induced by arterial pressure elevation such as in L-NAME-induced hypertension (Moreau *et al.*, 1995). The other, hypertrophic remodeling is due both to the increased ratio of media to lumen as well as to the increased cross-sectional area of the media and can occur in angiotensin II- or DOCA-salt-induced hypertension (Griffin *et al.*, 1991; Larivière *et al.*, 1993). Eutrophic and hypertrophic remodeling can occur simultaneously, as is the case in spontaneously hypertensive rats and several other models of hypertension (Baumbach and Heistad, 1989; Heagerty *et al.*, 1993).

Acknowledgement

Livius V. d'Uscio was a recipient of stipend from the ADUMED Foundation.

References

Aalkjaer, C. (1990) *J Hypertens.* **8**, 197–206.

Adams, M.A., Bobik, A. and Korner, P.I. (1989) *Hypertension* **14**, 191–202.

Alberts, G.F., Peifley, K.A., Johns, A., Kleha, J.F. and Winkles, J.A. (1994) *J. Biol. Chem.* **269**, 10112–10118.

Arai, H., Hori, S., Aramori, I., Ohkubo, H. and Nakanishi, S. (1990) *Nature* **348**, 730–732.

Arnal, J.F., Warin, L. and Michel, J.B. (1992) *J. Clin. Invest.* **90**, 647–652.

Barton, M., d'Uscio, L.V., Shaw, S., Meyer, P., Moreau, P. and Lüscher, T.F. (1998) *Hypertension* **31**, 499–504.

Baumbach, G.L. and Heistad, D.D. (1989) *Hypertension* **13**, 968–972.

Baylis, C., Mitruka, B. and Deng, A. (1992) *J. Clin. Invest.* **90**, 278–281.

Bloom, W. and Fawcett, D.W. (1968) *A Textbook of Histology.* Philadelphia, PA: Saunders.

Boonen, H.C.M. (1992) *Excitation–Contraction Coupling in Small Arteries: Role in Hypertension.* Den Haag: Cip-Gegevens Koninklijke Bibliotheek.

Brunner, H.R., Kirshman, J.O., Sealey, J.E. and Laragh, J.H. (1971) *Science* **174**, 1344–1346.

Busse, R., Lückhoff, A. and Bassenge, E. (1987) *Naunyn Schmiedebergs Arch. Pharmacol.* **336**, 566–562.

Campbell, D.J., Duncan, A.-M., Kladis, A. and Harrap, S.B. (1995) *Hypertension* **25**, 928–934.

Challiss, R.A.J. and Gray, D.W. (1994) In: Swales, J.D. (ed.) *Textbook of Hypertension,* pp. 131–138. London: Blackwell Scientific.

Chida, M. and Voelkel, N.F. (1996) *Am. J. Physiol.* **270**, L872–L878.

Cooke, R. (1986) *Crit. Rev. Biochem.* **21**, 53–118.

d'Uscio, L.V., Barton, M., Shaw, S., Moreau, P. and Lüscher, T.F. (1997) *Hypertension* **30**, 905–911.

Dagnino, L., Drouin, J. and Nemer, M. (1991) *Mol. Endocrinol.* **5**, 1292–1300.

Dahl, L.K., Heine, M. and Tassinair, L. (1962) *J. Exp. Med.* **115**, 1173–1190.

de Bold, A.J., Borenstein, H.B., Veress, A.T. and Sonnenberg, H.A. (1981) *Life Sci.* **28**, 89–94.

de Nucci, G., Thomas, R., D'Orleans-Juste, P. *et al.* (1988) *Proc. Natl Acad. Sci. USA* **85**, 9797–9800.

Dohi, Y., Thiel, M.A., Bühler, F.R. and Lüscher, T.F. (1990) *Hypertension* **16**, 170–179.

Dohi, Y., Criscione, L. and Lüscher, T.F. (1991) *Br. J. Pharmacol.* **104**, 349–354.

Dohi, Y., Hahn, A., Boulanger, C.M., Bühler, F.R. and Lüscher, T.F. (1992) *Hypertension* **19**, 131–137.

Drexler, H., Hanze, J., Finckh, M., Lu, W., Just, H. and Lang, R.E. (1989) *Circulation* **79**, 620–633.

Edwards, G., Dora, K.A., Gardener, M.J., Garland, C.J. and Weston, A.H. (1998) *Nature* **396**, 269–272.

Folkow, B. and Svanborg, A. (1993) *Physiol. Rev.* **73**, 725–758.

Fozzard, H.A. and Gibbons, W.R. (1973) *Am. J. Cardiol.* **31**, 182–192.

Frank, O. (1895) *Z. Biol.* **32**, 370–447.

Frank, O. (1959) *Am. Heart J.* **58**, 282–317.

Freeman, R.H., Davis, J.O. and Villarreal, D. (1984) *Circ. Res.* **54**, 1–9.

Fujii, K., Ohmori, S., Tominaga, M. *et al.* (1993) *Am. J. Physiol.* **265**, H509–H516.

Furchgott, R.F. and Zawadzki, J.V. (1980) *Nature* **288**, 373–376.

Gardiner, S.M., Compton, A.M., Bennett, T., Palmer, R.M.J. and Moncada, S. (1990) *Hypertension* **15**, 486–492.

Gardiner, S.M., Kemp, P.A., Bennett, T., Palmer, R.M.J. and Moncada, S. (1992) *Eur. J. Pharmacol.* **213**, 449–451.

Gaskell, W.H. (1881) *J. Physiol* **III**, 48–75.

Goldblatt, H., Lynch, J., Hanzal, R.F. and Summerville, W.W. (1934) *J. Exp. Med.* **59**, 347–379.

Gonzalez, E.R., Krieger, A.J. and Sapru, H.N. (1983) *Hypertension* **5**, 346–352.

Gray, S.D. (1984) *Biol. Neonate* **45**, 25–32.

Griffin, S.A., Brown, W.C.B., Macpherson, F. *et al.* (1991) *Hypertension* **17**, 626–635.

Hahn, A.W.A., Resink, T.J., Scott-Burden, T., Powell, J., Dohi, Y. and Buhler, F.R. (1990) *Cell Regul.* **1**, 649–659.

Halpern, W. and Kelley, M. (1991) *Blood Vessels* **28**, 245–251.

Halpern, W., Osol, G. and Coy, G.S. (1984) *Ann. Biomed. Eng.* **12**, 463–479.

Hayakawa, H. and Raij, L. (1997) *Hypertension* **29**, 235–241.

Heagerty, A.M., Aalkjaer, C., Bund, S.J., Korsgaard, N. and Mulvany, M.J. (1993) *Hypertension* **21**, 391–397.

Hilberd, M.G. and Trentham, D.R. (1986) *Ann. Rev. Biophys. Chem.* **15**, 119–161.

Hirata, Y., Takagi, Y., Fukuda, Y. and Marumo, F. (1989) *Atherosclerosis* **78**, 225–228.

Hwa, J.J., Ghibaudi, L., Williams, P. and Chatterjee, M. (1994) *Am. J. Physiol.* **266**, H952–H958.

Ichimaru, Y. and Kuwaki, T. (1998) *Psychiatr. Clin. Neurosci.* **52**, 169–172.

Ignarro, L.J., Byrns, R.E., Buga, G.M. and Woods, K.S. (1987) *Circ. Res.* **61**, 866–879.

Ikeda, M., Kohno, M., Horio, T. *et al.* (1995) *Clin. Exp. Pharmacol. Physiol.* **1**, S197–S198.

Imagawa, T., Miyauchi, T. and Satoh, S. (1985) *Renal Physiol.* **8**, 140–149.

Jaffe, D., Sutherland, L.E., Barker, D.M. and Dahl, L.K. (1970) *Arch. Pathol.* **90**, 1–16.

Jia, L., Bonaventura, J. and Stamler, J.S. (1996) *Nature* **380**, 221–226.

Judy, W.V., Watanabe, A., Henry, D., Besch, H., Murphy, W. and Hockel, G. (1976) *Circ. Res.* **38**, I121–II29.

Kauser, K. and Rubanyi, G.M. (1995) *Hypertension* **25**, 517–523.

Kim, S., Tokuyama, M., Hosoi, M. and Yamamoto, K. (1992) *Hypertension* **20**, 280–291.

Kramer, K., Grimbergen, J.A., van der Gracht, L., van Iperen, D.J., Jonker, R.J. and Bast, A. (1995) *Methods Find. Exp. Clin. Pharmacol.* **17**, 107–112.

Kukreja, R.C., Kontos, H.A., Hess, M.L. and Ellis, E.F. (1986) *Circ. Res.* **59**, 612–619.

Küng, C.F. and Lüscher, T.F. (1995) *Hypertension* **25**, 194–200.

Küng, C.F., Moreau, P., Takase, H. and Lüscher, T.F. (1995) *Hypertension* **26**, 744–751.

Kuwahara, M., Yayou, K., Ishii, K., Hashimoto, S., Tsubone, H. and Sugano, S. (1994) *J. Electrocardio.* **27**, 333–337.

Lang, M.G., Noll, G. and Lüscher, T.F. (1995) *Am. J. Physiol.* **269**, H837–H844.

Larivière, R., Thibault, G. and Schiffrin, E.L. (1993) *Hypertension* **21**, 294–300.

Lee, R.M.K.W. (1987) *Can. J. Physiol. Pharmacol.* **65**, 1528–1535.

Lüscher, T.F. and Vanhoutte, P.M. (1986) *Hypertension* **8**, 344–348.

Lüscher, T.F. and Vanhoutte, P.M. (1990) *The Endothelium: Modulator of Cardiovascular Function.* Boca Raton: CRC Press.

Lüscher, T.F., Raij, L. and Vanhoutte, P.M. (1987) *Hypertension* **9**, 157–163.

Lüscher, T.F., Boulanger, C.M., Dohi, Y. and Yang, Z. (1992) *Hypertension* **19**, 117–130.

Mercadier, J.J., Samuel, J.J., Michel, J.B. *et al.* (1989) *Am. J. Physiol.* **257**, H979–H987.

Moncada, S., Gryglewski, R., Bunting, S. and Vane, J.R. (1976) *Nature* **263**, 663–665.

Moncada, S., Herman, A.G., Higgs, E.A. and Vale, C. (1977) *Thromb. Res.* **11**, 323–344.

Moncada, S., Palmer, R.M.J. and Higgs, E.A. (1991) *Pharmacol. Rev.* **43**, 109–142.

Moreau, P., Takase, H., Küng, C.F., van Rooijen, M.M., Schaffner, T. and Lüscher, T.F. (1995) *Stroke* **26**, 1922–1928.

Moreau, P., d'Uscio, L.V., Shaw, S., Takase, H., Barton, M. and Lüscher, T.F. (1997) *Circulation* **96**, 1593–1597.

Moreau, P., d'Uscio, L.V. and Lüscher, T.F. (1998) *Cardiovasc. Res.* **37**, 247–253.

Morgan, D.A., Di Bona, G.F. and Mark, A.L. (1990) *Hypertension* **15**, 436–442.

Mortensen, L.H., Pawloski, C.M., Kanagy, N.L. and Fink, G.D. (1990) *Hypertension* **15**, 729–733.

Morton, J.J., Beattie, E.C., Griffin, S.A., MacPherson, F., Lyall, F. and Russo, D. (1990) *Clin. Sci.* **79**, 523–530.

Mueller, S.M. and Black, W.L., Jr. (1985) *Stroke* **16**, 73–75.

Mulvany, M.J. and Aalkjaer, C. (1990) *Physiol. Rev.* **70**, 921–961.

Murphy, R.A. (1994) In: Swales, J.D. (ed.). *Textbook of Hypertension*, pp. 139–145. London: Blackwell Scientific.

Nadaud, S., Philippe, M., Arnal, J.F., Michel, J.B. and Soubrier, F. (1996) *Circ. Res.* **79**, 857–863.

Nagao, T., Illiano, S. and Vanhoutte, P.M. (1992) *Am. J. Physiol.* **263**, H1090–H1094.

Nava, E., Noll, G. and Lüscher, T.F. (1995) *Circulation* **91**, 2310–2313.

Okamoto, K. and Aoki, K. (1963) *Jpn Circ. J.* **27**, 282–293.

Okamoto, K., Yamori, Y. and Nagaoka, A. (1974) *Circ. Res.* **34–35**, I143–I153.

Okamura, T., Myazcki, M., Inagemi, T. and Toda, N. (1986) *Hypertension* **8**, 560–565.

Ormsbee, H.S. and Ryan, C.F. (1973) Production of hypertension with deoxycorticosterone acetate-impregnated silicone rubber implants. *J. Pharmacol. Sci.*, **62**, 255–257.

Palmer, R.M.J., Ferrige, A.G. and Moncada, S. (1987) *Nature* **327**, 524–526.

Pocchiari, R.J., Hamlin, R.L. and McCune, S.A. (1993) *Am. J. Vet. Res.* **54**, 607–611.

Radomski, M.W., Rees, D.D., Dutra, A. and Moncada, S. (1992) *Br. J. Pharmacol.* **107**, 745–749.

Rapoport, R.M., Draznin, M.B. and Murad, F. (1983) *Nature* **306**, 174–176.

Rapp, J.P., McPartland, R.P. and Sustarsic, D.L. (1980) *Biochem. Genet.* **18**, 1087–1096.

Russell, G.I., Bing, R.F., Swales, J.D. and Thurston, H. (1983) *Am. J. Physiol.* **245**, H734–H740.

Sakurai, T., Yanagisawa, M., Takuwa, Y. *et al.* (1990) *Nature* **348**, 732–735.

Schlegel, P.A., Monney, M. and Brunner, H.R. (1985) *Clin. Exp. Hypertens.* **7**, 1583–1596.

Seo, B. and Lüscher, T.F. (1995) *Hypertension* **25**, 501–506.

Sessa, W.C., Harrison, J.K., Barber, C.M. *et al.* (1992) *J. Biol. Chem.* **267**, 15274–15276.

Sharp, P.E. and La Regina, M.C. (1998) *The Laboratory Rat.* New York: CRC Press.

Shepherd, J.T. (1990) *J. Hypertens.* **8**, S15–S27.

Shimokawa, H., Yasutake, H., Fujii, K. *et al.* (1996) *J. Cardiovasc. Pharmacol.* **28**, 703–711.

Smith, T.L. and Hutchins, P.M. (1979) *Hypertension* **1**, 508–517.

Starling, E.H. (1897) *Lancet* **1**, 569–572.

Stier, C.T., Jr, Benter, I.F., Ahmad, S. *et al.* (1989) *Hypertension* **13**, 115–121.

Takase, H., Moreau, P. and Lüscher, T.F. (1995) *Hypertension* **25**, 739–743.

Takase, H., Moreau, P., Küng, C.F., Nava, E. and Lüscher, T.F. (1996) *Hypertension* **27**, 25–31.

Takeda, K. and Bunag, R.D. (1980) *Hypertension* **2**, 97–101.

Takemoto, M., Egashira, K., Usui, M. *et al.* (1997) *J. Clin. Invest.* **99**, 278–287.

Thomas, D.D. (1987) *Annu. Rev. Physiol.* **49**, 691–709.

Tschudi, M.R., Criscione, L. and Lüscher, T.F. (1991) *J. Hypertens.* **9**, 164–165.

Tschudi, M.R. Mesaros, S., Lüscher, T.F. and Malinski, T. (1996) *Hypertension* **27**, 32–35.

Wagner, O.F., Christ, G., Wojta, J. *et al.* (1992) *J. Biol. Chem.* **267**, 16066–16068.

Walker, S.M., Bing, R.F. and Swales, J.D. (1986) *Clin. Sci.* **71**, 199–204.

Xiang, J., Linz, W., Becker, H. *et al.* (1984) *Eur. J. Pharmacol.* **113**, 215–223.

Yamada, H., Fabris, B., Allen, A.M., Jackson, B., Johnson, C.I. and Mendelsohn, F.A.O. (1991) *Circ. Res.* **68**, 141–149.

Yanagisawa, M., Kurihara, H., Kimura, S. *et al.* (1988) *Nature* **332**, 411–415.

Yang, B.C., Lawson, D.N. and Mehta, J.L. (1992) *Eicosanoids* **5**, 135–139.

Zanchi, A., Schaad, N.C., Osterheld, M.C. *et al.* (1995) *Am. J. Physiol.* **268**, H2267–H2273.

CHAPTER 18

Digestion, Metabolism

Haruki Senoo
Department of Anatomy, Akita University School of Medicine,
Akita, Japan

Digestion

Most foodstuffs are ingested in forms that are unavailable to the organism, since they cannot be absorbed from the digestive tract until they have been broken into smaller molecules. This disintegration of the naturally occurring foodstuffs into assimilable forms constitutes the process of digestion.

The rat is one of the most popular experimental animals for studying the physiology of digestion. It feeds mainly during the night and is also coprophagous, which means that some part of orally administered compounds and their metabolites remaining in the faeces is reingested.

The gastrointestinal tract is the portal through which nutritious substances, vitamins, electrolytes and fluids enter the body. Carbohydrates, proteins and lipids are degraded into absorbable units, mainly in the small intestine.

Digestion of major foodstuffs is an orderly process, involving the action of a large number of digestive enzymes. Enzymes from the salivary glands degrade carbohydrates and lipid; enzymes from the stomach degrade proteins and lipids; and enzymes from the exocrine pancreas degrade carbohydrates, proteins, lipids and nucleic acids such as DNA and RNA.

Other enzymes that complete the digestive process are found in the luminal membranes and the cytoplasm of the cells that line the small intestine. The action of the enzymes is assisted by hydrochloric acid secreted by the stomach and bile secreted by the liver.

Digestion of Carbohydrates

The main dietary carbohydrates are polysaccharides, such as starches (glucose polymers), disaccharides, and monosaccharides. In the oral cavity, starch is degraded by salivary α-amylase. The optimal pH for this enzyme is 6.7, so its action is suppressed by the acidic gastric juice when food enters the stomach. In the small intestine, both the salivary and the pancreatic α-amylases act on the ingested polysaccharides, the end product being oligosaccharides.

Enzymes responsible for further digestion of starch derivatives are located in the outer portion of the brush border, on the membrane of the microvilli of the small intestine. Hexoses and pentoses are rapidly absorbed across the wall of the small intestine. Essentially all of the hexoses are removed before the remains of a meal reach the terminal part of the ileum. The sugar molecules pass from the mucosal cells to the blood in the capillaries draining into the portal vein.

Digestion of Proteins and Nucleic Acids

Protein digestion begins in the stomach, where pepsins cleave some of the peptide linkages. Like many of the other enzymes concerned with protein digestion, pepsins are secreted in the form of inactive precursors and activated in the digestive tract. The pepsin precursors are called pepsinogens and are activated by gastric hydrochloric acid.

Pepsins hydrolyze the bonds between aromatic amino acids and a second amino acid, giving rise to polypeptides of diverse sizes. With a pH optimum of 1.6–3.2, the action of the pepsins is terminated when the gastric contents are mixed with the alkaline pancreatic juices in the duodenum and jejunum.

In the small intestine, the polypeptides are further digested by the powerful proteolytic enzymes of the pancreas and intestinal mucosa. Trypsin, chymotrypsin and elastase, which act on the interior peptide bonds in the peptide molecules, are called endopeptidases. The carboxypeptidases of the pancreas, the exopeptidases, hydrolyze the amino acids at the carboxy- and amino-terminals of the polypeptides. Some free amino acids are released into the intestinal lumen, but others are liberated at the cell surface by the enzymes in the brush border of the mucosal cells. Some di- and tripeptides are actively transported into the intestinal cells, hydrolyzed by intracellular peptidases, and the amino acids so produced then enter the bloodstream. Thus, the final stage of digestion of proteins to give amino acids occurs in the intestinal lumen, the brush border and the cytoplasm of the mucosal cells.

Digestion of Fat

Most lipid digestion begins in the duodenum, pancreatic lipase being one of the most important enzymes involved. This enzyme hydrolyzes the 1- and 3-bonds of triacylglycerol, and the main products of its action are free fatty acids and 2-monoacylglycerol. It acts on lipids that have been previously emulsified (see below).

The assimilation of dietary fats into the body requires predigestion by lipase. One lipase, pancreatic triacylglycerol lipase, is essential for the efficient digestion of dietary fats (Lowe, 1997). Most of the dietary cholesterol is in the form of cholesteryl esters, and these esters are also hydrolyzed by cholesteryl ester hydrolase in the intestinal lumen.

Lipids are finally emulsified in the small intestine by the detergent action of the bile salts, lecithin and monoacylglycerol. Lipids and bile salts interact spontaneously to form **micelles**. They contain fatty acids, monoacylglycerols and cholesterol in their hydrophobic centers. The lipids diffuse out of the micelles, and a saturated aqueous solution of the lipids is then maintained in contact with the brush border of the mucosal cells.

Lipids were thought to enter into the **enterocytes** by passive diffusion (Cardell et al., 1967). Fat is absorbed and transported through the epithelium very rapidly (Jersild, 1966). Within 1 minute, fat droplets can be seen in the endoplasmic reticulum and the Golgi apparatus. However, there is more recent evidence that carriers, such as fatty acid-binding protein (Ockner and Manning, 1974), are involved. The intestinal fatty acid-binding protein concentration is significantly greater in animals kept on a high fat rather than a low fat diet; saturated and unsaturated fat diets do not differ greatly in this respect. The preponderance of intestinal fatty acid-binding protein is in the villi from the proximal and middle intestine. Its ability to bind fatty acids *in vivo* as well as *in vitro*, and its response to changes in dietary fat intake support the concept that this protein participates in cellular fatty acid transport during fat absorption. The fate of the fatty acids in the enterocytes depends on their size. Fatty acids containing less than 10–12 carbon atoms pass from the mucosal cells directly into the portal blood, where they are transported as free fatty acids. The fatty acids containing more than 10–12 carbon atoms are reesterified to triacylglycerols in the mucosal cells. The triacylglycerols are then converted to **chylomicrons** and released by exocytosis. From the extracellular space, they enter the lymph (Leak and Burke, 1966). Cholesterol is readily absorbed from the small intestine if bile, fatty acids and pancreatic juice are present.

Absorption of Vitamins and Electrolytes

Absorption of water-soluble vitamins is rapid, but absorption of the fat-soluble vitamins A (Goodman et al., 1965), D, E and K is deficient if lipid absorption is depressed because of lack of pancreatic enzymes or if excluded from the intestine by obstruction of the bile duct. Most vitamins are absorbed in the upper small intestine.

Vitamin A is known to regulate diverse cellular activities such as cell proliferation, differentiation, morphogenesis and tumorigenesis (Blomhoff et al., 1990). The mechanism of action of vitamin A in these processes involves nuclear receptors that are specific for vitamin A metabolites.

The main dietary sources of vitamin A are retinyl esters from animal tissues and carotenoids from vegetables (Blomhoff et al., 1992a,b). All of the retinyl esters are enzymatically changed to retinol in the intestinal lymph and then pass into the general circulation, where several processes such as triacylglycerol hydrolysis and apolipoprotein exchange result in the formation of chylomicron remnants. Almost all retinyl esters present in the chylomicron remain within the particle during conversion to chylomicron remnants (Blomhoff, 1994).

The liver consists of parenchymal cells and nonparenchymal cells (endothelial cells, Kupffer cells and stellate cells) (Figure 18.2) of which two (parenchymal and stellate cells) are particularly important for the handling of vitamin A (Senoo et al.,

1997). Most of the absorbed dietary vitamin A is delivered to hepatic parenchymal cells when chylomicron remnants are metabolized by the liver. Constituents of chylomicron remnants, including retinyl esters, are taken up by the hepatic parenchymal cells, and hydrolyzed to retinol. Retinol is transported from parenchymal cells to stellate cells by a paracrine pathway (Blomhoff et al., 1992c).

By receptor-mediated endocytosis, the stellate cells also take up retinol from the blood, where it circulates as a complex of retinol and a specific binding protein, retinol-binding protein (RBP) (Senoo et al., 1993). The in vivo uptake of RBP in rat liver cells was demonstrated by biochemistry (Gyoen et al., 1987) and immunocytochemistry at the electron microscopic level using ultrathin cryosections (Senoo et al., 1990).

Once inside the cell, free retinol has several fates, one of which is the reformation of the complex with RBP and its return to the bloodstream (Figure 18.3). Thus, the stellate cells are important for the regulation of homeostasis of vitamin A.

Under physiological conditions, stellate cells store 80–90% of the total vitamin A in the whole body as retinyl palmitate in lipid droplets in the cytoplasm. When [^{3}H] retinol was injected via the portal vein, most of the labeled retinol was taken up by the liver within 90 minutes after injection, although labeled material was detected in all organs examined (Senoo et al., 1984). The radioactivity of the retinol in the liver did not change until 6 days after the injection. These results are consistent with the reports that the main storage site of vitamin A in mammals is the liver (Wake, 1971, 1980).

The intestines are faced each day with ingested fluid and secretions from the mucosa of the gastrointestinal tract and associated glands. More than 90% of this fluid is reabsorbed and fluid loss in the stool is scanty. Some Na^+ diffuses into or out of the small intestine depending on the concentration gradient. Na^+ is also actively absorbed throughout the small and large intestines, because the luminal membranes of all enterocytes in the small intestine and colon are permeable to Na^+ and their basolateral membranes contain Na^+,K^+-ATPase (Agnusdei and Civitelli, 1996; Turvill and Farthing, 1996, 1997; Licato and Brenner, 1997).

Cl^- normally enters enterocytes from the intestinal fluid via Na^+, K^+-$2Cl^-$ cotransporters in their basolateral membranes, and is then secreted into the intestinal membrane via channels that are regulated by various protein kinases. The movement of K^+

Chylomicrons incorporate carotenoids, retinyl esters and other fat-soluble vitamins (Figure 18.1). These huge lipoproteins (100–2000 nm in diameter) are **exocytosed** into the intestinal lymph and then pass into the general circulation, where several processes such as triacylglycerol hydrolysis and apolipoprotein exchange result in the formation of chylomicron remnants. Almost all retinyl esters present in the chylomicron remain within the particle during conversion to chylomicron remnants (Blomhoff, 1994).

Carotenoids, on the other hand, are internalized unchanged by the absorptive cells, where they are partially converted to retinol. In the absorptive cells, retinol complexed to a specific cellular retinol-binding protein, type 2 (CRBP II) is esterified by an enzyme called lecithin:retinol acyltransferase (LRAT) (Ong, 1994). The resulting retinyl esters are incorporated into chylomicrons in the absorptive cells.

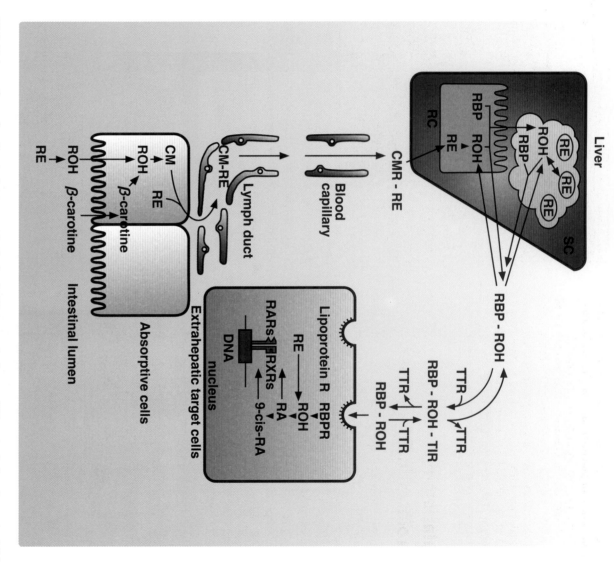

Figure 18.1 Major pathway for vitamin A transport in the body. Dietary retinyl esters (RE) are hydrolyzed to retinol (ROH) in the intestinal lumen before absorption by absorptive cells, and carotenoids are absorbed and then partially converted to retinol in the cells. In the absorptive cells, retinol reacts with fatty acid to form esters before incorporation into chylomicrons (CM). Chylomicrons reach the general circulation by way of the intestinal lymph, and chylomicron remnants (CMR) are formed in blood capillaries. Chylomicron remnants that contain almost all the absorbed retinol are mainly cleared by the hepatic parenchymal cells (PC) and to some extent also by cells in other organs (extrahepatic target cells). In hepatic parenchymal cells, retinyl esters are rapidly hydrolyzed to retinol, which then binds to retinol-binding protein (RBP). A complex of retinol-RBP (RBP-ROH) is secreted and transported to hepatic stellate cells (SC). Stellate cells store vitamin A mainly as retinyl ester. Most retinol-RBP in the bloodstream is reversibly complexed with transthyretin (TTR). The uncomplexed retinol-RBP is presumably taken up in a variety of cells by cell surface receptors specific for RBP (RBPR). Lipoprotein R, lipoprotein receptor; RA, retinoic acid; RARs, nuclear retinoic acid receptors; RXRs, nuclear retinoid X receptors.

across the gastrointestinal mucosa is due to diffusion. On the other hand, there are K⁺ channels in the luminal membrane of the enterocytes of the colon, so K⁺ also is secreted into the colon. From 30% to 80% of ingested calcium is absorbed. Active transport of Ca²⁺ out of the intestinal lumen occurs

mainly in the upper small intestine, and there is also some absorption by passive diffusion.

Most of the iron is absorbed in the upper part of the small intestine. Other mucosal cells can transport iron, but the duodenum and adjacent jejunum contain most of the iron suitable for absorption.

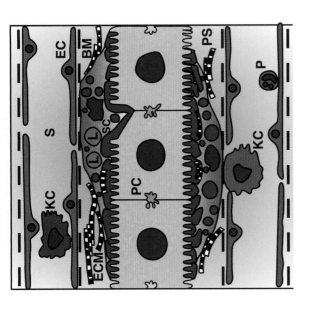

Figure 18.2 Structure of hepatic lobule. Hepatic cords of the lobule consist of parenchymal cells (PC). Endothelial cells (EC) form the thin lining of the sinusoids (S). Kupffer cells (KC) are tissue macrophages and belong to the monocyte–macrophage cell lineage. Pit cells (p) have natural killer activity. Stellate cells (SC) lie in the perisinusoidal space (PS) of Disse and store 80–90% of vitamin A of the whole body as retinyl palmitate in the lipid droplets (L) in the cytoplasm. BM, basement membrane components; ECM, extracellular matrix.

Regulation of Gastrointestinal Functions

The digestive and absorptive functions of the gastrointestinal tract (Figure 18.4) depend on a variety of mechanisms that soften the food, propel it through the gastrointestinal tract, and mix it with bile and digestive enzymes secreted by the salivary glands and pancreas. Some of these mechanisms depend on intrinsic properties of the intestinal smooth muscle. Others involve the operation of reflexes involving the neurons intrinsic to the gut, reflexes involving the central nervous system, paracrine effects of chemical messengers, and gastrointestinal hormones.

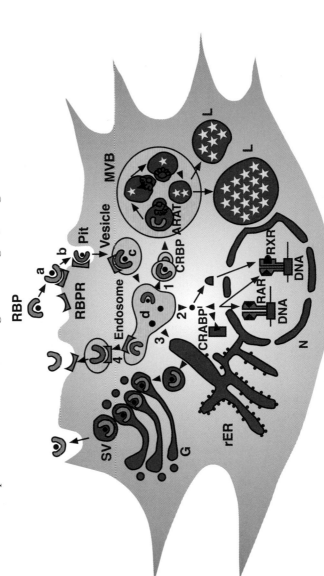

Figure 18.3 Uptake and storage of retinol and retinol-binding protein (RBP) by stellate cells. A complex of retinol and RBP circulates in the blood. The complex binds specifically to the receptor (RBPR) expressed on the cell surface of stellate cells (a), then reaches endosomes (d) through pits (b) and vesicles (c). From the endosomes, retinol can take three pathways: (1) Retinol binds to cellular retinol-binding protein (CRBP, MW 14 000–17 500) and is esterified with palmitic acid in multivesicular bodies (MVB) and stored in lipid droplets (L). (2) Retinol is oxidized to retinoic acid, which binds with cellular retinoic acid-binding protein (CRABP, MW 16 000) or is transported and binds with nuclear retinoic acid receptors (RAR) or retinoid X receptors (RXR). (3) Retinol is transported from endosomes to rough-surfaced endoplasmic reticulum (rER), binds with RBP, and is secreted to the outside of the cell through the Golgi apparatus (G) and secretory vesicles (sv). (4) RBP and its receptor are recycled and reutilized. ●, retinol; ★, retinyl palmitate; ▲, all-*trans*-retinoic acid; ●, 9-*cis*-retinoic acid; ◡, retinol-binding protein; ◠, specific receptor for RBP (RBPR); ◡, cellular retinol-binding protein; ⊡, cellular retinoic acid-binding protein; ∿, acyl CoA: retinol acyltransferase (ARAT); ◠, nuclear retinoic acid receptor (RAR) which binds all-*trans*-retinoic acid; ◡, nuclear retinoid X receptor (RXR) which binds 9-*cis*-retinoic acid; □, retinoic acid responsive element.

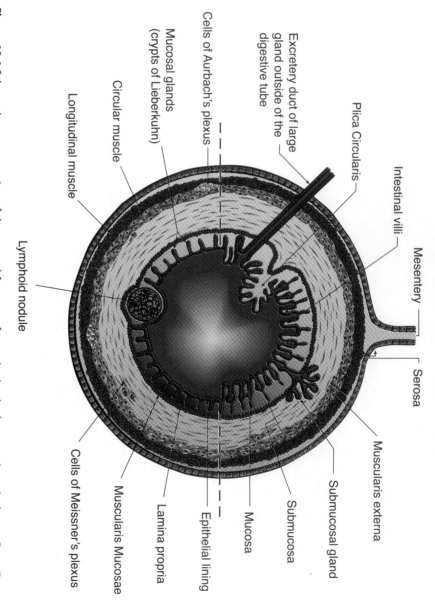

Figure 18.4 Schematic representation of the general features of organization in the gastrointestinal tract. From Fawcett (1994).

Labels on figure: Excretery duct of large gland outside of the digestive tube; Cells of Aurbach's plexus; Mucosal glands (crypts of Lieberkuhn); Circular muscle; Longitudinal muscle; Lymphoid nodule; Plica Circularis; Intestinal villi; Mesentery; Serosa; Muscularis externa; Submucosal gland; Submucosa; Mucosa; Epithelial lining; Lamina propria; Muscularis Mucosae; Cells of Meissner's plexus

Networks of **interstitial cells of Cajal** embedded in the musculature of the gastrointestinal tract are involved in the generation of electrical pacemaker activity for gastrointestinal motility (Faussone-Pellegrini *et al.*, 1977; Thuneberg, 1982; Thomsen *et al.*, 1998). This pacemaker activity manifests itself as rhythmic slow waves in membrane potential, and controls the frequency and propagation characteristics of gut contractile activity.

The hormones are humoral agents secreted by cells in the mucosa and transported in the circulation to influence the functions of the stomach, the intestine and the pancreas.

Oral cavity and esophagus

In the mouth, food is mixed with saliva and propelled into the esophagus (Brown and Hardisty, 1990). Peristaltic waves in the esophagus move the food into the stomach. Chewing (mastication) breaks up food particles and mixes the food with the secretions of the salivary glands. In the salivary glands, the secretory zymogen granules containing enzymes are discharged from the acinar cells into the ducts.

The decreased mastication effort required with a finely powdered or liquid diet has been associated with a marked reduction in mitotic rates in the oral epithelium and decreased saliva secretion with atrophy of the parotid gland. Proliferating cells in the oral mucosa originate from the stratum germinativum and cell turnover ranges from 3.2 to 5.8 days, being faster over the dorsal surface of the tongue.

The function of the salivary glands is to moisten food so as to begin the process of digestion (Neuenschwander and Elwell, 1990). Salivation is a complex function regulated by the autonomic nervous system, the salivatory nuclei, the appetite area within the hypothalamus, and reflexes within the stomach and upper intestine initiated by nausea or ingested irritants. Saliva is a mixture of amylase, mucin, electrolytes, immunoglobulin, water, and other components. The saliva produced by the rat parotid gland is unique in that it has a protein concentration of about 2%.

Salivary gland extirpation or ductal ligation shows that these glands have broader influences on a wide range of endocrine and exocrine functions than was previously recognized. The parotid gland produces a

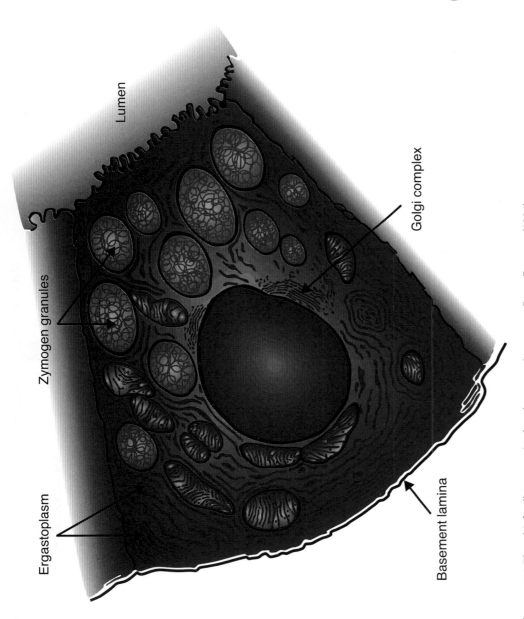

Figure 18.5 The chief cell as seen in the electron microscope. From Fawcett (1994).

Lumen

Golgi complex

Zymogen granules

Ergastoplasm

Basement lamina

hormone (parotid hormone) which stimulates dental fluid transport within the rat tooth and may prevent tooth decay.

The acini and ductular epithelium have the capacity to regenerate. The regenerative acinar and striated duct epithelium of the parotid gland arises from the intercalated duct cells. Swallowing is initiated by the voluntary action of collecting the oral contents on the tongue and propelling them backward into the pharynx. This starts a wave of involuntary contraction in the pharyngeal muscles that pushes the material into the esophagus.

Stomach

Food is stored in the stomach, mixed with acid, mucus and pepsin, and released at a regulated, steady rate into the duodenum. Storage of ingesta in the forestomach (which has a high pH and increased amylase activity) can result in a prolonged postprandial

hyperglycemia lasting 12–16 hours (Brown and Hardisty, 1990). Stress, alkaline materials, hyperosmolar solutions and prostaglandin E_2 increase gastric emptying time.

The hydrochloric acid secreted by the parietal cells kills many ingested bacteria, assists protein degradation, provides the necessary pH for pepsin to start protein digestion, and stimulates the flow of bile and pancreatic juice. It is concentrated enough to cause tissue damage, but in the normal rat the gastric mucosa does not become digested, in part because the gastric juice also contains mucus. The surface membranes of the mucosal cells and the tight junctions between the cells are also part of the mucosal barrier that protects the gastric epithelium from damage.

The **chief cells** (Figure 18.5) that secrete pepsinogens, the inactive precursors of the pepsins in gastric juice, contain zymogen granules. The secretory process is similar to that involved in the secretion of

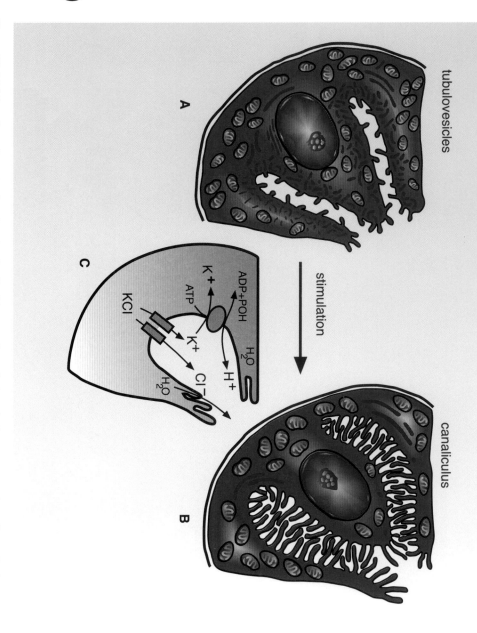

Figure 18.6 (a) Drawing of unstimulated parietal cell with extensive tubulovesicular system and small canaliculus. (b) Stimulated cell with long canaliculus, many microvilli and a depleted tubulovesicular system. (c) Fusion of tubulovesicles transfers H⁺, K⁺-ATPase to surface and conductive channels for K⁺ and Cl⁻. This permits movement of K⁺ and Cl⁻ into the canaliculus and the H⁺/K⁺ pump recycles K⁺ back into the cytoplasm, with the net effect of HCl secretion and ATP turnover. Flux of water into the canaliculus is driven osmotically by net solute flux. From Fawcett (1994).

trypsinogen and other pancreatic enzymes by the pancreas.

Four immunochemically distinguishable aspartic proteases, pepsinogen I (A), pepsinogen II (C), cathepsin D and cathepsin E, have been found in the mammalian gastric mucosa (Samloff *et al.*, 1987). The gastric mucosa of the rat, however, contains only three of the four enzymes (pepsinogen C and cathepsins D and E). Their specific endogenous inhibitors may play a role in gastric mucosal injury and protection (Nagy *et al.*, 1997).

The **parietal cells** (Figure 18.6) are polarized, with an apical membrane facing the lumen of the gastric glands and basolateral membrane in contact with the interstitial fluid. Canaliculi extend from the apical surface into the cell. H⁺,K⁺-ATPase in the apical

membrane of the parietal cells is responsible for the transfer of hydrogen ions into the glandular lumen. ATPase activity is controlled by the cytoplasmic levels of cyclic ATP and Ca²⁺, which act as intracellular messengers for a variety of receptors on the cell surface. The receptors form three physiological levels of control over acid secretion. The gastrin receptor is hormonally regulated by the gastric cells (G cells) (Figure 18.7) in the gastric antrum that respond to gastric digestion or the amino acid content.

Gastrin levels rise with food intake and fall with decreased pH, which then stimulates the D cells and induces somatostatin secretion, a negative feedback to gastrin secretion. Acid secretion is also modulated through the H₂ (histamine) receptor on parietal cells; blocking the H₂ receptor lowers acid secretion.

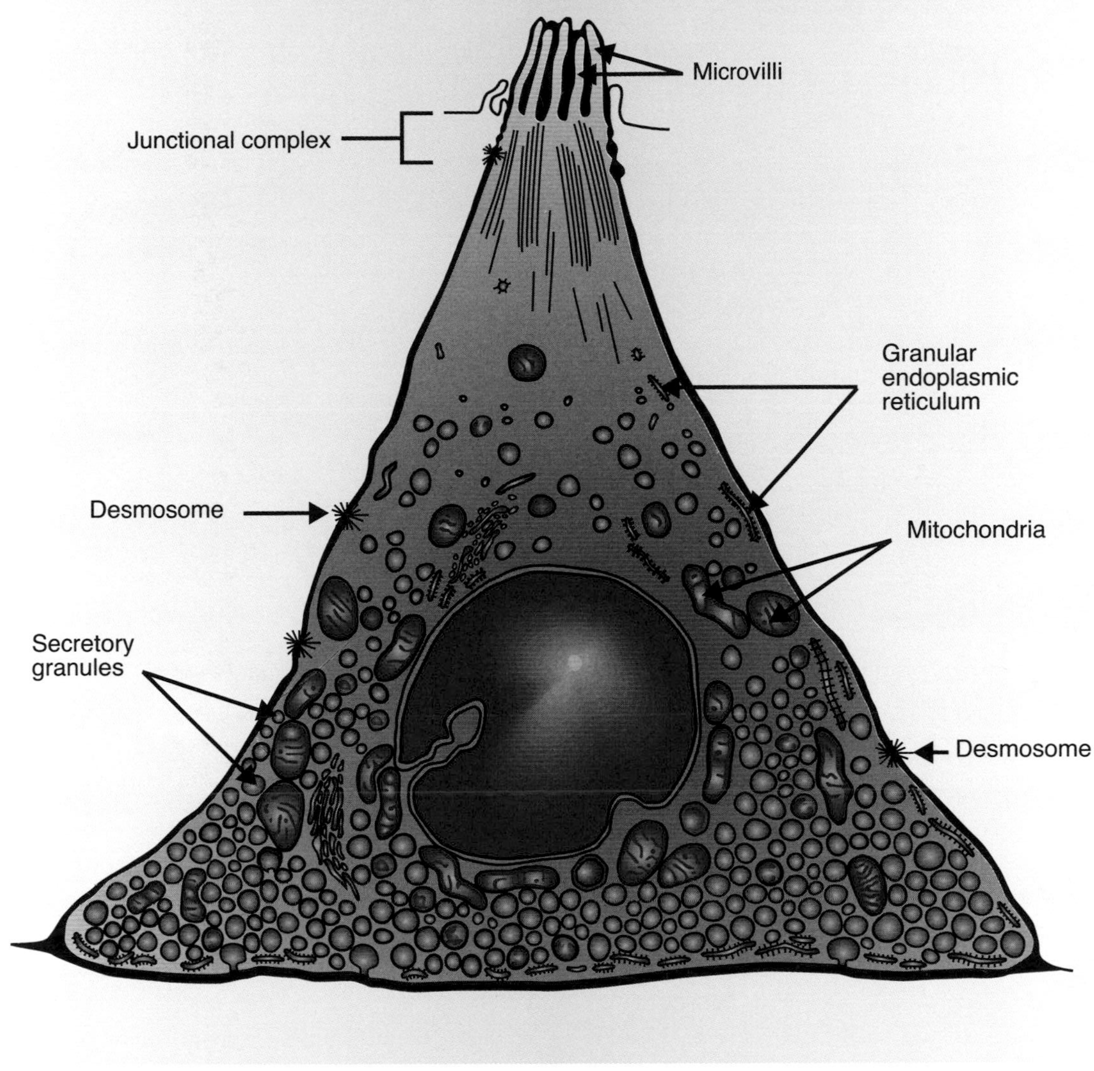

Figure 18.7 Schematic representation of the ultrastructure of the gastric cell (G cell). From Fawcett (1994).

A third parietal cell receptor, for muscarinic acid, responds to vagal stimulation, increasing acid secretion secondary to central nervous system influences. This type of acid secretion may be important; for example, the parietal cell mass increases in actively lactating rats secondary to elevated prolactin levels, and epinephrine potentiates histamine-stimulated acid production.

The parietal cell in most mammalian species is the source of **intrinsic factor**, a 49-Da glycoprotein necessary for the absorption of cyanocobalamin (vitamin B_{12}) from the small intestine. A deficiency of this vitamin is difficult to produce in the rat but may result in pernicious anemia. The chief cell is the source of pepsinogen for protein hydrolysis. Cell kinetics of the glandular stomach are altered by

gastrin levels, thyroxine, growth hormone, somatostatin and epidermal growth factor (EGF) as well as E_2 prostaglandins. Gastrin stimulates proliferation and cytoplasmic granulation of enterochromaffin-like cells (after prolonged elevation of basal gastrin levels) and release of somatostatin by the D cells. Type E prostaglandins increase mucous cells and foveolar epithelium and decrease chief and endocrine cells. EGF activates mucosal ornithine decarboxylase activity, leading to restitution of the mucosa after certain types of injury. This restitution does not involve the normal regeneration zone of the isthmus but takes place by direct migration of mucosal cells at the edges of the lesion. The time required to replace the surface epithelium is about 3 days.

When food enters the stomach, peristalsis begins,

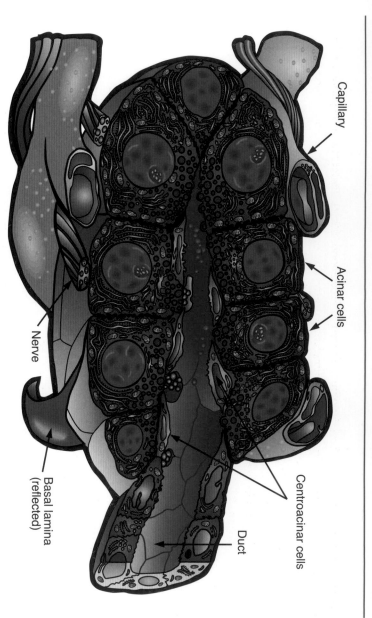

Figure 18.8 Drawing of a pancreatic acinus and its associated capillaries and nerve. From Fawcett (1994).

Capillary

Acinar cells

Nerve

Centroacinar cells

Basal lamina (reflected)

Duct

leading to mixing and grinding of the food and small, semiliquid portions of this then being permitted to pass through the pylorus and enter the duodenum. Gastric motility and secretion are regulated by neural and humoral mechanisms. The neural components are local autonomic reflexes, involving cholinergic neurons, and impulses from the central nervous system by way of the vagus nerves.

Exocrine portion of the pancreas

The pancreatic juice contains enzymes that are of major importance in digestion. Its secretion is regulated in part by a reflex mechanism and in part by the gastrointestinal hormones, secretin and cholecystokinin (CCK). The part of the pancreas that secretes pancreatic juice is a compound alveolar gland (Figure 18.8) resembling the salivary glands. Granules containing the digestive enzymes (zymogen granules) are formed in the cell and discharged by exocytosis from the apices of the cells into the lumina of the pancreatic ducts. The number of pancreatic ducts differs among individual rats. Fifteen to 40 excretory ducts join to form at least two and as many as eight main ducts, which open into the common bile duct where it traverses the pancreas and enters the duodenum. Some ducts may enter the duodenum directly.

The primary function of the exocrine pancreas is

synthesis and secretion of the enzymes necessary to digest food. The digestive enzymes are synthesized in acinar cells and stored as proenzymes within the zymogen granules; most of the enzymes (including trypsinogen, chymotrypsinogen and procarboxypeptidase A and B) are secreted as proenzymes which are enzymatically inert. Trypsinogen is converted to trypsin by the intestinal brush border enzyme enterokinase. Trypsin then activates the other inactive proteases.

The functional reserve capacity of the exocrine pancreas is large; as little as 5% of the total exocrine glandular tissue is adequate to maintain nearly normal digestion and absorption of purified diets fed to rats. The pancreas also secretes fluid and bicarbonate which neutralize the acid in the chyle entering the duodenum from the stomach. The epithelial cells of the ducts appear to be the major site of water and bicarbonate secretion.

Secretion of enzymes and bicarbonate-rich fluid by the exocrine pancreas is regulated by interacting neurohormonal and hormonal mechanisms. A basal rate of secretion (e.g. that which occurs in the absence of all intestinal stimulation) seems to be controlled by the release of acetylcholine from extrinsic and intrinsic nerves of the gland.

Following ingestion of food, stimulation of the pancreas begins with visual, olfactory and gustatory stimuli acting on the brain and mediated by efferent fibers in the vagus nerve. Acetylcholine released from vagal postganglionic fibers directly stimulates the pancreatic acinar cells to secrete enzymes. Similar cholinergic impulses from vagal postganglionic fibers in the stomach stimulate acid secretion and the release of gastrin from enterochromaffin cells in the pyloric antrum. Gastrin is a polypeptide similar in structure to CCK that stimulates the secretion of acid from the gastric mucosa and the secretion of enzymes from the pancreas. Distension of the stomach also stimulates the release of gastrin and acid from the gastric mucosa by short and long reflex pathways involving postganglionic fibers, the intramural plexuses and the vagus nerve.

The entry of acid and digestion products (fatty acids, amino acids, peptides) into the duodenum from the stomach provides the major stimulus to pancreatic secretion by causing the release of secretin and CCK from enterochromaffin cells in the intestinal mucosa. Secretin, released mainly in response to acid, stimulates the secretion of water and electrolytes from the pancreatic duct cells while inhibiting gastrin-stimulated acid secretion from the stomach. CCK strongly stimulates the secretion of enzymes from acinar cells and only weakly stimulates the secretion of water and electrolytes from the ducts. Gastropancreatic, enteropancreatic, and vago-vagal cholinergic reflexes interact to amplify and modify the pancreatic response to these hormones.

Varying the carbohydrate, protein or fat content of the diet alters the mixture of digestive enzymes found in the pancreatic secretions. The relative proportion of specific enzymes may be regulated at the level of their synthesis (long-term dietary changes) or selective secretion from the acinar cells (short-term changes from meal to meal). For short-term changes, the substrates and end products of digestion (amino acids, fatty acids, glucose) are believed to modify the enzyme content of the pancreatic secretions by release of hormonal substances (other than CCK or secretin) from the intestinal mucosa and by acting directly at the level of the acinar cell by positive and negative feedback mechanisms. Trypsin and chymotrypsin in the duodenum suppress pancreatic enzyme secretion, apparently by inhibiting the release of CCK from the intestinal mucosa. An intramural cholinergic pathway appears to be involved in the enzyme feedback regulation of CCK release.

Pancreatic polypeptide is a 36 amino acid hormone found in highest concentrations in the islets of Langerhans within the pancreas (Taylor, 1989;

Hazelwood, 1993). Pancreatic polypeptide released into the circulation after a meal through vagal cholinergic-dependent mechanisms specifically and potentially inhibits centrally mediated pancreatic exocrine secretion (Putnam et al., 1989; Okumura et al., 1995). The receptors for pancreatic polypeptide are distributed widely throughout the rat brain (Whitcomb et al., 1997). The distribution of many of these pancreatic polypeptide-binding sites corresponds to brain regions regulating digestion and autonomic function. Based on the pattern of binding in the olfactory and limbic system, the receptors for pancreatic polypeptide might be involved in positive reinforcement of ingestion behavior as well as modulation of gastrointestinal function.

Liver and biliary system

Traditionally, the liver lobule has been described in relation to the central vein. However, Rappaport developed the concept of a liver lobule having the portal triad as its center (Rappaport et al., 1954; Rappaport, 1957) (Figure 18.9). Many of the pathological processes in the liver are consistent with the concept developed by Rappaport. Different organizational units within the liver such as the classical lobule or portal lobule are thoroughly discussed in the literature (Fawcett, 1994).

The liver lobule of Rappaport (acinus) can be divided into three zones which vary with respect to blood pressure, oxygen, supply of nutrients, metabolism and degree of enzyme activity. Variation in these factors explains why many toxic lesions have a zonal distribution. The periportal zone (zone 1 of the acinus) is exposed to the most highly oxygenated blood and the highest level of nutrients, while the perivenous zone (zone 3 of the acinus) has the least available oxygen and substrate. Hepatic parenchymal cells in zone 1 have more mitochondria, while zone 3 parenchymal cells have a higher content of cytochrome P-450, epoxide hydrolase and glutathione transferase.

The hepatic parenchymal cells first come in contact with many of the amino acids, lipids, carbohydrates, vitamins, minerals and xenobiotics that are absorbed through the gastrointestinal tract. Nutrients are metabolized and distributed to the blood and bile. Glucose and acetoacetate are the principal energy sources secreted by the liver. However, the liver also synthesizes lipid for storage. It plays an important role in the metabolism and storage of vitamins and minerals, especially iron, copper and

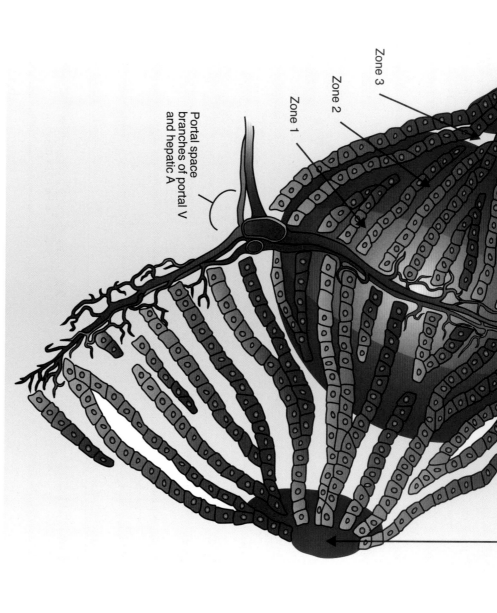

Figure 18.9 Diagram of the liver acinus, consisting of parenchyma centered around the terminal branches of the hepatic artery and portal vein. The cells in zone 1 have first call on the incoming oxygen and nutrients. The cells of zone 2 are less favored, and those of zone 3 are least favorably situated. From Fawcett (1994).

Terminal hepatic V (central V)

Zone 3

Zone 2

Zone 1

Portal space branches of portal V and hepatic A

Terminal hepatic V (central V)

zinc. The liver, central to bile acid metabolism, converts cholesterol to bile acids, secretes bile acids into the bile, and removes bile acids from the portal venous and hepatic arterial blood. The formation of bile by the liver assists in absorption and digestion of essential nutrients.

Xenobiotics are metabolized via two types of reaction: phase I metabolic reactions result in oxidation, reduction or hydrolysis; phase II reactions result in conjugation of xenobiotics. Since many of the phase I reactions result in increased reactivity of

the compounds, it is not surprising that metabolized compounds are frequently more toxic. Toxic metabolites or their harmless conjugates often are excreted in the bile.

Immune complexes entering the liver primarily from the spleen and endotoxins from the gastrointestinal tract are phagocytosed or inactivated by sinusoidal lining cells, primarily Kupffer cells. The liver synthesizes many important proteins including components of blood plasma such as albumin and α_2-globulin.

Small intestine

In the small intestine, the intestinal contents are mixed with the secretions of the mucosal cells and with pancreatic juice and bile (Elwell and McConnell, 1990). Digestion, which begins in the mouth and stomach, is completed in the small intestine, and the products of digestion of the small intestine, and the products of digestion are absorbed, along with most of the vitamins and fluid. Major physiological functions of the intestinal tract include motility, secretion and digestion, absorption, and metabolism. These functions are regulated in part by glucocorticoids, thyroid hormones and gastrointestinal peptide hormones such as secretin, gastrin, vasoactive intestinal polypeptide, gastric inhibitory polypeptides and somatostatin. Most of the bioactive polypeptides are in enterochromaffin cells or nerves of the intestine as well as other tissues.

Absorption through the intestinal mucosa can be through active transport, pinocytosis or diffusion. By gestation day 19–20 the fetus can absorb macromolecules by pinocytosis; absorption of immunoglobulins is primarily in the jejunum, and absorption of other proteins occurs in the ileum. This process occurs through the first 2 weeks of life before extracellular digestion is well developed; pinocytic activity begins to decrease during the third week following the birth. In the adults, the process of passive diffusion is the most common route for absorption of xenobiotics.

In the adult rat, absorption of macromolecules and some particles occurs through the M cells which cover the lymphoid tissue of the Peyer's patch. Metabolism of compounds may occur in the intestinal epithelium, or the absorbed compounds may enter the venous or lymphatic systems. Changes in the gut microflora and their role in activation or deactivation of a xenobiotic can also be an important consideration in toxicity/carcinogenesis studies.

It has been reported that in the F-344 rat a chemically defined liquid diet altered the small intestinal microflora and enhanced the toxicity of methotrexate. In addition to developmental changes in mechanisms of intestinal absorption, there are differences between the neonate and adult in intestinal enzymatic activity. At birth, hydrolytic activity in the intestine is directed toward the components of milk; lactase activity is high in the suckling rat but declines by one month, while the enzymatic activity for digestion of carbohydrates in solid food increases.

The small intestinal epithelium differentiates, in a migration-dependent manner, into four different lineages. Each of these cell types produces characteristic gene products and structure essential for its particular function (Licato and Brenner, 1997). Enterocytes produce brush border hydrolases, goblet cells release mucins and trefoil peptides, enterochromaffin cells secrete chromaffins, and Paneth cells make lysozyme, criptidins and defensins (Ouellette and Selsted, 1996). In the adult rat the intestinal epithelial crypt cells divide every 10–14 hours and the cell transit time from crypt to villus tip is 48 hours. The Paneth cell remains at the base of the crypt and is replaced about every 4 weeks. This cell produces lysozyme, and it has been postulated that it may function in the regulation of the gut microflora. In the normal rat the epithelial cells differentiate as they move along the villus surface toward the tip. In comparison to the young adult, there is delayed differentiation of enterocytes during passage from crypt to villus in the aged F-344 rat.

There is a significant increase in the mucosal mass of the ileum in the aged rat, which may be a compensatory hypertrophy in response to decreased efficiency in the function of the epithelium.

Colon

The main function of the colon is absorption of water, Na^+ and other minerals.

Metabolism

Over the last 15 years, a large number of animal models for human diseases have been discovered in laboratory rats. Such model animals have become an indispensable tool in many fields of biological and medical research. The rat is a suitable model for the investigation of metabolism.

The end products of the digestive processes are, for the most part, hexoses, fructoses, galactoses, glucose, amino acids and fat derivatives. These compounds are absorbed and metabolized in the organism in various ways (Figure 18.10).

Intermediary Metabolism

The fate of dietary components after digestion and absorption constitutes intermediary metabolism (Mayers, 1996). The short-chain fragments produced

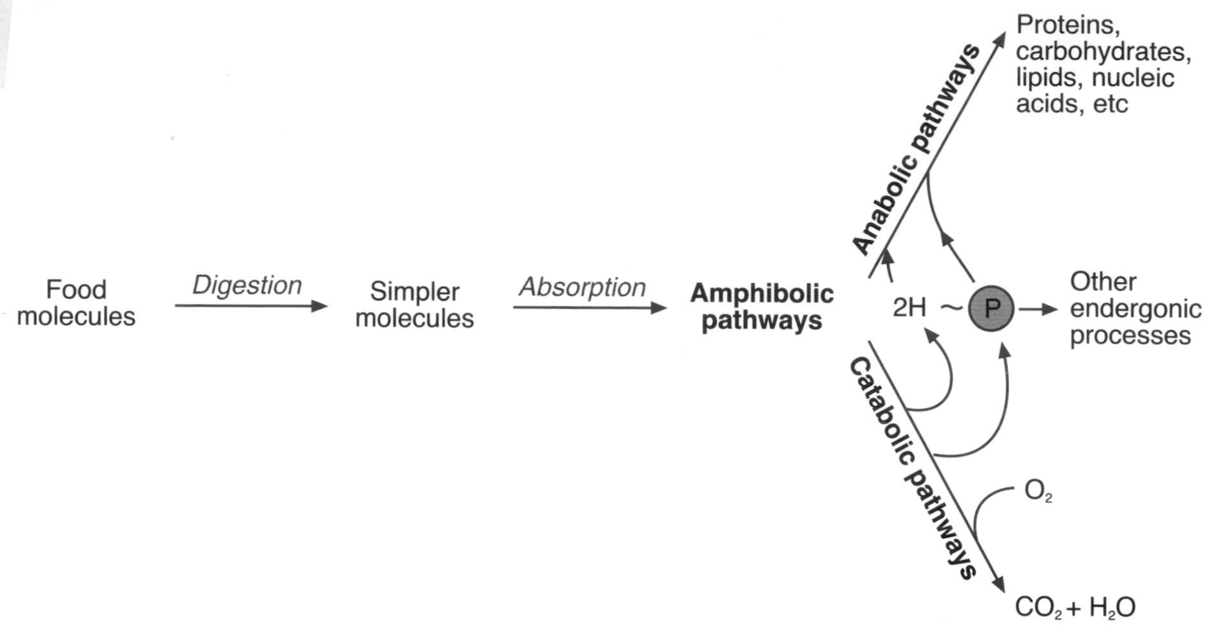

Figure 18.10 The three major categories of metabolic pathways. Catabolic pathways release free energy in the form of reducing equivalents (2H) or high-energy phosphate to power the anabolic pathways. Amphibolic pathways act as links between the other two categories of pathways. From Mayers (1996).

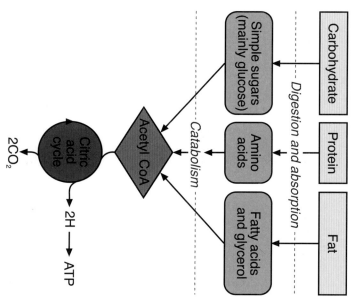

Food molecules — *Digestion* → Simpler molecules — *Absorption* → **Amphibolic pathways**

Catabolic pathways → 2H, O_2 → $CO_2 + H_2O$

$2H \sim P$ → Other endergonic processes

Anabolic pathways → Proteins, carbohydrates, lipids, nucleic acids, etc

by hexose, amino acid and fat catabolism are similar. From this common metabolic pool of intermediates, carbohydrates, proteins and fats can be synthesized, or the fragments can enter the citric acid cycle, a kind of final common pathway of catabolism, in which they are degraded to hydrogen atoms and CO_2. The hydrogen atoms are oxidized to form water by a chain of flavoprotein and cytochrome enzymes (Figure 18.11).

Much of the energy released by catabolism is not utilized directly by cells but is applied to the formation of bonds between phosphoric acid residues and certain organic compounds. Because the energy of bond formation in some of these phosphates is very high, relatively large amounts of energy (10–12 kcal/mol) are released when the bond is hydrolyzed. Compounds containing such bonds are called high-energy phosphate compounds but not all organic phosphates are of the high-energy type.

Some of the intermediates formed in carbohydrate metabolism are high-energy phosphates, but the most important high-energy phosphate compound is adenosine triphosphate (ATP) (Figure 18.12). This ubiquitous molecule is the energy storehouse of the organism. When hydrolyzed to adenosine diphosphate (ADP), it releases energy directly to such processes as muscle contraction, active transport and the synthesis of many chemical compounds. Loss of another phosphate to form adeno-

sine monophosphate (AMP) releases more energy (Figure 18.13).

Another energy-rich phosphate compound found in muscle is creatine phosphate. Other important phosphorylated compounds, at least some of which

Figure 18.11 Outline of the pathways for the catabolism of dietary carbohydrate, protein and fat. From Mayers (1996).

Carbohydrate → Simple sugars (mainly glucose)
Protein → Amino acids
Fat → Fatty acids and glycerol

Digestion and absorption

Catabolism

→ Acetyl CoA → Citric acid cycle → 2CO$_2$

2H → ATP

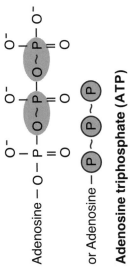

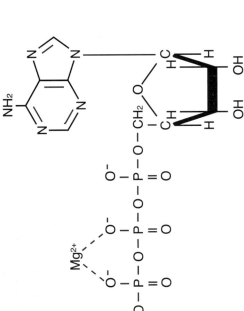

Figure 18.12 Adenosine triphosphate (ATP) as the magnesium complex. From Mayers (1996).

can serve as energy donors, include the triphosphate derivatives of pyrimidine or purine bases other than adenine. These include the guanine derivative, guanosine triphosphate (GTP), an important compound in signal transduction; the cytosine derivative, cytidine triphosphate (CTP); the uracil derivative, uridine triphosphate (UTP); and the hypoxanthine derivative, inosine triphosphate (ITP). Many catabolic reactions are associated with the formation of energy-rich phosphates.

Another group of high-energy compounds are the thioesters, the acyl derivatives of mercaptans. Coenzyme A (CoA) (Figure 18.14) is a ubiquitously distributed mercaptan containing adenine, ribose, pantothenic acid and thioethanolamine.

Adenosine triphosphate (ATP)

Adenosine diphosphate (ADP)

Adenosine monophosphate (AMP)

Figure 18.13 Structure of ATP, ADP and AMP, showing the position and the number of high-energy phosphates. From Mayers (1996).

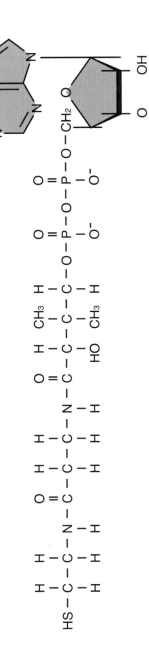

Coenzyme A (CoA)

Figure 18.14 Structure of coenzyme A (CoA). From Alberts et al. (1998).

Biological oxidations

Oxidation is the combination of a substance with O_2, or loss of hydrogen, or loss of electrons (Ganong, 1997). The corresponding reverse processes are called reduction. Biological oxidations are catalyzed by specific enzymes. Coenzymes are supplementary substances that usually act as carriers for products of the reaction.

A number of coenzymes serve as hydrogen acceptors, such as nicotinamide adenine dinucleotide (NAD$^+$) and nicotinamide adenine dinucleotide phosphate (NADP$^+$), forming dihydronicotinamide adenine dinucleotide (NADH) and dihydronicotinamide adenine dinucleotide phosphate (NADPH), respectively. The hydrogen is then transferred to the flavoprotein–cytochrome system. The flavoprotein–cytochrome system is a chain of enzymes that transfers hydrogen to oxygen, forming water. This process occurs in the mitochondria. Each enzyme in the chain is reduced and then reoxidized as the hydrogen is passed down the line. Each of the enzymes is a protein with a linked nonprotein prosthetic group. Cytochrome oxidase, which transfers hydrogens to O_2, forming H_2O, is the final enzyme in the chain.

Oxidative phosphorylation

Production of ATP associated with oxidation by the flavoprotein–cytochrome system is called oxidative phosphorylation. Oxidative phosphorylation involves the transfer of protons across the inner membrane that forms the cristae of the mitochondria, the transfer being driven by oxidation in the respiratory chain. This creates an electrochemical potential difference across the membrane, and transport of protons from the intracristal space back into the matrix space drives a reversible ATPase in the membrane in the direction that converts ADP and inorganic phosphate to ATP.

Metabolism of Carbohydrate

Dietary carbohydrates are, for the most part, polymers of hexoses, of which the most important are glucose, galactose and fructose. The main product of carbohydrate digestion and the principal circulating sugar is glucose (Figure 18.15).

Once it enters the cell, glucose is normally phosphorylated to form glucose 6-phosphate. The glucose 6-phosphate is either polymerized into glycogen or catabolized. The process of glycogen formation is called glycogenesis, and glycogen formation is called glycogenolysis. The liver and skeletal muscle are the major storage sites for glycogen, the storage form of glucose. The degradation of glucose to pyruvate or lactate is called glycolysis. Glucose catabolism proceeds via cleavage through fructose to trioses or via oxidation and decarboxylation to pentoses. The pathway to pyruvate through the trioses is the Embden–Meyerhof pathway, and that through 6-phosphogluconate and the pentoses is the direct oxidative pathway. Pyruvate is converted to acetyl CoA. Interconversions between carbohydrate, protein and fat include conversion of the glycerol from fats to dihydroxyacetone phosphate and conversion of a number of amino acids with carbon skeletons resembling intermediates in the Embden–Meyerhof pathway and citric acid cycle to these intermediates by deamination. In this way, and by conversion of lactate to glucose, nonglucose molecules can be converted to glucose (gluconeogenesis). Glucose can be converted to fats through acetyl CoA.

Citric acid cycle

The citric acid cycle (Krebs cycle, tricarboxylic acid cycle) is a sequence of reactions in which acetyl CoA is metabolized to CO_2 and H atoms (Figure 18.16). Acetyl CoA is first condensed with the anion of a four-carbon acid, oxaloacetate, to form citric acid and reduced CoA. In a series of seven subsequent reactions, 2CO_2 molecules are liberated. Four pairs of H atoms are transferred to the flavoprotein–cytochrome chain, forming 12ATP and 4H_2O, of which 2H_2O is used in the cycle. The citric acid cycle is the common pathway for oxidation to CO_2 and H_2O of carbohydrate, fat and some amino acids. The major entry into it is through acetyl CoA, but a number of amino acids can be converted to citric acid cycle intermediates by deamination.

Glycolysis to pyruvate occurs outside the mitochondria. Pyruvate then enters the mitochondria and is metabolized. Oxidative phosphorylation occurs only in the mitochondria. Within the mitochondria, the enzymes involved in this process are arranged in orderly sequences.

Phosphorylase

Degradation of glycogen is regulated by several hormones. Glycogen is synthesized from glucose 1-phosphate through uridine diphosphoglucose

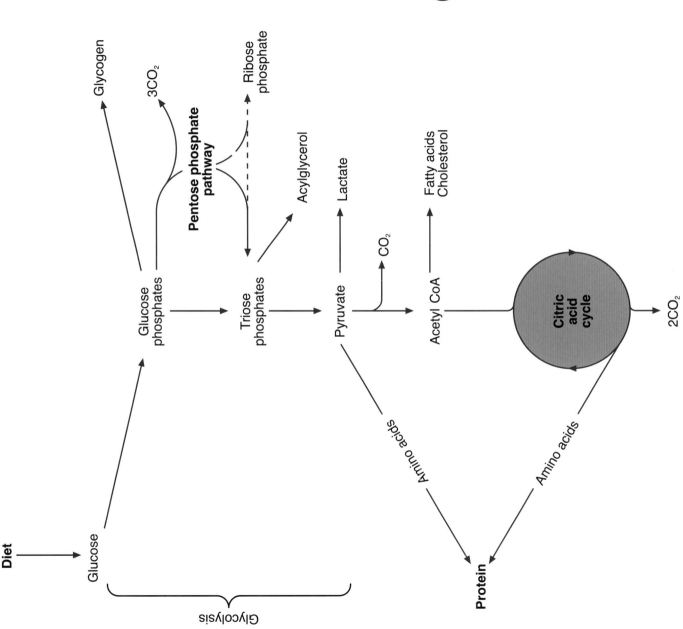

Figure 18.15 Overview of carbohydrate metabolism showing the major pathways and end products. From Mayers (1996).

(UDPG), with the enzyme glycogen synthase catalyzing the final step. Glycogen is a branched glucose polymer with two types of glucoside linkage. Cleavage of the 1:4α linkage in the polymer chain is catalyzed by phosphorylase.

Phosphorylase is activated in part by the action of epinephrine on β₂-adrenergic receptors in the liver. This initiates a sequence of reaction that provides a hormonal action through cyclic AMP. Protein kinase

A is activated by cyclic AMP and catalyzes the transfer of a phosphate group to phosphorylase kinase, converting it to its active form. The phosphorylase kinase in turn catalyzes the phosphorylation and consequent activation of phosphorylase.

Because the liver contains the enzyme glucose 6-phosphatase, much of the glucose 6-phosphate that is formed in this organ can be converted to glucose and can enter the circulation, increasing the serum

Figure 18.16 The citric acid cycle. From Alberts et al. (1994).

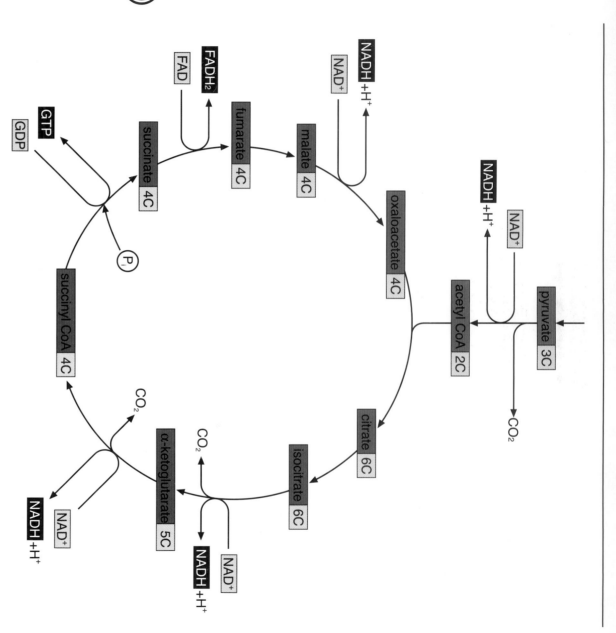

glucose level. By stimulating adenyl cyclase, epi-nephrine causes activation of the phosphorylase in the liver and skeletal muscle. The consequences of this activation are a rise in the glucose and lactate levels in the blood. There is a net uptake of glucose by the liver when the serum glucose is high and a net discharge when it is low. The liver regulates a constant circulating glucose level. This function is not automatic; glucose uptake and glucose release are regulated by the actions of numerous hormones.

The serum glucose level at any given time is determined by the balance between the amount of glucose entering the circulation and the amount of glucose leaving it. The main determinants are the dietary intake; the rate of entry into the cells of muscle,

adipose tissue and other organs; and the regulation by the liver. Other hexoses that are absorbed from the intestine include galactose, which is released by the digestion of lactose and converted to glucose in the organism; and fructose, part of which is ingested and part produced by hydrolysis of sucrose. After phosphorylation, galactose is converted to uridine diphosphogalactose. The uridine diphosphogalactose is converted to uridine diphosphoglucose, which is involved in glycogen synthesis.

Metabolism of Protein

Proteins are composed of large numbers of amino acids linked into chains by peptide bonds joining the

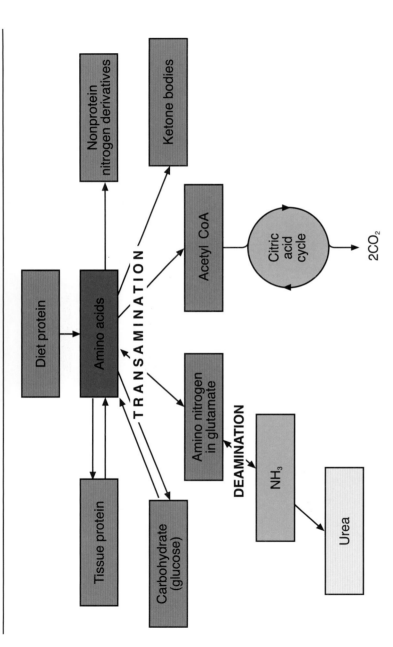

Figure 18.17 Overview of amino acid metabolism showing the major pathways and end products. From Mayers (1996).

amino group of one amino acid to the carboxyl group of the next. In addition, some proteins contain carbohydrates and lipids. Smaller chains of amino acids are called peptides or polypeptides.

Although small amounts of proteins are absorbed from the gastrointestinal tract and some peptides are also absorbed, most ingested proteins are first digested and then their constituent amino acids absorbed. The body's own proteins are being continuously hydrolyzed to amino acids and resynthesized (Figure 18.17).

Thyroid hormones, catecholamines, histamine, serotonin, melatonin and intermediates in the urea cycle are formed from specific amino acids. Methionine and cysteine provide the sulfur contained in proteins, CoA, taurine and other biologically important compounds. Methionine is converted into S-adenosyl-methionine, which is the active methylating agent in the synthesis of compounds such as epinephrine, acetylcholine and creatinine. It is a major donor of biologically labile methyl groups.

Mammalian S-adenosyl-methionine synthetase exists as two isozymes, liver-type and nonhepatic-type enzymes, which are the products of two different genes. The liver-type isozyme is only expressed in adult rat liver, whereas the nonhepatic-type isozyme is widely distributed in various tissues.

In addition to the liver-type isozyme, a minor amount of the nonhepatic-type isozyme is also detected in adult rat liver. In the hepatic parenchymal cells, the liver-type isozyme protein is predominantly expressed, and a small amount of the nonhepatic-type isozyme protein is also detected (Shimizu-Saito et al., 1997). In hepatic stellate cells (vitamin A-storing cells), the nonhepatic-type isozyme is exclusively or only expressed. Large amounts of both isozymes are present in endothelial and Kupffer cells.

Interconversions between amino acids and the products of carbohydrate and fat catabolism at the level of the common metabolic pool and the citric acid cycle involve transfer, removal or formation of amino groups. Transamination reactions, conversion of one amino acid to the corresponding keto acid with simultaneous conversion of another keto acid to an amino acid, occur in many tissues.

The transaminases involved are also present in the circulation. When injury to many active cells occurs as a result of a pathological process, the serum transaminase level rises. One example is the rise in serum glutamic-oxaloacetic transaminase (SGOT). Most of the NH_3 formed by deamination of amino acids in the liver is converted to urea, and the urea is excreted in the urine. Creatinine is synthesized in the liver from methionine, glycine and arginine. In skeletal muscle, it is phosphorylated to form phosphorylcreatinine, which is an important energy store for ATP synthesis.

Nucleosides are components not only of a variety of coenzymes and related substances but of RNA and DNA as well. Nucleic acids in the diet are digested and their constituent purines and pyrimidines absorbed, but most of the purines and pyrimidines are synthesized from amino acids, mainly in the liver. The nucleotides, RNA and DNA are then synthesized. RNA is in dynamic equilibrium with the amino acid pool, but DNA, once formed, is metabolically stable throughout life. The purines and pyrimidines released by the degradation of nucleotides may be reused or catabolized.

Protein degradation is a carefully regulated, complex process. The degradation of proteins starts after conjugation to the 74-amino acid polypeptide ubiquitin. This polypeptide is highly conserved and is present in species ranging from bacteria to humans. Protein degradation following conjugation to ubiquitin plays an important regulatory role in the cell cycle.

Metabolism of Fat

The biologically important lipids are the fatty acids and their derivatives, the triacylglycerols, the phospholipids and related compounds, and the sterols. The triacylglycerols are composed of three fatty acids bound to glycerol. Naturally occurring fatty acids contain an even number of carbon atoms. They may be saturated or unsaturated. The phospholipids are constituents of cell membranes. The sterols include the various steroid hormones and cholesterol.

During the isolating of substrains with different coat colors from noninbred Long-Evans rats, a new mutant Long-Evans cinnamon-like colored (LEC) strain causing hereditary hepatitis was established (Sasaki et al., 1985; Yoshida et al., 1987). The clinical signs of hepatitis in LEC rats are similar to human liver disease. Furthermore, liver cancer appears in long-surviving rats after recovery from jaundice. Therefore, LEC rats provide a pertinent model useful for basic and clinical studies of hepatitis and liver cancer (Yoshida et al., 1991). Abnormal lipid metabolism has been observed in the LEC rats (Taniguchi et al., 1991). The lipid patterns of the LEC rats are similar to those of choline-deficient

rats, in which the liver may fail to transfer the newly formed triacylglycerols and cholesterol into the plasma with a resultant increase in liver triacylglycerol content and a decrease in serum lipid levels. The LEC rats appear to be a useful model for the study of lipid metabolism in hepatocellular diseases, including hepatitis and hepatoma.

Fatty acid oxidation and synthesis

Fatty acids are degraded to acetyl CoA, which then enters the citric acid cycle in the organism. The main degradation occurs in the mitochondria by β-oxidation (Figure 18.18). Fatty acid oxidation begins with activation of the fatty acid by acyl CoA. Acyl CoA-binding protein is a highly conserved, 10-kDa cytosolic protein found in a wide variety of organisms ranging from plants to yeast and mammals (Gossett et al., 1996). Acyl CoA-binding protein is one of several families of cytosolic proteins that bind fatty acyl CoA and via this interaction may be involved in regulation of the intracellular acyl CoA pool size,

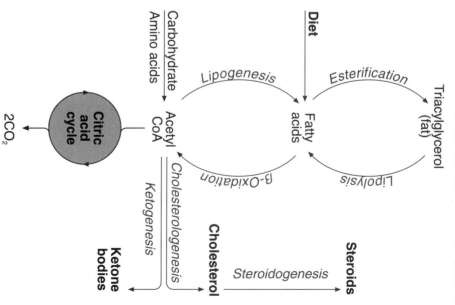

Figure 18.18 Overview of fatty acid metabolism showing the major pathways and end products. From Mayers (1996).

transport of acyl CoA, stimulation of enzymes involved in lipid metabolism, and protection of acyl CoA from intracellular hydrolysis (Mandrup et al., 1993; Rasmussen et al., 1993, 1994; Schjerling et al., 1996; Gossett et al., 1998).

Medium- and short-chain fatty acids can enter the mitochondria easily, but long-chain fatty acids must be bound to carnitine in ester linkage before they can enter mitochondria. Carnitine is β-hydroxy-γ-trimethylammonium butyrate, and is synthesized from lysine and methionine. A translocase moves the fatty acid-carnitine ester into the matrix space in exchange for free carnitine. In the matrix space, the ester is hydrolyzed, making the activated fatty acid molecule available for β-oxidation and providing free carnitine for further exchange. β-Oxidation proceeds by serial removal of two carbon fragments from the fatty acid. The energy yield of this process is large.

Many tissues can synthesize fatty acids from acetyl CoA. Blocking the metabolism of fats by inhibiting the oxidation of fatty acids with 2-mercaptoacetate or methyl palmorixate can produce an increase in food intake of rats (Friedman and Tordoff, 1986; Friedman et al., 1986; Scharrer and Langhans, 1986; Langhans and Scharrer, 1987) In addition, simultaneous blockade of both fat and glucose metabolism produces synergistic effects on food intake (Friedman and Tordoff, 1986; Friedman et al. 1986; Tordoff et al., 1988), suggesting that these signals are integrated to regulate intake. Studies of the mechanisms by which changes in energy utilization affect food intake suggest that signals related to glucose regulation may have direct central effects, whereas signals related to fat utilization are conveyed centrally by vagal fibers (Langhans and Scharrer, 1987; Ritter and Taylor, 1989, 1990). The primary source of energy for a rat pup is mother's milk, which provides 60–70% of its calories from fat (Fernando-Warnakulasuriya et al., 1981; Wells, 1985). Compared with adult rats, pups have higher capacities for the oxidation of fatty acids and appear to preferentially use products of fatty acid oxidation in the brain (Lockwood and Bailey, 1970, 1971; Wells, 1985; Yeh and Sheehan, 1985; Swithers, 1997).

In animals, the conversion of malonyl CoA into fatty acid is catalyzed by a single multifunctional protein, fatty acid synthetase. Expression of the fatty acid synthetase gene is regulated in a tissue-specific manner in response to various developmental, nutritional and hormonal signals (Smith and Ryan, 1979; Pope et al., 1988; Moustaïd and Sul, 1991).

Many of these tissue-specific changes in the concentration of fatty acid synthetase mRNA and protein result from changes of the level of transcription of the fatty acid synthetase gene. Several hormones, including insulin, glucagon, thyroid hormone and glucocorticoids, have been implicated as agents capable of influencing the expression (Paulauskis and Sul, 1989; Swierczynski et al., 1991; Iritani, 1992; Moustaïd et al., 1993; Oskouian et al., 1997).

Ketone bodies

Acetyl CoA units condense to form acetoacetyl CoA in many tissues. In the liver, which contains a deacylase, free acetoacetate is formed. This β-keto acid is converted to β-hydroxybutyrate and acetone, and because these compounds are metabolized with difficulty in the liver, they diffuse into the circulation. Acetoacetate is also formed in the liver through the formation of β-hydroxy-β-methylglutaryl CoA, and this pathway is quantitatively more important than deacylation. Acetoacetate, β-hydroxybutyrate and acetone are called ketone bodies. Tissues other than liver transfer CoA from succinyl CoA to acetoacetate and metabolize the active acetoacetate to CO_2 and H_2O through the citric acid cycle. The ketone bodies are an important source of energy in some conditions such as starvation.

Cellular lipids

The lipids in cells are of two main types: structural lipids, which are an inherent part of the membranes and other parts of cells; and neutral fat, stored in the fat droplets of the adipose cells. Neutral fat is mobilized during starvation, but structural lipid is preserved. The fat droplets are not inert, but active and dynamic, undergoing continuous degradation and resynthesis in tissues.

Brown fat

In brown fat depots, the fat cells as well as the blood vessels have an extensive sympathetic innervation. This is in contrast to white fat depots, in which there may be innervation to some adipocytes but the main sympathetic innervation is solely on blood vessels. In addition, ordinary adipocytes have only a single large lipid droplet of white fat, whereas brown fat cells contain several small fat droplets. Brown fat cells also contain many mitochondria. In these mitochondria, there is the usual inward proton

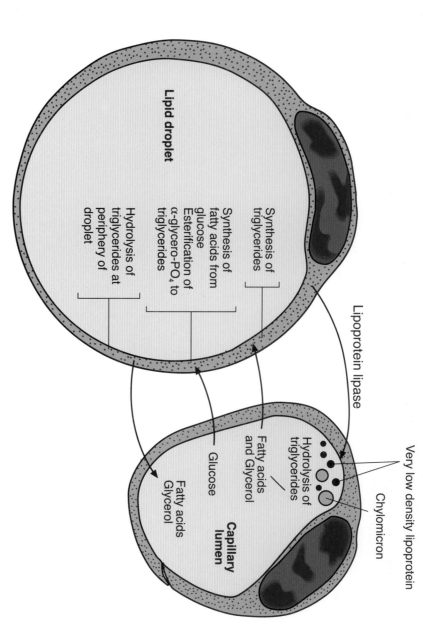

Figure 18.19 Schematic representation of lipid transport between the blood in a capillary and an adipose cell (at left). From Fawcett (1994).

conductance that generates ATP, but there is, in addition, a second proton conductance that does not generate ATP. This short-circuit conductance, which is associated with a polypeptide of molecular weight 32 000 in the membrane, causes uncoupling of metabolism and generation of ATP, so more heat is produced.

Plasma lipids and lipid transport

The major lipids in plasma do not circulate in the free form. Free fatty acids are bound to albumin, whereas cholesterol, triacylglycerols and phospholipids are transported in the form of lipoprotein complexes (Figure 18.19) The complexes greatly increase the solubility of the lipids. There are six families of lipoproteins, which are classified in size and lipid content. In general, the lipoproteins consist of a hydrophobic core of cholesteryl esters and triacylglycerols surrounded by protein and phospholipids. These lipoproteins are organized into an exogenous pathway that transports lipids from the intestine to the liver and an endogenous pathway that transports lipids to and from the tissues.

The protein constituents of the lipoproteins are called **apoproteins.** The major apoproteins are called apo E, apo C and apo B. Chylomicrons are formed in the intestinal mucosa during the absorption of the products of fat digestion. They are very large lipoprotein complexes that enter the circulation through the lymphatic ducts (vas lymphaticum centrale). These chylomicrons are cleared from the circulation by lipoprotein lipase, which is located on the surface of the endothelium of the capillaries. The enzyme catalyzes the degradation of the triacylglycerol in the chylomicrons to free fatty acids and glycerol, which then enter adipose cells and are reesterified. Alternatively, the free fatty acids remain in the circulation bound to albumin.

Lipoprotein lipase is a 110-kDa heparin-binding enzyme that hydrolyzes core triacylglycerols in circulating chylomicrons and very-low-density lipoproteins (VLDLs) to generate chylomicron remnants, which are 30–80 nm in diameter (Goldberg, 1996). Lipoproteins are synthesized by many cell types, including vascular smooth muscle cells and macrophages. Weaver et al. (1997) reported that internalization of lipoprotein lipase-associated VLDL by vascular smooth muscle cells is mediated by two pathways, one involving LDL receptor families and a second that is independent of the families, probably involving direct uptake by heparan sulfate proteoglycans. The LDL receptor family-dependent pathway leads to less cellular storage of cholesteryl ester.

Both lipoprotein lipase and hepatic lipase are under nutritional control. Lipoprotein lipase is increased in white adipose tissue but is decreased in heart of fasted rats (Eckel, 1987; Borensztajn, 1987), although some of the data reported in the literature are in conflict (Cherkes and Gordon, 1959; Robinson, 1965; Tan *et al.*, 1977; Grinberg *et al.*, 1985; Vilaró *et al.*, 1988). Recently, Galan *et al.* (1993, 1994) reported that the effect of fasting on the activity of lipoprotein lipase in the liver of neonatal rats depends on the rat strain used as a model.

The remnants are carried to the liver, where they bind to chylomicron remnants and VLDL receptors, are readily internalized by receptor-mediated endocytosis and are degraded in the lysosomes. The chylomicrons and their remnants constitute a transport system for ingested exogenous lipids. There is also an endogenous system composed ot VLDLs, intermediate-density lipoproteins (IDLs), low-density lipoproteins (LDLs), and high-density lipoproteins (HDLs), which transports triacylglycerols and cholesterol throughout the body. VLDLs are formed in the liver and transport triacylglycerols formed from fatty acids and carbohydrates in the liver to extrahepatic tissues. After their triacylglycerol is removed by the action of lipoprotein lipase, they become IDLs. The IDLs give up phospholipids and, through the action of the plasma enzyme lecithin-cholesterol acyltransferase (LCAT), take up cholesteryl esters formed from cholesterol in the HDLs. Some IDLs are taken up by the liver. The remaining IDLs then lose more triacylglycerol and protein and become LDLs.

LDLs provide cholesterol to the tissues. Cholesterol is an essential constituent of cell membranes and is used by gland cells to synthesize steroid hormones. In the liver and most extrahepatic tissues, LDLs are taken up by receptor-mediated endocytosis in coated pits. During receptor-mediated endocytosis, each coated pit is pinched off to form a coated vesicle and then an endosome. Protein pumps in the membranes of the endosomes lower the pH in the endosome. In the case of LDL receptor, but not the chylomicron remnants receptor, this triggers release of the LDL receptors, which recycle

to the cell membrane. The endosome then fuses with a lysosome, where cholesterol formed from the cholesteryl esters by the acid lipase in the lysosomes becomes available to meet the cell's needs. The cholesterol in the cells also suppresses intracellular synthesis of cholesterol by inhibiting esterification of any excess cholesterol that is released, and inhibits synthesis of new LDL receptors. All of these reactions provide feedback control of the amount of cholesterol in the cell.

It is apparent that in the steady state, cholesterol leaves as well as enters cells. The cholesterol leaving the cells is absorbed in HDLs, lipoproteins that are synthesized in the liver and the intestine. Some of the HDLs contain apo E and bind to LDL receptors on other cells, thus transporting cholesterol from one cell to another.

Free fatty acid metabolism

Free fatty acids are provided to adipocytes and other cells by chylomicrons and VLDLs. They are also synthesized in the fat depots in which they are stored. They circulate bound to albumin and are a major source of energy for many organs. They are used extensively in the heart, but probably all tissues, including the brain.

The supply of free fatty acid to the tissues is regulated by two lipases. Lipoprotein lipase on the surface of the endothelium of the capillaries hydrolyzes the triacylglycerols in chylomicrons and VLDLs, providing free fatty acid and glycerol, which are reassembled into new triacylglycerols in the adipocytes. The intracellular hormone-sensitive lipase of adipocytes catalyzes the degradation of stored triacylglycerols into glycerol and fatty acids, with the latter entering the circulation.

Cholesterol metabolism

Cholesterol is the major precursor of the steroid hormones and bile acids and is an essential constituent of cell membranes. It is absorbed from the intestine and incorporated into the chylomicrons formed in the mucosa. The intestinal mucosa plays a key regulatory role in cholesterol homeostasis in the body (Stange *et al.*, 1988; Field *et al.*, 1990). Events that occur in this tissue, such as cholesterol absorption, synthesis, esterification and exchange between mucosal and plasma sterol, contribute significantly to the subsequent metabolic processes that occur in the liver and other organs as well as plasma. In experiments using normocholesterolemic (SW) or genetically hypercholesterolemic (RICO) rats, bile cholesterol absorption has been demonstrated to be greater and more proximal than dietary cholesterol absorption, both taking place mainly in the top cells of the duodenum or the proximal jejunum (Lutton, 1996). Esterification of cholesterol also takes place mainly in the villus cells, while cholesterol synthesis is predominantly carried out in the crypt cells of the proximal duodenum and distal ileum. After the chylomicrons discharge their triacylglycerol in adipose tissue, the chylomicron remnants bring cholesterol to the liver. The liver and other tissues also synthesize cholesterol. Some of the cholesterol in the liver is excreted in the bile. Some of the biliary cholesterol is reabsorbed from the intestine. Most of the cholesterol in the liver is incorporated into VLDLs, and all of it circulates in lipoprotein complexes.

References

Agnusdei, D. and Civitelli, R. (1996) *Curr. Opin. Gastroenterol.* **12**, 190–198.

Alberts, B., Bray, D., Lewis, J., Raff, M., Roberts, K. and Watson, J.D. (1994) *Molecular Biology of the Cell*. New York: Garland Publishing.

Alberts, B., Bray, D., Johnson, A. *et al.* (1998) *Essential Cell Biology*. New York: Garland Publishing.

Blomhoff, R. (1994) In: Blomhoff, R. (ed.) *Vitamin A in Health and Disease*, pp. 1–35. New York: Marcel Dekker.

Blomhoff, R., Green, M.H., Berg, T. and Norum, K.R. (1990) *Science* **250**, 399–404.

Blomhoff, R., Green, M.H., Green, J.B., Berg, T. and Norum, K.R. (1992a) *Physiol. Rev.* **71**, 951–990.

Blomhoff, R., Green, M.H. and Norum, K.R. (1992b) *Annu. Rev. Nutr.* **12**, 37–57.

Blomhoff, R., Senoo, H., Smeland, S., Bjerknes, T. and Norum, K.R. (1992c) *J. Nutr. Sci. Vitam.* **38**, 327–330.

Borensztajn, J. (1987) In: Borensztajn, J. (ed.) *Lipoprotein Lipase*, pp. 133–148. Chicago: Evener.

Brown, H.R. and Hardisty, J.F. (1990) In: Boorman, G.A., Eustis, S.L., Elwell, M.R., Montgomery, Jr, C.A. and MacKenzie, W.F. (eds) *Pathology of the Fischer Rat*, pp. 9–30. San Diego: Academic Press.

Cardell, Jr, R.R., Badenhausen, S. and Porter K.R. (1967) *J. Cell Biol.* **34**, 123–155.

Cherkes, A. and Gordon, Jr, R.S. (1959) *J. Lipid Res.* **1**, 97–101.

Eckel, R.H. (1987) In: Borensztajn, J. (ed.) *Lipoprotein Lipase*, pp. 79–132. Chicago: Evener.

Elwell, M.R. and McConnell, E.E. (1990) In: Boorman, G.A., Eustis, S.L., Elwell, M.R., Montgomery, Jr, C.A. and MacKenzie, W.F. (eds) *Pathology of the Fischer Rat*, pp. 31–42. San Diego: Academic Press.

Faussone-Pellegrini, M.S., Cortesini, C. and Romagnoli, P. (1977) *Arch. Ital. Anat. Embriol.* **82**, 157–177.

Fawcett, D.W. (1994) *Bloom and Fawcett A Textbook of Histology*, 12th edn. New York: Chapman & Hall.

Fernando-Warnakulasuriya, G.J.P., Staggers, J.E., Frost, S.C. and Wells, M.A. (1981) *J. Lipid Res.* **22**, 668–674.

Field, F.J., Kam, N.T.P. and Mathur, S.N. (1990) *Gastroenterology* **99**, 539–551.

Friedman, M.I. and Tordoff, M.G. (1986) *Am. J. Physiol.* **251**, R840–R845.

Friedman, M.I., Tordoff, M.G. and Ramirez, I. (1986) *Brain Res. Bull.* **17**, 855–859.

Galan, X., Llobera, M. and Ramirez, I. (1993) *Biol. Neonate* **64**, 295–303.

Galan, X., Llobera, M. and Ramirez, I. (1994) *Lipids* **29**, 333–336.

Ganong, W.F. (1997) *Review of Medical Physiology*, 18th edn. New York: Prentice-Hall.

Goldberg, I.J. (1996) *J. Lipid Res.* **37**, 693–707.

Goodman, D.W., Huang, H.S. and Shiratori, T. (1965) *J. Lipid Res.* **6**, 390–396.

Gossett, R.E., Frolov, A.A., Roths, J.B., Behnke, W.D., Kier, A.B. and Schroeder, F. (1996) *Lipids* **31**, 895–918.

Gossett, R.E., Edmondson, R.D., Jolly, C.A. *et al.* (1998) *Arch. Biochem. Biophys.* **350**, 201–213.

Grinberg, D.R., Ramirez, I., Vilaró, M.S., Reina, M., Llobera, M. and Herrera, E. (1985) *Biochim. Biophys. Acta* **833**, 217–222.

Gyoen, T., Bjerkelund, T., Blomhoff, H.K., Norum, K.R., Berg, T. and Blomhoff, R. (1987) *J. Biol. Chem.* **262**, 10926–10930.

Hazelwood, R.L. (1993) *Proc. Soc. Exp. Biol. Med.* **202**, 44–63.

Iritani, N. (1992) *Eur. J. Biochem.* **205**, 433–442.

Jersild, Jr, R.A. (1966) *Am. J. Anat.* **118**, 135–162.

Langhans, W. and Scharrer, E. (1987) *J. Auton. Nerv. Syst.* **18**, 13–18.

Leak, L.V. and Burke, J.F. (1966) *Am. J. Anat.* **118**, 785–810.

Licato, L.L. and Brenner, D.A. (1997) *Curr. Opin. Gastroenterol.* **13**, 90–93.

Lockwood, E.A. and Bailey, E. (1970) *Biochem. J.* **120**, 49–54.

Lockwood, E.A. and Bailey, E. (1971) *Biochem. J.* **124**, 249–254.

Lowe, M.E. (1997) *J. Nutr.* **127**, 549–557.

Lutton, C. (1996) *Digestion* **57**, 1–10.

Mandrup, S., Jepsen, R., Skott, H. *et al.* (1993) *Biochem. J.* **290**, 369–374.

Mayes, P.A. (1996) In: Murray, R.K., Granner, D.K., Mayes, P.A. and Rodwell, V.W. (eds) *Harper's*

Biochemistry, 24th edn, pp. 158–167. Stamford: Appleton & Lange.

Moustaïd, S. and Ryan, P. (1979) *J. Biol. Chem.* **254**, 8932–8936.

Moustaïd, N. and Sul, H.S. (1991) *J. Biol. Chem.* **266**, 18550–18554.

Moustaïd, N., Sakamoto, K., Clarke, S., Beyer, R.S. and Sul, H.S. (1993) *Biochem. J.* **292**, 767–772.

Nagy, L., Johnson, B.R., Hauschka, P. and Szabo, S. (1997) *Am. J. Physiol.* **35**, G1151–G1158.

Neuenschwander, S.B. and Elwell, M.R. (1990) In: Boorman, G.A., Eustis, S.L., Elwell, M.R., Montgomery, Jr., C.A. and MacKenzie, W.F. (eds) *Pathology of the Fischer Rat*, pp. 31–42. San Diego: Academic Press.

Ockner, R.K. and Manning, J.A. (1974) *J. Clin. Invest.* **54**, 326–338.

Okumura, T., Pappas, T.N. and Taylor, I.L. (1995) *Gastroenterology* **108**, 1517–1525.

Ong, D.E. (1994) In: Blomhoff, R. (ed.) *Vitamin A in Health and Disease*, pp. 37–72. New York: Marcel Dekker.

Oskouian, B., Rangan, V.S. and Smith, S. (1997) *Biochem. J.* **324**, 113–121.

Ouellette, A.J. and Selsted, M.E. (1996) *FASEB J.* **10**, 1280–1289.

Paulauskis, J.D. and Sul, H.S. (1989) *J. Biol. Chem.* **264**, 574–577.

Pope, T.S., Smart, D.A. and Roonet, S.A. (1988) *Biochim. Biophys. Acta* **959**, 169–177.

Putnam, W.S., Liddle, R.A. and Williams, J.A. (1989) *Am. J. Physiol.* **256**, G698–G703.

Rappaport, A.M. (1957) *Anat. Rec.* **130**, 673–690.

Rappaport, A.M., Borowy, Z.J., Lougheed, W.M. and Lotto, W.N. (1954) *Anat. Rec.* **119**, 11–33.

Rasmussen, J.T., Rosendal, J. and Knudsen, J. (1993) *Biochem. J.* **292**, 907–913.

Rasmussen, J.T., Faergeman, N.J., Kristiansen, K. and Knudsen, J. (1994) *Biochem. J.* **299**, 165–170.

Ritter, S. and Taylor, J.S. (1989) *Am. J. Physiol.* **256**, R1232–R1239.

Ritter, S. and Taylor, J.S. (1990) *Am. J. Physiol.* **258**, R1395–R1401.

Robinson, D.S. (1965) *J. Lipid Res.* **6**, 222–227.

Samloff, I.M., Taggart, R.T., Shiraishi, T. et al. (1987) *Gastroenterology* **93**, 77–84.

Sasaki, M., Yoshida, M.C., Kagami, K. et al. (1985) *Rat News Lett.* **14**, 4–6.

Scharrer, E. and Langhans, W. (1986) *Am. J. Physiol.* **250**, R1003–R1006.

Schjerling, C.K., Hummel, R., Hansen, J.K. et al. (1996) *J. Biol. Chem.* **271**, 22514–22521.

Senoo, H., Hata, R., Nagai, Y. and Wake, K. (1984) *Biomed. Res.* **5**, 451–458.

Senoo, H., Stang, E., Nilsson, A. et al. (1990) *J. Lipid Res.* **31**, 1229–1239.

Senoo, H., Smeland, S., Malaba, L. et al. (1993) *Proc. Natl Acad. Sci. USA* **90**, 3616–3620.

Senoo, H., Sato, M. and Imai, K. (1997) *Acta Anat. Nippon* **72**, 79–94.

Shimizu-Saito, K., Horikawa, S., Kojima, N., Shiga, J., Senoo, H. and Tsukada, K. (1997) *Hepatology* **26**, 424–431.

Smith, S. and Ryan, P. (1979) *J. Biol. Chem.* **254**, 8932–8936.

Stange, E.F., Preclik, G., Schneider, A. and Reinmann, F. (1988) *Scand. J. Gastroenterol.* **23**, 79–85.

Swierczynski, J., Mitchell, D.A., Reinhold, D.S. et al. (1991) *J. Biol. Chem.* **266**, 17459–17466.

Swithers, S.E. (1997) *Am. J. Physiol.* **273**, R1649–R1656.

Tan, M.H., Sata, T. and Havel, R.J. (1977) *J. Lipid Res.* **18**, 363–370.

Taniguchi, M., Sugiyama, T. and Taniguchi, N. (1991) In: Mori, M., Yoshida, M.C., Takeichi, N. and Taniguchi, N. (eds) *The LEC Rat*, pp. 169–174. Berlin: Springer-Verlag.

Taylor, I.L. (1989) In: Schultz, S.T.S.T. (ed.) *Handbook of Physiology, The Gastrointestinal System*, Vol. 2, pp. 475–544. Bethesda: American Physiological Society.

Thomsen, L., Robinson, T.I., Lee, J.C.F. et al. (1998) *Nature Med.* **4**, 848–851.

Thuneberg, L. (1982) *Adv. Anat. Embryol. Cell Biol.* **71**, 1–130.

Tordoff, M.G., Flynn, F.W., Grill, H.J. and Friedman, M.I. (1988) *Brain Res.* **445**, 216–221.

Turvill, J.L. and Farthing, M.J.G. (1996) *Curr. Opin. Gastroenterol.* **12**, 129–133.

Turvill, J.L. and Farthing, M.J.G. (1997) *Curr. Opin. Gastroenterol.* **13**, 94–98.

Vilaró, M.S., Llobera, M., Bengtsson-Olivecrona, G. and Olivecrona, T. (1988) *Biochem. J.* **249**, 549–556.

Wake, K. (1971) *Am. J. Anat.* **132**, 429–462.

Wake, K. (1980) *Int. Rev. Cytol.* **66**, 303–353.

Weaver, A.M., Lysiak, J.J. and Gonias, S.L. (1997) *J. Lipid Res.* **38**, 1841–1850.

Wells, M.A. (1985) *Fedn Proc.* **44**, 2365–2368.

Whitcomb, D.C., Puccio, A.M., Vigna, S.R., Taylor, I.L. and Hoffman, G.E. (1997) *Brain Res.* **760**, 137–149.

Yeh, Y.-Y. and Sheehan, P.M. (1985) *Fedn Proc.* **44**, 2352–2358.

Yoshida, M.C., Masuda, R. Sasaki, M. et al. (1987) *J. Hered.* **78**, 361–365.

Yoshida, M.C., Sasaki, M. and Masuda, R. (1991) In: Mori, M., Yoshida, M.C., Takeichi, N. and Taniguchi, N. (eds) *The LEC Rat*, pp. 3–10. Berlin: Springer-Verlag.

CHAPTER 19

The Urinary System

Rudolf P Wüthrich
Physiological Institute, University Zürich-Irchel, Zürich, Switzerland

Introduction

As a laboratory animal, the rat has been extensively used to study the physiology of mammalian renal function. Whereas earlier researchers have used larger animals such as dogs and rabbits to elucidate the physiology of the urinary system, the rat has become the focus of these investigations more recently. Therefore, most of the modern knowledge on the function of the kidney has been derived from rat studies, and indeed a vast body of information is available. In this chapter the main functions of the rat kidney will be reviewed. For detailed reference the reader may consult standard references such as the American Physiological Society's textbook on *Renal Physiology* edited by E.E. Windhager (1992).

The principal role of the urinary system is to excrete the waste products which are derived from protein metabolism, and to regulate **electrolyte and water homeostasis** (control of the internal milieu). Additional roles are summarized in Table 19.1 and

include the regulation of red blood cell mass via erythropoietin, the control of blood pressure through the renin-angiotensin-aldosterone system, and the regulation of calcium and phosphate metabolism via $1,25(OH)_2$-vitamin D and parathyroid hormone (PTH).

A variety of pathophysiological alterations can cause perturbations in renal function. Acute or chronic injury to the kidneys results in renal failure which, when progressive, leads to a state of endogenous intoxication termed uremia. The 5/6th nephrectomy model, for example, has been used extensively to study the mechanisms of progression of renal failure in the rat (Brenner, 1985), and valuable therapeutic strategies for human renal diseases could be derived from these experiments (Anderson *et al.*, 1986; Meyer *et al.*, 1987). For reference, Table 19.2 lists some of the spontaneous models and experimental approaches that have been used to investigate the pathophysiological mechanisms of renal disease. A more detailed description of these examples is beyond the scope of the present

Table 19.1 Main physiological functions of the rat kidney

General functions
Clearance of waste products of protein metabolism
Regulation of salt and water metabolism
Regulation of potassium excretion
Regulation of acid–base homeostasis
Regulation of calcium and phosphate metabolism
Regulation of magnesium excretion
Regulation of blood pressure
Regulation of erythropoiesis

Production of hormones
Erythropoietin
Renin and angiotensin II
1,25(OH)$_2$-vitamin D (1α-hydroxylation of 25(OH)-vitamin D)
Prostaglandins
Kinins

Site of action of hormones
Angiotensin II
Aldosterone
Atrial natriuretic peptide (ANP); urodilatin
Endothelin and nitric oxide (NO)
Parathyroid hormone (PTH)
Vasopressin (antidiuretic hormone, ADH)
Uroguanylin

Basic Anatomical Considerations

The rat kidney occurs as a paired organ system which is located in the **retroperitoneal space** in the posterior part of the abdomen. Each adult kidney weighs approximately 0.8–1.4 g. Both kidneys are surrounded by a firm fibrous capsule which can easily be dissected and removed from the kidney. On the concave side of the kidneys lies the hilum through which vessels (renal artery, renal vein, lymphatics) and nerves pass into the renal sinus. On a bisected kidney, a pale outer region (cortex) and a darker inner region (medulla) can be identified (Figure 19.1). The cortex is subdivided into the cortical labyrinth and the medullary rays. The medulla displays three macroscopically recognizable concentric layers. The two external layers are formed by the outer medulla (OM), which is subdivided into outer (OS) and inner stripe (IS); the internal layer is formed by the inner medulla (IM). Internal to the IM lies a single papilla, the rat kidney is therefore also termed unipapillate. The tip of the papilla projects into the cavity of the renal pelvis which

chapter, and the reader may refer to major textbooks on renal disease (Brenner, 1996).

The architecture of the kidney is complex, and renal structure is critical in determining the various aspects of kidney functions. The basic anatomy and histology of the rat urinary system can be found in Chapters 13 to 15, and we will only briefly review here some general anatomical features. Detailed structural aspects of the rat kidney will be discussed below in the context of physiological functions.

Table 19.2 Rat models of renal dysfunction used to study experimental medical problems

Rat model	Corresponding human disease
Hypertension	
Spontaneously hypertensive rat (SHR)	Hypertension
Dahl salt-sensitive/resistant strains	
DOCA-salt treated rat	
1-clip 2 kidney renal artery clamping	Renal artery stenosis (Goldblatt model)
Metabolic disorders	
Brattleboro rat	Diabetes insipidus
Ammonium chloride administration	Metabolic acidosis
Inflammation	
Anti-Thy-1 antibody nephritis	Mesangio-proliferative glomerulonephritis
Heymann nephritis	Membranous glomerulonephritis
Puromycin nephrosis	Minimal change glomerulonephritis
Fisher → Lewis renal transplantation	Chronic renal transplant rejection
Toxicity	
Cyclosporine administration	Cyclosporine nephropathy
Renal cystic diseases	
Han:SPRD rat	Autosomal dominant polycystic kidney disease
Glomerulosclerosis	
5/6 nephrectomy	Chronic renal failure, focal and segmental glomerulosclerosis

collects the final urine and conveys it to the ureter (Kaissling and Dorup, 1995).

The functional units of the kidney are the nephrons. Each rat kidney is composed of approximately 30 000–40 000 nephrons (Baines and de Rouffignac, 1969). Each nephron is composed of a renal (malpighian) corpuscle, which contains the glomerulus, and a tubule (Figure 19.2). Glomeruli are highly vascularized structures whose main function is to produce the ultrafiltrate, which is also termed the primary urine. The tubules are polarized epithelia which can be subdivided anatomically and functionally into various segments. The main function of the tubules is to modify the primary urine by reabsorption, secretion and concentration to produce the final urine, the volume of which is generally <1% of the ultrafiltrate.

Vascularization of the Rat Kidney and Regulation of Renal Blood Flow

Both rat kidneys derive their vascularization from the abdominal aorta via the renal arteries (Figure 19.3). After dividing into interlobar and then into arcuate arteries, the vasculature then gives off the cortical radial arteries which provide the blood to perfuse the glomerular capillaries in the renal cortex via the afferent arteriole. Approximately 30–40% of the renal plasma volume is filtered at

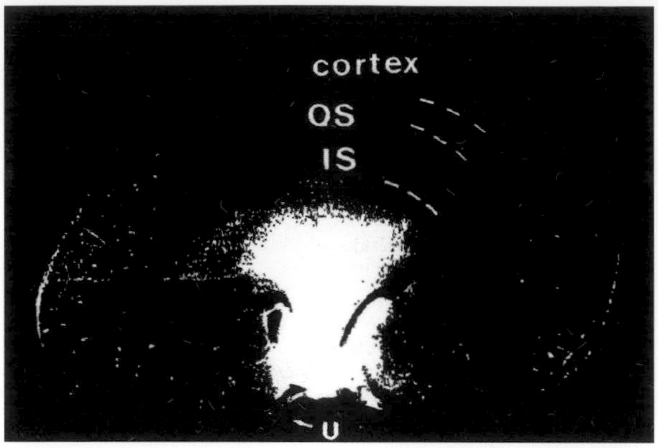

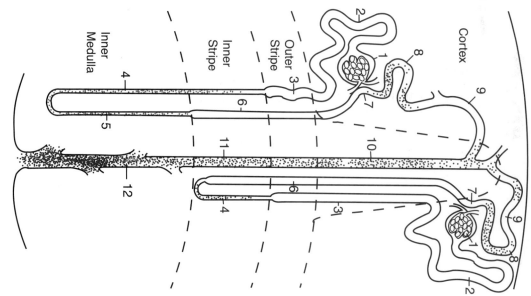

Figure 19.1 Longitudinal section through a unipapillary rat kidney. The cortex overlays the outer medulla (outer stripe (OS) and inner stripe (IS)) and the inner medulla (IM). The papilla (P) belongs to the IM. The ureter (U) leaves the kidney at the hilum. Borders between zones are indicated with broken lines. Arrowheads demonstrate the arcuate vessels which run along the corticomedullary border; small arrows indicate the vascular bundles within the IS. Figure kindly provided by Professor B. Kaissling.

this site through the glomerular barrier, producing a protein-free ultrafiltrate. The blood then leaves the glomerular capillary loops via the efferent arteriole. Blood flow is then **arborized** again into the peritubular capillaries, or it descends the vasa recta into the renal medullary and papillary region. Blood flow finally collects in the renal medullary and papillary region. Blood flow finally collects in the renal venous circulation to leave the kidneys via the renal veins which are draining into the inferior vena cava (Kriz and Bankir, 1988).

Rat renal blood flow (RBF) amounts to approximately 5 mL/min/g kidney weight in the adult rat, corresponding to a renal plasma flow (RPF) of 3 mL/min/g kidney weight. Approximately 30–40% of the RPF is filtered in the glomeruli, corresponding to 0.9–1.2 mL/min/g kidney weight. This represents the glomerular filtration rate (GFR) (Table 19.3).

It may be of practical importance to determine the GFR in the rat. Based on the principle that the clearance of a substance which is freely filtered and not reabsorbed nor secreted is identical to the GFR, one can use plasma creatinine (an endogenous substance which is filtered, not reabsorbed and only slightly secreted) to obtain an estimation of the GFR in the rat. A more precise but also more laborious method is to infuse rats with inulin, a fructose polymer that is also freely filtered and not reabsorbed nor secreted. The clearance of creatinine or

inulin is defined as the volume of plasma required to supply a given amount of these substances in the urine over any time unit. Clearances are calculated by the formula $U \times V / P$ where U and P reflect the plasma and urinary concentrations of creatinine or inulin (same units), and V the urinary flow rate in millilitres per minute (Harvey and Malvin, 1965).

The ability of the kidney to maintain constancy of RBF and GFR over a wide range of perfusion

Figure 19.2 General scheme of nephrons, depicting a short-looped (right side) and a long-looped nephron (left side) together with the collecting system. 1, glomerulus; 2, proximal convoluted tubule; 3, proximal straight tubule; 4, thin descending limb; 5, thin ascending limb; 6, thick ascending limb; 7, macula densa; 8, distal convoluted tubule; 9, connecting tubule; 10, cortical collecting duct; 11, outer medullary collecting duct; 12, inner medullary collecting duct. Reproduced with permission from Kriz and Bankir (1988).

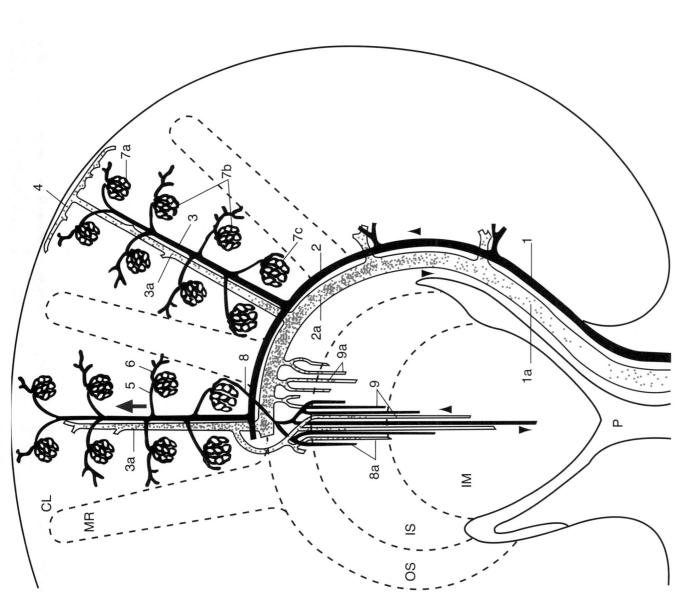

Figure 19.3 Schematic representation of rat renal circulation. Arteries are shown in black, veins in gray. CL, cortical labyrinth; MR, medullary ray; OS, IS, outer and inner stripe of the outer medulla; IM, inner medulla; P, renal pelvis. 1, 1a, Interlobar artery and vein; 2, 2a, arcuate artery and vein; 3, 3a, cortical radial artery and vein; 4, stellate vein; 5, afferent arteriole; 6, efferent arteriole; 7a, 7b, 7c, superficial, midcortical, and juxtamedullary glomeruli; 8, 8a, juxtamedullary efferent arteriole, and descending vasa recta; 9, 9a, ascending vasa recta (ascending within a vascular bundle, and ascending independent from a bundle). Reproduced with permission from Kriz and Bankir (1988).

pressures is called **autoregulation**. This autoregulatory response ensures that both RBF and GFR are held relatively constant when the blood pressure drops or increases (Figure 19.4). This autoregulatory response is mediated by the ability of arterioles to respond to tangential wall tension (**myogenic reflex**), the tubuloglomerular feedback mechanism (see below), as well as the influence of a number of vasoactive hormones such as angiotensin II (Navar et al., 1982).

Table 19.3 Main anatomical and physiological parameters of adult rat kidney function

Anatomy	
Kidney weight	0.8–1.4 g
Kidney dimensions	10 × 6 × 4 mm
Nephron number	30 000–40 000
Hemodynamic and filtration parameters	
Mean arterial blood pressure (BP)	100–120 mmHg
Renal blood flow (RBF)	5 mL/min/g kidney weight
Renal plasma flow (RPF)	3 mL/min/g kidney weight
Glomerular filtration rate (GFR)	0.9–1.2 mL/min/g kidney weight
	1 mL/min/100 g body weight
Filtration fraction (FF)	35–40%
SNGFR	30–40 nL/min
Max. urinary concentrating ability	ca. 2000 mOsm/kg H_2O
Min. urinary concentrating ability	ca. 10 mOsm/kg H_2O
Blood parameters relevant for renal function	
BUN	6.9 mmol/L
Creatinine	42.5 μmol/L
Sodium	135 mmol/L
Potassium	4.9 mmol/L
Calcium	2.6 mmol/L
Phosphate	2.3 mmol/L
Magnesium	1.3 mmol/L
Urinary parameters	
24-hour urine volume	15–30 mL
Urine rate flow	10–20 μL/min
Sodium	200 mmol/L
Potassium	150 mmol/L
Calcium	0.7 mmol/L
Phosphate	25 mmol/L
Creatinine	6 μmol/L
Protein	Trace amounts

This table indicates some of the main parameters of renal function in the rat, including blood and urine values of the most relevant solutes and electrolytes. Data are only approximations and vary significantly from strain to strain, and depend also on the age, sex and diet of the rats. Chemical data are from Waynforth (1980).

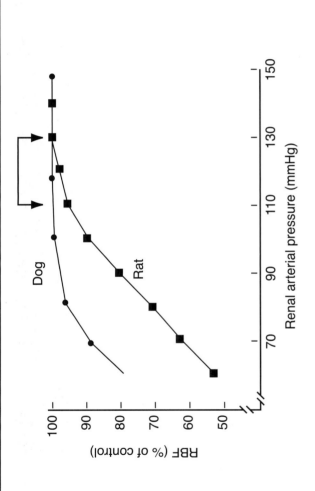

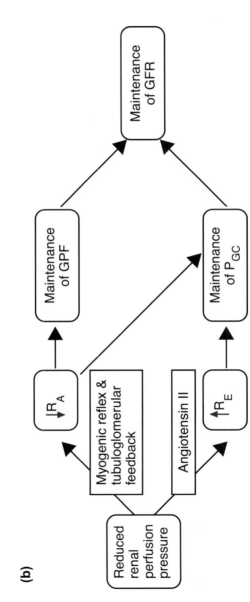

Figure 19.4 Mechanisms of renal autoregulation in the rat. **(a)** Autoregulatory response of renal blood flow (RBF) to lower renal arterial pressure in the rat and dog. The rat has a lower autoregulatory reserve compared with the dog. **(b)** In response to reduced renal perfusion pressure, glomerular plasma flow (GPF), glomerular capillary hydraulic pressure (P_{GC}) and glomerular filtration rate (GFR) are maintained. This occurs via a marked reduction in afferent arteriolar resistance (R_A) and an increase in efferent arteriolar resistance (R_E), by virtue of myogenic reflex, tubuloglomerular feedback and the effect of angiotensin II. Reproduced with permission from Badr and Ichikawa (1988).

Glomerular Structure and Mechanisms of Glomerular Filtration

The renal corpuscles are composed of the glomeruli and Bowman's capsule (Figure 19.5). They are the filtration units where the primary urine is produced and conveyed into Bowman's space. Rat glomeruli measure approximately 120–140 μm in diameter. The glomerular capillaries are composed of thin and fenestrated endothelial cells which are surrounded by a glomerular basement membrane. The latter is covered by visceral epithelial cells, the podocytes. The podocytes form a complex pattern of interdigitating foot processes which are separated

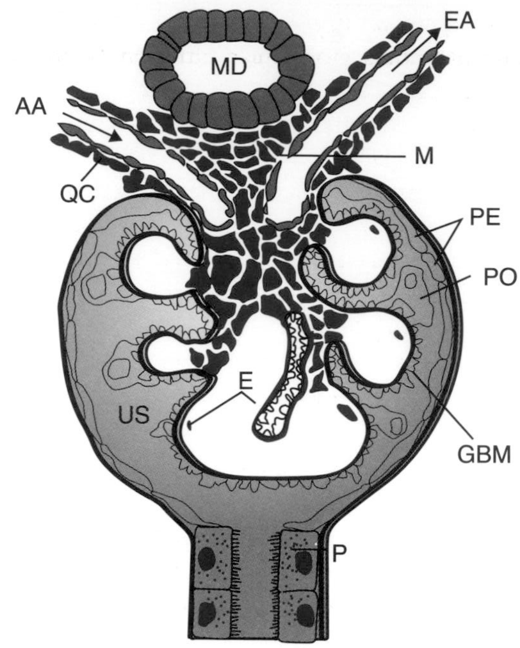

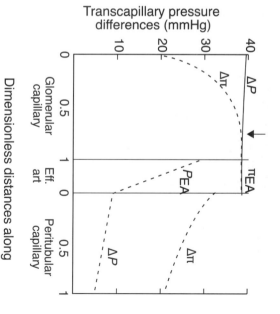

Dimensionless distances along capillary segments

Figure 19.5 Diagram of a longitudinal section of a renal corpuscle and the juxtaglomerular apparatus. Afferent (AA) and efferent arterioles (EA) enter and leave the tuft at the vascular pole. The distal tubule with the macula densa (MD), and the granular cells (GC) which secrete renin are also depicted at the vascular pole. The capillary tuft of the glomerulus consists of a network of specialized fenestrated endothelial cells (E) which are covered by the glomerular basement membrane (GBM). Visceral epithelial cells (podocytes, PO) cover the GBM at the outside of the glomerular capillaries with their numerous extensions, the foot processes, whereas parietal epithelial cells (PE) cover Bowman's capsule to form the urinary space (US) which is continuous with the lumen of the proximal tubule (P). Mesangial cells (M) secreting the mesangial matrix are supporting the glomerular tuft. Modified from Kriz et al. (1998) and Rose and Rennke (1994).

from each other by the slit diaphragm. The glomerular capillaries are supported by the mesangium which is composed of the mesangial cells and the mesangial matrix. The urinary space is delimited by the parietal epithelial cells which are overlying Bowman's capsule, a fibrous structure (Kriz *et al.*, 1998).

The glomerulus is responsible for the production of an ultrafiltrate of plasma. The mean area of filtration surface has been reported to be 0.184 mm² per glomerulus in the rat kidney (Shea and Morrison, 1975). Through this surface, each nephron ultrafiltrates approximately 30–40 nL/min, this is the single nephron glomerular filtration rate (SNGFR). When multiplied by the total nephron number in the rat (ca. 70 000) this amounts to approximately 3–4 liters per day. Considering a final daily urine volume of 15–30 mL in the rat, more than 99% of volume is reabsorbed by the tubular segments.

The driving force for the glomerular filtration is derived from the hydraulic pressure created by the pumping action of the heart. The filtration rate is proportional to the net ultrafiltration pressure (P_{UF}) which exists across the capillary wall. This pressure is determined by the balance of **hydraulic** and **oncotic pressures** that act between the glomerular capillary lumen and Bowman's space (Figure 19.6). In the glomerular capillaries of the rat, the hydraulic pressure gradient (ΔP) is high and relatively constant along the entire length of the glomerular capillaries (ca. 40 mmHg), whereas the oncotic pressure gradient ($\Delta \Pi$) opposing filtration is lower initially (ca. 20 mmHg) but rising along the length of the capillary as protein-free fluid is filtered. Thus, P_{UF} is positive but decreases progressively towards the efferent end of the capillary. When ΔP balances $\Delta \Pi$, filtration pressure equilibrium is said to occur, which means that ultrafiltration becomes zero. In

Figure 19.6 Transcapillary pressure profiles in the rat. The imbalance of hydraulic (ΔP) and oncotic pressures ($\Delta \Pi$) is responsible for filtration in the glomerular capillaries, and for fluid absorption in the peritubular capillaries. Efferent arteriolar oncotic (Π_{EA}) and hydraulic pressures (P_{EA}) are also depicted. In glomeruli, filtration equilibrium occurs towards the efferent end of the glomerular capillaries when $\Delta \Pi$ rises due to the volume contraction of plasma in the lumen (arrow). In peritubular capillaries, the low transcapillary hydraulic pressure is opposed by a much higher oncotic pressure, causing net fluid absorption. Modified from Deen et al. (1973).

pressure upstream in the glomerular capillaries and thereby promotes glomerular filtration. Third, the ultrafiltration coefficient K_f and hence the GFR is influenced by a number of factors, including the state of mesangial cell contraction and the available filtration surface. Fourth, the rate of fluid and electrolyte delivery to the macula densa region of the early distal tubule regulates the GFR via the so-called tubuloglomerular feedback (see below).

Despite a very high permeability of the glomerular capillary wall to water, plasma proteins are excluded almost completely from the primary urine. Whereas molecules with a molecular radius <20 Å are freely filtered, molecules >40 Å in size are completely excluded. This size selectivity is consistent with the presence within the GBM of 'pores' which limit the passage of macromolecules. Size alone does not regulate the passage of macromolecules, however. Negatively charged molecules are impeded and positively charged molecules are facilitated in their transport across the capillary wall (Bohrer et al, 1978). This is due to the presence within the glomerular capillary wall of negatively charged glycoproteins which are rich in sialic acid residues, conferring the so-called charge selectivity to the filtration process (Figure 19.7).

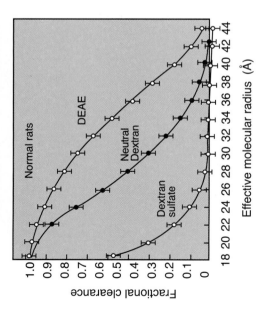

Figure 19.7 The principles of size and charge selectivity of the glomerular barrier are illustrated in the rat. Cationic dextran (DEAE), neutral dextran or anionic dextran sulfate of variable size (18–44 Å) are infused and recovered in the urine. Fractional clearances are calculated as the clearances of the dextrans over inulin (C_{DEAE}/C_{In}). A fractional clearance of 1 means that all dextran molecules are filtered, whereas a fractional clearance of 0 means that nothing is filtered. Both size and charge of the dextran molecules influence C_{DEAE}/C_{In}. Modified from Bohrer et al. (1978).

the normal rat this filtration pressure equilibrium is reached towards the efferent end of the glomerular capillaries (Deen et al, 1973).

An **ultrafiltration coefficient (K_f)** has been defined as a proportionality constant which relates P_{UF} to the filtration rate. K_f depends on the intrinsic water permeability properties of the capillary wall (k) and the available surface (A). Thus,

$$SNGFR = K_f \times P_{UF} = k \times A \times (\Delta P - \Delta \Pi)$$

Each of these determinants can change the SNGFR. A reduction in ΔP, as occurs for example in **hypovolemia**, or a reduction in the filtration surface which develops in various glomerular diseases will decrease SNGFR.

Under normal circumstances, glomerular filtration is a tightly regulated process, and is maintained constant by several mechanisms. First, the flow rate (single nephron RPF) influences the filtration rate, such that higher flow rates increase the SNGFR. Second, various vasoactive hormones, vascular tone and neural stimulation influence the resistance to flow provided by the afferent and efferent arterioles, and thereby determine the hydraulic pressure gradient ΔP. Angiotensin II, for example, is known to increase efferent arteriolar resistance and raises the

Cortical Peritubular Microcirculation and Fluid Reabsorption

Approximately two-thirds of the filtered fluid is reabsorbed at the level of the proximal tubules. This occurs in two phases: (1) translocation of fluid across the tubular epithelium into the peritubular interstitium, and (2) uptake in the peritubular capillary blood. The flux of fluid from the interstitium across the capillary wall is governed by the same interplay of hydraulic and oncotic forces as those that determine glomerular filtration (Figure 19.6).

The oncotic pressure is high in the peritubular capillaries but low in the interstitium, yielding a high $\Delta \Pi$. The peritubular capillaries are nourished by the efferent arteriole, and the hydraulic pressure (ΔP) is always low in this portal type of circulation. The oncotic pressure difference across the peritubular capillary wall therefore always exceeds the hydraulic pressure difference, favoring fluid movement into the capillaries. The pressure gradient is approximately 20–25 mmHg at the beginning of the peritubular capillary and declines to values of 10–15 mmHg towards the end of the peritubular capillary network, due to a dilution of plasma proteins by the reabsorbed fluid. Filtration equilibrium is not reached in this capillary bed, and fluid reabsorption into the peritubular capillaries is always favored (Deen et al., 1973).

Juxtaglomerular Apparatus (JGA) and Tubuloglomerular Feedback (TGF)

In the rat, as in other species, each nephron returns to its glomerulus at the level of a specialized structure termed the juxtaglomerular apparatus (JGA) (Figure 19.5). Specialized cells at the end of the thick ascending limb of the loop of Henle (the macula densa) lie in close proximity to the afferent and efferent arteriole. These cells sense changes in the distal fluid composition. A fall in NaCl concentration will be detected and will cause vasoconstriction of the afferent arteriole, resulting in a reduction of the GFR. This tightly regulated mechanism is termed **tubuloglomerular feedback (TGF)** and helps to preserve volume when distal fluid delivery is excessive. The tubuloglomerular feedback mechanism operates through the secretion of renin by specialized myoepithelial cells in the wall of the afferent arteriole, termed juxtaglomerular cells. In these cells, renin is stored in specific granules. Increased renin will convert angiotensinogen into angiotensin I, generating the vasoconstrictor angiotensin II via angiotensin-converting enzyme (ACE). This results in increased afferent (and efferent) arteriolar vasoconstriction (Figure 19.b). Renin secretion is also controlled by renal nerves which have abundant adrenergic terminals at the vascular pole of each glomerulus.

Tubular Structure and Function

The tubular part of the nephron is composed of a single-layered epithelium. The apical side is in contact with the tubular fluid, whereas the basal side is in contact to a tubular basement membrane which supports the tubules. Individual epithelial cells are held tightly together through a continuous layer of tight junctions. Figure 19.2 shows the various segments of the tubule. Originating from the urinary pole is the proximal tubule, which can be subdivided into a convoluted and a straight part. Following the proximal tubule is the loop of Henle, which is composed of a thin descending part, a thin ascending part and a thick ascending part. The loop of Henle is then followed by the distal convoluted tubule, the connecting segment and finally the collecting duct which drains the final urine into the renal pelvis at the level of the papilla.

The main function of the tubular epithelium is to modify the glomerular ultrafiltrate by reabsorption, secretion and concentration in such a way that the final urine contains a balanced amount of water, salt (NaCl), electrolytes (K^+, Ca^{2+}, Mg^{2+}, PO_4^{3-}, SO_4^{2-}), and waste products of protein metabolism (urea, ammonium) and other metabolic end-products. The rat kidney filters approximately 4 liters of protein-free ultrafiltrate per day. The tubules reabsorb this large amount of filtrate in order to conserve essential nutrients and to reduce the quantity of salt and water in the final urine to less than 1% of the filtered amount, while waste products are still being eliminated.

As a consequence of the unique anatomy of the kidney, two different transepithelial transport pathways must be distinguished in renal epithelium: an active transcellular pathway which uses metabolic energy; and a passive paracellular pathway which does not use energy. The primary active transport mechanism in the rat renal epithelium involves the ubiquitous Na^+, K^+-ATPase pump, which is located on the basolateral side of the epithelium. The Na^+, K^+-ATPase pumps Na^+ out of the cell into the peritubular space in exchange for K^+, with a ratio of 3 Na^+ for 2 K^+. This also generates a negative potential difference of approximately -60 mV for the cell interior. The generation by the Na^+, K^+-ATPase of a low Na^+ concentration within the epithelial cells couples transepithelial transport

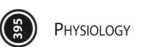

directly with metabolic energy (Lang and Busch, 1995).

Each tubular segment has unique functions in the reabsorption, secretion and concentration process. We will review here the most important functions of each tubular segment.

Proximal Tubular Function

The proximal tubule reabsorbs two-thirds of the tubular fluid and electrolytes, and almost all of the filtered organic compounds such as glucose and amino acids. The total volume of the proximal tubules within the rat kidney cortex amounts to approximately 50% of total cortex volume (Baines and de Rouffignac, 1969). This highlights the abundance of this tubular segment and its major role in fluid reabsorption. The proximal tubule can be subdivided into three different segments termed S1 (convoluted part), S2 (convoluted and straight) and S3 (straight part). The transport capacity decreases from S1 to S3.

The apical side of the proximal tubules possesses a well-developed brush border (formed of microvilli), generating a large surface for reabsorption. Numerous transport systems are located within the plasma membrane of the brush border, including the Na^+/H^+ antiporter (NHE3), Na^+/P_i, $Na^+/$ glucose and $Na^+/$amino acid cotransporters to name a few. At the basolateral side, large interdigitating lateral cell processes and membrane infoldings are developed which contain large mitochondria to provide energy (ATP) for the Na^+,K^+-ATPase. In addition to a large number of specific transport proteins, the apical and basolateral membranes also contain massive amounts of the water channel **aquaporin 1** (Channel-forming integral membrane protein of 28 kDa, CHIP28), which causes a high water permeability of the proximal tubule.

The glomerular ultrafiltrate is reabsorbed at the level of the proximal tubule by a process which is essentially iso-osmotic. Most of the filtered solutes are transported from the tubule fluid into the proximal tubular cells by specific transporters which also combine with Na^+ and are thus sodium-coupled secondary active processes (secondary with respect to the Na^+,K^+-ATPase, which is the primary active transport process driving other transports in the proximal tubule). Figure 19.8a shows the most important transport systems that have been identified in the proximal tubular epithelium. For all these systems, specific rat transport proteins have been characterized at a molecular level.

The proximal tubule is also the site of organic ion secretion; this occurs mainly at the level of the S2 segment. Organic ions are mostly waste products generated by the liver. In addition, many drugs are organic ions (for example antibiotics and diuretics). In the circulation these organic ions are tightly bound to serum proteins such as albumin. Therefore, organic ions are almost not filtered at the glomerular level and need to be secreted by specific active transport mechanisms. Avid tubular secretion lowers the unbound fraction of organic ions in the circulation, leading to their dissociation from the plasma proteins and further secretion. Several basolateral transport systems have been identified in the rat, leading for example to the secretion of substances such as hippurate, oxalate and urate (anions), and creatinine and thiamine (cations).

The proximal tubule is also the site where parathyroid hormone PTH displays its phosphaturic action. PTH acts by inducing a rapid endocytosis of the Na^+/P_i cotransporter by vesicular transport, and this leads to decreased phosphate reabsorption (Murer et al, 1998). In addition, proximal tubules also contain 1α-hydroxylase, the enzyme which is converting inactive 25(OH)-vitamin D into 1,25(OH)$_2$-vitamin D, generating the active form of vitamin D. Proximal tubules therefore play an important role in mineral metabolism.

Loop of Henle

The loop of Henle is located between the proximal and the distal convoluted tubule segments. It comprises a thin descending part, a thin ascending part and a thick ascending part (Figure 19.2). The transition from the proximal tubule to the thin-walled descending limb occurs at the macroscopically discernible border between the inner and outer stripes of the outer medulla. The thin part of the loop of Henle has variable length, forming nephrons with short or long loops; the shorter the loops, the more superficial the corresponding glomerulus. Rats have more short- than long-looped nephrons.

The features of salt and water reabsorption in the different segments of the loop of Henle are as

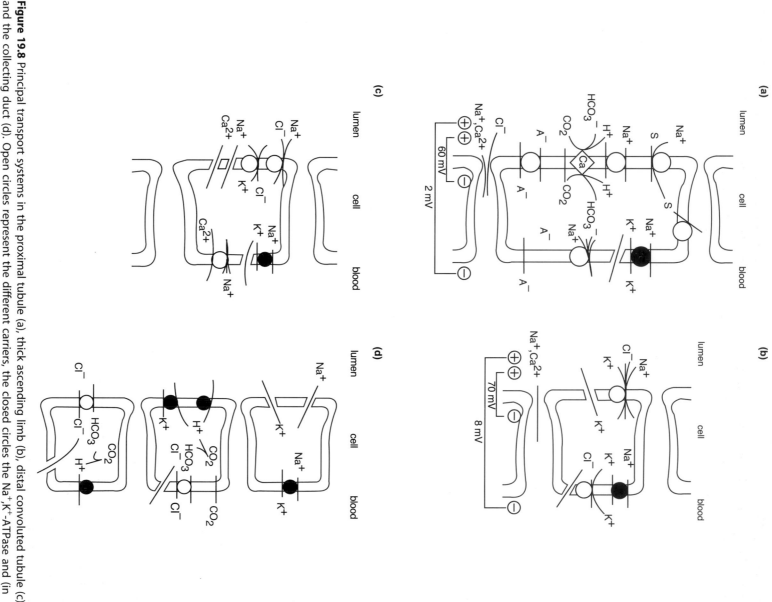

Figure 19.8 Principal transport systems in the proximal tubule (a), thick ascending limb (b), distal convoluted tubule (c) and the collecting duct (d). Open circles represent the different carriers, the closed circles the Na⁺,K⁺-ATPase and (in intercalated cells) the H⁺-ATPase and the H⁺,K⁺-ATPase. Channels are represented by interruptions in the cell membrane. (a) Principal proximal tubular transport systems. Many substrates (S) are translocated by Na⁺-dependent carriers in the apical membrane (glucose, amino acids, Pᵢ). Anions (A⁻) are exchanged apically and basolaterally. Carbonic anhydrase (Ca) generates HCO₃⁻ which is then extruded basolaterally via a Na⁺-dependent HCO₃⁻ transporter. Transtubular and transcellular potential differences are also indicated. (b) Principal transport systems in the TAL. The main transport system is the apically located Na⁺K⁺2Cl⁻ cotransporter. (c) Distal tubular transport systems. The main transporter is the apical Na⁺Cl⁻ cotransporter. Ca²⁺ is reabsorbed apically through channels and extruded basolaterally via a Na⁺/Ca²⁺ exchanger. (d) Transport systems in the collecting duct. Top, principal cell; middle type A intercalated cell; bottom, type B intercalated cell. Reproduced with permission from Lang and Busch (1995).

follows: (1) 25–35% of the filtered NaCl load is reabsorbed, primarily in the thick ascending limb; (2) reabsorption of NaCl occurs in excess of water, causing a fall in osmolality in the tubular fluid. This latter characteristic of transport is due to the relative impermeability of the thin and thick ascending limb (TAL) of the loop of Henle for water. This separation of NaCl and water movement is an essential part of the countercurrent exchange mechanism (see below).

As in the cortical peritubular circulation, the medullary microvasculature (vasa recta) serves two functions, namely to provide metabolic substrates and oxygen to tubule structures, and to remove waste products and water. The net medullary capillary pressure gradient P_{UF} ($\Delta P - \Delta \Pi$) amounts to approximately 20 mmHg, and therefore favors fluid reabsorption in the renal medulla.

In the rat renal medulla, a corticomedullary interstitial solute gradient is formed through the constant removal of solutes (primarily NaCl) in excess of water in the **TAL of Henle**. Osmolalities in the rat renal papilla can reach 2000 mOsm. The dissipation of this solute gradient is efficiently prevented in the medulla by a mechanism which is termed **countercurrent exchange.** Ascending and descending vessels (vasa recta) are arranged adjacent and in parallel, equilibrating osmotically because of their high solute and water permeability. Perfusion of iso-osmolar blood, therefore, does not dilute the concentration gradient along its descending direction along its osmotic gradient. A progressive rise in the osmolality of the descending blood ensues, reaching its maximum at the hairpin turn. When blood in the vasa recta ascends again, the opposite process occurs, and interstitial water is taken up again.

The descending thin segment of the loop of Henle is highly permeable for water but relatively impermeable for solutes, allowing water to be reabsorbed along the rising interstitial concentration gradient. The thin ascending limb is relatively impermeable to water but permeable to NaCl, which diffuses out of the tubule segment along its concentration gradient. Aquaporin 1 (CHIP28) is also present in the water-permeable segments of the loop of Henle, namely the thin descending loop, but it is absent from the thin and thick ascending segments, suggesting that

aquaporin 1 determines water permeabilities in the loop of Henle (Nielsen et al., 1993).

Figure 19.8b demonstrates the basic transport mechanisms that occur in the thick ascending limb of Henle. The TAL actively reabsorbs sodium chloride from the tubular fluid, mainly via the $Na^+K^+2Cl^-$ cotransporter. The absence of any water channels in the TAL probably explains the limited transcellular water flow in the TAL. Subtraction of solutes along this segment of the nephron progressively lowers tubular fluid salt content, and therefore this segment is also named the 'diluting segment'.

Distal Convoluted Tubule

The fine tuning of urinary composition takes place in the distal tubule and the collecting duct. Solute transport capacity is limited in these nephron segments. The tight junctions are poorly permeable, hence all solute transport has to pass the epithelial cells. The transition from the TAL to the distal convoluted tubule (DCT) is distinctly marked by an increase in epithelial height, and functionally coincides with the appearance of the Na^+Cl^- cotransporter in the apical membrane and the disappearance of the $Na^+K^+2Cl^-$ cotransporter. The distal tubule reabsorbs 5–8% of the filtered NaCl, mostly via the Na^+Cl^- cotransporter. The DCT is also the major site at which urinary calcium excretion is actively regulated under the influence of PTH and calcitriol. Ca^{2+} is able to enter the cell down a favorable electrochemical gradient. Within the cell it attaches to a calcium-binding protein and it is extruded at the basolateral membrane via a Ca^{2+}-ATPase and an Na^+/Ca^{2+} exchanger. Figure 19.8c demonstrates the different transport systems in the DCT. The DCT is followed by a short connecting tubule, several of which fuse together to form collecting ducts.

Collecting Duct

The collecting duct is composed of a variety of cell types. The principal cells in the collecting duct play an important role in Na^+ and water reabsorption and in K^+ secretion, whereas the intercalated cells are primarily involved in the regulation of acid–base balance.

Principal cells in the collecting duct are characterized by the presence of amiloride-sensitive luminal Na^+ channels, apical and basolateral K^+ channels, and a basolateral Na^+,K^+-ATPase (Figure 19.8d). Several hormones regulate Na^+ and water reabsorption in principal cells, including the mineralocorticoid hormone aldosterone, atrial natriuretic peptide (ANP) and antidiuretic hormone (ADH). Aldosterone enhances Na^+ reabsorption by increasing the number of open Na^+ channels, whereas ANP reduces the number of open Na^+ channels.

Water channels (mainly aquaporin 2) are abundant in principal cells and are involved in water transport across these cells. Under basal conditions, collecting tubules are relatively impermeable to water due to a low number of aquaporin 2 in the apical membrane. When ADH is released in a state of antidiuresis, it acts via the second messenger cAMP on V_2-receptors and promotes the insertion of preformed water channels in the apical membrane. This then enhances water reabsorption from the collecting tubule fluid. In the hyperosmotic environment of the renal medulla the urine is also concentrated in the presence of ADH. In the absence of ADH, the excreted urine is dilute and its volume is large due to a lack of water reabsorption in the collecting duct.

Intercalated cells are interspersed as single cells in the epithelium. These cells appear darker by light and electron microscopy and have a higher mitochondrial density. The number of intercalated cells decreases from the cortical to the inner medullary collecting duct. Intercalated cells contain very little Na^+,K^+-ATPase but large amounts of an electrogenic vacuolar type H^+-ATPase. They do not contain water channels. Together this explains the role for intercalated cells in acid–base homeostasis.

The intercalated cells can be subdivided morphologically and functionally into type A and type B cells. Morphologically, type A cells have a large apical pole with elaborate infolds, whereas type B cells contain narrowly arranged deep infoldings on the basolateral side. The principal functions of type A cells is to secrete H^+ in the tubular fluid, whereas type B intercalated cells secrete HCO_3^-. This functional difference is explained by the presence of large amounts of H^+-ATPase and H^+,K^+-ATPase on the apical side in type A cells. Alternatively large amounts of H^+-ATPase with subsequent H^+ extrusion on the basolateral side in type B cells promote the secretion of HCO_3^- apically through a Cl^-/HCO_3^- exchanger (Figure 19.8d).

Other Functions of the Rat Kidney

Erythropoietin

The rat kidney is also the main site of erythropoietin production, the most important hormone in the regulation of red blood cell production. Rat erythropoietin is produced by fibroblast-like cells in the peritubular interstitium. It is a circulating hormone that governs the rate of red blood cell production and hence the oxygen-carrying capacity of the blood. In response to anemia or hypoxemia, circulating levels of erythropoietin increase markedly.

Rat erythropoietin is a 34-kDa glycoprotein whose molecular structure has been elucidated (Nagao et al., 1992). It is a protein of 192 amino acids, containing a 26 amino acid signal peptide. A rat erythropoietin receptor has also been characterized (Masuda et al., 1993). It is a 68-kDa cell surface protein, present on the erythroid colony-forming units (E-CFU) in the bone marrow. The erythropoietin receptor is encoded by a single gene; the mRNA has a size of 2.1 kb. The transcript is translated into a 507 amino acid protein containing a 24 amino acid signal peptide. It belongs to the hemopoietin family of receptors, which includes the receptors for GM-CSF, G-CSF and several interleukins.

The erythropoietin gene is transcriptionally regulated. A number of transcription factor-binding sites, including a site for hypoxia-inducible factor (HIF-1) are present in the rat erythropoietin promoter. The precise mechanisms by which changes in oxygen tension regulate erythropoietin expression are still being investigated.

Regulation of Mineral Metabolism

The rat kidney also plays an important role in the regulation of calcium and phosphate homeostasis via the effects of parathyroid hormone (PTH) and vitamin D. PTH is stimulated by a fall in plasma Ca^{2+} and it acts to increase the plasma Ca^{2+} concentration. PTH stimulates Ca^{2+} reabsorption mainly in the distal tubule. The proximal tubule is another site of action for PTH, where it promotes phosphate excretion. PTH also enhances 1,25(OH)$_2$-vitamin D formation by stimulating 1α-hydroxylase activity in proximal tubules. Furthermore, PTH stimulates bone resorption in the presence of permissive amounts of 1,25(OH)$_2$-vitamin D, thereby releasing Ca^{2+} and P_i. The net effect is that PTH raises plasma Ca^{2+} concentrations, while having little effect on the plasma phosphate concentration.

Vitamin D may be regarded as the main hormonal regulator of phosphate homeostasis. Vitamin D is a fat-soluble sterol that is present in the diet. In the liver, vitamin D is converted into the inactive 25(OH)-vitamin D, and then in the kidney by 1α-hydroxylase into 1,25(OH)$_2$-vitamin D, also termed calcitriol. Calcitriol synthesis is promoted by PTH. Calcitriol enhances the absorption of Ca^{2+} and P_i from the intestine, promotes bone resorption in concert with PTH, and decreases Ca^{2+} and P_i excretion by the kidney. The net effects are elevations in both plasma Ca^{2+} and P_i concentrations. Calcitriol is also known to inhibit PTH production and release from the parathyroid gland. This represents an important negative feedback mechanism whereby an excessive elevation of the plasma Ca^{2+} concentration is prevented.

The kidney plays an important role in various complex physiological processes, including the regulation of mineral and electrolyte metabolism and of acid–base homeostasis, control of body water and of blood pressure. A more detailed description of various other physiological functions can be found in major textbooks on renal physiology, for example in Windhager (1992).

orifices of a female rat is nearly half that of a male rat, it is preferable to use anal cups only with the male rats (Waynforth, 1980). More details are given in Chapter 25.

The urinary output in the rat correlates closely with the drinking pattern. Normal urine production amounts to 15–30 ml daily. This may be much more in the Brattleboro rat (a model of diabetes insipidus), and much less in the case of water deprivation. The composition of the urine is also quite variable and depends on diet and metabolic state. Table 19.3 indicates some basic urinary findings solely to provide a guide because these values can vary significantly with strain, age and sex of the rat.

Acknowledgements

The author benefits from continued support by the Swiss National Science Foundation. The helpful comments by Professor B. Kaissling were greatly appreciated.

References

Anderson, S., Rennke, H.G. and Brenner, B.M. (1986) *J. Clin. Invest.* **77**, 1993–2000.

Badr, K.F. and Ichikawa, I. (1988) *New Engl. J. Med.* **319**, 623–629.

Baines, A.D. and de Rouffignac, C. (1969) *Pflügers Arch.* **308**, 260–276.

Bohrer, M.P., Baylis, C., Humes, H.D., Glassock, R.J., Robertson, C.R. and Brenner, B.M. (1978) *J. Clin. Invest.* **61**, 72–78.

Brenner, B.M. (1985) *Am. J. Physiol.* **249**, F324–F337.

Brenner, B.M. (1996) *The Kidney*, 5th edn. Philadelphia: W.B. Saunders.

Deen, W.M., Robertson, C.R. and Brenner, B.M. (1973) *Biophys. J.* **13**, 340–358.

Harvey, A.M. and Malvin, R.L. (1965) *Am. J. Physiol.* **209**, 849–852.

Kaissling, B. and Dorup, J. (1995) In: Greger, R.F., Knauf, H. and Mutschler, E. (eds) *Diuretics*, pp. 1–66. Berlin: Springer.

Kriz, W. and Bankir, L. (1988) *Kidney Int.* **33**, 1–7.

Kriz, W., Gretz, N. and Lemley, K.V. (1998) *Kidney Int.* **54**, 687–697.

Lang, F. and Busch, A. (1995) In: Greger, R.F., Knauf, H. and Mutschler, E. (eds) *Diuretics*, pp. 67–114. Berlin: Springer.

Masuda, S., Nago, M., Takahata, K. *et al.* (1993) *J. Biol. Chem.* **268**, 11208–11216.

Practical Urinary Collection and Analysis

Urine can be collected from rats with the use of metabolic cages. The rat must be confined in a cage with a wire grid floor for a defined interval of time, and urine plus feces can then be collected. Cages can be designed so as to allow separate collection of urine and feces and to prevent the contamination by food and water. To allow clean separation of urine and feces one can also use anal cups which are slipped over the rat's tail against its posterior. Because the distance between the anal and urethral

Meyer, T.W., Anderson, S., Rennke, H.G. and Brenner, B.M. (1987) *Kidney Int.* **31**, 752–759.

Murer, H., Forster, I., Hilfiker, H. *et al.* (1998) *Kidney Int.* **53** (suppl. 65), S2–S10.

Nagao, M., Suga, H., Okano, M. *et al.* (1992) *Biochim. Biophys. Acta* **1171**, 99–102.

Navar, L.G., Bell, P.D. and Burke, T.J. (1982) *Kidney Int.* **22** (suppl. 12), S157–S164.

Nielsen, S., Smith, B.L., Christensen, E.I., Knepper, M.A. and Agre, P. (1993) *J. Cell Biol.* **120**, 371–383.

Shea, S.M. and Morrison, A.B. (1975) *J. Cell Biol.* **67**, 436–443.

Waynforth, H.B. (1980) *Experimental and Surgical Technique in the Rat.* London: Academic Press.

Windhager, E.E. (1992) *Renal Physiology: Handbook of Physiology* (edited by the American Physiological Society). New York: Oxford University Press.

CHAPTER 20

Endocrinology

Satoshi Ohkura
Primate Research Institute, Kyoto University, Aichi, Japan

Hiroko Tsukamura
Graduate School of Bioagricultural Sciences, Nagoya University, Nagoya, Japan

Kei-ichiro Maeda
Graduate School of Bioagricultural Sciences, Nagoya University, Nagoya, Japan

Introduction

The rat is a good model for investigating the endocrine system, because the endocrine organs are of a reasonable size, being neither too small nor too big. This enables scientists to remove the organs or replace test substances easily at the laboratory level. Many different kinds of hormones have been isolated and identified in the rat, including hormones first identified in other animal species. This chapter reviews the functions of each endocrine organ, particularly their major hormones and the regulatory mechanisms for hormone release in the rat.

Hypothalamus

The hypothalamus is positioned at the base of the diencephalon and surrounds the third ventricle. Hypothalamic neuroendocrine cells synthesize hypothalamic hormones that stimulate or inhibit the secretion of hormones from the anterior pituitary gland. These releasing/inhibiting hormones are discharged from the neuronal terminals located in the median eminence and diffuse into the capillaries where they are carried to the anterior pituitary gland via the pituitary portal system to regulate synthesis and secretion of anterior pituitary hormones.

Neuroendocrinology began with Geoffrey Harris's famous experiments in the rat in which he cut the pituitary stalk with a small knife and found the atrophy of the endocrine organs (Harris, 1955). In this context, the rat is the major experimental animal in this field.

Gonadotropin-Releasing Hormone

Gonadotropin-releasing hormone (GnRH) is a polypeptide hormone of 10 amino acid residues which was originally isolated from the pig (Matsuo et al., 1971) and sheep (Burgus et al., 1972). The amino acid sequence of the GnRH molecule found in the rat hypothalamus is identical to that in other mammalian species (Sherwood et al., 1993). The decapeptide is synthesized by neurons which are mainly located in the regions anterior to the hypothalamus, such as the medial preoptic area, medial septum and the diagonal band of Broca in the rat (Kawano and Daikoku, 1981; Witkin et al., 1982; Silverman et al., 1994). GnRH stimulates the secretion and synthesis of two gonadotropins, luteinizing hormone (LH) and follicle-stimulating hormone (FSH), from the anterior pituitary gland. It binds to G protein-coupled receptors on pituitary gonadotrophs, and stimulates inositol triphosphate (IP$_3$) production and Ca^{2+} mobilization as a second messenger (Clayton, 1989). In almost all species, including the rat, GnRH is released into the pituitary portal vessels in a pulsatile manner (Clarke and Cummins, 1982; Moenter et al., 1992) and each GnRH pulse is the consequence of a synchronous burst of the GnRH neurons (Kawakami et al., 1982; Nishihara et al., 1994; O'Byrne and Knobil, 1994). Pulsatile GnRH release is believed to be regulated by the hypothalamic neural mechanism, called GnRH pulse generator (Dyer and Robinson, 1989; Maeda et al., 1995). GnRH is also known as LH-releasing hormone (LHRH). The existence of FSH-releasing hormone that exclusively stimulates FSH release is still under debate (Lumpkin et al., 1989).

Corticotropin-Releasing Hormone

Corticotropin-releasing hormone (CRH) is a 41 amino acid polypeptide (Vale et al., 1981, 1983) which is produced primarily in neurons in the PVN in the rat (Antoni, 1986). CRH stimulates the secretion of adrenocorticotropic hormone (ACTH), β-lipotropin (β-LPH), and β-endorphin from the anterior pituitary gland. All these hormones are processed from a common prohormone, proopiomelanocortin (POMC). CRH is also known to be an inhibitor of GnRH release at the hypothalamic level (Rivier et al., 1986; MacLusky et al., 1988). The release of CRH is augmented in response to stressful stimuli to activate the hypothalamo-pituitary-adrenal axis (Antoni, 1986; Maeda et al., 1994). There are two types of CRH receptors, CRF1 and 2 (Perrin et al., 1993; Lovenberg et al., 1995; Grigoriadis et al., 1996). A 40 amino acid peptide, urocortin, has been found in the rat brain and binds to CRF2 receptor with a higher affinity than CRH (Vaughan et al., 1995). α-Helical CRF is one of the most effective antagonists to the CRH receptors (Rivier et al., 1984), while several more potent antagonists have been reported (Gulyas et al., 1995).

Thyrotropin-Releasing Hormone

Thyrotropin-releasing hormone (TRH) is a three amino acid peptide hormone (O'Leary and O'Connor, 1995). The cell bodies of the neurons which synthesize and secrete TRH are located primarily in the hypothalamic paraventricular nucleus (PVN) in the rat (Lechan and Jackson, 1982). TRH regulates the synthesis and secretion of thyroid-stimulating hormone (TSH) from the anterior pituitary gland. It has also been reported that TRH has an activity as a potent prolactin-releasing factor (Bjoro et al., 1990; Lamberts and Macleod, 1990). The complementary DNAs of the TRH receptor have been cloned from several species including the rat, and the amino acid sequences show the TRH receptor is a seven transmembrane-spanning G protein-coupled receptor (Gershengorn and Osman, 1996).

Growth Hormone-Releasing Hormone and Somatostatin

Growth hormone-releasing hormone (GHRH) is a polypeptide which stimulates growth hormone (GH) secretion. In the rat, GHRH is composed of 43 amino acids, although the other mammalian GHRH (human, bovine, ovine, porcine) has 44 amino acid residues (Spiess et al., 1983). GHRH acts on pituitary **somatotrophs** through G protein-linked receptor and cyclic adenosine monophosphate (AMP), acting as a second messenger system (Mayo, 1992). The amino acid sequence homologies show that the rat GHRH receptor belongs to a family of seven membrane-spanning receptors for secretin, calcitonin, parathyroid hormone, vasoactive intestinal peptide (VIP), glucagon-like peptide 1 (GLP-1) and glucagon (Segre and Goldring, 1993). GHRH-producing neurons predominantly occur in the arcuate nucleus in the rat (Horvath and Palkovits, 1988).

On the other hand, somatostatin has an inhibitory action on GH release by preventing cyclic AMP generation in somatotrophs (Bluet-Pajot et al., 1998). The periventricular nucleus of the anterior hypothalamus and the amygdala are two major sites where somatostatin-containing neuronal cell bodies are found in the rat (Kawano and Daikoku, 1988; Epelbaum et al., 1994; Fodor et al., 1994). There are two forms of somatostatin in the median eminence, these being composed of 14 and 28 amino acid residues (Epelbaum et al., 1994). To date, five subtypes of the rat somatostatin receptor (sst1–5) have been cloned (Epelbaum et al., 1994; Meyerhof, 1998). These receptors belong to the superfamily of G protein-linked receptors with seven membrane-spanning domains and are assumed to serve distinct biological functions (Meyerhof, 1998).

Prolactin-Releasing and -Inhibiting Factors

It is currently accepted that the prolactin-inhibiting factor (PIF) is dopamine (Ben-Jonathan, 1985). Among the known dopaminergic neuronal cell groups, tuberoinfundibular dopaminergic (TIDA) neurons play an inhibiting role in prolactin secretion in the rat (Ben-Jonathan, 1985). With regard to the prolactin-releasing factor (PRF), TRH (Tashjian et al., 1971; Bjoro et al., 1990; Lamberts and Macleod, 1990), vasoactive intestinal peptide (VIP) (Kato et al., 1978; Bjoro et al., 1990; Lamberts and Macleod, 1990), neurotensin, substance P (Rivier et al., 1977) and oxytocin (Lumpkin et al., 1983) are considered as the candidates for the PRF from rat studies. Recently, a novel hypothalamic peptide with potent prolactin-releasing activity on rat anterior pituitary cells has been isolated and named prolactin-releasing peptide (PrRP) (Hinuma et al., 1998; Matsumoto et al., 1999), which has two molecular forms, one with 31 amino acid residues and another with 20 amino acids. PrRP neurons are widely distributed in the brain and might play a role as a neurotransmitter or neuromodulator (Maruyama et al., 1999).

Pituitary

The pituitary gland is located just beneath the hypothalamus (Imura, 1994). Developmentally, the adenohypophysis and neurohypophysis originate in the Rathke's pouch from the embryonic pharynx and neural tissues from the bottom of the third ventricle, respectively (Dubois and ElAmraoui, 1995). The pituitary gland can be divided into three: the anterior lobe, the intermediate lobe and the posterior lobe. The anterior pituitary has a humoral connection to the hypothalamus with the hypophysial portal system. On the other hand, the posterior pituitary gland is connected to the hypothalamus by the hypothalamo-hypophysial tract from the supraoptic nucleus (SON) and paraventricular nucleus (PVN) (Imura, 1994). Most of the rat anterior pituitary hormones, such as LH, FSH, TSH, prolactin, GH and ACTH, and their radioimmunoassay kits can be obtained from the National Hormone and Pituitary Program, USA for research purposes only.

Anterior Pituitary Hormones

Luteinizing hormone

Luteinizing hormone (LH) is a glycoprotein hormone (32 kDa) that consists of two polypeptide subunits, α and β, each of which has carbohydrate moieties (Combarnous, 1992). The α subunit is common to LH, FSH and TSH, which are all considered to have evolved from the same ancestral molecule. LH is produced by a specific type of secretory cell in the anterior pituitary called the **gonadotroph** (Imura, 1994). LH acts on testes and ovaries to stimulate synthesis of one kind of sex steroid hormones, the androgens, in both males and females (Norris, 1996). LH binds to a G protein-coupled receptor in the gonads and produces cyclic AMP as a second messenger (Norris, 1996). The LH receptor has a common feature of glycoprotein hormone (such as FSH and TSH) receptors: this subfamily of G protein-coupled receptors possesses a large extracellular domain in its structure (Combarnous, 1992).

In females, ovulation is induced by the massive release of LH (LH surge) (Karsch, 1984). Moreover, LH is also called luteotropin, because the glycoprotein causes formation of corpus luteum from the ruptured ovarian follicles after ovulation (luteinization) and is involved in progesterone synthesis by the corpus luteum, cooperating with prolactin in the rat (Norris, 1996). In almost all species, including the rat, the tonic mode of LH secretion shows a pulsatile manner (Gay and Sheth, 1972). Each LH pulse corresponds to a GnRH pulse generated by the putative hypothalamic mechanism in the rat (Maeda *et al.*, 1995). Changes in frequency of LH pulses is thought to be a most important factor controlling gonadal activity.

Follicle-stimulating hormone

Follicle-stimulating hormone (FSH) is a glycoprotein hormone (32 kDa) that consists of two subunits, α and β (Combarnous, 1992). The gonadotrophs in the anterior pituitary also produce FSH. FSH acts on gonads to stimulate follicular development in the female rat and spermatogenesis in the male (Sharpe, 1994; Norris, 1996). It is also involved in stimulating the activity of aromatase which converts androgens to estrogens in both genders. It acts through G protein linked-membrane receptors, in a similar manner to LH, to promote cyclic AMP production (Norris, 1996). The rat FSH receptor cDNA has been cloned and sequenced, and the FSH receptor belongs to a subfamily of glycoprotein hormone receptors which possess a large extracellular domain (Combarnous, 1992). The secretion of FSH is regulated not only by the release of GnRH from the hypothalamus, but also by the release of inhibin (inhibitory action) and activin (stimulatory action) from the gonad (see below).

Thyroid-stimulating hormone

Thyroid-stimulating hormone (TSH) is a glycoprotein hormone (32 kDa) that also consists of α and β subunits (Combarnous, 1992). The **thyrotroph** is the TSH secretory cell type in the anterior pituitary gland. The main role of TSH is in stimulating biosynthesis and release of the thyroid hormones stored in the thyroid gland (Magner, 1990). It acts through a subfamily of G protein-coupled receptors and the cyclic AMP second messenger system (Combarnous, 1992). TSH secretion from the pituitary gland is primarily controlled by hypothalamic TRH release.

Growth hormone

Growth hormone (GH) is a peptide hormone composed of 191 amino acids and synthesized by somatotrophs in the anterior pituitary gland (Imura, 1994). From the evolutionary point of view, GH is considered to share a common ancestral molecule with prolactin. It has general growth-promoting actions in the body (Norris, 1996) and stimulates the absorption of amino acids and their incorporation into proteins in muscle cells. In the liver and other tissues, GH stimulates the synthesis and secretion of insulin-like growth factors (IGFs), which induces cartilage and bone growth. The GH receptor molecule in the rat and other species has been identified as having one transmembrane domain and to lack kinase activity (Mathews, 1991). There is a strong sequence identity between the GH and the prolactin receptors in both the extracellular and cytoplasmic domains, suggesting that these two receptors evolved from a common ancestor (Boutin *et al.*, 1988). Moreover, both GH and prolactin receptors are members of a family of cytokine receptors, including the receptors for interleukins, colony-stimulating factors and interferons; this receptor family is defined by a striking homology of binding domains (Bazan, 1990; Kelly *et al.*, 1992). The basal GH secretion in the rat shows a pulsatile pattern which is under control of hypothalamic GHRH (stimulating factor) and somatostatin (inhibiting factor) release (Bertherat *et al.*, 1995; Bluet-Pajot *et al.*, 1998).

Prolactin

Prolactin is a peptide hormone composed of 198 amino acids and is produced by the lactotroph in the anterior pituitary gland (Imura, 1994). The prolactin molecule is a member of the lactogenic hormone (prolactin, GH and placental lactogens) gene family (Niall *et al.*, 1971). It is known that prolactin has a wide variety of actions on body functions in different species (Meites, 1988). These include effects related to reproduction, growth and development, water and electrolyte balance, and integumentary structures. In addition, it plays a key role first in the maintenance of luteal function and then on progesterone secretion during pseudopregnancy, pregnancy and lactation in the rat (Freeman, 1994). There have been reports suggesting that prolactin suppresses gonadotropin secretion in the rat (McNeilly, 1994). Two different forms (short and long) of the prolactin receptor have been identified by cloning their cDNAs in the rat (Kelly *et al.*, 1992). The structure of those prolactin receptors is similar to that of GH and cytokine receptors which do not have any kinase activity (Boutin *et al.*, 1988; Kelly *et al.*, 1992). The release of prolactin is mainly regulated by the hypothalamic inhibitory mechanism, i.e. the tuberoinfundibular dopaminergic (TIDA) system (Ben-Jonathan, 1985).

Adrenocorticotropic hormone

Adrenocorticotropic hormone (ACTH) is a single-chain peptide hormone composed of 39 amino acid residues. In the anterior pituitary, the ACTH molecule is produced in corticotrophs by cleavage of a prohormone known as proopiomelanocortin (POMC) (Norris, 1996). It stimulates secretion of the adrenal glucocorticoids and also has a variety of biological activities in other tissues, including the brain. The ACTH receptor is called the melanocortin 2 (MC2) receptor, a G protein-linked membrane receptor, which is a member of the melanocortin receptor family (MC1–5) (Mountjoy and Wong, 1997). MC2 receptors are expressed in the adrenal cortex (Mountjoy et al., 1992) and adipocytes (Boston and Cone, 1996). ACTH can bind to the other members of the MC receptor family with less affinity and its secretion is controlled by CRH release from the hypothalamus. It is known to increase in response to stress stimuli.

Intermediate Lobe Hormones

Melanocyte-stimulating hormone

Melanocyte-stimulating hormone (MSH) is a polypeptide hormone. Three different molecules (α, β and γ) have been found to date. MSHs are processed from a prohormone, POMC, by enzymatic cleavage (Norris, 1996). In reptiles, amphibians and fishes, MSH causes diffusion of melanin granules contained in the melanophore, so enabling animals to turn their skins darker when required. In the mouse, circulating α-MSH binds to the MC1 receptor expressed in the melanocyte of the hair follicle in order to control hair color (Mountjoy et al., 1992). α-MSH has been found to be widely distributed in the brain (Umegaki et al., 1983) and is involved in feeding behavior in the rat (Friedman, 1997; Mountjoy and Wong, 1997). Melanocortin 3 (MC3) and 4 (MC4) receptors are located in the various regions of the brain and mediate MSH action in the brain overall (Mountjoy et al., 1994).

Proopiomelanocortin

Proopiomelanocortin (POMC) is a prohormone for ACTH, MSH, lipotropin (LPH), corticotropin-like peptide (CLIP), and β-endorphin and is synthesized in the anterior and intermediate lobes (Norris, 1996). POMC is cleaved by proteolytic enzymes to yield the above-mentioned hormones in anterior or intermediate pituitary cells.

Posterior Pituitary Hormones

Oxytocin

Oxytocin is a peptide neurohormone composed of nine amino acid residues (Norris, 1996). This nonapeptide is produced by magnocellular neurons in the paraventricular nucleus (PVN) and the supraoptic nucleus (SON) of the hypothalamus in the rat (Jirikowski et al., 1988). The peptide is released into the circulation from the nerve terminals in the posterior pituitary. The action and regulatory mechanism of oxytocin have been well established by experiments in the rat. Oxytocin stimulates contraction of the myoepithelial cells, aligning the mammary alveoli and ducts of the mammary gland, and induces milk ejection. Oxytocin release during milk ejection is maintained through a neuroendocrine reflex known as the milk-ejection reflex: the suckling stimulus of the newborns on the nipples of the mother is transmitted to the hypothalamus, which induces oxytocin release from the posterior pituitary (Wakerley et al., 1994).

Another particular action of oxytocin is the induction of uterine smooth muscle contraction during labor (Challis and Lye, 1994). In this case, oxytocin secretion is induced by the stimulation of the vaginal cervix, known as the Ferguson reflex. It is also produced locally in the uterus during labor probably for the induction of uterine contraction (Zingg et al., 1995). Oxytocin causes the contraction of the smooth muscles of the reproductive tract in both male and female rats (Norris, 1996).

The cDNA encoding rat oxytocin receptor has been cloned and sequenced (Rozen et al., 1995). The receptor belongs to the group of G protein-coupled receptors with seven transmembrane domains and forms a receptor family together with the vasopressin V1a, V1b and V2 receptors due to the similarities of their amino acid sequences (Peter et al., 1995; Barberis et al., 1998).

Arginine vasopressin

The other posterior pituitary hormone, arginine vasopressin (AVP), also has nine amino acid residues and is synthesized by magnocellular neurons in the SON and PVN in the rat (Norris, 1996). Brattleboro rats, an AVP-deficient rat strain, has been used to elucidate the physiological roles of the AVP (Kim et al., 1997).

The principal role of AVP is an antidiuretic action on the kidney (Robertson, 1995). AVP increases reuptake of water from the glomerular filtrate and reduces the volume of urine produced. The peptide is therefore also called the antidiuretic hormone. AVP also increases blood pressure through contraction of vascular smooth muscle (Szczepanska-Sadowska, 1996). Stimulation of thirst at the level of the central nervous system is yet another property of AVP (Szczepanska-Sadowska, 1996). An increase in blood osmolality and a decrease in blood pressure stimulates AVP release (Norris, 1996). It is also known as a corticotropic factor cooperating with the CRH (Makara, 1992).

Three subtypes of rat AVP receptors, V1a (Morel et al., 1992), V1b (Lolait et al., 1995) and V2 (Lolait et al., 1992), have been identified. These G protein-coupled receptor subtypes form a receptor family including the oxytocin receptor and each type of receptor is linked to a different cellular mechanism depending on the tissue (Peter et al., 1995; Barberis et al., 1998).

Testis and Ovary

The gonads synthesize and secrete sex steroid hormones such as androgens, estrogens and progestins. These gonadal steroids have a variety of actions, including stimulation of gamete production, development of reproductive organs and expression of secondary sex characters and sexual behavior. In addition, the gonads produce a great variety of nonsteroidal hormones that can also influence gonadal functions.

Gonadal Steroids

Steroid hormones possess a common structure of four carbon rings called the steroid nucleus (Gore-Langton and Armstrong, 1994). They are synthesized

from cholesterol (Figure 20.1). Although steroidogenic tissues synthesize cholesterol from acetate *de novo*, the major source of cholesterol is high-density lipoproteins (HDL) found in the plasma in rats (Gwynne and Strauss III, 1982), but this is not the case for humans. At the first biosynthetic step, cholesterol is converted to pregnenolone with side-chain cleavage. Subsequently, pregnenolone is enzymatically processed via two different transforming pathways, the Δ4 pathway and the Δ5 pathway, transformation to androstenedione occurring through progesterone in the Δ4 pathway and through dehydroepiandrosterone (DHEA) in the Δ5 pathway (Miller, 1988). The dominant biosynthetic pathway is dependent upon species, or secretory cells in the gonads. In the rat, androgen is reported to be synthesized dominantly via the Δ4 pathway in the testis (Hall, 1994).

The synthesis of gonadal steroids is principally under the control of both LH and FSH secretion in both sexes. In the blood, gonadal steroids exist in either a free state or bound to sex steroid-binding proteins in the plasma. These proteins include albumin, gonadal steroid-binding globulin, and corticosteroid-binding globulin (Rosner, 1990). In addition, α-fetoprotein is present in the fetal and neonatal blood (Nunez, 1994). The binding of circulating steroids with plasma proteins may result in the retention of steroids at higher blood concentrations for longer periods.

The mechanism of gonadal steroid action in target cells is as follows. The steroid passes through the cell membranes, diffuses into the nucleus, and finally binds to its specific nuclear receptor to produce a cellular effect (O'Malley, 1984). The steroid-receptor complex binds to a specific hormone-responsive element on DNA as a transcription factor and promotes mRNA synthesis. The steroid receptors together form a large nuclear receptor superfamily including the receptors for estrogen, androgen, progestin, glucocorticoid, thyroid hormones, retinoic acids, etc. (Evans, 1988; Carson-Jurica et al., 1990).

Androgens

Androgens are defined as steroids that stimulate male secondary sexual characteristics (Norris, 1996). Androgens stimulate the development and function of male accessory reproductive organs, and are required for spermatogenesis. They also stimulate the expression of male sexual behavior and

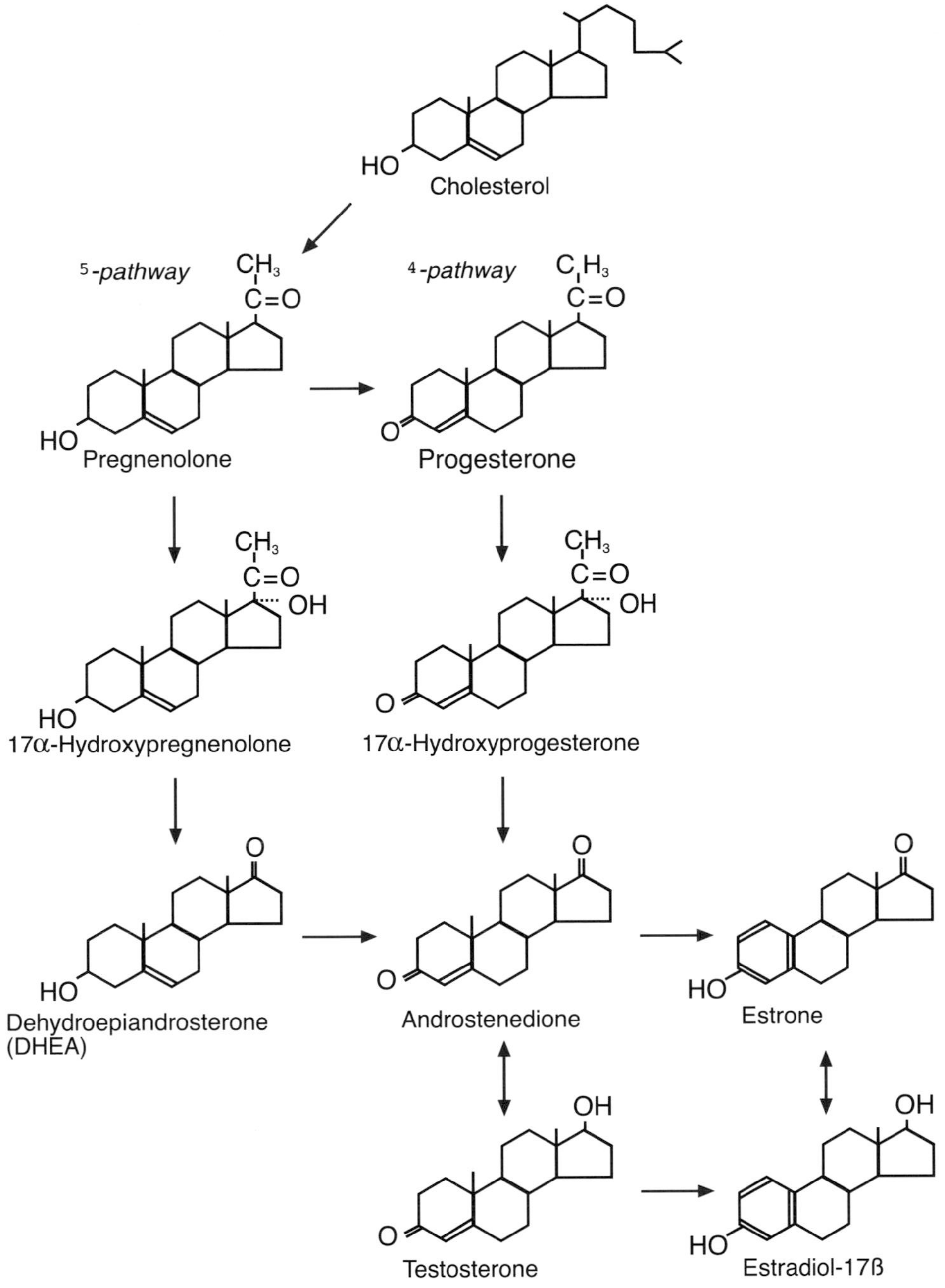

Figure 20.1 Pathways of gonadal steroid biosynthesis from cholesterol.

protein anabolism (Meisel and Sachs, 1994). Moreover, androgens exert a negative feedback effect on gonadotropin secretion.

In the rat, the principal androgen is testosterone. In the male rat, testosterone is mainly synthesized in the Leydig cells predominantly via the Δ4 pathway (Hall, 1994) and its synthesis and secretion is stimulated by LH. The ovary and adrenal cortex are minor sources for testosterone secretion in females (Baird, 1984). The action of testosterone in target organs,

such as external genitalia, is expressed after conversion to 5α-dihydrotestosterone (DHT) by 5α-reductase (Miller, 1988).

Estrogens

Estrogens are defined as compounds that induce estrus and female secondary sexual characteristics (Norris, 1996). In the rat ovary, estrogens are synthesized from androgens by an enzymatic reaction called aromatization (Miller, 1988). LH and FSH stimulate the synthesis of androgens in follicular thecal cells and their conversion into estrogens in the granulosa cells of the follicle, respectively. Estrogens stimulate development and function of female accessory reproductive organs, follicular growth and development, and growth of mammary glands. In the rat, cornification of the epidermal cells of the vagina is apparently under the influence of estrogens, so that the rat estrous cycle can be readily identified from vaginal smears. Estrogens also induce the brain to produce estrous behavior: in the rat, females have to be exposed to estrogens before progesterone exposure in order to enhance the induction of 'lordosis' behavior (Pfaff et al., 1994). They also exert a negative feedback effect on tonic GnRH/gonadotropin release as well as a positive feedback on GnRH release in order to induce a preovulatory gonadotropin surge (Karsch, 1984). There are three forms of natural estrogens: estrone, estradiol-17β and estriol. Among them, the most potent estrogen secreted by the ovary is estradiol-17β.

Progestins

Progestins are responsible for the maintenance of pregnancy, a major progestin being progesterone. The latter is secreted primarily from the corpus luteum in the ovary and a small amount from the adrenal cortex. In contrast to humans, nonhuman primates and sheep, the rat placenta produces little progesterone throughout pregnancy (Heap and Flint, 1984). In the rat, LH and prolactin are the luteotropic factors which stimulate the synthesis and release of progesterone. Progesterone causes relaxation of uterine smooth muscle leading to reduced excitability of the myometrium during pregnancy (Heap and Flint, 1984). The uterine secretion from the endometrium before implantation is maintained by progesterone as well: for expression of this effect, tissues must first be exposed to estrogens (Baird, 1984). Together with estrogens, progesterone also stimulates the development of the mammary glands. In the rat, it plays a positive role during the periovulatory period and a negative role during pregnancy and lactation in regulating gonadotropin secretion. In lactating rats in particular, progesterone secreted from the lactational corpus luteum, developed from postpartum ovulation, inhibits LH secretion in cooperation with the suckling stimulus given by pups (McNeilly, 1994).

Nonsteroidal Ovarian Hormones

Inhibin and activin

Glycoproteins which selectively regulate FSH release from anterior pituitary gland, but not LH secretion, have been isolated from granulosa cells of the ovary and Sertoli cells of the testis in the rat. One is inhibin, the inhibitor of FSH secretion, and the other is activin which is a potent releaser of FSH (Vale et al., 1988; Taya et al., 1991; Mayo, 1994). There are two forms of the inhibin molecule which are heterodimers composed of a common α subunit (18 kDa) and either βA (inhibin A) or βB (inhibin B) subunits (14 kDa). Activins are dimers of the two β subunits and therefore exist in three different forms (activin A, βA/βA; activin AB, βA/βB; activin B, βB/βB) have been isolated (Ying, 1989). The precursor proteins and mature subunits are structurally related, and both inhibins and activins belong to the transforming growth factor β (TGF β) superfamily (Kingsley, 1994). Activin may act on the pituitary to stimulate FSH release as well as within gonads to enhance FSH action, acting as a local regulator (Vale et al., 1988; Findlay, 1993). Inhibin or activin bind to their specific membrane receptors (type I and type II) which both possess serine/threonine kinase activity (Mathews and Vale, 1993).

Follistatin

Follistatin was first isolated from porcine follicular fluid and selectively inhibits FSH secretion (Ueno et al., 1987). Follistatins are single-chain glycosylated polypeptides which have different molecular sizes (31, 32, 35 and 39 kDa) both in porcine (Shimasaki et al., 1988) and bovine (Robertson et al., 1987) follicular fluid. Follistatin inhibits FSH release from rat pituitary cells in vitro (Ying et al., 1987) via binding to and inactivation of activin, as revealed from the rat study of Nakamura et al. (1990).

Uterus

Prostaglandins

Prostaglandins are a group of small lipids derived from arachidonic acid and found in many tissues of the body (Smith *et al.*, 1991; Mitchell and Trautman, 1993). They can be classified into several subgroups on the basis of their structure. Prostaglandins are involved in the physiological events influencing ovarian cellular function in mammalian species. Prostaglandins are synthesized in the uterus in sheep and cows or in the ovary in nonhuman primates and women and have been reported to be closely associated with **luteolysis** during the estrous cycle (Auletta and Flint, 1988). In the rat, the role of prostaglandins in luteolysis during pseudopregnancy or pregnancy has been open to question. There are several reports suggesting that prostaglandin F$_{2\alpha}$ (PGF$_{2\alpha}$) of luteal origin is involved in the spontaneous demise of the corpus luteum in the rat (Olofsson and Norjavaara, 1990; Olofsson *et al.*, 1990; Olofsson *et al.*, 1992). Prostaglandins also play an important role in parturition in the rat (Poyser, 1995). In addition, PGF$_{2\alpha}$ and prostaglandin E$_2$ (PGE$_2$) may be involved in the mechanism for ovulation (Olofsson and Leung, 1996). Prostaglandin receptors are classified as several subtypes: they are termed DP, EP, FP, IP and TP, and a further subdivision for the EP receptor has been reported as EP1–4 (Negishi *et al.*, 1995; Woodward *et al.*, 1997). They are G protein-coupled receptors and are linked to different signal transduction systems.

Placenta

Placental Lactogen

The placenta of mammals has an endocrine role in pregnant females. In rat placenta, several molecules similar to pituitary prolactin are produced, these being known as placental lactogens. There are two forms of placental lactogens in the rat, placental lactogen I (PL-I) and II (PL-II) (Soares *et al.*, 1991). PL-I, which is a glycoprotein secreted as a heterogeneous complex (36–42 kDa), is found in plasma mainly during midgestation (Robertson *et al.*, 1982). On the other hand, PL-II (25 kDa) is not glycosylated and is secreted predominantly during the latter half of pregnancy (Robertson *et al.*, 1982). Rat placental lactogens secreted during pregnancy stimulate the corpus luteum to maintain progesterone secretion, which in turn supports the progress of pregnancy, particularly after midgestation (Soares *et al.*, 1991). Another important action of placental lactogens is to stimulate insulin secretion and the proliferation of pancreatic β-cells during pregnancy in the rat (Brelje *et al.*, 1993; Kawai and Kishi, 1997). Several studies in mouse liver and ovary demonstrate that both types of placental lactogens bind to the same receptors as prolactin (Harigaya *et al.*, 1988; MacLeod *et al.*, 1989) with greater affinity than prolactin. Studies in sheep have suggested the possibility that placental lactogens may have their own unique receptor (Freemark *et al.*, 1987, 1988).

Oxytocin

Oxytocin gene expression has been demonstrated not only in the hypothalamus, but also in the uterus (Lefebvre *et al.*, 1992a), placenta (Lefebvre *et al.*, 1992b), and fetal membranes (Lefebvre *et al.*, 1993) in the rat. Expression of the oxytocin gene in rat uterus appears to increase in late gestation (Lefebvre *et al.*, 1992a) or during pseudopregnancy (Lefebvre *et al.*, 1994b). In contrast, the levels of oxytocin mRNA in rat placenta and fetal membranes decrease as pregnancy progresses during late gestation (Lefebvre *et al.*, 1992b, 1993). These findings in the rat suggest that oxytocin produced by these tissues plays a role in initiating parturition as a **paracrine modulator.** Uterine, but not hypothalamic, oxytocin gene expression also increases between diestrus and proestrus and remains elevated at estrus of the rat estrous cycle (Lefebvre *et al.*, 1994b). It has been suggested that an elevation of oxytocin gene expression during the estrous phase is caused by the synergistic action of ovarian steroids (Lefebvre *et al.*, 1994a).

Heart

Atrial Natriuretic Peptide

Atrial natriuretic peptide (ANP), consisting of 28 amino acid residues in the rat, is known to act at the level of the kidney to increase sodium excretion into the urine (de Bold, 1985). ANP also inhibits aldosterone release from the adrenal cortex. Moreover, ANP suppresses vasopressin release to promote diuresis. Chronic high blood pressure causes ANP release from the atrium of the heart (Rosenzweig and Seidman, 1991). Three types of membrane-bound receptors have been isolated for ANP (Maack, 1992). ANP activates guanylyl cyclase activity after interaction with those receptors and increases cyclic guanosine monophosphate (GMP) levels as a second messenger (Wong and Garbers, 1992). Two additional natriuretic peptides have been found: brain natriuretic peptide (BNP) is a peptide of 45 (rat) or 32 (human) amino acids isolated from the brain and then from the heart; the other is a 22 amino acid peptide called type C natriuretic peptide (CNP) (Rosenzweig and Seidman, 1991).

Adipose Tissue

Leptin

Leptin, a 16-kDa protein, has been identified as an *obese* (*ob/ob*) gene product in the mouse. It is produced in the adipose cells and secreted into the general circulation (Zhang et al., 1994). In recent years, the physiological roles of leptin have been extensively studied in mice and humans rather than rats and it has been attracting clinical and pharmaceutical interests for the potential control of appetite and therefore obesity (Halaas et al., 1995). Intracerebroventricular injection of recombinant leptin decreases food intake at low doses, indicating that leptin exerts its effect on appetite control centrally (Campfield et al., 1995). Plasma levels of leptin are highly correlated with body adiposity in obese humans and rodents (Maffei et al., 1995).

Interest in its reproductive function began with the finding that exogenous leptin injections into normally infertile adult *ob/ob* mice can induce fertility (Barash et al., 1996; Chehab et al., 1996). In particular, leptin has received widespread attention as a metabolic cue to modulate the timing of puberty onset in the mouse (Chehab et al., 1997) and rat (Cheung et al., 1997). Moreover, the short-term regulation of reproductive activity by leptin has been demonstrated in the adult female mouse and rat (Ahima et al., 1996; Nagatani et al., 1998).

The structure of the leptin receptor has been determined as a single membrane-spanning receptor and belongs to a family of prolactin/GH and cytokine receptors (Tartaglia et al., 1995). The receptor itself does not have any kinase activity in the intracellular domain (Bazan, 1990; Miller and Bell, 1996). Leptin receptor mRNA is expressed in the hypothalamus as well as the choroid plexus in the mouse (Tartaglia et al., 1995). In the rat, it has also been reported that leptin receptors are localized in the hypothalamus (Schwartz et al., 1996).

Thyroid Gland

Thyroid Hormones

The thyroid gland produces two separate thyroid hormones called thyroxine/tetraiodothyronine (T4) and triiodothyronine (T3) under the control of TSH. T4 and T3 are synthesized from two iodinated tyrosines by coupling with each other in the follicular cells of the thyroid gland, and have 4 or 3 iodine atoms per molecule, respectively (McNabb, 1993). Thyroid hormones are conjugated with thyroglobulins and stored in the lumen of thyroid follicles which is filled with a protein-rich fluid termed colloid. In general, T4 is the major circulating compound and is deiodinated enzymatically in the liver or target cells to form T3 (McNabb, 1993).

Most of the circulating thyroid hormones are transported to target tissues by binding to plasma proteins, thyroid hormone binding proteins, such as thyroxine-binding globulin and thyroxine-binding prealbumin and albumin. Thyroid hormones are important for the metabolism, reproduction, growth, and development in mammals including the rat (McNabb, 1993). These actions are mostly exerted in cooperation with other hormones. At the target tissues, thyroid hormones enter the cells and bind to their nuclear receptors which belong to the steroid/thyroid hormone receptor superfamily (Yen and Chin, 1994). There are two major thyroid hormone receptor isoforms, TRα-1 and TRβ-1, but several other isoforms have been discovered as well (Lazar, 1993). Following the binding to receptors, thyroid hormones interact with nuclear DNA to initiate gene transcription. Since these receptors have greater affinity for T3 than T4, T3 has more potent effect on metabolism and preconversion of T4 to T3 is required for the thyroid hormone action (Norris, 1996).

Calcitonin

Parafollicular cells of the thyroid gland, called the C cells, secrete the hypocalcemic hormone calcitonin. Rat calcitonin is a single-chain polypeptide of 32 amino acid residues (Azria, 1989). Calcitonin is released in response to high plasma calcium concentrations and promotes the deposition of calcium into bone to decrease plasma calcium levels (Azria, 1989). This hypocalcemic effect of calcitonin is ascribed to the prevention of bone resorption by inhibiting the activity of osteoclasts. Calcitonin is known to enhance cyclic AMP accumulation in target cells through the G protein-coupled calcitonin receptor (Lin et al., 1991), whose amino acid sequence is similar to a receptor family for GHRH, secretin, parathyroid hormone, VIP and glucagon (Segre and Goldring, 1993).

Parathyroid Gland

The main function of the parathyroid gland is to synthesize and release parathyroid hormone (PTH) from chief cells. Rat PTH is a polypeptide composed of 84 amino acids and plays an indispensable role in calcium homeostasis as a hypercalcemic factor (Mallette, 1991). PTH causes calcium mobilization from bones and enhances calcium reabsorption by the kidneys: these actions cause an elevation in plasma calcium concentrations (Mallette, 1991; Dempster et al., 1993). The secretion of PTH is stimulated by a low level of plasma calcium and is inhibited by high plasma calcium concentrations (Mallette, 1991). Calcitonin secreted from the thyroid gland antagonizes the action of PTH on bone. The rat PTH receptor has been cloned (Juppner et al., 1991) and its amino acid sequence indicates that it belongs to the same family as the calcitonin receptor (Segre and Goldring, 1993).

Adrenal Gland

The adrenal gland consists of two separate endocrine glands, the medulla and the cortex, which secrete several adrenal hormones. Adrenal hormones promote changes in metabolism and ionic regulation.

Adrenal Medulla

Catecholamines

The medullary portion of the adrenal gland is composed of secretory cells which are ontogenically homologous to postganglionic sympathetic neurons (Mulrow, 1986). These secretory cells, which are called chromaffin cells, release either epinephrine or norepinephrine directly into the blood circulation.

Small amounts of dopamine are also released from the adrenal medulla. The release of adrenal catecholamines is primarily under the direct neural control of ganglionic cholinergic sympathetic neurons innervating the adrenal medulla (Mulrow, 1986). A variety of stressful stimuli induce adrenal catecholamine release to the general circulation (Brown et al., 1990). In addition, ACTH and glucocorticoids also exert a stimulatory effect on the secretion of epinephrine and norepinephrine (Mulrow, 1986). All adrenal catecholamines are enzymatically synthesized from the common amino acid tyrosine. Both epinephrine and norepinephrine promote the breakdown of glycogen to glucose in liver or muscle cells (Mulrow, 1986). Adrenal catecholamines also stimulate the contraction of cardiac muscle cells. Adrenergic receptors are categorized as α and β receptors. Both are further divided into two subtypes of receptors, i.e. $\alpha1$ and $\alpha2$ receptors, and $\beta1$ and $\beta2$ receptors (Caron and Lefkowitz, 1993; Strosberg, 1993).

Adrenal Cortex

The adrenal cortex, which surrounds the adrenal medulla, is composed of lipid-containing, steroidogenic adrenocortical cells that secrete adrenal steroid hormones. Adrenal steroid hormones include glucocorticoids, mineralocorticoids and androgens that have weak potency, such as dehydroepiandrosterone (DHEA). Adrenal steroids are synthesized from cholesterol through the same pathway as the sex steroid hormones (Miller, 1988). The adrenal cortex is divided into the following three regions according to their histological characteristics: the zona glomerulosa, zona fasciculata and zona reticularis (Mulrow, 1986).

Glucocorticoids

Glucocorticoids are generally defined as steroids that affect glucose metabolism. The major glucocorticoids in mammals are cortisol and corticosterone. These glucocorticoids are secreted from the zona fasciculata and zona reticularis of the adrenal cortex under the primary control of ACTH from the anterior pituitary (Mulrow, 1986). In the rat, the primary glucocorticoid is corticosterone, while the other species, such as human and sheep have cortisol as a primary glucocorticoid (Norris, 1996). Corticosterone is one of the key hormones in energy metabolism, since it raises blood glucose levels by inhibiting glucose utilization by peripheral tissues and by enhancing the conversion of amino acids into glucose (gluconeogenesis) (Mulrow, 1986). In addition, adaptations to a certain kind of stressor can be obtained by the mediation of glucocorticoids. There are many glucocorticoid receptors in various regions of the brain, implying that the steroid is involved in regulating brain function in response to stressful stimuli. The glucocorticoid receptor is a member of the nuclear receptor superfamily (Evans, 1988; Carson-Jurica et al., 1990).

Mineralocorticoids

Mineralocorticoids regulate Na^+ and K^+ balance in the body fluids. The major ones in the rat are aldosterone and deoxycorticosterone (Funder, 1993). Aldosterone is the most potent mineralocorticoid and is released from the zona glomerulosa of the adrenal cortex. Release of aldosterone is regulated mainly by the renin-angiotensin system (see below). The primary action of aldosterone is to maintain the normal Na^+–K^+ balance by promoting Na^+ reabsorption into the blood and K^+ excretion into the urine in the kidney (Funder, 1993). Aldosterone also exerts an effect on regulation of the volume of extracellular fluid. It binds to the nuclear receptor, which is also a member of the nuclear receptor superfamily (Funder, 1993).

Binding proteins

Most of the glucocorticoids, but not mineralocorticoids, exist in the blood as a form bound to a specific plasma transport protein known as the corticosteroid-binding globulin (Rosner, 1990), which is synthesized by the liver. Some glucocorticoids also bind to albumin in the blood. These binding proteins are considered to play a role as a buffer reservoir for free steroid hormones: free hormones are available for movement out of capillaries and into target cells.

Kidney

Renin-Angiotensin

The renin-angiotensin system is a feedback control mechanism for the synthesis and release of

aldosterone, a mineralocorticoid (Vallotton et al., 1990). Renin, which is a glycoprotein enzyme (40 kDa), is released from the juxtaglomerular apparatus in the kidney in response to a decrease in sodium concentrations of extracellular fluids or in blood pressure (Norris, 1996). Renin converts the angiotensinogen to angiotensin I in the blood. Then angiotensin I is converted by the angiotensin-converting enzyme (ACE) to an octapeptide, angiotensin II, which in turn stimulates aldosterone release from the adrenal cortex. Angiotensin II also has a potent vasoconstricting effect and raises blood pressure (Vallotton et al., 1990). In addition, it stimulates drinking by acting on the subfornical organ in the brain and induces vasopressin release from the posterior pituitary (Wong et al., 1992).

Two forms of angiotensin II receptor subtypes, AT_1 and AT_2, have been identified (Wong et al., 1992). The AT_1 receptor is found in most of the vascular tissues. The AT_2 receptor is found in the adrenal medulla and ovarian granulosa cells in the rat and in the uterus in human. In the adrenal cortex, kidney and heart, both AT_1 and AT_2 receptors are present. In the rat brain, both AT_1 and AT_2 receptor subtypes have been found with distinct distributions (Rowe et al., 1992).

Pineal Gland

Melatonin, an indoleamine, is secreted by the pineal gland in the rat as in other mammalian species. It is synthesized from the amino acid tryptophan by several steps of enzymatic conversion. N-Acetyltransferase (NAT) is considered to be the rate-limiting enzyme for melatonin synthesis (Reiter, 1991b). The pineal gland has an important role in mediating daily or seasonal endocrine activity at the central level. Pineal melatonin secretion is controlled by the circadian rhythm with the blood level being high during the dark period and low during the light period (Reiter, 1991a). This daily secretory profile of plasma melatonin depends on the activity of NAT, and this enzymatic activity rhythm is regulated by neural signals from the hypothalamic suprachiasmatic nucleus (SCN) (Reiter, 1991b). The pineal gland is innervated by the sympathetic system which is controlled by two retinal pathways both passing through the superior cervical ganglion

(SCG) (Lincoln, 1984). One of these pathways, called the retinohypothalamic pathway, involves the SCN. In the rat, melatonin is involved in mediating various biological rhythms (Armstrong and Redman, 1985; Kennaway, 1997). In addition, melatonin could be involved in regulating mechanisms of prolactin release (Reiter, 1980). Melatonin-binding sites or receptors have been found in the hypothalamus and pars tuberalis in the rat (Stankov *et al.*, 1991). The receptor is a membrane-associated receptor which is coupled to a G protein (Reppert, 1997).

Pancreas

The mammalian pancreas plays an essential role in metabolism and digestion. It is a mixed glandular organ consisting of both endocrine and exocrine glands (Norris, 1996). The endocrine pancreas secretes hormones, such as insulin, glucagon, somatostatin and pancreatic polypeptide, which regulate glucose and lipid metabolism, whereas the exocrine pancreas produces critical digestive enzymes into the small intestine through the pancreatic duct. The endocrine pancreas consists of groups of endocrine cells which are scattered throughout the gland. These groups of cells are known as the islets of Langerhans. Several different types of cells have been identified in the islets of Langerhans: A, B, D and pancreatic polypeptide cells (Samols, 1991).

Pancreatic Hormones

Insulin

Insulin is a hypoglycemic and antilipolytic hormone secreted by B cells of the pancreatic islets. The rat insulin molecule is composed of two different polypeptide chains (21 amino acid A chain and 30 amino acid B chain) linked by disulfide bonds (Norris, 1996). Proinsulin is cleaved by a specific enzyme, carboxypeptidase E (Naggert *et al.*, 1995), and converted to insulin and C-peptide in the B cell.

Insulin causes hypoglycemia through increasing the uptake of blood glucose mainly into adipose or muscle cells (Cheatham and Kahn, 1995). After insulin binds to a tyrosine kinase transmembrane receptor in the target cell membrane, it facilitates the cellular uptake of glucose by mobilizing insulin-dependent glucose transporter (GLUT 4) in muscle and fat cells (Sargeant *et al.*, 1993). The transport of amino acids, fatty acids or various ions from the blood into the cells is also stimulated by insulin. Moreover, insulin enhances the activity of hexokinase that stimulates glucose oxidation. Hyperglycemia stimulates synthesis and release of insulin through a direct action of glucose on B cells (Samols, 1991). On the other hand, decreases in blood glucose cause a reduction of insulin secretion. Regulation of insulin secretion by the autonomic nervous system also occurs. Acetylcholine or activation of parasympathetic nerves stimulates insulin secretion, whereas norepinephrine from the sympathetic nerves and also epinephrine inhibit it (Samols, 1991). Somatostatin from the pancreatic D cells inhibits insulin release through a direct action on the B cells as a paracrine regulator within the pancreas (Samols, 1991).

The insulin receptor is a heterotetrameric glycoprotein consisting of two α and two β subunits (Quon *et al.*, 1994; Holman and Kasuga, 1997). The α subunit is located entirely in the extracellular space and contains the insulin-binding domain. The β subunit is a transmembrane peptide and possesses tyrosine-specific protein kinase activity in the intracellular domain. The β subunit also contains tyrosine residues which are autophosphorylated in response to insulin binding to the α subunit.

Glucagon

Pancreatic A cells in the islets are the source of the hyperglycemic hormone glucagon. Rat glucagon is a single-chain polypeptide composed of 29 amino acid residues and is similar to the gastrointestinal hormones such as secretin and cholecystokinin (Samols, 1991). Glucagon stimulates glycogenolysis in the liver to raise blood glucose concentrations (Samols, 1991). Lipolysis is also promoted by glucagon. These hyperglycemic effects of glucagon are mediated through stimulation of adenylate cyclase activity and production of cyclic AMP after binding to its membrane receptors (Jelinek *et al.*, 1993). The rat glucagon receptor also transduces a signal leading to an increase in the intracellular concentration of calcium (Jelinek *et al.*, 1993). The homologies of amino acid sequence in this receptor show that it belongs to a family of seven membrane-spanning receptors for GHRH, secretin, calcitonin, parathyroid hormone, VIP and GLP-1 (Segre and Goldring, 1993).

Somatostatin

Pancreatic D cells of islets produce somatostatin. In mammals, two types of pancreatic somatostatin are discovered, one of which is composed of 14 amino acid residues and is identical to the hypothalamic somatostatin in the rat (Samols, 1991). The other somatostatin molecule has 28 amino acids. Both somatostatins are reported to inhibit insulin, glucagon and pancreatic polypeptide secretion in a paracrine mechanism (Samols, 1991). However, the regulatory mechanism of pancreatic somatostatin secretion is not fully understood.

Pancreatic polypeptide

The mammalian pancreas also produces pancreatic polypeptide in cells other than A, B and D cells. Isolated rat pancreatic polypeptide is a peptide hormone consisting of 36 amino acid residues and is similar to neuropeptide Y and peptide YY structurally (Samols, 1991). Although pancreatic polypeptide may regulate insulin and glucagon secretion locally as a paracrine regulator, its detailed action is still obscure.

Gastrointestinal Hormones

Secretin

Secretin was the first molecule to be termed a 'hormone' by Bayliss and Starling in 1902 (Bayliss and Starling, 1902). Rat secretin is a polypeptide consisting of 27 amino acid residues and is secreted by S cells in the duodenal mucosa (Norris, 1996). The presence of acidic chyme in the duodenum is the potent stimulant for the release of secretin into the blood. Secretin stimulates the pancreas to secrete HCO_3^--rich alkaline juice and neutralize the acidic chyme which has been forwarded to the small intestine (Thompson, 1990). Secretin binds to a G protein-coupled receptor to generate cyclic AMP production and then stimulate pancreatic HCO_3^- secretion (Segre and Goldring, 1993). The amino acid sequence homologies show that the rat secretin receptor belongs to a receptor family for GHRH, calcitonin, parathyroid hormone, VIP and glucagon.

Gastrin

Gastrin is a peptide hormone secreted from G cells in the mucosa of the antral portion of the stomach. There are two forms of gastrin molecules composed of 17 amino acids: gastrin I and sulfated gastrin II (Norris, 1996). A larger form of gastrin (34 amino acids) termed big gastrin is also present in the blood. Gastrin secretion is stimulated by digested contents in the stomach, particularly by amino acids and its release is also induced by parasympathetic stimulation. Gastrin stimulates gastric acid secretion from the gastric gland (Thompson, 1990). This action is mediated by G protein-linked gastrin receptors through IP_3 production and phosphokinase C activation (Wank, 1998).

Motilin

Motilin is a peptide (22 amino acids) that was first found in M cells of the duodenum in the dog (Itoh, 1997). It was so named because the peptide stimulates motility in the gastrointestinal tract in the dog. The episodic secretion of the peptide is well associated with the motility of the gastrointestinal tract in the dog. In the rat, the amino acid sequence of this hormone has not yet been determined, but motilin immunoreactivities have been found both in the duodenum and in the brain (Jacobowitz et al., 1981; O'Donohue et al., 1981; Sakai et al., 1994). Motilin stimulates the migrating motor complex to cause intestinal contraction. This stimulatory action of motilin on smooth muscles of intestine increases the passage of the contents through the small intestine. Motilin secretion from the M cells is stimulated under alkaline conditions in the duodenum (Itoh, 1997) and is regulated by the vagus nerve and blood glucose level (Funakoshi et al., 1982). A heterotrimeric G-protein-coupled receptor for motilin has recently been isolated from human stomach (Feighner et al., 1999). The rat motilin receptor has not been identified yet.

Cholecystokinin

Cholecystokinin (CCK) is a peptide hormone which has effects on pancreatic enzyme and bile release (Reeve Jr. et al., 1994). Several CCK molecules have been isolated, including peptides composed of 8, 33, 39 and 58 amino acid residues (Walsh and Dockray,

1994). Proteins, amino acids and lipids in the gastric effluent forwarded into the duodenum are the direct stimulators of CCK secretion from the intestinal I cells (Thompson, 1990). CCK induces contraction of smooth muscles in the walls of the gallbladder to expel the bile. CCK also acts on the stomach to decrease the rate of gastric evacuation through relaxation of gastric smooth muscles and contraction of the pyloric sphincter. CCK receptors are classified into four types: CCK$_A$, CCK$_B$ gastrin receptor and CG-4 (Wank *et al.*, 1994; Wank, 1998).

Acknowledgements

We thank Drs A. Yokoyama, K. Yamanouchi, S. Hayashi, M. Kawai, K. Kishi, F. Maekawa and S. Tsukahara for their great help in writing this manuscript and to Ms. Niwa for her secretarial assistance.

References

Ahima, R.S., Prabakaran, D., Mantzoros, C. *et al.* (1996) *Nature* **382**, 250–252.

Antoni, F.A. (1986) *Endocr. Rev.* **7**, 351–378.

Armstrong, S.M. and Redman, J. (1985) In: Evered, D. and Clark, S. (eds) *Photoperiodism, Melatonin and the Pineal*, pp. 188–207. Newark: Pitman.

Auletta, F.J. and Flint, A.P.F. (1988) *Endocr. Rev.* **9**, 88–105.

Azria, M. (1989) *The Calcitonins*. Basel: Karger.

Baird, D.T. (1984) In: Austin, C.R. and Short, R.V. (eds) *Hormonal Control of Reproduction*, pp. 91–114. Cambridge: Cambridge University Press.

Barash, I.A., Cheung, C.C., Weigle, D.S. *et al.* (1996) *Endocrinology* **137**, 3144–3147.

Barberis, C., Mouillac, B. and Durroux, T. (1998) *J. Endocrinol.* **156**, 223–229.

Bayliss, W.M. and Starling, E.H. (1902) *J. Physiol. (Lond.)* **28**, 325–353.

Bazan, J.F. (1990) *Proc. Natl Acad. Sci. USA* **87**, 6934–6938.

Ben-Jonathan, N. (1985) *Endocr. Rev.* **6**, 564–589.

Bertherat, J., Bluet-Pajot, M.T. and Epelbaum, J. (1995) *Eur. J. Endocrinol.* **132**, 12–24.

Bjoro, T., Sand, O., Ostberg, B.C. *et al.* (1990) *Biosci. Rep.* **10**, 189–199.

Bluet-Pajot, M.T., Epelbaum, J., Gourdji, D., Hammond, C. and Kordon, C. (1998) *Cell. Mol. Neurobiol.* **18**, 101–123.

Boston, B.A. and Cone, R. (1996) *Endocrinology* **137**, 2043–2050.

Boutin, J.-M., Jolicoeur, C., Okamura, H. *et al.* (1988) *Cell* **53**, 69–77.

Brelje, T.C., Scharp, D.W., Lacy, P.E. *et al.* (1993) *Endocrinology* **132**, 879–887.

Brown, M.R., Koob, G.F. and Rivier, C. (1990) *Stress: Neurobiology and Neuroendocrinology*. New York: Dekker.

Burgus, R., Butcher, M., Amoss, M. *et al.* (1972) *Proc. Natl Acad. Sci. USA* **69**, 278–282.

Campfield, L.A., Smith, F.J., Guisez, Y., Dovos, R. and Burn, P. (1995) *Science* **269**, 546–549.

Caron, M.G. and Lefkowitz, R.J. (1993) *Recent Prog. Horm. Res.* **48**, 277–290.

Carson-Jurica, M.A., Schrader, W.T. and O'Malley, B.W. (1990) *Endocr. Rev.* **11**, 201–220.

Challis, J.R.G. and Lye, S.J. (1994) In: Knobil, E. and Neill, J.D., (eds) *The Physiology of Reproduction*, pp. 985–1031. New York: Raven Press.

Cheatham, B. and Kahn, C.R. (1995) *Endocr. Rev.* **16**, 117–142.

Chehab, F.F., Lim, M.E. and Lu, R. (1996) *Nature Genet.* **12**, 318–320.

Chehab, F.F., Mounzih, K., Lu, R. and Lim, M.E. (1997) *Science* **275**, 88–90.

Cheung, C.C., Thornton, J.E., Kuijper, J.L., Weigle, D.S., Clifton, D.K. and Steiner, R.A. (1997) *Endocrinology* **138**, 855–858.

Clarke, I.J. and Cummins, J.T. (1982) *Endocrinology* **111**, 1737–1739.

Clayton, R.N. (1989) *J. Endocrinol.* **120**, 11–19.

Combarnous, Y. (1992) *Endocr. Rev.* **13**, 670–691.

de Bold, A.J. (1985) *Science* **230**, 767–770.

Dempster, D.W., Cosman, F., Parisien, M., Shen, V. and Lindsay, R. (1993) *Endocr. Rev.* **14**, 690–709.

Dubois, P.M. and ElAmraoui, A. (1995) *Trends Endocrinol. Metab.* **6**, 1–7.

Dyer, R.G. and Robinson, J.E. (1989) *J. Endocrinol.* **123**, 1–2.

Epelbaum, J., Dournaud, P., Fodor, M. and Viollet, C. (1994) *Crit. Rev. Neurobiol.* **8**, 25–44.

Epelbaum, J., Briard, N., Djordijevic, D. *et al.* (1998) *Ann. NY Acad. Sci.* **839**, 249–253.

Evans, R.M. (1988) *Science* **240**, 889–895.

Feighner, S.D., Tan, C.P., McKee, K.K., Palyha, O.C., Hreniuk, D.L., Pong, S.-S., Austin, C.P., Figueroa, D., MacNeil, D., Cascieri, M.A., Nargund, R., Bakshi, R., Abramovitz, M., Stocco, R., Kargman, S., O'Neill, G., Van Der Ploeg, L.H.T., Evans, J., Patchett, A.A., Smith, R.G. and Howard, A.D. (1999) *Science* **284**, 2184–2188.

Findlay, J.K. (1993) *Biol. Reprod.* **48**, 15–23.

Fodor, M., Csaba, Z., Kordon, C. and Epelbaum, J. (1994) *J. Chem. Neuroanat.* **8**, 61–73.

Freeman, M.E. (1994) In: Knobil, E. and Neill, J.D. (eds) *The Physiology of Reproduction*, pp. 613–658. New York: Raven Press.

Freemark, M., Comer, M., Korner, G. and Handwerger, S. (1987) *Endocrinology* **120**, 1865–1872.

Freemark, M., Comer, M. and Korner, G. (1988) *Endocrinology* **122**, 2771–2779.

Friedman, J.M. (1997) *Nature* **385**, 119–120.

Funakoshi, A., Glowniak, J., Owyang, C. and Vinik, A.I. (1982) *J. Clin. Endocrinol. Metab.* **54**, 1129–1134.

Funder, J.W. (1993) *Ann. Rev. Physiol.* **55**, 115–130.

Gay, V.L. and Sheth, N.A. (1972) *Endocrinology* **90**, 158–162.

Gershengorn, M.C. and Osman, R. (1996) *Physiol. Rev.* **76**, 175–191.

Gore-Langton, R.E. and Armstrong, D.T. (1994) In: Knobil, E. and Neill, J.D. (eds) *The Physiology of Reproduction*, pp. 571–627. New York: Raven Press.

Grigoriadis, D.E., Lovenberg, T.W., Chalmers, D.T., Liaw, C. and De Souza, E.B. (1996) *Ann. NY Acad. Sci.* **780**, 60–80.

Gulyas, J., Rivier, C., Perrin, M., Koerber, S.C., Sutton, S., Corrigan, A., Lahrichi, S.L., Craig, A.G., Vale, W. and Rivier, J. (1995) *Proc. Natl Acad. Sci. USA* **92**, 10575–10579.

Gwynne, J.T. and Strauss III, J.F. (1982) *Endocr. Rev.* **3**, 299–329.

Halaas, J.L., Gajiwala, K.S, Maffei, M. *et al.* (1995) *Science* **269**, 543–546.

Hall, P.F. (1994) In: Knobil, E. and Neill, J.D. (eds) *The Physiology of Reproduction*, pp. 1335–1362. New York: Raven Press.

Harigaya, T., Smith, W.C. and Talamantes, F. (1988) *Endocrinology* **122**, 1366–1372.

Harris, G.W. (1955) *Neural Control of the Pituitary Gland*. London: Edward Arnold.

Heap, R.B. and Flint, A.P.F. (1984) In: Austin, C.R. and Short, R.V. (eds) *Hormonal Control of Reproduction*, pp. 153–194. Cambridge: Cambridge University Press.

Hinuma, S., Habata, Y., Fujii, R., Kawamata, Y., Hosoya, M., Fukusumi, S., Kitada, C., Masuo, Y., Asano, T., Matsumoto, H., Sekiguchi, M., Kurokawa, T., Nishimura, O., Onda, H. and Fujino, M. (1998) *Nature* **393**, 272–276.

Holman, G.D. and Kasuga, M. (1997) *Diabetologia* **40**, 991–1003.

Horvath, S. and Palkovits, M. (1988) *Neuroendocrinology* **48**, 471–476.

Imura, H. (1994) *The Pituitary Gland*. New York: Raven Press.

Itoh, Z. (1997) *Peptides* **18**, 593–608.

Jacobowitz, D.M., O'Donohue, T.L., Chey, W.Y. and Chang, T.-M. (1981) *Peptides* **2**, 479–487.

Jelinek, L.J., Lok, S., Rosenberg, G.B. *et al.* (1993) *Science* **259**, 1614–1616.

Jirikowski, G.F., Caldwell, J.D., Pedersen, C.A. and Stumpf, W.E. (1988) *Neuroscience* **25**, 237–248.

Juppner, H., Abou-Samra, A.-B., Freeman, M. *et al.* (1991) *Science* **254**, 1024–1026.

Karsch, F.J. (1984) In: Austin, C.R. and Short, R.V. (eds) *Hormonal Control of Reproduction*, pp. 1–20. Cambridge: Cambridge University Press.

Kato, Y., Iwasaki, Y., Iwasaki, J., Abe, H., Yanaihara, N. and Imura, H. (1978) *Endocrinology* **103**, 554–558.

Kawai, M. and Kishi, K. (1997) *J. Reprod. Fertil.* **109**, 145–152.

Kawakami, M., Uemura, T. and Hayashi, R. (1982) *Neuroendocrinology* **35**, 63–67.

Kawano, H. and Daikoku, S. (1981) *Neuroendocrinology* **32**, 179–186.

Kawano, H. and Daikoku, S. (1988) *J. Comp. Neurol.* **271**, 293–299.

Kelly, P.A., Djiane, J. and Edery, M. (1992) *Trends Endocrinol. Metab.* **3**, 54–59.

Kennaway, D.J. (1997) *Biol. Signals* **6**, 247–254.

Kim, J.K., Summer, S.N., Wood, W.M., Brown, J.L. and Schrier, R.W. (1997) *J. Am. Soc. Nephrol.* **8**, 1863–1869.

Kingsley, D.M. (1994) *Genes Dev.* **8**, 133–146.

Lamberts, S.W.J. and Macleod, R.M. (1990) *Physiol. Rev.* **70**, 279–318.

Lazar, M.A. (1993) *Endocr. Rev.* **14**, 184–193.

Lechan, R.M. and Jackson, I.M. (1982) *Endocrinology* **111**, 55–65.

Lefebvre, D.L., Giaid, A., Bennett, H., Lariviere, R. and Zingg, H.H. (1992a) *Science* **256**, 1553–1555.

Lefebvre, D.L., Giaid, A. and Zingg, H.H. (1992b) *Endocrinology* **130**, 1185–1192.

Lefebvre, D.L., Lariviere, R. and Zingg, H.H. (1993) *Biol. Reprod.* **48**, 632–639.

Lefebvre, D.L., Farookhi, R., Giaid, A., Neculcea, J. and Zingg, H.H. (1994a) *Endocrinology* **134**, 2562–2566.

Lefebvre, D.L., Farookhi, R., Larcher, A., Neculcea, J. and Zingg, H.H. (1994b) *Endocrinology* **134**, 2556–2561.

Lin, H.Y., Harris, T.L., Flannery, M.S. *et al.* (1991) *Science* **254**, 1022–1024.

Lincoln, G.A. (1984) In: Austin, C.R. and Short, R.V. (eds) *Hormonal Control of Reproduction*, pp. 52–75. Cambridge: Cambridge University Press.

Lolait, S.J., O'Carroll, A.M., Mahan, L.C. *et al.* (1995) *Proc. Natl Acad. Sci. USA* **92**, 6783–6787.

Lolait, S.J., O'Carroll, A.M., McBride, O.W., Konig, M., Morel, A. and Brownstein, M.J. (1992) *Nature* **357**, 336–339.

Lovenberg, T.W., Liaw, C.W., Grigoriadis, D.E. *et al.* (1995) *Proc. Natl Acad. Sci. USA* **92**, 836–840.

Lumpkin, M.D., McDonald, J.K., Samson, W.K. and McCann, S.M. (1989) *Neuroendocrinology* **50**, 229–235.

Lumpkin, M.D., Samson, W.K. and McCann, S.M. (1983) *Endocrinology* **112**, 1711–1717.

Maack, T. (1992) *Annu. Rev. Physiol.* **54**, 11–27.

MacLeod, K.R., Smith, W.C., Ogren, L. and Talamantes, F. (1989) *Endocrinology* **125**, 2258–2266.

MacLusky, N.J., Naftolin, F. and Leranth, C. (1988) *Brain Res.* **439**, 391–395.

Maeda, K.-I., Cagampang, F.R.A., Coen, C.W. and Tsukamura, H. (1994) *Endocrinology* **134**, 1718–1722.

Maeda, K.-I., Tsukamura, H., Ohkura, S., Kawakami, S.,

Nagabukuro, H. and Yokoyama, A. (1995) *Neurosci. Biobehav. Rev.* **19**, 427–437.

Maffei, M., Halaas, J., Ravussin, E. *et al.* (1995) *Nature Med.* **1**, 1155–1161.

Magner, J.A. (1990) *Endocr. Rev.* **11**, 354–381.

Makara, G.B. (1992) *Ciba Found. Symp.* **168**, 43–51.

Mallette, L.E. (1991) *Endocr. Rev.* **12**, 110–117.

Maruyama, M., Matsumoto, H., Fujiwara, K., Kitada, C., Hinuma, S., Onda, H., Fujino, M. and Inoue, K. (1999) *Endocrinology* **140**, 2326–2333.

Mathews, L.S. (1991) *Trends Endocrinol. Metab.* **2**, 176–180.

Mathews, L.S. and Vale, W.W. (1993) *Receptor* **3**, 173–181.

Matsumoto, H., Noguchi, J., Horikoshi, Y., Kawamata, Y., Kitada, C., Hinuma, S., Onda, H., Nishimura, O. and Fujino, M. (1999) *Biochem. Biophys. Res. Commun.* **259**, 321–324.

Matsuo, H., Baba, Y., Nair, R.M.G., Arimura, A. and Schally, A.V. (1971) *Biochem. Biophys. Res. Commun.* **43**, 1334–1339.

Mayo, K.E. (1992) *Mol. Endocrinol.* **6**, 1734–1744.

Mayo, K.E. (1994) *Trends Endocrinol. Metab.* **5**, 407–415.

McNabb, F.M.A. (1993) *Thyroid Hormones.* Englewood Cliffs: Prentice-Hall.

McNeilly, A.S. (1994) In: Knobil, E. and Neill, J.D. (eds) *The Physiology of Reproduction*, pp. 1179–1212. New York: Raven Press.

Meisel, R.L. and Sachs, B.D. (1994) In: Knobil, E. and Neill, J.D. (eds) *The Physiology of Reproduction*, pp. 3–105. New York: Raven Press.

Meites, J. (1988) In: Hoshino, K. (ed.) *PRL Gene Family and its Receptors*, pp. 123–130. Amsterdam: Elsevier.

Meyerhof, W. (1998) *Rev. Physiol. Biochem. Pharmacol.* **133**, 55–108.

Miller, R.J. and Bell, G.I. (1996) *Trends Neurosci.* **19**, 159–161.

Miller, W.L. (1988) *Endocr. Rev.* **9**, 295–318.

Mitchell, M.D. and Trautman, M.S. (1993) *Mol. Cell. Endocrinol.* **93**, C7–C10.

Moenter, S.M., Brand, R.M., Midgley, A.R. and Karsch, F.J. (1992) *Endocrinology* **130**, 503–510.

Morel, A., O'Carroll, A.M., Brownstein, M.J. and Lolait, S.J. (1992) *Nature* **356**, 523–526.

Mountjoy, K.G. and Wong, J. (1997) *Mol. Cell. Endocrinol.* **128**, 171–177.

Mountjoy, K.G., Robbins, L.S., Mortrud, M.T. and Cone, R.D. (1992) *Science* **257**, 1248–1251.

Mountjoy, K.G., Mortrud, M.T., Low, M.J., Simerly, R.B. and Cone, R.D. (1994) *Mol. Endocrinol.* **8**, 1298–1308.

Mulrow, P.J. (1986) *The Adrenal Gland.* New York: Elsevier.

Nagatani, S., Guthikonda, P, Thompson, R.C., Tsuka-mura, H., Maeda, K.-I. and Foster, D.L. (1998) *Neuroendocrinology* **67**, 370–376.

Naggert, J.K., Fricker, L.D., Varlamov, O. *et al.* (1995) *Nature Genet.* **10**, 135–142.

Nakamura, T., Takio, K., Eto, Y., Shibai, H., Titani, K. *et al.* (1990) *Science* **247**, 836–838.

Negishi, M., Sugimoto, Y. and Ichikawa, A. (1995) *Biochim. Biophys. Acta* **1259**, 109–119.

Niall, H.D., Hogan, M.L., Sayer, R., Rosenblum, I.Y. and Greenwood, I. (1971) *Proc. Natl Acad. Sci. USA* **68**, 866–869.

Nishihara, M., Mori, Y., Yoo, M.J. and Takahashi, M. (1994) In: Levine, J.E. (ed.) *Pulsatility in Neuroendocrine Systems*, pp. 114–126. San Diego: Academic Press.

Norris, D.O. (1996) *Vertebrate Endocrinology.* San Diego: Academic Press.

Nunez, E.A. (1994) *Tumor Biol.* **15**, 63–72.

O'Byrne, K.T. and Knobil, E. (1994) In: Levine, J.E. (ed.) *Pulsatility in Neuroendocrine Systems*, pp. 100–113. San Diego: Academic Press.

O'Donohue, T.L., Beinfeld, M.C., Chey, W.Y. *et al.* (1981) *Peptides* **2**, 467–477.

O'Leary, R. and O'Connor, B. (1995) *J. Neurochem.* **65**, 953–963.

O'Malley, B.W. (1984) *J. Clin. Invest.* **74**, 307–312.

Olofsson, J.I. and Leung, P.C. (1996) *Biol. Signals* **5**, 90–100.

Olofsson, J. and Norjavaara, E. (1990) *Biol. Reprod.* **43**, 762–768.

Olofsson, J., Norjavaara, E. and Selstam, G. (1990) *Biol. Reprod.* **42**, 792–800.

Olofsson, J., Norjavaara, E. and Selstam, G. (1992) *Prostaglandins Leukot. Essent. Fatty Acids* **46**, 151–161.

Perrin, M.H., Donaldson, C.J., Chen, R., Lewis, K.A. and Vale, W.W. (1993) *Endocrinology* **133**, 3058–3061.

Peter, J., Burbach, H., Adan, R.A. *et al.* (1995) *Cell. Mol. Neurobiol.* **15**, 573–595.

Pfaff, D.W., Schwartz-Giblin, S., McCarthy, M.M. and Kow, L.-M. (1994) In: Knobil, E. and Neill, J.D. (eds) *The Physiology of Reproduction*, pp. 107–220. New York: Raven Press.

Poyser, N.L. (1995) *Prostaglandins Leukot. Essent. Fatty Acids* **53**, 147–195.

Quon, M.J., Butte, A.J. and Taylor, S.I. (1994) *Trends Endocrinol. Metab.* **5**, 369–376.

Reeve Jr., J.R., Eysselein, V., Solomon, T.E. and Go, V.L.W. (1994) *Ann. NY Acad. Sci.* **713**.

Reiter, R.J. (1980) *Endocr. Rev.* **1**, 109–131.

Reiter, R.J. (1991a) *Trends Endocrinol. Metab.* **2**, 13–19.

Reiter, R.J. (1991b) *Endocr. Rev.* **12**, 151–180.

Reppert, S.M. (1997) *J. Biol. Rhythms* **12**, 528–531.

Rivier, C., Brown, M. and Vale, W. (1977) *Endocrinology* **100**, 751–754.

Rivier, C., Rivier, J. and Vale, W. (1986) *Science* **231**, 607–609.

Rivier, J., Rivier, C. and Vale, W. (1984) *Science* **224**, 889–891.

Robertson, D.M., Klein, R., de Vos, F.L. *et al.* (1987) *Biochem. Biophys. Res. Commun.* **149**, 744–749.

Robertson, G.L. (1995) *Endocrinol. Metab. Clin. North Am.* **24**, 549–572.

Robertson, M.C., Gillespie, B. and Friesen, H.G. (1982) *Endocrinology* **111**, 1862–1866.

Rosenzweig, A. and Seidman, C.E. (1991) *Annu. Rev. Biochem.* **60**, 229–255.

Rosner, W. (1990) *Endocr. Rev.* **11**, 80–91.

Rowe, B.P., Saylor, D.L. and Speth, R.C. (1992) *Neuroendocrinology* **55**, 563–573.

Rozen, F., Russo, C., Banville, D. and Zingg, H.H. (1995) *Proc. Natl Acad. Sci. USA* **92**, 200–204.

Sakai, T., Satoh, M., Koyama, H. *et al.* (1994) *Peptides* **15**, 987–991.

Samols, E. (1991) *The Endocrine Pancreas.* New York: Raven Press.

Sargeant, R., Mitsumoto, Y., Sarabia, V., Shillabeer, G. and Klip, A. (1993) *J. Endocrinol. Invest.* **16**, 147–162.

Schwartz, M.W., Seeley, R.J., Campfield, L.A., Burn, P. and Baskin, D.G. (1996) *J. Clin. Invest.* **98**, 1101–1106.

Segre, G.V. and Goldring, S.R. (1993) *Trends Endocrinol. Metab.* **4**, 309–314.

Sharpe, R.M. (1994) In: Knobil, E. and Neill, D.J. (eds) *The Physiology of Reproduction*, 2nd edn, pp. 1363–1434. New York: Raven Press.

Sherwood, N.M., Lovejoy, D.A. and Coe, I.R. (1993) *Endocr. Rev.* **14**, 241–254.

Shimasaki, S., Koga, M., Esch, F. *et al.* (1988) *Biochem. Biophys. Res. Commun.* **152**, 717–723.

Silverman, A.-J., Livne, I. and Witkin, J.W. (1994) In: Knobil, E. and Neill, J.D. (eds) *The Physiology of Reproduction.* New York: Raven Press.

Smith, W.L., Marnett, L.J. and DeWitt, D.L. (1991) *Pharmacol. Ther.* **49**, 153–179.

Soares, M.J., Faria, T.N., Roby, K.F. and Deb, S. (1991) *Endocr. Rev.* **12**, 402–423.

Spiess, J., Rivier, J. and Vale, W. (1983) *Nature* **303**, 532–535.

Stankov, B., Fraschini, F. and Reiter, R.J. (1991) *Brain Res. Rev.* **16**, 245–256.

Strosberg, A.D. (1993) *Protein Sci.* **2**, 1198–1209.

Szczepanska-Sadowska, E. (1996) *Reg. Peptides* **66**, 65–71.

Tartaglia, L.A., Dembski, M., Weng, X. *et al.* (1995) *Cell* **83**, 1263–1271.

Tashjian, Jr., A.H., Barowsky, N.J. and Jensen, D.K. (1971) *Biochem. Biophys. Res. Commun.* **43**, 516–253.

Taya, K., Kaneko, H., Watanabe, G. and Sasamoto, S. (1991) *J. Reprod. Fertil.* (suppl.) **43**, 151–162.

Thompson, J.C. (1990) *Gastrointestinal Endocrinology.* San Diego: Academic Press.

Tucker, H.A. (1994) In: Knobil, E. and Neill, J.D. (eds) *The Physiology of Reproduction*, pp. 1065–1098. New York: Raven Press.

Ueno, N., Ling, N., S.Y., Esch, F., Shimasaki, S. and Guillemin, R. (1987) *Proc. Natl Acad. Sci. USA* **84**, 8282–8286.

Umezaki, K., Shiosaka, S., Kawai, Y. *et al.* (1983) *Cell Mol. Biol.* **29**, 377–386.

Vale, W., Spiess, J., Rivier, C. and Rivier, J. (1981) *Science* **213**, 1394–1397.

Vale, W., Rivier, C., Brown, M.R. *et al.* (1983) *Recent Prog. Horm. Res.* **39**, 245–270.

Vale, W., Rivier, C., Hsueh, A. *et al.* (1988) *Recent Prog. Horm. Res.* **44**, 1–34.

Vallotton, M.B., Capponi, A.M., Johnson, E.I. and Lang, U. (1990) *Horm. Res.* **34**, 105–110.

Vaughan, J., Donaldson, C., Bittencourt, J. *et al.* (1995) *Nature* **378**, 287–292.

Wakerley, J.B., Clarke, G. and Summerlee, A.J.S. (1994) In: Knobil, E. and Neill, J.D. (eds) *The Physiology of Reproduction*, pp. 1131–1177. New York: Raven Press.

Walsh, J.H. and Dockray, G.J. (1994) *Gut Peptides.* New York: Raven Press.

Wank, S.A. (1998) *Am. J. Physiol.* **274**, G607–G613.

Wank, S.A., Pisegna, J.R. and de Weerth, A. (1994) *Ann. NY Acad. Sci.* **713**, 49–66.

Witkin, J.W., Paden, C.M. and Silverman, A.-J. (1982) *Neuroendocrinology* **35**, 429–438.

Wong, P.C., Chiu, A.T., Duncia, J.V. Herblin, W.F., Smith, R.D. and Timmermans, P.B.M.W.M. (1992) *Trends Endocrinol. Metab.* **3**, 211–217.

Wong, S.K.-F. and Garbers, D.L. (1992) *J. Clin. Invest.* **90**, 299–305.

Woodward, D.F., Regan, J.W., Lake, S. and Ocklind, A. (1997) *Surv. Ophthalmol.* (suppl. 2) **41**, S15–S21.

Yen, P.M. and Chin, W.W. (1994) *Trends Endocrinol. Metab.* **5**, 65–72.

Ying, S.-Y. (1989) *J. Steroid Biochem.* **33**, 705–713.

Ying, S.-Y., Becker, A., Swanson, G. *et al.* (1987) *Biochem. Biophys. Res. Commun.* **149**, 133–139.

Zhang, Y., Proenca, R., Maffei, M., Barone, M., Leopold, L. and Freidman, J.M. (1994) *Nature* **372**, 425–432.

Zingg, H.H., Rozen, F., Chu, K. *et al.* (1995) *Recent Prog. Horm. Res.* **50**, 255–273.

CHAPTER 21

Behaviour, Neurology and Electrophysiology

Werner Classen
Novartis Crop Protection AG, Stein, Switzerland

General Aspects

The rat is a group-living, nocturnal, omnivorous mammal which can walk, climb, jump and swim. It is adapted to live in holes or tunnels. Rats mainly rely on auditory, olfactory and tactile information for orientation with visual information being used when available. Their behaviour is only partially inherited and to some extent can be modified by learning and thus is adapted to different environmental conditions. This makes the rat a good model for studying the basic principles of behaviour.

Depending on the information looked for, different techniques are used for the evaluation of behaviour. When looking for the health status of

an animal or for pharmacological effects induced by a chemical, clinically relevant changes in spontaneous behaviour are rated. Analysing behavioural components of spontaneous behaviour by counting the frequency or measuring the duration of specific behaviours provides information on the animal's needs or interests. Such an ethological approach is used, e.g. to analyse social behaviour of group-housed animals, but can also be used to control instrumental behaviour for the validity of the parameters measured or simply as endpoints in an instrumental test. Instrumental techniques are used to modify spontaneous behaviour or its frequency in order to gain information on some underlying mechanisms of mood, learning or memory or to measure specific sensorimotor functions.

Clinical Approach

The main goal of the clinical approach is to identify abnormal neural functions and/or changes in behaviour that point to a potential illness. Observations are used as a diagnostic tool to identify diseases and, if possible, to localize underlying causes. In toxicological experiments the clinical approach is used as the first line approach, while in pharmacological or behavioural experiments it may provide hints regarding side-effects or toxic effects that may be important for correct interpretation of the results. This aspect is crucial in all experiments as animal welfare regulations require anxiety, pain or distress in such animals to be avoided or at least minimized. In behavioural studies this is also important because anxiety or distress may influence the outcome of the experiment.

Individual animals do not necessarily show identical behaviour when in the same situation nor do animals exhibit all the signs of a behavioural complex. Furthermore, signs may have different causes. Therefore evaluation of clinical signs should always include a step during which the likelihood of the different interpretations is evaluated, as is as done in differential diagnosis.

Behavioural Stimulation

One of the most common behavioural changes observed is related to the animal's drive or state of arousal. Behavioural stimulation or inhibition in their mild forms reflect the normal physiological variability in arousal but may also be influenced by the animal's health status, pain, distress or anxiety. As rats are nocturnal animals they sleep throughout most of the day when we usually perform the experiments and when awake show some exploratory behaviour, groom themselves, may nibble some food or drink. The arousal level extends from this range of normal or baseline activity up to a state of extreme activity which may encompass almost continuous exploration, sniffing, rearing or locomotion. Even during such extreme states of behavioural stimulation, conduct of individual movements is normal. Depending on the neurotransmitter systems stimulated and/or the extent of stimulation, animals show either predominantly increased locomotion or stereotyped movements (endless, apparently meaningless repetition of a part of a larger behavioural complex).

Behavioural Inhibition

Behavioural inhibition is a continuum that begins with near normal behaviour at one end and extends to the extreme where animals are no longer capable of standing or moving. As the baseline activity differs between rat strains, is subjected to a circadian cycle, and depends on the animals' history (environmental or housing conditions), mild behavioural inhibition is difficult to detect. Besides reduced rearing, muscle tone and/or responsiveness to stimuli, exploration and locomotor activity are reduced compared with normal animals. When an animal is stimulated by placing it into an unfamiliar environment, behavioural inhibition is reversed for a limited period of time. Often, behavioural inhibition is related to distress, malaise or sickness. Although differentiation is not always that simple and clear, nonspecific changes in behaviour should be discriminated from specific or directly induced behavioural effects.

CNS Overexcitation

Neurophysiologically, increased excitatory activity in the CNS reflects an imbalance of excitatory and inhibitory neuronal activity. Increased excitatory activity often begins in the hippocampo-amygdaloid area and from there spreads throughout the entire brain. The first signs associated with excitatory activity are usually eye blinking, twitching of ear lobes or facial muscles (see Table 21.1). With continuous growth of the epileptic focus, these uncontrollable fasciculations will gradually involve neck muscles (bobbing of head), forelimbs (forelimb clonus) and finally encompass most skeletal muscles of the body (generalized clonic convulsion). Autonomic functions may be stimulated as well. CNS overexcitation is not accompanied by behavioural stimulation but rather preceded by a period of mild behavioural inhibition.

Autonomic Stimulation

The most prominent signs related to stimulation of the autonomic nervous system are salivation, lacrimation, chromodacryorrhoea (secretion of a dark red fluid by the Harderian gland) and piloerection. Other signs such as loose stool or diarrhoea, micturition, laboured respiration (due to bronchoconstriction) or

Table 21.1 Signs associated with arousal and mild CNS overexcitation

Signs	Behavioural		CNS overexcitation	
	Inhibition	Stimulation	Mild	Severe
Exploration	↓	↑	↓/0	↓
Rearing	↓	↑	↓/0	↓
Locomotion	↓	↑	↓/0	↓
Responsiveness to stimuli	↓	0/↑	0/↑	0/↑
Muscle tone	↓	0/↑	0/↑	0/↑
Stereotypies	a	0/p	a	a
Fasciculations	a	a	p	p
Head bobbing	a	a	p	p
Fore limb clonus	a	a	a	p
Clonic convulsion	a	a	a	p

↑ increase; ↓ decrease; 0, not changed; a, absent; p, present.

Some common signs occur during both increased arousal and mild CNS overexcitation. These two states can be differentiated when considering the entire complex of signs exhibited. More pronounced CNS overexcitation is indicated by signs such as head bobbing, fore limb clonus or clonic convulsions.

miosis also belong to this functional domain. A mild autonomic stimulation is not always easy to recognize as the slightly increased amount of saliva is swallowed and the lacrimal fluid is voided via the lacrimal ducts. With increasing stimulation, fluid leaks or pours out of the mouth and eyes, wetting the surrounding fur. Increased defecation up to diarrhoea and/or frequent micturition all belong to the picture of pharmacological stimulation of autonomic functions and may occur under stressful conditions as well.

Neuromotor Dysfunction

Neurophysiologically, locomotion is a complex phenomenon involving different sensory modalities (proprioceptive, vestibular, visual, tactile), as well as neuromuscular (reflex circuits) and CNS functions. It is thus not surprising that the nervous circuits involved are widespread and their functions are not yet fully understood. Different hierarchically structured neuronal circuits, located in the spinal cord, pons/cerebellum, basal ganglia and the cortex are responsible for the control of movements (Kelly, 1985).

Disturbances in neuromotor functions may be detected by mere observation of the moving animal: rats may rear less often, exhibit an abnormal gait or

ataxia or may even be unable to walk. A normal gait is characterized by smooth movements, regular and symmetrical position of legs during walking or standing and the absence of stumbling or falling. As rats have a low centre of gravity, slight neuromotor dysfunctions are not seen easily.

A prerequisite for normal neuromotor function is a muscle tone within a normal range. With a reduced muscle tone the animal stands or walks on the entire foot pad with the abdomen almost touching the ground (creeping movement). Increased muscle tone, on the other hand, results in an elevated position of the body, seen especially at the abdomen, with the weight put on the toes only and hind limbs increasingly spread outwards when standing or walking. Movements may appear stiff or uncoordinated. Increased muscle tone may be induced by dysfunctions of the extrapyramidal motor system, spinal cord or neuromuscular junction. Diffuse or toxic CNS damage in general impairs fine motor control and results in altered muscle tone, staggering or dysmetric gait, uncoordinated leg movements, etc. Vestibular defects typically induce gait asymmetries indicated by a drift or circling in the direction of the affected side and of course induce nystagmus. In cases of damage localized either to the spinal cord, peripheral nerve or the muscle(s), movement of individual legs is no longer possible (paralysis) or movement is impaired (paresis) resulting in abnormal placing of the foot or the limited strength or control of the leg does not allow the full weight of the body to be supported. Lesions involving the peripheral motor nerve (lower motor neuron) invariably result in reduced muscle tone (flaccid paresis), while a lesion of the upper motor neuron (efferent motor pathway cranial to lower motor neuron) results in increased muscle tone (spastic paresis). In case of a sudden damage to the upper motor neuron a flaccid paresis (spinal shock) is followed days or weeks later by spastic paresis. Alterations in gait resembling that of paresis may also be seen in cases of pain of orthopaedic origin.

Signs of Systemic Effects

A compound may be given inadvertently at a dose level that induces toxicity in animals or may induce changes in particular organ systems. Such effects can be reflected by changes on parts of the nervous system and result in clinical signs which in general are not specific. Nonetheless, it is important that the experimenter keeps in mind that such effects may occur. Signs often associated with systemic effects are reduced activity, piloerection, hunched posture and/or palpebral closure and are usually accompanied by reduced food intake and reduced body weight development.

Pain

Painful situations may occur in any experiment. Pain may be caused by the experimental procedure itself, such as surgery or inflammatory reactions, or as a result of unexpected toxicity or accidents. To minimize the animals' suffering it is important to know the behavioural changes manifesting pain or distress. Such changes vary with the duration of pain. For example, acute pain is signalled by guarding (protection of painful body parts), licking, scratching or biting of the painful part, abnormal posture, vocalization, restlessness or recumbency; whereas chronic pain leads to reduced activity, licking of the painful part, dysuria or unkempt fur and often is accompanied by reduced food intake and body weight development (Norton and Griffiths, 1985; Wright et al., 1985). Signs of chronic pain in particular are not specific and most of them are common signs of intoxication.

Neurological Examination

In cases where the animal's movements are disturbed, the question arises as to whether this is due to dysfunction or damage to the nervous system, to other parts of the locomotor system such as bone, joints or muscles or if it is secondary to systemic toxicity or pain. A diagnostic tool for identifying potential neural involvement is the neurological examination which provides information on the functional integrity of the nervous system or parts of it. As a result of such an examination, neural circuits with altered or impaired function may be identified. In case of normal neural function, the cause for the disturbed movements has to be of muscular, orthopaedic or systemic origin.

General Approach

The first step in a neurological examination is careful observation of the animal's gait and arousal state. Thereafter, specific sensory receptors are stimulated and the motor responses induced by these stimuli are observed. Such motor responses may be exaggerated, normal, reduced or absent. In the case of a normal or exaggerated sensorimotor response, peripheral neurons involved in the sensorimotor response tested are intact. In the case of a reduced or absent response, damage within the sensory and/or motor branch of the peripheral circuit tested or of the effector muscle has to be assumed. To confirm and further localize a neuronal defect, another sensorimotor response has to be tested which uses a neuronal circuit that partially overlaps with that involved in the first response. As rats are rather small animals, testing of reflexes such as the patellar reflex is not easy to perform and thus sensorimotor function tests have been developed that are easier to conduct with small animals. These tests, however, do not allow such a precise localization of the lesions as the classical reflex tests do.

Localization of damage in the peripheral nerves or spinal cord is possible because of the hierarchical structure of the nervous system with reflex arches at spinal cord level and further sensorimotor connections at cerebellar, subthalamic and cortical levels. In the case of damage to the central nervous system, exact localization is more difficult due to the limited

In contrast to diffuse CNS damage, localized, circumscribed brain lesions often cannot be detected using neurological techniques as only functions other than neuromotor may be affected (Thompson, 1978). Some common neurological tests are described below. For further information see also Irwin (1968), Tupper and Wallace (1980), Goldberger *et al.* (1990), and Redding and Braund (1978). For regulatory toxicity studies such an approach had been standardized and is known as the Functional Observational Battery (Moser *et al.*, 1997).

Gait Analysis

Due to the low centre of gravity in rats only severe sensorimotor defects result in abnormal gait, with mild damages not being manifested when observing the animal. Such mild deficits may be identified by analysing the rat's gait. Changes in the conduct of individual leg movements and/or lack of coordination is reflected in altered geometry of footprints. A normal rat produces a narrow trace with the footprints of the hind feet at regular distances apart. To quantify changes in gait the width, distance between footprints and their regularity can be analysed (Figure 21.1) (De Medinacely *et al.*, 1982; Parker and Clarke, 1990).

Landing Foot Splay

Another way to detect sensorimotor dysfunction is to test the limits of the system. This is done when dropping the animal in the prone position from about 30 cm on to a table. In order to land on its feet, the rat balances its body in a vertical position. In cases of sensorimotor deficits this task is increasingly difficult and the animal needs larger balancing movements to control its position and therefore spreads its hind legs. As a consequence of this, the distance between the imprints of the hind feet is larger (Figure 21.2) (Edwards and Parker, 1977).

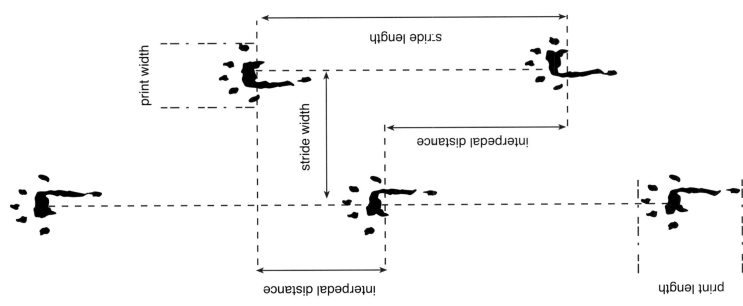

Figure 21.1 Gait analysis. Footprints can be described by their length and width; while the gait can be characterized by stride length, interpedal distance or stride width.

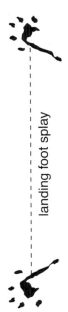

landing foot splay

Figure 21.2 Landing foot splay. The distance between two characteristic points of the hind footprints is measured. Landing foot splay is increased with increasing sensorimotor deficit.

number of central pathways involved in the sensorimotor responses usually tested in rats. When brain damage is not circumscribed and therefore affects more than one function, identification and rough localization of a damage within the CNS is possible.

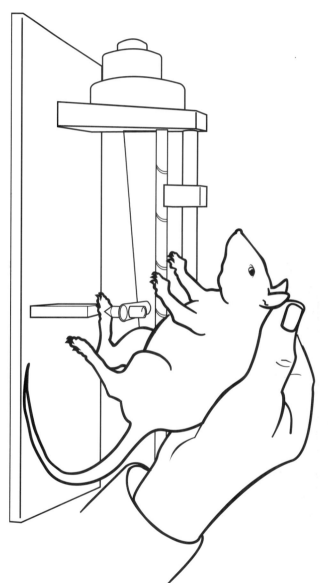

Figure 21.3 Randall–Sellito paw pressure test. This test was originally designed to measure oedema-related increases in pain sensitivity and its reduction by antiflogistic compounds. Pain is induced by a mechanical stimulus and pain perception is measured as the delay in withdrawing the paw.

Landing foot splay involves vestibular and proprioceptive sensory input to the sensory cortex and motor efferents from the motor cortex via corticospinal and extrapyramidal system to the muscles of body and legs.

Grip Strength

With reduced use or denervation of muscles their strength rapidly declines. The strength of some limb muscle groups can be measured easily as the force needed to pull the animal off a bar (Meyer et al., 1979) or a grid (Mattsson et al., 1986). Grip strength is a voluntary response which involves touch and proprioceptive sensation, sensory afferents to the thalamus and sensory cortex and motor efferents from the motor cortex via the efferent motor system to the leg muscles involved in the response. Grip strength has been demonstrated as a sensitive indicator for peripheral neuropathy (Classen et al., 1994), but can also be influenced by pharmacologically active compounds (Nevins et al., 1993).

Extensor Reflex

This voluntary response assesses the integrity of the peripheral and central parts of the sensorimotor response involved. The rat is suspended by the scruff skin and its hind feet slowly placed onto a

surface. The animal will extend its legs to support the weight of its body as soon as the feet touch the ground. The nervous circuit tested in this case includes the touch receptors in the feet, afferent sensory neurons to the thalamus and sensory cortex. From there the information travels to the motor cortex and via the efferent motor system to the muscles of the hind limbs.

Pain Response

Pinching the tip of the tail with a forceps results in vocalization, a defensive movement or a flight response of the animal. The wide range of possible reactions already indicates that the response is voluntary. Except for the muscles involved, which depend on the animal's response, the same efferent motor systems are needed as for the extensor reflex. The afferent branch includes pain receptors and their afferents to the thalamus and sensory cortex. For a quantification of pain perception the intensity of the stimulus provoking a response is measured. Typically this is done by measuring the weight with which a pen with a defined point presses onto the foot pad until the animal withdraws the foot (Randall–Sellito paw pressure test; Figure 21.3) or by measuring the time taken until the rat reacts to a thermal stimulus (hot plate test, tail flick test; Figure 21.4).

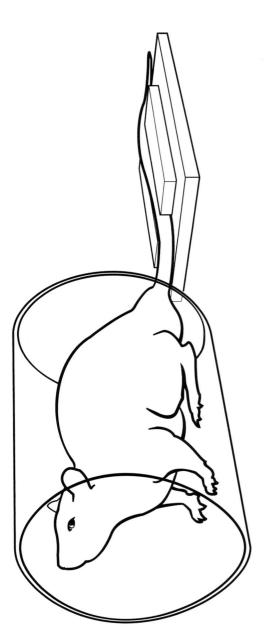

Figure 21.4 Tail flick test. In this test, the latency to withdraw the tail from a heat source is measured. Either a focused light or a water bath is used as a heat source to induce pain.

Touch Response

Touching the skin of the rat usually results in a movement directed towards the site where the body was touched. Depending on the strain used and/or the housing conditions (group-housed rats often respond less than single-housed ones) this response can be limited to a short direction of sensory attention towards the site of touch and thus may be difficult to see. This shift in attention is indicated by a short backward turn of the ipsilateral ear lobe. To improve detection of such a minimal response the attention of the animal first has to be attracted and directed frontally. The nervous circuits involved in this response includes touch receptors in the skin, afferent, sensory neurons to the thalamus and sensory cortex and motor efferents to the muscles involved with parts of the limbic system also playing a role in this response (Marshall *et al.*, 1971; Ljungberg and Ungerstedt, 1976).

Vestibular Responses

The vestibular system provides essential sensory information about the position of the body within space in order to balance the body correctly in a vertical plane and, when falling or jumping, ascertain that the rat will land on its feet. Except when climbing, the rat tries to keep its head in a horizontal position with the dorsal part of the head in the direction opposite to that of gravitation. Vestibular functions can be tested by bringing the animal out of

this 'ideal' position. This can be achieved, for example, by holding a rat by the tail: the rat will raise its head, especially when getting closer to a surface. Another test is done by holding the rat from the back side around its thorax and turning it on its back. When released, the animal turns back onto its feet. A more demanding test is the mid-air righting test. The rat is held upside down and dropped from about 30 cm above a table. During the fall the animal will turn and land on all four feet. To dampen the impact in the case of a vestibular or motor deficit the table should be covered with a sufficiently thick piece of rubber foam (Figures 21.5 and 21.6).

Pupillary Reflex

This is a very simple reflex to assess. When a light touches the retina of a dark-adapted rat, the pupil of this eye and to a lesser extent that of the contralateral eye will constrict. This reflex involves the sensory receptors in the retina, the afferent optic neuron to the pretectal nucleus and from there via the nucleus of Edinger-Westphal and N. oculomotorius to the ciliary muscle. As the iris is not pigmented in albino rats the pupillary reflex is best seen using a direct ophthalmoscope.

Visual Placing

This is a simple but crude test for visual function in rats. The animal is lifted by the tail and slowly moved

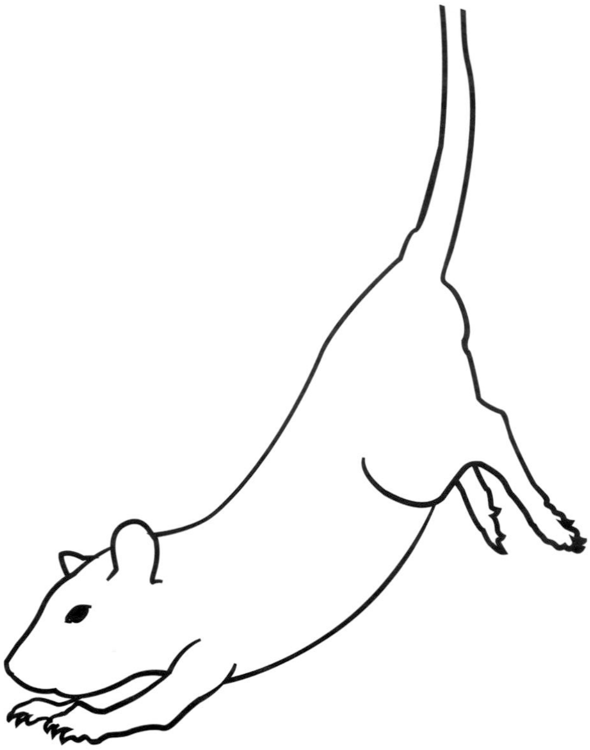

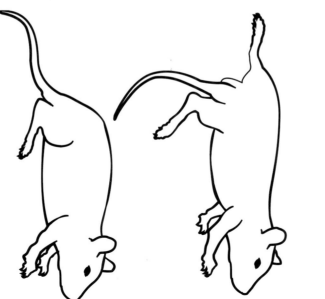

Figure 21.5 Vestibular response. Dorsoflexion of the back and lifting of the head is measured as the vestibular response shown by rats when held by the tail.

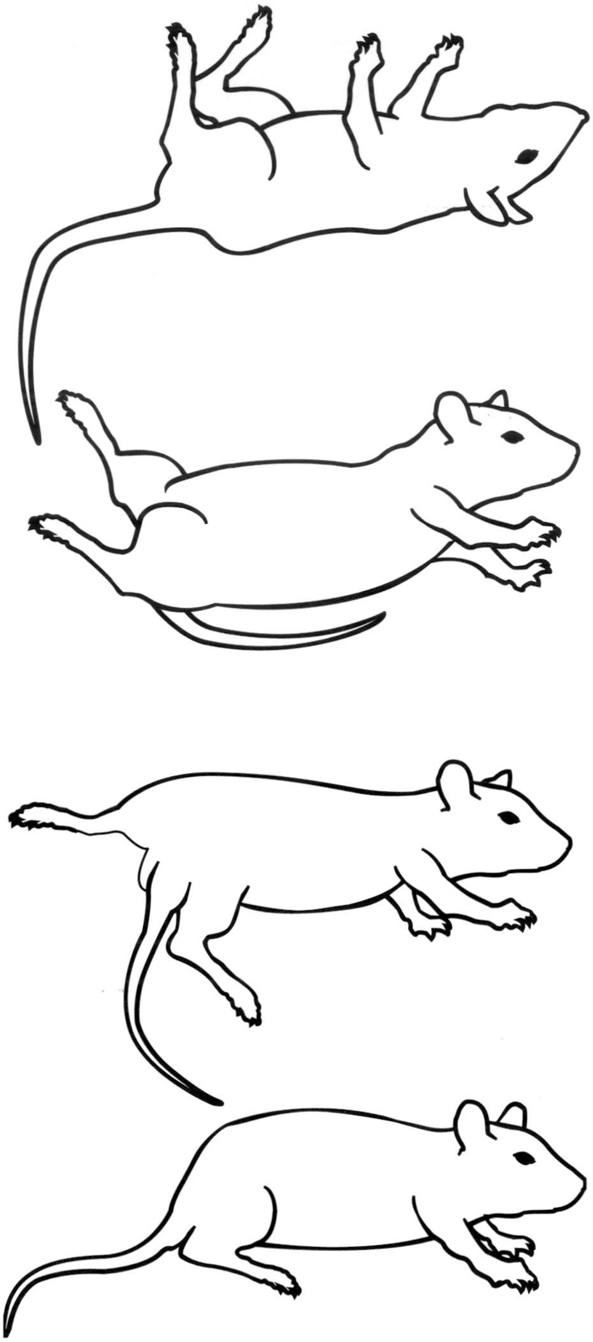

Figure 21.6 Mid-air righting. When dropped backside down the rat turns during the fall to land on its feet. This sensorimotor response is acquired around postnatal day 15.

Neurophysiological Techniques

In order to extend the diagnosis of a neurological deficit, such examinations may be complemented by neurophysiological techniques. Measuring nerve conduction velocity allows more precise quantitation/characterization and location of the lesion or

horizontally towards the edge of a table, a beam or a metal grid. When the rat approaches the surface it extends its front legs in order to get hold or support the body. This response depends on visual input and, as a voluntary response, involves visual and motor cortices and efferent motor tracts (corticospinal and extrapyramidal), spinal cord and peripheral nerves to the muscles involved.

differentiation between sensory, neural or muscular deficits. Furthermore, recording the CNS activity using electroencephalographic techniques may allow better characterization of CNS deficits. The different techniques and methodological aspects have been described in detail (Cracco and Bodis-Wollner, 1986; Hughes, 1994).

Peripheral Nerve Conduction Velocity

The velocity with which a nerve signal travels along the nerve fibres in a peripheral nerve, i.e. the nerve conduction velocity (NCV), can be measured *in vitro* on excised nerves (Birren and Wall, 1956), *in vivo* using surgically exposed nerves (McDonald, 1963; DeJesus *et al.*, 1978) or in intact animals (Glatt *et al.*, 1979). To measure the NCV, the selected nerve segment must be long enough to permit accurate measurement and as the NCV greatly depends on the temperature, it is important to control this variable carefully in the tissue or bath surrounding the nerve (Birren and Wall, 1956; DeJong *et al.*, 1966). Using pairs of two closely spaced stimuli and varying the interval between these stimuli allows measurement of the time needed by the nerve to restore the ionic equilibrium and to generate the second action potential, the refractory period.

Evoked Potentials

Electrical potentials recorded from the brain in response to external stimuli are called evoked potentials (EPs). As there is continuous brain activity even in the absence of peripheral stimuli, the evoked potential has to be filtered out of the background activity. This is achieved by averaging the electrical activity recorded after a train of 50 or more identical stimuli presented at a rate of about 1 Hz. The averaged signal obtained is characteristic for the sensory modality and stimulus used, and the individual peaks may be traced back to nerve activity in specific areas along the afferent sensory pathway.

Visually evoked potentials (VEPs)

These are recorded epidurally from above the primary visual cortex (e.g. 7 mm posterior of Bregma, 3 mm lateral to midline) and can be generated using stimuli ranging from diffuse light flashes (flash evoked potentials; FEPs) to complex patterns of shape and colour (pattern reversal evoked potentials; PREPs). PREPs are indicators of the ability to perceive patterns, and can be elicited by shifting patterns on a television screen or computer monitor. Their testing requires proper accommodation of the stimulus on the retina, and placing the fully aware animal in front of the screen (Mattsson *et al.*, 1992).

Auditory evoked potentials (AEPs)

These may be recorded epidurally from above the cortex (same site as for VEP) or the brainstem (BAEP) in response to brief auditory stimuli (clicks or pips) and can be used to detect specific losses in the auditory system (Figure 21.7). BAEPs can be obtained with subcutaneous electrodes above the cerebellum and brainstem (hypodermic needles placed subcutaneously at the vertex) in awake restrained or anaesthetized animals. When using pure tone stimuli and measuring the stimulus intensity needed to induce a predefined minimal signal, an audiogram is obtained which shows the hearing sensitivity across the frequency band tested (Rebert, 1983; Sullivan *et al.*, 1989).

Sensory evoked potentials (SEPs)

These are elicited by electrical stimulation of sensory receptors or peripheral nerves in the foot, tail or skin and are recorded from the somatosensory cortex (e.g. 1.5 mm posterior to the Bregma, 3 mm lateral to the midline). Recording from the cerebellum (e.g. 12 mm posterior of Bregma, at midline) can help to differentiate effects and/or localize lesions more precisely. SEPs are not without interpretational difficulties as they are sensitive to temperature changes (Rebert, 1983; Albee *et al.*, 1987; Sohmer, 1991).

Electroencephalography

The frequency, amplitude, variability and pattern of the EEG is a measure of the dynamic process of the instantaneously integrated activity of the brain. An EEG obtained using surface electrodes or epidural electrodes is a summation of the electrical activity mainly from neurons a few millimetres beneath the electrode and does not accurately reflect activity of deeper structures. By implanting electrodes into subcortical structures their activity can be recorded (Dyer *et al.*, 1979a,b; Naalsund, 1986).

The EEG reflects instantaneous changes in the state of CNS activity and thus primarily indicates the state of arousal, anaesthesia or excitatory activity characterized by spikes and spindles. It is composed of electrical signals of different frequencies. The contribution of the various frequencies can be determined using the technique of Fourier transformation. This allows determination of the energy in the specific frequency bands.

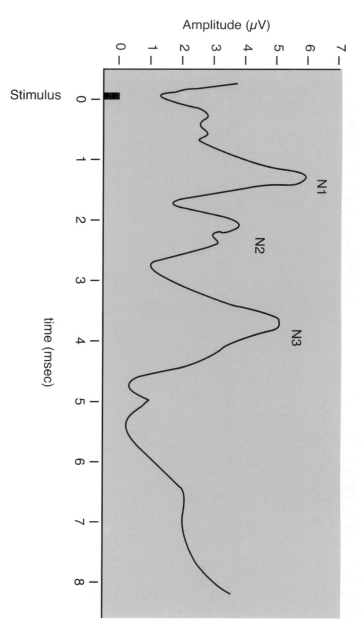

Figure 21.7 Evoked potentials. This schematic drawing of an auditory evoked potential recorded above the brainstem demonstrates the nomenclature used for the individual peaks. The individual peaks reflect activity in the acoustic nerve (N1), cochlear nucleus (N2) and lateral lemniscus (N3). To identify changes in the evoked potential, its amplitude and latency is quantified.

Ethological Approach

Behaviour may be regarded as the relationship between the organism and its environment and must be adjusted according to the requirements of either or both. During evolution, behaviour has been optimally adapted to the animals' environment. Although environmental conditions may dramatically change over a short time period, the animals' behavioural repertoire will change only marginally from one generation to the other. This allows the study of behaviour under different environmental conditions, including the conditions provided in the laboratory.

Besides observation of clinical signs as indicators of pharmacological effects or of toxicity, spontaneous behaviour can be quantified either by recording it periodically (e.g. every full minute), continuously or by measuring the duration of the behaviour over a predefined time period. To facilitate evaluation and interpretation of the data

behaviour such as investigation or sex-related, aggressive, submissive or escaping behaviour. When exposed to a chemical or to changes in environmental conditions, animals react very sensitively with shifts in their behavioural pattern. Although this approach is sensitive and in general does not require expensive test apparatus, purely ethological approaches are not often used. Some reasons for this may be that specific perceptual capabilities and/or extensive training are needed to recognize and interpret the behavioural sequences correctly. Furthermore, as the potential for automated analysis is limited, ethological studies are time consuming. In addition, behavioural changes are also induced by minor environmental alterations, thereby confounding such experiments. Therefore, ethological approaches are only mentioned in the context of other tests where this approach may support the correct interpretation of the endpoints evaluated in that test.

obtained, the different behavioural responses are usually x assigned to different categories such as nonsocial behaviour, e.g. residual behaviour, maintenance behaviour or exploration as well as social

Behavioural Tests

The fact that the animal's behaviour is influenced by its environment has been used to study basic mechanisms underlying behaviour, to localize the brain areas involved or to identify neurotransmitters which modulate this behaviour. By exposing rats to a standardized environment or to a defined change in these environmental conditions induces a specific behaviour or a behavioural change. Such test situations may be used to study effects of pharmacologically active compounds or brain lesions. Out of the plethora of behavioural tests only a few will be described briefly in order to give an impression of the broad range of aspects covered by these tests.

Open Field

The open field was first designed by Hall (1934) as the most simple maze possible, a large circular arena (2.4 m in diameter) surrounded by a wall. This design was expected to reduce environmental stimuli to a minimum, thereby facilitating interpretation of the behaviour shown by the rats. The floor of the open field was divided into several fields by concentric circles and radial lines. The rat was placed into the open field next to the wall and the movements and behaviour shown recorded. By modifying testing conditions it was recognized that, for example, a hungry rat walked further, but did not necessarily eat when food was provided in the arena. Rats that did not eat in the open field may be considered 'emotional'. Such animals in general entered the open, central area less often and were more likely to defecate. However, the evidence for the sign's validity as an indicator for emotional behaviour was found not to be that solid (Walsh and Cummins, 1976).

Plus Maze

The plus maze is a test for emotional behaviour or anxiety and was developed in order to screen for anxiolytic compounds other than those of the benzodiazepine type. The test apparatus consists of an elevated, plus-shaped maze. Two opposite arms of the maze have opaque walls, while the other two arms are open. As emotional rats prefer to stand under the shelter of a wall, the time spent on the open arms can be used as a measure for an animal's

emotional state or anxiety. Ethologically based endpoints such as rearing on open arms or reaching out of the enclosed arm have been used as well and may support the construct validity of endpoints (Cole and Rodgers, 1994).

Behavioural Despair and Learned Helplessness

These tests were developed to screen antidepressants by using effects other than the monoaminergic side-effects. For the behavioural despair test the animal is placed in a deep water tank from which it cannot escape. After an initial period during which the animal actively tries to escape from the water, the rat stops moving and floats just keeping its nose above the water. This inactivity was considered to reflect despair and was shown to be reduced by some antidepressants (Porsolt et al., 1978; Nomura et al., 1982). In the learned helplessness test the rats are exposed to inescapable foot shocks which induce passive endurance of foot shocks in a later shuttle box situation (Sherman et al., 1982; Martin et al., 1987).

Conditioned Behaviour

In addition to the spontaneous or innate behaviour that is observed using the techniques described, a variety of behavioural patterns are learned. Learning paradigms can be classified into three broad categories: habituation, respondent or classical (Pavlovian) conditioning, and operant or instrumental (Skinnerian) conditioning.

Habituation is considered to be a primitive form of learning due to its nonassociative characteristics (Overstreet, 1977).

Respondent or classical conditioning (Pavlovian conditioning) is based on the fact that the rat builds associations between successive events or stimuli. One of these events or stimuli, the unconditioned stimulus (UCS) is inducing a response, the unconditioned response (UCR). When the UCS is paired repetitively with another stimulus, the conditioned stimulus (CS), the rat will form an association between these two stimuli and finally the CS will elicit

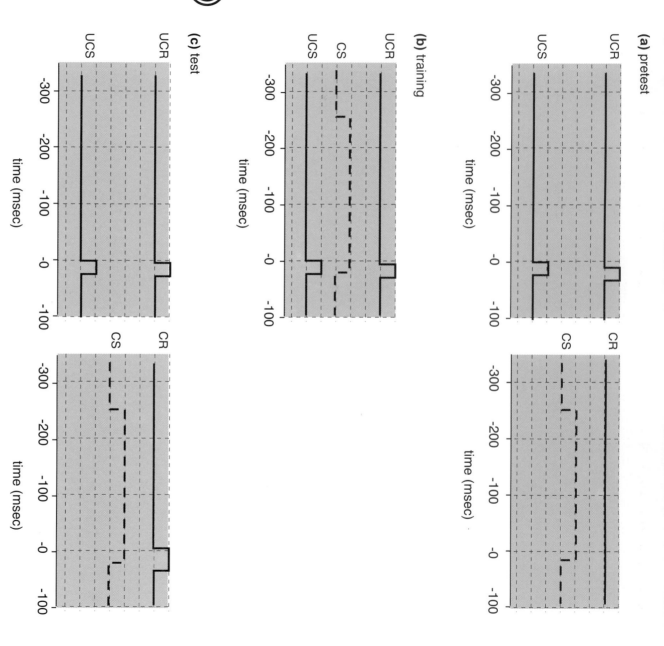

(a) pretest

(b) training

(c) test

Figure 21.8 Schematic representation of classical conditioning. (**a**) In the naive animal only the unconditioned stimulus (UCS) induces a response (unconditioned response, UCR). (**b**) During training the UCS and the conditioned stimulus (CS) are presented together for a number of trials. (**c**) After training (test trial) a response can be induced by the UCS as well as the CS.

the same response in the absence of the UCS; this response is called the conditioned response (CR) (Figure 21.8).

Operant or instrumental conditioning was first described by Skinner. When a particular response is followed by a reward or an adverse event, this behaviour occurs more frequently in the first situation and less often in the second one. When, for example, a rat in a Skinner box presses a lever and as

a consequence of this receives some food, a hungry rat will press this lever more frequently in order to get more food. Operant conditioning can be divided into two different domains: free operant conditioning and discrete-trial operant conditioning. Both are applications of the same principle, but they provide data of a different nature. Free operant conditioning is essentially a performance test and its main dependent variable is the rate of response that is normally evaluated at steady states using reinforcement schedules such as 'fixed ratio' or 'fixed interval' (MacPhail and Leander, 1981). Discrete trial operant conditioning reduces the importance of response rates to the benefit of an accuracy index or a learning index such as percentage correct responses or trials to criterion. Discrete trial operant conditioning can help to formulate specific questions about memory or learning.

Habituation

Habituation takes place during prolonged or repetitive exposure to the same experimental situation (Overstreet, 1977; Patel and Porsolt, 1982). The most common situations are habituation of motor activity, which largely depends on the size and complexity of the test apparatus, and habituation of the startle response, which depends on the stimulus intensity, duration and variability of interstimulus intervals (Davis, 1984).

Object discrimination

Another test involving habituation is the object discrimination test, a memory test which is generally used to measure short-term memory. When placing an object in an open field, a two-compartment box or a Y-maze, the rat will explore the object as it provides novel stimuli and, as it becomes more familiar, the time spent examining declines. When placing a new object next to the one to be familiarized in the test apparatus, the rat will direct its interest towards the new object with the familiar object being examined for only a short period. The difference in exploration times of the new and the familiar object thus indicates that the rat recognized the familiar object (Andrews et al., 1995; Dellu et al., 1992).

Classical Conditioning

Conditioned eye blink

For this test the animal is restrained with recording electrodes fixed to the eyelid. The CS, usually a tone stimulus, is followed by the UCS, an air puff directed to the cornea of the eye or an electric stimulus. The UCS elicits a rapid closure of the eyelid, an eye blink. Repetitive pairing of the tone stimulus and UCS will finally result in an eye blink induced by the tone stimulus alone (Skelton, 1988). Eye blinks can be conditioned in all species including humans and have been studied thoroughly. As this test measures a comparable endpoint in all species and as conditioning can be modified by the same procedures and compounds, it is an ideal test for the comparison of this type of learning across species.

Conditioned taste aversion

When consumption of a novel food is followed by sickness or a pharmacological effect, the rat will avoid this food in the future. In contrast to most other examples of conditioned behaviour, a single trial is sufficient for the rat to learn this conditioned avoidance response. Conditioned taste aversion is usually measured in a choice situation where the rat can select between a standard diet or fluid and the novel-tasting one which had been paired with exposure to a substance. The reduction in intake of novel food after the conditioning as compared with before conditioning is used as a measure of the acquisition of taste avoidance (Dragoin et al., 1971; Sakai and Yamamoto, 1998).

Instrumental Learning

There are two different test procedures used for operant conditioning: (1) the mazes where the animal has to go to a specific site in order or to get the reward and (2) the Skinner boxes where the rat has to perform a specific act such as pressing a lever or nose poke. Although at first glance these two test conditions seem to differ in principle, they both follow the rule that a specific behaviour is facilitated when followed by reinforcement.

Active/passive avoidance

Both adverse conditioning paradigms use a two-compartment test box in which the rat has to build an association between one side of the box and an aversive event, usually a foot shock. In the passive avoidance paradigm, the rat is placed into the safe compartment which is illuminated to stimulate the animal to cross over into the dark, preferred compartment where it will receive an unavoidable foot shock and is then removed from the apparatus. With a strong foot shock the rat learns the association between the dark compartment and foot shock in a single trial (one-trial passive avoidance test) (Jarvik and Kopp, 1967). With lower shock intensities, several trials are needed until the rat stays in the safe compartment for a predetermined time. One to several days after training the retention of this association is measured as the latency of the animal to enter the dark compartment.

In the active avoidance paradigm, the rat is placed into the dark, unsafe compartment. The upcoming foot shock may be signalled by a light and/or tone stimulus or simply indicated by placing the rat into the start box. Within a predefined time the animal has to cross to the other, safe compartment of the box in order to avoid the foot shock. As the door to the safe compartment remains open, the animal can escape the foot shock. After each trial the rat is removed from the box and after a delay placed back into the start compartment for a next trial. This procedure is repeated until the animal reaches a predefined level of avoidance.

Shuttle box

The shuttle box is an attempt to automate the active avoidance procedure. Instead of removing the animal after each trial, the rat is left in the box and after a predefined intertrial interval the compartment in which the rat stays is selected as the unsafe or start compartment. The opposite or safe compartment is signalled by a light whereas a tone indicates the upcoming foot shock. In this test both sides of the two-compartment box are safe or unsafe and the animal has to overcome its fear of entering the compartment in which it received a foot shock. It has been demonstrated that shuttle avoidance learning strongly depends on the animal's emotionality and less so on its cognitive ability (Roozendaal et al., 1992; Escorihuela et al., 1995).

Maze learning

As with punishment, the animal's behaviour can be modified using some reinforcement such as food. For food to be reinforcing, the rat has to be hungry and the animal has to feel safe and eat the food in the test box. Therefore, the animals have to be thoroughly acclimatized to the test conditions. A variety of mazes of different complexity have been designed, such as the T-maze, star maze, hole board or Hebb–William maze (Meunier et al., 1986; van der Staay et al., 1990). Less acclimatization is needed when escape from water is used as reinforcement, as in a Morris water maze. When providing the reinforcement always at the same site in the maze the animal's capability to memorize this site is tested ('reference memory'). On the other hand, when reinforcement depends on the last response (e.g. arm not yet visited in the T-maze or star maze) the animal's short-term memory or 'working memory' is tested (Brandeis et al., 1989).

Operant Conditioning

Operant conditioning requires the rat to behave in a specific way such as pressing a lever, or poking its nose into a hole in order to receive food as a reward or to avoid punishment.

Schedules used in free operant conditioning are based either on a time criterion or on the number of lever presses. On a fixed interval schedule, the first response after a predefined time interval is rewarded, while in the differential reinforcement of the low rates schedule the animal has to refrain from responding for a certain time and is reinforced for the first response made after this criterion has been met. Under a fixed ratio schedule every nth response is rewarded while under a variable ratio the reinforcements are delivered unpredictably. The different schedules produce characteristic response patterns which can be modified by pharmacologically active compounds. The change in these response patterns is the endpoint measured. These test situations are rather artificial and extrapolation to daily life situations in humans is rather difficult.

An almost unlimited number of discrete trial operant conditioning schedules have been designed in order to test sensory functions or different types and aspects of memory. Discrete-trial operant conditioning can help to formulate specific questions, whether about memory or about learning or other functions.

At the same time it reduces the importance of response rates to the benefit of an accuracy index or a learning index such as percentage correct responses or trials to criterion. Some examples of discrete trial operant conditioning are the delayed matching to sample (short-term memory), left–right discrimination (reference memory) or continuous learning paradigms (general cognitive capacity), which require the rats to learn new response sequences in a multi-lever test box (Pollard et al., 1981). To measure sensory functions the presence or absence of a sensory stimulus determines e.g. the lever to press. The perception threshold of, for example, a tone signal is then determined as the loudness at which the rat responds at chance level (Bushnell et al., 1994).

Regulatory Neurotoxicology

In order to identify, characterize and quantify a potential neurotoxic effect induced by a chemical, the methods described in this section are usually used. Details of potential approaches have been published by different groups (WHO-IPCS, 1986; ECETOC, 1992; US-EPA, 1994, 1998a; Eisenbrandt *et al.*, 1994). Test guidelines giving specific details on the conduct of such studies have been adopted or drafted by various countries (US-EPA, 1998b; MAFF, 1998) as well as by the OECD (1995, 1997). Tests suggested in these guidelines include clinical signs for detection of peripheral and central neurotoxic effects and autonomic dysfunction, neurological tests directed towards sensory and motor functions, as well as locomotor activity, an apical test affected by peripheral and/or central nervous system dysfunction and by systemic toxicity.

In toxicity studies, absence of toxicity has to be demonstrated for each organ by showing its function to be normal. In order to exclude a neurotoxic effect, the morphological and functional integrity of all parts of the nervous system has to be demonstrated using tests of sufficient sensitivity. For the efficient use of resources, a tiered approach is taken. In a first experiment in which animals are exposed to high dose levels a potential neurotoxic effect is identified using simpler and less time-consuming behavioural tests and standard histopathological techniques. Behavioural investigations usually conducted in this first-tier test include detailed clinical observations, neurological examination and measurement of locomotor activity. In the case of a clear or equivocal effect, a second study (tier 2) is conducted in which the spectrum of effects induced is better characterized and usually a dose level can be determined at which the effects are no longer seen. This tier 2 study is usually conducted at lower dose levels and thus allows differentiation between behavioural changes related to neurotoxicity and those secondary to severe systemic organ toxicity. As in the tier 1 study, clinical observations, neurological examination and measurement of locomotor activity are included as behavioural tests. Morphological changes are evaluated in perfusion-fixed tissues using standard or specific staining techniques and more sophisticated tests may be included such as specific electrophysiological measurements. In a further, tier 3 study

specific effects may be assessed using highly sensitive tests such as electrophysiology or tests measuring specific functions such as learning and memory.

After single or repeated administration, a chemical can induce either acute, pharmacological (neuroactive) effects that appear within hours after administration or a chronic or delayed effect that appears only after several days and may last for weeks or months. Often this delayed effect is accompanied by morphological changes in the nervous system.

Acute effects are best detected after a single, high dose using simple tests (e.g. clinical signs) that allow characterization of the effects and to determine their time course. In a second iteration using more sophisticated tests, the effects may be characterized better and a dose level can be determined at which the compound no longer induces an effect.

Chronic or delayed effects are best identified after repeated administration and as the effects last for days, also more sophisticated or more time-consuming behavioural or functional tests can be included in an initial experiment. As occurrence of neuropathy is a likely and critical endpoint associated with chronic or delayed effects, morphological changes are evaluated in perfusion-fixed tissues using standard or specific staining techniques. Depending on the effects observed, neurophysiological or specific behavioural tests may be conducted in a further study to assess specific functions that may be affected at lower doses.

References

Albee, R.R., Mattsson, J.L., Yano, B.L. and Chang, L.W. (1987) *Teratology* **9**, 203–211.

Andrews, J.S., Jansen, J.H., Linders, S., Princen, A. and Broekkamp, C.L. (1995) *Physiol. Behav.* **57**, 785–790.

Birren, J.E. and Wall, P.D. (1956) *J. Comp. Neurol.* **104**, 1–16.

Brandeis, R., Brandys, Y. and Yehuda, S. (1989) *Int. J. Neurosci.* **48**, 29–69.

Bushnell, P.J., Kelly, K.L. and Crofton, K.M. (1994) *Neurotoxicol. Teratol.* **16**, 149–160.

Classen, W., Gunson, D.E., Iverson, W.O., Traina, V.M., Vonau, M.H., and Krinke, G.J. (1994) *Exp. Toxic. Pathol.* **46**, 119–125.

Cole, J.C. and Rodgers, R.J. (1994) *Psychopharmacology (Berl.)* **114**, 288–296.

Cracco, R.Q. and Bodis-Wollner, I. (1986) *Frontiers of Clinical Neuroscience*, Vol. 3, *Evoked Potentials*. New York: Alan R. Liss.

Davis, M. (1984) In: Eaton, R.C. (ed.) *Neural Mechanisms of Startle Behavior*, pp. 287–351. New York: Plenum Press.

DeJesus, C.V.P., Towfighi, J., and Snyder, D.R. (1978) *Muscle Nerve* **1**, 162–167.

DeJong, R.H., Hershey, W.N. and Wagman, I.H. (1966) *Anesthesiology* **27**, 805–810.

Dellu, F., Mayo, W., Cherkaoui, J., Le Moal, M. and Simon, H. (1992) *Brain Res.* **588**, 132–139.

De Medinacely, I., Freed, W.J., and Wyatt R.J. (1982) *Exp. Neurol.* **77**, 634–643.

Dempster, J. (1992) *Computer Analysis of Electrophysiological Signals*. London: Academic Press.

Dragoin, W., McCleary, G.E. and McCleary, P. (1971) *Behav. Res. Meth. Instrum.* **3**, 309–310.

Dyer, R.S., Burden, E., Hulebak, K., Schulz, N., Swartzwelder, M.S. and Annau, Z. (1979a) *Neurobehav. Toxicol.* **1**, 21–25.

Dyer, R.S., Swartzwelder, H.S., Eccles, C.W. and Annau, Z. (1979b) *Neurobehav. Toxicol.* **1**, 5–19.

ECETOC (1992) European Chemical Industry Ecology and Toxicology Centre, Monograph no. 18: Evaluation of the neurotoxic potential of chemicals. Brussels, Belgium: ECETOC.

Edwards, P.M. and Parker, V.H. (1977) *Toxicol. Appl. Pharmacol.* **40**, 589–591.

Eisenbrandt, D.L., Allen, S.L. *et al.*, (1994) *Fd Chem. Toxic.* **32**, 655–669.

Escorihuela, R.M., Tobena, A., Driscoll, P. and Fernandez-Teruel, A. (1995) *Neurosci. Biobehav. Rev.* **19**, 353–367.

Glatt, A.F., Talaat, H.N. and Koella, W.P. (1979) *Therapy* **5**, 539–543.

Goldberger, M.E., Bregman, B.S., Vierck, C.J. and Brown, M. (1990) *Exp. Neurol.* **107**, 113–117.

Hall, C.S. (1934) *J. Comp. Psychol.* **18**, 385–403.

Hughes, J.R. (1994) EEG in clinical practice, 2nd edn, Butterworth-Heinemann, Boston.

Irwin, S. (1968) *Psychopharmacology* **13**, 222–225.

Jarvik, M.E. and Kopp, R. (1967) *Psychol. Rep.* **21**, 221–224.

Kelly, J.P. (1985) In: Kandel, E.R. and Schwartz, J.H. (eds) *Principles of Neural Science*, 2nd edn, pp. 222–243. New York: Elsevier.

Ljungberg, T. and Ungerstedt, U. (1976) *Exp. Neurol.* **53**, 585–600.

Lowitsch, K., Maurer, K. and Hopf, H.C. (1983) *Evozierte Potentiale in der klinischen Diagnostik, visuell, akustisch, somatosensibel.* Stuttgart: Georg Thieme Verlag.

McDonald, W.I. (1963) *Brain* **86**, 501.

MacPhail, R.C. and Leander, J.D. (1981) *Toxicol. Teratol.* **3**, 19–26.

MAFF (Ministry of Agriculture, Forestry and Fisheries, Japan) (1998) Agricultural Chemicals Inspection Station, Guidelines on the compiling of test results

on toxicity (draft): 'Acute neurotoxicity test' and 'Multiple dose oral neurotoxicity test'.

Marshall, J.F., Turner, B.H., and Teitelbaum, P. (1971) *Science* **174**, 523–525.

Martin, P., Soubrie-P. and Simon, P. (1987) *Prog. Neuropsychopharmacol. Biol. Psychiatry* **11**, 1–7.

Mattsson, J.L., Albee, R.R., and Brandt, L.M. (1984) *Fundam. Appl. Toxicol.* **4**, 944–948.

Mattsson, J.L., Albee, R.R., Johnson, K.A., and Quast, J.F. (1986) *Neurobehav. Toxicol. Teratol.* **8**, 255–263.

Mattsson, J.L., Albee, R.R. and Eisenbrandt, D.L. (1989) *J. Am. College Toxicol.* **8**, 271–286.

Mattsson, J.L., Boyes, W.K. and Ross, J.F. (1992) In: Tilson, H.A. and Mitchell, C.L. (eds) *Neurotoxicology*, pp. 125–145. New York: Raven Press.

Meunier, M., Saint-Marc, M. and Destrade, C. (1986) *Physiol. Behav.* **37**, 909–913.

Meyer, O.A., Tilson, H.A., Byrd, W.C. and Riley, M.T. (1979) *Neurobehav. Toxicol.* **1**, 233–236.

Moser, V.C., Tilson, H.A., MacPhail, R.C. *et al.* (1997) *Neurotoxicology* **18**, 929–938.

Naalsund, L.U. (1986) *Acta Pharmacol. Toxicol.* **59**, 325–331.

Nevins, M.E., Nash, S.A., and Beardsley, P.M. (1993) *Psychopharmacology* **110**, 92–96.

Nomura, S., Shimizu, J., Kinjo, M., Kametani, H. and Nakazawa, T. (1982) *Eur. J. Pharmacol.* **83**, 171–175.

Norton, D.B. and Griffiths, P.H.M. (1985) *Vet. Rec.* **116**, 431–436.

OECD (Organization for Economic Cooperation and Development) (1995) Guideline for the Testing of Chemicals no. 407: 'Repeated dose 28-day oral toxicity study in rodents', adopted 27 July 1995.

OECD (1997) Guideline for the Testing of Chemicals no. 424: 'Neurotoxicity study in rodents', adopted 21 July 1997.

Overstreet, D.H. (1977) *Physiol. Psychol.* **5**, 230–238.

Parker, A.J. and Clarke, K.A. (1990) *Physiol. Behav.* **48**, 41–47.

Patel, A. and Porsolt, R.D. (1982) *Psychopharmacol. (Berl)* **78**, 346–352.

Pollard, G.T., McBennett, S.T., Rohrbach, K.W. and Howard, J.L. (1981) *Drug Devel. Res.* **1**, 67–75.

Porsolt, R.D., Anton, G., Blavet, N. and Jalfre, M. (1978) *Eur. J. Pharmacol.* **47**, 379–391.

Rebert, C.S. (1983) *Neurobehav. Toxicol. Teratol.* **5**, 659.

Redding, R.W. and Braund, K.G. (1978) In: Hoerlein, B.F. (ed.) *Canine Neurology: Diagnosis and Treatment*, 3rd edn, pp. 53–70. Philadelphia: W.B. Saunders.

Roozendaal, B., Wiersma, A., Driscoll, P., Koolhaas, J.M. and Bohus, B. (1992) *Brain Res.* **596**, 35–40.

Sakai, N. and Yamamoto, T. (1998) *Behav. Brain Res.* **93**, 63–70.

Sherman, A.D., Sacquitne, J.L. and Petty, F. (1982) *Pharmacol. Biochem. Behav.* **16**, 449–454.

Skelton, R.W. (1988) *Behav. Neurosci.* **102**, 586–590.

Sohmer, H. (1991) *J. Basic Clin. Physiol. Pharmacol.* **2**, 243–255.

Stanley, E.F. (1981) *Exp. Neurol.* **71**, 497–506.

Sullivan, M.J., Rarey, K.E. and Conolly, R.B. (1989) *Neurotoxicol. Teratol.* **10**, 525–530.

Thompson, R. (1978) *A Behavioral Atlas of the Rat Brain.* New York: Oxford University Press.

Tupper, D.E. and Wallace, R.B. (1980) *Acta Neurobiol. Exp.* **40**, 999–1003.

US-EPA (United States Environmental Protection Agency) (1994) *Fed. Reg.* **59**, 42360–42404.

US-EPA (1998a) *Fed. Reg.* **63**, 26926–26954.

US-EPA (1998b) Office of Prevention, Pesticides and Toxic Substances: OPPTS Harmonized Test Guidelines 870.6200: 'Neurotoxicity Screening Battery'.

van der Staay, F.J., van Nies, J. and Raaijmakers, W. (1990) *Behav. Neurol. Biol.* **53**, 356–370.

Walsh, R.N. and Cummins, R.A. (1976) *Psychol. Bull.* **83**, 482–504.

WHO-IPCS (World Health Organization, International Program on Chemical Safety) (1986) *Environmental Health Criteria 60: Principles and methods for the assessment of neurotoxicity associated with exposure to chemicals.* Geneva: WHO.

Wright, E.M., Marcella, K.L. and Woodson, J.F. (1985) *Animal* **19**, 20–36.

CHAPTER 22

Immunology and Hematology

Hiroshi Matsuda
Department of Veterinary Clinic, Tokyo University of Agriculture and Technology, Tokyo, Japan

Akane Tanaka
Department of Veterinary Clinic, Tokyo University of Agriculture and Technology, Tokyo, Japan

Atsuko Itakura
Department of Veterinary Clinic, Tokyo University of Agriculture and Technology, Tokyo, Japan

Immunology

Immunogenetics

The major histocompatibility complex (MHC), called RT1 in rats, is located on chromosome 17 (Gill *et al.*, 1989). This MHC class I molecule is encoded by a large number of genes, such as *RT1.A*, *RT1.F*, pregnancy-associated locus, *RT1.C*, *RT1.E*, *RT1.N*, *RT.BM1* and *RT.1M*. *RT1.A* and *RT1.E* are closely related to murine *H-2K* and *H-2D*, respectively; and *RT1.N*, *RT.BM1* and *RT.1M* are very similar to murine *H-2T10/H-2T22*, *H-2T23* and *H-2M*, respectively (Gill *et al.*, 1989; Paker *et al.*, 1991; Wang *et al.*, 1995). A recent study has also

demonstrated the new loci, *RT1.S1* and *RT1.S2*, with five exons similar to other MHC class I loci (Salgar *et al.*, 1997). *RT1.B* and *RT1.D*, which encode the MHC class II molecule, have homology with murine *H-2A* and *H-2E*, respectively. In addition, *RT1.H* is also included in MHC class II loci (Watters *et al.*, 1987).

Immunoglobulins

The classes of immunoglobulins identified in rats are IgG, IgA, IgM, IgE and IgD, IgG being classified into four subclasses. Rat IgG1 and IgG2a are similar to murine IgG1; and rat IgG2b and IgG2c are homologs of murine IgG2a/IgG2b and IgG3 respectively (Bruggemann, 1988). Rat immunoglobulin allotypes have been described for κ chains and heavy chains of IgA, IgG2b, and IgG2c; and they are controlled by Igk, Igh-1, Igh-2, and Igh-3 loci, respectively. The immunoglobulin allotypes of rat inbred strains are well described by Gutman (1996).

Antigen-presenting Cells

Dendritic cells

Identification of dendritic cells (DCs) is mostly based on their morphology because of the lack of specific surface markers other than MHC class II. However, several important surface markers have been found on DCs. Some populations of rat DCs express an antigen (Ag) recognized by OX-62 monoclonal antibody (mAb), which has the biochemical properties of an **integrin** (Brenan and Puklavec, 1992), while CD11c and DEC-205 receptor (R) have been found on murine DC (Jiang et al., 1995).

In addition to the Ag-presenting activity of DCs, recent studies have demonstrated their cytotoxic activity, although the cytotoxic mechanism is different between rats and mice. DCs in the spleen and thymus express natural killer cell R (NKR) protein 1. In response to stimulation by NKR protein 1, killing activity is enhanced (Josien et al., 1997), suggesting that rat DC may exhibit NK cell-like activity.

Mononuclear phagocytes

A rat monocyte–macrophage lineage is recognized by three different mAbs, ED1, ED2 and ED3. ED1 recognizes the majority of monocyte–macrophage lineage cells. They are then classified further into subpopulations by binding patterns of ED2 and ED3 (Dijkstra et al., 1985).

Macrophages function as a source of **eicosanoids** and various cytokines which modulate inflammatory responses, and play a key role in the primary host defense against pathogens such as bacteria and viruses. Rat macrophages have the capacity to synthesize or secrete a variety of cytokines and chemokines, such as interleukin (IL) 1β, IL-6, IL-10, interferon γ (IFNγ), tumor necrosis factor α (TNFα), transforming growth factor β (TGFβ), platelet-derived growth factor (PDGF), monocyte chemoattractant protein 1 (MCP-1), and macrophage inflammatory proteins (MIP) 1α and 2 (Feng et al., 1993; Huang et al., 1992; Kovacs et al., 1994; Ogle et al., 1994; Shi et al., 1995).

Lymphocytes

T cells

Differentiation

The developmental stages of thymocytes are classified by the expression pattern of surface antigens, such as CD4, CD8 and T cell receptors (TCRs), and the signals necessary for their differentiation have been described. Several signals essential for rat thymocyte development have been demonstrated. Rat $CD4^-CD8^-$ cells can differentiate into $CD4^+CD8^+$ cells without any stimulation *in vitro* (Hunig and Mitnacht, 1991). However, stimulation of $CD4^-CD8^-$ cells with anti-αβ Ab is effective for the induction of the expression of the IL-2R β chain on rat $CD4^+CD8^+$ cells, and the addition of IL-2 leads to differentiation from $CD4^+CD8^+$ cells into $CD4^-CD8^+$ cells (Park et al., 1993). In relation to this point, IL-2 may be involved in T-cell development in rats, while an essential function of IL-2 in murine T-cell development was ruled out by a recent study using IL-2-deficient mice (Schorle et al., 1991). It is of interest to note that in mice, TCR ligation alone is able to induce $CD4^+$ T cells from $CD4^+CD8^+$ cells (Takahama et al., 1994), suggesting that murine $CD4^+CD8^+$ cells are committed to becoming $CD4^+$ T cells, while rat $CD4^+CD8^+$ cells are committed to becoming $CD8^+$ T cells (Park et al., 1993).

Subpopulations and cytokine profiles

Among some of the specific surface markers raised against T cells, the TCRs are the most relevant for defining T cells. In rats they are divided into two subpopulations, as in humans and mice, i.e. TCRαβ and TCRγδ. Although most of the peripheral T cells bear TCRαβ, a very small number of γδ-bearing cells can be identified among the T cells of the lymph nodes and intestinal intraepithelial lymphocytes in rats (Kuhnlein et al., 1994). In contrast to mice and humans, however, the majority of rat γδ T cells express CD8 but not CD4. McMenamin et al. (1995) have recently demonstrated the significant involvement of rat γδ T cells in the downregulation of IgE synthesis induced by inhaled soluble antigens.

The Th2-like cells of the rat, with a higher capacity for the production of IL-4 and IL-5, are generated by stimulation of splenocytes with IL-4 and anti-IFNγ, whereas the addition of IFNγ does not induce their differentiation into Th1 cells (Noble et al., 1993). CD4+ T cells are classified into two subpopulations depending on the expression of CD45R on the surface in humans, mice and rats. In rats, CD45RC+ T cells are considered to be memory T cells, which rapidly provide help for B cells to produce antibody (Powrie and Mason, 1989), and have a capacity to produce greater quantities of IL-4 than CD45RC+ T cells (McKnight et al., 1991). In contrast, CD45RC+ T cells are considered to be naive T cells, which produce more IL-2 and IFNγ than CD45RC− T cells. Rat CD8+ T cells may be involved in the production of some cytokines, such as IL-5, IL-10 and IFNγ (Noble et al., 1995).

B cells

Differentiation and surface markers

Rat B lineage cells are identified by three mAbs, HIS14, HIS22 and HIS24, directed against epitopes of CD45R similar to B220 in mice (Kroese et al., 1990, 1995; Opstelten et al., 1986). Their expression profiles differ at the different developmental stages of the B cells. Antigens recognized by HIS14 and HIS24 are expressed on terminal deoxynucleotidyl transferase+ pro-B cells in the bone marrow (Opstelten et al., 1986), and their expression is maintained throughout maturation. HIS24 antigen expression, however, is downregulated in the marginal zone of the spleen (Kroese et al., 1990, 1995). In contrast, the expression of HIS22 antigen is restricted to surface IgM− IgD+ mature B cells.

In addition, expression of Thy-1 also clearly reflects the developmental stages of rat B cells: Thy-1+ immature B cells differentiate into Thy-1− mature B cells in local tissues (Crawford and Goldschneider, 1980; Kroese et al., 1995). Differentiation of rat B cells must be regulated by some factors in a similar manner to mice, in which stromal cell- or T cell-derived factors, such as stem cell factor (SCF), IL-7 and flt3 ligand are required (Dorshkind, 1996). Exactly which essential factor(s) are required for B-cell differentiation remains unclear.

Natural killer cells

Rat NK cells are identified as large granular lymphocytes expressing asialo-GM1 and CD8 but not CD5 (Reynolds et al., 1981; Woda et al., 1984). NKR protein 1, a type II membrane receptor whose expression was originally reported on rat NK cells, is very involved in their functions of target cell recognition, cytotoxic activity and granule release (Giorda et al., 1990). NKR protein 1 is also expressed on granulated metrial gland cells (Head et al., 1994) which are the major cell population of the rodent decidua, suggesting that in rats as well as in mice, the cells similar to NK cells exert some regulatory effect during pregnancy by means of their killing activity (Linnemeyer and Pollack, 1991). Santoni et al. (1989) pointed out another molecule involved in cytotoxic activity: fibronectin. This is one of the components of the extracellular matrix, and it is expressed and released by rat NK cells. NK activity of large granular lymphocytes is upregulated by IFN or IL-2 in rats (Henney et al., 1981). In contrast to the results from mice, however, neither synergistic nor additive effects are observed when both cytokines were applied simultaneously (Vaage et al., 1989).

Hematology

Hematopoietic Stem Cells

All types of blood cells originate from a very minor cell population, called 'hematopoietic stem cells (HSC)' in the bone marrow (Figure 22.1). As shown in Figure 22.2, rat leukocytes in the peripheral blood are composed of five types of cells, similar to humans and other experimental animals. Although hematological data about the rat is limited, some fundamental values including serum levels of biochemical constituents are summarized in Tables 22.1 and 22.2.

As a result of the remarkable development of multiparameter cell-sorting techniques, major progress has been made in biological and/or medical research on cell surface marker expression on HSC and progenitor cells. In 1980, Goldschneider et al. (1980) reported that stem cells in rat bone marrow are positive for Thy-1 antigen using fluorescent activated cell sorting (FACS). An attempt to identify the phenotype of colony-forming units in spleen (CFU-S) was done in rat bone marrow using several mAbs (OX7, W3/13, and OX22) to cell surface molecules. OX7 recognizes an antigenic determinant expressed on the Thy-1 glycoprotein, W3/13 recognizes a determinant expressed on some sialoglycoproteins, and OX22 recognizes only the high molecular weight forms of leukocyte common antigen. Rat CFU-S

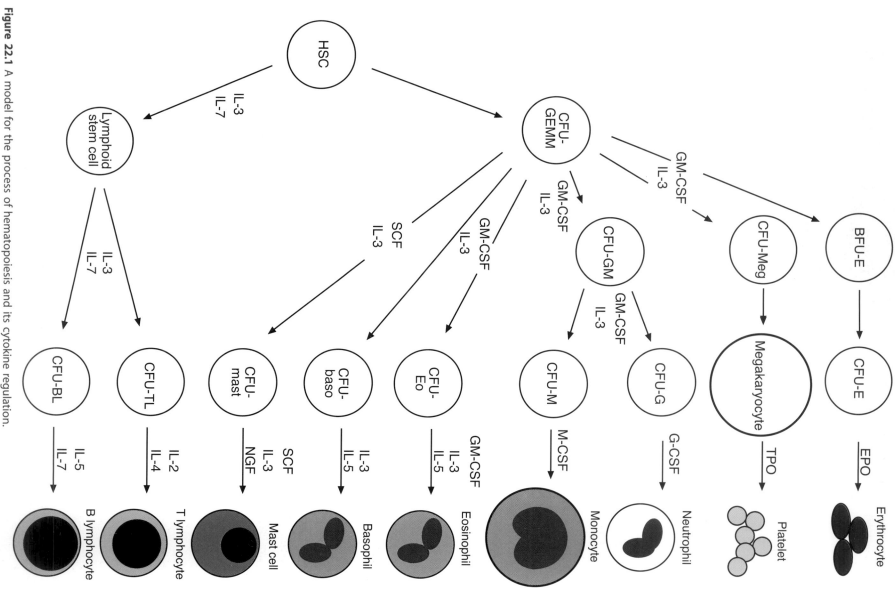

Figure 22.1 A model for the process of hematopoiesis and its cytokine regulation.

could be characterized as OX7 upper 20% positive, W3/13 lower 50% positive, and OX22 negative (McCarthy *et al.*, 1985, 1987).

Erythropoiesis

Committed precursors

The process of erythrocyte development from HSC is supported by three major events: first, the emergence of committed precursors from pluripotent HSC (CFU-GEMM); secondly, the formation of the burst-forming unit-erythroid (BFU-E), this being the most immature erythroid progenitor detected by an *in vitro* colony assay, whose growth is controlled by granulocyte–macrophage colony-stimulating factor (GM-CSF) and IL-3 but independent of erythropoietin (EPO); finally, the differentiation into colony-forming unit-erythroid (CFU-E), whose growth depends on EPO. Rolovic *et al.* (1990) studied the relationship between megakaryocytopoiesis, erythropoiesis and granulopoiesis at the level of progenitor cells in the bone marrow of rats exposed to hypoxia for 4 weeks, and found that hypomegakaryocytic thrombocytopenia was accompanied by decreased megakaryocytopoiesis and increased CFU-E, while granulopoiesis and a number of BFU-E were within normal levels. These findings suggest the existence of an inverse relationship between red blood cell and platelet production.

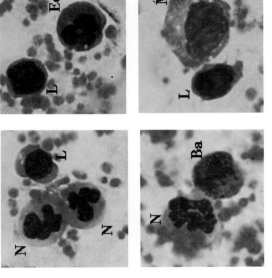

Figure 22.2 Microscopic features of rat leukocytes in the peripheral blood (Diff Quick stain, × 1000). N, neutrophils with coiled or twisted nucleus; L, small lymphocytes with round, densely stained nucleus and pale cytoplasm; Eo, an eosinophil filled with acidophilic granules; Mo, a monocyte with ameboid nucleus, abundant cytoplasm and some vacuoles in the cytoplasm. Ba, a basophilic filled with basophilic granules.

Erythropoietin

EPO is a glycoprotein secreted by kidney cells as a major regulator of erythropoiesis. At the stage of BFU-E, crythroid precursors do not express EPOR, while normal CFU-E cells become EPO-dependent. Using the RT-PCR method, the EPO mRNA was detected in the peritubular cells (capillary fraction:

Table 22.1 Blood properties in the rat

Age (weeks)	Sex	RBC ($\times 10^6/\mu L$)	WBC ($\times 10^3/\mu L$)	HCT (%)	Hb (g/dL)	Platelet ($\times 10^5/\mu L$)
7–10	M	7.69	11.6	45.1	16.6	12.91
	F	7.77	8.8	46.0	16.6	12.81
30–34	M	9.08	11.8	46.0	17.0	11.46
	F	7.95	7.4	44.0	16.5	11.89
56–60	M	9.28	9.9	47.5	16.6	11.02
	F	8.01	6.2	45.0	16.4	11.09
100–104	M	8.53	10.6	45.0	17.1	11.44
	F	7.00	7.3	40.5	15.5	10.48
115–140	M	7.54	11.7	41.2	15.5	12.36
	F	6.58	8.1	40.0	14.9	9.73

From Bailly and Duprat (1993).
RBC, red blood cells (erythrocytes); WBC, white blood cells; HCT, hematocrit; Hb, hemoglobin.

Table 22.2 Blood chemistry of the rat

	General normal range
Total protein (g/dL)	5.9–8.4
Albumin (g/dL)	3.2–4.3
Globulin (g/dL)	2.9–4.8
Glucose (mg/dL)	89.5–183.3
Total cholesterol (mg/dL)	50–100
Creatinine (mg/dL)	0.39–2.29
Urea nitrogen (mg/dL)	12–25.8
Sodium (mEq/L)	129–150
Potassium (mEq/L)	4.6–6.0
Calcium (mg/dL)	9.6–11.0
Chloride (mEq/L)	97–110
Phosphorus (mg/dL)	6.0–8.0

From Ringlar and Dabich (1979).

afferent/efferent arteriole, vasa recta) of the rat kidney (da Silva *et al.*, 1994).

Granulopoiesis

Committed precursors

All granulocytes originate from CFU-GEMM in the bone marrow. Progenitor cells committed to neutrophils and macrophages are confirmed as CFU-granulocytes and macrophages (CFU-GM), whose growth and differentiation are supported by GM-CSF and IL-3. Further progression separates CFU-GM into monopotent progenitors, CFU-granulocytes (CFU-G) and CFU-macrophages (CFU-M), which can be affected by granulocyte CSF (G-CSF) and macrophage CSF (M-CSF), respectively. Eosinophils are also bone marrow-derived granulocytes arising from CFU-GEMM, whose involvement in parasite infection and allergic disorders has been well documented (Weller, 1991). Not only the development of eosinophil precursors (CFU-Eo) but also the maintenance of mature eosinophils are supported by GM-CSF, IL-3 and IL-5. Basophils complete their differentiation within the bone marrow. Kasugai *et al.* (1993) showed that infection with *Nippostrongylus brasiliensis* led to an increase in the number of immature basophils in the bone marrow but not in nude-athymic rats, thus validating the idea that T cell-derived cytokines are indispensable for basophil development.

Growth factors

T cell-derived cytokines and stromal cell-derived growth factors act alone or synergistically with each other to expand primitive and committed hematopoietic progenitors. SCF has been shown to stimulate early hematopoietic progenitor cells, and to enhance proliferation of committed precursors in the presence of various kinds of lineage-specific CSF. In fact, coinjection of recombinant rat SCF and recombinant human G-CSF to rats for 1 week caused a synergistic increase in the number of mature neutrophils in the bone marrow and dramatic peripheral neutrophilia (Ulich *et al.*, 1991). IL-3 increased the CFU-GM pool in the bone marrow, while GM-CSF induced a significant increase in the number of peripheral neutrophils in rats (Cairo *et al.*, 1991a). The administration of recombinant human IL-6 in combination with G-CSF enhanced the CFU-GM pool in the bone marrow and liver/spleen and also increased the number of peripheral neutrophils (Cairo *et al.*, 1991b).

Thrombopoiesis

Committed precursors

When bone marrow cells were incubated in pokeweed mitogen-stimulated spleen cell-conditioned media or L cell-conditioned media, acetylcholinesterase-positive megakaryoblast colonies developed, and their progenitor cells were called CFU-megakaryocytes (CFU-Meg) (Hoffman, 1989). Jackson (1973) mentioned the existence of transient acetylcholinesterase-positive cells between CFU-Meg and megakaryoblasts in rodents. Megakaryoblasts lose their mitotic ability and increase their DNA contents by endomitosis to form polyploid cells. After enucleation, the process of thrombopoiesis culminates in the release of mature platelets into the circulation (Ellis *et al*, 1995).

Thrombopoietin

Blood plasma from animals with **thrombocytopenia** possesses the ability to enhance thrombopoiesis, and the existence of a certain humoral factor which induces the proliferation, differentiation and maturation of megakaryocyte progenitors and megakaryocytes has been postulated. The isolation and cloning of the long-sought-after regulator of platelet production was reported in 1994 (Kaushansky *et al*., 1994; Lok *et al*, 1994; de Sauvage *et al*, 1994; Wendling *et al*, 1994). This factor, thrombopoietin, was identified as a ligand for c-Mpl, a cytokine receptor encoded by the *c-mpl* proto-oncogene. Rat thrombopoietin was purified directly from the plasma from sublethally irradiated rats, and its ability to stimulate the production of megakaryocytes from CFU-Meg was confirmed (Kato *et al*, 1995).

Mast Cell Development

Heterogeneity

Mast cell precursors that are derived from the multipotential HMCs leave the bone marrow, circulate in the bloodstream, and invade local tissues where they differentiate into at least two phenotypically different subpopulations: connective tissue-type mast cells (CTMCs) and mucosal mast cells (MMCs). By their location, histochemical and biochemical characteristics, electron microscopic features, and T cell-derived growth factor-dependency, they are distinguishable. CTMCs are strongly stained with safranin and berberine sulfate, and possess many cytoplasmic granules which show metachromasia with toluidine blue-staining and contain high levels of histamine. In order to take the classification of heterogeneity further, the expression of murine mast cell proteases has been analyzed by many researchers. Mast cell

proteases represent more than 50% of the total protein content of mature mast cells in mice, rats, dogs and humans, and are enzymatically active at neutral pH. Rat mast cells have two types of proteases designated rat mast cell protease (RMCP) I and II. Because 90% of RMCPI-containing cells stained red and all RMCPII-containing cells stained blue after the Alcian blue/safranin sequences, RMCPI and RMCPII phenotypes are regarded as one of the criteria for typing CTMCs and MMCs, respectively (Gibson *et al*, 1987).

Growth factors

Murine bone marrow-derived cultured mast cells (BMCMCs) resemble MMCs in their phenotype, and their growth and survival are supported by T cell-derived cytokines, such as IL-3, IL-4, IL-9 and IL-10. IL-3 is able to induce proliferation of BMCMCs, while other interleukins work synergistically with other factors rather than having an independent effect. Recombinant rat IL-3 stimulated both the development of MMCs from rat bone marrow precursors and maintained the proliferation of rat MMC lines (Haig *et al*, 1988).

Mutations at the *W* or *Sl* loci cause serious hematopoietic defects and mast cell deficiency in mice. Since the *W* locus encodes *c-kit* receptor tyrosine kinase and the *Sl* locus encodes its ligand SCF, the signal mediated by SCF binding to the *c-kit* receptor has been thought to be essential for mast cell development. *Ws/Ws* rats have mast cell depletion and their phenotype is very similar to that of *W/Wᵛ* mast cell-deficient mice. Tsujimura *et al*. (1991) found that a small deletion at the tyrosine kinase domain of the *c-kit* gene led to a deficiency in mast cell production in *Ws/Ws* rats. Haig *et al*. (1994) reported that rat SCF stimulated the growth of both rat serosal mast cells and BMCMCs alone or synergistically with IL-3.

Nerve growth factor (NGF) is a well-characterized neurotropic polypeptide important for the survival, development and function of mast cells, as well as peripheral sympathetic and sensory neurones. Matsuda *et al*. (1991) demonstrated that addition of NGF to cultures resulted in the development of CTMCs from murine BMCMCs and bone marrow cells in the presence of IL-3. When IL-3 is not included in the medium, NGF as well as SCF can support survival of rat peritoneal mast cells by suppressing apoptosis (Kawamoto *et al*, 1995).

The Hematopoietic Microenvironment

Stromal cells supporting hematopoietic growth

Stromal cells of the bone marrow have been demonstrated to supply the growth-promoting and differentiation-inducing factors essential for the regulation of hematopoiesis. Using a liquid culture system, Dexter et al. (1990) managed to maintain HSCs in vitro for several months. Molecules of the extracellular matrix, such as heparan sulfate, laminin and fibronectin, are able to bind growth factors and in this way the stromal cells can form microenvironmental niches which preferentially promote development of multipotent and committed cells along discrete lineages.

Growth factor production

Zsebo et al. (1990a,b) cloned a partial cDNA encoding murine SCF and demonstrated that the gene was synthenic with the Sl locus. They also provided evidence that SCF is a ligand for the c-kit receptor. These findings indicate that stromal cell-derived SCF is essential for hematopoietic cell growth. Matsuda et al. (1988a,b) reported that NGF, a stromal cell (fibroblast)-derived growth factor, promotes human hematopoietic colony formation, and acts in a relatively selective way to induce the differentiation of eosinophils and histamine-containing cells (basophils and mast cells). They also found that production of NGF from fibroblasts is controlled by various inflammatory cytokines released from mast cells or other types of cells in the microenvironment (Matsuda et al., 1998).

GM-CSF and IL-6 are produced by bone marrow stromal cells derived from human and rodents. Derigs et al. (1994) reported that GM-CSF production of a murine marrow stromal cell line was enhanced synergistically by the addition of IL-1 and TNFα, but increased intracellular cAMP levels inhibited the effect. They also showed that acute formation of cAMP led to IL-6 production, suggesting that cAMP regulation is involved in the cytokine-directed marrow microenvironmental function.

Sudo et al. (1989) investigated the stromal cell-dependent B-cell development using two stromal cell clones, ST2 and PA6. ST2, unlike PA6, supported B lymphopoiesis by constitutive production

of IL-7, leading to speculation that the B-cell differentiation from early progenitors requires IL-7 derived from stromal cells.

IL-11, which was isolated from a primate stromal cell line, PU-34, has been shown to induce proliferation of early HSC synergistically with other cytokines. Cairo et al. (1993) investigated the effect of IL-11 in combination with G-CSF in neonatal rat hematopoiesis. They found that IL-11 alone stimulated thrombopoiesis, and that IL-11 and G-CSF caused a significant increase in the number of the neutrophils in the bone marrow and blood circulation.

References

Bailly, Y. and Duprat, P. (1993) In: Jones, T.C., Ward, J.M., Mohr, U. and Hunt, R.D. (eds) Hematopoietic System, pp. 27–38. New York: Springer-Verlag.

Brenan, M. and Puklavec, M. (1992) J. Exp. Med. 175, 1457–1465.

Bruggemann, M. (1988) Gene 74, 473–482.

Cairo, M.S., Mauss, D. and Plunkett, J. (1991a) Pediatr. Res. 29, 504–509.

Cairo, M.S., Plunkett, J.M., Nguyen, A., Clark, S. and van de Ven, C. (1991b) Pediatr. Res. 30, 554–559.

Cairo, M.S., Plunkett, J.M., Nguyen, A., Schendel, P. and van de Ven, C. (1993) Pediatr. Res. 34, 56–61.

Cramer, D.V. (1993) In: Jones, T.C., Ward, J.M., Mohr, U. and Hunt, R.D. (eds), Hematopoietic System, pp. 3–9. New York: Springer-Verlag.

Crawford, J.M. and Goldschneider I. (1980) J. Immunol. 124, 969–976.

da Silva, J.L., Schwartzman, M.L., Goodman, A., Levere, R.D. and Abraham, N.G. (1994) J. Cell. Biochem. 54, 239–246.

de Sauvage, F.J., Hass, P.E., Spencer, S.D. et al. (1994) Nature 369, 533–538.

Derigs, H.G., Reifel-Miller, A., Kaushansky, K., Hromas, R.A. and Boswell, H.S. (1994) Exp. Hematol. 22, 924–932.

Dexter, T.M., Coutinho, L.H., Spooncer, E. et al. (1990) Ciba Found. Symp. 148, 76–86.

Dijkstra, C.D., Döpp, E.A., Joling, P. and Kraal, G. (1985) Immunology 54, 589–599.

Dorshkind, K. (1996) In: Weir, D.M. (ed.) Handbook of Experimental Immunology, 5th edn, pp. 81.1–81.12. Massachusetts: Blackwell Science.

Ellis, M.H., Avraham, H. and Groopman, J.E. (1995) Blood Rev. 9, 1–6.

Feng, L., Tang, W.W., Chang, J.C. and Wilson, C.B. (1993) Biochem. Biophys. Res. Commun. 192, 452–458.

Gibson, S., Mackeller, A., Newlands, G.F. and Miller, H.R. (1987) *Immunology* **62**, 621–627.

Gill, T.J. III, Smith, G.J., Wissler, R.W. and Kunz, J.W. (1989) *Science* **245**, 269–275.

Giorda, R., Rudert, W.A., Vavassori, C., Chambers, W.H., Hiserodt, J.C. and Trucco, M. (1990) *Science* **249**, 1298–1300.

Goldschneider, I., Metcalf, D., Battye, F. and Mandel, T.J. (1980) *J. Exp. Med.* **152**, 419–437.

Gutman, G.A. (1996). In: Weir, D.M. (ed.) *Handbook of Experimental Immunology*, 5th edn, pp. 23.1–23.11. Massachusetts: Blackwell Science.

Haig, D.M., McMenamin, C., Redmond, J. *et al.* (1988) *Immunology* **65**, 205–211.

Haig, D.M., Huntley, J.F., MacKellar, A. *et al.* (1994) *Blood* **83**, 72–83.

Head, J.R., Kresge, C.K., Young, J.D. and Hiserodt, J.C. (1994) *Biol. Reprod.* **51**, 509–523.

Henney, C.S., Kuribayashi, K., D.E. and Gillis, S. (1981) *Nature* **291**, 335–338.

Hoffman, R. (1989) *Blood* **74**, 1196–1212.

Huang, S., Paulauskis, J.D., Godleski, J. and Kobzik, L. (1992) *Am. J. Pathol.* **141**, 981–988.

Hunig, T. and Mitnacht, R. (1991) *J. Exp. Med.* **173**, 561–568.

Jackson, C.W. (1973) *Blood* **42**, 413–421.

Jiang, W., Swiggard, W.J., Heufler, C., Peng, M., Mirza, A., Steinman, R.M. and Nussenzweig, M.C. (1995) *Nature* **375**, 151–155.

Josien, R., Heslan, M., Soulillou, J.-P. and Cuturi, M.-C. (1997) *J. Exp. Med.* **186**, 467–472.

Kasugai, T., Okada, M., Morimoto, M. *et al.* (1993) *Blood* **81**, 2521–2529.

Kato, T., Ogami, K., Shimada, Y. *et al.* (1995) *J. Biochem.* **118**, 229–236.

Kaushansky, K., Lok, S., Holly, R.D. *et al.* (1994) *Nature* **369**, 568–571.

Kawamoto, K., Okada, T., Kannan, Y., Ushio, H., Matsumoto, M. and Matsuda, H. (1995) *Blood* **86**, 4638–4644.

Kovacs, E.J., van Stedum, S. and Neuman, J.E. (1994) *Immunobiology* **190**, 263–274.

Kroese, F.G.M., Butcher, E.C., Lalor, P.A., Stall, A.M. and Herzenberg, L.A. (1990) *J. Immunol.* **20**, 1527–1534.

Kroese, F.G.M., de Boer, N.K., de Boer, T., Nieuwenhuis, P., Kantor, A.B. and Deenen, G.J. (1995) *Cell Immunol.* **162**, 185–193.

Kuhnlein, P., Park, J.-H., Herrmann, T., Elbe, A. and Hunig, T. (1994) *J. Immunol.* **153**, 979–986.

Linnemeyer, P.A. and Pollack, S.B. (1991) *J. Immunol.* **147**, 2530–2535.

Lok, S., Kaushansky, K., Holly, R.D. *et al.* (1994) *Nature* **369**, 565–568.

McCarthy, K.F., Hale, M.L. and Fehnel, P.L. (1985) *Exp. Hematol.* **13**, 847–854.

McCarthy, K.F., Hale, M.L. and Fehnel, P.L. (1987) *Cytometry* **8**, 296–305.

McKnight, A.J., Barclay, A.N. and Mason, D.W. (1991) *Eur. J. Immunol.* **21**, 1187–1194.

McMenamin, C., McKersey, M., Kuhnlein, P., Hunig, T. and Holt, P.G. (1995) *J. Immunol.* **154**, 4390–4394.

Matsuda, H., Coughlin, M.D., Bienenstock, J. and Denburg, J.A. (1988a) *Proc. Natl Acad. Sci. USA* **85**, 6508–6512.

Matsuda, H., Switzer, J., Coughlin, M.D., Bienenstock, J. and Denburg, J.A. (1988b) *Int. Arch. Allergy Appl. Immunol.* **86**, 453–457.

Matsuda, H., Kannan, Y., Ushio, H., Kiso, Y., Kanemoto, T., Suzuki, H. and Kitamura, Y. (1991) *J. Exp. Med.* **174**, 7–14.

Matsuda, H., Koyama, H., Sato, H. *et al.* (1998) *J. Exp. Med.* **187**, 297–306.

Noble, A., Staynov, D.Z. and Kemeny, D.M. (1993) *Immunology* **79**, 562–567.

Noble, A., Macary, P.A. and Kemeny, M. (1995) *J. Immunol.* **155**, 2928–2937.

Ogle, C.K., Wu, J.Z., Mao, X., Szczur, K., Alexander, J.W. and Ogle, J.D. (1994) *Inflammation* **18**, 511–523.

Opstelten, D., Deenen, G.J., Rozing, J. and Hunt, S.V. (1986) *J. Immunol.* **137**, 76–84.

Paker, K.E., Carter, C.A., Murphy, G. and Fabre, J.W. (1991) *Immunogenetics* **34**, 211–213.

Park, J.-H., Mitnacht, R., Torres-Nagel, N. and Hunig, T. (1993) *J. Exp. Med.* **177**, 541–546.

Powrie, F. and Mason, D. (1989) *J. Exp. Med.* **169**, 653–662.

Reynolds, C.W., Sharrow, S.O., Ortaldo, J.R. and Herberman, R.B. (1981) *J. Immunol.* **127**, 2204–2208.

Ringler, D.H. and Dabich, L. (1979) In: Baker, H.J., Lindsey, J.R. and Weisbroth, S.H. (eds) *The Laboratory Rat*, pp. 105–121. San Diego: Academic Press.

Rolovic, Z., Basara, N., Biljanovic, P.I., Stojanovic, N. and Pavlovic, K.V. (1990) *Exp. Hematol.* **18**, 190–194.

Salgar, S.K., Yuan, X., Kunz, H.W. and Gill, T.J. III. (1997) *Immunogenetics* **45**, 353–364.

Santoni, A., Gismondi, A., Morrone, S. *et al.* (1989) *J. Immunol.* **143**, 2415–2421.

Schorle, H., Holtschke, T., Hunig, T., Schimpl, A. and Horak, I. (1991) *Nature* **352**, 621–624.

Shi, M.M., Godleski, J. and Paulauskis, J.D. (1995) *Biochem. Biophys. Res. Commun.* **211**, 289–295.

Sudo, T., Ogawa, Y., Iizuka, M. *et al.* (1989) *J. Exp. Med.* **170**, 333–338.

Takahama, Y., Suzuki, H., Katz, K.S., Grusby, M.J. and Singer, A. (1994) *Nature* **371**, 67–70.

Tsujimura, T., Hirota, S., Nomura, S. *et al.* (1991) *Blood* **78**, 1942–1946.

Ulich, T.R., del Castillo, J., McNiece, I.K. *et al.* (1991) *Blood* **78**, 1954–1962.

Vaage, J.T., Reynolds, C.W., Reynolds, D., Fossum, S. and Rolstad, B. (1989) *Eur. J. Immunol.* **19**, 1895–1902.

Wang, C.-R., Lambracht, D., Wonigeit, K., Howard, J.C. and Lindahl, K.F. (1995) *Immunogenetics* **42**, 63–67.

Watters, J.W.F., Locker, J.D., Kunz, H.W. and Gill, T.J. III. (1987) *Immunogenetics* **26**, 220–229.

Weller, P.F.N. (1991) *N. Engl. J. Med.* **324**, 1110–1118.

Wendling, F., Maraskovsky, E., Debili, N. *et al.* (1994) *Nature* **369**, 571–574.

Woda, B.A., McFadden, M.L., Welsh, R.M. and Bain, K.M. (1984) *J. Immunol.* **132**, 2183–2184.

Zsebo, K.M., Wypych, J., McNiece, I.K. *et al.* (1990a) *Cell* **63**, 195–201.

Zsebo, K.M., Williams, D.A., Geissler, E.N. *et al.* (1990b) *Cell* **63**, 213–224.

CHAPTER 23

Physiology of Stress and Starvation-like Conditions

Haruki Senoo
Department of Anatomy, Akita University School of Medicine, Akita, Japan

Stress

Selye (1936a, 1943) reported that certain physiological changes occurred in experimental animals exposed to a wide variety of stresses, such as emotional excitement, toxic drugs, trauma and exhausting forced muscular exercise. These changes presented some of the classic signs of the stress syndrome: thymus involution, enlargement of the adrenal cortex, secretion of epinephrine from the adrenal medulla, and others.

Stress affects the central nervous system (CNS) leading indirectly to the modulation of the activity of steroid, catecholamine, peptide and opioid systems. It also affects other body systems: behavior, immune, cardiovascular and gastrointestinal systems. In response to stress, a cascade of neurohumoral events chiefly at the level of the hypothalamic-pituitary-adrenocortical (HPA) axis is triggered, the result of which is the termination of the stress reaction leading to normalization (Sutanto and de Kloet, 1994). Stress-induced events are complex. Laboratory animals have been indispensable in their roles as models in the study of stress, and consequently in shedding light on our understanding of stress.

Rats are the favored laboratory animals for such purposes and genetically selected strains have been developed as a consequence of this. These include spontaneously hypertensive rats and corresponding control Wistar Kyoto rats (SHR and WKY respectively), apomorphine-susceptible and apomorphine-unsusceptible rats (APO-SUS and APO-UNSUS), Roman Low and High Avoidance rats (RHA and RLA), immunologically altered Lewis (LEW/N) and the corresponding controls Fischer (F-344/N) and Wistar rats.

The Hypothalamic-Pituitary-Adrenocortical Axis

The concept of stress has evolved, in the past 45 years, from stimulus-induced organ responses to psychological influences on behavior in which the experience of stress and the handling of stressful information were emphasized. The hypothalamic-pituitary-adrenocortical (HPA) axis is the pivot for the animal's ability to adapt and cope with stress; its activity is under stringent regulation of the corticosteroid receptor systems in the CNS.

The activity of the HPA axis can be stimulated by psychological factors such as uncertainty, conflict, lack of control and information, or suppressed by factors such as consummatory behavior and sense of control (De Kloet et al., 1991). The activation and suppression of the HPA axis is modulated by corticosteroids. Neuroendocrine studies have shown that mineralocorticoids (MRs) are important for the sensitivity of the stress response system, while glucocorticoids (GRs) suppress stress-induced neuroendocrine activation (Ratka et al., 1989). The involvement of the hippocampus in the neuroendocrine feedback system and the subsequent behavioral adaptation is well established (McEwen et al., 1986; Meaney et al., 1992; Oitzl and de Kloet, 1992). In a series of electrophysiological studies, it has been shown that in the hippocampus, MR-mediated effects of corticosterone raise the excitability of neuronal cells; this excitability is suppressed by the steroid's action via GR. A balance between MR- and GR-mediated effects is of importance for the homeotic control of the animal's stress responsiveness and adaptation.

Various Responses to Stimuli

There are many sex- and age-dependent variations among individuals in response to various stressors and other exogenous stimuli as determined using a wide range of physiological and biochemical endpoints. The state and condition of the individuals also play a major part in this respect. The effect of housing, for instance, has been known for a long time (Barrett and Stockham, 1963).

Age is an important factor in determining individual responsiveness. Aging is characterized by a general diminution in organ functions associated with a decreased ability to maintain homeostasis, while at ontogeny, during the first 2 weeks of the rat's life, the neonate responds poorly to a stressor. Aged rats, compared to the young controls, exhibit less efficient HPA axis activity in response to a stressor, as reflected also in the animal's behavior.

Genetically Selected Rat Strains

It was proposed in the late 1960s that the need to understand possible physiological mechanisms underlying or accompanying individual differences in behavior among humans and animals was a good reason for the selection of various strains of rodents (Treiman and Levins, 1969). The use of genetically selected rats has been a useful approach in this respect since they serve as animal models for specific physiological conditions that exhibit different physiological and behavioral patterns in response to a stress stimulus. Numerous genetically selected animal models have been developed to assist in the study of endocrine and nonendocrine parameters. These models have been utilized for the study of the individuals' differences in responses to stress and other stimuli. The selection procedure for rat lines and strains started about 35 years ago (Bignami, 1965); such selection has been based on physiological, behavioral and pharmacological parameters and the selection characteristics have been maintained over generations.

Roman High Avoidance (RHA) and Roman Low Avoidance (RLA) rats are Wistar-derived rats, selected and bred for rapid versus nonacquisition of two-way, active avoidance behavior in the shuttle box (Bignami, 1965). RHA rats generally show a more active avoidance behavior than their RLA counterparts when exposed to various environmental challenges.

In the rat, another example of behavior-based rat strain selection is the pharmacogenetically selected APO-SUS and APO-UNSUS rat. The following rat strains have also been selected for various parameters of emotionality: the Maudsley Reactive and Nonreactive rats (Broadhurst, 1975); Syracuse High- and Low-Avoidance rats (Brush et al., 1988); the Swiss sublines RLA/Verh and RHA/Verh rats (Driscoll, 1986; Driscoll et al., 1990); the Canadian sublines RLA/Lu and RHA/Lu rats (Satinder, 1981). The central nucleus of the amygdala is known to be involved in the regulation of autonomic, neuroendocrine and behavioral responses to stress. Its involvement in the selection of coping strategies has been suggested by using RHA/Verh and RLA/Verh rats (Wiersma et al., 1997). Corticotropin-releasing hormone (CRH) seems to be the key neurohormone in the control of the central nucleus of the amygdala output.

Apomorphine-susceptible (APO-SUS) and apomorphine-unsusceptible (APO-UNSUS) rats are selected based on the different response to the dopamine agonist apomorphine (Cools et al., 1990). It was previously known that rats belonging to a single outbred colony of Wistar rats can show highly individually specific behavioral responses as exemplified in a defeat test where certain rats flee and others freeze. The fleeing response correlates with the amount of gnawing elicited by the dopamine agonist apomorphine. The breeding of the subsequent generations resulted in selection of APO-SUS and APO-UNSUS rats which have subsequently been used to examine the reactivity of the HPA axis in relation to central catecholaminergic systems.

The immunologically altered rat strain Lewis (LEW/N) is a prototype strain for the study of a number of experimental autoimmune diseases including experimental autoimmune encephalomyelitis, uveitis, orchitis and adjuvant-induced arthritis. These rats, which are Wistar-derived inbred animals, also develop arthritis in response to group A streptococcal cell wall peptidoglycan polysaccharide while the histocompatible Fischer (F-344/N) rats do not develop arthritis in response to the same polysaccharide stimulus. LEW/N rats have a blunted HPA axis reactivity. The susceptibility of LEW/N to arthritis is due to its inability to mount a steroid response compared to that in the disease-resistant strain. Corticosteroids seem to play a major influence in the genesis of arthritis in LEW/N rats.

In order to study the mechanisms involved in the regulation of the cardiovascular system and hypertension, various animal models for hypertension have been developed. In the early 1960s, Dahl and

co-workers selectively bred rats for susceptibility or resistance to the hypertensive effects of high salt intake (Rapp and Dene, 1985). Another type of genetically selected hypertensive rat is the spontaneously hypertensive rat (SHR). When SHRs are used to model hypertension, the normotensive Wistar Kyoto (WKY) rats are used as the control. Recently, two new strains of WKY rats have been developed as a result of a cross between WKY rats and SHRs (Hendley et al., 1991); one strain (WK-HT) is hypertensive but not hyperactive while the other (WK-HA) is hyperactive but normotensive.

The importance of central corticosteroid action in blood pressure regulation and salt appetite is a well-known phenomenon (McEwen et al., 1986; De Kloet et al., 1988; Grünfeld, 1990). These studies have shown that the effects of mineralocorticoids on this regulatory system are mediated via the central MRs which include those aldosterone-sensitive MRs located in the anterior hypothalamus and circumventricular organs (De Kloet et al., 1991).

These animal models have been used for the investigation of endocrine and nonendocrine stress-related phenomena. In this respect, alteration in the activity of the HPA axis is of importance since such an activity is a reflection of the animal's responsiveness to a stressful situation.

Various Stressors for Experimental Animals

The animal's response to stress depends not only upon the state and condition of the animal but on the nature or type of the stressor itself, as well as the various central and peripheral components, all of which affect the animal's neuroendocrine response and the stress-related behavioral patterns (Sutanto and de Kloet, 1994).

Acute stress

When animals are subjected to acute stress, a wide range of physiological alterations take place. These changes can occur rapidly, such as in the case of increased plasma corticosterone level within 5 minutes after ACTH injection or a 1-minute ether stress (Jones and Gillham, 1988; Jones and Stockham, 1966). Immobilization stress has been used to examine the activity of male rats in the forced swim-test (Armario et al., 1991) in three behavioral categories: struggling, mild swim and immobility.

Immobilization or restraint stress has a profound influence on the animal's immune system. Acute tail-shock in the rat causes increased plasma cholesterol levels (Brennan et al., 1992); it also enhances the secretory activity of goblet cells in the basal mucosa (Tachibana et al., 1991).

Ether has always been regarded as an anesthetic agent, however, ether anesthesia is by itself a stressor which causes dramatic alteration in the activity of the HPA axis components (Jones and Gillham, 1988). Ether anesthesia produces a marked endocrine response; it causes pronounced increases in plasma levels of corticosterone, epinephrine and norepinephrine. A short, single experience of stress can have long-term consequences for the animal's stress response. Rats exposed to a single, short session of inescapable foot shocks showed long-lasting alterations in behavioral responses to environmental stimuli, accompanied by alteration in the HPA activity, including changes in the corticosteroid receptor profile in the CNS. These data indicate that a single stress experience induces profound changes in stress responsiveness and behavior.

Chronic stress

Chronic stress has been connected to major physiological and psychological illnesses in humans. Evidence in the past has indicated that chronic stress is an important factor in the development of hypertension, gastrointestinal disorders, immune suppression, reproductive dysfunction and mental depression (Sutanto and de Kloet, 1994). The use of laboratory animals has been instrumental in investigating the consequences of chronic stress. Most chronic stress is in the form of repeated exposure on a daily basis to stressors such as cold, restraint or intermittent foot shock. One predominant feature of this type of regimen is the finding that repeated stress leads to adaptation or habituation, hence repeated exposure to the same stressor evokes less hormonal response to each stress session. This depends on the type of stress used (Jones and Gillham, 1988; Pitman et al., 1988; Natelson et al., 1988).

Chronic or repeated stress causes a wide range of physiological and neuroendocrine changes. For example, chronic stress in the form of constant illumination resulted in the disruption in the circadian patterns of corticosterone, progesterone and melatonin (Persengiev et al., 1991). When rats were given foot shock daily for 14 days, 7 days of this treatment

resulted in increased adrenal weight and decreased thymic weight (Kant et al., 1987). However, rats maintained on this paradigm for 14 days are able to maintain escape behavior, eat and drink, gain weight and groom. When the effects of this stressor on the levels of three stress-responsive hormones (corticosterone, ACTH and prolactin) were examined, it appeared that levels of plasma corticosterone were elevated during the first 7 days in the stressful environment, although the levels of plasma ACTH and prolactin were similar in stressed and control animals at all the time points measured.

Stress Proteins

When cells or organisms are exposed to stress, such as heat shock, hypoxia, cold, glucose starvation, heavy metals or infection with viruses, they respond to it by synthesizing a group of proteins called stress proteins (also called heat shock proteins (HSPs) or chaperones) (Craig, 1985; Lindquist and Craig, 1988). Although this stress response is universal, it was first observed in *Drosophila* (Ritossa, 1962). Stress proteins are the most highly conserved proteins during evolution, and the importance of their role has been clarified not only in stressed cells but also in cells under normal conditions (Nagata, 1996).

The folding of many newly synthesized proteins in the cell depends on HSPs. These prevent the formation of misfolded protein structures, both under normal conditions and when cells are exposed to stresses such as high temperature (Hartl, 1996). Recent evidence indicates that altered protein folding is the molecular basis of a growing list of human diseases (Thomas et al., 1995).

HSPs bind to denatured or unfolded proteins to prevent their aggregation and cellular damage. When mature proteins or newly synthesized proteins are denatured by heat shock, a major heat shock protein, HSP70 binds to the denatured proteins, and the concentration of the free HSP70 decreases (Figure 23.1). The heat shock factors (HSFs), which are inactivated when the concentrations of free HSP70 are relatively high, are activated, move into the nucleus and form trimers (Sorger, 1991; Westwood and Wu, 1993). HSF trimers bind to a conserved, 15-bp sequence, called the heat shock element (HSE), located upstream of the HSP70 gene and promote transcription. Thus, biosynthesized HSP can suppress HSFs in an autoregulatory manner.

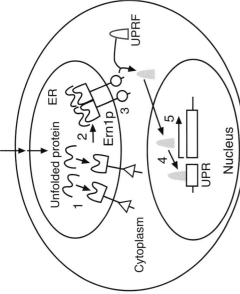

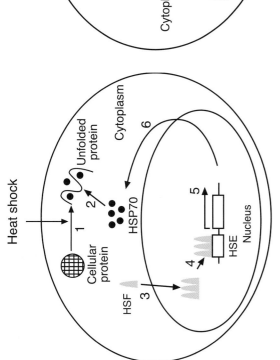

Figure 23.1 Pathway from heat shock signal to activation of transcription of heat shock protein. When mature proteins or newly synthesized proteins are denatured by heat shock, heat shock protein 70 (HSP70) binds to the denatured proteins (1), and the concentration of free HSP70 decreases (2). Heat shock factors (HSFs), inactivated by certain levels of free HSP70, are activated, move into the nucleus and form trimers (3). HSFs bind to the heat shock element (HSE) (4) and promote transcription of HSP70 (5), which then inactivates HSFs (6).

Figure 23.2 Pathway from the unfolded protein signal to activation of transcription of glucose-regulated protein (GRP). Unfolded proteins accumulated in the endoplasmic reticulum (ER) by glucose starvation bind to the N-terminal domain of Ern1p (1). Binding induces conformational changes in Ern1p that, together with oligomerization (2), activate the protein kinase domain (3). The signal is passed to cytosolic molecule(s). Modification of the unfolded protein response element factor (UPRF), allows the transcription factor to bind to the UPR element of the gene (4) and to activate transcription (5).

The content of two membrane proteins of molecular weights 78 000 and 94 000 respectively increases in cultured chick embryo fibroblasts when transformed by Rous sarcoma virus (Stone *et al*, 1974). These proteins belong to the HSF family. The increased content of the 94-kDa and 78-kDa proteins is not due directly to the onset of transformation but their induction is due to the rapid depletion of glucose from the culture medium by the rapidly growing transformed cells (Shiu *et al*, 1977). When glucose is maintained at high levels in the culture medium of such cells, the synthesis of the 94-kDa protein is arrested and that of the 78-kDa protein is suppressed. When glucose is removed from the culture medium of normal cells, these proteins increase to levels similar to those of transformed cells.

Since the amount of these two proteins is regulated by the concentration of glucose, these proteins are called glucose-regulated proteins or GRPs. They are found in the endoplasmic reticulum (ER). A variety of stresses, in addition to glucose starvation, can induce GRPs; these include tunicamycin, calcium ionophore and insulin. Depletion of glucose induces the accumulation of unfolded proteins in the ER, and triggers a signaling pathway from the

ER to the nucleus (Figure 23.2; Kozutsumi *et al*, 1988; Mori *et al*, 1992). The *ERN1* gene encodes a transmembrane protein (Ern1p) whose N-terminal portion is located inside the ER and whose cytoplasmic C-terminal portion carries a protein kinase activity (Mori *et al*, 1993). Accumulation of unfolded proteins in the ER leads to activation of the cytosolic domain of Ern1p. Ern1p is thought to be the sensor of events in the ER and it is suggested that binding of ligand causes transfer of information across the ER membrane, leading to activation of a specific set of transcription factors.

Stress Proteins in Rats

Several clinical studies have indicated a relationship between stress and pancreatitis (Kaplan, 1956; Nakai *et al*., 1983). Water-immersion stress induces a 60-kDa HSP in rat pancreas without any pathological changes (Otaka *et al*, 1993), while neither serum amylase levels nor pancreas weight show any increase. Intraperitoneal injection of caerulein (40 mg/kg body weight) can induce acute pancreatitis in rats. When the water-immersion stress is given following caerulein injection, acute pancreatitis develops (Yamaguchi et al., 1990). However, when the rats are pretreated with water-immersion and the 60-kDa HSP is induced, acute pancreatitis does not develop and no changes in serum amylase levels are seen following a caerulein injection (Otaka et al., 1994). Rats are good models for induction of HSPs and for the analysis of protection mechanisms against diseases.

When exposed to a forced walking stress for 2 weeks, some rats became persistently inactive (depression model rats), whereas others gradually recovered from exhaustion (spontaneous recovery rats). Cortical noradrenergic degeneration is involved in the pathogenesis of depression (Kitayama et al., 1997). While stress and sleep have been extensively studied individually, a few papers show good evidence of the stress–sleep relationship. In humans, the influence of stress on sleep is clearly suggested in relation to depression. In this respect it is reported that depressive patients generally exhibit a high cortisolemia, probably resulting from a chronic stress component. This impairment occurs together with a shortening of paradoxical sleep latency, a decrease in slow-wave sleep duration, an increase in the number of awakenings and a flattening of the sleep–waking rhythms (Appelboom-Fondu et al., 1988; Ross et al., 1989; Goldenberg, 1993). In animals, the stress–sleep relationship is more clearly defined. It is reported that an immobilization stress of 2 hours, applied just at the beginning of the dark phase, namely, when the animals begin to be active, induces a paradoxical sleep rebound 4 hours after the end of the restraint. Under such conditions, the amount of slow-wave sleep is not significantly modified (Rampin et al., 1991; Bonnet et al., 1997). Interindividual differences in the effects of acute stress on the sleep–wakefulness cycle have been demonstrated in the rat (Bouyer et al., 1997).

Nitric oxide is a gaseous neurotransmitter that may mediate a decrease in sympathetic output to the periphery. Krukoff and Khalili (1997) reported that more nitric oxide-producing neurons were activated in the rat brain during stress than during minimal or moderate levels of stimulation.

Physiological Impairments Associated with Stress

The neuroendocrine system

Corticotropin-releasing hormone (CRH) located in the paraventricular nucleus of the hypothalamus is the principal hypophysiotropic neuropeptide that stimulates synthesis and release of pituitary adrenocorticotropin (Vale et al., 1981). CRH is also widely distributed throughout the brain (Sawchenko and Swanson, 1990) where it may modulate autonomic function (Brown and Fisher, 1990) and behavioral activation (Takahashi and Kalin, 1989; Koob et al., 1993) associated with the response to stress. The central nucleus of the amygdala is an important extrahypothalamic CRH region that is a part of a neural circuit mediating stress-induced responses. The central nucleus of the amygdala contains the highest density of CRH-containing cell bodies within the amygdaloid complex (Sawchenko and Swanson, 1990). Stress rapidly induces elevations in CRH mRNA in the rat central amygdala nucleus and hypothalamic paraventricular nucleus (Hsu et al., 1998).

The efflux of 5-hydroxytryptamine (5-HT, brain serotonin) in the median raphe nucleus appears to respond to different forms of stress, whereas that in the dorsal raphe nucleus only increases after the injection of saline. The release of 5-HT in the forebrain is also dependent on the type of stress procedure and the region studied (Adell et al., 1997). Rating of behavior showed that fluoxetine treatment increased swimming behavior and decreased immobility during the test swim (Kirby and Lucki, 1997). Immobility was positively correlated and swimming was negatively correlated with changes in extracellular 5-HT in the lateral septum but not in the striatum. 5-HT exerts a differential regulation of stress-induced activation of proopiomelanocortin (the precursor of the adrenocorticotropin) gene expression in the anterior and intermediate lobes of the pituitary in male rats (Garcia-Garcia et al., 1997).

Stress-induced neuroendocrine and behavioral responses were inhibited in the rat by preprothyrotropin-releasing hormone 178-199, a 22-amino acid peptide (McGivern et al., 1997). Chronic social stress alters the levels of corticotropin-releasing hormone and arginine vasopressin mRNA in rat brain (Albeck et al., 1997). The heat shock protein 70 (HSP70) gene expression was reported in the medulla, after whole-body hyperthermia (Shimizu et al., 1997). Xie and McCobb (1998) reported that stress hormones regulate splicing of potassium channels. Expression of alternative splice variants of Slo, a gene encoding calcium- and voltage-activated potassium channels, was measured in rat adrenal chromaffin tissue from normal and hypophysectomized animals. Hyophysectomy triggered an abrupt decrease in the proportion of *Slo* transcripts containing a 'STREX' exon. The decrease was prevented by adrenocorticotropic hormone injections.

Gastrointestinal tract

Selye (1936b) noted that acute ulcers of the digestive tract were observed in rats exposed to nonspecific stresses. Since then, stress procedures including restraint have been used for induction of gastric ulcers in rats (Shay *et al.*, 1945; Takagi *et al.*, 1964; Senay and Levine, 1967; Paré and Glavin, 1986). Chronic stress as well as acute stress is a potent inducer of stress ulcers. The term 'stress ulcer' encompasses upper gastrointestinal hemorrhage and lesions as a consequence of a variety of factors including burns, intracranial trauma and systemic infections in humans. In experimental rat models for stress ulcer, the most commonly employed methods are cold restraint, water restraint, shock stress and food deprivation.

The animal's ulcerative response to a stressor depends on predisposing factors (age, sex, strains, lines, early experiences), the nature of the stress employed to induce the ulcer, and the post-stress events. In the study of stress-induced ulcers in several rat strains, it has been shown that RHA rats develop more starvation-induced ulcers than RLA rats. Maudsley reactive rats are more susceptible to restraint-induced ulcers than Maudsley nonreactive rats.

One concern in early stress experiments was the rather protracted starvation period often used prior to the actual stress, such as restraint. Most workers recognized then, as now, that experimental ulcers are more reliably produced if the gut is primed by emptying via food deprivation prior to the induction of stresses. Thus, stress and starvation conditions have been used in rats to get a considerable amount of information concerning drug effects on the stress syndrome, especially gastric ulcer.

The neuroendocrine basis of stress ulcerogenesis remains unclear; the existence of a brain–gut axis has been proposed. Hydroxy radicals have been reported to be the major causative factor in stress-induced gastric ulceration (Das *et al.*, 1997). The mechanical forces of gastric hypercontractility were also reported to be contributors to the gastric mucosal injury in rodent cold restraint models (Ephgrave *et al.*, 1997). Nitric oxide, derived from the gastric inducible type of nitric oxide synthese, may play an important role

in the suppression of stress-induced mucosal injury of the stomach (Yu *et al.*, 1997).

A few studies have reported stress-induced intestinal fluid secretion in humans and rats (Barclay and Turnberg, 1987; Empey and Fedorak, 1989). Acute stress alters intestinal transport physiology in Wistar-Kyoto rats, a stress-susceptible strain (Saunders *et al.*, 1994). The stress stimulates the release of acetylcholine, resulting in altered epithelial function in these genetically predisposed rats (Saunders *et al.*, 1997).

Cardiovascular system

It has been widely demonstrated that noise stress can induce both morphological and functional changes in several organs and systems (Bearwood *et al.*, 1975; Kraicer *et al.*, 1977; Griefahn and Muzet, 1978; Alario *et al.*, 1987; Gue *et al.*, 1987). In particular, the cardiovascular system is most affected following exposure to different kinds of stress, including noise. Both acute and subacute noise exposure induces modification in the cardiac β-adrenoceptor responsiveness and morphohistochemical changes, consisting of an increase in sympathetic fiber density (Paparelli *et al.*, 1992; Breschi *et al.*, 1994). After acute noise stress, cardiac ultrastructural damage has been observed at the mitochondrial level with lysis of the cristae and dissolution of the matrix (Papparelli *et al.*, 1995; Pellegrini *et al.*, 1996; Soldani *et al.*, 1997a).

Gender differences exist in noise stress-induced ultrastructural changes in rat myocardium (Soldani *et al.*, 1997b). Furthermore, changes in cardiovascular functions after noise have been described, such as constantly elevated arterial blood pressure and an increase in corticosterone plasma levels in experimental animals (Cohen *et al.*, 1981; De Boer *et al.*, 1988, 1989; Altura *et al.*, 1992).

Stress has been implicated as a risk factor for increased morbidity and mortality due either to myocardial ischemia or to malignant arrhythmia in the absence of ischemia (Ketterer, 1993; Merz *et al.*, 1993; Meerson, 1994; Tennant *et al.*, 1994; Krittayaphong *et al.*, 1995; Krantz *et al.*, 1996). In experimental animals, it has been shown that acute stress decreases the fibrillation threshold of the myocardium (Meerson, 1994) and also increases the risk for cardiac arrhythmias associated with myocardial ischemia (Verrier and Kovach, 1995; Wolf, 1995). Repeated intermittent stress exacerbates myocardial ischemia–reperfusion injury (Scheuer and Mifflin, 1998).

On the other hand, heat stress protects aged hypertrophied and nonhypertrophied rat hearts against ischemic damage (Cornelussen et al., 1997). Chronic heat improves mechanical and metabolic responses of trained rat heart on ischemia and reperfusion (Levy et al., 1997). Heat shock protects rat myocardial mitochondria (Borman et al., 1998).

The change in arterial blood pressure in response to presentation of an acute behavioral stress in rat includes an initial rapid rise followed by a delayed, but more sustained, pressor response. The autonomic nervous system organizes the cardiovascular response to a suddenly perceived behavioral stress (Li et al., 1998).

Other systems

Cold stress facilitates calcium mobilization from bone in an ovariectomized rat model of osteoporosis (Islam et al., 1998). Metallothionein, a low molecular weight, cysteine-rich metal-binding protein, is involved in zinc and copper metabolism and in heavy metal detoxification (Cousins, 1985; Bremner, 1987). Eighteen hours of immobilization stress, accompanied by food and water deprivation, increased liver metallothionein but decreased kidney metallothionein (Giralt et al., 1993).

Starvation-like Conditions

Protein-energy malnutrition (PEM), also called protein-calorie malnutrition (PCM), is present when insufficient energy or protein is available to meet metabolic demands, thereby leading to impairments in normal physiological processes (Mason and Rosenberg, 1994). Inadequate dietary intake is only one of several mechanisms by which this may occur. Increased metabolic demands due to disease and increased nutrient losses are two other common mechanisms by which the body's protein and energy economy may become disrupted enough to cause PEM. Protein deficiency may also arise in the face of adequate protein intake if the dietary protein is of poor quality.

During periods of protein and/or energy deficit, compensatory mechanisms serve to lessen the pathological impact of these deficiencies. To understand how malnutrition develops, it is important to understand the responses to such inadequate intake. During the first 24 hours of fasting, circulating glucose, fatty acids and triacylglycerols and liver and muscle glycogen are used as fuel sources. Triacylglycerols, derived mainly from adipose tissue, can be catabolized to fatty acids and ketone bodies by most tissues. However, over the short term, tissues such as the brain can only use glycolytic pathways to obtain energy. Since fatty acids are not converted to carbohydrate, these glycolytic tissues must utilize either glucose or substrates that can be converted to glucose. Amino acids, derived primarily from skeletal muscle, constitute the major endogenous substrate for glucose production for this purpose. Since there is no storage form of protein in the body, a fasting individual sustains a daily loss of functionally significant protein.

The provision of adequate fuel substrate to critical tissues, particularly the brain, has homeostatic priority during protein/energy deprivation. Brief starvation leads to acute adaptive responses that sustain the supply of glucose to tissues that require it and minimize the amount of protein degradation to meet this need. To accomplish this end, certain tissues, such as the heart, kidney and skeletal muscles, change their primary fuel substrate from glucose to fatty acids and ketone bodies.

Progressive starvation is associated with depletion of hepatic glycogen stores, followed by mobilization of adipose tissue triacylglycerol. Adipose tissue lipolysis produces glycerol and nonesterified free fatty acids. Glycerol serves as a substrate for hepatic gluconeogenesis, whereas free fatty acids serve as an alternative oxidative substrate to glucose and thereby promote glucose recycling through lactate production and gluconeogenesis. Although glucose utilization is rapidly suppressed in the rat heart, relatively high rates of glucose uptake and phosphorylation are maintained in oxidative skeletal muscle for at least 9–12 hours after food withdrawal (Holness and Sugden, 1990). Even after 24 hours of starvation, rates of glucose utilization by these latter muscles remain at 40% of those observed in the fed state (Holness and Sugden, 1990).

Because pyruvate oxidation is suppressed (Holness et al., 1989; Holness and Sugden, 1990), glucose is degraded to lactate, which is released into venous effluent. After very extended (48 to 72 hours) starvation, almost complete suppression of glucose utilization by oxidative skeletal muscle results in a decline in the availability of C-3 derivatives of glucose (e.g. lactate, pyruvate and alanine) to sustain hepatic gluconeogenesis and a significant reduction in whole-body glucose turnover (Holness and Sugden, 1990, 1997; Barzilai et al., 1985).

Fasting leads to a marked decrease in thermogenesis, a mechanism that is closely associated with reduced sympathetic and thyroidal activities (Landsberg and Young, 1978). Reduction of brown adipose tissue thermogenesis in response to starvation has been related to tissue atrophy and to a specific decrease in GDP-binding, UCP levels (Puigserver et al., 1991, 1992) and UCP mRNA levels (Champigny and Ricquier, 1990; Picó et al., 1994). Response to food deprivation of the rat brown adipose tissue mitochondrial uncoupling system diminishes with age (Garcia-Palmer et al., 1997).

It is well established that starvation followed by refeeding causes an increase in rat liver lipogenic enzyme activity in comparison to the levels obtained with the same diet fed ad libitum (Tepperman and Tepperman, 1958; Frenkel, 1975; Wakil et al., 1983; Goodridge, 1987). Rat white adipose tissue lipogenesis occurs after the multiple cycles of the starvation–refeeding protocol (Kochan et al., 1997). Zara and Gnoni (1995) investigated the effect of starvation on the activity of the tricarboxylate carrier in intact rat liver mitochondria and in a reconstituted system. In both experimental conditions, the rate of citrate transport, when compared to the controls, is greatly reduced in starved rats. These data suggest that the starvation-induced decrease of citrate carrier activity could be due to a change in the intrinsic properties of the transport protein.

During short-term starvation, degradation of newly synthesized lipoprotein lipase is an important determinant for its secretion from the adipocytes and hence its functional activity in the capillary endothelium (Lee et al., 1998). Starvation induces insulin-dependent tyrosine phosphorylation of the 195-kDa protein in the rat liver (Ito et al., 1997).

With extended starvation, other adaptations appear. The brain, which ordinarily obtains energy only by glucose oxidation, acquires the ability to use keto acids for its fuel requirements, and this contributes further to protein conservation. Animal studies suggest that protein that is consumed during relative protein starvation is utilized more efficiently. Moreover, chronic protein deprivation leads to a reduced rate of protein turnover, and amino acids are reutilized more efficiently for the synthesis of new proteins, contributing to savings in both energy and amino acid requirements.

During relative or total caloric starvation, such adaptations allow the body to provide the energy necessary for metabolism and to minimize the obligatory loss of protein, which appears primarily as nitrogen-containing compounds in the urine. After long periods of starvation, nitrogen loss in the urine may decrease. However, these homeostatic mechanisms do not compensate entirely for the imposed deficits, and eventually the negative caloric and/or protein balance leads to pathological consequences.

Physiological Impairments Associated with Starvation-like Conditions

Gastrointestinal system

Alterations in the gastrointestinal structure and function with PEM arise partially from undernutrition and partially from decreased stimulation of the gut by ingested nutrients (Mason and Rosenberg, 1994). Overnight fasting causes hemorrhagic lesions in the stomach of streptozotocin-induced diabetic rats (Takeuchi et al., 1994). These results suggest that gastric lesions induced in the rats by fasting are insulin-sensitive and may be associated with a profound hyperglycemic response to food deprivation.

The sustained absence of nutrients in the intestine results in structural and functional atrophy of the intestine. Marked blunting, or total absence, of the intestinal villi is associated with decreased levels of disaccharidases and aminopepidases in the mucosa. Experimental and clinical studies have shown that prolonged starvation leads to serious metabolic disturbances as well as morphological and functional alterations of the intestinal tract (Dugue et al., 1975). Following starvation, ultrastructural alteration was demonstrated in the rat intestinal epithelium fed with polymeric, oligopeptidic or elementary full diet (Botsios et al., 1993). It is shown that several physiological and pathological conditions such as protein malnutrition, intestinal resection, postnatal maturation, abetalipoproteinemia, sickle cell disease and diabetes are associated with selective alteration in the fluidity and/or lipid composition of the enterocyte membrane (Menge et al., 1983; Brasitus and Dudeja, 1985; Brasitus et al., 1986; Livshin et al., 1987; Hubner et al., 1988; Dudeja et al., 1991).

Goodlad et al. (1988) reported that 4 days starvation significantly decreases the crypt cell production rate, small intestinal length, crypt cell population and absorption. Starvation brings about increased transport of glucose across the membrane of intestinal epithelial cells of rat (Gupta and Waheed, 1992). Transport of L-proline, glycine and L-glutamic acid, which represent imino, glycine and acidic systems respectively, increased significantly in the Na^+-dependent pathway, whereas transport of L-lysine, representing the basic system, increased significantly in the Na^+-independent pathway during starvation (Waheed and Gupta, 1997).

The adaptive changes that occur in the small intestine during fasting include mucosal hypoplasia and a reduction in the rate of cell proliferation (Karasov et al., 1983). Fasting and refeeding modulate putrescine transport in rat intestinal brush-border membrane vesicles (Brachet et al., 1996). Gastric and pancreatic secretions are reduced in volume and contain decreased concentrations of acid and digestive enzymes. The volume of bile and the concentration of conjugated bile acids in bile are reduced.

Antwi et al. (1988) demonstrated that fasting for 48 hours increased phosphorylation of adipose tissue, which is considered to be the rate-limiting step for glycogen synthesis, but not of muscle glycogen synthase. The effects of starvation on the level of glycogen synthase gene expression were examined in rat liver during starvation (Nur et al., 1995). Depletion of hepatic glycogen store by 72 hours of starvation was supercompensated by 24 hours of refeeding a standard laboratory diet. These data indicate that the efficiency of glycogen synthase mRNA translation, rather than its abundance, decreases during starvation.

Differences in hepatic glutaminase activity in rats starved or fed different levels of protein are mainly due to differences in the rate of transcription of the gene (Watford et al., 1994). Lysosomal uptake and degradation of polypeptides such as glyceraldehyde-3-phosphate dehydrogenase, ribonuclease, and ribonuclease S-peptide are progressively activated in rat liver by starvation (Mortimore et al., 1989; Kopitz et al., 1990; Wing et al., 1991; Dunn, 1994; Cuervo et al., 1995).

It is well known that starvation can result in a post-starvation anorexia both in rats and in humans (Duncan et al., 1962; Hamilton, 1969; Nelson and Ksir, 1975). Furthermore, the pattern of nutrient self-selection is also altered, with starvation resulting in a post-starvation increase in fat or carbohydrate uptake (Piquard et al., 1978, 1979; Bligh et al., 1990; Hunsicker et al., 1992). The activation of the serotoninergic system abolishes the increase in carbohydrate intake and potentiates post-starving anorexia (Duhault et al., 1993).

Immunological functions, Hematopoiesis

PEM impairs the cell-mediated and humoral immune systems. The functional integrity of T lymphocytes, polymorphonuclear leukocytes, and the complement system is uniformly blunted, and B-lymphocyte function may be impaired (Mason and Rosenberg, 1994). Feed restriction results in decreased hematopoietic tissue (Levin et al., 1993).

Endocrine system

Hormonal alterations are common in PEM; most appear to be physiological adaptations to the undernourished state. The inadequate intake of food leads to a decrease in the availability of circulating glucose and amino acids, low circulating levels of insulin, and increased levels of growth hormone. These alterations, in conjunction with the decreased levels of somatomedins and increased levels of cortisol in PEM, promote muscle protein catabolism and at the same time enhance incorporation of the liberated amino acids into visceral organs.

Elevated plasma glucocorticoids are frequently associated with malnutrition in disease or injury, and high levels of exogenous glucocorticoids can cause immune suppression and protein wasting (Watters and Wilmore, 1989; Quan and Walser, 1992; Reaich et al., 1993; Hill et al., 1995). Protein malnutrition increases plasma adrenocorticotropin and anterior pituitary proopiomelanocortin mRNA in the rat (Jacobson et al., 1997). Urea synthesis is inhibited, decreasing nitrogen loss and enhancing the reutilization of amino acids. The enhancement of lipolysis and gluconeogenesis provides substrates for energy. The serum levels of triiodothyronine and thyroxine are commonly decreased.

Starvation induces the increase in the parathyroid hormone/parathyroid hormone-related protein receptor mRNA of bone and kidney in sham-operated and thyroidparathyroidectomized rats (Kawane et al., 1997). Primary gonadal dysfunction is common, including decreased levels of circulating testosterone and estrogen and impairment in reproductive potential.

Cardiovascular system

Moderate to severe PEM produces both quantitative and qualitative alterations in the heart. Myocardial mass is decreased, although proportionately less than the loss in body weight. Microscopic analysis of the myocardium reveals myofibrillar atrophy, edema and, less commonly, patchy necrosis and infiltration with chronic inflammatory cells. These structural changes are associated with alterations in myocardial performance, most evident under conditions of increased demand, as a decrease in cardiac output, stroke volume and maximal work capacity. The cardiac alterations associated with PEM are reversible. Starvation increases the amount of pyruvate dehydrogenase kinase isozyme 4 in the rat heart (Wu et al., 1998).

Respiratory system

All muscles, including the diaphragm and other respiratory muscles, undergo structural and functional atrophy, causing decreases in the inspiratory and expiratory pressures and in the vital capacity. Decreased respiratory muscle strength and a blunted ventilatory drive impair the ability to sustain ventilation in the severely malnourished individual.

Acute nutritional deprivation in adult rats produces no significant atrophy of either type I or type II diaphragm muscle fibers, despite a 20% reduction in body weight (Lewis and Sieck, 1990). In contrast, an identical experimental protocol of acute nutritional deprivation in rapidly growing adolescent rats reduced body weight by 32% and the cross-sectional areas of type I and type II diaphragm fibers by 22% and 44%, respectively (Lewis and Sieck, 1992; Lewis et al., 1997).

Skeletal muscle

Muscle size is determined by the balance between the rates of protein synthesis and degradation. Accelerated degradation is an important factor contributing to the loss of muscle weight in various physiological and pathological conditions, including starvation (Li and Goldberg, 1976; Goodman and Ruderman, 1980; Li et al., 1978). Ubiquitin–protein conjugates increase concomitantly with the increase in proteolysis in rat skeletal muscle during starvation (Wing et al., 1995). Refeeding after starvation involves a temporal shift in the control site of glycogen synthesis in rat muscle (James et al., 1998).

Urological system

Short-term starvation increases calciferol-24-hydroxylase activity and mRNA level in rat kidney (Hagenfeldt-Pernow et al., 1994). Starvation also has effects on rat kidney peroxisomal and microsomal fatty acid oxidation (Orellana et al., 1993).

References

Adell, A., Casanovas, J.M. and Artigas, F. (1997) Neuropharmacology 36, 735–741.

Alario, P., Gamallo, A., Beato, M.J. and Trancho, G. (1987) Physiol. Behav. 40, 29–32.

Albeck, D.S., McKittrick, C.R., Blanchard, D.C. et al. (1997) J. Neurosci. 17, 4895–4903.

Altura, B.M., Altura, B.T., Gebrewold, A., Ising, H. and Gunther, T. (1992) J. Appl. Physiol. 72, 194–202.

Antwi, D., Young, J.H., Shargill, N.S., Lesikar, D.D. and Kaslow, H.R. (1988) Am. J. Physiol. 254, E720–E725.

Appelboom-Fondu, J., Kerkhops, M. and Mendelwick, J. (1988) J. Affect. Dis. 4, 35–40.

Armario, A., Gil, M., Marti, J. Pol, O. and Balasch, J.A.F. (1991) Pharmacol. Biochem. Behav. 39, 373–377.

Barclay, G.R. and Turnberg, L.A. (1987) Gastroenterology 93, 91–97.

Barrett, A.M. and Stockham, M.A. (1963) J. Endocrinol. 26, 97–105.

Barzilai, N., Massillon, D. and Rossetti, L. (1995) Biochem. J. 310, 819–826.

Bearwood, C.J., Mundell, C.A. and Utian, W.H. (1975) Am. J. Obstet. Gynaecol. 121, 682–687.

Bignami, G. (1965) Anim. Behav. 13, 221–227.

Bligh, M.E., DeStefano, M.B., Kramlik, S.K., Douglass, L.W., Dubuc, P. and Castonguay, T.W. (1990) Physiol. Behav. 48, 373–381.

Bonnet, C., Léger, L., Baubet, V., Debilly, G. and Cespuglio, R. (1997) Brain Res. 751, 54–63.

Borman, L., Steinmann, C.M.I., Gericke, G.S. and Polla, B.S. (1998) Biochem. Biophys. Res. Commun. 246, 836–840.

Botsios, D., Economou, L., Manthos, A. et al. (1993) Histol. Histopath. 8, 527–535.

Bouyer, J.J., Deminiére, J.M., Mayo, W. and Le Moal, M. (1997) Neurosci. Lett. 225, 193–196.

Brachet, P., Prévoteau, H., Mathé, V. and Tomé, D. (1996) Digestion 57, 374–381.

Brasitus, T.A. and Dudeja, P.K. (1985) J. Biol. Chem. 260, 12405–12409.

Brasitus, T.A., Dudeja, P.K., Worman, H.J. and Foster, E.S. (1986) Biochim. Biophys. Acta. 855, 16–24.

Bremner, I. (1987) Prog. Food Nutr. Sci. 11, 1–37.

Brennan, Jr., F.X., Job, R.F., Watkins, L.R. and Maier, S.F.A.F. (1992) *Life Sci.* **50**, 945–950.

Breschi, M.C., Scatizzi, R., Martinotti, E., Pellegrini, A., Soldani, P. and Paparelli, A. (1994) *Int. J. Neurosci.* **75**, 73–81.

Broadhurst, P.L. (1975) *Behav. Genet.* **5**, 299–319.

Brown, M.R. and Fisher, L.A. (1990) In: DeSouza, E.B. and Nemeroff, C.B. (eds) *Corticotropin-releasing Factor: Basic and Clinical Studies of a Neuropeptide*, pp. 291–298. Boca Raton: CRC Press.

Brush, F.R., Del Paine, S.N., Pellegrino, L.J., Rykaszewski, I.M., Dess, N.K. and Collins, P.Y. (1988) *J. Comp. Psychol.* **102**, 337–349.

Champigny, O. and Ricquier, D. (1990) *J. Nutr.* **120**, 1730–1736.

Cohen, S., Krantz, D.S., Evans, G.W. and Stokols, D. (1981) *Am. Sci.* **69**, 528–535.

Cools, A., Brachten, R., Heeren, D. and Willemen, A. (1990) *Brain Res. Bull.* **24**, 49–69.

Cornelussen, R.N., Garnier, A.V., Geurten, M.M.V., Reneman, R.S., Van der Vusse, G.J. and Snoeckx, L.H.E.H. (1997) *Am. J. Physiol.* **273**, H1333–H1341.

Cousins, R.J. (1985) *Physiol. Rev.* **65**, 238–309.

Craig, E.A. (1985) *CRC Crit. Rev. Biochem.* **18**, 239–280.

Cuervo, A.M., Knecht, E., Terlecky, S.R. and Dice, J.F. (1995) *Am. J. Physiol.* **269**, C1200–C1208.

Das, D., Bandyopadhyay, D., Bhattacharjee, M. and Banerjee, R.K. (1997) *Free Radic. Biol. Med.* **23**, 8–18.

De Boer, S.F., Slangen, J.L. and Van der Gugten, J. (1988) *Physiol. Behav.* **44**, 273–280.

De Boer, S.F., Van der Gugten, J. and Slangen, J.L. (1989) *Physiol. Behav.* **45**, 789–795.

De Kloet, E.R., Rosenfeld, P. van Eekelen, J.A.M., Sutanto, W. and Levine, S. (1988) In: Boer, G.J., Feenstra, M.G.P., Mirmiran, M., Swaab, D.F. and van Haaren, F. (eds) *Progress in Brain Research*, Vol. 73, pp. 101–120. Amsterdam: Elsevier.

De Kloet, E.R., Joels, M., Oitzl, M., S. and Sutanto, W. (1991) In: Jasmin, G. and Cantin, M. (eds) *Stress Revisited; Methods and Achievements in Experimental Pathology*, 14th edn, pp. 104–132. Basel: Karger.

Driscoll, P. (1986) *Behav. Gen.* **16**, 355–364.

Driscoll, P., Dedek, J., D'Angio, M., Claustre, Y. and Scatton, B. (1990) *Adv. Anim. Breed. Gen.* **5** (suppl.), 97–107.

Dudeja, P.K., Harig, J.M., Wali, R.K., Knaup, S.M., Ramaswamy, K. and Brasitus, T.A. (1991) *Arch. Biochem. Biophys.* **284**, 338–345.

Dugue, E., Bolanos, O. and Loreto, H. (1975) *Am. J. Clin. Nutr.* **28**, 901–909.

Duhault, J., Lacour, F., Espinal, J. and Rolland, Y. (1993) *Appetite* **20**, 135–144.

Duncan, G.G., Jensen, W.K., Fraser, R.J. and Cristofori, F.C. (1962) *J. Am. Med. Assoc.* **181**, 99–102.

Dunn, Jr., W.A. (1994) *Trends Cell Biol.* **4**, 139–143.

Empey, L.R. and Fedorak, R.N. (1989) *Prostaglandins Leukot. Essent. Fatty Acids* **38**, 43–48.

Ephgrave, K.S., Cullen, J.J., Broadhurst, K., Kleiman-Wexler, R., Shirazi, S.S. and Schulze-Delrieu, K. (1997) *Neurogastroenterol. Mot.* **9**, 187–192.

Frenkel, R. (1975) *Curr. Top. Cell Regul.* **9**, 157–181.

Garcia-Garcia, L., Fuentes, J.A. and Manzanares, J. (1997) *Brain Res.* **772**, 115–120.

Garcia-Palmer, F.J., Pericas, J., Matamala, J.C. et al. (1997) *Biochem. Mol. Int.* **42**, 1151–1161.

Giralt, M., Gasull, T., Hernandez, J., Garcia, A. and Hidalgo, J. (1993) *BioMetals* **6**, 171–178.

Goldenberg, F. (1993) *Rev. Neurophysiol. Clin.* **23**, 487–515.

Goodlad, R.A., Plumb, J.A. and Wright, N.A. (1988) *Clin. Sci.* **74**, 301–306.

Goodman, M.N. and Ruderman, N.B. (1980) *Am. J. Physiol.* **239**, E269–E276.

Goodridge, A.G. (1987) *Annu. Rev. Nutr.* **7**, 157–185.

Griefahn, B. and Muzet, A. (1978) *J. Sound Vibrat.* **59**, 99–101.

Grünfeld, J.-P. (1990) *Horm. Res.* **34**, 111–113.

Gue, M., Fioramonti, J., Frexinos, J., Alvinerie, M. and Bueno, L. (1987) *Dig. Dis. Sci.* **32**, 1411–1417.

Gupta, P.D. and Waheed, A.A. (1992) *FEBS Lett.* **300**, 263–267.

Hagenfeldt-Pernow, Y., Ohyama, Y., Sudjana-Sugiaman, E., Okuda, K. and Björkhem, I. (1994) *Eur. J. Endocrinol.* **130**, 608–611.

Hamilton, C.L. (1969) *Am. N.Y. Acad. Sci.* **157**, 1004–1017.

Hartl, F.U. (1996) *Nature* **381**, 571–580.

Hendley, E.D., Holets, V.R., McKeon, T.W. and McCarty, R.A.F. (1991) *Clin. Exp. Hypertension (A)* **13**, 939–945.

Hill, A.D.K., Naama, H.A. Gallagher, H.J., Shou, J., Calvano, S.E. and Daly, J.M. (1995) *Surgery* **118**, 130–137.

Holness, M.J. and Sugden, M.C. (1990) *Biochem. J.* **270**, 245–249.

Holness, M.J. and Sugden, M.C. (1997) *Am. J. Physiol.* **272**, E556–E561.

Holness, M.J., Liu, Y.L. and Sugden, M.C. (1989) *Biochem. J.* **264**, 771–776.

Hsu, D.T., Chen, F.-L., Takahashi, L.K. and Kalin, N.H. (1998) *Brain Res.* **788**, 305–310.

Hubner, C., Lindner, S.G., Stern, M., Claussen, M. and Kohlschutter, A. (1988) *Biochim. Biophys. Acta* **939**, 145–150.

Hunsicker, K.D., Mullen, B.J. and Martin, R.J. (1992) *Physiol. Behav.* **51**, 325–330.

Islam, N., Chanda, S., Ghosh, T.K. and Mitra, C. (1998) *Jpn J. Physiol.* **48**, 49–55.

Ito, Y., Takahashi, S., Takenaka, A., Hidaka, T. and Noguchi, T. (1997) *Biosci. Biotech. Biochem.* **61**, 2122–2124.

Jacobson, L., Zurakowski, D. and Majzoub, J.A. (1997) *Endocrinology* **138**, 1048–1057.

James, A.P., Flynn, C.B., Jones, S.L., Palmer, T.N. and Fournier, P.A. (1998) *Biochem J.* **329**, 341–347.

Jones, M.T. and Gillham, B. (1988) *Physiol. Rev.* **68**, 743–818.

Jones, M.T. and Stockham, M.A. (1966) *J. Physiol.* **184**, 741–750.

Kant, G.J., Leu, J.R., Anderson, S.M. and Mougey, E.H. (1987) *Physiol. Behav.* **40**, 775–779.

Kaplan, M.H. (1956) *Am. J. Gastroenterol.* **25**, 234–252.

Karasov, W.H., Pond, R.S., Solberg, D.H. and Diamond, J.M. (1983) *Proc. Natl Acad. Sci. USA* **80**, 7674–7677.

Kawane, T., Saikatsu, S., Akeno, N., Abe, M. and Horiuchi, N. (1997) *Eur. J. Endocrinol.* **137**, 273–280.

Ketterer, M.W. (1993) *Psychosomatics* **34**, 478–484.

Kirby, L.G. and Lucki, I. (1997) *J. Pharmacol. Exp. Ther.* **282**, 967–976.

Kitayama, I., Yaga, T., Kayahara, T. *et al.* (1997) *Biol. Psychiatry* **42**, 687–696.

Kochan, Z., Karbowska, J. and Swierczynski, J. (1997) *Metabolism* **46**, 10–17.

Koob, G.F., Heinrichs, S.C., Pich, E.M. *et al.* (1993) *Ciba Found. Symp.* **172**, 277–289.

Kopitz, J., Kisen, G.O., Gordon, P.B., Bohley, P. and Seglen, P.O. (1990) *J. Cell Biol.* **111**, 941–953.

Kozutsumi, Y., Segal, M., Normington, K., Gething, M.-J. and Sambrook, J. (1988) *Nature* **332**, 462–464.

Kraicer, J., Betaud, G. and Lywood, D.W. (1977) *Neuroendocrinology* **23**, 352–367.

Krantz, D.S., Kop, W.J., Santiago, H.T. and Gottdiener, J.S. (1996) *Cardiol. Clin.* **14**, 271–287.

Krittayaphong, R., Light, K.C., Biles, P.L., Ballenger, M.N. and Sheps, D.S. (1995) *Am. J. Cardiol.* **76**, 657–660.

Krukoff, T.L. and Khalili, P. (1997) *J. Comp. Neurol.* **377**, 509–519.

Landsberg, L. and Young, J.B. (1978) *N. Engl. J. Med.* **298**, 1295–1301.

Lee, J.-J., Smith, P.J. and Fried, S.K. (1998) *J. Nutr.* **128**, 940–946.

Levin, S., Semler, D. and Ruben, Z. (1993) *Toxicologic Pathology* **21**, 1–14.

Levy, E., Hasin, Y., Navon, G. and Horowitz, M. (1997) *Am. J. Physiol.* **272**, H2085–H2094.

Lewis, M.I. and Sieck, G.C. (1990) *J. Appl. Physiol.* **68**, 1938–1944.

Lewis, M.I. and Sieck, G.C. (1992) *J. Appl. Physiol.* **73**, 974–978.

Lewis, M.I., LoRusso, T.J. and Fournier, M. (1997) *J. Appl. Physiol.* **82**, 1064–1070.

Li, J.B. and Goldberg, A.L. (1976) *Am. J. Physiol.* **231**, 441–448.

Li, J.B., Higgins, J.E. and Jefferson, L.S. (1978) *Am. J. Physiol.* **236**, E222–E228.

Li, S.-G., Randall, D.C. and Brown, D.R. (1998) *Am. J. Physiol.* **274**, R1065–R1069.

Lindquist, S. and Craig, E.A. (1988) *Annu. Rev. Genet.* **22**, 631–677.

Livshin, L., Mokady, S. and Cogan, U. (1987) *J. Nutr.* **117**, 684–688.

McEwen, B.S., de Kloet, E.R. and Rostene, W. (1986) *Physiol. Rev.* **66**, 1121–1188.

McGivern, R.F., Rittenhouse, P., Aird, F., Van de Kar, L.D. and Redel, E. (1997) *J. Neurosci.* **17**, 4886–4894.

Mason, J.B. and Rosenberg, I.H. (1994) In: Isselbacher, K.J., Braunwald, E., Wilson, J.D., Martin, J.B., Fauci, A.S. and Kasper, D.L. (eds) *Harrison's Principles of Internal Medicine*, 13th edn, pp. 440–446. New York: McGraw-Hill.

Meaney, M.J., Aitken, D.H., Sharma, S. and Viau, V. (1992) *Neuroendocrinology* **55**, 204–213.

Meerson, F.Z. (1994) *Clin. Cardiol.* **17**, 362–371.

Menge, H., Sepulveda, F.V. and Smith, M.W. (1983) *J. Physiol.* **334**, 213–223.

Merz, C.N.B., Krantz, D.S. and Rozanski, A. (1993) *Tex. Heart Inst. J.* **20**, 152–157.

Mori, K, Sant, A., Kohno, K., Normington, K., Gething, M.-J. and Sambrook, J.F. (1992) *EMBO J.* **11**, 2583–2593.

Mori, K., Ma, W., Gething, M.-J. and Sambrook, J. (1993) *Cell* **74**, 743–756.

Mortimore, G.E., Pösö, A.R. and Lardeux, B.R. (1989) *Diabetes Metab. Rev.* **5**, 49–70.

Nagata, K. (1996) In: Feige, U., Morimoto, R.I., Yahara, I. and Polla, B. (eds) *Stress-inducible Cellular Responses.* Basel: Birkäuser Verlag.

Nakai, Y., Araki, T., Takahashi, S., Shimada, A. and Nakagawa, 'I'. (1983) *Psychother. Psychosom.* **39**, 201–212.

Natelson, B.H., Ottenweller, J.E., Cook, J.A., Pitman, D., McCarty, R. and Tapp, W.N. (1988) *Physiol. Behav.* **43**, 41–46.

Nelson, S. and Ksir, C. (1975) *Physiol. Behav.* **14**, 673–675.

Nur, T., Sela, I., Webster, N.J.G. and Madar, Z. (1995) *J. Nutr.* **125**, 2457–2462.

Oitzl, M.S. and de Kloet, E.R. (1992) *Behav. Neurosci.* **106**, 62–71.

Orellana, M., Fuentes, O. and Valdés, E. (1993) *FEBS Lett.* **322**, 61–64.

Otaka, M., Itoh, H., Kuwabara, T. *et al.* (1993) *Int. J. Biochem.* **25**, 1769–1773.

Otaka, M., Itoh, H., Kuwabara, T. *et al.* (1994) *Int. J. Biochem.* **26**, 805–811.

Paparelli, A., Soldani, P., Breschi, M.C. *et al.* (1992) *J. Neural Transm.* **88**, 105–113.

Paparelli, A., Pellegrini, A., Lenzi, P., Gesi, M. and Soldani, P. (1995) *J. Submicrosc. Cytol. Pathol.* **27**, 137–142.

Paré, W.P. and Glavin, G.B. (1986) *Neurosci. Biobehav. Rev.* **10**, 339–370.

Pellegrini, A., Soldani, P., Gesi, M., Lenzi, P. and Paparelli, A. (1996) *J. Submicrosc. Cytol. Pathol.* **28**, 507–512.

Persengiev, S., Kanchev, L. and Vezenkova, G.A.F. (1991) *J. Pineal Res.* **11**, 57–62.

Picó, M.C., Herron, D., Palou, A., Jacobson, A., Cannon, B. and Nedergard, J. (1994) *Biochem. J.* **302**, 81–86.

Piquard, F., Schaefer, A. and Habesey, P. (1978) *Physiol. Behav.* **20**, 771–778.

Piquard, F., Schaefer, A., Haberey, P., Chanez, M. and Peret, J. (1979) *J. Nutr.* **109**, 1035–1044.

Pitman, D.L., Ottenweller, J.E. and Natelson, B.H. (1988) *Physiol. Behav.* **43**, 47–55.

Puigserver, P., Lladó, I., Palou, A and Gianotti, M. (1991) *Biochem. J.* **279**, 575–579.

Puigserver, P., Gianotti, M. and Palou, A. (1992) *Int. J. Obes.* **16**, 255–261.

Quan, Z.Y. and Walser, M. (1992) *Am. J. Clin. Nutr.* **55**, 695–700.

Rampin, C., Cespuglio, R., Chastrette, N. and Jouvet, M. (1991) *Neurosci. Lett.* **126**, 113–118.

Rapp, J.P. and Dene, H. (1985) *Hypertension* 7, 340–346.

Ratka, A., Sutanto, W., Bloemers, M.M. and de Kloet, E.R. (1989) *Neuroendocrinology* 50, 117–123.

Reaich, D., Channon, S.M., Scrimgeour, C.M., Daley, S.E., Wilkinson, R. and Goodship, T.H.J. (1993) *Am. J. Physiol.* **265**, E230–E235.

Ritossa, F. (1962) *Experientia* **18**, 571–573.

Ross, R.J., Ball, W.A. and Sullivan, K.A. (1989) *Am. J. Psychiatry* **146**, 697–707.

Satinder, K.P. (1981) *J. Comp. Physiol. Psychol.* **95**, 175–187.

Saunders, P.R., Kosecka, U., McKay, D.M. and Perdue, M.H. (1994) *Am. J. Physiol.* **267**, G794–G799.

Saunders, P.R., Hanssen, N.P.M. and Perdue, M.H. (1997) *Am. J. Physiol.* **273**, G486–G490.

Sawchenko, P.E. and Swanson, L.S. (1990) In: DeSouza, E.B. and Nemeroff, C.B. (eds) *Corticotropin-releasing Factor: Basic and Clinical Studies of a Neuropeptide*, pp. 29–51. Boca Raton, FL: CRC Press.

Scheuer, D.A. and Mifflin, S.W. (1998) *Am. J. Physiol.* **274**, R470–R475.

Selye, H. (1936a) *Br. J. Exp. Pathol.* **17**, 234–248.

Selye, H. (1936b) *Can. Med. Assoc. J.* **34**, 706.

Selye, H. (1943) *Lancet* **244**, 252.

Senay, E.C. and Levine, R.J. (1967) *Proc. Soc. Exp. Biol. Med.* **124**, 1221–1223.

Shay, H., Komarov, S.A., Fels, S.S., Meranze, D., Gruenstein, M. and Siplet, H. (1945) *Gastroenterology* **5**, 43–61.

Shimizu, K., Nomoto, M., Ueta, Y. *et al.* (1997) *Biochem. Biophys. Res. Commun.* **233**, 550–554.

Shiu, R.P.C., Pouyssegur, J. and Pastan, I. (1977) *Proc. Natl Acad. Sci. USA* **74**, 3840–3844.

Soldani, P., Pellegrini, A., Gesi, M., Lenzi, P., Cristofani, R. and Paparelli, A. (1997a) *Anat. Rec.* **248**, 521–532.

Soldani, P., Pellegrini, A., Gesi, M. *et al.* (1997b) *J. Submicrosc. Cytol. Pathol.* **29**, 527–536.

Sorger, P.K. (1991) *Cell* **65**, 363–366.

Stone, K.R., Smith, R.E. and Joklik, W.K. (1974) *Virology* **58**, 86–100.

Sutanto, W. and de Kloet, E.R. (1994) *Lab. Anim.* **28**, 293–306.

Tachibana, M., Senuma, H., Ebara, T. and Kumamoto, K.A.F. (1991) *Commun. Chem. Pathol. Pharmacol.* **73**, 153–158.

Takagi, K., Kasuya, Y. and Watanabe, K. (1964) *Chem. Pharmacol. Bull.* **12**, 465–472.

Takahashi, L.K. and Kalin, N.H. (1989) In: Blanchard, R.J., Brain, P.F., Blanchard, D.C. and Parmigiani, S. (eds) *Ethoexperimental Approaches to the Study of Behavior*, pp. 580–594. Norwell, MA: Kluwer Academic Publishers.

Takeuchi, K., Ueshima, K., Ohuchi, T. and Okabe, S. (1994) *Dig. Dis. Sci.* **39**, 626–634.

Tennant, C.C., Palmer, K.J., Langeluddecke, P.M., Jones, M.P. and Nelson, G. (1994) *Eur. Heart J.* **15**, 472–478.

Tepperman, H.M. and Tepperman, J. (1958) *Diabetes* 7, 478–485.

Thomas, P.J., Qu, B.-H. and Pedersen, P.L. (1995) *Trends Biochem. Sci.* **20**, 456–459.

Treiman, D.M. and Levins, E. (1969) *Endocrinology* **84**, 676–680.

Vale, W., Speiss, J., Rivier, C. and Rivier, J. (1981) *Science*, **213**, 1394–1397.

Verrier, R.L. and Kovach, J.A. (1995) In: Podrid, P.J. and Kowey, P.R. (eds) *Cardiac Arrythmia. Mechanisms, Diagnosis and Management*, pp. 151–168. Baltimore: Williams and Wilkins.

Waheed, A.A. and Gupta, P.D. (1997) *Life Sci.* **61**, 2425–2433.

Wakil, S.J., Stoops, J.K. and Joshi, V.C. (1983) *Annu. Rev. Biochem.* **52**, 537–579.

Watford, M., Vincent, N., Zhan, Z., Fannelli, J., Kowalski, T. and Kovacevic, Z. (1994) *J. Nutr.*, **124**, 493–499.

Watters, J.M. and Wilmore, D.W. (1989) In: DeGroot, L.J. (ed.) *Endocrinology*, pp. 2367–2393. Philadelphia: Saunders.

Westwood, J.T. and Wu, C. (1993) *Mol. Cell. Biol.* **13**, 3481–3486.

Wiersma, A., Knollema, S., Konsman, J.P., Bohus, B. and Koolhaas, J.M. (1997) *Behav. Genet.* **27**, 547–555.

Wing, S.S., Chiang, H.-L., Goldberg, A.L. and Dice, J.F. (1991) *Biochem. J.* **275**, 165–169.

Wing, S.S., Haas, A.L. and Goldberg, A.L. (1995) *Biochem. J.* **307**, 639–645.

Wolf, S. (1995) *Integr. Physiol. Behav. Sci.* **30**, 215–225.

Wu, P., Sato, J., Zhao, Y., Jaskiewicz, J., Popov, K.M. and Harris, R.A. (1998) *Biochem. J.* **329**, 197–201.

Xie, J. and McCobb, D.P. (1998) *Science* **280**, 443–446.

Yamaguchi, H., Kimura, T. and Nawata, H. (1990) *Gastroenterology* **98**, 1682–1688.

Yu, H., Sato, E.F., Minamiyama, Y., Arakawa, T., Kobayashi, K. and Inoue, M. (1997) *Digestion* **58**, 311–318.

Zara, V. and Gnoni, G.V. (1995) *Biochim. Biophys. Acta* **1239**, 33–38.

CHAPTER 24

Routes of Administration

Klaus Nebendahl
University of Göttingen, Göttingen, Germany

General

Substances such as chemical elements, compounds, drugs, antibodies, cells or other agents may be administered by different routes. Numerous routes have been well documented in the literature. As every route has both advantages as well as disadvantages and as, for instance, the absorption, bioavailability and metabolism of the substance are factors which should be considered carefully, a knowledge of available methods and techniques of administration and of the disposition and fate of the administered substance will aid the scientist in choosing the most suitable route for his/her purpose. The exact details of any administration must be checked prior to any experiment.

A complete review of all methods used for administration would go far beyond the scope of this chapter. For a full discussion of all administration routes available, the reader is referred to the periodical literature. Only some administration routes, techniques and guidelines for safe injection volumes,

sites of administration, preparation of sites, injection techniques etc. will be described here. As a number of questions frequently arise concerning the suitability of solutions for injection and precise answers are often not forthcoming (Waynforth and Flecknell, 1992), some remarks are made with respect to volume and rate of injection, absorption of the administered substance, bioavailability and distribution of substances in the body, as well as factors that may modify the dosage etc.

An introduction to this topic would be incomplete without a reference to the humane treatment of laboratory rats which are, beside mice, the most frequently used animals in experimental studies. Nearly every route of administration can be performed relatively painlessly if attention is given to the proper restraint of the rat and adequate technical skill is employed. The European Convention for the Protection of Vertrebrate Animals Used for Experimental and Other Scientific Purpose states that persons carrying out such procedures should be well trained in handling and restraining experimental animals, should have the foundation for responsible use of the animals and should have a scientifically high standard, in order to protect the animals used in those procedures which may possibly cause pain, suffering or distress and to ensure that, where unavoidable, they shall be kept to a minimum. (ETS 123, 1986).

Principles of Administration

Handling and Restraining

Rats can be trained to accept handling and restraining and can become familiar with their handlers. Though time-consuming, it is essential to minimize distress. All procedures should therefore be carried out only by persons well known to the animal. Sedation or general anaesthesia is generally only required if the technique involved is more than a pinprick or the administered substances are known to cause pain etc.

Site of Administration

Numerous sites have been described in the literature for the administration of substances to rats, but some of these sites are unacceptable nowadays (e.g. foot-pad injection of Freund's Complete Adjuvant) (CCAC, 1989).

Preparation of the Site

Sometimes the area must be clipped or cleaned with warm water. Afterwards the skin should be swabbed with disinfectant or alcohol. In some cases it may be necessary to apply local analgesics to the site before administration to prevent pain.

Safety and Solubility of Substances

All parenteral administration must be done using an aseptic technique and the substances or injection solutions must be sterile and free from pyrogenous material. In order to administer an accurate dosage and to avoid causing tissue damage the toxicity of the substance, the volume and the way of administration has to be considered. If the substance has to be diluted, the diluent selected must be safe. Physiological saline (0.9% sodium chloride) or other physiological solvents like phosphate buffered saline (PBS) or various culture media are suitable vehicles. Although distilled water can under certain conditions be used, saline should be preferred because water *ad injectionem* injected subcutaneously causes pain and intravenous injection produces haemolysis.

For reasons of solubility or rate of absorption some substances require a more complex solvent to render them suitable for administration. Many solvents, for example water, water with 0.85% sodium chloride, 60% polyethylene glycol, 10% Tween 80, 0.5% methylcellulose, have been found suitable in most instances and do not greatly affect the activity of interest of the substances to be investigated due to their own inherent properties (Woodard, 1965). All of these vehicles can be administered by any of the injection routes available, but the concentrations mentioned are the maximum practicable, and in many cases it is possible and indeed desirable that lower concentrations should be used (Waynforth and Flecknell, 1992). When administering drugs, the solvent should ideally be the same as the one in which the drug is normally formulated.

Lipid-soluble substances can only be dissolved in oil, but their absorption is delayed when administered. As oil cannot be injected intravenously, lipophilic substances must be injected in a 15% oil-water emulsion. Oil-based adjuvants or oil-water emulsions given intraperitoneally may cause acute peritonitis. They should only be administered by this mode when all other routes have proved ineffective.

Substances can be injected in the form of a suspension. Since suspended particles have the tendency to sediment, these particles should be evenly distributed before the suspension is injected intravenously. If injected intravenously it should be noted that the particles will be filtered out in the capillary beds of the extremities and the lung, modifying the distribution of the injected material and sometimes causing pulmonary distress to the animal (Waynforth and Flecknell, 1992).

pH of the Injected Solution

Rats, like humans, tolerate the injection of solutions within a fairly wide range of pH. For all routes of administration, a working range is in the range of pH 4.5–8.0 (Woodard, 1965). The widest tolerance to pH is shown by the intravenous route because of the buffering capacity of the blood and of the very quick dilution through the side-on flow of venous blood, followed by the intramuscular and then the subcutaneous route. Nevertheless, the rate of intravenous injection must be kept slow and precautions taken to avoid irritating solutions getting outside the vein.

Volume and Frequency of Administration

Though volume and frequency of administration are mainly determined by the requirements of the experiment, the animal should not be strained or stressed. The volume of substances given is limited by their toxicity and by the size of the rat and should be as small as possible. Likewise the frequency of administration should be restricted to a minimum, to avoid unnecessary stress. The volume and rate of injection have to be considered, particularly if solutions are given intravenously, because haemodynamic changes and pulmonary oedema may occur and very rapid injections can produce cardiovascular failure and be lethal.

The Rate of Absorption and Distribution of Administered Substances

The rate of absorption is influenced by the blood flow to the site of administration, the nature of the substances and the manner and concentration in which they are presented (Wolfensohn and Lloyd, 1994). The rate influences the time-course of the effect of the substance and is an important factor in determining substance dosage (Waynforth and Flecknell, 1992). Only in a few cases is it possible to inject substances at the place where they should be effective. Normally they must be absorbed from the site of administration into the blood. Therefore, the size of the absorbing surface, the blood flow to the site of administration and the solubility of the substance in the tissue fluids are important factors that will determine the rate of absorption. Whilst endogenous compounds normally pass through biological membranes by special transport mechanisms, the penetration of xenobiotics follows physical

principles, such as passive diffusion according to the concentration gradient (Frimmer and Lämmler, 1977). Lipid solubility, physicochemical properties, degree of ionization and molecular size of substances are important factors in respect to the rate of absorption. Compounds which are highly soluble in the body fluids will be absorbed quickly. Substances which are ionized and are not lipid soluble will only be absorbed if a specific carrier exists (Wolfensohn and Lloyd, 1994). As absorption of administered substances mostly happens by diffusion down a concentration gradient, the absorption of substances is dependent on the dosage.

Enteral Administration

Enteral administration involves the introduction of substances into the gastrointestinal tract via the mouth or through the anus using a suppository. The latter method is not very practical when working with rats (Baumans et al., 1993). The advantage of enteral administration is the fact that it is possible to give comparatively large amounts of nonsterile substances or solutions. For oral preparations, a pH as low as 3 can be tolerated for a solution of fairly high buffer capacity. On the other hand, alkaline solutions are very poorly tolerated by the mouth (Woodard, 1965).

In principle, gastrointestinal absorption takes place over the whole length of the digestive tract. Absorption of most orally given substances occurs by diffusion of their nonionized forms, since the mucosal lining of the gastrointestinal tract is almost impermeable to ionized molecules. Consequently, absorption of substances will be enhanced in the acid stomach or in the nearly neutral intestine depending on the ionic character of the compound. The far larger surface area of the intestinal villi, however, makes intestinal absorption dominant (Claassen, 1994a).

Buccal or sublingual administration avoids the destructive effects that may be encountered in the stomach following oral administration (Woodard, 1965). Consequently this route is sometimes required in animal experimentation. The absorption rate of substances has not been investigated to any considerable extent and is probably insignificant in rats. It is known that the mucosa of the mouth cavity can only absorb hydrophobic, nonionized substances.

The gastric juice of rats is highly acidic (pH 2.0–4.0) (Dittmer, 1961). For substances given orally the stomach is a significant site of absorption for many acidic or neutral compounds, whereas only the weakest bases are absorbed to any appreciable extent at normal gastric pH values (Baggot, 1977). All other substances are absorbed only at a very low rate.

Using the oral administration route it should be understood that substances can be destroyed by the gastric juice, that the food content of the stomach influences both the rate and order of gastric emptying and that the rate of substance absorption is markedly influenced by its residence time in the stomach and is directly related to the rate at which substances are passed from the stomach into the intestine (Levine, 1970).

Because of its extensive surface area (total length 1020–1385 mm, average diameter 9.5–13 mm) (Hebel, 1969) and rich blood supply, the upper small intestine of the rat is the major site of absorption for all substances after oral administration. Absorption in the intestine is dependent on: (1) the physicochemical state of the substances, (2) the nonabsorptive physiological function and state of the intestine, (3) the metabolic activity and function of the absorbing cells, and (4) the structure of the absorbing surface (Levine, 1970). Through the efflux of intestinal juice, pancreatic juice and bile the intestinal content becomes nearly neutral. This will reduce the degree of ionization and the absorption rate of substances will increase. Lipid-soluble substances of the digestive content are rapidly absorbed, whereas, dependent on size, the absorption of solids is moderate.

The absorbing surface of the large intestine (length 220–270 mm, average diameter 23 mm) (Hebel, 1969) is much smaller than the surface of the small intestine; the large bowel is therefore not so important for absorption.

Using the oral administration routes it has to be kept in mind that enzymes of the microflora of the digestive tract can metabolize substances. Under physiological conditions, microorganisms are only to be found in the large intestine and normally such enzymic metabolism applies only to those substances not yet absorbed in the upper tract. This means that oral administration has the disadvantage that the enzymic activity of microorganisms may alter substances before they are absorbed in the bowel. If the metabolites are not biologically active, the administration of these substances may be without any effect. On the other hand, some insoluble substances become soluble as the result of enzymic activity during their passage through the stomach and the small intestine and hence their absorption then becomes possible in the large intestine.

Excluding those absorbed in the mouth and rectum, all substances given and absorbed through the gastrointestinal tract are transported by the portal vein to the liver. Some substances can be metabolized there to a large extent, before reaching the systemic circulation and/or the site of action. This phenomenon is called the 'first-pass effect' and has to be considered in selecting routes of administration. Note that similar, but slightly different lengths of the small and large intestine are quoted in Chapter 15.

Oral Administration (per os)

The simplest method for administering substances is to mix them with food or drinking water. However, this is not practicable with substances which are unpalatable, insoluble or chemically unstable in drinking water or when they irritate the mucosa of the gastrointestinal tract.

Giving substances with food or drink is an easy method of administration. It is not necessary to train the rat for the procedure because no handling or restraining is required. The animal is not disturbed, the administration takes place without any stress, and eating, drinking or digestion happens under normal physiological conditions and only the substances are rapidly metabolized. With compounds that are rapidly metabolized, it is possible to administer in the diet quantities of some chemicals over 24 hours that would be lethal in a single intubation dosage (Woodard, 1965).

Mixing substances into food must be done carefully and decomposition must be prevented otherwise the animal might refuse to eat the substances. Some technical equipment for preparing an accurate mixture is necessary. In most cases it is best to involve a foodstuff company to produce an exact mixture pressed in pellets. When feeding pellets decomposition of the food is prevented.

The daily food and water intake of the rat must be known before starting so that the quantity of substance to be mixed with the food or drinking water can be calculated (Table 24.1). Other factors may also come into play. If, for instance, the circadian rhythm influences the effect of a substance then the feeding behaviour of the rat should be

Table 24.1 Food intake of rats and specification of common diets

	Intake (g/rat/day)	ME content of standard diets[a] (kJ ME/g diet)
Growing rat	8.0–20.0	12.6–14.6
Fully grown rat	15.0–20.0	11.7
Nursing or pregnant rat	up to 65	12.6–14.6

ME, metabolizable energy.
[a] NB: Food intake can vary dependent on strain, body weight, activity, conditions of holding (temperature or humidity) and other factors. See also Table 4.1.

known. It is well known that rats eat only a small part of their food during the day itself and consume 80% of their total daily food intake at night, taking 5–8 meals during this period (Claassen, 1994a) (see also Chapter 4 about food intake).

Some substances are better absorbed when given orally on an empty stomach (Woodard, 1965). In consideration of this fact, it must be known how long the animal can be starved without any harm to its welfare. For instance, Jeffrey et al. (1987) observed variable amounts of food in the stomachs of male rats following an overnight fast and noted that the diet type and diet regimen can result in variable quantities of food being retained in the stomach after fasting overnight. However, Schlingmann et al. (1997) found that the stomach of rats fasting 6, 12 and 18 hours was almost empty and that only rats fasted for 6 hours did not show any distress. Prolonged food deprivation with water available *ad libitum* leads to a gradual increase of the haematocrit value, with a corresponding decrease in plasma volume. A decrease of the plasma and interstitial volume may result in a significant decrease of substance distribution volume (Claassen, 1994b). Therefore, the duration of food deprivation should be as short as possible.

Oral administration by diet or drinking water is not suitable when an exact amount of substance intake is required. Because food and water wastage happens all the time, it is, for instance, impossible to determine the exact amount of diet or water intake of rats. Therefore, neither the precise food or water intake nor the correct intake of substances with food or water is normally feasible. The only way this can be done is by keeping the animals in metabolic cages and recording the wastage.

The feeding or drinking intake is influenced by

the conditions of housing and especially by the environment. Normally the temperature in rooms for laboratory animals is well controlled by air conditioning. It should be noted that high temperatures will decrease the intake of food and increase the consumption of water. For instance, the water intake at 22°C is about 20% higher than the food intake, while at 30°C water intake is more than double (Weihe, 1987). For this reason the temperature and humidity must be recorded during the experiment.

The substances in food or drinking water can cause the rat to refuse to eat or drink and the animal may lose weight or become dehydrated. If the substances increase the metabolic rate, overeating must be prevented to avoid an overdose. For these reasons the animal and its food and water intake must be observed carefully.

Another disadvantage is that rats must be caged singly for observing or measuring food or water intake. This housing condition may cause stress to rats and will reduce the success of this route of administration.

Intragastric Administration by Gavage

Gavage makes it possible to administer substances directly into the stomach with accurate dosages and reliable timing. When a liquid volume is administered by gavage a substantial amount of the dose passes rapidly through the stomach to the small intestine. This occurs both in fasted and in fed animals (Claassen, 1994a) and results in the substances being absorbed very rapidly. For example, within one minute after quinine solution administration to the fasting rat, 24% is absorbed (Watanabe et al,

Table 24.2 Recommended sizes of bulbs for oral dosing needle and administration volume for rats of different body weights

Body weight (g)	Diameter of bulb (mm)	Volume (mL)
30	1.0	1.0
50	1.0	2.0
100	1.5	3.0
200	2.0	4.0
300	2.0	5.0

1977). Absorption is much faster than that with dietary administration, leading to a peak rather than a slow and prolonged gradient in the blood. Using this technique there is a risk of introducing trauma or a fatal accident; only trained and experienced personnel should carry out intragastric administration. Training can be done with dead animals or with a rat model (e.g. Koken Rat, Koken Co. Ltd, Tokyo, Japan). When training with anaesthetized rats it is important to choose an anaesthetic that allows the animal to retain its swallowing reflex (e.g. ketamine/xylazine).

Knowledge of the rat's drinking or feeding habits will also help to determine whether or not a substance should be given on a full stomach or an empty one. When fed *ad libitum*, rats never have an empty stomach at any time of the day. The stomach has its maximum content at the end of the dark period and a minimum is found at the end of the light period. Therefore, only very small volumes should be administered and rats must not be starved

prior to gavage in the afternoon. In the morning, rats should not receive any food before intragastric administration, because it is not possible to determine how full the stomach is if the rats are getting food and water *ad libitum*.

Numerous methods have been devised to administer materials into or through the oral cavity and ultimately into the stomach of rodents (Kraus, 1980). Ferrill and Hill (1943) published a simplified method for feeding. Although described many years ago and only minimally modified over the years, this method for administration of liquid substances is probably even nowadays the mostly frequently used technique as it is both easy to learn and to perform.

Intragastric administration of solutions

This route of administration is carried out using a special blunt-ended, curved or straight needle with a ball tip. The ball tip helps to prevent the needle from damaging the oesophagus and from passing through the glottal opening into the trachea. The diameter of the bulb and the length of the needle will depend on the size of the rat to be gavaged (Table 24.2) Before starting administration, it is checked that the probe is of a suitable length, i.e. reaching from the mouth to the caudal end of the breastbone (outside the rat) and this should be noted on the tube (Figure 24.1). If much more than this length protrudes during administration then it indicates that the trachea has been entered and the needle must be removed for a fresh try (Waynforth and Flecknell, 1992).

The chosen needle and the appropriate syringe filled with the desired amount of solution are linked together and the needle can be moistened with water or oil to make it slippery. For administration, the conscious rat must be restrained very firmly by

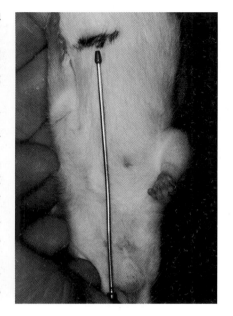

Figure 24.1 Measuring the suitable length of a probe for intragastric administration, i.e. reaching from the mouth to the end of the breastbone, and noting the length of the probe.

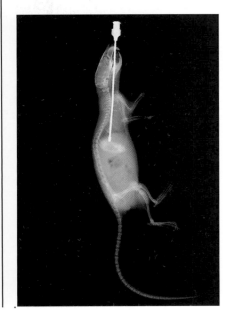

Figure 24.2 Radiograph of gavage of a rat with a straight, blunt-ended stainless steel needle. The stomach is filled with X-ray contrast medium.

gripping a fold of skin from the scruff of the neck down the back so that the head of the rat is kept immobile. Its position is vertical with the head tipped slightly forward. No mouth gag is necessary. To force the jaw open, pressure can be applied to the mandible. The ball tip is inserted behind the incisors into the back of the mouth. Using the tube as a lever, the head of the rat is tipped back. When the needle and the rat are in a straight line the probe is pushed gently along the groove of the hard palate through the very short pharynx (Hebel, 1969) into the oesophagus. Swallowing movements can help so that the probe slips through the oesophageal opening. If any obstruction is felt, no force must be exerted, but another try must be made to find the oesophageal opening (D'Amour et al., 1965). As it is important to prevent the tube from entering the trachea, the rat must be watched carefully. The needle can usually be seen passing down the oesophagus on the left side of the neck (Wolfensohn and Lloyd, 1994). If it is in the trachea, the animal will cough and it is possible to feel the tube touching the cartilage rings of the trachea (Baumans et al., 1993). Once in the oesophagus, the tube is gently pushed down into the stomach. The passage may be obstructed at the sphincter to the entrance of the stomach. Manipulation of the syringe to produce a gentle thrusting movement combined with a gentle backward and forward movement will often overcome this difficulty.

When the tube is in position the solution must be given slowly at first to ascertain that the needle is truly intragastric. If the rat struggles severely, coughs or the injected solution appears in the mouth or at the nose, then the injection is being made erroneously into the lungs. If this happens administration must stop immediately, and the animal must be observed very carefully. If there is any sign of lung damage, it should be killed humanely. Once it has been ascertained that the needle is in the right position, the solution can be given fairly rapidly (Figure 24.2). As soon as administration is finished, the tube must be withdrawn. When administering a corrosive solution the needle must be flushed with saline before pulling back to make sure that the mucosa of the upper gastric tract is not irritated or even damaged.

Intragastric administration by this procedure can be performed very rapidly. One person can feed as many as 120 animals per hour after very little training (Ferrill and Hill, 1943). When properly performed, accidental tracheal infusion is rare (Kraus, 1980).

Intragastric administration of solid materials in capsules

The administration tube for capsules is very similar to the stainless steel needles used for soluble or liquid substances but has a cup for the capsule in place of the bulb. The internal diameter of the cup is in accordance with the external diameter of commercially available capsules. Further details about the needle and the gelatine miniature capsules are described by Lax et al. (1983). The filled capsule is placed firmly into the cup with the capsule cover facing the interior. The rat is held and the prepared tube is inserted in the same way and with the same care and caution as in the previously described intragastric method. Normally the tube is only inserted at the distal end of the oesophagus. The capsule is either ejected by air, which is forced through the cannula and the cup by depressing the plunger of the syringe, which was partly withdrawn before being attached to the tube (Waynforth and Flecknell, 1992) or by water (using 0.3 mL) (Lax et al., 1983) or by pushing a steel rod with a plate on one side. The length of the rod is designed in such a way that when introduced into the tube the free end of the rod does not reach the distal end of the tube (Stanislaus et al., 1979). After ejection of the capsule, the feeder is quickly pulled out. The rat's mouth may have to be held shut until it swallows. Regardless of the location of the capsule in the oesophagus or the method of ejection the capsule will reach the stomach providing normal peristaltic action occurs, and will discharge its contents within a few minutes.

Parenteral Administration

Parenteral administration involves application of a substance to the body in a manner that passes the gastrointestinal tract. Giving small amounts of solutions is called an injection, while administration of larger quantities of solutions is named an infusion. In both cases the skin must be penetrated by a needle. Other methods of parenteral administration include subcutaneous or intraperitoneal implantation of an osmotic pump and, without penetrating the skin, inhalation or topical application. Substances are transported by the blood from the site of administration to the target tissues. The rate of absorption is dependent on the route of administration.

For parenteral application all animals must be properly handled and restrained in order that injection procedures can be carried out without endangering either the rat or the operator. Various proper restraining techniques and many commercially available mechanical restraining devices have been described in the literature (see Chapter 3). The duration and extent of handling or restraining will depend, among other factors, on the method chosen for vascular access and the requirements of the experiment. Over the years, many routes and methods of administration have been used and documented in the literature. Some of the recommended techniques for injection are the same as for venous blood collection or bleeding procedures. To avoid repetition they are not described here but in Chapter 25.

Although injections should normally be given without anaesthesia, this is not a general rule. For instance, if the person carrying out the injection is not well trained, or if the substances are irritating, it is sometimes better to anaesthetize the rat with a short-acting narcotic.

When using injection or infusion techniques, several points deserve special attention. Parenteral administrations require strict asepsis to be maintained. Sharp needles of a size appropriate to be maintained. Sharp needles of a size appropriate to the administrations require strict asepsis to be maintained. Sharp needles of a size appropriate to the size of the rat must always be used. As a general rule, the smallest possible gauge of needle should be selected. It should be kept in mind that a thin needle prevents leakage of fluids and, as an injection may cause pain, helps to minimize discomfort to the rat. The viscosity of the solution must be considered relative to the size of needle used and the thickness of the cannula must be compatible with the viscosity

of the solution to be injected. On the other hand, using too thin needles may risk snapping the needle from the syringe. Because of the risk of embolism, air bubbles in fluids must be avoided. The injection of cold fluids is painful (Baumans et al., 1993), so the fluid must be brought at least to room temperature or better still up to body temperature before use. Substances injected into the circulation must be soluble in suitable solvents. The solution should always be injected slowly and aspiration must be done to ensure that the tip of the needle is in the right place.

The physiological principles of fluid administration are not discussed here and only some recommendations are given with respect to volume.

Intradermal Injection (i.d.)

The most usual sites are the skin covering the back or the abdomen. When not using hairless or nude rats the hair must be removed. This can be done either with a depilatory or with an electric clipper or wet shaver. Depilatories are chemical substances and they could interfere with the study. Their use should therefore be considered carefully (Waynforth and Flecknell, 1992). If possible, the animal should be prepared several days in advance because of the effect on the experiment. Shaving should be done at least one day ahead because of the risk of microinjuries. Before starting the injection the site must be clean and swabbed with an antiseptic.

Only very small quantities of solutions (0.05–0.1 mL per injection site) can be deposited intradermally. For injection, a special short-bevelled hypodermic needle (Shick needle) or an ordinary 26-G needle is held bevel down almost parallel to the skin and is pierced into the skin only for 2–3 mm (Figure 24.3). An intradermal injection results in a small bleb at the injection site; no bleb is formed when the injection is done subcutaneously by mistake.

Topical Application

The skin is also a convenient site for the administration of drugs. The absorption of substances through the skin is an area of research that has been extensively studied for a number of years (Hughes and Hall, 1997). Dermal absorption represents a pathway for substances to enter the body, particularly in cases of occupational and environmental exposure.

subcutaneous injection is the best option when a relatively long period of absorption from a repository injection site is desired. Sensitivity of the tissues to irritant substances limits the application of this route. As stated by Woodard (1965), this route is less tolerant of nonphysiological pH and of chemical irritation than the intravenous or intramuscular routes. Substances or solutions which have such adverse characteristics should be diluted with suitable fluids before being administered subcutaneously. On the other hand, oil suspensions can be given subcutaneously. An increased rate of absorption can be achieved by the injection of hyaluronidase into the same site (Woodard, 1965).

Subcutaneous injection is the preferred method for the administration of substances into rats. This is due to the simplicity of injection technique, greater choice of injection sites and the possibility of depositing large volumes. The maximum volume at each site should be 1 mL per 100 g body weight (Iwarsson et al., 1994).

Recommended injection volumes and suggested hypodermic needle sizes for aqueous solutions are given in Table 24.3. Viscous solutions or suspensions require a needle of 2–4 wire gauge number.

In general, the dorsolateral areas of the neck and shoulder are the preferred sites (CCAC, 1980). Other recommended sites are the back or the flank. As subcutaneous injections are rarely painful (Wolfensohn and Lloyd, 1994), a conscious rat can usually be used.

A fold of loose skin is lifted between the thumb and the forefinger and at the base of the fold the needle, attached to the syringe, is passed in an anterior direction through the skin parallel to the body of the rat, to avoid penetrating deeper tissues. Ideally, the whole of the needle shaft should lie subcutaneously as this prevents leakage of the injected fluid. When in position, the tip of the needle should be moved up and down to reveal its whereabouts and also to ascertain that the needle is truly subcutaneous. If the tip cannot be discerned then the needle could be in an intraperitoneal or intramuscular position and must be slightly withdrawn to lie subcutaneously (Figure 24.4). Before injecting the substance, aspiration has to be done to ensure that the needle has not entered a blood vessel or has moved out of the skin again. When injecting a large volume subcutaneously (e.g. more then 2 mL), leakback and hence loss of fluid can be minimized further by changing the needle path after the needle has been pushed in half way (Waynforth and Flecknell, 1992).

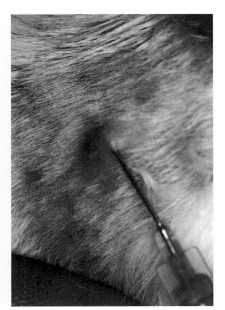

Figure 24.3 Intradermal injection using a 26-G needle.

Numerous factors can affect the extent of percutaneous absorption of a substance. These include the physicochemical properties of the substance, the attributes of the vehicle and the permeability of the skin (Wester and Maibach, 1986; Franklin et al., 1989). Important factors affecting dermal absorption are the water and lipid solubility properties of the substances used for topical application. The outermost layer of the skin is essentially a lipid barrier, whereas the viable epidermis, which lies below the stratum corneum, is basically an aqueous environment (Guy and Hadgraft, 1991). Thus, the ability of a substance to be absorbed through the skin and enter the systemic circulation is determined by the ability to partition into both lipid and water phases.

The usual sites and the preparation of the skin are the same as for intradermal injection. After clipping hair for topical administration, the hairless area should be cleaned of any fat and grease and other debris. The substances should be dissolved in a volatile solvent or mixed in a suitable cream before application and then applied with a dropper or smeared onto the skin with a swab.

As active hair growth or the age of the skin will influence absorption of topically applied substances, the state of the hair cycle should be taken into consideration.

Subcutaneous Injection (s.c.)

In comparison with other routes of administration, the subcutaneous injection has several advantages. The subcutaneous area is well supplied with capillaries but their number may differ at various sites of injection and this may lead to differences in the rate of substance absorption. Nevertheless, as this method of administration will produce a substance depot,

Table 24.3 Recommended administration volumes and suggested hypodermic needle sizes

	Intravenous Volume (mL)	G	Intraperitoneal Volume (mL)	G	Intramuscular Volume (mL/site)[b]	G	Subcutaneous Volume (mL/site)[b]	G
Baumans et al. (1993)	0.5	23–25	5.0	24	0.1	25	1–5	24
Bauck and Bihun (1997)	slowly 0.5–3	≤22	max. 10	≤22	0.2–0.3	≤22	5–10	≤21
Waynforth and Flecknell (1972)	2[a]	–	up to 10	–	0.2	–	up to 5	–
Weiss et al. (1996)	max. 2	–	max. 5	–	max 0.5	–	max. 5	–
Wolfensohn and Lloyd (1994)	1	25–27	5–10	23–25	0.1	25	1–2[b]	25

[a] Injected over 1–2 min.
[b] Maximum of 2–4 sites.

Intramuscular Injection (i.m.)

This route usually results in more rapid absorption than from the subcutaneous route (Woodard, 1965). Absorption usually takes 45–60 minutes for most fluids. Repository forms are available which remain for days and weeks (Moreland, 1965). Small muscle masses of the rat restrict the number of practical injection sites and consequently the volume that can safely be given by the intramuscular route (Bauck and Bihun, 1997). Intramuscular injections are frequently painful due to the distension of muscle fibres which occurs, and therefore good technique and restraint are required (Wolfensohn and Lloyd, 1994).

Recommended injection volumes and suggested hypodermic needle sizes are given in Table 24.3.

Intramuscular injections for rats are usually given into the muscles of the thigh. Large volumes and potentially irritant compounds should be injected into the quadriceps muscle group, which covers the anterior aspect of the thigh. In rats, the quadriceps feels like a small peanut on the front of the thigh, and can be immobilized with the thumb and forefinger of one hand whilst injecting with the other (Wolfensohn and Lloyd, 1994). The muscles of the posterior thigh area should be avoided because the sciatic nerve runs along the back of the femur. Irritant substances that are inadvertently injected in close proximity to this nerve may result in lameness or in the animal's self-mutilation of the affected limb (Bauck and Bihun, 1997). Intramuscular injections can also be given into the area of the gluteal muscles of the hind leg.

Penetration by the needle of 5 mm is sufficient for a deep intramuscular injection and also avoids the risk of damaging the periost of the femur. It is not easy to be sure that the needle is truly intramuscular. However, it should not be possible to feel the tip of the needle through the skin if it is indeed in the muscle and not subcutaneous. Sometimes an intramuscular injection will fail, even though the needle is felt to be in the muscle mass, because it actually lies in one of the fascial planes (Waynforth and Flecknell, 1992).

Before injecting, aspiration must be done to rule out accidental injection into a blood vessel. After the injection the site should be massaged to disperse the dose (Wolfensohn and Lloyd, 1994).

Because of the difficulties described, intramuscular administration should only be used if

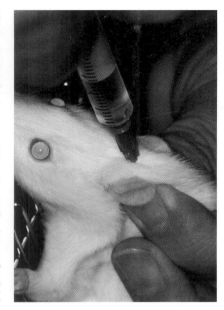

Figure 24.4 Subcutaneous injection at the base of a fold of loose skin (area at the neck) using a 26-G needle.

At the start of an intraperitoneal injection, some workers tilt the rat so that the head is lower than the abdomen in an attempt to slide the viscera cranially and away from the needle. However, the viscera are quite immobile because of the slight vacuum in the abdomen and this manipulation is of questionable value (Fallon, 1996). Small rats can be properly restrained and injected by one person. When injecting larger animals, it is advisable to have an assistant. The hindquarters and tail are restrained by the assistant, and the operator extends one of the animal's hind legs and carries out the injection (Waynforth and Flecknell, 1992).

Because of the risk that the injection is made between the skin and the abdomen muscles or the risk of damage to the kidney, the needle should be inserted neither horizontally nor vertically (Baumans et al., 1993). The needle should enter the skin at an angle of 20–45°. To avoid intestine or urinary bladder injection, it is essential to insert only the tip of the cannula into the peritoneal cavity. No resistance should be encountered to the passage of the needle (Wolfensohn and Lloyd, 1994).

It is often assumed that an intraperitoneal injection always delivers the substances to the peritoneal cavity. There are only a few references to incorrect intraperitoneal injections and it is probable that the error is not always noticed. A significant number of injections are actually made intragastrically, intra-intestinally, subcutaneously, retroperitoneally or intracytically (Claassen, 1994c). The frequency of erroneous injections by skilled investigators has been reported to be from 11% to 20% (Lewis et al., 1966). But even the well-controlled use of a standardized injection technique can only reduce the number of erroneous injections, for example as

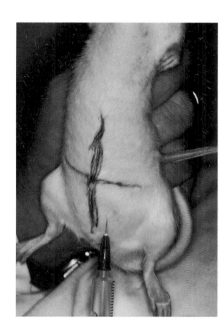

Figure 24.6 Intraperitonael injection into the lower left quadrant using a 26-G needle.

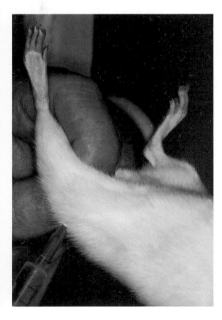

Figure 24.5 Intramuscular injection into the quadriceps muscle group using a 26-G needle.

there is no alternative and should only be performed by well-trained persons (Figure 24.5).

Intraperitoneal Injection (i.p.)

This is the most frequently used parenteral route of administration in rats. The large surface area of the abdominal cavity and its abundant blood supply facilitate rapid absorption. Absorption from this route is usually one-half to one-quarter as rapid as that from the intravenous route (Woodard, 1965). However, for long-term studies, repeated injections may lead to tissue reaction and adhesions. As relatively large volumes can be given intraperitoneally, potentially irritant substances can be generously diluted. When using this method it has to be kept in mind that substances given intraperitoneally are first absorbed into the portal circulation. Biotransformation of the injected substances may take place in the liver before they reach the general circulation, so that their bioavailability is quite different to that of an intravenous injection.

Intraperitoneal injections are generally undertaken without anaesthesia (CCAC, 1980). Recommended injection volumes and suggested hypodermic needle sizes are given in Table 24.3.

The abdomen can be divided into four quadrants by the midline and a line perpendicular to it passing through the umbilicus. Intraperitoneal injections should be given into the lower left quadrant of the abdomen (Figure 24.6). In this area of the rat there are no vital organs except for the small intestine. In contrast, the lower right quadrant contains much of the large bowel, and the upper abdomen is a hazardous area to inject because the liver, stomach and spleen are situated here.

reported by Schneider and Schneider (1970) to 5.5%. Sometimes it is possible to recognize the error; for instance, when the injection is made into the intestine, fluid will often be seen issuing from the rectum immediately after the injection (Waynforth and Flecknell, 1992), or the rat will defecate.

For these reasons it is essential that aspiration is done before the injection to ensure that neither the intestine nor the urinary bladder nor a blood vessel has been entered.

If an injected fluid needs to be diluted quickly in the blood, then the intravenous rather than the intraperitoneal route should be given preference, thus also avoiding the risk of peritonitis.

Intravenous Injection (i.v.)

Intravenous administration offers various advantages over the other routes of injection. For example, it gives control over the rate of introduction into the general circulation, rapid response, etc. and it provides the most complete availability of substances with minimal delay. By controlling the administration rate, constant plasma concentrations can be obtained at the required level. Unexpected side-effects during administration can be halted by stopping the injection. Compounds that are poorly absorbed by the digestive tract or are unacceptably painful when given intramuscularly or subcutaneously may be administered intravenously when given carefully into the vein without leaks into the surrounding tissues.

Several general points on intravenous injection or infusion deserve special attention. Except in terminal experiments, reasonable aseptic techniques with sterile equipment must be employed, particularly when rats are being used in long-term studies and frequent injections are required. The syringe plus needle or the catheter must first be filled with the liquid so that no air bubbles are injected. When using large veins it should be easy to aspirate blood if the cannula lies correctly but it is not always possible to do so with small veins. After injecting a small amount of the solution into a small vein the injected fluid should be washed away by the blood in the vessel. If this does not happen the position of the needle is doubtful. If a bleb should arise, the position of the needle is certainly not in the vein but in the surrounding tissue. A fresh attempt must be made or the needle should be moved in the surrounding tissue in such a way that it then enters the

vein. When finishing the intravenous injection, a swab must always be pressed on to the injection site while pulling out the cannula to prevent backflow of administered fluid and/or blood.

If the vessel has to be used several times the first injection should be made as distal as possible in relation to the heart and subsequent administrations should be placed progressively more proximal. This procedure is necessary because venipuncture and the injection of substances can damage and/or block the vein and the distal part of the vessel may no longer be used for subsequent administrations.

When selecting the site of injection the consequences of a possible intravascular thrombosis, or a possible extravascular administration of substances etc. have to be considered. As injected substances can be metabolized by the liver it is important to know whether the selected vein is part of the portal or general circulation. While the intravenous route has many advantages, it is potentially the most dangerous route of substance administration, for instance with anaesthetics, and great care must be exercised in calculation of the total dose to be administered (Baggot, 1977).

The rat, although an extremely useful and widely used experimental animal, has no readily accessible veins of sufficient size for venipuncture. Therefore many methods for vascular access have been described in the literature (Moreland, 1965; Kraus, 1980; Petty, 1982; Cocchetto and Bjornsson, 1983; Waynforth and Flecknell, 1992). Percutaneous injections are made with conscious rats into the lateral tail vein, lateral marginal vein (v. saphena) or dorsal metatarsal vein, and with anaesthetized animals into the sublingual vein or penile vein. Some techniques are difficult to perform so many methods have been developed to make this task easier, including the use of a wide range of hypodermic needle sizes, improving visibility of the injection site by magnification, transillumination, shaving, surgical incision and the application of heat, tourniquets and chemicals for vasodilatation. After making a skin incision and surgical exposition administrations can be made into the external jugular vein or femoral vein. Both routes require the use of anaesthesia.

Different restraint devices and other equipment have been recommended for immobilizing the rat and thus facilitating injection (Waynforth and Flecknell, 1992). Anaesthetizing the animal is considered helpful, but may be contraindicated for some experiments. Use of these methods or equipment cannot guarantee a successful injection. For instance the vein can be deflected by the needle, an inserted needle can dislodge or perforate the vein whenever the syringe is manipulated or the restrained rat flinches (Nachtman *et al*, 1988).

The same vein can be used for intravenous administration or for blood collection, and intravenous injections, in general, can be performed using one of the numerous techniques as for bleeding. These are described in Chapter 25. For some routes a certain amount of technical skill is required and these are therefore not advisable for people who rarely use them.

In order to avoid pain and shock, injections must always be given slowly, especially when administering large volumes. Recommended intravenous injection volumes and the suggested hypodermic cannula size (gauges) are given in Table 24.3.

Lateral tail vein

If anaesthesia is not used, a restraint device is usually necessary because the tail is sensitive. Several types of clear plastic restraint devices that allow tail access are commercially available for rats (Waynforth and Flecknell, 1992; Fallon, 1996).

From the tip to the root of the tail the lateral vein lies immediately beneath the skin but the vein narrows from the root to the tip. Because of very small vessels at the tip of the tail the whole length of the vein cannot be used for intravenous injection. Videm (1980) presented a simple and relatively rapid method using the lateral tail vein at the root of the tail where the skin, after being shaved, is thin and smooth and where the vessels are superficial and accessible for intravenous injection.

Young rats are easier to inject into the tail vein than older ones whose tail skin is exceedingly tough and covered by scales, making it quite difficult to pierce and enter the vessels.

Since the tail of the rat is a major thermoregulatory organ with a large surface available for heat loss, an enhanced blood flow in the dilated veins and hence a successful venipuncture can be ensured by warming prior to injection. Warming the whole rat to a temperature around 40°C by placing the animal into a thermostatically warmed 'hot-box' (Conybeare *et al*, 1988), warming the tail under a heating lamp (Waynforth and Flecknell, 1992) or holding the tail in warm water for 1–2 minutes (Fallon, 1996) can induce tail vein dilation. When placing rats in a warmed box, it is essential that the animal should be kept under constant observation

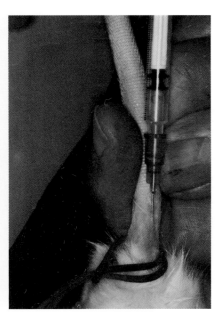

Figure 24.7 Lateral tail vein injection using a 24-G 'over the needle' catheter.

in order to prevent hyperthermia as indicated by rapid breathing, panting or salivating (Joint Working Group, 1993). Another method for obtaining good venous filling is constriction. There are several methods described using finger pressure (Barrow, 1968) and/or a tourniquet (Videm, 1980; Petty, 1982; Waynforth and Flecknell, 1992). The pressure or the tourniquet must be released just before the injection is made.

For injection, the tail should be bent down with one hand while the vein is punctured at the angle of the bend with the needle and syringe held in the other hand (Figure 24.7). The vessel must be entered at a very small angle almost parallel to the vein. After injection is started, failure of injection is identified by swelling of the tail or blanching of the skin. A useful aid is to fit a tube between the needle and the syringe, so that the needle can be controlled better and not pulled out or allowed to penetrate through the vessel during infusions.

The injection is carried out using a 23–25-G needle.

Lateral marginal vein (saphenous vein)

In the opinion of Grice (1963) injection into this vein is the method of choice. The rat may be anaesthetized or placed in a restrainer, leaving one hind limb free. The posterior and lateral surface of the thigh and leg of the hind limb are shaved. The rat is held firmly by an assistant placing the right hand over the hips of the animal, with the free limb positioned between the first and second fingers and applying sufficient pressure to cause this vein to become quite prominent without the use of any

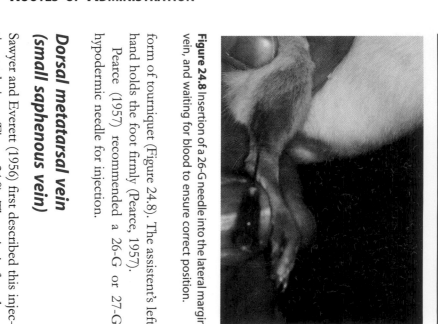

Figure 24.8 Insertion of a 26-G needle into the lateral marginal vein, and waiting for blood to ensure correct position.

form of tourniquet (Figure 24.8). The assistent's left hand holds the foot firmly (Pearce, 1957).

Pearce (1957) recommended a 26-G or 27-G hypodermic needle for injection.

Dorsal metatarsal vein (small saphenous vein)

Sawyer and Everett (1956) first described this injection technique (Figure 24.9). The vein is found on the dorsal surface of the foot. The skin over the lateral plantar surface is shaved and swabbed with antiseptic. The operator holds the foot by the toes during the procedure, and an assistant aids by holding the knee in such a manner that sudden flexion and withdrawal of the foot are prevented. A 26-G hypodermic needle kept almost horizontal to the surface and directed toward the ankle is inserted through the skin and into the vein at a point where it just starts to travel up the foot after first crossing the foot and supplying the toes with blood.

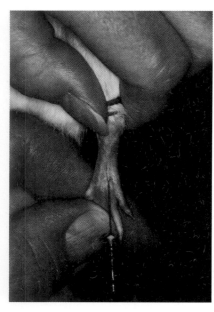

Figure 24.9 Dorsal metatarsal vein injection using a 26-G needle.

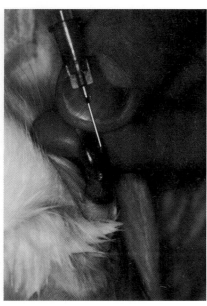

Figure 24.10 Dorsal penis vein injection using a 26-G needle.

Sawyer and Everett (1956) recommended a 26-G hypodermic needle for injection.

Dorsal penis vein

Petty (1982) maintained that the dorsal penis vein injection for male rats is much simpler, more rapid, more reproducible and easier to accomplish than tail vein injection and the technique can be learned easily. Waynforth and Flecknell (1992), who described the method in detail, stated that this route should only be used under special circumstances, because of the consequences of damage to the vein.

Nightingale and Mouravieff (1973) investigated whether the penile vein is part of the portal or general circulation. Based on these experiments, they concluded that injection into this vein leads to the general circulation and that a first-pass effect on metabolism is not to be expected.

The rat is either restrained by an assistant or may be anaesthetized by a short-acting narcotic agent and its penis extruded while pressing at the base of the penis downwards while pressing at the base of the penis (Figure 24.10). The penis is held at the very tip. The large penile veins are seen along both sides of the penis. Once the vein is pierced, aspiration of blood is virtually impossible, therefore only a very small volume has to be injected first to see if it flows freely. After the injection, the injection site is pressed with a swab for a few seconds and the gland is encouraged to retract to prevent further bleeding.

For rats from weaning age and older, Waynforth and Flecknell, (1992) recommended a 24-G hypodermic needle and 30-G for smaller animals.

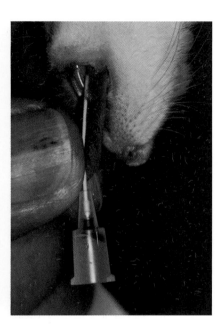

Figure 24.11 Sublingual vein injection using a 24-G 'over the needle' catheter.

Sublingual vein

As the entire procedure, namely, anaesthesia, suture and injection, can be done in less than 5 minutes, Petty (1982) recommended the sublingual vein which is frequently overlooked as an injection site (Figure 24.11). Any differences in the eating or drinking habits of the rat were noted after injection. As the injection technique is described in detail by Petty (1982) or Waynforth and Flecknell (1992) the reader is referred to these articles.

Waynforth and Flecknell (1992) recommended a 25-G or 30-G hypodermic needle for injection.

Without special experience, access to the jugular vein or the femoral vein is only possible after surgical exposure of these vessels. As injection via a needle and infusion via a catheter require similar preparation, more details in respect to these injection techniques are given later.

Intravenous Injection or Infusion by Catheter

Chronic venous cannulation or implantation of indwelling vascular catheters in rats are an accepted and extremely useful experimental technique for repeated injection or permanent infusion, since they reduce the stress of multiple injection associated with, for example, restraint and discomfort of repeated needle pricks. A number of authors have described techniques for chronic catheterization of different blood vessels of the rat. Each technique has its own individuality and the investigator must adapt to meet the needs of the experimental design (Petty, 1982). The procedures described differ also in the different protection devices employed to prevent the rat from manipulating the catheter through pushing, pulling away or biting, in the methods of maintaining proper catheter placement and of exteriorizing the catheter, in the use of different surgical techniques and in the techniques used to maintain the patency of the catheter.

The procedures used to fit rats with an indwelling vascular catheter fall into two general categories using either direct access or remote access.

Direct access is accomplished by attaching a syringe or a piece of tubing to the exteriorized distal end of the catheter just before injection or infusion. This requires some form of handling or restraint of the rat. The duration and extent of these

manipulations will, of course, depend on the method chosen for implantation, on the type of catheter, on the requirement of the study and in particular on the experience of the operator.

Remote access involves tethering the rat, usually by a protecting device, as the catheter is extended beyond the rat's home cage. This method permits access to the vascular system of otherwise undisturbed, freely moving rats housed singly.

Tubing for catheters is available with various internal and external diameters. Advances in the polymer industry have led to the production of many synthetic materials with acceptable indices of biocompatibility. Vascular acceptance of extracorporeal devices is far more difficult to achieve than with other tissues *in vivo*. Two fundamental properties of the vascular system cause problems when foreign materials are placed in the bloodstream. First, rejection of intravascular implants is rapid due to the immediacy of thrombogenic reactions. Second, the surface properties of synthetic polymers differ from those of blood vessels, a feature favouring the accumulation of platelets and other thrombogenic agents. Hence, the physicochemical properties of intravascular materials are important factors influencing the long-term success of vascular implants (Desjardins, 1986). Intravascular catheters differ with respect to physical properties and biocompatibility and are available in a wide variety of synthetic materials. Silicon rubber (Silastic) tubing is adequate for many catheters used for rats, since it seems to cause little reaction, even after 18 months, whereas nonsilicon rubber materials tend to cause fibrotic reactions over time. The problem with Silastic is that it is too flexible and, therefore, predisposed to kinking, especially in smaller tubes (Joint Working Group, 1993).

Various methods have been used to minimize the incidence of thrombotic occlusion of the intravascular catheter and to remove existing thrombotic obstructions to prolong the patent lifetime of catheters. Schedules for routine catheter care of rats have not been compared or standardized. To prevent clotting in the catheter, it should be flushed with heparinized saline or another anticoagulant after placement and between infusions or injections at least twice a week, if not daily. The dead space in the cannula is then replaced by a carefully calculated amount of fresh anticoagulant. A concentration of 10–1000 IU heparin per mL saline is recommended (Joint Working Group, 1993). If the catheter still becomes blocked, it may be possible to dissolve the thrombotic occlusion by filling the catheter with a solution of urokinase or streptokinase (Hurtubise et al., 1980). Cannulas without heparin form small clots at the tip, which, if dislodged, may cause pulmonary, renal or heart infarcts.

Numerous procedures for the insertion of catheters into different arteries and veins of rats by percutaneous or surgical techniques have been described.

Percutaneous insertion

Percutaneous methods involve the implantation of the catheter into a blood vessel by piercing the vessel with a needle and pushing the catheter through the needle into the vessel.

In a nonsurgical approach, catheters are inserted into the tail vein of the rat. For instance, Little et al. (1962) and Rhodes and Patterson (1972) inserted the needle through the intact skin into the tail vein. When blood flowed freely, the catheter was guided through the trough of the needle into the vein. Nachtman et al. (1988) and Waynforth and Flecknell (1992) used a commercially available over-the-needle catheter, comprising a short cannula fitted over the needle which is only a few millimetres longer than the cannula. This unit has two distinct advantages over hypodermic needles. It provides a visual check that the vein has been entered as blood fills the needle chamber, and once the cannula is established intravenously, any movement by the rat or the operator does not lead to penetration or laceration of the vessel wall as easily as a hypodermic needle because its cannula is pliable and blunt. After positioning the tip of the needle and cannula into the vein, the needle is withdrawn whilst holding the cannula firmly in place. Once the cannula has been filled with blood, the needle can be withdrawn completely.

Surgical implantation

Detailed procedures for the preparation of catheter equipment and inserting the catheter have been described by Weeks and Davis (1964) and Harms and Ojeda (1974), who described an easy-to-prepare cannula and a simple procedure for cannulation of the jugular vein.

Numerous methods are available for implantation of catheters in different veins and/or arteries of rats (Petty, 1982). Cocchetto and Bjornsson (1983) reviewed many articles on arterial and venous implantations, gave methodological notes as well as procedural comments. The tail vein, right jugular vein and femoral vein or the left carotid artery and the aorta are mostly used for cannulation. Surgical techniques for the permanent catheterization of the jugular vein (Remie et al., 1990a), femoral vein (D'Amour et al., 1965), tail vein (Born and Moller, 1974), carotid artery (Waynforth and Flecknell, 1992) and femoral artery (Yoburn et al., 1984) are comprehensively described in the literature. The reader is referred to these articles.

As it is not easy to get a tube into a surgically exposed, small vessel of a rat, a small vessel cannulator is sometimes recommended (Pope, 1968; Rezek and Havlicek, 1975). There are various techniques for fixing the extravascular or intravascular portion of a catheter with the vessel and the surrounding tissue or within the lumen of the blood vessel. Details can be found in the article by Cocchetto and Bjornsson (1983). With rats, intravascular catheters are commonly exteriorized by subcutaneous tunnelling from the vascular incision site to the back of the neck or between the shoulder blades (Cocchetto and Bjornsson, 1983), and sometimes also to the root of the tail (Jones and Hynd, 1981).

The various procedures for protecting the catheter differ in the protective device used to prevent the animal from manipulating the free end of the catheter and/or the connection to the infusion pump. Many authors (Kleinman et al., 1965; Dalton et al., 1969; Edmonds and Thompson, 1970; Cox and Beazley, 1975; Rhodes and Patterson, 1979; Jones and Hynd, 1981; Kanz et al., 1989) have addressed the problem of the protection of the catheter from kinking and chewing by the animal.

As a general rule, infusion of about 1% of the blood volume per hour will not affect fluid disposition. Infusion of larger volumes should be based on preliminary studies designed to determine whether the cellular and ionic components of blood are maintained in a normal range (Desjardins, 1986). For example, for long-term feeding of rats (140–250 g) Steiger *et al.* (1972) infused a specially formulated solution intravenously at a rate of 30–60 mL/day. However, at low flow rates of less than 0.5 mL per hour, catheter occlusion by thrombosis may be observed (Cox and Beazley, 1975).

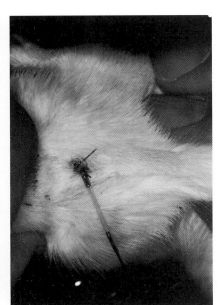

Figure 24.12 Free end of a jugularis catheter exteriorized by subcutaneous tunnelling from the vascular incision site to the back of the neck. Catheter is sealed with a steel rod.

A number of authors (Little *et al.*, 1962; Popovic and Popovic, 1960; Engberg, 1969) have described techniques for proper catheter placement. Other writers (e.g. Wittgenstein and Rowe, 1965) have directed their attention towards minimal restraint or towards methods of compensation for rotational movement of the animal in the cage (Eve and Robinson, 1963).

It catheters are implanted for continuous infusion over long periods and the use of a portable pump is not practical, the tube must be connected with an infusion pump. Therefore, it is necessary to take special precautions to prevent twisting and kinking of the delivery tubing through movements of the rat. The freedom of the animal must be inhibited as little as possible by the protective device and must allow the animal to move in an unrestricted manner within its cage. If the implanted tube is to be used for multiple injection the free end of the tube must also be protected from biting or pulling out. For this purpose the same protective device as for long-term infusion can be used. If the catheter is exteriorized in the neck area and only a short piece is outside the body, it is not necessary to protect the catheter if the animal is housed singly (Figure 24.12).

Rats are not only stressed by the operative procedure but also by the fact that the animal has to wear a protecting device, is housed singly and is limited in movement (Birkhahn *et al.*, 1976; O'Neill and Kaufman, 1990). In general, rats require a period of several days to recover from the procedures for the implantation of chronic catheters. During the first 4 postoperative days the normal weight gain is disturbed and even weight loss can occur (Popovic and Popovic, 1960; Kleinman *et al.*, 1965; Claassen, 1994d).

Other Methods for Parenteral Administration

Osmotic Minipump

Commercially available implantable osmotic minipumps are designed to deliver microlitre quantities of semisolid or liquid formulations of substances as a continuous infusion of precise volumes for a period of up to 6 weeks without the need for external connection or frequent animal handling (Waynforth and Flecknell, 1992). This small device has been used very successfully in laboratory rats and 3315 reports about the use of osmotic minipumps can be ordered from the Alzet® bibliography (ALZA Corp, Palo Alto, CA, USA).

The minipump system is composed of three concentric layers: the substance reservoir, the osmotic sleeve and the rate-controlling, semipermeable membrane. An additional component, called the 'flow moderator', is a 21-G stainless steel tube with a plastic end-cup (Figure 24.13). For more details and principle of operation see the technical information manual of the manufacturer.

Eleven different pumps are available, varying in size from 1.5 × 0.6 cm to 5.1 × 1.4 cm, with a nominal pumping rate from 0.25 μL/h to 10.0 μL/h, a nominal duration from 1 day to 6 weeks and a nominal reservoir volume from 100 μL to 2 mL (Figure 24.14).

Because of the mechanism by which the pumps operate, their delivery profile is independent of the chemical and physical properties of the agent

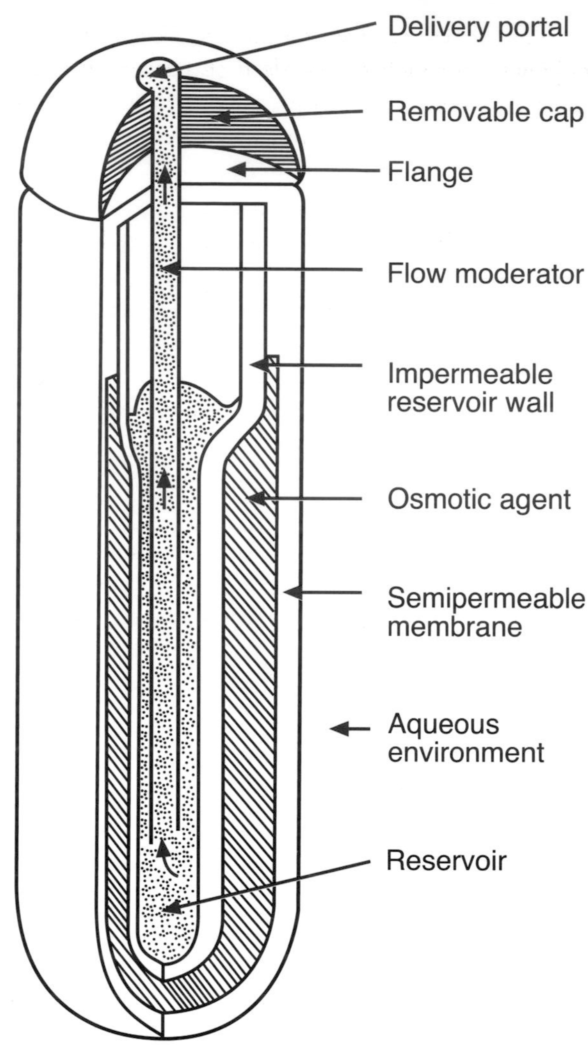
Delivery portal
Removable cap
Flange
Flow moderator
Impermeable reservoir wall
Osmotic agent
Semipermeable membrane
Aqueous environment
Reservoir

Figure 24.13 Cross-section of an Alzet® osmotic pump, demonstrating design components, working method and nominal performance.

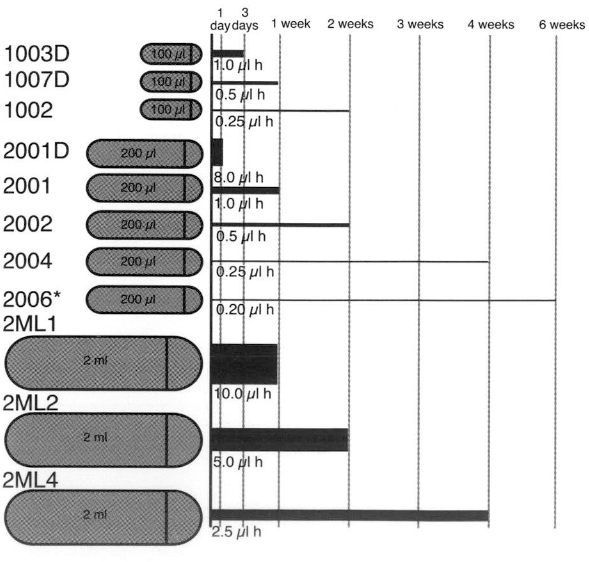
1 day
3 days
1 week
2 weeks
3 weeks
4 weeks
6 weeks
1003D
1007D
1002
2001D
2001
2002
2004
2006*
2ML1
2ML2
2ML4
100 µl
200 µl
2 ml
1.0 µl h
0.5 µl h
0.25 µl h
8.0 µl h
1.0 µl h
0.5 µl h
0.25 µl h
0.20 µl h
10.0 µl h
5.0 µl h
2.5 µl h

Figure 24.14 Available Alzet® osmotic pump models.

dispensed. Substances of various molecular configuration, including ionized substances and macromolecules, can be dispensed continuously in a variety of vehicles at constant rates. The average pumping rate should be calibrated and correct performance should be checked before implantation. In rats, pumps can be implanted subcutaneously or intraperitoneally following the animal size guidelines of the manufacturer. A kit for performing brain infusion is also available. As the attachment to a catheter does not alter the delivery rate of the pump, infusion into the venous or arterial circulation via a catheter is also possible. Full instructions for the correct use of the minipumps are given by the manufacturer.

The compelling advantage of these minipumps is that they can be placed *in situ* without further need for infusion equipment and that a large number of animals can be treated effectively with a uniform infusion rate. However, infusion is limited to specific volumes for restricted time periods (Desjardins, 1965). This disadvantage can perhaps be solved by implanting a new pump.

Oro-endotracheal Intubation

With the expanding use of rats in research involving surgery of increasing complexity, there is an increasing need for improvements in rat anaesthesia techniques. A free airway is useful in reducing mortality during and after operations. Inhalation anaesthetics provide excellent control over induction and maintenance of anaesthesia but are difficult to use because of the mode of delivery and miniaturizing the standard anaesthetic protocol. Numerous reports (Dudley *et al.*, 1975; McGarrick and Thexton, 1979; Levy *et al.*, 1980) using a mask for administration of volatile anaesthetics in spontaneously breathing rats have been published. However there is the problem of adequately fitting masks, lack of control of ventilation, waste of anaesthetic gases and hazardous pollution of the operating room. Tracheostomy is unacceptable for the recovery of the rat. Therefore, intubation has to be selected for further consideration. Acceptable techniques for endotracheal intubation of the rat are reported including blind intubation (Stark *et al.*, 1981), laryngoscopic techniques with specially designed (Proctor and Fernando, 1973; Nicholson and Kinkead, 1982; Costa *et al.*, 1986) or human laryngoscopes (Schaefer *et al.*, 1984) and direct tracheal visualization by a fibre-optic illuminator (Thet, 1983), a surgical microscope

Fernando (1973) inserted under direct vision a guidewire through the cords first, passed an endotracheal cannula over the wire and between the cords into the trachea without difficulty and then removed the wire (Figure 24.15). A guidewire from a Seldinger catheter is ideal as its tip is soft and flexible. Both techniques are also described in detail by Flecknell (1996).

After connecting the tube to the ventilator the rat must be ventilated and chest movement and air exchange must be checked for correct cannula placement. If the tube becomes plugged with mucus secretion during ventilation and causes respiratory difficulties, the cannula must be exchanged with a new one.

As some experimental protocols require that substances be given intratracheally, intubation techniques can also be used for these studies.

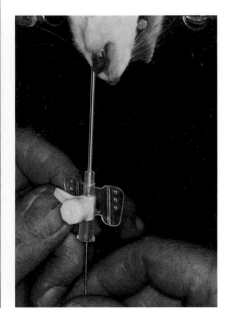

Figure 24.15 Insertion of an endotracheal tube ('over the needle' catheter) into the trachea using the Seldinger technique.

(Peña and Cabrera, 1980) or a head-mounted, mirror-reflected, adjustable-focus light (Alpert *et al.*, 1982).

For starting the intubation, an endotracheal cannula of suitable size (internal diameter of the trachea 2–3 mm) must be prepared and a careful examination of the pharynx and larynx carried out. The use of an endotracheal tube with an inflatable cuff is impossible because the lumen/cuff ratio is unrealistic and the deflated cuff makes insertion extremely difficult (Proctor and Fernando, 1973). For intubation a 16- or 12-G arterial cannula can be used. Some authors recommend modification of the introductory end of the tube to facilitate penetration of the tracheal lumen or to prevent unintentional intubation of a bronchus and the Luer fitting to provide connection to an anaesthetic circulation (Proctor and Fernando, 1973; Costa *et al.*, 1986; Flecknell, 1996).

Intubation of rats is possible using a purpose-made laryngoscope (Costa *et al.*, 1986) or an otoscope (Tran and Lawson, 1986; Remie *et al.*, 1990b). Prior to intubation, the animal is anaesthetized to a sufficient depth to abolish the cough and swallowing reflex. Atropine (0.01 mg) is useful in reducing mucus secretion and helps to prevent tube blockage. Laryngospasm may be prevented or alleviated by spraying a local anaesthetic solution on the cannula or on to the vocal cords before intubation. If the laryngeal region is covered with mucus, the area must be cleared with a cotton-tipped applicator to allow visualization. The technique of intubation using a laryngoscope and insertion of the tracheal tube between the vocal cords during the next inspiration into the lumen of the trachea is well described by Costa *et al.* (1986). By adopting the Seldiger vessel cannulation technique for intubation, Proctor and

References

Alpert, M., Goldstein, D. and Triner, L. (1982) *Lab. Anim. Sci.* **32**, 78–79.

Baggot, J.D. (1977) In: Meyer Jones, I., Booth, N.H. and McDonald L.E. (eds) *Veterinary Pharmacology and Therapeutics*, 5th edn, pp. 43–78. Ames: Iowa State University Press.

Barrow, R.H. (1968) *Lab. Anim. Care* **18**, 570–571.

Bauck, L. and Bihun, C. (1997) In: Hillyer, E.V. and Quesenberry, K.E. (eds) *Ferrets, Rabbits, and Rodents: Clinical Medicine and Surgery*, pp. 291–306. Philadelphia: W.B. Saunders Company.

Baumans, V., ten Berg, R.G.H., Bertens, A.P.M.G., Hackbarth, H.J. and Timmermann, A. (1993) In: van Zutphen, L.F.M., Baumans, V. and Beynen, A.C. (eds) *Principles of Laboratory Animal Science*, pp. 299–318. Amsterdam: Elsevier.

Birkhahn, R.H., Bellinger, L.L., Bernardis, I. and Border, J.R. (1976) *J. Surg. Res.* **21**, 185–190.

Born, C.T. and Moller, M.L. (1974) *Lab. Anim. Sci.* **24**, 355–358.

CCAC (Canadian Council on Animal Care) (1980) In: *Guide to the Care and Use of Experimental Animals*, Vol. 1, pp. 53–54. Ottawa: CCAC.

CCAC (1989) *CCAC Guidelines on Acceptable Immunological Procedures*. Ottawa: CCAC.

Claassen, V. (1994a) In: Claassen, V. (ed.) *Neglected Factors in Pharmacology and Neuroscience Research*, pp. 59–115. Amsterdam: Elsevier.

Claassen, V. (1994b) In: Claassen, V. (ed.) *Neglected Factors in Pharmacology and Neuroscience Research*, pp. 321–334. Amsterdam: Elsevier.

Claassen, V. (1994c) In: Claassen, V. (ed.) *Neglected Factors in Pharmacology and Neuroscience Research*, pp. 46–58. Amsterdam: Elsevier.

Claassen, V. (1994d) In: Claassen, V. (ed.) *Neglected Factors in Pharmacology and Neuroscience Research*, pp. 5–22. Amsterdam: Elsevier.

Cocchetto, D.M. and Bjornsson, T.D. (1983) *J. Pharmacol. Sci.* **72**, 465–492.

Conybeare, G., Leslie, G.B., Angles, K., Barrett, R.J., Luke, J.S.H. and Gask, D.R. (1988) *Lab. Anim.* **22**, 177–182.

Costa, D.L, Lehmann, J.R., Harold, W.M. and Drew, R.T. (1986) *Lab. Anim. Sci.* **36**, 256–261.

Cox, C.E. and Beazley, R.M. (1975) *J. Surg. Res.* **18**, 607–610.

D'Amour, F.E., Blood, F.R. and Beldin, D.A. (1965) In: D'Amour, F.E., Blood, F.R. and Beldin, D.A. (eds) *Manual for Laboratory Work in Mammalian Physiology*, 3rd edn. Chicago: University of Chicago Press.

Dalton, R.G., Touraine, J.L. and Wilson, T.R. (1969) *J. Lab. Clin. Med.* **74**, 169–174.

Desjardins, C. (1986) In: Gay, W.J. and Heavner, J.E. (eds) *Methods of Animal Experimentation*, Vol. VII, Part A, pp. 143–194. Orlando: Academic Press.

Dittmer, D.S. (1961) In: Dittmer, D.S. (ed.) *Biological Handbooks: Blood and other Body Fluids*, p. 408. Washington D.C.: Federation of American Society of Experimental Biology.

Dudley, W.R., Soma, R.A., Barnes, C., Smith, T.C. and Marshall, B.E. (1975) *Lab. Anim. Sci.* **25**, 481–482.

Edmonds, C.J. and Thompson, B.D. (1970) *J. Physiol.* **207**, 41P–42P.

Engberg, A. (1969) *Acta Physiol. Scand.* **75**, 170–175.

ETS 123 (1986) European Convention for the Protection of Vertebrate animals used for Experimental and other Scientific Purpose. Strasbourg: Council of Europe.

Eve, C. and Robinson, S.H. (1963) *J. Lab. Clin. Med.* **62**, 169–174.

Fallon, M.T. (1996) In: Laber-Laird, K., Swindle, M.M. and Flecknell, P. (eds) *Handbook of Rodent and Rabbit Medicine*, pp. 1–38. Oxford: Pergamon.

Flecknell, P. (1996) In: Flecknell, P. (ed.) *Laboratory Animal Anaesthesia*, 2nd edn, pp. 15–73. London: Academic Press.

Ferrill, H.W. and Hill, C. (1943) *J. Lab. Clin. Med.* **28**, 1624–1625.

Franklin, C.A., Somers, D.A. and Chu I. (1989) *J. Am. Coll. Toxicol.* **8**, 815–827.

Frimmer, M. and Länmler, G. (1977) In: Frimmer, M. and Länmler, G. (eds) *Pharmakologie und Toxikologie*, 2nd edn, pp. 9–31. Stuttgart: Schattauer Verlag.

Grice, H.C. (1963) *Lab. Anim. Care* **14**, 483–493.

Guy, R.H. and Hadgraft, J. (1991) In: Hobson, D.W. (ed.) *Dermal and Ocular Toxicology. Fundamentals and Methods*, pp. 221–246. Boca Raton: CRC Press.

Harms, P.G. and Ojeda, S.R. (1974) *J. Appl. Physiol.* **36**, 391–392.

Hebel, R. (1969) *Säugetierkundliche Mitteilungen* **17**, 247–270.

Hughes, M.F. and Hall, L.L. (1997) *Food Chem. Toxicol.* **35**, 697–704.

Hurtubise, M.R., Bottino, J.C., Lawson, M. and McCredie, B. (1980) *Arch. Surg.* **115**, 212–213.

Ivarsson, K., Lindberg, L. and Waller T. (1994) In: Svendsen, P. and Hau, J. (eds) *Handbook of Laboratory Animal Science*, pp. 229–272. Boca Raton: CRC Press.

Jeffrey, P., Burrows, M. and Bye, A. (1987) *Lab. Anim.* **21**, 330–334.

Joint Working Group on Refinement (1993) *Lab. Anim.* **27**, 1–22.

Jones, P.A. and Hynd, J.W. (1981) *Lab. Anim.* **15**, 29–33.

Kanz, M.F., Vanoye, C. and Moslen, M.T. (1989) *Lab. Anim.* **23**, 36–38.

Kleinman, L.I., Radford, E.P. and Torelli, G. (1965) *Am. J. Physiol.* **208**, 578–584.

Kraus, A.L. (1980) In: Baker, H.J., Lindsey, J.R. and Weisbroth, S.H. (eds) *The Laboratory Rat*, Vol.2, pp. 1–92. New York: Academic Press.

Lax, E.R., Militzer, K. and Trausche, A. (1983) *Lab. Anim.* **17**, 50–54.

Levine, R.R. (1970) *Am. J. Dig. Dis.* **15**, 171–188.

Levy, D.E., Zwies, A. and Duffy, T.E. (1980) *Lab. Anim. Sci.* **30**, 868–870.

Lewis, R.E., Kynz, A.L. and Bell, R.E. (1966) *Lab. Anim. Care* **16**, 505–509.

Little, J.R., Brecher, G., Bradley, T.R. and Rose, S. (1962) *Blood* **19**, 236–242.

Löscher, W. and Kroker, R. (1994) In: Löscher, W., Ungemach, F.R. and Kroker, R. (eds) *Grundlage der Pharmakotherapie bei Haus- und Nutztieren*, 2nd edn, pp. 19–22. Berlin: Paul Parey.

McGarrick, J. and Thexton, A. (1979) *J. Physiol.* **289**, 15P–16P.

Moreland, A.F. (1965) In: Gay, W.T. (ed.) *Methods of Animal Experimentation*, Vol. 1, pp. 1–42. New York: Academic Press.

Nachtman, R.G. Driscoll, T.B., Gibson, L.A. and Johnson, P.C. (1988) *Lab. Anim. Sci.* **38**, 629–630.

Nicholson, J.W. and Kinkead, E.R. (1982) *Lab. Anim. Sci.* **32**, 509–510.

Nightingale, C.H. and Mouravieff, M. (1973) *J. Pharmacol. Sci.* **62**, 860–861.

O'Neill, P.J. and Kaufman, L.N. (1990) *Lab. Anim. Sci.* **40**, 641–643.

Peña, H. and Cabrera, C. (1980) *Lab. Anim. Sci.* **30**, 712–713.

Pearce, K.A. (1957) *Nature* **178**, 709.

Petty, C. (1982) In: Petty, C. (ed.) *Research Techniques in the Rat*, pp. 66–107. Springfield: Charles C. Thomas.

Pope, R.S. (1968) *J. Appl. Physiol.* **24**, 276.

Popovic, V. and Popovic, P. (1960) *J. Appl. Physiol.* **15**, 727–728.

Proctor, E. and Fernando, A.R. (1973) *Br. J. Anaesth.* **45**, 139–142.

Remie, R., van Dongen, J.J. and Rensema, J.W. (1990a) In: van Dongen, J.J., Remie, R., Rensema, J.W. and van Wunnik, G.H.J. (eds) *Manual of Microsurgery on the Rat*, pp. 159–169. Amsterdam: Elsevier.

Remie, R., Bertens, A.P.M.G., van Dongen, J.J., Rensema, J.W. and van Wunnik, G.H.J. (1990b) In: van Dongen, J.J., Remie, J.J., Rensema, J.W. and van Wunnik, G.H.J. (eds) *Manual of Microsurgery on the Rat*, pp. 61–80. Amsterdam: Elsevier.

Rezek, M. and Havlicek, V. (1975) *Physiol. Behav.* **15**, 623–626.

Rhodes, M.L. and Patterson, C.E. (1979) *Lab. Anim. Sci.* **29**, 82–84.

Sawyer, C.H. and Everett, J.W. (1956) *Nature* **178**, 268–269.

Schaefer, C.F., Brackett, D.J., Downs, P., Tomkins, P. and Wilson, M.F. (1984) *J. Appl. Physiol.* **56**, 533–535.

Schlingmann, F., Vermeulen, J.K., deVries, A., Tolboom, J. and Remie, R. (1997) In: O'Donoghue, P.N. (ed.) *Harmonization of Laboratory Animal Husbandry. Proceedings of the 6th FELASA Symposium*, pp. 89–92. London: Royal Society of Medicine Press.

Schneider, G. and Schneider, G. (1970) *Z. Versuchstierk.* **12**, 16–19.

Stanislaus, F., Schneider, G.F. and Hofrichter, H. (1979) *Arzneim.-Forsch./Drug Res.* **29**, 186–187.

Stark, R.A., Nahrwold, M.L. and Cohen, P.J. (1981) *J. Appl. Physiol.* **51**, 1355–1356.

Steiger, E., Vars, H.M. and Dudrick, S.J. (1972) *Arch. Surg.* **104**, 330–332.

Thet, L.A. (1983) *Lab. Anim. Sci.* **33**, 368–369.

Tran, D.Q. and Lawson, D. (1986) *Lab. Anim. Sci.* **36**, 540–541.

Videm, S. (1980) *Z. Versuchstier Kunde* **22**, 101–104.

Waynforth, H.B. and Flecknell, P.A. (1992) In: Waynforth, H.B. and Flecknell, P.A. (eds) *Experimental and Surgical Technique in the Rat*, pp. 1–67. London: Academic Press.

Watanabe, J., Okabe, H., Ichihashi, T., Mizzojiri, K., Yamada, H. and Yomamoto, R. (1977) *Chem. Pram. Bull. (Tokyo)* **25**, 2147–2155.

Weeks, J.R. and Davis, J.D. (1964) *J. Appl. Physiol.* **19**, 540–541.

Weihe, W.H. (1987) In: Poole, T.B. (ed.) *The UFAW Handbook on the Care & Management of Laboratory Animals*, 6th edn, pp. 309–330. Essex: Longman.

Weiss, J., Maess, J., Nebendahl, K. and Rossbach, W. (1996) In: Weiss, J., Maess, J., Nebendahl, K. and Rossbach, W. (eds) *Haus- und Versuchstierpflege*, pp. 296–310. Stuttgart: Gustav Fischer Verlag.

Wester, R.C. and Maibach, H.I. (1986) In: Bridges, J.W. and Chasseaud, L.F. (eds) *Progress in Drug Metabolism*, Vol. 9, pp. 95–109. London: Taylor & Francis.

Williams, C.S.F. (1976) In: Williams, C.S.F. (ed.) *Practical Guide to Laboratory Animals*, pp. 52–62. Saint Louis: Mosby Company.

Wittgenstein, E. and Rowe, K.W. (1965) *Lab. Anim. Care* **15**, 375–378.

Wolfensohn, S. and Lloyd, M. (1994) In: Wolfensohn, S. and Lloyd, M. (eds) *Handbook of Laboratory Animals Management and Welfare*, pp. 143–173. Oxford: Oxford University Press.

Woodard, G. (1965) In: Gay, W.J. (ed.) *Methods of Animal Experimentation*, Vol.1, pp. 343–359. New York: Academic Press.

Yoburn, B.C., Morales, R. and Inturrisi, C.E. (1984) *Physiol. Behav.* **33**, 89–94.

CHAPTER 25

Collection of Body Fluids

Jürgen Weiss
University of Heidelberg, Heidelberg, Germany

George R Taylor
University of Missouri-St. Louis, St. Louis, MO USA

Frank Zimmermann
University of Heidelberg, Heidelberg, Germany

Klaus Nebendahl
University of Göttingen, Göttingen, Germany

Blood

General Remarks

Blood is taken from rats for a wide variety of scientific purposes, and many blood collection techniques have been developed and described over the past decades. Today, there are two notable outcomes. One is that the techniques have been greatly refined and improved, and, second, much more is known about the reactions of the animals to blood collection and the consequent, inevitable hemorrhaging. It is commonly accepted that an animal's response to intrusive blood sampling involves more than simply the loss of a volume of blood. Also important are the rate of blood loss, the site and method of collection, the skill of the technician, the use and type of anesthesia, the age and sex of the animal, and its nutritional and health status.

Stress to the animal associated with the procedure selected for blood sampling can influence circulating levels of glucose (Klinger et al., 1965; Beauzeville, 1968), corticosteroids, prolactin, epinephrine, growth hormone, insulin, plasma renin (Joint Working Group on Refinement, 1993; Brown and Martin, 1974; Oates and Stokes, 1974; Bellinger and Mendel, 1975), and serum enzymes (Friedel et al., 1974), as well as counts for red and white blood cells and platelets, and packed cell volume (Wright, 1970). Such physiological changes may even invalidate experimental results (Ajika et al., 1972). The Joint Working Group on Refinement

(1993), as well as McGuill and Rowan (1989), have reviewed the effects on the animal of the various methods of blood sampling. A series of important recommendations emerged from those reviews.

The initial decision by a researcher is the volume of blood to be collected. That decision will depend, basically, on the analyses to be made of the blood or its contents, for example, bloodborne antibodies, under the limitations imposed by the whole blood volume of the animal that defines the amount of blood that can be withdrawn without endangering the animal. With minor blood losses of <10% of the whole blood volume, the animals may be asymptomatic. Indeed, compensatory mechanisms will be instigated in the animal to replace lost volumes of blood. With moderate (ca. 15–20%) blood losses the animal will suffer decreases in arterial pressure and cardiac output despite the compensatory mechanisms. With further blood loss, decreases in cardiac output, blood pressure and tissue perfusion may become life threatening. Clinical signs of hemorrhagic shock include pallor, skin and extremities that are cold to the touch, a fast pulse, suppressed activity or restlessness, hyperventilation, muscular weakness and subnormal body temperature.

The Joint Working Group on Refinement (1993) indicated that a rat has a total volume of 50–70 mL blood per kg body weight, and McGuill and Rowan (1989) reported the range to be 58–70 mL/kg. The latter authors suggested that the whole blood volume, using the mean average of 64 mL/kg, calculates as 6.4% of an animal's body weight. Thus, a 200-g rat would have an absolute blood volume of 19.2 mL. It should be noted, however, that this percentage will be lower in older or heavier, and certainly obese, animals. To ensure a safe volume of blood is withdrawn from these animals, the estimate of blood volume should be based on the animal's expected normal weight. For a single blood sample, McGuill and Rowan (1989) recommended an upper limit of 15%, while the Joint Working Group on Refinement (1993) suggested a maximum of 10% of total blood volume be taken from a normal sized, healthy animal. Considering the recent literature and practical experience on special needs and estimated adverse impact on the animals, the Society for Experimental Animal Science (1998) suggested an even more conservative approach to decisions on percentage of the total blood volume to be collected, sampling frequency, and sampling technique (Table 25.1).

The rule of thumb common in laboratories is the so-called 10%–10% rule. That is, total volume of blood is 10% of the animal's body weight and 10% of the blood volume is a safe amount to be collected. According to the rule, a 400-g rat, for example, would have 40 mL of total blood and an investigator may take 4 mL of blood in one sampling. However, the initial 10% of the rule overestimates the blood volume of most laboratory animals. Actually, the volume of blood in a 400-g rat is closer to 6% than to 10% of its body weight. Using the 6% figure, the calculation is a more accurate total blood volume of 24 mL, and 10% of this volume is 2.4 mL that could be withdrawn without visible effects on the animal.

If repeated samplings are necessary or, especially, with multiple sampling in a single session, the bleeding should be followed by a rest of a minimal period of time. According to McGuill and Rowan (1989), Cornell University uses a 10% weekly limit rule. But, the authors argue for a 7.5% weekly limit as being more judicious. This is based on findings that collecting 8% weekly requires many weeks for hemoglobin concentrations to return to normal. Although the Joint Working Group on Refinement (1993) stated that 10% of the circulating blood volume can be removed, they advise a 3–4-week respite before the procedure is repeated and the same volume is collected. As reported by this group, a maximum of 1% of an animal's circulating blood volume can be removed in repeat samplings at shorter intervals. That is, for sampling every 24 h the maximum should be roughly 0.6 mL/kg/day.

As is now obvious, there is a considerable potential for error in determining blood volumes. Investigators should, therefore, be cautious when estimating limits on blood sampling volumes. If possible, they should use the lower, more conservative values.

Cardiac Puncture

Cardiac puncture is best used for terminal blood sampling, because of the risk of **cardiac tamponade**. However, the procedure should be carried out with the animal under anesthesia. The rat is placed in right lateral recumbancy, i.e. on its side with the left side of the body accessible. The apex heartbeat can be detected with the finger and thumb placed on either side of the chest, in the region of the fourth to sixth ribs. If the protocol is for survival of the rat after cardiac puncture, it is necessary to maintain asepsis by shaving the hairs over the area and treating the exposed skin with a suitable antiseptic, e.g. a

Table 25.1 Blood sampling in rats: recommended methods and sites, volumes and frequencies

Volume and frequency	Sampling method/site	Specific requirements	Estimated adverse impact
1 Small volume 0.02–0.05 mL	(a) Puncture of tail vessels (b) Incision of the tip of the tail (c) Retroorbital puncture	(a) Needle: 23 G–26 G (c) Anesthesia (e.g. inhalation); use of heparinized glass capillaries, e.g. hematocrit capillary (75 µL vol., 75 mm length, 1.5 mm o.d.)	(a–b) Low, < 1 day (c) Low-moderate, <1 day
2 Maximal volume 1.8 mL/300 g rat Recovery: 2 weeks	(a) Puncture of tail vessels (b) Retroorbital puncture (c) Cardiac puncture (d) V. jugularis	(a) Needle: 23 G–26 G (b) Anesthesia (see also 1c) (c) Anesthesia; needle: 26 G (d) Anesthesia; needle: 23–25 G	(a) Low (b–d) Low-moderate, <1 day
3 Repeated sampling daily: max. 0.2 mL/ 300 g rat weekly: max. 0.9 mL/300 g rat	(a) Permanent catheter in A. femoralis, V. jugularis (b) Retroorbital puncture	(a) Anesthesia, polyethylene catheter, o.d. ca. 0.61 mm, Portsystem (b) Anesthesia (see also 1c)	(a) Low-moderate, depending on duration of catheterization (b) Low-moderate, <1 day
4 Terminal collection	(a) Cardiac puncture (b) Puncture of aorta abdominalis (c) Puncture of V. cava (d) Retroorbital puncture (e) Decapitation	(a) Anesthesia; needle: 26 G (b) Anesthesia (c) Anesthesia (d) Anesthesia (see also 1c)	(a–e) Low

From Society for Experimental Animal Science (1998).

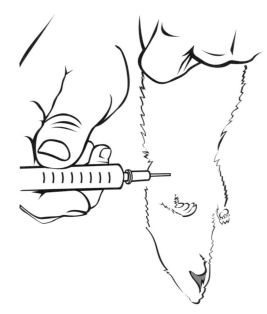

Figure 25.1 Cardiac puncture through the left side of the chest wall of the rat. From Kraus (1980).

70% ethanol solution. A 2-mL syringe with a needle no larger than 23 G is recommended in order to minimize damage to the myocardium.

The needle is introduced into the left side of the thoracic cavity, perpendicular to the chest wall, and directly over the area where the apex heartbeat is most easily detected. Once the needle is introduced into the left ventricle, gentle suction is applied with the syringe until blood is obtained (Figure 25.1). The needle should be fixed at this point with the fingers so that it is not inadvertently moved out of the ventricle, either during withdrawal or in the event that the syringe is exchanged for a second syringe. Filling and changing syringes is best done with the help of a second person. This person can free the filled syringe, remove it, and attach a fresh syringe as the first person maintains the needle in its fixed position. Withdrawal of blood from the heart should be slow and steady, at a rate of about 2 mL or less per min, to maximize the volume collected without risk of cardiovascular failure. Cardiac puncture and its potential effects on various hematological and other parameters has also been investigated and compared with alternative techniques by Carlberg and Alvin (1992), Jimenez et al. (1985), Plas-Roser et al. (1982), and Mock and Frankel (1978).

If applying suction to the syringe yields little blood, the needle tip may have been positioned within the myocardium, the heart may have been completely penetrated, or the tip may be in the atrium. Gently retracting the needle and repositioning the tip for proper penetration of the left ventricle may be required. No more than two or three fresh attempts should be made to enter the heart as each attempt causes some hemorrhaging in the heart, which could prove fatal.

Alternative approaches for cardiac puncture have been described, defined mainly by position of the anesthetized rat, such as in dorsal recumbancy, i.e. on its back rather than on its side (Kraus, 1980; Flecknell, 1987; Iwarsson et al., 1994). A detailed and illustrated description of the various modifications of cardiac puncture has been published by Waynforth and Flecknell (1992).

Gupta (1973) used a special Vacutainer system for obtaining cardiac blood from neonatal rats. The neonate is placed on its back with its head pointing downward. A 21-G needle is slowly and gradually inserted into the thorax through the thoracic inlet (Figure 25.2) until blood appears within the collecting tube. Neonate and needle must be held in this

Figure 25.2 Cardiac puncture in the newborn rat using a Vacutainer system. From Kraus (1980).

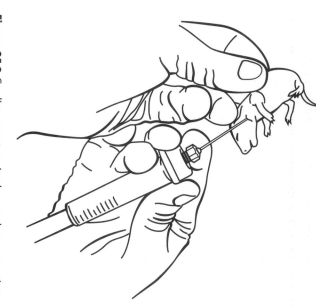

position for the entire collection procedure. The author reported that 0.2 mL can be obtained from rats 3–5-days old and, using a similar procedure, a volume of 0.7 mL from pups ca. 2 weeks old.

Retroorbital Puncture

Though first described by Pettit in 1913 and successfully used in many laboratories, retroorbital puncture has become more and more controversial. It is argued that there are too many adverse side-effects associated with the procedure. Some researchers have concluded that retroorbital puncture (Figure 25.3) should not be used at all (Van Herck et al., 1992; Iwarsson et al., 1994) or only when no suitable alternative is available (Waynforth and Flecknell, 1992). The Joint Working Group on Refinement (1993) and McGee and Maropot (1979) report a series of possible serious insults caused by incorrect use of the technique. For instance, it can result in a retroorbital hematoma with excess, painful pressure on the eye. Damage to the optic nerve and other intraorbital structures can lead to visual deficits, including blindness. Admittedly, the retroorbital technique may require more experience and personal skills for successful application than other methods. In that event, retroorbital puncture can be a suitable method for single and, even, repeated blood sampling from the rat (Neptun et al., 1985; Smith et al., 1986).

The proper application is the following. Rats should be anesthetized with an inhalation anesthetic.

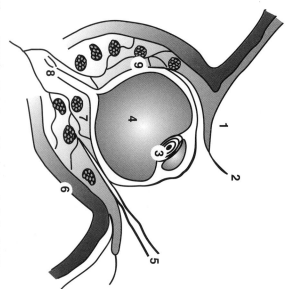

Figure 25.3 Sagittal view of the rat eyeball. Eyelid (1), eyelash (2), lens (3), vitreous body (4), puncturing capillary (5), skull bone (osseous orbita) (6), retroorbital venous plexus (7), optic nerve (8), retina (9). From Weiss et al. (1996).

back the skin, the eyeball is made to protrude (Figure 25.4). The thumb should be placed so that it is also occluding the jugular vein. A sterile hematocrit tube or a Pasteur pipette containing heparin is used. The tube is pushed through the conjunctiva medially (inner side) of the ocular cavity while the tube is gently rotated until the plexus is reached, and it fills with blood. If no blood is obtained, the pipette should be withdrawn a short distance and rotated at the same time. If the rat is held so that the capillary tube is facing downwards, blood can be allowed to drip into a collecting vessel. Depending on age and weight of the rat, 1–2 mL of blood can be obtained easily without the suction required in cardiac punctures. Once the collection is completed, the nape of the neck should be released momentarily before withdrawal of the pipette to minimize hemorrhage from the puncture site. Care should also be taken not to abrade the cornea whilst continuing to apply pressure on the eyeball to limit hemorrhaging after the tube is removed. Bleeding usually stops immediately, particularly if the eyelids are closed. Any excess blood can be removed with gauze.

Jugular Vein

Puncture of the jugular vein in the rat without anesthesia and incision of the skin is possible, but the technique requires experience and skill (Figure 25.5).

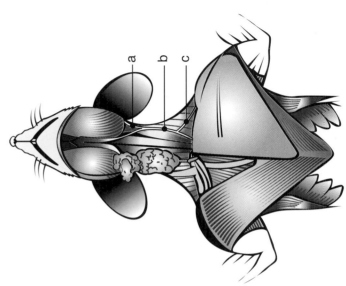

Figure 25.5 View of the ventral surface of the rat's neck and chest with the maxillary vein (a), external jugular vein (b), and the cephalic vein (c). Redrawn from Popesko et al. (1992).

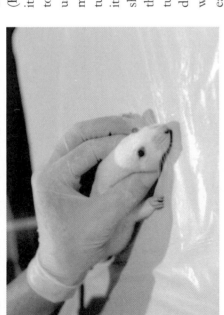

(a)

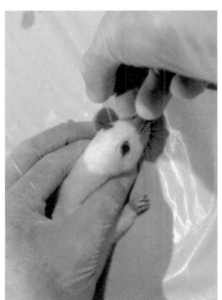

(b)

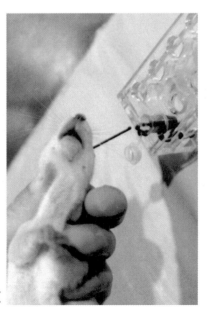

(c)

Figure 25.4 For retroorbital puncture the eyeball is made to protrude (a), the tube is pushed through the conjunctiva medially (b), and once the plexus is reached, the tube fills with blood which can be collected (c).

Once the rat has been removed from the inhalation chamber, the puncture should be performed without delay. While the anesthetized animal is resting on a solid surface, the animal is held gently but firmly by the nape of the neck. By pressing down with the thumb and forefinger just behind the eye and pulling

Rawlings *et al.* (1994) compared data from blood obtained by tail vein puncture with that collected from chronically implanted catheters inserted in tethered rats. The authors concluded that blood from jugular vein cannulated rats is more suitable for kinetic-based research, when compounds are used which exhibit multicompartmental elimination kinetics.

Saphenous Vein

Blood collection from the saphenous vein in the leg is usually reserved for larger animals, such as monkeys (Dang *et al.*, 1989; Phillipi-Falkenstein and Clarke, 1992), cows (Benoit and Dailey, 1991) and horses (Pethick *et al.*, 1993). But this method has been modified for blood collection in the smaller laboratory animals, for example with guinea-pigs (Carraway and Gray, 1989). Recently, a method has been described for mice, rats, hamsters, gerbils, minks and ferrets (Hem and Smith, 1998).

As adapted for rats, the procedure is to place a nonanesthetized animal into a restrainer that allows access to one of the hind legs. The leg is extended and held in place by grasping the fold of skin located between the tail and thigh. The thigh is shaved and swabbed with a 70% alcohol solution, revealing the saphenous vein that can then be seen through the skin. A 23-G needle is used to puncture the vein and the drop of blood that appears will flow freely into the tip of a Microvette or, alternatively, the blood can be pipetted (Figure 25.6). Approximately 200 μL can be obtained with this method. Repeated samples can be taken from the same site by removing the scab and inducing new blood flow.

If repeated samplings are required, a cannula can be implanted in the jugular vein, although the researcher may want to consider a different collection technique (Yoburn *et al.*, 1984; Korber and Flye, 1987; Paulose and Dakshinamurti, 1987; Rabinovici *et al.*, 1994; Kurata *et al.*, 1997). Hutchaleelaha *et al.* (1997) presented a simple apparatus for serial blood sampling from cannulated external jugular vein with simultaneous measurement of locomotor activity. Results of the study suggest the applicability of the device in facilitating pharmacokinetic/pharmacodynamic modeling of drugs that affect locomotor activity. Verbaeys *et al.* (1995) investigated the influence of feeding, blood sampling method and type of anesthesia on renal function parameters in rats. Finally,

For others, the procedure is for the rat to be anesthetized, the fur on the ventral portion of the neck is shaved and the skin swabbed with 70% ethanol. A skin incision is made parallel to the midline, and the jugular vein is exposed. In larger animals the overlaying fat layers should be cleared first by blunt dissection. Using a 25-G needle, the jugular vein is penetrated through the pectoral muscle which covers part of the vein. Blood is withdrawn slowly. After removal of the needle, the overlying pectoral muscle may help prevent hemorrhage. The skin incision is closed with one or two skin clips or sutures. According to Phillips *et al.* (1973) and Renaud (1969), 1–2 mL blood per 100 g body weight can be obtained using this method. Kurata *et al.* (1997) investigated the effect of blood collection on rat hematological parameters and reported that collection of less than 0.9 mL of blood from the jugular vein per day is conceivable as the volume without causing changes in hematologic parameters.

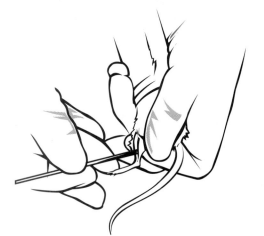

Figure 25.6 Puncture of the saphenous vein. The animal is placed in a suitable restrainer with a hindleg being extended. The puncture site is shaved, swabbed with 70% alcohol and the saphenous vein is punctured using a 22-G needle. Blood sampling is performed by holding a microcapillary tube against the blood drop that forms on the skin (redrawn with permission from Hem and Smith, 1998).

Tail

Ventral tail artery

The rat tail contains a dorsal vein, two lateral veins, and a ventral artery (Figure 25.7). A major advantage of collecting blood from the ventral tail artery is that the arterial pressure provides a good blood flow without the need for adjunct suction or vacuum devices. Gerecke (1971) recommended this method for repeated blood sampling in the rat, whereas Fejes-Toth *et al.* (1984) used the tail artery as an entrance for cannulization of the abdominal aorta. For the collection of blood the rat is lightly anesthetized with ether and placed in dorsal recumbancy. (Ether is used in preference to pentobarbital, chloralose or urethane, which decrease blood pressure and thus diminish blood flow.) The tail is dipped in warm water (ca. 45°C) for a few minutes to dilate the artery and to soften the skin. If a 'hot box' is used for whole body warming, the animals must be observed for signs of heat stress, manifested by salivation or collapse. The index finger is firmly pressed against the tail ca. 5 cm from the tip of the tail to make the artery visible. The artery is then punctured ca. 1–2 cm in front of the index finger using a 1-inch 24-G needle (0.7 mm o.d.). Further bleeding is stopped by firmly pressing a gauze on the puncture site. A volume of 1 mL blood can be obtained by this technique without problems. Puncture of the tail artery is thus a comparably convenient and safe technique, which provides blood with minimal hemolysis (Hurwitz, 1971).

Dorsal and lateral tail veins

For puncture of the dorsal tail vein, the animal is placed in a suitable restrainer and the tail is dipped in warm water (ca. 45°C; see also Furuhama and Onodera, 1983) for a few minutes to dilate the vessels and make them more visible. Pressure is put on the dorsal vein by either using the index finger or applying a rubberband or piece of string to the base of the tail as a tourniquet. (A simple tourniquet, to be passed round the tail and to be tightened by gently withdrawing the plunger of a modified syringe has been described by Minasian (1980).) A 23- or 21-G needle is inserted into the vein and the tourniquet is released to allow the blood to flow freely. (Blood flow can be improved by using a 21-G × 1-inch butterfly needle which is modified by removing all but 5 mm of its plastic cannula.) In most cases it may be useful to let the blood drip into a collecting vessel rather than using a syringe connected to the needle. Once the collection procedure is completed, the needle is removed from the vein and further bleeding is stopped by applying light finger pressure on the vessel. Samples of at least 0.5 mL blood can be obtained using this technique. Omaye *et al.* (1987) used a special tourniquet, developed by Minasian (1980), to induce hemostasis and collected up to 5 mL blood by puncturing the dorsal tail vein.

If blood is collected from one of the lateral veins (Figure 25.8), the same procedure can be performed as described for the dorsal vein. The only difference is that the animal may be anesthetized, so that it can

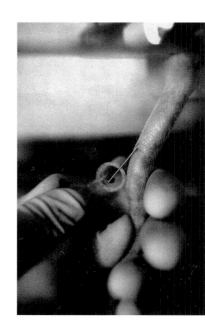

Figure 25.8 Puncture of the left lateral vein of the rat using a 22-G needle with scab removed to prevent coagulation.

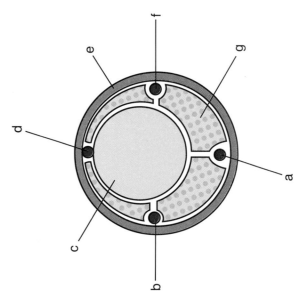

Figure 25.7 Transverse sectional view of the rat tail: ventral artery (a), the lateral veins (b, f), vertebra (c), dorsal vein (d), skin (e), and tendon bundles (g).

be kept in a lateral recumbancy. If repeated blood sampling is necessary, the vessel should be punctured in a slightly more anterior portion of the vein or using a different vein. Information concerning a comparison of tail vein puncture and chronically implanted catheters inserted in tethered rats has been given by Rawlings *et al.* (1994).

Incision of a tail vein

A tail vein in the distal end of the tail is incised longitudinally about 1 cm from the tip, continuing for ca. 1 cm in length using a scalpel blade. A small blood sample (0.1–0.2 mL) can be collected by letting it drip into a suitable receptacle. Gentle pressure is usually sufficient to induce haemostasis, though chemical cauterization may be necessary, using potassium permanganate or ferric chloride.

Nerenberg and Zedler (1975) collected blood from the lateral tail veins using a vacuum-assisted method. The authors incised the vein after coating the area to be incised with petroleum jelly. The tail was then placed into a modified Liebig condensor jacket which was connected to a vacuum system (Figure 25.9). Repeated blood sampling of up to several milliliters can be performed with this method.

Cannulation of tail vessels

For certain studies, cannulation of the ventral artery or the lateral veins is necessary (Frank *et al.*, 1991). Implantation of the cannula has to be performed under anesthesia and, once implanted, cannulae can be used for repeated samplings or even injections over a certain period of time (ca. 5–6 h), while the animals have to be restrained in a suitable apparatus. If larger amounts of blood are withdrawn, the loss of volume should be compensated by infusion of appropriate fluids or heparinized blood from a donor rat.

Amputation or tail clipping

An alternative technique for obtaining smaller amounts of blood (<0.5 mL) involves complete transection of the tail, ca. 5 mm anterior to its tip. Blood flow can be increased by warming the tail in warm water (ca. 45°C) for a few minutes and massaging it gently from the severed end. However, massaging ('milking') the tail may set up an inflammatory leukocytosis resulting in an abnormal increase in the number of white blood cells in the sample collected (Waynforth and Flecknell, 1992).

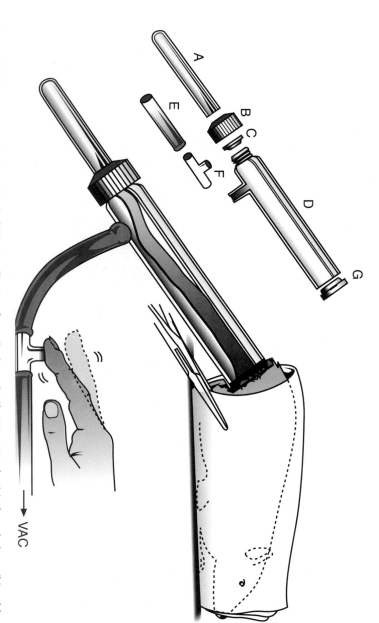

Figure 25.9 Vacuum-assisted method of blood collection from the lateral tail vein: test tube (a), threaded cap (b), rubber grommet (c), modified Leibig condensor jacket (d), plastic chamber connecting bleeding apparatus to vacuum line (e), T-connector (f), and rubber grommet (g). From Kraus (1980).

If repeated blood sampling is required, more anterior portions of the tail can be cut off. However, it has to be considered that repeated cutting of the tail tip may result in trauma to cartilage and eventually to the coccygeal vertebrae, which would represent a painful and unnecessary injury of the animal. It also has to be stated that repeated amputations of the rat tail may cause granulomata and – in excessive cases – may remove the animal's natural ability to control its body temperature and balance.

Carotid Artery

The main reason for tapping into arteries is that a large volume of blood can be obtained rapidly and relatively easily. Often the carotid artery is chosen (Fitzgerald *et al.*, 1997). Leal *et al.* (1988) developed a method to obtain maternal–fetal plasma samples from rats. Using a microsampling technique blood is collected from the carotid artery of the dam and from the umbilical vein of the fetus. In most instances, access to the carotid artery is accessed by implanting a cannula. Methods for vascular access have been described in detail by Cocchetto and Bjornsson (1983). Samples using this method have been compared with blood obtained from other catheterized blood vessels by Rabinovici *et al.* (1994), Ishikawa *et al.* (1993), Korber and Flye (1987), Yoburn *et al.* (1984), Rozenberg *et al.* (1984), and Jarrige *et al.* (1978).

The considerable blood pressure in arteries is an important consideration when introducing an arterial cannula. Any unsecured lesion in an artery will bleed profusely. The Joint Working Group on Refinement (1993) recommended the general use of small, nontraumatic haemostats or vascular clamps, the so-called 'bulldog' clamps, applied to the vessel to occlude the blood flow as the cannula is being introduced. When possible, the cannula should be placed in the same direction as the flow of blood. It is also important to take care that a dislodged particle or thrombus does not find its way into circulation. Should the fragment lodge in the artery that supplies it, the result could be a blocked artery and the blood flow to the organ supplied by the artery interrupted.

Aorta

Accessing the dorsal aorta is a method for obtaining large volumes of blood when the experimental protocol is for nonrecovery surgery, i.e. the animal is to be euthanized. The method of blood collection from the dorsal aorta is the same as that described below for the posterior vena cava. The only difference is that the aorta is entered just anterior to its distal bifurcation into the common arteries (Figure 25.10). Waynforth and Flecknell (1992) have detailed the technique of terminal blood sampling from the dorsal aorta. Upton and Morgan (1975) and Friedel *et al.* (1974) delivered detailed comparisons of collecting blood from the abdominal aorta to other blood sampling techniques.

More recently, Fitzgerald *et al.* (1997) developed an animal model for blood transfusion and sterile blood sampling from rats. The authors reported that puncture of the abdominal aorta is a simple and reliable method for the collection of sterile blood.

Vena Cava

Winsett *et al.* (1985) developed a method for obtaining repeated blood samples from conscious rats by translumbar vena cava puncture. The conscious rat

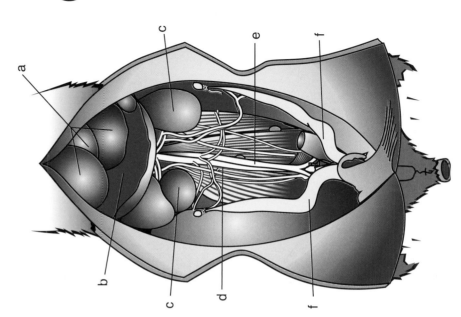

Figure 25.10 Abdominal cavity of a female rat after removal of the alimentary tract. Liver (a), stomach (b), kidneys (c), vena cava (d), abdominal aorta (e), and uterus horns (f). Redrawn from Popesko *et al.* (1992).

was held prone by an assistant, and the 5/8-inch 25-G needle was inserted at the level of the first lumbar vertebra in the coronal plane at an angle of 45° from the vertical plane. The authors reported performing the procedure a remarkable total of 350 times in 30 rats (100–300 g body weights); 2 mL were obtained from each rat at weekly intervals over 8 weeks of sampling. The time required to obtain 30 samples was 15–20 min.

The more common methods involve anesthetizing the animal and implanting indwelling catheters either for withdrawal of blood from the inferior or superior vena cava or for administration of substances into one of these vessels (Kaufmann, 1980; Fejes-Toth *et al.*, 1984; Berthoud *et al.*, 1986; Sugihara *et al.*, 1988; Yang *et al.*, 1997). Along these lines, Moslen *et al.* (1988) described a two-cannula method, one for parenteral infusion and the other for serial blood sampling in a freely moving rat. The latter cannula was inserted into the superior vena cava (Figure 25.10) and 'exteriorized' in the scapular region, that is, a segment of the cannula was routed to the external surface of the animal. The cannula for infusion of substances was inserted in the inferior vena cava via the femoral vein and exteriorized at the tail.

Waynforth and Flecknell (1992) suggested a method for obtaining blood from the posterior vena cava. The chest cavity of an anesthetized rat is exposed by ventral surgical cut. After pushing aside the organs, the widest section of the posterior vena cava can be located at about the level of the kidneys. A 19-G or 21-G needle is used to enter the vessel. Blood must be withdrawn slowly until the vessel wall collapses. It is best to stop the withdrawal temporarily while the vessel refills with blood before continuing. This method can only be used in the rat for nonsurvival surgery.

Exsanguination

Most frequently used methods for euthanizing rats in this research area are cardiac puncture, bleeding from dorsal aorta or decapitation. The latter is often performed with a guillotine, which may seem at first a barbaric and esthetically unpleasant procedure. If performed by trained personnel, however, decapitation can be a humane method of sacrificing animals without anesthesia. Moreover, it is an effective means of collecting large quantities of mixed venous and arterial blood from animals without potential confusion from anesthetizing drugs.

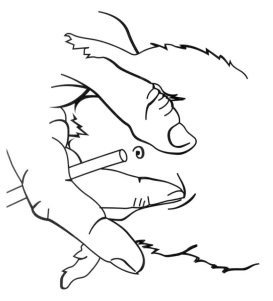

Figure 25.11 Urine sampling in the rat: manual pressure and collection into capillary tube. From Kraus (1980).

Blood obtained with decapitation has been used as a standard by which other blood-sampling methods have been compared. That is, the blood obtained with decapitation has been used as a control to determine the effects of blood sampling on various parameters (Carlberg and Alvin, 1992; Paulose and Dakshinamurti, 1987; Jimenez *et al.*, 1985; Wiersma and Kasteljin, 1985; Laakso *et al.*, 1984). It is interesting to note that Messow (1991) reported that few features of the stress response were activated with decapitation, provided decapitation is performed in a proper manner and within 120 seconds, beginning with the moment the cage and animal are taken from the rack.

Urine

Voluntary and Induced Urination

When rats are taken from their cages, they frequently urinate, indicating a mild form of stress with the restraint of being handled by a human. Nelson *et al.* (1966) report that waving a small cotton ball moistened with diethyl ether under the nose of a rat can stimulate a specific form of induced urination known as **micturation**. This provides the opportunity to collect small volumes (30–100 μL) of urine in a suitable receptacle for later analysis.

Micturation also may be stimulated by applying gentle but firm suprapubic pressure in rats (Figure 25.11). An average of 150–200 μl urine can then be collected in capillary pipettes or other suitable receptacles (Draper and Robbins, 1956; Hayashi and Sakaguchi, 1975).

Since it is difficult to estimate the volume of urine obtained by both methods, the actual volume excreted can be determined by weighing the urine and calculating its volume by means of the specific gravity of 0.85 (Kraus, 1980).

Metabolism Cage Systems

If larger volumes of urine output are to be collected or if experimental effects over long-term periods are of interest to the investigator, an appropriately designed metabolic cage should be used. Its principal virtue is allowing urine and feces to be collected and separated from food, water, hair, exfoliated skin or other contaminants. Although most metabolism cages are merely urine–feces separators, some special cage types are designed also to regulate and collect both inhaled and exhaled gases.

The principle of a metabolism cage (Figure 25.12) is the confinement of a rat in an enclosure with a wire grid floor. The cage is placed on top of a funnel device so that urine falling on the sides of the funnel is channeled via a side arm into a collection vial, while the fecal pellets drop separately into another vial. In the more sophisticated designs, feeding and watering compartments of the metabolism cage are incorporated in such a way that food and water do not significantly contaminate the urine and feces.

Haas et al. (1997) investigated the feasibility of metabolism cage conditions for the study of short-term manipulations on renal output. For the study, a metabolism cage with a wire mesh floor was placed above a fraction collector. The times were recorded, and the individual voidings of the freely moving rats were collected separately using computer communication. Surprisingly, during normal diuresis, the volume of urine voided and collection times appeared to be highly variable and poorly correlated. However, creatinine excretion could be used for correction of incomplete bladder emptying since creatinine is constantly produced throughout the body's musculature and subsequently excreted via the kidney (Thomson and Olesen, 1986; Shirley et al., 1989). The method of creatinine correction makes this animal model suitable both for assessing short-term renal interventions and for detecting subtle pharmacological manipulations.

It has been argued (Cocchetto and Bjornsson, 1983) that the design of a metabolism cage, such as

its limited floor space and social isolation, could induce stress in the animals. One solution is to ensure the animals have adequate time to adapt to the unfamiliar environment before experimental measurements are initiated.

Economic considerations or the need for special environments for a study have led to the development of a variety of noncommercial systems (Plummer and Wright, 1970; Vries et al., 1977; Black and Claxton, 1979; Wesslau et al., 1989; Fenske, 1989; Waynforth and Flecknell, 1992).

More recently, Badiani et al. (1995) designed a system for the analysis of liquid and solid food intake over time in rats, that at the same time monitors locomotor activity and **diuresis.** The apparatus consists of rat cages equipped with photocells, bottles, electronic balances and a funnel to collect urine with computer interfaces, an AT-compatible microcomputer for data collection, and a VAX system for analysis. The system may be useful for the study of differential effects of drugs on various parameters of feeding and drinking. Because it allows for the monitoring of all behavior for periods of 24 consecutive hours without disturbing the animals, it can be applied to the study of light/dark cycles of ingestive behavior.

Cystostomy and Cannulation

Cystostomy, or direct puncture of the bladder through the abdomen, is a routine procedure in larger animal species. Its usefulness in smaller species common in the laboratory is less practical. Hoy and Adolph (1956), however, surgically implanted a plastic cannula in the urinary bladder to obtain a continuous flow of urine (Figure 25.13). The authors measured a continuous urine flow of ca. 0.3–0.5 mL/h in healthy, conscious adult rats. The cannulation method can be used in both male and female rats of all ages.

More recently, Xu and Melethil (1990) described a method for serial sampling of various body fluids from anesthetized rats. Cannulae were implanted into the right jugular and left femoral veins, the bile duct and bladder. The special silicon polymer bladder catheter was attached via a ca. 2-mm incision at the tip of the bottom of the organ. Dosing with aluminum was followed by serial collection of blood, bile and urine. Urine flow remained steady at 0.5–0.7 mL/h during the 12-hour collection period, which is slightly higher than the values reported by Hoy and Adolph (1956).

The TECNIPLAST Metabolic Cage

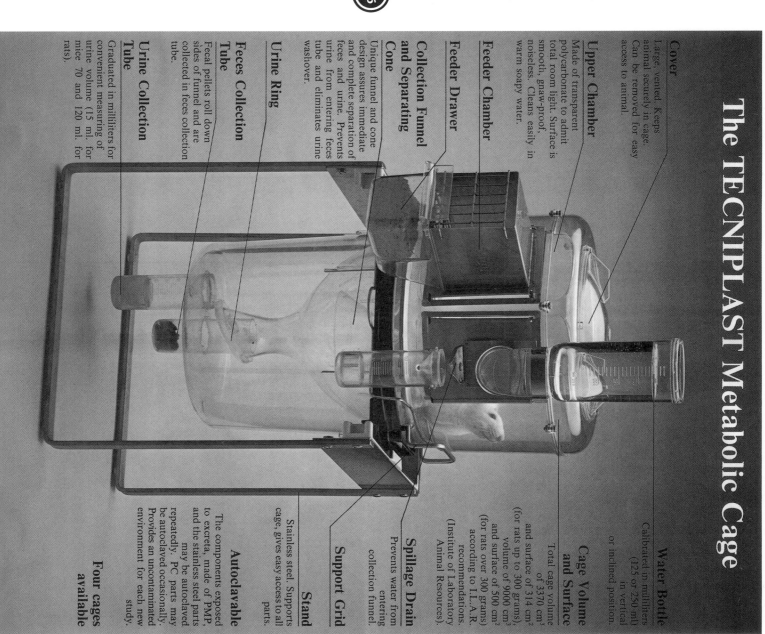

Cover
Large, vented. Keeps animal securely in cage. Can be removed for easy access to animal.

Upper Chamber
Made of transparent polycarbonate to admit total room light. Surface is smooth, gnaw-proof, noiseless. Cleans easily in warm soapy water.

Feeder Chamber

Feeder Drawer

Collection Funnel and Separating Cone
Unique funnel and cone design assures immediate and complete separation of feces and urine. Prevents urine from entering feces tube and eliminates urine washover.

Urine Ring

Feces Collection Tube
Fecal pellets roll down sides of funnel and are collected in feces collection tube.

Urine Collection Tube
Graduated in milliliters for convenient measuring of urine volume (15 ml. for mice 70 and 120 ml. for rats).

Water Bottle
Calibrated in milliliters (125 or 250 ml) in vertical or inclined position.

Cage Volume and Surface
Total cage volume and surface of 3370 cm³ of 314 cm² (for rats up to 300 grams), volume of 9000 cm³ and surface of 500 cm² (for rats over 300 grams) according to I.L.A.R. recommendations. (Institute of Laboratory Animal Resources).

Spillage Drain
Prevents water from entering collection funnel.

Support Grid

Stand
Stainless steel. Supports cage, gives easy access to all parts.

Autoclavable
The components exposed to excreta, made of PMP, and the stainless steel parts may be autoclaved repeatedly. PC parts may be autoclaved occasionally. Provides an uncontaminated environment for each new study.

Four cages available

Figure 25.12 Commercial metabolism cage with floor surface of 500 cm² for rats up to 500 g body weight.

For male rats, an external drainage catheter is used. According to White (1971), a modified polyethylene catheter (Leur-End Intramedic polyethylene catheter; Clay Adams, Parsippany, NY, USA) can be slipped over the tip of the penis of an anesthetized male rat, tucked under the foreskin and secured in place by tying the foreskin around the catheter with a single silk ligature. Although a special 'loading' technique is required, the author reported a urine flow rate of 6–10 mL/h was obtained.

Other Methods

Jackson and Sutherland (1984) described a reusable urinary collection device suitable for quantitative collection of uncontaminated urinary samples from rats without the requirement of a metabolism cage. The device can be attached quickly (5 min) to the pelvic skin using an adhesive that requires a minimum of handling and discomfort to the conscious rat. Compared with animals housed in traditional metabolism cages, there were no statistically significant differences in food and water consumption, or urinary output for rats with the adhesive collection device.

Some experimental designs require special restraining systems, particularly for studies using

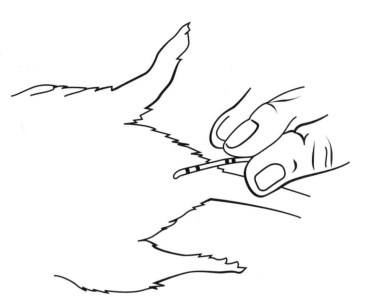

Figure 25.14 Urine sampling in the rat: catheterization of female rats with a No. 4 coude catheter. From Kraus (1980).

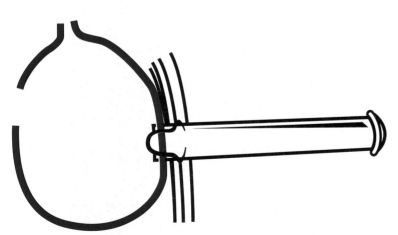

Figure 25.13 Urine sampling in the rat: urine cystostomy technique. From Kraus (1980).

Bladder Puncture

Because it is difficult to reliably hit the small bladder in rodents such as rats, it is recommended that bladder puncture, or **centesis**, is used only at necropsy. Urine can be withdrawn easily from the bladder with a needle and syringe.

Catheterization

Urethral catheterization is only applied routinely in larger species. Use of the method in rats is possible only under general anesthesia (Mulder et al., 1981; Intengan and Smyth, 1997). Special care must be taken to minimize the risk of introducing infection into the urinary tract during the procedure. Catheters must be sterilized before use, as should any other material such as lubricating gels and speculums. Moreover, different forms of catheters must be used for the two genders.

In female rats, repeated short-term urethral catheterization can be done using a No. 4 coude urethral catheter (Figure 25.14; Cohen and Oliver, 1964). The authors reported a continuous urinary flow for up to 4 hours while the rat was maintained under anesthesia.

chronic cannulae implants. Lewis *et al.* (1989) introduced a restrainer that accommodated rats of different body weights and maximized the convenience in procedures to collect blood, feces and urine. Roerig *et al.* (1980) described a similar, inexpensive restraining device, made of commonly found items such as a plastic dinner plate and smoking pipe cleaners.

Lacrimal Fluid

According to Kraus (1980) secretions from tear glands, or lacrimal fluid, may be obtained at the medial canthus. For this purpose a pharmacologic stimulation of tearing with parasympathomimetic drugs such as pilocarpine is recommended. Fluid may be collected into suitable capillary micropipettes.

Saliva

Saliva has become an increasingly exploited substance for studies, for example, of oral fluid immunology, circadian rhythms of salivary flow and electrolyte discharge. Expanding points of interest are transepithelial electrolyte transport in various pathophysiological situations, such as different forms of experimental hypertension and end-stage renal failure (Stahlin *et al.*, 1978).

Pilocarpine and isoproterenol, both injected intraperitoneally, are the two major agents used to stimulate salivation. Pilocarpine at a dosage of 0.1–10 mg/kg body weight promotes saliva flow in rats (Holloway and Williams, 1965; Robinovitch and Sreebny, 1969; Menaker *et al.*, 1974; Martinez and Camden, 1983; Abe *et al.*, 1987; Scott and Berry, 1989; Damas, 1994). Isoproterenol was also successful at dosages of 10–250 mg/kg body weight (Robinovitch and Sreebny, 1969; Martinez and Camden, 1983; Scott and Berry, 1989; Damas, 1994). In contrast, salivary secretion can be inhibited by administration of hyoscine hydrobromide (Schneyer and Hall, 1965).

The basal salivary flow in a nonanesthetized rat in the absence of drug stimulation is reported by Wolf and Kakehashi (1966) to be 0.84 mL/4 h. Martinez and Camden (1983) obtained an average total volume of 120 µL/h saliva from juvenile (3 weeks old) rats using a procedure in which a cannula is attached to the main excretory ducts of individual glands.

Intraperitoneal administration of pilocarpine and isoproterenol, both of 10 mg/kg body weight, were used to induce salivation.

Collection of saliva may be performed by one of four different procedures. (1) Saliva can be obtained from the rat's oral cavity (Holloway and Williams, 1965; Menaker *et al.*, 1974; Tatevossian and Wright, 1974; Vissink *et al.*, 1989). Recently, Guhad and Hau (1996) investigated the concentration of salivary sIgA as a possible marker for stress in rats. The animals were trained to release saliva as a conditioned response by presenting a chocolate reward stimulus. Discs of filter paper were used to soak up saliva directly from the animal's oral cavity. (2) Intraoral duct cannulation has been employed with some frequency (Hellekant and Kasahara, 1973; Schneyer and Flatland, 1975; Martinez and Camden, 1983; Abe *et al.*, 1987). For instance, Scott and Berry (1989) were interested in the effects of chronic ethanol administration on stimulated secretion from the parotid gland of rats. Under Valium-Hypnorm anesthesia, parotid saliva was collected by inserting an intraoral duct cannula and administering pilocarpine or isoprenaline. (3) Direct collection of saliva has been obtained from the cut end of a surgically isolated duct. Saliva may be obtained from the proximal end of the transected salivary gland ducts. Collection is usually made into a suitable receptacle after administration of pilocarpine or isoprenaline (Kraus, 1980). (4) Finally, the entire gland can be excised at necropsy (Nagler *et al.*, 1993).

Peritoneal Fluids

Nashed (1975) described a simple method for the collection of peritoneal cells from rats using a glass pipette (Figure 25.15). Cell collection within 30–60 s was possible on an intact unanesthetized animal using lavage with a specially designed and constructed peritoneal cell glass pipette, through which 30–35 mL of warmed Hank's solution was inserted into the abdominal cavity. The solution was aspirated, allowing collection of 5–20 million peritoneal cells per suspension. According to the author, this procedure can be repeated on different occasions in the same animal without apparent adverse effects. Similar procedures have been reported by Friend and Lock (1979), Casciato *et al.* (1976) and Chambers (1975).

Bile

The biliary system can be an important route of elimination for many xenobiotics. Investigation of bile contents is, therefore, important for many pharmacokinetic, material balance, and metabolism studies. Numerous techniques for chronic bile duct cannulation have been developed, but choice of method depends upon several factors.

Unlike humans, rats have no gallbladder. Bile flows directly through the common bile duct into the duodenum of the rat (Figure 25.16). Pancreatic juices join the common bile duct distal to the site where the bile enters. Thus, bile, pancreatic fluid or a mixture of the two can be collected depending upon the site at which the cannula is placed and ligatures are made. Electrolytes depleted by chronic bile diversion must be replenished by parenteral or oral fluid administration of either filtered control bile or commercial bile salts solution (e.g. 0.005% of B-8756, Sigma, St Louis, USA). Free access to drinking water containing certain amounts of glucose, sodium chloride, potassium chloride and Ringer's solution reportedly supply adequate electrolyte replacement (Cocchetto and Bjornsson, 1983). Because the volume of bile flow depends upon body temperature (Roberts and Plaa, 1966; Roberts *et al.*, 1967), the procedure must be performed under stable temperature conditions. Drugs can be used to change biliary release. Phenobarbital, depending on the mode of administration, can induce a ca. 50% increase in bile

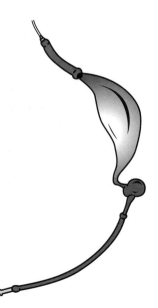

Figure 25.15 Specially constructed peritoneal cell glass pipette (50 mL volume). The left end is fitted with a mouthpiece, the right end terminating with a 15-G hypodermic needle. The needle is inserted into the abdominal cavity and Hank's solution is instilled from the pipette. Hank's solution is then aspirated again, containing 5–20 million peritoneal cells. From Kraus (1980).

Collection of ascitic fluid, for instance, from rats inoculated intraperitoneally with hybridoma cells, may be performed at necropsy. To prevent unnecessary pain with the procedure, animals should be killed during a moderate stage of ascite development. Ascitic fluid can be aspirated with a syringe and a 20-G needle. If the needle becomes obstructed by the intestines or the omentum, the needle can be removed from the syringe and the fluid allowed to flow freely into a suitable receptacle. Nagel *et al.* (1989) reported a method of repeated sampling of ascitic fluid from the same rat. Two silicon tubes were implanted into the abdominal cavity, one for drug administration and regulation of pressure, the other tube enabled ascitic fluid to be withdrawn.

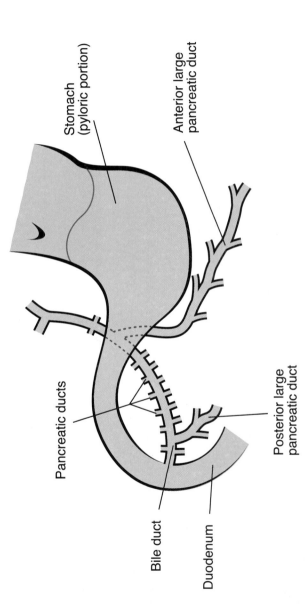

Figure 25.16 The bile duct and its anatomical relationships. From Waynforth and Flecknell (1992).

flow rate (Klaassen, 1970; Manzo et al., 1980), whereas cycloheximide can reduce it to ca. 30–50% of the flow rate of control rats (Lock et al., 1979).

Waynforth and Flecknell (1992) presented a detailed and illustrated description of the various bile duct catheterization methods. The techniques appearing in the literature can be classified into the following categories.

1 *T-cannula.* Using tubing shaped as a T, Chipman and Cropper (1977) inserted a T-piece into the bile duct so that bile flow to the duodenum was not disturbed except during sampling. The disadvantage of this technique is that it does not allow total collections of bile. Xu et al. (1992) and Klauda et al. (1973) used similar T-cannulae methods.

2 *Extracorporeal reservoir.* Rath and Hutchison (1989) described a method of bile duct cannulation allowing bile to be collected and reinfused into conscious rats. A bile duct cannula was inserted at a (proximal) site towards the hilum and a second cannula was inserted at the (distal) duodenum using a PE-loop. The loop was placed externally to the abdomen, being protected in a Perspex housing anchored to the abdominal wall. After surgery, the animals were given a postoperative recovery period of 7 days. For the experiment the Perspex cap was removed, and the loop was disconnected. Bile was collected from the proximal cannula, while the distal cannula was used for reinfusion of bile from a control rat or infusion of a commercial bile salt solution. Bile flow rates were within the range of 1–3 mL per hour with both of these methods.

3 *Intracorporeal reservoir.* Heitmeyer and Powers (1992) modified a technique described by Johnson and Rising (1978) for continuous collection of bile from unrestrained rats. The authors implanted an externally accessible, continuous-loop cannula at the same time that a cannula was attached to the common bile duct. The rats were allowed full recovery from anesthesia, and a normal bile salt pool was maintained until the experiment began. Then the cannula loop was cut, and bile was diverted into a surgically implanted glass collection vial that was removed periodically via an externalized sampling port. In this study an average bile flow rate of 0.98 ± 0.04 mL/h was reported over a 24-hour collection period. See Chapter 27 about permanent double bill fistula with intact enterohepatic circulation.

Pancreatic Juice

In rats a number of the pancreatic ducts join the bile duct to form the common bile duct. It is therefore necessary to stop or divert biliary flow into the lower segment of the common duct to collect pancreatic juice uncontaminated by bile. Reviews of surgery of the pancreatic ducts and of materials and methods for the collection of pancreatic fluids have been published by Lambert (1965), Kraus (1980) and, most recently, by Zabielski et al. (1997).

Waynforth and Flecknell (1992) described the collection of pancreatic secretions in the rat using a procedure that separates pancreatic from biliary secretions. The authors tied one ligature around the bile duct where it enters the duodenum and a second on the hilum of the liver prior to the point where the duct bifurcates. A catheter was placed into the duct near these ligatures and pure pancreatic secretion was obtained through the external catheter. The flow rate of pancreatic secretion was variable but usually was 0.5–1 mL/h. The serious limitation of this technique, as in many of the other published techniques, was that the ligated hilum duct caused biliary obstruction. The resulting development of jaundice reduced the survival time of the animals to only a few weeks.

Colwell (1951) described another cannulation method. The proximal end of the common bile duct between pancreas and liver free from hepatic radicals was ligated, hemisected and a cannula was implanted and fixed in place with a ligature. The distal portion of the cannula was threaded through the ligated duodenal end of the bile duct into the duodenum acting as an 'artificial bile duct' and thus re-established the enterohepatic circulation. A second cannula was placed just beyond the openings of the most distal pancreatic ducts. The volume of pancreatic secretion obtained was 1.6–3.5 mL per 100 g body weight/24 h.

However, Zabielski et al. (1997) argue that the collected pancreatic juice, or at least a portion of it, must be reintroduced into the duodenum. Pancreatic juice does not only have a crucial enzymatic and homeostatic activity, it also seems to be an important regulator of intestinal microflora (Pierzynowski et al., 1992). To accomplish reintroduction of pancreatic juice into the duodenum, Onaga et al. (1993) kept rats in metabolic cages, and a peristaltic pump was used to pump juices back into the animal at a slow, constant rate. These latter authors emphasized

Since spontaneous ejaculations seldom occur in rats (Agmo *et al.*, 1977; Brown *et al.*, 1984) and because artificial vaginas have not proved useful in this species, special technical procedures were developed to obtain rat semen. Currently, there are a number of sperm collection methods for rats, each with different influences on the numbers and motility of sperm.

Perhaps the earliest method was described by Blandau and Jordan (1941), who obtained sperm samples from various portions of the female reproductive tract following mating. The primary disadvantage of this method is the lack of quantitative evidence, because there is no way to confirm that all sperm ejaculated have been harvested. Another problem is that too many of them are clotted together and therefore cannot be used for artificial insemination or *in vitro* fertilization.

Later, Vreeburg *et al.* (1974) developed a technique where the vas deferens was surgically attached (anastomosed) to the urinary bladder to permit harvesting of sperm by collecting urine over a 24-hour time period. The problem is that sperm obtained with this method cannot be used for artificial insemination.

Electroejaculation

Electroejaculation allows the collection of sperm by multiple samplings over time in the same male. However, Scott and Dzuik (1959) experienced difficulties when applying electroejaculation to their rats. Electrical stimulation caused the ejaculate to coagulate and the spermatozoa were entrapped in the hardened coagulum. The coagulum blocked the urethra, resulting in death from uremia in ca. 10% of the rats within 4 days. The solution (Scott and Dzuik, 1959) was to surgically remove both the seminal vesicle and coagulating gland (anterior prostate). Subsequent electroejaculation produced an ejaculate consisting almost entirely of sperm with little accompanying fluid. Birnbaum and Hall (1961) applied electroejaculation to males with surgically removed coagulating glands, leaving the seminal vesicles intact. They usually obtained coagulum-free sperm samples, but some specimens still formed a coagulum. On the other hand, Lawson *et al.* (1967) used the same method and report problems with coagulated semen.

Waynforth and Flecknell (1992) reported that removal of the coagulating gland is not necessary in

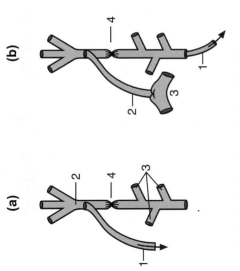

Figure 25.17 Technique for collecting bile (**a**) and pancreatic juice (**b**). (**a**) Cannula (1), placed into the common bile duct (2), proximal to entrance of pancreatic ducts (3), and ligature (4), distal to cannula and proximal to pancreatic ducts. (**b**) Cannula (1) into common duct distal to entrance of pancreatic ducts, second cannula (2) ('artificial bile duct') into proximal common duct and also into duodenum (3), ligature distal to 'artificial bile duct' and proximal to pancreatic ducts (4). From Kraus (1980).

the importance that reintroduction of pancreatic juices is performed at approximately the rate of endogenous secretions. Although there have been many methodological improvements over the years, Zabielski *et al.* (1997) state that there is not yet a single, ideal model for chronic collection of pancreatic juice. The methods published to date are notable for both their advantages and serious limitations (Figure 25.17).

Semen

General Remarks

Semen refers to the complete discharge ejaculated by the male rat. It has two major components: the spermatozoa, or cellular component, and the seminal plasma, or liquid portion. Variations in the volume of semen ejaculated are due largely to the amount of secretory products contributed by the sex accessory glands. However, many factors such as strain, age, frequency and most recent occurrence of ejaculation, season of the year, environmental conditions, nutritional state, and general health of the animal all play important roles in semen production (Taylor *et al.*, 1985).

electroejaculation if carefully controlled conditions are used. The equipment used by these authors that is required include (1) a single bipolar rectal electrode measuring 4.8 mm diameter at the tip and with ring electrode contacts 2.5 cm apart, (2) an audio oscillator with a capacity to supply sine waves of frequencies anywhere between 10 and 60 cycles/s and a voltage up to 20 V into a load of 600 Ω or more. With the animal anesthetized, the rectal probe was inserted slowly until the rear ring electrode was in a position just inside the rectum. The following electrical sequence was then performed to induce ejaculation in the animal. While the oscillator was set to 30 cycles/s, the voltage was increased from 0 to 2 V maximum within 1–2 s, remained at this level for ca. 5 s and, then, reduced to 0 V in 1–2 s, remaining at 0 for ca. 10 s. This specific sequence of stimulation was repeated until ejaculation occurred, or for a maximum of 25 times. The authors reported that this electroejaculation method can be performed many times on the same rat, provided that the stimulus is kept below 3 V and 60 cycles/s.

Excising of Cauda Epididymis

Numbers of sperm, of course, are only one feature of ejaculate integrity, an observation of particular importance for reproductive toxicologists. Percentage of sperm in the sample showing motility is also of considerable interest, as well as other measures of sperm movement such as percentage progressive motility, progressive velocity and path velocity. For these analyses, it is common for the studies to collect the sperm by surgically exposing the vas deferens or cauda epididymis. Samples are taken from the proximal and the distal parts of the cauda epididymis and are collected using either a 'diffusion' or an 'aspiration' method (Slott et al., 1991; Klinefelter et al., 1991).

For the aspiration method, according to Klinefelter et al. (1991), the epididymis was placed on a paper towel and the vas deferens was clamped with a hemostat to create pressure in the epididymal tubule. A small incision was made into the midproximal part of the cauda and a certain amount of the epididymal contents was aspirated into a capillary tube. The sample was diluted with medium and held at 34°C for ca. 15 min until sperm dispersed. In the diffusion method according to Klinefelter et al. (1991), the epididymis was excised and placed in a Petri dish containing an aliquot of medium. Using a

scalpel blade, the lumen of the midproximal cauda epididymal tubule was pierced, taking care to avoid cutting blood vessels. Sperm were allowed to diffuse into the medium for ca. 15 min. The tissue is removed, and the sperm are incubated until they are to be analyzed.

Samples obtained from the distal portion of the cauda epididymis (Figure 25.18) are reported to have higher motility and higher percentages of forward-moving sperm with greater velocities than sperm sampled from the proximal cauda epididymis (Slott et al., 1991). Moreover, compared with samples obtained by aspiration, sperm samples collected by the diffusion method were less variable and more highly correlated with an experimental treatment for the percentage motile and progressively motile sperm motion parameters (Klinefelter et al., 1991). If samples are taken from the whole cauda epididymis, the values can be expected to lie somewhere

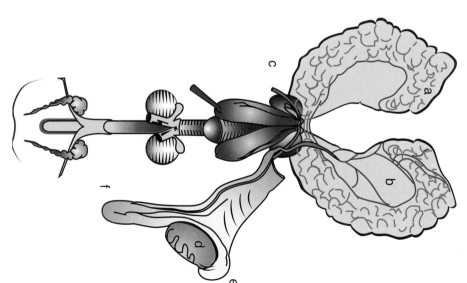

Figure 25.18 Genital organs of the male rat: seminal vesicle (a), coagulating gland (b), vas deferens (c), testis (d), caput epididymidis (e), and cauda epididymidis (f). Redrawn from Popesko (1992).

between, and with somewhat greater variability, the values for the distal and proximal cauda (Slott et al., 1991).

Seed et al. (1996) have summarized recent efforts to reduce interlaboratory variability. One recommendation is that, regardless of the specific site chosen for sperm sampling, conditions should be optimized so that values of 70% motility or greater are achieved consistently in control animals within a laboratory. Finally, sperm numbers per ejaculate are reported in the literature as being 50–350 × 10[6] (Bennett and Vickery, 1970; Taylor et al., 1985; Waynforth and Flecknell, 1992), while Slott et al. (1991) found 1–2 × 10[5] sperm/L (dilute sperm). These data make clear that results such as number and motility of sperm do not only depend upon factors such as rat strain, age, general health and so forth, but also upon the method of preparation utilized.

Female Reproductive Products

Long and Evans (1922) first described and correlated the cellular changes with ovarian activity of the rat. Later, authors described methods of collecting vaginal fluids and staining of the various cells for microscopy (Clarkson and Kalnins, 1959; Gregoire et al., 1967; Hafez, 1970; Bernardis et al., 1994, 1995, 1997; Cassone et al., 1995).

Today, there are two primary sampling methods used with female rats: collection of vaginal fluids for investigation of rat models of vaginal inflammation (vaginitis) and collection of materials for the preparation of vaginal smears for determination of the stage of the estrus cycle.

Collection of Vaginal Fluids

In a recent series of studies, Bernardis et al. (1994, 1995) described a procedure for obtaining vaginal fluids using a calibrated (1-μL samples) plastic loop (Disponoic, PBI) inserted into the vagina of rats. Fluid removed was divided into two portions either to be stained by the periodic acid Schiff–van Gieson method for microscopic examination or to be used

for culturing vaginal cells. For the latter, the contents of each loop were shaken vigorously to suspend the cells in a 0.1 mL PBS solution, and aliquots of the suspension were streaked onto plates containing Sabouraud-dextrose agar with chloramphenicol (20 mg/mL). Following incubation of the plates at 30°C for 48 hours, the CFU per milliliter was calculated (Bernardis et al., 1994).

Flecknell (1987) recommended a method that involved simply inserting a small volume of saline solution into the vagina using a blunt-ended pipette, followed by aspiration of the liquid to obtain a suspension of cellular debris.

Atherton et al. (1986) described a similar method in which vaginal fluids were collected using calibrated eye droppers. Sterile 0.9% w/v NaCl at pH 7.5 was introduced into the vagina, and the contents were flushed twice. Fluids were then centrifuged and the cellular pellet was removed and stained with 0.5% methylene blue to determine the stage of estrus. Supernatants could be frozen and used for other analyses of interest. Gregoire et al. (1967) investigated the appearance of labeled ^{14}C-glucose in rat vaginal fluid and genital tract tissue. For this purpose vaginal fluids were collected from female rats following subcutaneous injection of 10 mL of uniformly labelled glucose. A preweighed cotton-tipped applicator was inserted into the vagina, rotated about the vaginal walls, and the sticks were removed and reweighed. The samples were placed in vials, and the radioactive labeled product was quantified.

Vaginal Smears

The copulation rate of naturally cycling females can be markedly increased by mating only those females which appear to be in proestrus according to the external appearance of the genital region or according to vaginal cytological findings. As described by Baker (1979), such rats of the proestric stage are characterized by their slightly swollen vulva and by their dry vagina. For identification of the respective stage, vaginal smears can be produced by cautiously inserting a sterile swab, a glass rod, or a platinum loop into the vagina and transferring the adhering material onto a glass slide. These smears are fixed and stained with Hema® staining solution (Heiland, Stuttgart, Germany). As depicted in Figure 25.19, the critical phase for mating is characterized by nucleated epithelial cells, few cornified epithelial cells and few leukocytes.

Figure 25.19 Assessment of estrous cycle stage of rats by investigating vaginal smears. Characteristic features are cornified epithelial cells (a), nucleated epithelial cells (b), leukocytes (c), and mucus (d). Proestrus (upper left): predominantly nucleated epithelial cells, few cornified epithelial cells, and few leukocytes. Estrus (upper right): almost exclusively cornified epithelial cells, most of them cornified with pycnotic nuclei. Metestrus (lower left): predominantly leukocytes and cornified epithelial cells. Diestrus (lower right): predominantly leukocytes, few epithelial cells, and mucus.

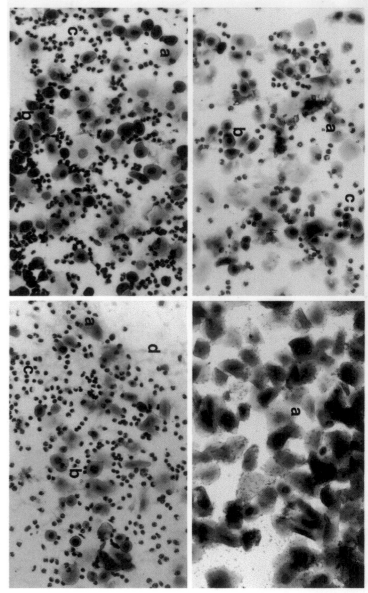

Milk

As part of the safety evaluation of new compounds, an important measurement is the potential for the compound, or its bioactive metabolites, to be transferred from a lactating dam to its litter. Consequently, several methods have been developed for the collection of milk from female rats. Some are direct methods such as using hand-milking or milking machines, whereas others use indirect methods such as taking milk from the stomachs of euthanized pups. Finally, Brake (1979) recommended the cannulation of mammary tissue following intraperitoneal oxytocin administration as the most efficient and productive method for the collection of milk from lactating rats.

Manual Ejection

A common procedure, known as 'stripping', consists of manual kneading of the teat (Luckey *et al.*, 1954; Galef and Sherry, 1973) with repetitive, bottom-to-

top stroking motions. Expressed milk is collected in graduated cylinders. Milk yield is dependent upon the time between separating the dam from her pups and the stripping procedure. Brake (1979) reported an average yield of ca. 0.4 mL milk per nipple of an anesthetized female for 22–24 hour separation periods and 0.1 mL for 4–6 hour separation times. Intraperitoneal injection of 0.4 mL oxytocin to a female increased milk yield to 0.5 mL milk for the longer separation time and to ca. 0.4 mL for the shorter separation period (Brake, 1979).

Milking Machines

Various types of milking devices have been developed for use with rats. Cox and Mueller (1937) described an early version of a milking machine for rats and guinea-pigs. Depending on the stage of lactation, 3.0–8.0 mL milk have been obtained. Various modified and improved models have been developed subsequently (Temple and Kon, 1937; Goole and Taylor, 1974; Keen *et al.* 1980; Fisher *et al.*, 1981; Waynforth and Flecknell, 1992). Rodgers (1995) described direct and indirect methods of

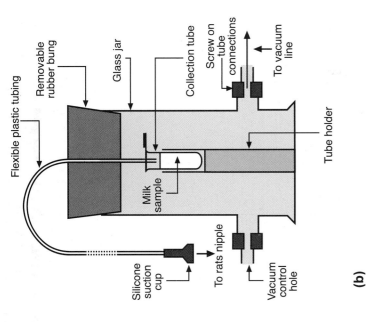

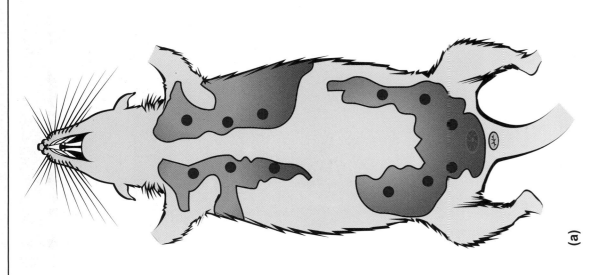

Figure 25.20 (a) Ventral view of a female rat with six pectoral and six inguinal nipples. From Weiss *et al.* (1996). **(b)** Diagrammatic representation of rat milking equipment. From Rodgers (1995).

milk collection in rats, discussed the methods, and made the following recommendations:

1 Reduction of litter size to six pups per litter within 48 hours of parturition to increase the milk yield.

2 Fourteen days postpartum is the highest production period for lactating rats and, consequently, is the optimum time for milk collection.

3 Removal of the dam from the litter only for ca. 5 min prior to milking. Longer periods did not appreciably increase milk yield (although cf. Brake, 1978).

4 Intraperitoneal administration of 4 IU oxytocin/kg body weight (prepared as a 4 IU/mL solution and administered at a dose level of 4 IU/kg body weight, at a standard dose volume of 1 mL/kg body weight) to a dam 5 min prior to milking will stimulate milk 'let down'.

5 Milk collection using a vacuum system (Figure 25.20) required no anesthesia. Milk could be obtained from all the dam's nipples, ca. 0.5 mL per nipple. Vacuum was controlled at 200 mbar. A pulsation was created by placing a finger on the control hole; repeated slight movements of the finger off the control hole would allow small amounts of air into the flask, therefore increasing and decreasing the vacuum.

6 The dam can be returned to to its litter immediately after milking. Although the method described by Rodgers (1995) appears to require a great deal of patience and manual dexterity to achieve competence, it causes less stress to the animal than other methods and samples can be obtained without the use of continuous restraint or anesthesia.

Lymph

The first method for cannulation of the thoracic duct and collection of lymph fluid in the anesthetized rat was described by Reinhardt (1945). He injected 0.5 mL of trypan blue intraperitoneally 30 min prior to cannulation to enable easy identification of the main lymphatic trunks. The author found a lymph flow rate of an average of 0.45 mL/h. Later on Bollmann et al. (1948) extended the method for collection of lymph from either the liver, intestine, or thoracic duct of the rat by inserting a plastic cannula in the duct lymphatic vessels, using Evans blue as contrast medium. Up to 5 mL lymph were obtained daily from the hepatic duct, 20 mL from the intestinal and 25 mL from the thoracic duct respectively.

Gowans (1957) cannulated the abdominal thoracic duct using the procedure of Bollmann et al. (1948) to collect lymph continuously from unanesthetized, but restrained rats. The collected lymph was reinfused into the femoral vein of the cannulated rat. The devices allowed quantitation of lymph output, at the same time maintaining lymphatic volume since reinfusion was continually in progress. Gallo-Torres (1977) published a well-illustrated review about the application of lymphatic vessel, bile duct, and portal vein cannulation in the rat. Waynforth and Flecknell (1992) provided the most recent and detailed description of catheterization of the thoracic and the mesenteric lymph ducts in the adult rat. Catheterization of other lymphatic channels was described by Lambert (1965); Steer (1980) and Lee (1984) made some modifications of the methods mentioned above.

Cerebrospinal Fluid (CSF)

Methods for ventricular access developed in the past are suitable for withdrawal of CSF fluid as well as for administration of substances. A review of the various procedures has been presented by Myers et al. (1988) and a well-illustrated description was given by Avery (1975).

For most procedures applied, the anesthetized rat is placed in a sternal recumbency over a special stand (Griffith and Farris, 1942; Waynforth and Flecknell, 1992) while its head is allowed to hang over the upper part of the stand and is freely moveable. In most recent applications a stereotaxic apparatus is used, instead of the simple stand, for fixing the rat to make sure that contact is made with the necessary brain structures. A common problem with the

collection of cerebrospinal fluid is contamination with blood due to inadvertent puncture of small dural blood vessels. To avoid significant red cell contamination, about 3–7 days should be allowed to elapse between successive punctures (Waynforth and Flecknell, 1992).

Noble et al. (1967) have developed a simple, rapid and atraumatic method for application of substances directly to the lateral ventricles of the rat brain. Through a skin incision and a small hole (0.5 mm i.d.) lateral to the sagittal and caudal of the coronal structures (Figure 25.21) substances could be injected or CSF could be withdrawn. deBalbian-Verster et al. (1971) described a freehand cerebroventricular injection technique for unanesthetized rats. They implanted a special chronic polyethylene cannula in the lateral ventricle according to the coordinates of Noble et al. (1967); a second hole was drilled nearby for a stainless steel retaining screw. The advantage over the technique described by Noble et al. (1967) is that repeated specimens can be collected from the unanesthetized rat after recovery from anesthesia.

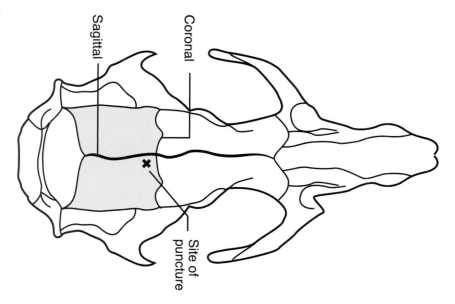

Figure 25.21 Dorsal view of a rat skull indicating location for insertion of a needle into the lateral ventricle. From Kraus (1980).

Sagittal

Coronal

Site of puncture

Hayden et al. (1966) and Hilliard et al. (1968) described detailed procedures for constructing and implanting a chronic cannula into the lateral ventricle of the rat brain using a stereotaxic apparatus.

Takara et al. (1977) reported a new technique for collecting CSF using a capillary phenomenon technique. Through a small hole in the atlanto-occipital dura mater 0.05–0.1 mL of the fluid could be obtained from the cisterna magna. Waynforth and Flecknell (1992) applied a method for cisternal puncture and obtained approximately 0.1–0.15 mL of cerebrospinal fluid within 3 min; the method was adapted from the technique of Griffith and Farris (1942). However, Withyachumnarnkul and Knigge (1980) obtained as much as 0.3–0.5 mL within 5–10 min from the cisterna magna, using a 27-G needle connected to a withdrawal pump.

More recently, artificial cerebrospinal fluids (aCSF) were used for perfusion of spinal cord and brain to collect material resulting from a reaction of the rat body to certain treatments, such as application of drugs (Sen and Phillis, 1993; Benoliel et al., 1992; Myers et al., 1988; Cesselin et al., 1985). Pohl et al. (1992) perfused the spinal cord of rats with an artificial fluid containing (in mM): NaCl 126.5; NaHCO$_3$ 27.5; KCl 2.4; KH$_2$PO$_4$ 0.5; CaCl$_2$ 1.1 MgCl$_2$ 0.85; Na$_2$SO$_4$ 0.5; glucose 5.9; adjusted to pH 7.3 with an O$_2$–CO$_2$ mixture, 95/5, v/v. For proper application and subsequent collection of the aCSF, Xin et al. (1997) implanted, as a first step, a guide cannula unilaterally by using a stereotaxic apparatus. For the actual experiment a special microdialysis probe was inserted into the guide cannula. The aCSF was continually perfused into the dialysis probe at a certain rate and after at least 1 hour perfusion for equilibrium, dialysate samples were collected and frozen for later analyses.

Acknowledgements

The authors thank S. Wayss and C. Weiss-Niedenthal for technical assistance in preparing this manuscript.

References

Abe, K., Hidake, S., Ishibashi, K. et al. (1987) J. Dent. Res. **66**, 745–750.

Agmo, A., Soulairac, M.L. and Soulairac, A. (1977) Scand. J. Psychol. **18**(4), 345–347.

Ajika, K., Kalra, S.P., Fawcett, C.P., Krulich, L. and McCann, S.M. (1972) Endocrinology **90**, 707–715.

Akrawi, S.H. and Wedlung, P. (1987) J. Pharmacol. Meth. **17**, 67–74.

Atherton, R.W., Culver, B., Seitz, J., Khatoon, S. and Gern, W. (1986) Arch. Androl. **16**, 215–226.

Avery, D.D. (1975) In: Singh, D. and Avery, D.D. (eds) Physiological Techniques in Behavioral Research. New York: Plenum.

Badiani, A., Mundl, W.J. and Cabilio, S. (1995) Physiol. Behav. **57**, 973–981.

Baker, D.E.J. (1979) In: Baker, H.J., Lindsey, J.R. and Weisbroth, S.H. (eds) The Laboratory Rat, Vol. 1, pp. 153–168. New York: Academic Press.

Beauzeville, C. (1968) Proc. Soc. Exp. Biol. Med. **129**, 932–936.

Bellinger, L.L. and Mendel, V.E. (1975) Proc. Soc. Exp. Biol. Med. **148**, 5–8.

Bennett, J.P. and Vickery, B.H. (1970) In: Hafez, E.S.E. (ed.) Reproduction and Breeding Techniques for Laboratory Animals, pp. 299–315. Philadelphia: Lea & Febiger.

Benoit, A.M. and Dailey, R.A. (1991) J. Anim. Sci. **69**, 2971–2979.

Benoliel, J.J., Bourgoin, S., Mauborgne, A. et al. (1992) Brain Res. **590**, 255–262.

Bernardis, F. de, Molinari, A., Boccanera, M. et al. (1994) Infect. Immun. **62**, 509–519.

Bernardis, F. de, Cassone, A., Sturtevant, J. and Calderone, R. (1995) Infect. Immun. **63**, 1887–1892.

Bernardis, F. de, Boccanera, M., Adriani, D., Spreghini, E., Santoni, G. and Cassone, A. (1997) Infect. Immun. **65**, 3399–3405.

Berthoud, H.R., Laughton, W.B. and Powley, T.L. (1986) Am. J. Physiol. **250**, E331–337.

Bickhardt, K., Buttner, D., Muschen, U. and Plonait, H. (1983) Lab. Anim. **17**, 161–165.

Birnbaum, D. and Hall, T. (1961) Anat. Rec. **140**, 49–50.

Black, W.D. and Claxton, M.J. (1979) Lab. Anim. Sci. **29**, 253–254.

Blandau, R.J. and Jordan, E.S. (1941) J. Lab. Clin. Med. **26**, 1361–1362.

Boeber, R. (1988) Lab. Anim. **33**,

Bollmann, J.L., Cain, J.C. and Grindlay, J.H. (1948) J. Lab. Clin. Med. **33**, 1349–1352.

Brake, S.C. (1979) Physiol. Behav. **22**, 795–797.

Brown, G.M. and Martin, J.B. (1974) Psychosom. Med. **36**, 241–247.

Brown, R.D., Shepherd, B.A. and Martan, J. (1984) J. Exp. Zool. **231**, 117–119.

Carlberg, K.A. and Alvin, B.L. (1992) Med. Sci. Sports Exerc. **24**, 610–614.

Carraway, J.H. and Gray, L.D. (1989) Lab. Anim. Sci. **39**, 623–624.

Casciato, D.A., Goldberg, L.S. and Bluestone, R. (1976) Vox. Sang. **31** (1 suppl.), 25–31.

Cassone, A.M., Boccanera, D., Adriani, G., Santoni, G.

and DeBernardis, F. (1995) *Infect. Immun.* **63**, 2619–2624.

Cesselin, F., LeBars, D., Bourgoin, S. *et al.* (1985) *Brain Res.* **339**, 305–313.

Chambers, T.R. (1975) *Lab. Anim. Sci.* **25**, 619–620.

Chang, S.L., Emmick, K. and Wedlund, P.J. (1986) *J. Pharm. Sci.* **75**, 456–458.

Chipman, J.K. and Cropper, M.C. (1977) *Res. Vet. Sci.* **22**, 366–368.

Clarkson, T.B. and Kalnins, P. (1959) *Proc. Anim. Care Panel* **9**, 35–37.

Cocchetto, D.M. and Bjornsson, T.D. (1983) *J. Pharm. Sci.* **72**, 465–492.

Cohen, A.E. and Oliver, H.M. (1964) *Lab. Anim. Care* **14**, 471–473.

Colwell, A.R. (1951) *Am. J. Physiol.* **164**, 812–821.

Cox, W.M. and Mueller, A.J. (1937) *Nutrition* 249–261.

Damas, J. (1994) *Arch. Int. Physiol. Biochim. Biophys.* **102**, 103–105.

Dang, D.C., Hidden, G. and Rombauts, P. (1989) *Reprod. Nutr. Dev.* **29**, 449–459.

DeBalbian-Verster, F., Robinson, C.A., Hengeveld, C.A. and Bush, E.S. (1971) *Life Sci.* **10**, 1395–1402.

Deringer, M.K. (1963) In: Burdette, W.J. (ed.) *Methodology in Mammalian Genetics*, pp. 563–564. San Francisco: Holden-Day.

Doris, P.A., Harvey, S. and Pang, P.K. (1987) *Life Sci.* **41**, 1383–1389.

Draper, H.H. and Robbins, A.F. (1956) *Proc. Soc. Exp. Biol. Med.* **91**, 174–175.

Fejes-Toth, G., Naray-Fejes-Toth, A., Ratge, D. and Frolich, J.C. (1984) *Hypertension* **6**, 926–930.

Fenske, M. (1989) *Z. Versuchstierkd.* **32**, 65–70.

Fisher, A.N., Neale, M.G. and Smith, D.A. (1981) *Xenobiotica* **11**, 871–877.

Fitzgerald, R.D., Potter, R.F., Dietz, G.E., and Sibbald, W.J. (1997) *Acta Anaesthesiol. Scand. Suppl.* **111**, 253–256.

Flecknell, P.A. (1987) In: Tuffery, A.A. (ed.) *Laboratory Animals – An Introduction for New Experimenters*, pp. 225–260. Chichester: Wiley-Interscience.

Frank, P., Schoenhard, G.L. and Burton, E. (1991) *J. Pharmacol. Meth.* **26**, 233–238.

Friedel, R., Trautschold, I., Gaertner, K., Helle-Feldmann, M. and Gaudssuhn, D. (1974) *Z. Klin. Chem. Klin. Biochem.* **13**, 499–505.

Friend, J.V. and Lock, S.O. (1979) *Med. Lab. Sci.* **36**, 387–389.

Furuhama, K. and Onodera, T. (1983) *J. Toxicol. Sci.* **8**, 161–163.

Galef, B.G.-J. and Sherry, D.F. (1973) *J. Comp. Physiol. Psychol.* **83**, 374–379.

Gallo-Torres, H.E. (1977) *J. Toxicol. Environ. Health*, **2**, 827.

Gerecke, D. (1971) *Z. Gesamte Exp. Med.* **154**, 339–340.

Goole, J.A. and Taylor, J.C. (1974) *J. Physiol.* **242**, 5–7.

Gowans, J.L. (1957) *Br. J. Exp. Pathol.* **38**, 67–78.

Gregoire, A.T., Driscoll, D.H. and Adams, A. (1967) *J. Reprod. Fertil.* **14**, 313–316.

Griffith, Jr., J.Q. and Farris, E.J. (eds) (1942) In: *The Rat in Laboratory Investigation*, Ch. 9. Philadelphia: J.B. Lippincott.

Guhad, F.A. and Hau, J. (1996) *Neurosci. Lett.* **216**, 137–140.

Gupta, B.N. (1973) *Lab. Anim. Sci.* **23**, 559.

Haas, M., Kluppel, A.C., Moolenaar, F., Meijer, D.K., de Jong, P.E. and de Zeeuw, D. (1997) *J. Pharmacol. Toxicol. Meth.* **38**, 47–51.

Hafez, E.S.E. (ed.) (1970) In: *Reproduction and Breeding Techniques for Laboratory Animals*. Philadelphia: Lea & Febiger.

Hall, W.G. and Rosenblatt, J.S. (1977) *J. Comp. Physiol. Psychol.* **91**, 1232–1247.

Hammer, C.E. (1970) In: Hafez, E.S.E. (ed.) *Reproduction and Breeding Techniques for Laboratory Animals*, pp. 56–73. Philadelphia: Lea & Febiger.

Hayashi, S. and Sakaguchi, T. (1975) *Lab. Anim. Sci.* **25**, 781–782.

Hayden, J.F., Johnson, L.R. and Maikel, R.F. (1966) *Life Sci.* **5**, 1509–1515.

Heitmeyer, S.A. and Powers, J.F. (1992) *Lab. Anim. Sci.* **42**, 312–315.

Hellekant, G. and Kasahara, Y. (1973) *Acta Physiol. Scand.* **89**, 198–207.

Hem, A. and Smith, A. (1998) The manuscript is available via Internet at Laboratory Animal Veterinary Services, Vivarium, University of Bergen, Norway.

Hilliard, W.G., Dillistone, E.J. and Oliver, W.T. (1968) *Can. J. Comp. Med.* **32**, 368–371.

Holloway, P.J. and Williams, R.A.D. (1965) *Arch. Oral Biol.* **10**, 237–244.

Horton, M.L., Olson, C.T. and Hobson, D.W. (1986) *Am. J. Vet. Res.* **47**, 1781–1782.

Hoy, P.A. and Adolph, P.F. (1956) *Am. J. Physiol.* **187**, 32–40.

Hurwitz, A. (1971) *J. Lab. Clin. Med.* **78**, 172–174.

Hutchaleelaha, A., Sukbuntherng, J. and Mayersohn, M. (1997) *J. Pharmacol. Toxicol. Meth.* **37**, 9–14.

Intengan, H.D. and Smyth, D.D. (1997) *Br. J. Pharmacol.* **121**, 861–866.

Ishikawa, I., Shikura, N., Takada, K. and Sato, Y. (1993) *Nephron* **64**, 605–608.

Iwarsson, K., Lindberg, L. and Waller, T. (1994) In: Svendsen, P. and Hau, J. (eds) *Handbook of Laboratory Animal Science*, pp. 256–272. Boca Raton: CRC Press.

Jackson, A.J. and Sutherland, J.C. (1984) *J. Pharm. Sci.* **73**, 816–818.

Jansen, R.D. and Moorehead, H.C. (1986) *Diabetologia* **29**, 388–391.

Jarrige, J.F., Boucher, D. and Leinot, M. (1978) C. R. *Seances Soc. Biol. Fil.* **172**, 919–926.

Jimenez, W., Martinez-Pardo, A., Arroyo, V. *et al.* (1985) *Rev. Esp. Fisiol.* **41**, 299–303.

Johnson, P. and Rising, P.A. (1978) *Xenobiotica* **8**, 27–30.

Joint Working Group on Refinement (1993) *Lab. Anim.* **17**, 1–22.

Kaufmann, S. (1980) *Am. J. Physiol.* **239**, R123–125.

Keen, C.L., Lonnerdal, B. Sloan, M.V. and Hurley, L.S. (1980) *Physiol. Behav.* **24**, 613–615.

Klaassen, C.D. (1970) *J. Pharmacol. Exp. Ther.* **175**, 289–294.

Klauda, H.C., McGovern, R.F. and Quackenbush, F.W. (1973) *Lipids* **8**, 459–463.

Klinefelter, G.R., Gray, L.E. and Suarez, J.D. (1991) *Reprod. Toxicol.* **5**, 39–44.

Klinger, W., Kersten, L. and Melhorn, G. (1965) *Z. Versuchstierkd.* **6**, 35–47.

Korber, K.E. and Flye, M.W. (1987) *Microsurgery* **8**, 245–246.

Kraus, A.L. (1980) In: Baker, H.J., Lindsey, J.R. and Weisbroth, S.H. (eds) *The Laboratory Rat*, Vol. II, *Research Applications*. London: Academic Press.

Kurata, M., Misawa, K., Noguchi, N., Kasuga, Y. and Matsumoto, K. (1997) *J. Toxicol. Sci.* **22**, 231–238.

Kvetnansky, R., Sun, C.L., Lake, C.R., Thoa, N., Torda, T. and Kopin, I.J. (1978) *Endocrinology* **103**, 1868–1874.

Laakso, M.L., Johannson, G., Porkka-Heiskanen, T. and Peder, M. (1984) *Acta Physiol. Scand.* **121**, 233–239.

Lambert, R. (1965) In: *Surgery of the Digestive System in the Rat*. Chicago: Charles C. Thomas.

Lawson, R.L., Krise, G.M. and Sorensen, A.M. (1967) *J. Appl. Physiol.* **22**, 174–176.

Leal, M., Carson, S., Bidanset, J.H., Balkon, J., Barletta, M. and Hyland, M.D. (1988) *Reprod. Toxicol.* **1**, 111–116.

Lee, J.S. (1984) *Microvasc. Res.* **27**, 370–378.

Lewis, A., Long, A. and Griffiths, R. (1989) *J. Pharmacol. Meth.* **22**, 59–63.

Lock, S., Witschi, H. and Plaa, G.L. (1979) *Proc. Soc. Exp. Biol. Med.* **161**, 546–550.

Long, J.A. and Evans, H.M. (1922) *Mem. Univ. Calif.* **6**, 1–148.

Luckey, T.D., Mende, T.J. and Pleasants, J. (1954) *J. Nutr.* **54**, 345–359.

McGee, M.A. and Maronpot, R.R. (1979) *Lab. Anim. Sci.* **29**, 639–642.

McGuill, M.W. and Rowan, A.N. (1989) *ILAR NEWS* **31**, 5–20.

Manzo, L., Gregotti, C., Richelmi, P., DiNucci, A. and Berte, F. (1980) *Chemotherapy* **26**, 164–166.

Martinez, J.R. and Camden, J. (1983) *J. Dent. Res.* **62**, 543–547.

Menaker, L., Sheetz, J.H., Cobb, C.M. and Navia, J. (1974) *Lab. Invest.* **30**, 341–349.

Messow, C. (1991) In: K. Gaertner, (ed.) *Qualitaetskriter-ien der Versuchstierforschung*, pp. 239–269. Weinheim: VCH.

Minasian, H. (1980) *Lab. Anim.* **14**, 205–208.

Mock, E.J. and Frankel, A.I. (1978) *Neuroendocrinology* **26**, 202–207.

Moslen, M.T., Kanz, M.F., Bhatia, J. and Catarau, E.M. (1988) *J. Parent. Ent. Nutr.* **12**, 633–638.

Mulder, G.J., Scholtens, E. and Meijer, D.K. (1981) *Methods Enzymol.* **77**, 21–30.

Myers, R.D., Privette, T.H., Hornsby, R.L. and Swartzwelder, H.S. (1988) *Neurochem. Res.* **13**, 989–995.

Nagel, J.D., Kort, W.J., Varossieau, F. and McVie, J.G. (1989) *Lab. Anim.* **23**, 179–199.

Nagler, R.M., Baum, B.J. and Fox, P.C. (1993) *Radiat. Res.* **136**, 392–396.

Nashed, N. (1975) *Lab. Anim. Sci.* **25**, 225–227.

Nelson, E., Hanano, M. and Levy, G. (1966) *J. Pharmacol. Exp. Ther.* **153**, 159.

Neptun, D.A., Smith, C.N. and Irons, R.D. (1985) *Fundam. Appl. Toxicol.* **5**, 1180–1185.

Nerenberg, S.T. and Zedler, P. (1975) *J. Lab. Clin. Med.* **85**, 523–526.

Nicholas, J.S. and Barron, D.H. (1932) *J. Pharmacol. Exp. Ther.* **46**, 125–129.

Noble, E.S., Wortmann, R.J. and Axelrod, J.A. (1967) *Life Sci.* **6**, 281–291.

Oates, H.F. and Stokes, G.S. (1974) *Clin. Exp. Pharmacol. Physiol.* **6**, 495–501.

Omaye, S.T., Skala, J.H., Gretz, M.D, Schaus, E.E. and Wade, C.E. (1987) *Lab. Anim.* **21**, 261–264.

Unaga, I., Zabielski, K., Minco, H. and Kato, S. (1993) XXXII Congress Int. Union Physiol. Sci., Glasgow, GB, 95, I/P, 83.

Pages, T., Fernandez, J.A., Adan, C., Gamez, A., Viscor, G. and Palacios, L. (1993) *Lab. Anim.* **27**, 171–175.

Paulose, C.S. and Dakshinamurti, K. (1987) *J. Neurosci. Methods* **22**, 141–146.

Pethick, D.W., Rose, R.J., Bryden, W.L. and Gooden, J.M. (1993) *Equine Vet. J.* **25**, 41–44.

Phillipi-Falkenstein, K. and Clarke, M.R. (1992) *Lab. Anim. Sci.* **42**, 83–85.

Phillips, W.A., Stafford, W.W. and Stuut, J. (1973) *Proc. Soc. Exp. Biol. Med.* **143**, 733–735.

Pierzynowski, S.G., Sharma, P., Sobcyk, J., Garwacki, S. and Barej, W. (1992) *Int. J. Pancreatol.* **12**, 121–125.

Plas-Roser, S., Boehm, N. and Aron, C. (1982) *Ann. Endocrinol. Paris* **43**, 53–59.

Plummer, D.T., and Wright, P.J. (1970) *J. Physiol. Lond.* **209** (suppl.), 16P+.

Pohl, M., Collin, E., Bourgoin, S., Clot, A.M., Hamon, M., Cesselin, F. and LeBars, D. (1992) *Neuroscience* **50**, 697–706.

Poole, T. (ed.) (1987) *The UFAW Handbook on The Care & Management of Laboratory Animals*, 6th edn. Essex: Longman Scientific & Technical.

Rabinovici, R., Rudolph, A.S., Vernick, J. and Feuerstein, G. (1994) *Crit. Care Med.* **22**, 480–485.

Rath, L. and Hutchison, M. (1989) *Lab. Anim.* **23**, 163–168.

Rawlings, J.M., Provan, W.M., Wilks, M.F. and Batten, P.L. (1994) *Hum. Exp. Toxicol.* **13**, 123–129.

Reinhardt, W.O. (1945) *Proc. Soc. Exp. Biol. Med.* **58**, 123.

Renaud, S. (1969) *Lab. Anim. Care* **19**, 664–665.

Riley, V. (1960) *Proc. Soc. Exp. Biol. Med.* **104**, 751–754.

Roberts, R.J. and Plaa, G.L. (1966) *Gastroenterology* **50**, 768–771.

Roberts, R.J., Klaassen, C.D. and Plaa, G.L. (1967) *Proc. Soc. Exp. Biol. Med.* **125**, 313–317.

Robinovitch, M.R. and Sreebny, L.M. (1969) *Arch. Oral Biol.* **14**, 935–949.

Rodgers, C.T. (1995) *Lab. Anim.* **29**, 450–455.

Roerig, D.L., Hasegawa, A.T. and Wang, R.I. (1980) *Lab. Anim. Sci.* **30**, 549–551.

Rozenberg, A.E., Bordiukova, I.L. and Markov, Kh.M. (1984) *Bull. Eksp. Biol. Med.* **98**, 121–122.

Salem, H., Grossman, M.H. and Bilbey, D.J. (1963) *J. Pharm. Sci.* **52**, 794–795.

Schneyer, L.H. and Flatland, R.F. (1975) *J. Appl. Physiol. Toxicol.* **10**, 237–244.

Schneyer, C.A. and Hall, H.D. (1965) *Am. J. Physiol.* **209**, 484–488.

Scott, J. and Berry, M.R. (1989) *Alcohol.* **24**, 145–152.

Scott, J.V. and Dzuik, P.J. (1959) *Anat. Rec.* **133**, 655–666.

Seed, J., Chapin, R.E., Clegg, E.D. *et al.* (1996) *Reprod. Toxicol.* **5**, 449–458.

Sen, S. and Phillis, J.W. (1993) *Free Radic. Res. Commun.* **19**, 255–265.

Shirley, D.G., Walter, S.J. and Zewde, T. (1989) *J. Physiol. Lond.* **408**, 833–836.

Slott, V.L., Suarez, J.D. and Parreault, S.D. (1991) *Reprod. Toxicol.* **5**, 449–458.

Smith, C.N., Neptun, D.A. and Irons, R.D. (1986) *Fundam. Appl. Toxicol.* **7**, 658–663.

Society for Experimental Animal Science (1998). Submitted to *Der Tierschutzbeauftragte.*

Stahlin, F.O., Schmid, G., Hempel and Heidland, A. (1978) *Res. Exp. Med. Berl.* **172**, 247–253.

Steer, H.W. (1980) *J. Immunol.* **125**, 1845–1848.

Sugihara, H., Wakabayashi, I., Minami, S., Takahashi, F., Shibasaki, T. and Ling, N. (1988) *Brain Res.* **475**, 128–133.

Takara, E., Takeyama, E., Jimbo, M. and Kitamura, K. (1977) *No. T. Shinkei* **29**, 804–806.

Tatevossian, A. and Wright, W.G. (1966) *J. Dent. Res.* **45**, 979.

Tatevossian, A. and Wright, W.G. (1974) *Arch. Oral Biol.* **19**, 825–827.

Taylor, G.T., Weiss, J., Frechmann, T. and Haller, J. (1985) *J. Reprod. Fertil.* **73**, 323–327.

Temple, P.L. and Kon, S.K. (1937) *Biochem. J.* **31**, 2197–2198.

Thomson, K. and Olesen, O.V. (1986) *Acta Pharmacol. Toxicol. Copenhagen* **59**, 242–248.

Upton, P.K. and Morgan, D.J. (1975) *Lab. Anim.* **9**, 85–91.

Van Herck, H., Baumans, V., Van der Craats, N.R. *et al.* (1992) *Lab. Anim.* **26**, 53–58.

Verbaeys, A., Ringor, S., van Maele, G. and Lameire, N. (1995) *Urol. Res.* **22**, 377–382.

Vissink, A., s-Gravenmade, E.J., Konings, A.W. and Ligeon, E.E. (1989) *Arch. Oral Biol.* **34**, 577–578.

Vreeburg, J.T., VanAndel, M.V., Kort, W.J. and Westbroek, D.L. (1974) *J. Reprod. Fertil.* **41**, 355–359.

Vries, de, J., Verboom, C.N., Bast, A., Pieterse, H. and Stouthamer, A.H. (1977) *Xenobiotica* **7**, 517–520.

Wakerley, J.B. and Drewett, R.F. (1975) *Physiol. Behav.* **15**, 277–281.

Waynforth, H.B. and Flecknell, P.A. (1992) In: *Experimental and Surgical Technique in the Rat*, 2nd edn, pp. 68–99. London: Academic Press.

Weiss, J., Maess, J., Nebendahl, K. and Rossbach, W. (eds) (1996) *Haus- und Versuchstierpflege.* Stuttgart: Gustav Fischer.

Wesslau, C., Jung, K., Fritsch, W. and Kreuschner, H. (1989) *Z. Exp. Chir. Transplant. Kunstliche Organe* **22**, 59–61.

Wiersma, J. and Kastelijn, J. (1985) *J. Endocrinol.* **107**, 285–292.

Winder, W.W. and Yang, H.T. (1987) *J. Appl. Physiol.* **63**, 418–420.

Winsett, O.E., Townsend, C.M. and Thomson, J.C. (1985) *Am. J. Physiol.* **249**, G145–146.

White, W.A. (1971) *Lab. Anim. Sci.* **21**, 401–402.

Withyachumnarnkul, B. and Knigge K.M. (1980) *Neuroendocrinology* **30**, 382–388.

Wolf, R.O. and Kakehashi, S. (1966) *J. Dent. Res.* **45**, 979.

Wolfensohn, S. and Lloyd, M. (1994) In: *Handbook of Laboratory Animal Management and Welfare*, pp. 168–169. Oxford: Oxford University Press.

Wright, B.A. (1970) *Lab. Anim. Care* **20**, 274.

Xin, L., Geller, E.B., Liu-Chen, L.Y., Chen, C. and Adler, M.W. (1997) *J. Pharmacol. Exp. Ther.* **282**, 1055–1063.

Xu, Z.X. and Melethil, S. (1990) *J. Pharmacol. Methods* **24**, 203–208.

Xu, Z.X., Rosenlof, L.K., Selby, J.B. and Jones, R.S. (1992) *J. Surg. Res.* **53**, 520–523.

Yang, H., Wang, Q. and Elmquist, W.F. (1997) *Pharm. Res.* **14**, 1455–1460.

Yoburn, B.C., Morales, R. and Inturrisi, C.E. (1984) *Physiol. Behav.* **33**, 89–94.

Zabielski, R., Lesniewska, V. and Guilloteau, P. (1997) *Reprod. Nutr. Dev.* **37**, 385–399.

CHAPTER 26

Anesthesia, Artificial Ventilation and Perfusion Fixation

Makoto Shibutani
National Institute of Health Sciences, Tokyo, Japan

Anesthesia

Anesthesia in experimental animals is essential for reducing or eliminating the pain and anxiety derived from physiological examination or surgical procedures. Moreover, anesthesia immobilizes the animal and minimizes the risk of injurious animal movements that could affect the outcome of experiment.

For clarity, the following terms are defined: *sedation/tranquilization* refers to a state of mild depression in which the animal is awake and calm; *analgesia* refers to the temporal reduction of pain sensation accompanied by a trance-like neurolepsis, which is a state of depressed awareness of the surroundings; and *anesthesia* refers to the temporal and reversible reduction or elimination of sensory and motor responses. The purpose and extent of treatment should be evaluated in order to determine whether analgesia, sedation or surgical anesthesia would be appropriate for a given procedure.

Full surgical anesthesia includes (1) sedation with decreased perception of external stimuli, (2) analgesia, and (3) suppression of reflex activity and skeletal muscle tone. It is achieved by combining several different drugs, for example a sedative with an analgesic. This type of anesthesia is a balanced combination of sedation, analgesia, hypnosis and muscle relaxation. Because many anesthetic drugs act synergistically on the central nervous system (CNS), drug combinations often allow a reduction of the dose of each agent (anesthetic potentiation) to decrease the risk of toxic reactions and minimize unwanted side-effects.

While anesthetic methods include local and systemic anesthesia, local anesthesia is not usually common in rodents. The depth of anesthesia can be determined empirically by monitoring the depth

Table 26.1 Commonly used preanesthetic agents in rats

Agent	Dosage
Anticholinergic	
Atropine	0.04 mg/kg, i.p., s.c.
Glycopyrrolate	0.5 mg/kg, i.m.
Sedative agent	
Acepromazine	2.5 mg/kg, i.m., i.p.
Diazepam	2.5–5.0 mg/kg i.m., i.p.
Midazolam	3.75 mg/kg, i.p.

Anticholinergics, such as atropine, are useful for increasing the heart rate as a protection against anesthesia-derived **bradycardia**, and for suppressing excess salivation or bronchial mucus secretion. Sedative agents, such as diazepam or other benzodiazepines, are often the choice for calming the animals. This reduces catecholamine release and thus the anesthetic dose needed to promote a more successful induction of anesthesia (Svendsen, 1994). Table 26.1 outlines the representative preanesthetic agents used in rats. Atropine sulfate should always be given to rats 20–30 minutes before anesthesia. Diazepam (Valium, Aposepam, Diazemuls) is the most common benzodiazepine used in rats for its efficient sedative and muscle relaxing properties. Midazolam is a water-soluble benzodiazepine. Xylazine is the most common sedative for veterinary and laboratory animals, but it is not recommended for rats (Green, 1975).

Analgesia

Analgesics are used to produce balanced anesthesia, **neuroleptanalgesia** and relief of postoperative pain. Analgesic application before surgery is particularly useful for potentially invasive procedures. There are three major types of analgesics (Sharp and La Regina, 1997): (1) opiates, such as buprenorphine, butorphanol, morphine, pentazocine and meperidine, which act on the CNS via stimulation of opioid receptors; (2) peripherally acting compounds, such as antihistamines or local anesthetics, which block **nociceptor impulses**; and (3) nonsteroidal anti-inflammatory drugs, such as aspirin or acetaminophen. Opiates are the most effective analgesics and can stimulate or depress the CNS, depending on the dose administered. Depression of the CNS includes analgesia, respiratory depression and sedation. However, overdosing causes excitement.

and rate of breathing, or by simple sensory tests. Breathing should be deep and regular. Eye blinking when the eyelid is touched, foot withdrawal when pinched or a movement in response to a skin pinch are indications of inadequate depth of anesthesia for surgical treatment. Systemic anesthesia affects the body temperature control of the animal, and heat loss from the surgical field may result in a fall in body temperature. Therefore, the animal's body temperature should always be monitored, and application of a heat generator, such as a heating pad, is necessary to maintain the animal's body temperature near to the normal level.

The anesthetic agent is delivered either by injection or inhalation. When working on a metabolism/toxicity study, the rate and species of liver cell microsomal enzymes which may be induced by the anesthetics should be considered before starting the experiment.

Before anesthetic treatment, it is often beneficial to apply preoperative medications including antibiotics and preanesthetic agents; these will serve to lessen the severity of side-effects and to promote xthe anesthetic response. When inhalation anesthesia is required, sedative preanesthetics must be administered before endotracheal intubation.

Preoperative Medication

If there is a real risk of postoperative infection, antibiotics should be administered sufficiently in advance of a surgical procedure in order to obtain optimal blood levels. It is noteworthy that rats are highly resistant to postoperative infection and may require only a single **bolus** dose of antibiotics.

Injectable Anesthesia

The advantage of injectable anesthetics is derived from the simplicity of equipment—only a syringe and needle are required. One caveat, however, involves the slow onset of drug effects, which may lead to difficulty in controlling the level of anesthesia.

Small animals such as rodents have relatively high metabolic rates, and thus require relatively large doses of anesthetics compared to large animals.

When administering an injectable agent to rats, the route of administration, volume and discomfort level to the animal should be considered. Dilution to reduce the discomfort level is necessary when an irritating agent is applied. In rats, intraperitoneal (i.p.) injection is the most common method of administration, although intramuscular (i.m.), subcutaneous (s.c.) and intravenous (i.v.) injections are preferable in certain situations. The rates of absorption and anesthetic effect vary considerably depending on the route of drug delivery. When choosing i.m. or i.p. administration, drugs with a wide safety margin are preferable. When compared to other routes of delivery, the i.v. route usually produces the most rapid and predictable dose/time response of anesthetic action.

Gender differences in anesthetic action are also common, depending upon the rodent species and type of drug. In particular, female rats are more susceptible to drugs like pentobarbital than male rats (Svendsen, 1994). Such gender differences could have profound effects on drug effects and surgical outcomes and must be appropriately compensated for.

Balanced anesthesia, a combination of two or more drugs or anesthetic regimens, is a common procedure when working with injectable anesthesia. Table 26.2 provides information about dosages and anesthetic time for representative anesthetic agents used in rats. There is a long period of unconsciousness following anesthesia, and in this period, the effect of the anesthetic will gradually wear off. In this state, the animals may become excitable and should be administered additional anesthetic if they appear to be waking up.

Thiopental (Pentothal) is classified as a very short-time acting barbiturate, and is the most common induction compound. Due to its alkaline nature, thiopental solution should only be administered intravenously. Because of its highly lipid-soluble nature, a small amount injected rapidly produces a high concentration in the brain and an almost immediate state of deep **narcosis**. The agent is soon redistributed, however, to the nonfat tissues of the body, resulting in a rapid decrease in the depth of narcosis. Thiamylal and hexobarbital are both thiopental analogues.

Pentobarbital (Nembutal, Somnopentyl, Mebumal), a short-acting barbiturate, is the most widely used anesthetic agent in laboratory animals. However, a single application of this drug shows a narrow dose–response range of surgical anesthesia and respiratory depression (Buelke-Sam *et al*., 1978). Moreover, pentobarbital causes hypothermia in rats, and temperature control is always required when using this anesthesia (Wixson *et al.*, 1987).

Neuroleptanalgesia using fentanyl-fluanisone (Hypnorm) (0.3 mL/kg) or fentanyl-droperidol (Innovar vet) (0.2–0.4 mg/kg) in combination with diazepam provides superior anesthesia and muscle relaxation in rats (Svendsen, 1994). The medetomidine/fentanyl cocktail acts to lengthen the duration of anesthesia (Sharp and La Regina, 1997).

Alpha-chloralose and urethane should only be used in experiments involving nonsurvival procedures. Both compounds produce light hypnosis and muscle relaxation without analgesia, and are sometimes used in combination (Svendsen, 1994). In addition, α-chloralose is a valuable choice for

Table 26.2 Agents used for injectable anesthesia in rats

Agent(s)	Dosage	Anesthesia time
Thiopental	20 mg/kg, i.v.	<10 min
Pentobarbital	50 mg/kg (male),	15 min
	25 mg/kg (female), i.v. or i.p.	
Fentanyl-fluanisone +	0.3 ml/kg, i.p.	20 min
diazepam	2.5 mg/kg, i.p.	
Chloral hydrate	300–400 mg/kg, i.p.	1 h
Fentanyl +	0.3 mg/kg, i.p.	>1 h
Medetomidine	0.2–0.3 mg/kg, i.p.	
Urethane	1000–1200 mg/kg, i.p.	>6 h
α-Chloralose	55–65 mg/kg i.p.	8 h

PROCEDURES 514 ANESTHESIA AND PERFUSION FIXATION

Inhalation Anesthesia

Inhalation anesthesia controls the depth of anesthesia precisely by changing the level of gas exposure. The equipment may consist of an air-sealed anesthetic chamber or a sophisticated anesthetic delivery system. An important concept in inhalation anesthesia is the minimum alveolar concentration (MAC). MAC is the alveolar concentration of a given compound at a pressure of 1 atm, which will prevent response to painful stimuli in 50% of the animals/patients in a group. The lower the MAC, the more potent the anesthetic drug. Generally, levels around 1.2–1.3 MAC are suitable if no preanesthetic analgesics have been administered.

The use of the anesthetic chamber gives only minimal control over anesthetic administration. The system involves placing the animals in an isolated environment where the volatile anesthetic agent evaporates. The anesthetic agent and the rat should be separated to avoid direct contact with the irritating agent. This technique provides very short-term anesthesia applicable primarily to quick procedures. An anesthetic chamber can be assembled using a large transparent container, anesthetic-absorbent material, and a wire mesh barrier between the animal and the liquid phase anesthetic (Figure 26.1). The rat is placed in the container where it becomes anesthetized as it inhales the volatized anesthetic. After removal from the anesthetic chamber, additional anesthetic can be administered during treatment by placing the 50-mL conical tube stuffed with anesthetic-soaked material, such as cotton wool or a paper towel, over the rat's face. The rat will inhale the supplementary anesthetic as it breathes. Prolonging anesthesia with this method is not recommended because of the difficulty in controlling the depth of anesthesia and of risk to personnel by exposure to the anesthetic gas.

Endotracheal intubation must be applied in order to deliver adequate anesthetic gas for longer durations. Endotracheal catheters with adapters for breathing tubes are commercially available. Otherwise, a 16-gauge intravenous polyethylene catheter can be used with a flexible guidewire for intubation (Alpert et al., 1982; Thet, 1983). Start with the rat on its back, its nose extended slightly over the edge of the table, then fix the nose on the table by pulling the upper jaw from below with an elastic band behind the incisors. The guidewire can then be placed in the trachea over the epiglottis. The intravenous catheter is threaded over the guidewire.

physiological experiments which require a stable cardiovascular parameters (Brown et al., 1989). Urethane is a **carcinogen**, and therefore may present a health risk to the personnel. It lengthens **thrombin** and **activated partial thromboplastin times** (Sharp and La Regina, 1997).

Ketamine is a **dissociative anesthetic** and is not recommended as an anesthetic for rats (Svendsen, 1994). Although subcutaneous application of etorphine hydrochloride (0.0125–0.05 mg/kg), acepromazine (0.04–0.16 mg/kg) and atrophine sulfate (0.075–0.3 mg/kg), could be effective in rats, possibly severe respiratory depression may occur, inducing unacceptable hypoxia and **acidosis** (Svendsen and Carter, 1985).

A number of anesthetic antagonists are available for controlling the magnitude of anesthetic effects in animals that appear to be overdosed. Butorphanol or nalbuphine act as antagonist of fentanyl. Yohimbine or atipamizole antagonize medetomidine (Sharp and La Regina, 1997).

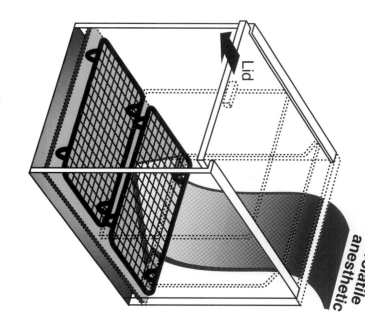

Figure 26.1 Anesthetic chamber, consisting of a transparent container, anesthetic absorbent material, and a wire mesh barrier between the animal and the liquid phase anesthetic.

While holding the catheter in place, the guidewire is removed and the catheter is attached to the anesthetic circuit. Illumination with fiberoptic lights is helpful for successful intubation. The anesthetic circuit deadspace must be minimized by placing the adapter close to the mouth, since the deadspace will result in insufficient gas exchange, which can cause suffocation.

Essentially, anesthesia with a gas delivery system requires the supply of O_2 to the lung alveolar membrane, the removal of CO_2 from the lungs, and the supply of anesthetic gas at a controlled pressure to the alveolar membrane. Since most anesthetics depress the respiratory center and therefore cause a reduction in alveolar ventilation, artificial ventilation is crucial in order to provide stable alveolar ventilation with normal oxygenation and acid–base balance.

Anesthetic delivery systems are classified as: (1) to and fro systems; (2) open systems; (3) semi-open systems; and (4) closed systems. The to and fro system consists of a soda-lime CO_2 absorber with a pop-off valve and a closed rebreathing bag into which the inspired gas is introduced. This system provides a minimized supply of anesthetic gas. The open or semi-open system vents a large waste of anesthetic gas into the atmosphere with considerable risks to personnel. In addition, if respiratory arrest of the animal occurs, assisted ventilation is difficult to give with this system. The closed circle absorption system is most widely used, because it removes CO_2 efficiently and it is easy to control inspired anesthetic concentrations. Assisted ventilation can also be applied by manually compressing the rebreathing bag.

The agents used for inhalation anesthesia are listed in Table 26.3.

Halothane is a fluorinated hydrocarbon which is a nonirritating, clear liquid. It is a most popular volatile anesthetic for surgery. Anesthesia can be induced initially with 2–3% vapor in sedated rats, and can then be maintained with a 0.5% concentration. Rats will recover 10–20 minutes after removal of halothane. It causes immediate respiratory depression, hypotension and sometimes induces ventricular fibrillation due to an increase in myocardial sensitivity to epinephrine. Inhaled halothane is metabolized in the liver, resulting in a marked induction of liver cell microsomal enzymes. Therefore, this anesthetic is not recommended for drug metabolism/toxicity studies. Also halothane should never be used with an open system anesthetic machine.

Enflurane is a chemically stable fluorinated ether with physical properties similar to those of halothane. Anesthesia can be induced with 3–5% vapor, and can be maintained at a concentration of 1–3%. Respiratory depression and acidosis are the main risks with this anesthesic. Liver metabolism of enflurane is very poor, and this agent is largely eliminated via the lung. This could be of advantage in studies on drug metabolism and toxicity.

Isoflurane is related chemically to enflurane. Respiratory depression is slightly more severe than with halothane, but there is less cardiovascular depression (Eisele *et al.*, 1986). This anesthetic is even less well metabolized by the liver than enflurane, and therefore, it is suitable for the metabolism/toxicity studies.

Methoxyflurane is a halogenated ethyl methyl ether. Respiratory and cardiovascular suppression is less remarkable than with halothane. This

Table 26.3 Agents for inhalation anesthesia

Agent	Vapor pressure	% Saturation at 22°C	MAC (v/v %)	Blood–gas partition coefficient	Induction/ recovery	% to be metabolized
Halothane	242	32	0.95	2.3	Fast	15
Enflurane	171	23	2.21	1.9	Fast	2–5
Isoflurane	240	32	1.20–1.57	1.3	Fast	<1
Methoxyflurane	23	3	0.22	13	Slow	50–70
Diethyl ether	443	58	3.0	15	Slow	5–10
Nitrous oxide	39 500	100	250	0.4	Fast	–

compound has very potent analgesic properties but a slow rate of induction, and therefore is best used after induction with a short-acting injectable agent or in combination with halothane. Anesthesia using an inhalation chamber is not recommended with this compound (Heidt, 1978; Watson and McLeod, 1978; Bett et al., 1980).

Diethyl ether is a colorless volatile fluid. Its vapor is very inflammable and much heavier than air, and is therefore likely to accumulate on the floor. It is irritable to the respiratory tract. The blood sugar concentration rises due to the increase in epinephrine release (Svendsen, 1994). Although diethyl ether is a safe anesthetic, its inflammable nature diminishes its usefulness.

Nitrous oxide is a colorless gas at normal air pressure. Its anesthetic potential is poor, but it characteristically reduces the MAC for halothane, methoxyflurane, isoflurane and the dose of pentobarbital. Nitrous oxide has little or no adverse effects on any organ, and is therefore useful in combination with other anesthetics. It should be used in a mixture with oxygen not exceeding 50%.

Fluovac (International Market Supply, UK) is a system that both supplies the anesthetic and scavenges excess vapors simultaneously by the application of a specially designed double coaxial mask. This system does not require tracheal intubation, and its anesthetic scavenging unit enables the efficient adsorption of anesthetic vapors from the work area, thus protecting personnel from exposure. This system also allows optimal access to the animal and is especially valuable for microsurgery.

Recovery from Anesthesia

There are several risks for animals recovering from anesthesia. At the transition between the unconscious and conscious levels, rats may undergo a period of excitement, which may itself result in self-inflicted injury if they are left unattended. It is important to put each anesthetized animal in a separate cage/room, otherwise a recovering animal may attack the unconscious animals and kill them. The external temperature should be controlled as anesthetic treatment often causes hypothermia. A temperature control unit or cabinet is commercially available. For rats, the optimum recovery temperature should be about 35°C.

Artificial Ventilation

Artificial ventilation is essential for maintaining the normal pO_2, pCO_2, and acid–base balance of the blood. Artificial ventilation in laboratory animals is useful for sequential analyses of biological parameters, especially for the investigation of kinetic analyses such as in brain metabolism. As a rule, artificial ventilation should be used whenever physiological experiments are performed on anesthetized animals. Anesthetic gas inhalation can also be applicable for the ventilation system. A basic system of artificial ventilation consists of a ventilator and a single breathing tube. The breathing tube is connected to the animal's airway via an endotracheal tube, and the distal end of the breathing tube is connected to the inspiratory/expiratory ports of the ventilator in order to supply/exhaust gases via a T-piece adapter. The airway pressure monitor tube is connected with the breathing tube/endotracheal tube nearest to the animal airway.

The ventilator system is designed to control respiration by adjusting the respiration frequency of breathing, the inspiratory:expiratory (I:E) ratio, and the tidal volume. The inspired fresh gas can be from any source, such as an anesthetic gas, or air/O_2 mixture, depending on the anesthetic method selected. This gas can be warmed and humidified before reaching the animal. Intrapulmonary exposure of some test chemicals/compounds is also possible when using a vaporizer unit.

Procedure for Setting Up a Ventilation System

There are several different types of ventilator systems available for setting up a common system, such as that shown in Figure 26.2.

1 Connect a high-pressure (normally 4 bar) gas source (piped gas, air compressor or cylinder air or O_2) to the inlet port of the ventilator. If the ventilator uses an air pump to produce high pressure, reduce the pressure of the source gas using a Douglas bag before connecting the inlet port.

2 Connect the breathing tube with the gas outlet port of the ventilator using a T-piece adapter. Connect the anesthetic gas vaporizer (or anesthetic machine) between the outlet port and the breathing tube.

Table 26.4 Ventilator settings for rats

Body weight (g)	Tidal volume (mL)	Rate (breaths/min)	Flow (L/min)	Inspiratory time (s)
100	0.90	70	0.13	0.4
200	1.50	60	0.18	0.5
400	3.00	50	0.30	0.6

Table 26.4 shows the representative ventilator settings for rats. The setting values such as flow rate and inspiratory time may be determined using the calculation chart included in the instruction manual.

7   Block the outlet port of the T-piece adapter and adjust the airway pressure control (tidal volume) until the peak airway pressure display reads approximately 10–15 cmH₂O. Wait for a couple of breaths between adjustments to allow the airway pressure to stabilize.

8   Connect the animal to the ventilator using an endotracheal tube. (Details concerning tracheal intubation are described in Anesthesia.)

9   Observe the chest movement and adjust the maximum airway pressure control for normal and adequate chest movement.

Procedure for Weaning an Animal from Anesthesia

Weaning an animal off artificial ventilation can be a harmful experience for both animal and personnel. The following procedure describes a typical weaning process:

1   Remove any anesthetic agent in the respiratory gas flow until only oxygen is flowing.

2   Slowly decrease the airway pressure by adjusting the maximum airway control (tidal volume control) for several minutes, or slowly decrease the rate of ventilation (frequency).

3   When spontaneous breathing starts, the airway pressure or frequency can be further reduced until full spontaneous breathing is observed. The fresh gas supply should be increased to twice the minute volume to prevent it from being breathed in again. When an adequate level of spontaneous breathing is observed, the ventilator can be disconnected. After a few minutes of sustained spontaneous breathing the endotracheal tube may be removed.

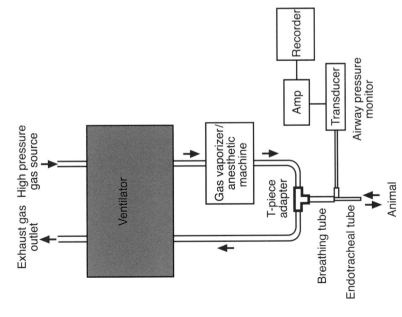

Figure 26.2 Simplified circuit of the ventilator system.

3   Connect the other side of the T-adapter with the gas-scavenging unit, such as the inlet port of the ventilator. Gas scavenging minimizes harm to personnel when using chemical or anesthetic gases.

4   Connect the airway pressure monitoring line from the top of the breathing tube to the signal transducer unit.

5   Turn on the ventilator and set the gas flow using either the ventilator flowmeter or the flowmeter located on the anesthetic machine.

6   Adjust the frequency and I:E ratio control to match the breathing rate of the animal. An I:E ratio of 1:1 or 1:2 will normally be sufficient.

Perfusion Fixation

Perfusion fixation refers to the preservation and stabilization of macromolecular structures within animal tissues by the perfusion throughout the vasculature system of a chemical fixative. Perfusion is essential for the ultrastructural study of fragile tissues, particularly central and peripheral nervous tissues. The removal of tissues without prior perfusion fixation almost invariably produces artifacts, which can adversely affect further scientific analyses. For example, nonperfused CNS tissue may undergo **anoxic artifacts** and **'dark cell'** formation. Typically, the animals are anesthetized and perfused intracardially (through the left ventricle) with an exsanguinating solution, followed by an appropriate fixative.

A number of fixatives and concentrations are available. Because different fixatives preserve molecular or structural components of tissues to varying degrees, it is usually necessary to optimize the choice of fixative depending upon the type of tissue and the components of that tissue to be analyzed. We have always preferred to use ice-cold exsanguinating and fixative solutions in order to preserve subcellular structures, although many laboratories prefer to use solutions at room temperature as penetration into the tissue is more rapid. This latter has some disadvantages, including evaporation of the fixative and consequent risk to personnel and should be performed under a fume hood if possible. Hayat (1981) has given a comprehensive overview of the advantages of perfusion fixation and its availability in electron microscopic study.

In general, 3.75% formalin (stock formalin diluted 1:9) or sometimes 4% (stock diluted 1:8.4) in 0.1 M phosphate buffer is the fixative of choice for

light microscopic observation. For electron microscopy studies, 1–3% formaldehyde (prepared from paraformaldehyde powder) mixed with 0.1–4% glutaraldehyde in 0.1 M phosphate or cacodylate buffer improves the preservation of membrane structures. The concentration required for each fixative may vary, especially for immunohistochemical labeling, where the characteristics of the primary antibody selected as well as the target antigen to be labeled become critical.

Perfusion of fixative without prior flushing with exsanguinating solution may risk intravascular coagulation of the blood which will then ruin the perfusion. Anticoagulants, such as heparin (1000 units/L), are often included in the exsanguinating solution to improve perfusion efficiency. For electron microscopic studies, 0.1 M phosphate buffer is superior to physiological saline (0.9% NaCl) as an exsanguinating solution. Furthermore, the addition of 7% sucrose to the solution is recommended for the fixation of nervous tissues. Perfusion should be performed under physiological pressure (approximately 90–120 mmHg) perfusion pumps are also commercially available). Too little pressure or too much may lead to incomplete perfusion or perfusion-derived artifacts respectively.

Materials

The following materials are required for perfusion fixation:

- Suitable chemical fume hood or vented necropsy table.
- Exsanguinating solution, usually saline (0.9% NaCl) or 0.1 M phosphate buffer.
- Fixative for perfusion.
- Two perfusion bottles, for the exsanguinating solution or fixative. Peristaltic pumps are also available; their flow rate can be calibrated and set for 35–40 mL/min (adult rat) or 5–10 mL/min (neonatal rat).
- Chemically resistant tubings (Tygon or equivalent), each leading from the bottom of the exsanguinating and fixing solution bottles to a three-way (Y-piece) adapter. The outlet side of the adapter leads to the perfusion catheter by tubing. A stopcock valve is connected between the bottle and the inlet side of the Y-piece adapter. When using a peristaltic pump, it is connected between the outlet side of the adapter and the perfusion catheter.

There is an unique ventilator system (Zoovent CWC600AP, International Market Supply, UK) by which the animal can breathe spontaneously at any time without the stress of 'fighting' the ventilator. The principle is to use a pressure driven single breathing tube in which the respiratory gas is introduced near to the animal's airway while a jet gas outlet in a more distal part of the tube drives the respiratory gas into the lungs. The jet driving gas is independent of the respiratory gas, and therefore, the breathing system is open to the atmosphere at all times.

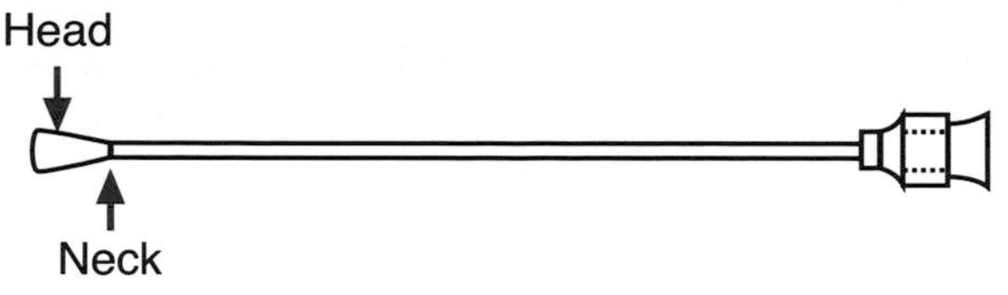

Head

Neck

Figure 26.3 Intragastric catheter valuable as a perfusion catheter.

3 Wipe the thoracic and abdominal regions with water or alcohol to reduce the inconvenience of loose hair.

4 Pinch up the skin overlying the sternal xyphoid process with the forceps and cut through the skin on both thoracic and abdominal cavity with surgical scissors.

5 Cut the abdominal wall laterally along both posterior margins of the rib bones, and then cut the diaphragm muscle along the ventral line of attachment to the thoracic wall.

6 Disclose the thoracic cavity by cutting upwards bilaterally along the rib wall.

7 Remove the mediastinal tissue between heart and sternum, and expose the heart from the pericardium.

8 Clamp the xyphoid process to hold the free rib wall out of the way using a hemostat.

9 Separate the aorta from the pulmonary trunk at the base of the heart using electron microscopic forceps with vented tips, and bring a surgical thread to encircle the aorta close to its origin.

10 Make a small incision through the apex of the left ventricle to make a cannulation hole into the ventricle. The ventricular septum should be kept intact.

11 Insert the perfusion catheter through the ventricular hole into the proximal portion of the aorta and fix it by clamping its neck over the aortic wall with a previously inserted surgical thread. It is important to locate the tip of the catheter just above the aortic opening. When inserted too far into the aorta, the tip may become blocked. For neonatal rats, a sharp needle may be used to introduce the perfusion media, this being inserted into the left ventricle instead of the aorta and then either held in place or clamped.

12 Make a small incision in the right auricle to let the perfusate escape.

Perfusion Procedure

1 The perfusion apparatus must be checked prior to surgery by first running fixative through the tubing to remove any air bubbles from the circuit, then switching the valve to the exsanguinating solution until the fixative is completely flushed out of the tubing leading to the perfusion catheter. Bubbles or fixative in the initial flush will obstruct the vascular bed of the subject, giving poor perfusion.

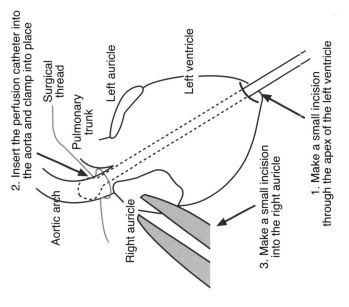

Aortic arch

Pulmonary trunk

Left auricle

Left ventricle

Surgical thread

Right auricle

1. Make a small incision through the apex of the left ventricle

3. Make a small incision into the right auricle

Figure 26.4 Simplified surgical scheme of perfusion fixation.

2. Insert the perfusion catheter into the aorta and clamp into place

- Surgical scissors, iris scissors, surgical forceps, electron microscopic forceps with vented tips, hemostats, etc.
- Perfusion catheters, 18–22 gauge for adult rats; 26–28 gauge for neonatal rats. An intragastric catheter with a spherical head is recommended as a perfusion catheter (Figure 26.3).
- Surgical thread.

Surgical Preparation of Subject
(Figure 26.4)

1 Administer sodium pentobarbital, 25–50 mg/kg of body weight by intraperitoneal injection. Verify that the animal is in deep anesthesia before proceeding with the surgical preparation.

2 Place and fix the anesthetized rat on its back on a cork plate in a stainless steel tray. The tray should be tilted slightly with a drain hole over a collection vessel for disposal of perfusates as hazardous waste.

Table 26.5 Fixing agents used in perfusion fixation

Agent	Concentration	Fixing speed	Constituent to be preserved
Glutaraldehyde	2–4%	0.5 mm/h	Proteins Carbohydrates Nucleic acids
Formalin	3.5–4%	~2.5 mm/h	Proteins Nucleic acids

2 When the perfusion catheter is secured in the heart, flush it for up to 1 minute to exsanguinate the animal (usually about 40–50 mL of solution for an adult rat; 10 mL for a neonatal rat). Excessive flushing risks loss of water-soluble antigens.

3 Turn the valve so that the fixative flows through the line.

4 Perfuse for 10–15 min with fixative: 400–600 mL (adult rat), 50–100 mL (neonatal rat).

5 Remove the tissue to be analyzed and postfix in the fixative or other solution as desired. For electron microscopy, brain tissue can be left in the skull overnight before removing it.

6 Turn the valve back to the setting for exsanguinating solution and flush thoroughly.

Fixatives

Fixatives are composed of fixing agent(s), a buffer, and sometimes additives. Fixing agents used in perfusion fixation are usually aldehydes, which act by binding the aldehydic part of the molecule with tissue components, particularly proteins, by cross-linking and thus stabilizing them. Table 26.5 lists aldehydes commonly used in perfusion fixation.

Because of its dialdehydic nature, glutaraldehyde cross-links protein molecules effectively, but as a result penetration into the tissue is relatively slow. On the other hand, formaldehyde cross-links less strongly due to its monoaldehyde nature and, being a much smaller molecule than glutaraldehyde, it penetrates tissue more quickly. For this reason, it is preferable to use a mixture of both glutaraldehyde and formalin (frequently referred to as formaldehyde which is, in fact, a gas) in the correct buffer for electron microscopic analysis. Yet another alternative is to use the two fixatives sequentially. Formalin from a 40% stock solution is not suitable for ultrastructural analysis because the methanol, included in the solution as a stabilizing agent, destroys the ultrastructural conformation.

The buffer solution determines the pH and osmolarity of the fixative. The fixative pH should be maintained in the range 7.2–7.4, and the osmotic pressure of the buffer should be isotonic with that of the tissues. The average osmolarity of mammalian tissues is 400 mOsm. For the rat nervous system, this is 320 mOsm (Karlsson and Schultz, 1965; Glauert, 1975). The tonicity of the fixative can be judged by examining the mitochondrial structure, which is particularly sensitive to osmotic changes (Bagnell et al., 1995). Nonelectrolytes, such as sucrose, polyvinyl-pyrrolidone or dextran, may be added to the buffer to adjust osmolarity. Hayat (1981, 1986) provided useful tables of osmolarities for buffers, fixatives, and additives. Use of an osmometer is strongly recommended as mistakes can be made in dilutions as well as in checking the actual measurement.

Secondary fixation with ice-cold osmium tetroxide is necessary to improve contrast. In practice, the tissue is cut into small pieces (1–2 mm cubes) after perfusion fixation, and then put into fresh fixative for a further hour at 4°C or room temperature depending on normal lab practice. After washing with ice-cold buffer solution, postfix the tissue blocks with 1–2% osmium tetroxide for 1–2 hours at 4°C.

References

Alpert, M., Goldstein, D. and Triner, L. (1982) Lab. Anim. Sci. 32, 78–79.

Bagnell, R., Madden, V., Langaman, C. and Suzuki, K. (1995) In: Chang, L.W. and Slikker, W. Jr. (eds) Approaches and Methods, pp. 81–98.

Bett, N.J., Hynd, J.W. and Green, C.J. (1980) *Lab. Anim.* **14**, 225–228.

Brown, J.N., Thorne, P.R. and Nuttall, A.L. (1989) *Lab. Anim. Sci.* **39**, 142–148.

Buelke-Sam, J., Holson, J.F., Bazare, J.J. and Young, J.F. (1978) *Lab. Anim. Sci.* **28**, 157–162.

Eisele, P.H., Woodle, E.S., Hunter, G.C., Talken, L. and Ward, R.E. (1986) *Lab. Anim. Sci.* **36**, 402–405.

Glauert, A.M. (1975) In: Glauert, A.M. (ed.) *Practical Methods in Electron Microscopy.* New York: North-Holland.

Green, C.J. (1975) *Lab. Anim.* **9**, 161–178.

Hayat, M.A. (1981) *Fixation for Electron Microscopy.* New York: Academic Press.

Hayat, M.A. (1986) *Basic Techniques for Transmission Electron Microscopy.* New York: Academic Press.

Heidt, G.A. (1978) *Lab. Anim. Sci.* **28**, 212–213.

Karlsson, U.L. and Schultz, R.L. (1965) *J. Ultrastruct. Res.* **12**, 160–186.

Sharp, P.E. and La Regina, M.C. (1997) In: Suckow, M.A. (ed.) *A Volume in The Laboratory Animal Pocket Reference Series, The Laboratory Rat,* pp. 101–113. Boca Raton: CRC Press.

Svendsen, P. (1994) In: Svendsen, P. and Hau, J. (eds) *Handbook of Laboratory Animal Science,* Vol. 1, *Selection and Handling of Animals in Biomedical Research,* pp. 311–337. Boca Raton: CRC Press.

Svendsen, P. and Carter, A.M. (1985) *Acta Pharmacol. Toxicol. Copenhagen* **57**, 1–7.

Thet, L.A. (1983) *Lab. Anim. Sci.* **33**, 368–369.

Watson, R.T. and McLeod, K. (1978) *Arch. Otolaryngol.* **104**, 179–180.

Wixson, S.K., White, W.J., Hughes, H.C., Jr., Lang, C.M. and Marshall, W.K. (1987) *Lab. Anim. Sci.* **37**, 743.

CHAPTER 27

Experimental Surgery

René Remie
Department of Laboratory Animal Science, Solvay Pharmaceuticals, Weesp and University Center for Pharmacy, Groningen University, Groningen, The Netherlands

General Principles

The Surgeon

From the outset, the study of surgical and especially microsurgical techniques makes many mental and physical demands on the personnel involved. Attention to detail and intense concentration are extremely important when learning new techniques. The surgeon must develop the ability to concentrate on the visual image, as seen through the microscope, and become familiar with the magnified objects. Normally direct eye-to-hand contact is used but under these circumstances an awareness is needed of the fact that even simple movements in a significantly smaller world are more complex than they are 'life-size'. Under the operating microscope not only are the objects enlarged, but at the same time any movements are magnified between 8 and 40 times. In addition, the physical ability required to coordinate hand movement decreases in proportion to the magnification.

Individual preparation

Some tips for the novice surgeon are listed here.

- Make sure that the environment is quiet. A dedicated operating theatre is ideal.
- Try to avoid any mental stress.
- Make sure that the operating table is at the correct height, giving adequate support to your arms. Sit upright to avoid strain injury to shoulders, neck and back.
- Plan your exercises. You need to be able to devote all your time to the exercise. Make sure that you have no appointments, and that you cannot be disturbed by telephone calls etc. It is unrealistic to expect to perform well when your attention is divided or you act hastily.
- Try to avoid heavy physical exertion during the 24 hours preceding the surgical exercise, as this will interfere with your fine muscular control and will probably increase your tremor.
- Do not change any habits relating to your intake of coffee; a radical increase or decrease will increase your tremor.

- Do not become discouraged when something has gone wrong. If you encounter a difficulty, evaluate it and try to correct it before you continue. Do not let frustration become your greatest enemy.

- Do not work for too long at a stretch. Micro-surgery is very fatiguing. If possible, take a 10-minute break every hour, otherwise you will lose concentration and your coordination and learning ability will be reduced.

Planning

Planning and preparation of an operation are important, and often underestimated. Ideally, an operation should commence in the morning, in order to provide optimal postoperative care. The same is true for surgery at the end of the week, unless proper attention can be provided over the weekend.

Before starting an operation, make sure that everything needed is at your disposal. It is most frustrating to have to leave the operating theatre to search for things you require, not to mention the break it causes in the aseptic technique. For detailed instructions the reader is referred to Acland (1980) and Remie et al. (1990b).

Anatomy

A thorough knowledge of the rat's anatomy is essential. Do not start an operation until you are familiar with all the structures in the area of interest. Use the operating microscope to look in detail at all kinds of tissue and learn how to handle the tissues with your instruments. Animals killed after an experiment make good learning material. For example, try dissecting some blood vessels to see how much tension they can withhold. As you will see, the majority of functions during microdissection are performed by slight pronation and supination movements of the fingers and forearm. Small spreading movements parallel to the blood vessel (or other structures) will prevent tearing of branches. During dissection, try to use atraumatic techniques, i.e. do not grab the whole thickness of the blood vessel between the jaws of your forceps as this will cause irreparable damage. Try to pick up vessels only by their outer layer, the adventitia. The less damage you cause to the blood vessels and the surrounding tissues the better. In addition to the work on the anatomy that you will find in this handbook (Chapters 13 to 15), it may be useful to study Greene's work (1963) and the work of Hebel and Stromberg (1986).

Surgical asepsis

Considering the ubiquity of microorganisms, it is fortunate that only a small percentage are capable of causing diseases. It is against these pathogens that numerous methods of sanitization, disinfection and sterilization have been developed. Although the rat has a remarkable resistance to the development of wound infection it is, however, important not to neglect aseptic technique for surgical procedures.

Surgery in the laboratory rat should be governed by the same basic principles as those for surgery on human beings. Surgical asepsis can be defined as the body of techniques designed to maintain an object or area in a condition as free of all microorganisms as possible. Unfortunately, the opinion among researchers that aseptic technique is a waste of time and money is still widespread.

Surgery on laboratory animals nowadays is often characterized by the use of so-called 'clean technique', meaning that the principles of aseptic surgery are completely neglected during procedures on small rodents. Most researchers gloss over these shortcomings by saying that a high percentage of animals remains alive after the operation. However, it is not the fact that the animals stay alive but rather the fact that they can be used as reliable models giving useful results that should be the argument.

Asepsis during surgery is far more important than is generally realized (Bradfield et al., 1992). Unfortunately, the literature about this topic is limited (Waynforth, 1993), probably due to the fact that the untimely death of an animal is seldom connected to the surgical conditions. As a consequence, more animals than is strictly necessary are often used. Furthermore, the consequences on the welfare aspects of the animals are unknown.

Another outcome of bad aseptic technique is the reduction of long-term patency rates of inserted cannulae (Popp and Brennan, 1981). In our hands, permanent jugular vein cannulae can remain patent for up to six months when both cannulae and surgical instruments are sterilized before use, in addition to some standard precautions (see below). When using nonsterile cannulae and instruments, the patency is drastically reduced to between 1 and 2 weeks. In addition, the recovery of the animal is delayed and the time needed to return to the preoperative weight is extended.

A high level of aseptic technique can be achieved using the following procedures:

- Sterilization (generally achieved by autoclaving) of surgical instruments and all materials to be permanently implanted in the animal.
- The use of an assistant to help you during surgery.
- The use of proper scrub when washing hands, e.g. Betadine scrub (a polyvinylpyrolidone-iodine solution), Hibi-scrub (chlorhexidine solution).
- Subsequent disinfection with Sterillium (isopropanol, *n*-propanol and ethylhexadecyl-dimethyl-ammoniumethylsulfate).
- The use of sterile suture materials, hypodermic needles and syringes and sterile solutions (saline and heparin).
- A clean operating area, including a silicon rubber plate (30 × 25 × 1 cm) which can easily be sterilized or disinfected using 0.5% of an aqueous chlorhexidine solution or 70% ethanol.
- The avoidance of talking, sneezing and coughing, and unnecessary body movements during surgery.

It is also important to be aware of what is sterile and what is nonsterile. Needless to say, only sterile things may be touched by the surgeon. In case of doubt, consider the object as contaminated.

A wealth of information concerning good surgical practice (GSP) can be found in the work of Tracy (1994).

In addition to the above mentioned precautions, animals can be administered an antibiotic in case a break of aseptic technique is likely to occur or when the total operating time exceeds 180 minutes. A single dosage of 150 mg/kg amoxycillin subcutaneously (s.c.) or ampicillin (150 mg/kg s.c.) given 10 min prior to the operation will give adequate protection against possible infections.

Surgical instruments

In order to proceed with surgery on the rat, it is essential to possess your own set of instruments. These should be of a good quality and must be well maintained. Do not begin with old, worn-out or obsolete equipment. Once you have acquired your set, do not lend it out.

A set should consist of the following:

Microsurgical instruments

- Two jeweller's forceps (No. 5, Dumont)
- One jeweller's forceps 45°-angled (Dumont)
- A vessel stretcher or vessel dilator

- A needle holder (Barraquer-type), without a lock
- A pair of ring-handled dissecting scissors with gently curved blades
- A pair of fine 45°-angled iridectomy scissors (Wecker-type)
- Vessel clamps including a clamp applicator:
  One 10-mm double approximator (Acland)
  Two 12-mm single clamps (Acland, Biemer or Heifetz)

Other instruments

- Anatomical or dissecting forceps (straight)
- Anatomical or dissecting forceps (90°-angled)
- A pair of fine-toothed forceps
- A pair of ring-handled scissors (straight, sharp/sharp or sharp/blunt)
- A needle holder (Matthieu or Castroviejo)
- An artery forceps, baby-Mosquito or micro-Halsted clamp
- Towel clips (Backhaus)
- Baby Dieffenbach Serrefines (bulldog hemostatic clamps)
- Bulldog clamp, modified to resemble a Satinsky vascular clamp
- An instrument case.

Microsurgical instruments should not be too long, 11–12 cm is suitable. An advantage of the Barraquer needle holder is that the round grips allow easy rotating movements. Clamps can be divided into venous and arterial types, the latter having a higher shutting strength. It is necessary to be careful with clips that have a very high shutting strength, as they may damage the vessel wall.

Microsurgical instruments are very delicate and require careful handling and cleaning. Always clean your instruments immediately after surgery with tapwater. Every now and then you should clean your instruments by placing them in an ultrasonicator. Before the instruments are stored they must be dried and oiled using standard instrument oil.

Holding the instrument

The instruments should be held in a pencil grip. The relative positions of the hands to the instruments are shown in Figure 27.1. Remember that only your fingertips move, while the rest of your hand should rest on the operating table. If you neglect these basic rules you will soon find out that you make unwanted movements, inhibiting your work.

For further information about the handling of the

Table 27.1 Types of cannula

Cannula type	Length (cm)	Inner and outer diameters (mm)	Rings (cm from tip)	Tip inner and outer diameters (mm)
Jugular vein cannula	10	0.51 × 0.94	4.2	
Bile cannula (prox.)	18	0.51 × 0.94	0.7 and 5	
Bile cannula (dist.)	18	0.51 × 0.94	0.7 and 5	0.30 × 0.64
Duodenum cannula	18	0.51 × 0.94	0.5, 0.7 and 5	
Iliolumbar cannula	18	0.51 × 0.94	0.7 and 5	0.30 × 0.64
Portal vein cannula	18	0.51 × 0.94	0.7 and 5	

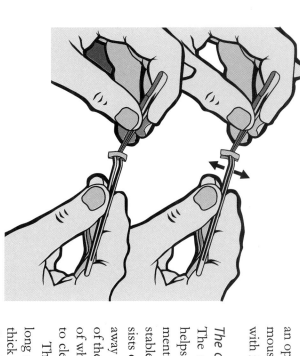

Figure 27.1 The tissue is dissected by repeatedly spreading the tips of the forceps.

General Techniques

Preparation of Cannulae and Other Materials

Cannulae

Permanent cannulae used in the rat are preferably made of silicon rubber. Silicon tubing is rather flexible, causes hardly any immunity problems, and can be sterilized easily. As a routine we use Silastic or Siliclear Medical-Grade tubing from Dow Corning or Degania Silicone respectively. These tubings are available in various sizes. Table 27.1 lists the types of

nonmicrosurgical instruments, the reader is referred to the works of Anderson and Romfh (1980), Kirk (1978) and Wind and Rich (1987).

Standby equipment

The electrical clipper

Rats have very thin hairs and not all electrical clippers can be used to shave them. An efficient and reliable clipper is the one from Aesculap, the Favorita 11 (GT 104). This clipper has a large range of cutter-heads, of which the most suitable for rats is the one with 1/20 mm clipping height.

The light source

A portable cold-illumination lighting system will be very effective in case you can do without the use of

an operating microscope. Proper lighting is of enormous help for surgery. Do not start an operation with inadequate lighting.

The operating table

The operating table is of major importance as it helps you in your struggle against unwanted movements. The table should be placed on an extremely stable frame to minimize vibrations. Our table consists of a main part in which two half circles are cut away in order to give maximum support to the arms of the surgeon(s), and two small panels. The material of which the table is made must be smooth and easy to clean (e.g. PVC).

The rat board should be approximately 30 cm long and 25 cm wide. It is best made of 7–10-mm-thick silicon rubber, as this is easily cleaned and disinfected, sterilized if necessary, and it readily accepts needles to secure the instruments and clamps.

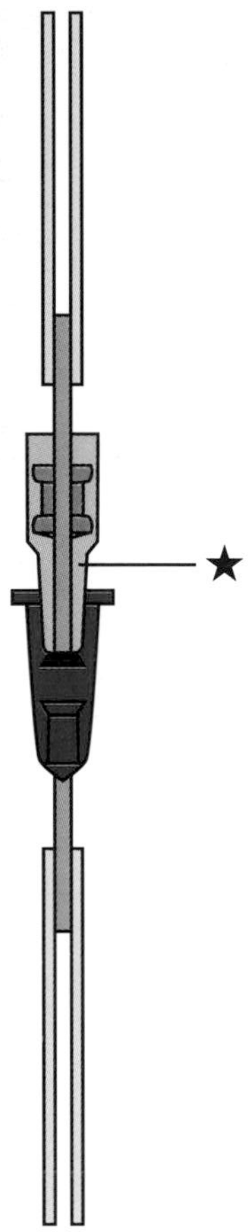

Figure 27.2 A swivel made out of a 1-mL syringe and two hypodermic 20-G needles. The space marked with an asterisk should be filled with high vacuum grease, to prevent leakage and allow for easy rotation.

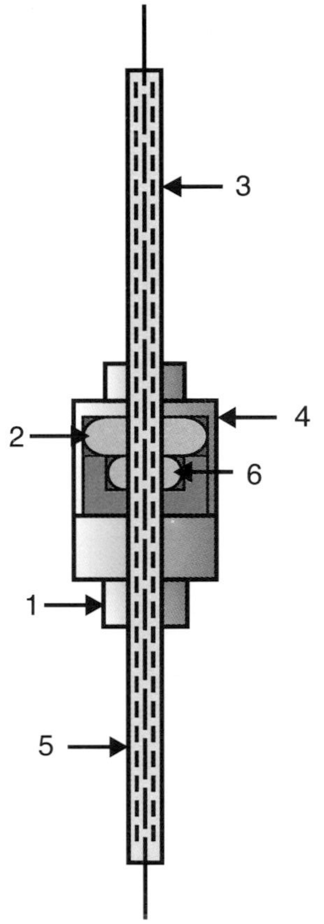

Swivels

Swivels are used when, for example, infusions are given to a freely moving animal, or when fluids, such as bile, are collected over a longer period of time. Several types have been described (Thomas and Mayer, 1968; Strubbe, 1974; Darracq et al., 1980). We routinely use a modification of the one described by Darracq. This swivel is made of a 1-mL syringe and two hypodermic needles as shown in Figure 27.2. The swivel described by Strubbe (1974) is extremely useful for the infusion of fluids as it has a very low dead-volume.

Another useful swivel is shown in Figure 27.3. This was developed by E. Schut and S. ten Have, University of Groningen.

Figure 27.3 Schematic diagram of the small stainless steel swivel used to allow free movement to the rats during collection of bile. The swivel can also be applied for long-term infusion of fluids into unanesthetized animals. (1) Ferrule, (2) flange, (3) tube (diameter 0.8 mm), (4) closing ferrule, (5) tube (diameter 0.8 mm), (6) rubber O-ring. Actual length is 2.5 cm.

cannula, their lengths, the diameter used for each cannula and the positioning of the silicon rings which are wrapped around the tubing.

L-shaped adapters

Fixation of a cannula to the skull is achieved using a stainless steel needle bent to a 90° angle (L-shaped adapter). The point should be removed from a 20-G needle, and the surface polished with emery paper. Subsequently the needle is bent to a 90° angle. The L-shaped adapter has one short and one longer end, 8 and 12 mm respectively.

Sutures

In 1957 the microneedle, swaged on a 7-0 silk suture was introduced. The two main factors in the development of microsutures have been the material used and the needles. Both resorbable (polydioxanone, polyglycolic acid and polylactic acid or a combination thereof) and nonresorbable materials are used today. In microvascular surgery a great deal of experience has been gained with silk, nylon and polyester. Today suture materials are of high quality, they cause hardly any reactions, they pull easily through tissue and can be knotted securely. The mechanical performance of knotted sutures is generally measured by knot break load, minimum numbers of throws required for knot security, knot rundown force, first throw holding force and tissue drag force (Faulkner et al., 1996).

Together with suture diameter, needle size has diminished. Sutures used in microvascular surgery should be atraumatic. The needles must be round-bodied with a flattened end and for better control. The most frequently used arch length for the needle is 3/8. Apart from the microsutures there is an overwhelming supply of macrosutures.

As a rule of thumb always use resorbable material. Only where it is necessary to secure something (a cannula or electrode) should nonresorbable sutures be used.

Tying knots

Knot tying starts with picking up the suture with the forceps. A loop (throw) is made on the tip of the needle holder placed just above the wound edges. Depending on the tension between the wound edges, single or double throws are made around the tip of the needle holder. Next the short end of the suture is grasped with the needle holder and the loop is pulled off and tightened (gently). This is the first half of the knot. Do not let go of the suture held with the forceps, but immediately make a second loop around the needle holder which again should be just above the wound edges in the middle of the 'V' formed by the draw strings of the suture. Pull off the loop and tighten the knot. You will see that the first half of the knot is progressively tightened during this procedure.

The configuration of a knot can be classified into two general types by the relation between the ears of the knot and the loop. When the right ear and loop of two throws exit on the same side of the knot (parallel to each other), the knot is judged to be square or reef. Where the right ear and loop exit on or cross on different sides of the knot, it is called a granny knot. The above described knot with two throws to overcome tension on the wound edges is called a friction or surgeon's knot.

Tera and Åberg (1976) devised a simple description of a knot's configuration. The number of wraps for each throw is indicated by the appropriate Arabic number. The relationship between each throw, being either cross or parallel, is given by the symbols × or =, respectively. In accordance with this code, the square knot is designated 1=1, and the granny knot as 1×1, while the surgeon's knot is 2=1. A surgeon's knot with an extra half knot for security is represented by 2=1=1. By following the above mentioned sequence you will always tie 1=1 or 2=1 knots.

Preparation of the Crown of the Head

The majority of cannulation techniques start with the preparation of the crown of the head. To start with, the animal's head should be shaved and disinfected with a chlorhexidine solution. An incision approximately 1 cm in length should be made in the crown of the head. This will provide enough space to mount three stainless steel screws (1.0 mm in diameter and 4.2 mm in length) in the crown of the skull which are used for additional anchoring. The membranous tissue should be removed, using curved jeweller's forceps, and the bregma (the point on the top of the skull where the coronal and sagittal sutures meet) is then exposed. Using a 3/0-round dental drill, three holes are made, two on the left and one on the right of the bregma (Figure 27.4). The stainless steel dental drill is held loosely between the thumb and forefinger to allow rotating movements. To ensure that underlying tissues such as the dura, the rostral sagittal sinus or the transverse sinus are not punctured, the conical end of the drill is covered with a piece of

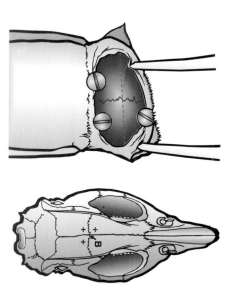

Figure 27.4 The position of three stainless steel screws relative to the bregma (B).

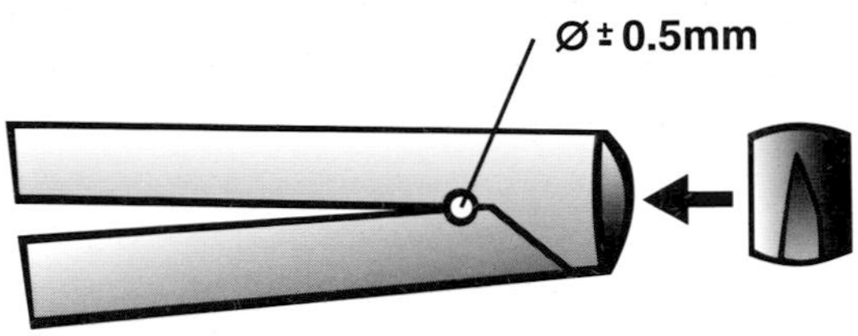

xiphoid cartilage, using a sharp-blunt pair of scissors. The skin should be slightly elevated to avoid unwanted damage to the underlying tissues. Subsequently, the abdominal muscles are lifted and a small transverse incision is made. The tissue should be spread to allow air to enter the peritoneal cavity. The abdomen is then opened over the linea alba towards the sternum (Figure 27.6), thus exposing the xiphoid cartilage. Sometimes, small incisions in the connective tissue on the left side of the xiphoid cartilage help, after retraction and fixation of the left lateral lobe of the liver together with the intestines, to expose the portal area.

The abdominal wall is closed in two layers, using a continuous suture technique with a resorbable 4-0 suture. The second layer is the skin, which should be closed using the running suture technique with either a 4-0 resorbable or nonresorbable suture, making use of the same method. The sutures in the skin should be removed after 7 days.

Subcutaneous Tunneling

Before you pass the cannula(e) to the head, you must have sutured the total abdominal muscle layer and the abdominal skin, leaving only about 1 cm open. Artery forceps can be used to secure the suture during the tunneling procedure. Figure 27.7 shows how the animal is held and how a slender needle holder (e.g. Ryder) is pushed subcutaneously in a caudal direction through the connective tissue over a distance of about 8–10 cm. Subsequently, the point of the needle holder is turned towards the opening in the abdominal skin and is pushed out. During this

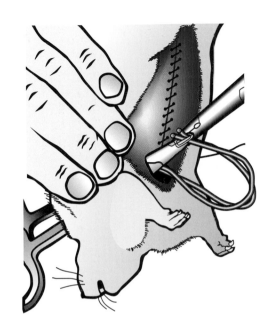

Figure 27.7 Subcutaneous tunneling of cannulae.

polyethylene (PE) tubing, leaving about 2 mm of the tip uncovered. If you have access to a mechanical drill, this procedure can be carried out very quickly. The screws are fitted into the holes using specially prepared surgical forceps and a small screwdriver (Figure 27.5). They are tightened to such an extent, that approximately 2 mm is left between the skull and the head of the screws.

Opening and Closure of the Abdominal Wall

After shaving and disinfecting the abdominal wall, the rat is turned in a supine position and, when necessary, secured to the operating table with adhesive tape. The abdomen is opened through a midline incision from the level of the pubic bones to the

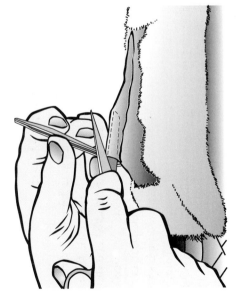

Figure 27.6 Opening of the abdominal cavity using a sharp-blunt straight pair of scissors. The scissors are pushed in the cranial direction over the linea alba just past the xiphoid cartilage. Always make sure that you see the blunt part of the scissors passing directly under the skin, thus avoiding cutting the intestines.

Ø ± 0.5mm

Figure 27.5 The head of surgical forceps with a 0.5-mm hole drilled in it for easy fixation of the screws during insertion.

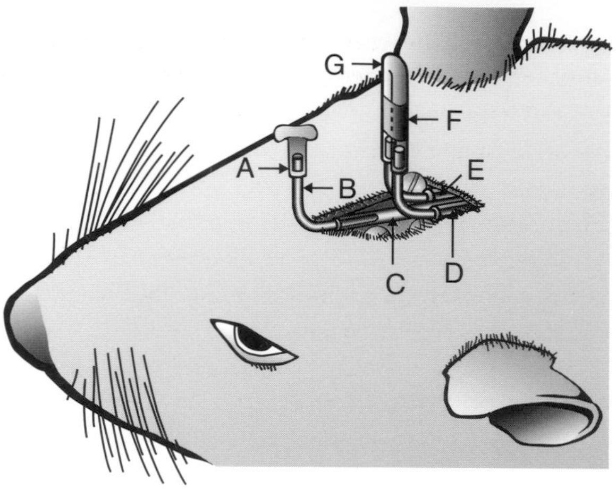

procedure the point of the needle holder should be as near to the skin as possible, thus preventing it from entering any muscle layer. The cannula(e) or electrodes can now be grasped and pulled through to emerge at the crown of the head.

A similar procedure can be used to subcutaneously pass the permanent jugular vein cannula from the neck to the crown of the head. Always make sure that the cannula makes a smooth curve, ensuring that the animal can move freely without tearing the cannula (for details see Remie et al., 1990d).

Fixation of Cannulae

Prior to fixation, the cannula has to be slid over the short end of the L-shaped adapter. To serve this purpose you may use some diethyl-ether to make the silicon tubing even more supple and the cannula will slide smoothly over the stainless steel tubing.

Catheters placed in blood vessels should now be flushed with saline (0.5 mL) and filled with a 60% polyvinylpyrrolidone (mol.wt 10 000) solution in saline with 500 IU/mL heparin (PVP solution). The long end of the L-shaped stainless steel adapter should be closed with a piece of heat-sealed PE-tubing (PE-cap).

Next, the cannula together with the angled adapter should be fixed to the skull with acrylic glue or bone cement. Make sure the glue flows properly under the heads of the screws and that it is wrapped

Figure 27.8 Situation on the crown of the head after cannulation of the bile duct (double) and the jugular vein. (A) Polyethylene cap, (B) L-shaped adapters, (C) jugular vein cannula, (D) proximal bile cannula, (E) distal bile cannula, (F) adhesive tape, (G) U-shaped piece of polyethylene tubing.

around the vertical part of the adapter as this will prevent any movement. Figure 27.8 shows the combination of a jugular vein cannula and a double bile cannula before the glue is applied.

Note that between the PVP solution and the methylmethacrylate an insoluble precipitate may be formed. Therefore you must flush the cannula and refill it with PVP solution one day after the operation, during your routine check of the animal's condition.

Permanent Cannulation of the Jugular Vein

Introduction

Blood plays a central role in biomedical research. There are numerous ways in which blood can be sampled from the laboratory rat (see also Chapters 25 and 28). For example:

- puncture of the ophthalmic venous plexus
- puncture of the heart
- cutting the tail
- decapitation.

In all these methods, the animal is either anesthetized, handled or restrained before the sample is taken. This inevitably causes adverse reactions in the animal, such as a rise of glucose, prolactin, catecholamine and corticosteroid levels. Needless to say, these changes may interfere with the results of experiments. Several techniques have been put forward to take blood samples from an animal without disturbing it. Permanent cannulation of the jugular vein was described in the rat and the ground squirrel by Popovic et al. in 1963. Cannulation of the jugular vein in combination with a head attachment apparatus allowing easy connection of cannulae was first introduced by Steffens (1969). These techniques enable continuous blood sampling from the general circulation and even infusion of fluids in the freely moving rat. During sampling or infusion the animal remains undisturbed, which is of vital importance in experiments monitoring behavior or where stress factors are expected to influence results. Several modifications have been introduced, for example and between the chin and its right armpit. Using blunt forceps, connective and adipose tissue are pushed aside and the jugular vein is exposed. The division of the external jugular into the maxillary vein, and the linguofacial vein should be identified. This bifurcation is recognizable by the presence of a small lymph node. At this point the largest vessel is chosen for cannulation and mobilized over a distance of about 5 mm.

Small artery forceps (Micro Halstead or baby-Mosquito) are used to clamp the vessel 3 mm rostral from the bifurcation. The vein should then be ligated rostral to the clamp using 6-0 silk. A second ligature is put loosely around the vessel (Figure 27.10). Using iridectomy scissors, a V-shaped hole is then cut in the vein 2 mm rostral from the bifurcation. Prior to its insertion into the vessel, the sterile cannula must be connected via a 23-G needle to a 1-mL syringe filled with a heparinized saline solution (50 IU/mL). No air bubbles should be left in the cannula.

Using sharp-pointed jeweller's forceps to dilate the vessel, the cannula is slid between the legs of the

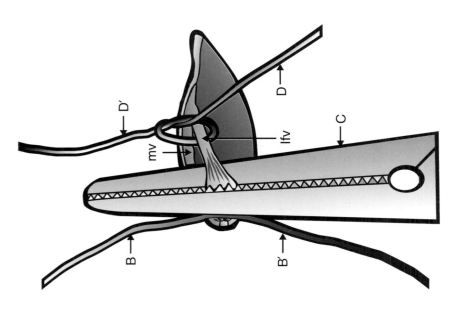

Figure 27.10 Clamping and ligation of the vessel. (B–B') Rostral ligature, (C) artery forceps (baby mosquito), (D–D') caudal ligature. mv, Maxillary vein; lfv, linguofacial vein.

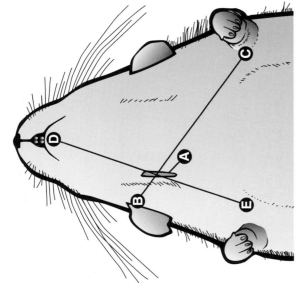

Figure 27.9 Imaginary lines to determine the exact location of the jugular vein bifurcation. (A) Incision, (B–C) line between the left arm pit and the right ear, (D–E) line between the right arm pit and the chin.

by Brown and Hedge (1972), who introduced the L-shaped adapter, Nicolaidis *et al.* (1974), who used an additional stainless steel head bolt, and Dons and Havlik (1986), who used a multilayered cannula. A nice overview of methods for vascular access and collection of body fluids from the laboratory rat has been given by Cocchetto and Bjornsson (1983).

The technique described below is one of the most simple and reliable, and it should be regarded as one of the basic techniques in cannulation of blood vessels (Remie *et al.*, 1990e).

The Operation

The operation can be divided into four parts:

● Preparation of the crown of the head
● Cannulation of the jugular vein
● Subcutaneous tunneling of the cannula
● Fixing of the cannula.

Cannulation of the jugular vein

After the neck of the animal has been shaved on the right side, the skin should be disinfected with chlorhexidine solution. An incision is then made just above the right clavicle (Figure 27.9). This place can be found easily by drawing imaginary lines between the animal's right ear and its left armpit,

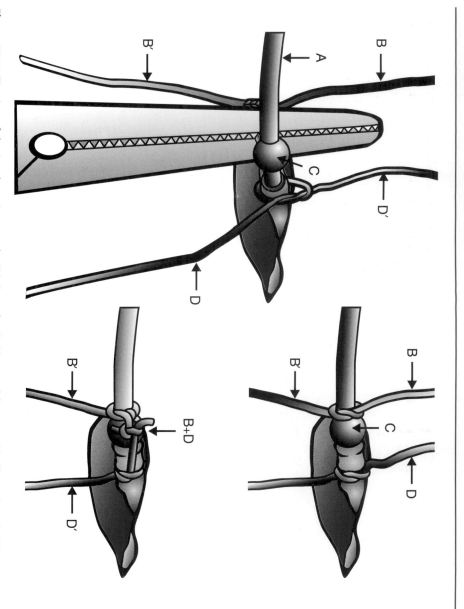

Figure 27.11 Fixation of the jugular vein cannula. (A) Cannula, (B–B') rostral ligature, (C) silicon ring, (D–D') caudal ligature.

forceps and gently pushed into the vessel until the silicon ring reaches the V-shaped hole. Sometimes, when trying to push the cannula gently into the vessel it bounces on release. If this happens the cannula has almost certainly entered the subclavicular vein. This can be remedied by pulling the cannula back, leaving it inside the vessel, then pushing it back in gently while lifting the animal's chest by the skin. When the silicon ring has reached the vessel, the tip of the cannula should now be at the level of the right atrium. This can be checked by removing the needle and the syringe and looking at the fluid in the free end of the cannula. During inspiration the fluid should be sucked into the cannula, while during expiration the fluid should be pushed back (intrathoracic pressure). Moreover, the heart frequency should be superimposed on the respiratory-induced fluid movements. The catheter should be further checked by aspirating some blood, and the cannula flushed gently with heparinized saline solution. The artery forceps are now removed, the caudal ligature gently tied, and the rostral ligature used to anchor the cannula to the

vessel. Subsequently, the syringe should be removed and the cannula gently clamped using a small microvascular clamp. To ensure that the cannula cannot move, one drawstring of each ligature should be cross-tied (Figure 27.11).

Subcutaneous tunneling of the cannula

In Figure 27.12 the small artery forceps are shown just before they are pushed in longitudinally under the skin in a caudal direction to a distance of about 3 cm. Subsequently, the forceps should be turned anticlockwise through an angle of 90°, and pushed in the direction of the incision in the neck. The cannula should be grasped by the forceps and pulled back. Care must be taken not to twist the cannula during this procedure. The forceps are then removed and replaced by the small microvascular clamp.

Flushing and filling of the cannula with PVP-solution is described earlier. Finally, the wound in the neck of the animal should be closed with two resorbable sutures (Figure 27.13).

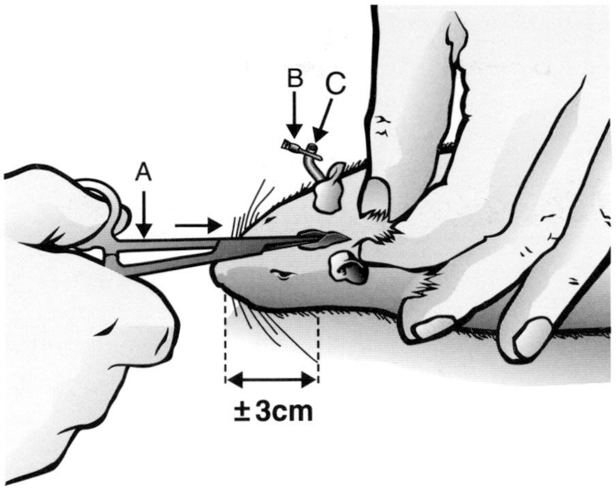

0.2 mL of saline should be pushed in, to clear the tube, followed by 2 µL of heparinized saline (500 IU/mL). Next a small air bubble should be introduced by opening the tube briefly. More saline is then injected until the first air bubble reaches the stainless steel tubing. A second air bubble is introduced as 'marker', and injected over a distance of approximately 4 cm. The first air bubble should now be almost at the end of the catheter and is separated from the circulation by the 2 µL heparin solution (Figure 27.14).

When a sample is taken, the content of the polyethylene tube is aspirated until blood just enters the nozzle of the syringe. The air bubbles make sure that there is no mixture of blood from the preceding sample with the new sample to be taken. A clean syringe is used to take the sample. At the end of the experiment the polyethylene tubing is removed, and the cannula is refilled with 100 µL of PVP solution.

The sampling procedure can also be applied to other cannulae. However, the distance to which the marker air bubble has to be pushed into the polyethylene tubing must be recalculated, depending on the internal diameter and the length of the Silastic tubing used for the cannulation of the vessel.

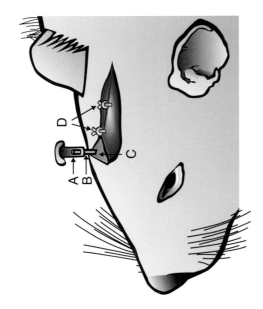

Figure 27.12 Subcutaneous tunneling of the jugular vein cannula. (A) Artery forceps, (B) small vascular clip (Heifetz), (C) cannula.

Figure 27.13 Situation on the crown of the head at the end of the operation. (A) Polyethylene cap, (B) L-shaped adapter, (C) dental acrylic cement, (D) sutures.

Permanent Double Bile Fistula with Intact Enterohepatic Circulation

Introduction

Techniques described in the literature for the collection of bile from various experimental animal species are numerous. In most of these techniques either restrained or anesthetized animals are used in which the common bile duct is cannulated. However, it has been known for quite some time that factors such as anesthesia, surgical intervention, the way of sampling and immobilization may strongly influence the results. These factors may therefore be responsible for many inconsistencies in the literature regarding data on bile excretion (Light et al., 1959; Lambert, 1965; Kuipers et al., 1985b). Besides the above mentioned effects, most of the experimental set-ups

Blood Sampling from the Permanent Jugular Vein Cannula

To take blood samples from the general circulation, a 40-cm-long polyethylene tube (o.d. 1.45 mm, i.d. 0.75 mm) should be filled with saline and stoppered with a small nail. After removing the PE-cap, the tubing should be attached to the L-shaped adapter at the top of the animal's head. During the sampling procedure, the tube is clamped with curved forceps. A 1-mL syringe is connected to the polyethylene tube and a few drops of blood mixed with PVP-solution are aspirated and discarded. Subsequently,

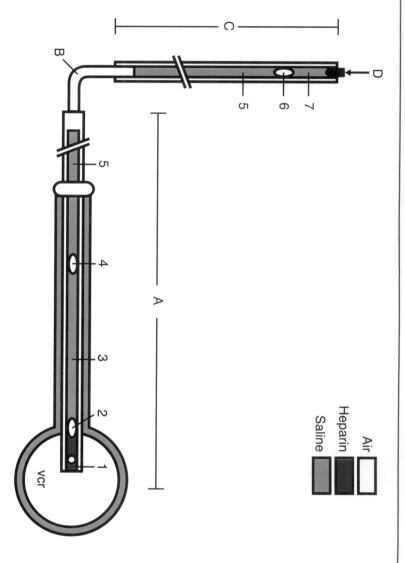

Figure 27.14 Schematic presentation of the jugular vein sampling procedure. Numbers 1–7 indicate the sequence of the procedure. (A) The cannula inside the animal, (B) L-shaped adapter on the crown of the head, (C) polyethylene tubing (0.75 × 1.45 mm), (D) a copper nail of approximately 0.85 mm in diameter. vcr, Vena cava rostralis at the level of the right atrium. (2) first air droplet, (6) second air droplet, (7) additional air droplet for extra cleaning of the tube.

are reabsorbed in the gut, transported back to the liver via the portal blood where they participate in liver metabolism, and are re-excreted into the bile and so on. This phenomenon is called the enterohepatic circulation (EHC). In this way an optimal concentration of, for example, bile acids, is guaranteed.

Historical Overview

In 1935, Sawyer and Lepkovsky (1934) provided an overview of the techniques used for the collection of bile at that time, and they described the cannulation of the lower bile duct (a biliary-pancreatic fistula). Bile together with pancreatic juice was collected in a glass bulb (6 mL) with two side-arms, which was placed in the abdominal cavity. A second cannula which emerged from the animal's back was used to empty the glass bulb twice a day. However, they reported that the animals died within 90 hours due to tremendous weight loss. Johnson and Rising (1978) modified the Sawyer and Lepkovsky (1934) technique and reported that the animals were in better condition and could be used for up to 6 days.

allow only short-term collection of bile. For the pharmacokinetic profiling of drugs it is often necessary to follow the elimination over a longer period of time. This dictates the need for models that allow long-term collection of bile, preferably without restraining or anesthetizing the animal. In the past 50 years a number of techniques have been developed for prolonged bile collection in rats with the aim of approaching physiologically normal or close to normal conditions (Sawyer and Lepkovsky, 1934; Fisher and Vars, 1955; Light *et al.*, 1959; Zyl, 1959; Chipman and Cropper, 1977; Enderlin and Honohan, 1977; Johnson and Rising, 1978; Vonk *et al.*, 1978a,b; Weis and Barth, 1978; Balabaud *et al.*, 1981; Tomlinson *et al.*, 1981; Tse *et al.*, 1982; Kuipers *et al.*, 1985a,b; Rath and Hutchison, 1989; Remie *et al.*, 1990f).

The common bile duct is fairly translucent and has a diameter of about 1 mm. It runs from the hilum of the liver, where the hepatic ducts meet, through the pancreatic tissue, where it collects the excretory ducts of the pancreas, into the duodenum. At this point the duct is surrounded by a muscular structure, the sphincter of Oddi. The laboratory rat has no gall bladder. Substances excreted by the liver

Air
Heparin
Saline

Fisher and Vars (1955) modified this technique further, using a rubber balloon protected by a plastic cylinder, which was fixed on the animal's back with adhesive tape. These animals could be used for up to 9 weeks. Zyl (1959) was the first to describe a double cannulation technique of the bile duct to restore the enterohepatic circulation. He used polyethylene catheters, which were exteriorized in the middle of the animal's back. Bile was collected in glass containers strapped on to the back of the animal with adhesive tape.

Light et al. (1959) used a cannula for restoration of the EHC. It was introduced via an opening in the greater curvature of the stomach and pushed through the pylorus into the duodenum, until the tip reached the point of entrance of the common bile duct. Enderlin and Honohan (1977) were the first to collect bile from the rat's upper bile duct from outside its cage via a long piece of polyethylene tubing, which was externalized at the interscapular region. They reported a success rate of about 66%. Chipman and Cropper (1977) used vinyl tubing with Silastic tips to cannulate the common bile duct in the direction of the liver and the duodenum. Both cannulae were connected to a T-piece situated at the flank of the animal. The sampling arm was taken subcutaneously from the T-piece to emerge at the neck, just cranial to the scapulae.

Vonk et al. (1978a,b) used a flexible silicon cannula for the cannulation of the upper bile duct, which was run subcutaneously to emerge at the crown of the head. Bile could be collected at the outside of the animal's cage, using polyethylene tubing and a small swivel joint to allow free movement of the animal during sampling. Animals could be kept alive producing bile for several months while their general condition, as indicated by weight gain and food intake, was good.

The technique described by Weis and Barth (1978) resembles the technique of Zyl (1959) with regard to the cannulae insertion. The cannulae were exteriorized in the animal's lower right flank and were protected by a steel wire mosquito net. Although the animals were not restrained, their movement was limited due to the protective net. Bile flow could be measured by injecting air bubbles into the loop connecting both cannulae, and small bile samples could be collected from the loop. The enterohepatic circulation was intact and the sphincter of Oddi functioned physiologically.

Balabaud et al. (1981) modified the technique described by Vonk et al. (1978a,b) as they experienced

difficulties such as cessation of the bile flow probably caused by kinking of the silicon cannula. To overcome this problem they used a rigid polyethylene cannula which was sharply bent into a U-shape. Furthermore, they used a swivel joint with a larger diameter, which allowed bile precipitates to pass more easily.

Tomlinson et al. (1981) modified the technique of Enderlin and Honohan (1977) by using a silicon cannula with a polyethylene tip for easy insertion, but they placed the cannula in the lower bile duct at approximately 1.5 cm from the duodenum. They also mentioned that it was possible to study the enterohepatic circulation in these unrestrained conscious rats and described a technique similar to Zyl's (1959) technique.

Tse et al. (1982) described a cascade model to study the enterohepatic circulation of a radioactive labeled drug, using unrestrained awake rats. The bile duct of donor rats was cannulated with a Silastic cannula, and the recipient rats were equipped with an additional cannula in the duodenum opposite the sphincter of Oddi. The cannulae were exteriorized through a stab incision at the back, and fixed to the animal's back with a special adapter plate, kept in place by adhesive tape.

Kuipers et al. (1985a) modified and extended their own technique (Vonk et al., 1978a,b), by introducing a second cannula through a pursestring suture placed in the wall of the duodenum at about 1 cm proximal to the sphincter of Oddi. An additional permanent jugular vein cannula (Remie et al., 1990e) was placed during the same operation session, to allow sampling of blood and intravenous administration of compounds. Details of this bile fistula technique will be given below.

Rath and Hutchison (1989) modified the technique of Chipman and Cropper (1977). They also used the para-lumbar region of the animal for the exteriorization of the cannulae (vinyl tubing with a silicon tip).

The technique described in this section is based upon the technique by Vonk et al. (1978a). The method used by Kuipers et al. (1985a), varies only in the area where the bile is led back into the body (approximately 2 cm distally from the pylorus, directly into the duodenum).

Kuipers et al. (1985b) describe the effects of interruption and restoration of the EHC on several parameters, such as food intake, body weight, plasma glycocholate and cholesterol concentration, and concluded that their model was an excellent tool for studying the biliary excretion process and the effects of bile on intestinal absorption. Using the technique described below we were able, amongst other things, to study the pharmacokinetic properties of compounds that are cleared or metabolized by the liver and excreted into the bile. The animals can be followed for several weeks or even months. In combination with the permanent jugular vein cannula, the model enables excellent kinetic profiling of drugs and other substances of course, in the absence of anesthetics, which are known to affect the process of bile formation as well as bile acid absorption (Kuipers et al., 1985a).

The Operation

The operation can be divided into the following parts:

- Preparation of the crown of the head
- Opening of the abdominal wall
- Double cannulation of the bile duct
- Cannulation of the duodenum
- Closure of the abdominal wall
- Subcutaneous tunneling to the head
- Fixation of the cannulae.

Double cannulation of the bile duct

After opening the abdominal wall, the intestines are lifted out and laid on the right side of the animal (as viewed by the surgeon) on gauze moistened with warm (37°C) saline solution. Using jeweller's forceps the bile duct is then ligated with a 7-0 silk suture. Subsequently, the duct is placed under tension, (in the caudal direction) using artery forceps. This enables easy handling during cannulation. A second 7-0 silk ligature is loosely placed around the duct just cranial to the first ligature. With the aid of an operation microscope, a V-shaped hole should be made just cranial of the first ligature using jeweller's forceps and iridectomy scissors.

A sterile (proximal) cannula is inserted into the bile duct. The duct wall is lifted using jeweller's forceps, thereby facilitating easy cannulation. The second ligature is then tied and pulled taut, making sure that the cannula is not obstructed. If this part of the operation has been completed successfully, the bile will be driven into the cannula. Subsequently, the first ligature should be released from the artery forceps, and the threads tied behind the silicon ring, again ensuring the free passage of bile through the cannula. The rat should then be turned clockwise through a 90° angle, and the ligature reclamped and placed in the cranial direction, thereby putting the distal part of the duct under tension. A third ligature should now be loosely introduced around the duct, just distal to the first ligature. Following the procedure described above another V-shaped aperture should be made between the third and the first ligature, again using jeweller's forceps and iridectomy scissors. The distal bile cannula should now be inserted into the bile duct. During cannulation a cotton wool stick can be very useful in absorbing pancreatic juice, thus allowing an unimpeded view of the place of insertion. The third ligature should be tied and pulled taut, and the first ligature should be re-released from the artery forceps and tied around the second cannula behind the silicon ring (Figure 27.15, insert). All the loose threads should now be cut close to the knots. The animal is returned to its original position and the sections of the cannulae that lie between the silicon rings should be placed smoothly in the abdominal cavity. The cannulae are fixed using 7-0 silk suture to the abdominal muscle near the xiphoid cartilage (Figure 27.15).

Cannulation of the duodenum

When the second procedure is to be applied, cannulation of the bile duct is followed by cannulation of the duodenum. After location of the place where the bile duct enters the duodenum (the sphincter of Oddi), a four fine-stitch pursestring suture (7-0) should be made in the wall of the duodenum at the outer border at about 1 cm proximal to the sphincter. Before an incision is made inside the pursestring, using a 20-G needle, some iodine solution should be put on this spot. The cannula should be inserted into the duodenum until the first, smaller silicon ring has entered the lumen, and the purse-string tightened between the first and the second ring (Figure 27.16). This cannula, together with the bile cannula, should be placed, kink-free in the abdominal cavity and anchored to the internal muscle wall as described above.

Subsequently, the abdomen should be closed in two layers, and the cannulae should be tunneled subcutaneously. With a 5-cm piece of polyethylene tubing (0.75 × 1.45 mm), the two long ends of the 20-G, L-shaped stainless steel adapters should be connected. Using a piece of adhesive tape, the polyethylene tube should be fixed. The short ends

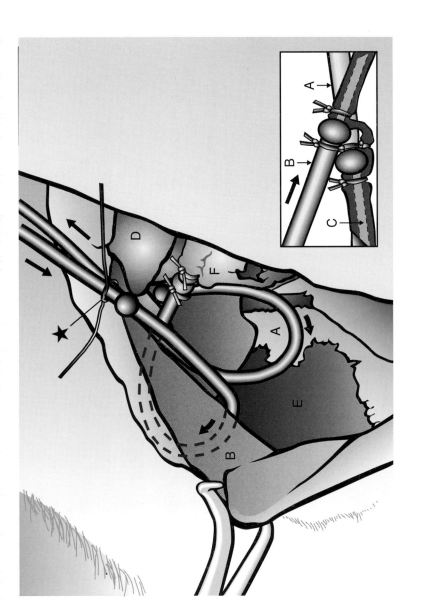

Figure 27.15 Position of the cannulae in the abdominal cavity after a double bile fistula. The insert shows a detail of the common bile duct (C) into which the proximal (A) and distal (B) cannulae have been inserted. Arrows indicate the direction of the bile flow. The asterisk marks the place of the 7-0 silk suture used to anchor the cannula to the internal abdominal muscle. (D) Liver, (E) right kidney, (F) pancreas.

of the L-shaped adapters are then connected to the bile cannulae. It is good to form the habit of always having the proximal bile cannula (the one taking the bile from the liver) on the same side of the head. This will prevent you from making mistakes when you connect the animals to the swiveled sampling cannula prior to the experiment. The cannulae, together with the angled tubing, should be fixed to the skull as described, earlier.

Collection of bile

The animals should be housed in individual cages. When bile has to be collected, they are attached to long swivelled PE-cannulae (0.75 × 1.45 mm) (Figure 27.17). A stainless steel coil may be used to protect the rats from gnawing the tubing. The end of the cannula must be just below the bottom of the cage as this will provide enough under-pressure to

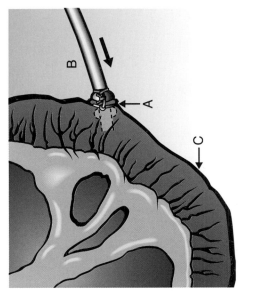

Figure 27.16 The duodenal cannula (B) inserted in the pursestring suture (A) and anchored behind the silicon ring. The arrow indicates the direction of the bile flow. (C) Outer border of the duodenum.

Permanent Cannulation of the Portal Vein

Introduction

Sampling or infusion in the general circulation is often carried out using a jugular vein cannula. However, it may be of major interest for pharmacological and physiological studies to have access to the portal vein in the unanesthetized, freely moving rat. Several cannulation techniques have been described (Hyun et al., 1967; Pelzmann and Havemeyer, 1971; Suzuki et al., 1973; Russell and Mogenson, 1975; Sable-Amplis and Abadie, 1975; Helman et al., 1984). The majority of these techniques use a side branch of the portal vein for cannulation. Sable-Amplis and Abadie (1975), however, described a T-shaped cannula of polyethylene tubing that was inserted in the portal vein between the gastroduodenal vein and the splenic vein. Helman et al. (1984) used the left portal branch to enter the vein, because they were unsuccessful with the T-shaped cannula. Russell and Mogenson (1975) used another side branch (the rostral mesenteric vein) to accomplish cannulation of the portal vein. All these methods suffered from a limited long-term patency of the catheter being a maximal 14 days.

In this section a technique will be described in which the patency is significantly improved. Post-operative weight loss was kept low between 3% and 5% on the third day. After 5–7 days the preoperative weight was reached. After two months, sampling was still feasible in 60% of the animals. Some animals could be used in experiments for over five months.

We used this technique in combination with two platinum electrodes around the portal vein in close proximity to the catheter tip in the same freely moving animals. This resulted in a model highly suited to the in vivo study of presynaptic regulation of neurotransmitter release from noradrenergic nerve terminals (Remie and Zaagsma, 1986; Remie et al., 1988a,b, 1989, 1990a).

Applications

It is generally appreciated that the stress of restraint as well as various anaesthetic agents affects hepatic functioning. Yet the pentobarbital-anesthetized rat fitted with a bile fistula is probably still the most widely used (Remie et al., 1991) experimental model for the study of bile formation and biliary excretion of drugs, xenobiotics and endogenous compounds in vivo. The experimental rat model described herein allows us to investigate these processes without interference from anesthesia or restraint-induced stress. Long-term experiments can be performed under steady-state conditions in rats with normal feeding behavior (Kuipers et al., 1985b). Small bile samples can be collected from rats with an intact enterohepatic circulation after disconnection of both cannulae; alternatively, studies can be performed in rats with chronic bile diversion, in which hepatic synthetic and excretory processes as well as bile flow have stabilized at new steady-state levels (Smit et al., 1990).

let the bile flow into the cannula. For continuous collection of bile, the cannula can be connected to a fraction collector.

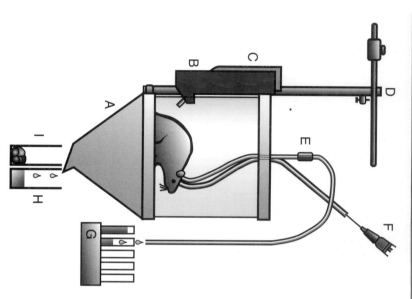

Figure 27.17 Simultaneous sampling of blood and bile from a freely moving rat. Feces and urine may be collected separately. (A) Metabolic cage, (B) food container, (C) water flask, (D) lever with counter weight, (E) swivel, (F) syringe with blood sample, (G) fraction collector, (H) urine, (I) feces.

Single Cannulation of the Portal Vein

The operation can be divided into seven parts:

- Preparation of the crown of the head
- Opening of the abdominal wall
- The pursestring suture
- Cannulation of the portal vein
- Closure of the abdominal wall
- Subcutaneous tunneling to the head
- Fixation of the cannula.

Some remarks will be made on the use of a portal sample and infusion cannula combined with stimulation electrodes.

The pursestring suture

After opening the abdominal wall, the intestines are lifted out and laid on the right side of the animal (as viewed by the surgeon) on gauze moistened with warm (37°C) saline solution. This will provide an excellent view of the portal area.

Using a micro needle holder and a cotton wool stick, a four or five, fine-stitch pursestring suture

(7-0 silk suture armed with a BV-1 needle) are placed in the wall of the portal vein just opposite the gastroduodenal vein. The needle and thread should be guided through the vessel carefully, to avoid tearing the very delicate portal wall. As you enter the lumen of the portal vein, bleeding may occur after each stitch. By applying light pressure on the bleeding spot using the cotton-wool stick, bleeding will soon be arrested. The diameter of the pursestring should be approximately 1 mm. After the suture has been completed a single knot is tied.

Cannulation of the portal vein

The portal vein should be clamped with a small curved bulldog clamp modified to resemble a Satinsky vascular clamp. Using iridectomy scissors and a pair of jeweller's forceps the center of the pursestring should be cut. Subsequently, the cannula, which is filled with heparinized saline (50 IU/mL), should be inserted into the vessel and pushed in until the silicon ring reaches the vein (Figure 27.18). Next the pursestring should be gently tightened, taking care not to obstruct the cannula. This can be controlled by flushing through the cannula with some heparinized saline solution. The drawstrings

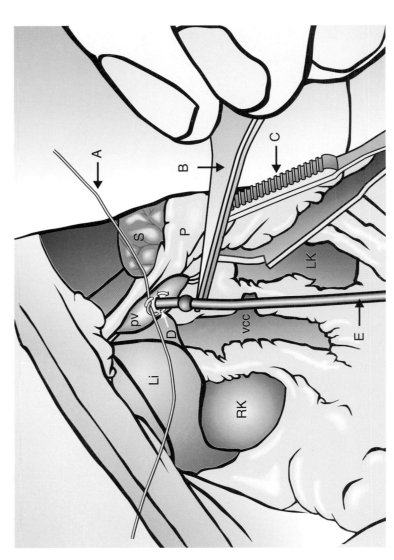

Figure 27.18 Placement of the portal vein cannula. (A) Drawstring of the pursestring suture, (B) anatomical forceps, (C) modified bulldog clamp (according to Satinsky), (D) the pursestring suture, (E) the portal vein cannula. pv, portal vein; vcc, vena cava caudalis; Li, liver; LK, left kidney; RK, right kidney; P, pancreas; S, stomach.

of the suture are used to anchor the cannula behind the first silicon ring.

In experienced hands the total clamping time is less than 1 min (when the surgeon has assistance, the clamping time can be reduced to 20–30 s). The second silicon ring is used to anchor the cannula to the internal abdominal muscle, near the xiphoid cartilage. To complete the operation, the abdomen is closed, the cannula is tunneled subcutaneously to emerge at the crown of the head where it is fixed to the skull using dental glue.

Portal sample and infusion cannula combined with stimulation electrodes

An additional cannula used for the infusion of drugs can be placed into the portal vein 10 mm distally from the first, using a similar technique. Using an 8-0 monofilament suture, a three to four fine-stitch pursestring is made in the wall of the portal vein. The vessel should be clamped with the same clamp as used for the first cannula. In order to make the hole as small as possible, the portal wall in the

pursestring suture should be punctured with a 23-G needle. The cannula is now pushed into the lumen of the portal vein and the pursestring suture closed. Again the drawstrings of the pursestring suture are used to anchor the cannula in the same way as described above.

After both cannulations have been completed, the stimulation electrodes should be placed around the portal vein. The electrode is made of platinum wire (0.50 mm) which is bent into a circle (3.0 mm diameter) with one end free to make a connection with a flexible Teflon-coated wire. A two-pin male microplug, made of an IC foot (integrated circuit) is soldered on to the other end.

The portal vein should be mobilized by blunt dissection, between the gastroduodenal vein and the rostral pancreaticoduodenal vein. This segment should be lifted using straight forceps, and the electrodes put in place. The circles should then be closed to give an optimal vessel fit (Figure 27.19). The electrodes may be anchored to the portal vein with two 9-0 Ethilon sutures (not shown).

Before the second layer of the abdominal wall is closed, the free end of the cannulae and the

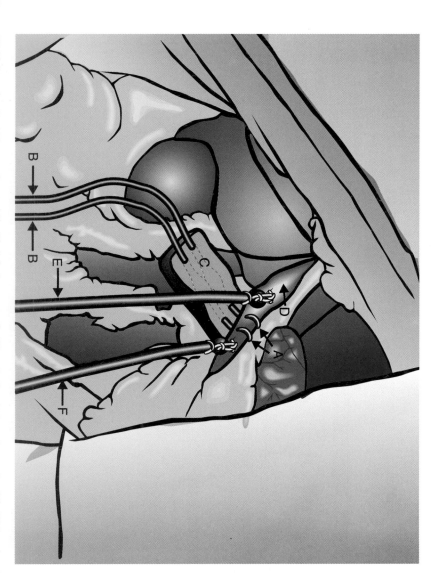

Figure 27.19 Portal vein with sample cannula (E), infusion cannula (F) and stimulation electrodes (A). (B) Insulated wire, (C) dental acrylic cement, (D) portal vein.

hemodynamic parameters. In several areas, for example the study of the relationship between social behavior and blood pressure, it is simply impossible to use either restrained or anesthetized rats. Restraining the animal, or restricting its freedom of movement by technical means is a very strong stressor that will influence the parameters to be measured. Standard techniques such as plethysmographic, or cuff methods have several limitations. The animals have to be handled, restrained and trained before experiments can be performed. Moreover, the method itself introduces variations in blood pressure, and there seems to be an inconsistency between the direct blood pressure value and the one measured by the cuff method (Bunag, 1971; Bunag *et al.*, 1971).

Direct measurement of blood pressure is usually done by cannulation of one of the carotid arteries. This, however, can interfere with the proper functioning of the pressure receptors in the carotid sinus. Several techniques have been described (Weeks and Jones, 1960; Buckingham, 1976; Sloop and Krause, 1981; most of them, however, are unclear about the percentage of success, and/or the long-term patency of the cannula.

We have been using the following technique for several years, and in its final form it has proved to have a low (less than 5%) mortality rate during surgery, a high patency rate of more than 85% after 2 weeks, and more than 65% after 4 weeks. Some animals could be used for up to three months. Apart from measuring blood pressure, sampling of arterial blood or infusion into the arterial system is also feasible.

More recently, small implantable telemetric transducers have become available. The cannula connected to these transducers can be implanted similar to the cannulation technique described below.

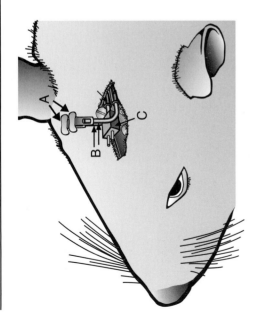

Figure 27.20 Situation on the crown of the head at the end of the operation. (A) Polyethylene caps, (B) L-shaped adapters, (C) miniature connector made of an IC foot.

insulated wire should be driven subcutaneously to emerge at the crown of the head. Each cannula should be slid over the short end of a 20-G stainless steel L-shaped adapter. The heparinized saline should now be replaced by the viscous PVP solution. The L-shaped adapters together with the IC foot are anchored to the skull with the three small stainless steel screws and dental acrylic glue (Figure 27.20).

Permanent Cannulation of the Iliolumbar Artery

Introduction

Much of the knowledge about blood pressure, its regulation and the influence of drugs on the cardiovascular system, has been derived from experiments with acutely prepared, anesthetized or immobilized animals. Although valuable, this information is obscured by the direct effects of anesthetics and surgical intervention. It is well known that general anesthesia has a considerable impact on base-line blood flow and myocardial function. Surgery can, among other things, introduce local vasomotion, thus disturbing the normal

The Operation

The operation can be divided into six parts:

- Preparation of the crown of the head
- Opening of the abdominal wall
- Cannulation of the iliolumbar artery
- Closure of the abdominal wall
- Subcutaneous tunneling to the head
- Fixation of the cannula.

Cannulation of the iliolumbar artery

After opening the abdominal wall, the intestines are lifted out and laid on the left side of the animal (as viewed by the surgeon) on gauze moistened with warm (37°C) saline solution. This will provide a good view of the lower abdominal region. For easy cannulation, the aorta and the iliolumbar artery should be dissected free from the iliolumbar vein and vena cava, to a distance of 1 and 2 cm respectively. This is done using standard sharp preparation technique. Figure 27.21 shows the ligatures that are placed around the iliolumbar artery. The first ligature (7-0 silk) is placed approximately 6 mm from the bifurcation. A second ligature (7-0 silk) is then placed about 2 mm proximal to the first. Both ligatures should be drawn tight. Subsequently, two clamps are placed on the abdominal aorta. When you place the distal clamp first, the segment will be filled with blood under pressure, making it easier to

place the third ligature. This ligature is an 8-0 monofilament suture, which should be applied in the muscular layer (not in the lumen) of the iliolumbar artery at the place shown in Figure 27.22. Subsequently using angled jeweller's forceps and iridectomy scissors, a V-shaped hole should be made in the wall of the artery.

The sterile cannula which is filled with heparinized saline solution (50 IU/mL) should now be inserted into the aorta (Figure 27.23). Next the 8-0 Ethilon suture should be pulled taut, but not tight, thus avoiding obstruction of the cannula. The second ligature should be tightened just behind the silicon ring, making it impossible for the cannula to be pushed out of the vessel. After the iliolumbar artery has been cut, between the first and the second ligature (Figure 27.24), allowing for the cannula to be placed in line with the aorta, the clamps should be released. The distal clamp should be released first (lower pressure), followed by the proximal clamp. The cannula should be laid kink-free in the abdominal cavity and then sutured to the internal abdominal muscle, near the xiphoid cartilage. Subsequently, the abdomen should be closed in two layers, and the cannula tunneled subcutaneously. The cannula, together with the L-shaped adapter, should be fixed to the skull.

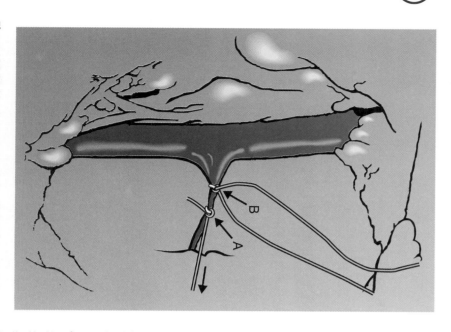

Figure 27.21 Ligatures around the iliolumbar artery. (A) First ligature put under tension in the direction of the arrow. (B) Second ligature.

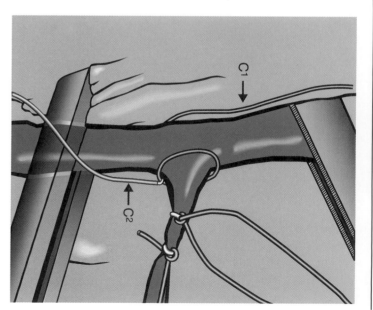

Figure 27.22 The drawstrings (C¹ and C²) are turned around the vessel and a single knot is placed.

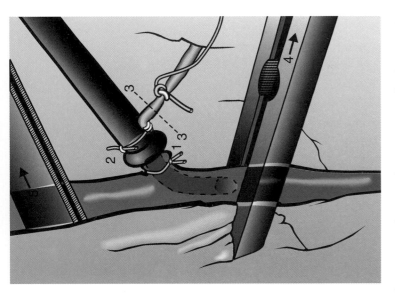

Figure 27.23 Insertion of the iliolumbar cannula into the small hole in the artery. (C) Cannula, (C') silicon ring, (D) jeweller's forceps.

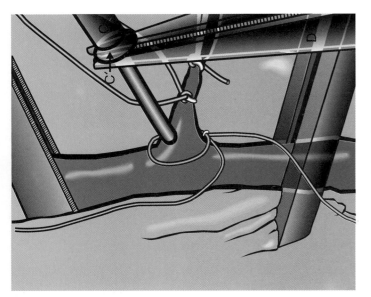

Figure 27.24 The cannulation is almost finished. (1) The vessel is closed around the cannula. (2) The second ligature is tied behind the silicon ring to anchor the cannula. (3) The iliolumbar artery is cut between the first and the second ligature. (4) The distal (low-pressure) clamp is removed. (5) The proximal (high-pressure) clamp is removed.

Transplantation of the Heart

Introduction

In cardiac transplantation models in rats we can differentiate between orthotopic and heterotopic techniques. Although desirable from a physiological point of view, orthotopic transplantation is rather troublesome to perform due to technical difficulties with the extracorporeal circulation. In transplantation research, heterotopic models with empty beating hearts are preferred. In these models blood flows into the donor aorta, perfuses the coronary arteries and the myocardium leading to ventricular contractions. Blood returning from the coronary veins drains into the right atrium, the right ventricle and flows through the pulmonary artery out into the vena cava of the recipient. This nonphysiological approach is not functionally comparable to a normal beating heart and has still unknown effects on the immunological functioning of both graft and recipient.

Two heterotopic heart transplant techniques are conventionally used. The first, being the simplest, uses the abdominal aorta and the vena cava. The second one uses the carotid artery and the jugular vein (Heron, 1971).

Abbott and Lindsey (1964) described a technique for heterotopic heart transplantation in the rat, connecting the recipient's abdominal aorta and the donor's ascending aorta using end-to-end technique. Bui-Mong-Hung and Vigano (1966) developed a rat model also using the abdominal vessels. Tomita (1966) and Ono and Lindsey (1969) modified this technique. The main modification was the use of end-to-side anastomoses between the graft and the recipient. This modification prevented the development of severe hind-leg ischemia.

In 1970 Lee *et al.* developed a technique for auxiliary heterotopic heart–lung transplantation, followed by a nonsuture heart transplantation technique by Heron in 1971.

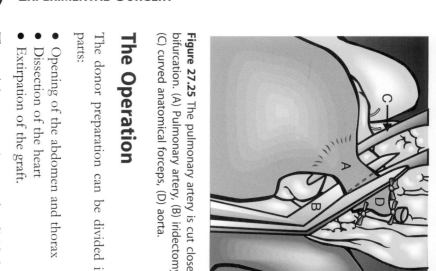

Figure 27.25 The pulmonary artery is cut close to the bifurcation. (A) Pulmonary artery, (B) iridectomy scissors, (C) curved anatomical forceps, (D) aorta.

The Operation

The donor preparation can be divided into three parts:

- Opening of the abdomen and thorax
- Dissection of the heart
- Extirpation of the graft.

The recipient operation can be divided into four parts:

- Opening of the abdominal cavity
- Dissection of vessels, exposure of the graft and placing the clamps
- The anastomoses and the removal of the clamp
- Closure of the abdominal cavity.

Donor preparation

Opening of the abdomen and thorax

After the rat has been anesthetized, the abdomen and the chest are shaven and disinfected. The abdomen is opened as described earlier. The anterior chest wall should be separated from the diaphragm, thus allowing the rib cage to be cut 1.5 cm left and right from the sternum up to the clavicles. The xiphoid cartilage is lifted and the anterior chest wall is cut near the clavicles.

Dissection of the heart

In order to prevent the blood from clotting, 50 IU heparin is injected via the infrahepatic vena cava. Since the ischemic time for the rat heart is approximately one hour, the following steps must be carried out in a short period of time (less than 10 minutes). To prevent blurred vision by excessive bleeding in the thoracic cavity, the infrarenal abdominal aorta

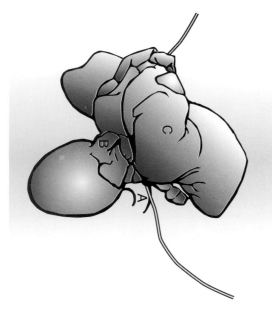

Figure 27.26 The extirpated heart together with the lungs. (A) Aorta, (B) pulmonary artery, (C) lung.

and the vena cava are cut and the animal is bled off. Blood can be quickly absorbed using gauze.

The superior and inferior vena cava are ligated close to the heart with 6-0 silk and separated. The thymic lobes are dissected and removed in the rostral direction. The ascending aorta and the pulmonary trunk are transected. Subsequently the innominate artery and the left carotid artery are ligated and cut. The aorta is cut just before the bifurcation of the left subclavian artery. The common pulmonary artery is transected near its bifurcation in order to preserve maximum vessel length (Figure 27.25).

Extirpation of the graft

The vessels from the left atrium and the pulmonary veins are ligated using 4-0 silk. Heart and lungs are extirpated. Subsequently, the lungs are removed from the heart by cutting next to the ligature. The heart should be placed in cold sterile Ringer's solution and kept on ice (Figure 27.26).

Recipient preparation

After the animal has been anesthetized, shaven and disinfected, it is placed in a supine position with the head away from the surgeon.

Dissection of vessels, exposure of the graft and placing the clamp

The aorta and vena cava
After the abdomen is opened, the intestines are packed in sterile gauze moistened with warm (37°C) saline solution and are put to the right side

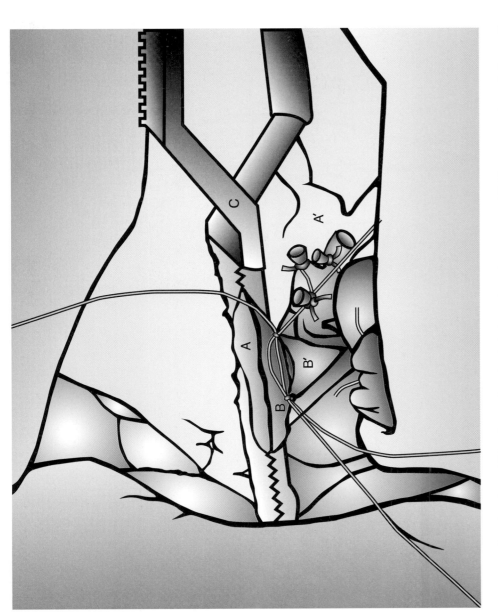

Figure 27.27 After the clamp (C) has been placed, a hole is cut into the vena cava (B). The corner sutures between the vena cava (B) and the pulmonary artery (B') are placed. A and A' are the recipient and donor aorta respectively.

as viewed by the surgeon. Subsequently the infrarenal abdominal aorta and vena cava are freed from peritoneum and are separated over a length of approximately 2 cm. This will provide enough space for the application of a small bulldog clamp modified according to Satinsky.

Exposure of the graft

The graft is positioned transversely in the right side of the abdominal cavity of the recipient. Before the clamp is applied, the aorta and pulmonary artery should be exposed.

Placing the clamp

The modified bulldog clamp is brought in position while the aorta and vena cava are slightly lifted using anatomical forceps. It is of utmost importance to match the pedicle diameter of both the aorta and pulmonary artery of the donor, with the elliptical incisions in the infrarenal abdominal aorta and the longitudinal incision in the vena cava of the recipient.

In cases where the diameters do not match, this will cause all sorts of problems, varying from stenosis due to thrombosis, to excessive bleeding after clamp removal. After the holes have been cut, the vessels are irrigated to dislodge adherent clots from the lumen.

Anastomoses – pulmonary artery to the vena cava

For this anastomosis we also use a continuous end-to-side technique. First the corner stay sutures are placed and some traction is applied (Figure 27.27). The anterior wall of the anastomosis should now be completed. Let the tip of the needle penetrate the venous wall from the outside to the inside, close to the corner stay suture. Subsequently it should penetrate the opposite wall of the pedicle from the inside to the outside, again as close to the corner stay suture as possible. Next, the suture is pulled through carefully until the vessel edges just meet. A series of stitches should be made and again the final stitch should be placed as close to the corner stay suture as possible. After placing the final stitch the suture should be tied. Try to pull the suture taut, thus avoiding a pursestring effect.

The heart should now be turned over and the posterior wall (now anterior) should be sutured using standard technique.

Anastomoses – the graft aorta to the abdominal aorta

Next we start with the corner sutures of the aorta anastomosis. After carefully exposing the pedicle, first the cranial corner stay suture is put in place. The pedicle is gently supported at the inside using jeweller's forceps. The needle penetrates the wall between the legs of the forceps from the outside to the inside. Leave one end of the suture long enough so that it can be used as a traction stay suture. The needle should then be inserted in the aorta from the inside to the outside. Subsequently a surgical knot is

tied. You should now check the size of the holes in the vessels. In case of an arteriotomy being too small, you may insert a closed jeweller's forceps into the lumen. By opening them slowly lengthwise along the vessel, the hole may be stretched to the required size. Now the second corner stay suture is placed at 180°. This time the needle is passed from outside the artery to inside thence inside the pedicle to outside. Again the suture is gently tied, leaving one end longer for traction. Small bulldog clamps may be used to obtain this traction, thus providing easy exposure during completion of the anastomosis.

Over-and-over stitches, as shown in Figure 27.28 should be placed in the anterior wall. Care should be taken when applying the first and the final stitch close to the corner sutures. On the one hand through-stitches are easily made and on the other hand these stitches should be as close to the corner sutures as possible since this will prevent excessive bleeding afterwards.

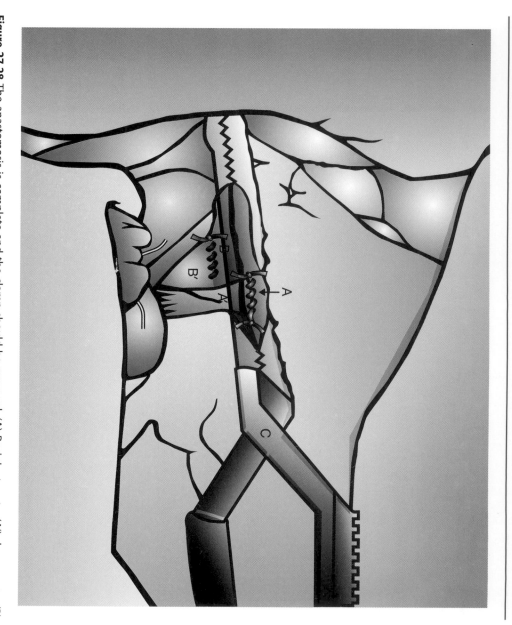

Figure 27.28 The anastomosis is complete and the clamp should be removed. (A) Recipient aorta, (A') donor aorta, (B) recipient vena cava, (B') donor pulmonary artery, (C) modified bulldog clamp (according to Satinsky).

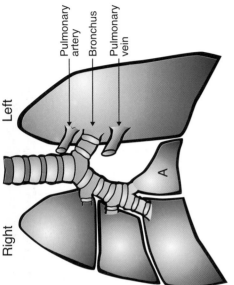

Right

Left

Pulmonary artery

Bronchus

Pulmonary vein

A

Figure 27.29 Anatomy of the rat lungs. (A) The postcaval lobe.

The heart should now be turned over and the posterior wall (now anterior) sutured using the same technique.

Releasing the Satinsky clamp

After the anastomosis has been completed, the Satinsky clamp should be removed. This is best done by slightly opening the clamp, allowing blood to enter both pedicles. The clamp is then released and the anastomosis left alone for one minute, allowing fibrin webs to be formed thus diminishing hemorrhagic risk. The clamp should now be removed completely. Use a cotton-wool stick to slightly press the anastomosis. Keep the cotton-wool stick in place until the bleeding has stopped.

Closure of the abdomen

Before replacing the intestines, the transplanted heart should be checked for leakage on the anastomoses and, if possible, corrected. The intestines are replaced into the abdominal cavity and the abdominal wall should be closed in two layers.

Orthotopic Lung Transplantation

Introduction

In the rat, the history of lung transplantation goes back to 1970. It was Lee *et al.* (1970) who first described an auxiliary nonfunctional heterotopic heart–lung transplantation. In this technique the aorta and the right atrium of the transplant were connected to the abdominal aorta and vena cava of the recipient respectively. In this model ventilation was not possible and perfusion was nonphysiological. A year later Herr (1971) described an orthotopic nonauxiliary heart–lung transplantation technique. This technique was rather troublesome as it took 300 transplants to get one surviving animal. In the same year, Asimacopoulos (1971) accomplished an orthotopic transplantation of the left lung in the rat. For his technique he used rather heavy rats with a body weight between 400 and 600 g. However, mortality rate was extremely high (80%), and the article lacked any discussion about the survivors.

Several investigators tried to improve the technique of lung transplantation in the rat. An important step forward was the simplified technique of

endotracheal intubation by Bartels (1979). Using this technique combined with a Keuskamp infant ventilator, Marck *et al.* (1979) devised a modification of the orthotopic left lung transplantation in the rat based on the technique of Asimacopoulos (1971). Subsequently, this technique was followed by a modification of Prop *et al.* in 1980 (Marck, 1983; Prop, 1984; Prop and Marck, 1984). Konertz (1985) modified the technique of Marck by avoiding a direct end-to-end anastomosis of the pulmonary vein. Instead they connected the pulmonary vein of the graft directly to the left appendage.

The left lung was selected for the transplantation because it consists of one big lobe. The right lung consists of four smaller lobes (see Figure 27.29).

Prop (1984) reported an 85% overall survival rate for the operation and the 168 days follow-up period.

The Operation

Two surgeons should carry out the operation, allowing simultaneous preparation of the donor graft and the recipient.

Anesthesia

To inhibit mucus secretion, atropine should be administered in a dosage of 0.25 mg/kg, i.m. Both the donor and the recipient should be intubated and artificially ventilated. For the endotracheal intubation a powerful light source is used to transilluminate the neck of the animal. The light penetrating the tissues will illuminate the larynx and the vocal cords, which facilitates rapid intubation (Bartels, 1979;

Remie et al., 1990c). The rats are anesthetized using N_2O and O_2 (2:1) with 0.5–1.0% halothane. The ventilator was set to 2–3.5 mL tidal volume at a frequency of 40–60 breaths/min. Peak airway pressure should be limited to 20 cmH_2O. Positive end expiratory pressure (PEEP) should be adjusted to 2 cmH_2O.

The donor operation can be divided into four parts:

- Opening of the abdomen and the thorax
- Dissection of the vessels and bronchus of the left lung
- Perfusion of the graft
- Removal of the graft.

The recipient operation can be divided into six parts:

- Thoracotomy
- Extirpation of the host's postcaval lobe and the left lung
- Placing of the Blalock pulmonary clamp
- Arterial and venous anastomoses
- Bronchial anastomosis
- Closure of the thorax with negative pressure drainage.

Donor preparation

Opening of the abdomen and thorax

After the induction of anesthesia, the abdomen and thorax of the animal are shaved and disinfected. The animal is placed on its back on a silicone rubber plate. Prior to the donor organ preparation 1000 IU of heparin are to be injected intravenously. This can be done directly into the ventricle of the heart after the thorax has been opened. First, the abdomen is opened following the linea alba towards the xiphoid cartilage and subsequently transversely alongside the false ribs, thus providing a good view of the diaphragm. Next the ribs are divided on both sides of the spine, i.e. on both sides of the thoracic vertebral column. The xiphoid cartilage is pulled in the cranial direction. Since ventilation is continuous during dissection, attention should be paid to avoiding damage to the vulnerable lung tissue by the sharp rib ends. They are best covered with moist gauze.

Dissection of the vessels and bronchus of the left lung

We start with the dissection of the ascending aorta followed by the cranial and the caudal part of the vena cava. Next the assistant surgeon exposes the hilus of the left lung. Using wet cotton-wool sticks, the lung is manipulated carefully to expose the underlying vessels. The vessels are freed from their surrounding tissue. Next the bronchus should be dissected.

Perfusion of the graft

Clamps are placed on the ascending aorta and vena cava (cranial and caudal) (Figure 27.30). A needle connected to a perfusion system (containing cold saline solution) is introduced into the right ventricle of the heart. Before perfusion, the left pulmonary artery is cut to avoid congestion of the lung during perfusion.

Removal of the graft

Before the removal of the lung a small piece of a sterile surgical glove 8 × 8 cm is cut out and the magnesium powder removed. The piece is folded in such a way that a hole of 0.5 cm in diameter is cut in the center point. The vessel pedicle as well as the bronchial stump is pushed carefully through the hole after which the glove is wrapped around the lung to cover it completely. Every now and then fluid should be injected into the artificial pouch in order to prevent the lung from dehydrating. By covering the lung this way, it can be handled more easily and the tissue is protected against damage during the operation.

For the removal of the donor lung, the pulmonary artery and vein should both be cut. Using small scissors, the bronchus is cut between two cartilage rings about three to four rings from the lung. During transplantation the lung remains uninflated.

Recipient preparation

Thoracotomy

The chest is shaved and the animal is placed on its right side on the operating table, the operating area is disinfected and covered with sterile incision foil (Steri-Drape, 3M, nr. 2035). A left-side thoracotomy in the third or fourth intercostal space is performed (Figure 27.31). The intercostal space is located and opened carefully, avoiding any penetration of lung tissue underneath. The blunt tip of a pair of scissors is inserted into the thoracic cavity and the intercostal muscles are cut in the dorsal direction as far as possible. A small part of the latissimus dorsi muscle is cut. Next, the intercostal muscle is cut in the direction of the sternum. After the pleural space has been opened, a 7-cm Alm retractor is placed in the wound and the ribs are spread. Now the left lung is properly exposed and ready for extirpation.

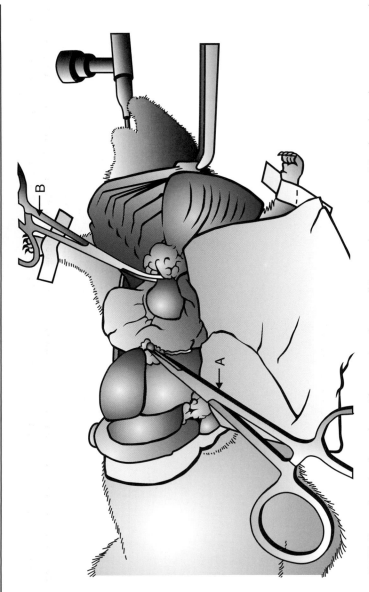

Figure 27.30 Harvesting the donor lung. The anterior chest wall is turned over, clamp A is placed on the vena cava and clamp B on the ascending aorta. The graft is ready for perfusion.

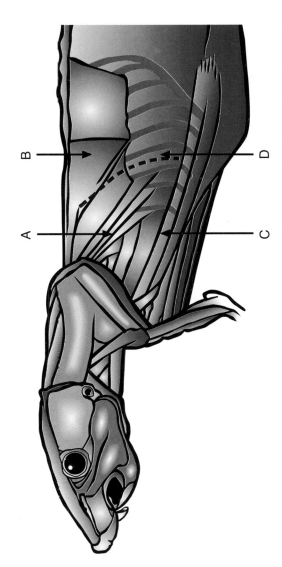

Figure 27.31 Deep muscles. (A) Musculus serratus ventralis, (B) musculus serratus dorsalis cranialis, (C) musculus rectus thoracis et abdominis, (D) musculus intercostalis externus.

Extirpation of the host's postcaval lobe and the left lung

First the postcaval lobe of the right lung (Figure 27.32) is ligated and resected. It may be of help for the assistant to wrap the lung in a small, saline-moistened strip of gauze. When necessary the assistant can expose the vessels properly by retracting the lung in different directions. The bronchus and the left pulmonary artery and vein must be freed from surrounding tissue. Moving the lung (by the assistant) facilitates the procedure. After the bronchus is freed from the pulmonary artery and vein, it is ligated close to the bifurcation using 4-0 nonabsorbable suture. The ligature should not be cut too short, as after trans-section of the bronchus it may retract a little underneath the vena cava.

Placing of the Blalock pulmonary clamp

After the bronchus has been cut, the pulmonary vein and artery are clamped using a Blalock pulmonary vessel clamp (Figure 27.33). The clamp is turned over and laid on the same holder as the Alm retractor. The clamp is provided with two small eyes for suture fixation, while the yaws are covered with silicon tubing for smooth occlusion of the vessels without damage. Both vessels can now be transected and the left lung removed. The vessel stumps should now be carefully flushed with saline to remove all blood (clots). Next the graft is placed on the shaft of the Blalock clamp. In this way movements of the beating heart or the ventilated lungs will not disturb the suturing.

Arterial and venous anastomoses

We start with the arterial anastomosis and a continuous technique is used. The corner stay sutures are inserted and the first half of a surgical knot can be made. Both knots can be tightened, while the vessels of the graft and the recipient are matched up. The stay sutures can be fixed to the eyes of the Blalock clamp and the anastomosis may be kept under slight tension (Figure 27.34). The end-to-end anastomoses are completed using standard technique. After the venous anastomosis has been completed, the Blalock clamp is removed and circulation through the graft is restored.

Bronchial anastomosis

The bronchus stumps are cut to the desired length (as short as possible on the donor side). A telescopic technique is used for the anastomosis (Figure 27.35). The first stitch (9-0 monofilament) is placed

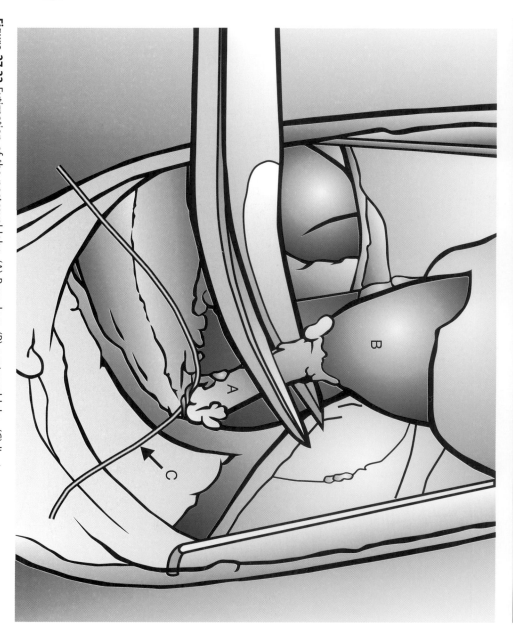

Figure 27.32 Extirpation of the postcaval lobe. (A) Bronchus, (B) postcaval lobe, (C) ligature.

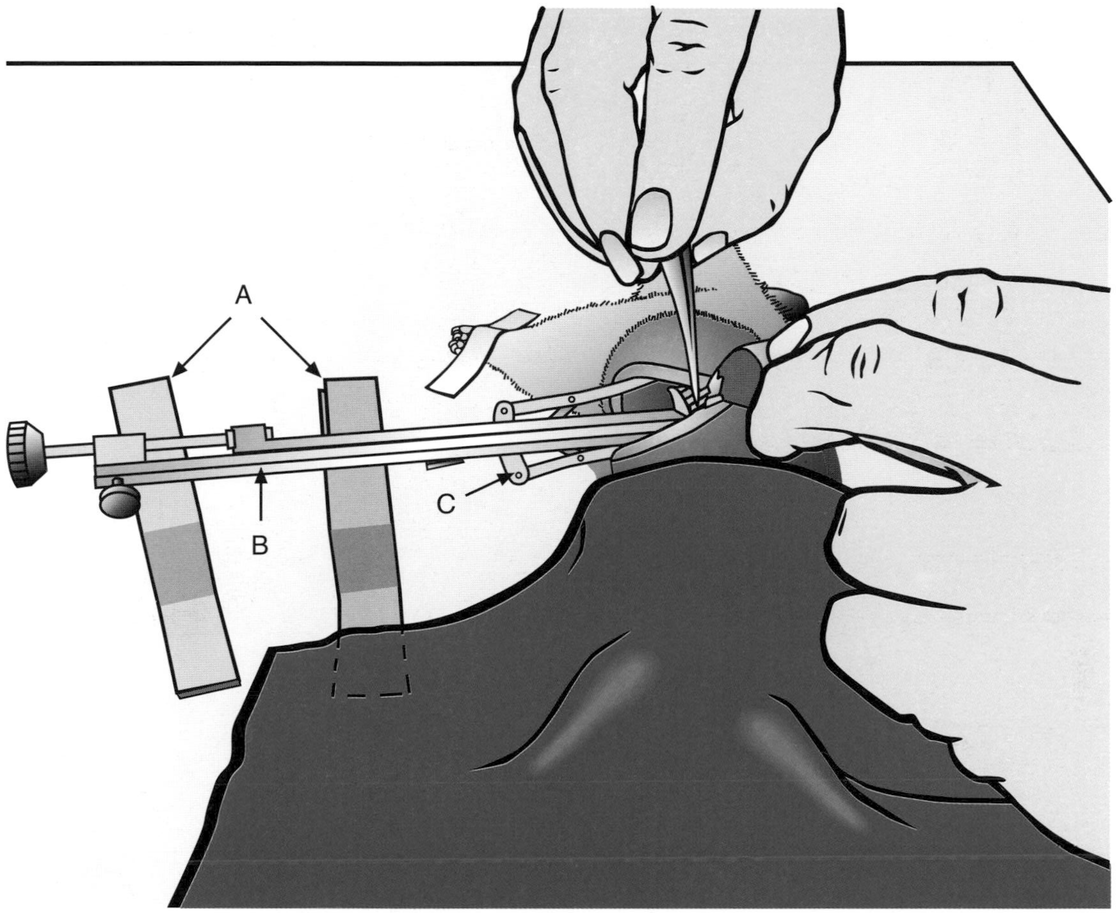

Figure 27.33 Position of the animal and instruments during removal of the recipient left lung. (A) Small bars to support the Blalock pulmonary clamp, (B) the Blalock pulmonary clamp, (C) the Alm retractor.

between the first and second cartilage ring from the edge of both the recipient and the donor stump. The membranous part of the anastomosis can be closed with interrupted knots (Figure 27.35), as a continuous suture could cause stenosis of the anastomosis. After completion the constricting ligature can be removed which induces immediate ventilation of the graft. Next the animal is shortly hyperinflated (maximum of $30\,cmH_2O$) to remove partial atelectasis. Air leakage through the anastomosis can also be checked during hyperinflation.

Closure of the thorax with negative-pressure drainage

A drain is brought into the thoracic cavity with the tip against the dorsal part of the diaphragm and a 2-mL syringe is connected. The Alm retractor should now be removed carefully. Using 4-0 absorbable sutures three to four stitches are used to close the thorax. Next the muscular layer is closed again using 4-0 absorbable suture. Subsequently, the skin is

closed and negative pressure drainage performed. The animal is now disconnected from the ventilator and should start breathing spontaneously.

Intracranial Surgery

Introduction

In the ever expanding field of brain research the rat continues to play a prominent role. As with other areas of biomedical research, an understanding of the metabolic processes occurring in the brain involves a wide range of specialties, e.g. neurophysiology, neurobiology, biochemistry, genetics, molecular and cell biology.

Surgery on the head is easier than surgery on other parts of the body, because there is little risk of excessive hemorrhage and the area is easily exposed.

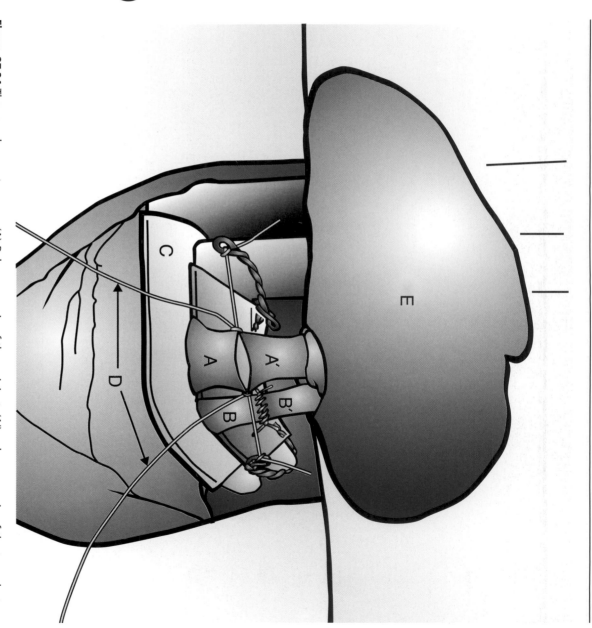

Figure 27.34 The vascular anastomoses. (A) Pulmonary vein of the recipient, (A') pulmonary vein of the transplant, (B) pulmonary artery of the recipient, (B') pulmonary artery of the transplant, (C) Blalock pulmonary clamp, (D) suture, (E) donor lung.

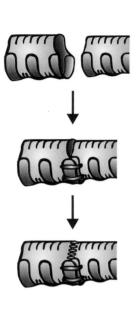

Figure 27.35 The bronchus anastomosis using the telescopic technique. Interrupted sutures are used.

Stereotaxic brain surgery is one of the techniques used to apply mono- or bipolar needle-shaped electrodes, infusion cannulae or sample cannulae for the collection of liquor. In this section some

basic principles in the use of stereotaxic equipment will be discussed. Furthermore some frequently used techniques will be described.

Anatomy

As with all surgery, a thorough knowledge of the anatomy of the area of interest is of vital importance. Fortunately there are a number of atlases available describing different aspects of the rat brain (Table 27.2). More information on stereotaxic atlases can be found on: http://www-cajal.ucsd.edu/Pages/AtlasDocs/Kopf Atlas Dir Unified.html.

Table 27.2 Atlases describing areas of the rat brain		
Authors	Year of publication	Brain area described
Krieg	1946a,b	Cortex
De Groot	1959a	Forebrain
De Groot	1959b	Hypothalamus
Massopust	1961	Diencephalon
Konig and Klippel	1963	Forebrain and lower brainstem
Wunscher et al.	1965	Brainstem
Albe-Fressard et al.	1966, 1971	Diencephalon
Pellegrino and Cushman	1967	Total brain
Pellegrino et al.	1979	Total brain
Valenstein et al.	1969	Hypothalamus (young rat)
Sherwood and Timiras	1970	Developing brain
Scremin	1970	Hypothalamus
Hurt et al.	1971	Mesencephalon
Abad-Alegria	1971, 1973	Brainstem
Peters	1974	Cerebellum
Abad-Alegria	1974	Cortex
Jansco and Kiraly	1980	Primary sensory chemosensory distribution
Simson et al.	1981	Total brain
Nieuwenhuys et al.	1982	Median forebrain bundle
Paxinos and Watson	1982, 1986	Total brain
Altman and Bayer	1994	Developing brain
Paxinos and Watson	1998	Total brain (also on CD-ROM)

For details on the anatomy of the rat brain, the reader is referred to references in Table 27.2.

Spatial Relationships

In anatomy, the basis defining all spatial relationships is the imaginary median plane, which runs from the head to the tail (Figure 27.36). This plane divides the body into two equal (right and left) halves. Another imaginary plane is the sagittal plane, which runs parallel to the median plane. The sagittal plane also divides the animal into two, not necessarily equal (left and right) sections. So there can be many sagittal planes but, by definition, only one median plane. The transverse plane lies perpendicular to the median plane; it divides the animal into a rostral part, to define structures that are lying in the direction of the head, and a caudal part, which defines structures situated in the direction of the tail.

The transverse planes are traversed in turn by the coronal planes; these divide the body into a ventral and a dorsal component. The terms 'proximal' and 'distal' respectively relate to the anatomical definition of towards and away from the center, the median line or point of attachment or origin.

On the head itself we use the terms rostral and caudal, while in the rest of the body we use cranial and caudal (see van Dongen et al., 1990 for more details). In the brain we use the term anterior instead of rostral and posterior instead of caudal.

Figure 27.37 shows the skull diagram of a 290-g Wistar rat in dorsal and lateral view (Paxinos and Watson, 1998). Important landmarks are: bregma, lambda and the interaural line. Note that lambda is 0.3 mm anterior to the coronal plane passing through the interaural line.

The principle of stereotaxic surgery is based upon the constant relationship between these landmarks on the skull and parts of the brain. A system of three coordinates is used to pinpoint a specific location in the brain relative to one of these landmarks:

Stereotaxic Brain Surgery

Preparation of the animal

Animals should preferably weigh between 250 and 350 g for adult Wistar rats of either sex (Kline and Reid, 1984; Paxinos *et al.*, 1985) although there may be some differences in craniometric and stereotaxic data for rats of different strain, sex and weight. No substantial stereotaxic error, however, will occur when rats of 290 g of different strain and sex are used (see Paxinos and Watson, 1998 for details). For the use of stereotaxis in newborn rats, the reader is referred to Cunningham and McKay (1993).

After the animal has been anesthetized, the head is shaved and disinfected. The rat is placed in a Kopf small-animal stereotaxic instrument. The head will be fixed in three places, the two bony ear canals and the upper jaw (Figures 27.37 and 27.38). Start by inserting the ear bars into both ear canals. The head should pivot freely about the interaural axis and should have little lateral movement. Move the incisor bar under the upper incisors. Place the nose clamp over the nose, gently retract the incisor bar anteriorly and tighten it. Next the incisor bar should be adjusted vertically until the heights of lambda and bregma are equal (both in a coronal

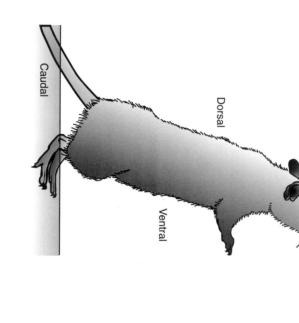

Figure 27.36 The spatial relationships.

1 Anterior–posterior (A-P)
2 Dorsal–ventral (D-V)
3 Lateral (Lat).

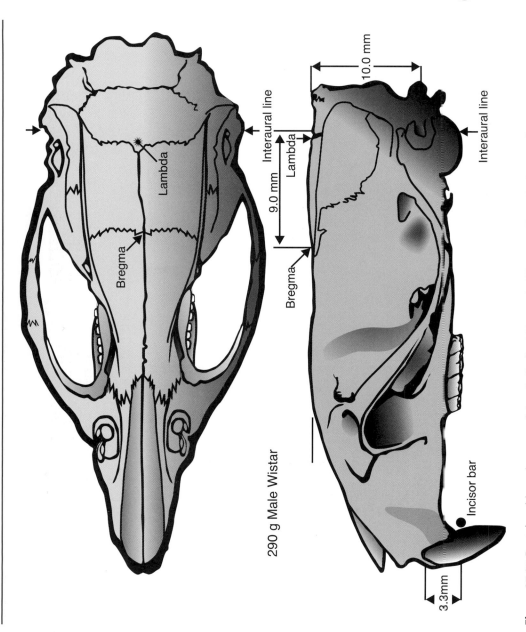

290 g Male Wistar

Figure 27.37 Dorsal and lateral aspect of the skull of a 290-g male Wistar rat. From Paxinos and Watson (1998).

plane), resulting in a flat-skull position (Paxinos and Watson, 1998).

For the implantation procedure it is imperative that all the periosteum is removed from the crown of the head, ensuring that the acrylic dental cement will adhere properly to the skull. After positioning of the implantable device, three additional holes should be drilled in the skull as described earlier.

Positioning of implantable devices

To determine the exact position of an implantable device (electrode, cannula, microdialysis probe, etc.) you have to use one of the stereotaxic atlases listed before. That of Paxinos and Watson (1986, 1998) comes highly recommended. After the animal has been placed in the stereotaxic instrument, the implantable device is clamped into the electrode carrier. Make sure that the device is straight and has a 90° angle to the coronal plane. Next the tip of the

device is adjusted directly above the bregma and the reading for the A-P and the Lat zero point are taken. Subsequently, calculate the readings after the distances given in the stereotaxic atlas are added or subtracted from the A-P and Lat zero readings. The device should now be moved to the newly calculated A-P and Lat position. The device is lowered until it just touches the skull, giving the vertical zero reading. Calculate what the final reading must be in order for the device tip to penetrate the brain to the specific depth. When the device is in the newly calculated position, it should be slightly raised and the place on the skull where the hole has to be drilled should be marked with a sharp pencil. Move the electrode aside and drill a hole of sufficient diameter in the skull at the pencil mark (Figure 27.39a,b). Next the device should again be positioned in the A-P and Lat planes, according to the previous calculation. Now the device is lowered over the required distance to the reading of the calculated vertical placement (D-V value).

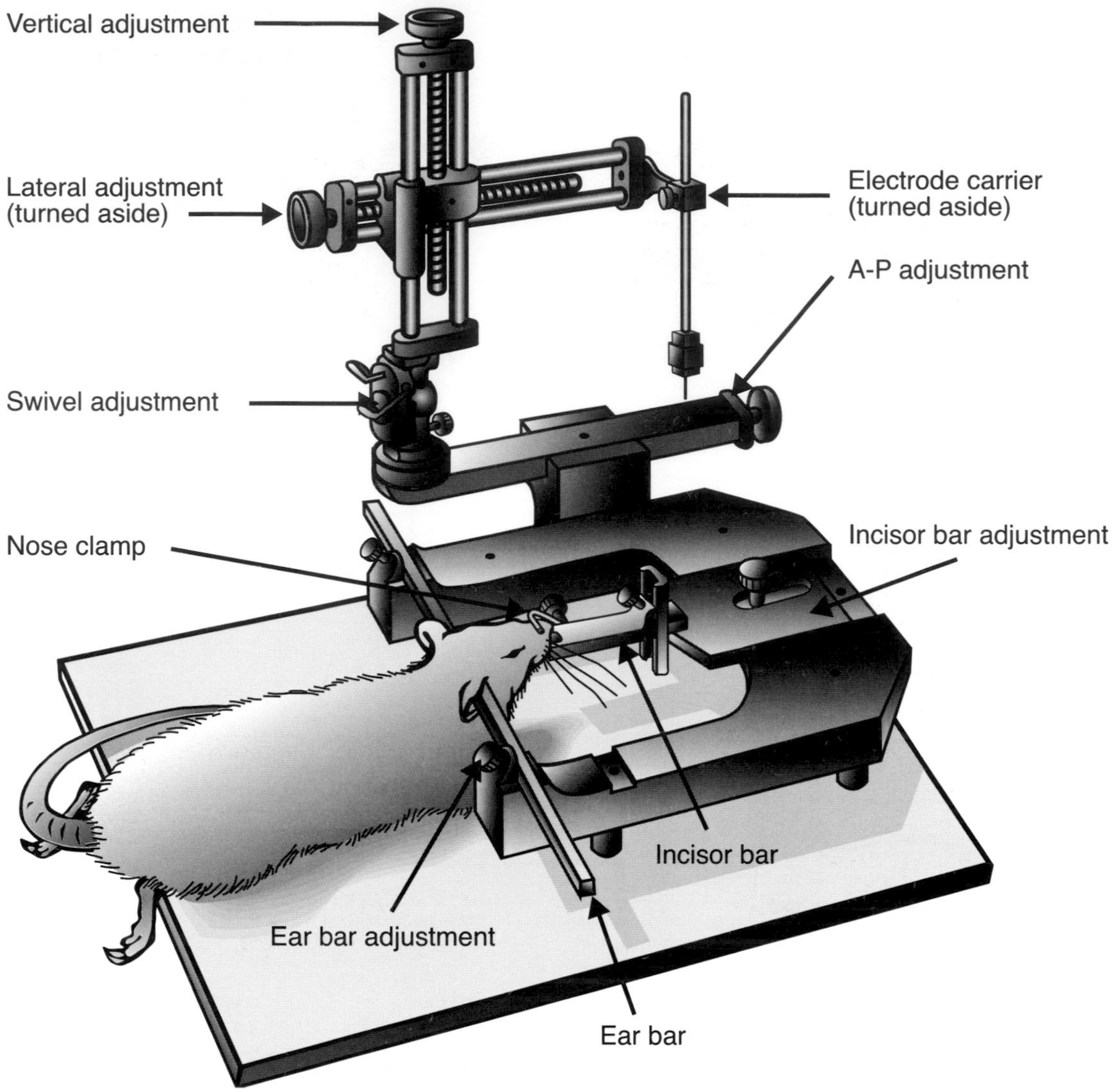

Figure 27.38 Anesthetized rat fixated in the Kopf stereotaxic instrument.

Lesion or stimulation using electrodes

Monopolar electrodes can be used to injure or stimulate brain areas by passing an electrical current between the relatively small surface area on the tip of the electrode, to a relatively large amount of body tissue acting as a ground terminal. Electrodes are preferably made of platinum, and should be insulated. A two-component epoxy resin can be used for insulation. Simply dip in the electrode once or twice and let the resin cure. Next 0.5 mm of the tip is freed of its insulation using a scalpel blade.

Always connect the positive terminal (anode) of the current source to the electrode, thus preventing the formation of hydrogen and oxygen. The cathode should be clamped on a muscular layer on the head. After the lesion has been made, the electrode is removed and the hole in the skull is closed with bone wax. Next the skin is closed using the interrupted suture technique (Figure 27.39c,d).

For stereotaxic electrode placement in neonatal rats, the reader is referred to the work of Heller *et al.* (1979).

Bipolar electrodes are very similar to the monopolar ones. They are commercially available but you can also build them yourself. Before implantation of the bipolar electrode, it should be soldered to a miniature connector (e.g. an IC foot).

Technically, the bipolar electrode is implanted in the same way as the monopolar electrode. After the electrode has been placed in a specific brain region, according to the calculated A-P, Lat and D-V values, the electrode, together with the small IC foot connector, is glued to the skull using acrylic dental

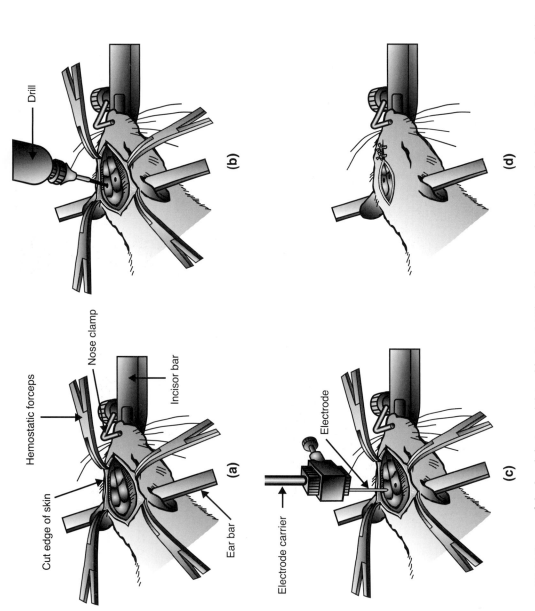

(a)

Cut edge of skin

Hemostatic forceps

Nose clamp

Incisor bar

Ear bar

(b)

Drill

(c)

Electrode carrier

Electrode

(d)

Figure 27.39 Crown of the head during a bilateral lesion. (a) The skull exposed and the calculated positions marked. (b) The holes are drilled. (c) The electrode is inserted to the calculated depth. (d) The skin is closed using interrupted sutures.

cement. Note that the electrode carrier is still holding the electrode during this process. After the dental cement has cured, the skin should be closed around the connector.

Electroencephalography

Electroencephalography recording (EEG) requires specialized equipment and techniques. The signals picked up from the cortex are of very low voltage and should be derived from as close to the source as possible. Electrode placement therefore is of vital importance (Rosenberg *et al*, 1976). We routinely use 1-mm stainless steel screws. The screws are equipped with 2-cm-long small-diameter noninsulated stainless steel wires, which are point-welded to the top of the screw. The screws are placed on the crown of the head, the first 2mm posterior and 2mm lateral to

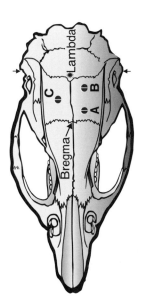

Lambda

Bregma

C

A B

Figure 27.40 Dorsal aspect of the skull with screws for EEG measurement. A and B are measuring electrodes while C can be used as ground.

bregma and a second one 2mm anterior and 2mm lateral to lambda (Figure 27.40). A third screw is used for additional anchoring and can also be used as a ground electrode. The wires of all three screws are soldered (*in situ*) to a small connector.

Signals may be registered via a multichannel electrical swivel while the animal is kept in a slowly rotating cage (to keep it awake) placed in a Faraday cage. The use of a telemetric device that can be magnetically switched on and off, ensuring a long lifespan of the battery (approximately 1 year) is more sophisticated.

Central nervous system injections and infusions

Several techniques have been described for placement of cannulae in one of the ventricles of the rat for injection, sampling and infusion. Most techniques are rather simple and use a combination of an external guide cannula and an internal cannula (Myers, 1963, 1970; Hoebel, 1964; Grunden and Linburn, 1969; Myers et al., 1967; Khavari, 1970; Chisholm and Singer, 1970). Using a stereotaxic procedure Myers (1963) implanted a 26-G needle in the ventricle. The needle was secured to the skull with four stainless steel screws and epoxy glue. A 32-G infusion cannula was passed through the 26-G needle. Coupling with the external cannula was troublesome. Grunden and Linburn (1969) modified a 23-G hypodermic needle to serve as a guide cannula for ventricular injection and used a mandril to close the system and keep it from getting obstructed when not in use.

A very reliable and inexpensive cannula and injection system for local chemical brain stimulation with small volumes of fluids has been described by Strubbe (1975). This system, which will be described below, has several advantages over those mentioned in the literature. Its construction is very simple, it is inexpensive and therefore disposable, it allows bilateral infusions without disturbing the animal and it gives you a direct visual check of the rate at which the fluid enters the brain.

The system consists of a permanent guide (outer) cannula, made from a disposable hypodermic 23-G needle. The colored plastic is removed with the exception of the white fixed inner ring. The thin plastic layer above the ring is removed using a sharp knife. The needle is cut to a length depending on the depth of the brain area to be stimulated (Figure 27.41). After disinfection in chlorhexidine solution, the cannula tip is placed stereotaxically as described above. The plastic ring being just above the surface of the skull is now fixed using acrylic dental cement and three screws to anchor the cement to the skull. A polythene cap (i.d. 0.58 mm, o.d. 0.96 mm) is placed on the outer cannula. If bilateral cannulae are wanted, they can be mounted in a brass bar with holes at the required distance and glued together with dental cement.

The inner cannula consists of a stainless steel tube (i.d. 0.1 mm, o.d. 0.29 mm) and should be exactly 3 mm longer than the guide cannula. Over these 3 mm a polythene tube (PE) is slipped (i.d. 0.29 mm, o.d. 0.61 mm). A silicon cuff (i.d. 0.5 mm, o.d. 1.0 mm) is then slid over this connection.

On the other end of the PE tube a silicon cuff (i.d. 0.5 mm, o.d. 1.0 mm) is placed. Over this cuff a second silicon tube (i.d. 1.0 mm, o.d. 3.0 mm) is slipped. A small nail with a head of suitable size (plunger) is pushed into the silicon tube and the injection system is ready (Figure 27.41).

The injection system is first filled completely with methylene blue (1% in saline). Subsequently the nail is pushed down and slightly pulled back again until an air bubble can just be perceived above the inner cannula. Now the tip of the inner cannula is placed in the fluid to be injected. The nail is pulled up so that the infusion tube is filled with that fluid. The inner cannula is then placed into the outer cannula. The silicon cuff on the lower end of the injection tube serves to attach it firmly to the guide cannula. The injection can now be made by pushing down the nail. The air bubble, separating the methylene blue from the injection fluid, may serve as a marker for reading the volume administered. This volume can be calculated from the diameter of the PE tubing. Figure 27.42 shows the rat attached to the infusion system (Strubbe, 1975).

Microdialysis

Chemical interplay between cells occurs in the extracellular fluid, a compartment usually overlooked due to the fact that it is hard to access experimentally. Many experimental approaches have been suggested to get information about the extracellular environment of the intact brain, for example ventricular perfusion, cortical cup perfusion and push-pull cannulae (Gaddum, 1961). The introduction of a dialysis membrane into the tissue (Bito et al., 1966) has provided the first generally applicable way of interacting with the extracellular compartment.

Brain dialysis is a relatively new technique for the investigation of in vivo release of neurotransmitters and amino acids (Zetterström et al., 1983; Ungersted, 1984, 1991; Imperato and Di Chiara, 1984; Westerink and De Vries, 1988). It has some

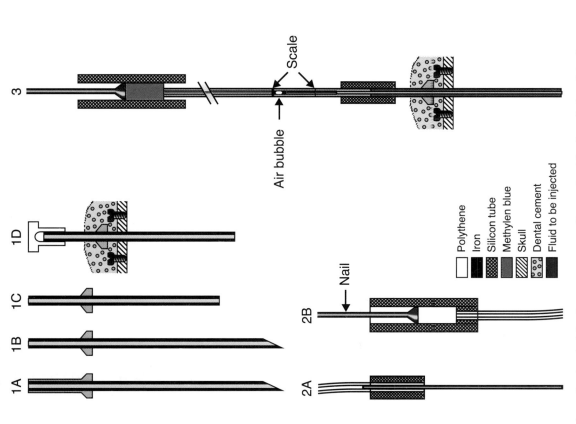

Figure 27.41 Preparation of a simple injection system according to Strubbe (1975). Detail in the text.

Polythene
Iron
Silicon tube
Methylen blue
Skull
Dental cement
Fluid to be injected

advantages over other techniques such as push–pull perfusion, which have the risk of doing mechanical damage to the tissue, and *in vivo* voltammetry (Gonon *et al.*, 1980; Ewing *et al.*, 1982) where it is often uncertain what the chemical identity of the detected material is (see Ungerstedt, 1991; Westerink and Justice, 1991, for more details). Today a range of different probes is used, for example the trans-striatal, the U-shaped, the I-shaped and the commercially available Carnegie cannulae.

Four different types of intracerebral microdialysis probes (Figure 27.43) were characterized by Santiago and Westerink (1990). They concluded that every type of dialysis probe causes a certain amount of damage when implanted into the brain. In acute

experiments the best results were obtained using the I-shaped probe. In the chronic situation (24 hours after implantation) all probes performed well. During the second day after implantation, conditions were optimal to carry out dialysis experiments. After 48 hours certain restrictions are to be expected due to elevated K^+ levels in the neuronal tissue. The trans-striatal probe displayed a high output as it perfuses bilateral brain structures, but from an animal welfare point of view, too much discomfort is produced due to damage to the temporal muscles.

Implantation of these devices has been described earlier. Details about perfusion fluids and other practical aspects can be found in the work of Robinson and Justice (1991).

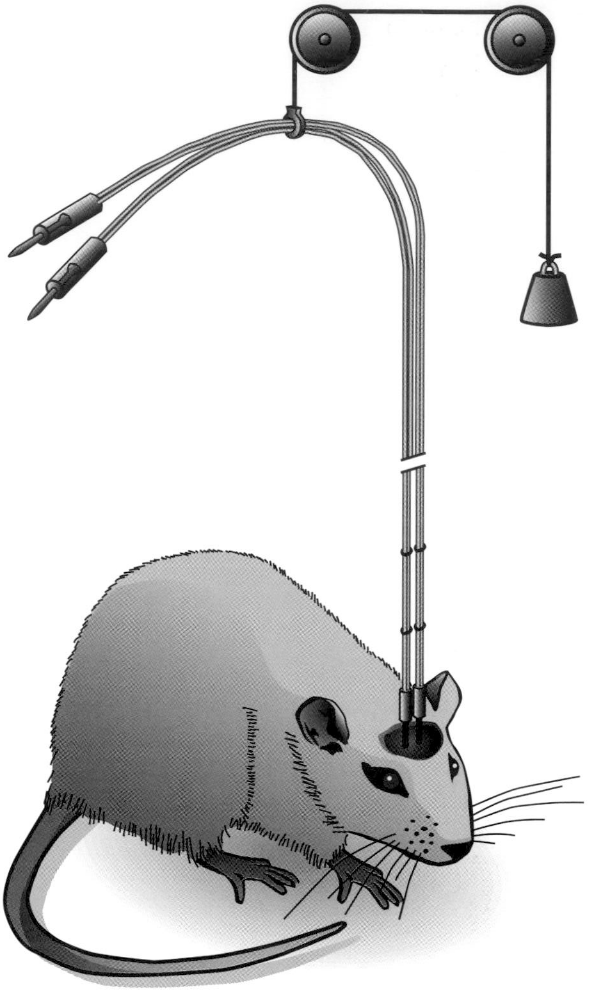

Figure 27.42 Freely moving rat during local brain injection.

Basic Surgical Procedures

point where the needle enters the heart. Next cut a hole in the right atrium to allow blood to be drained from the head. Keep on flushing with saline solution until the effluent is clear and then switch to formaldehyde perfusion (250 mL). Next the brain can be removed.

Make an incision from behind the ears to the nose. Cut the skin from the skull down to the nose. Remove the temporal muscles from the skull and the first two vertebrae. Next remove the cranial bone using small bone cutters until the olfactory bulbs are visible. Cut the dura and lift the brain, starting with the anterior part. Cut the cranial nerves, lift the rest of the brain and cut the spinal cord. Continue the fixation process by placing the brain in fresh formaldehyde for 3 days.

Note that perfusion fixation is also described in Chapter 26.

Cesarian section

Cesarian section is a commonly used technique to perpetuate a rat strain as a specific pathogen-free colony (SPF). Therefore the procedure must be carried out under strict aseptic conditions. The operation should be carried out just before the natural birth process commences and two surgical methods can be used. First the hysterectomy, which involves the complete removal of the gravid uterus from the mother animal. The second technique is called hysterotomy, and involves the removal of the fetuses from the mother.

Anatomy

The rat uterus is bicornuate, with the uterine horns located on either side of the abdominal cavity. The horns extend to the lower pole of the kidney. Blood is supplied to the ovary, the uterus, and the cervix by the ovarian artery that runs along the entire length of the inner side of each uterine horn. The two ovaries are small, almost round organs attached to the uterine horns via convoluted Fallopian tubes.

Perfusion of the brain

In most experimental work on the brain it is necessary to perfuse and remove the brain after the experiment(s), to see the exact location of electrodes, lesions, infusion cannulae or dialysis probes. Therefore we have to perfuse the brain with saline and formaldehyde fixative (10%) respectively. Perfusion can be performed simply using two reservoirs, one filled with saline and the other with 10% formaldehyde. Using a three-way stopcock both fluids may be perfused through the same needle (19-G).

The animal is deeply anesthetized using twice the amount of barbiturate needed for surgical anesthesia. Open the abdomen and the thorax as described earlier. Insert a perfusion needle into the left ventricle of the heart. Keep the needle in place by clamping it with hemostatic forceps onto the

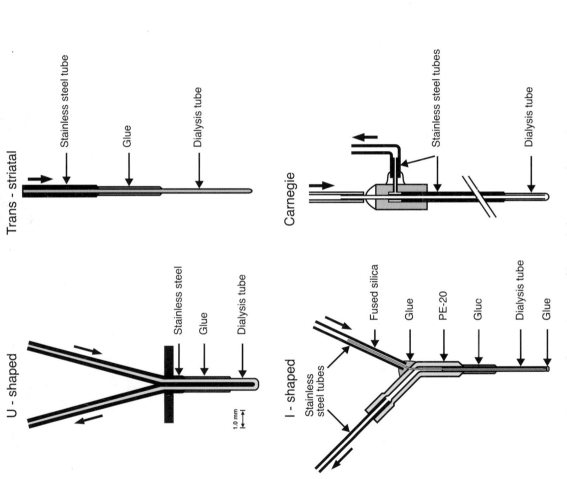

Figure 27.43 Dimensions and shapes of several types of brain dialysis cannulae.

The operations

Hysterectomy

If the animal is not supposed to recover after the operation, it should be killed humanely. After removal of the fur the animal should be submersed in an antiseptic solution (chlorhexidine/ethanol) and laid on its back with the tail pointing towards the surgeon. The abdominal cavity is opened as described earlier. The uterine horns are pulled out, removed, and immediately placed in a box containing warm (38°C) antiseptic solution. This box is then quickly brought into an isolator in the usual way, and the young are liberated from the uterus. As soon as the animals start breathing, the umbilical cords should be ligated and cut.

If the animal should survive the operation, one may choose to leave the ovaries and their blood supply intact. The ovarian artery should then be ligated just caudal to the bifurcation (Figure 27.44).

Hysterotomy

During this procedure one or more fetuses may be removed from the uterus. The pregnant animal is anesthetized using isoflurane O_2/N_2O. The abdominal cavity is opened as described earlier. One uterine horn is pulled out and laid on sterile, warm, saline-moistened gauze. Depending on the number of young to be removed, an incision of 2 cm is made alongside the outer wall of the uterus. If all the fetuses are to be removed, the whole horn should be opened.

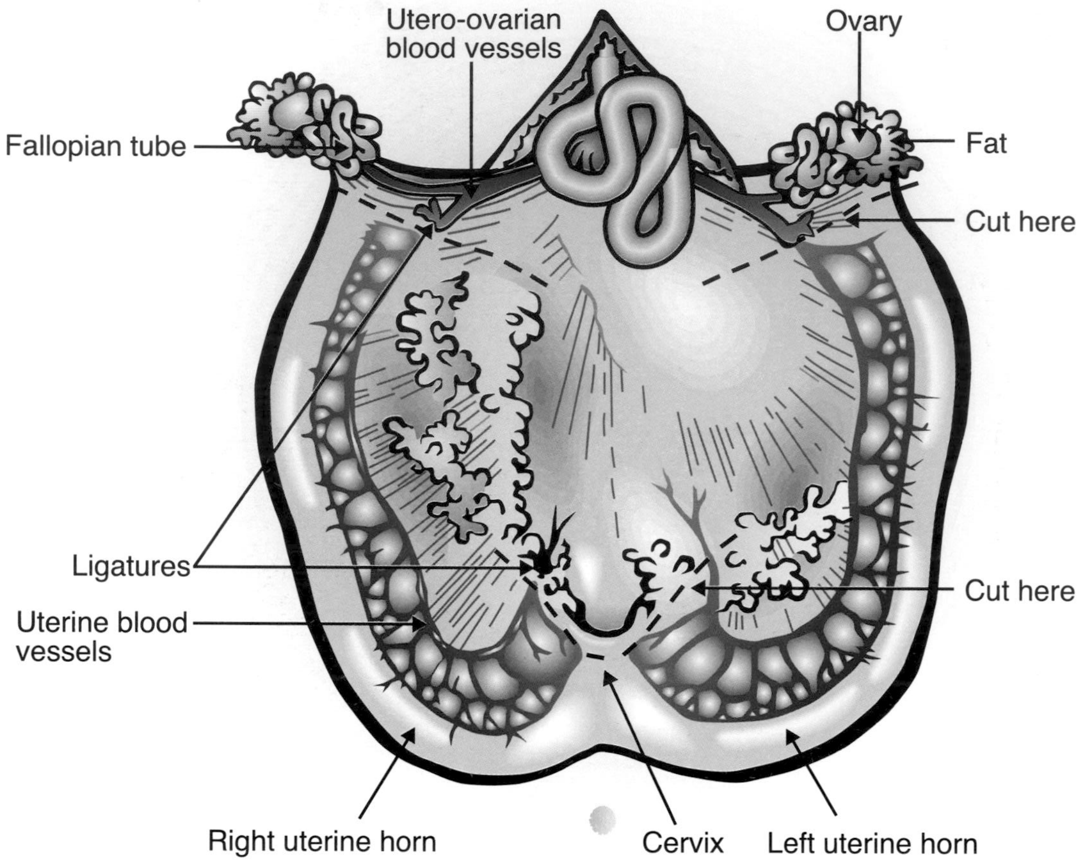

Figure 27.44 Anatomy of the rat uterus. During hysterectomy, the uterus is ligated as indicated and cut on the dotted lines.

Subsequently the blood vessels between the placental disc and the uterus should be ligated before the disc is removed. Next the young should be liberated from the amniotic sac. As soon as the animals start breathing, the umbilical cord together with the blood vessels should be ligated and the animals kept in a dry and warm place (Figure 27.45). The uterus should be closed using a 5-0 resorbable suture. Next the abdominal muscle and the skin are closed as described earlier.

Female Castration (Ovariectomy)

The back of the anesthetised animal should be shaven and disinfected. Placed on its ventral surface with its tail pointing to the surgeon, a small 2-cm midline

dorsal skin incision is made about half way between the hump and the tail base. Using speading movements with a pair of scissors the connective tissue between the skin and the muscular layer is bluntly dissected on both sides in a ventral direction over a distance of about 3 cm. The skin is pulled to one side and the muscular layers are opened half way down the side of the animal. The ovary, surrounded by a considerable amount of fat, can be found underneath in the abdominal cavity. The fat tissue should be grasped and the ovary pulled out through the incision (Figure 27.46). A ligature should be placed around the uterine horn together with some fat tissue just below the Fallopian tube. The ovary, together with the fat tissue, can be safely cut off. The uterine horn should be pushed back into the abdominal cavity. Depending on the size of the muscular incision, one or two 5-0 resorbable sutures should be used to close it.

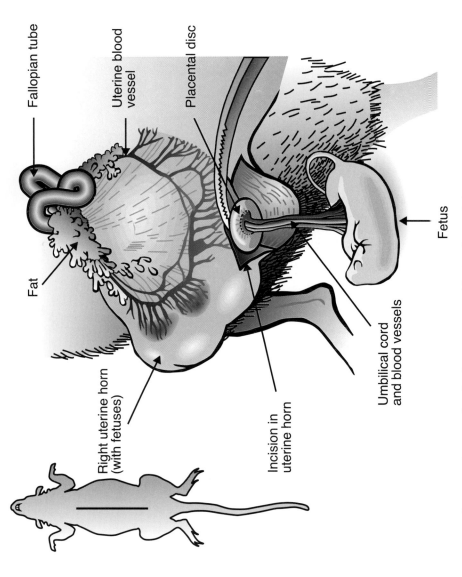

Figure 27.45 The uterus is opened and a fetus is removed by its placental disc.

Fallopian tube

Uterine blood vessel

Placental disc

Fat

Right uterine horn (with fetuses)

Incision in uterine horn

Umbilical cord and blood vessels

Fetus

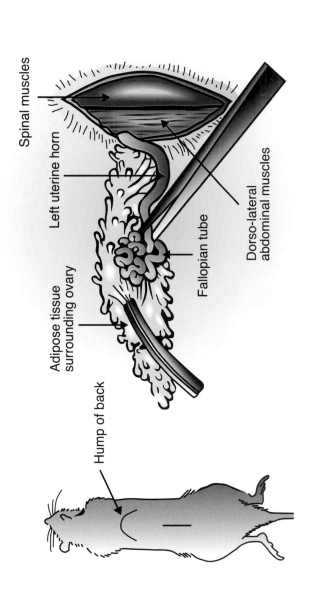

Figure 27.46 Uterine horn pulled out of the abdominal cavity through the dorsolateral abdominal muscles.

Spinal muscles

Left uterine horn

Dorso-lateral abdominal muscles

Adipose tissue surrounding ovary

Fallopian tube

Hump of back

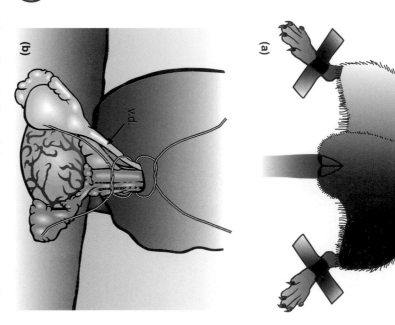

when the rat is about 40 days old. In adult rats the testes and epididymis are easily palpable through the wall of the scrotum. Each testis is connected to an epididymis that can be divided into a caput and a cauda epididymidis. The epididymis consists of a mass of tubules in which spermatozoa are stored while they become mature and motile. Spermatozoa leave the epididymis through the vasa deferentia. Each vas (ductus) deferens loops over the corresponding ureter, penetrates the dorsolateral lobe of the prostate, and opens into the beginning of the urethra.

The operation

After anesthetizing the animal, the skin of the scrotal sac should be shaven, cleaned and disinfected. A small 1-cm median incision should be made through the skin at the tip of the scrotum (Figure 27.47). The cremaster muscles are opened with a small 7-mm incision on each side. The cauda epididymidis is pulled out together with the testis, followed by the caput epididymidis, the vas deferens and the testicular blood vessels. A single ligature is placed around the vas deferens and the blood vessels. The testis can now be removed.

After both testes have been removed, the remaining pieces of the vas deferens, the fat and the blood vessels are pushed back into the sac. The incisions in the cremaster muscles are closed using two resorbable 5-0 sutures and the skin is closed with a 4-0 suture.

Figure 27.47 (a) Place of the skin incision at the tip of the scrotum. (b) A ligature is placed around the vas deferens and the blood vessels. For safety reasons sometimes two ligatures are placed. v.d., Vas deferens.

The procedure is repeated on the other side and finally the skin is closed with a 4-0 suture.

Female sterilization

If one only wants to sterilize the female rat, the above mentioned procedure should be followed to the point where the ligature is placed around the uterine horn. For sterilization a small ligature should be placed around the junction between the Fallopian tube and the uterine horn. The tube should be severed just distal to the ligature.

Male Castration (Orchidectomy)

Anatomy

The scrotum is located ventrolateral to the anus. The testes are ovoid bodies that develop in the abdominal region and descend to the scrotal sac

Vasectomy

Sometimes male rats should remain sexually active but not fertile. In these cases the animals should be vasectomized. The above mentioned procedure should be followed to the point where the testis is pulled out of the cremaster muscle. Next the vas deferens should be exposed and severed between two 4-0 ligatures. Each testis should be returned in its sac and the incisions closed as described above.

Splenectomy

The abdominal cavity is opened as described earlier. The spleen lies in the left dorsal part of the abdominal cavity. Beneath the rib cage its cranial pole is related to the dorsal margin of the left lateral lobe of the liver. From this point it extends in a curve

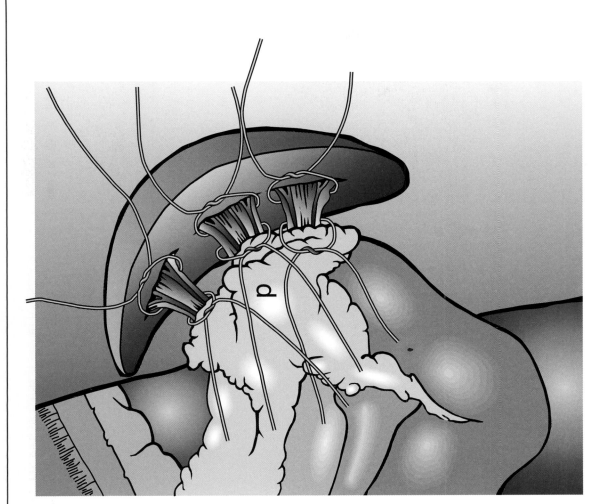

caudoventrally between the left kidney and the greater curvature of the stomach. The spleen should be pulled out of the abdominal cavity and placed on sterile, warm, saline-moistened gauze. Before entering the splenic artery (a. lienalis) it splits into five to eight branches. The number of veins coming from the spleen corresponds to the number of arteries. Figure 27.48 shows the ligatures that are placed around the blood vessels. After tying the ligatures the blood vessel can be cut and the spleen removed. Alternatively, only the proximal ligatures can be placed and tied; this, however, may lead to blood flowing out of the spleen into the abdominal cavity.

After the spleen has been removed the abdominal cavity is closed as described earlier.

Adrenalectomy

The adrenal glands are small, round organs located slightly rostral of the anterior pole of the kidney. The glands are often attached to the kidney by means of adipose tissue. The approach to the removal of the adrenal glands is similar to that for the removal of the ovaries. The back of the anesthetized animal should be shaven and disinfected. Placed on its ventral surface with its tail pointing to the surgeon, a small 2 cm midline dorsal skin incision is made just below the hump. Using spreading movements with a pair of scissors the connective tissue between the skin and the muscular layer is bluntly dissected on both sides in a ventral direction over a distance of about 3 cm. The skin is pulled to one side and the muscular layers are opened just posterior to the last rib and a few millimetres below the spinal muscles. This is approximately one-third the way down the side of the rat. Make sure that the incision is only 3–4 mm as this is enough to allow the passage of the adrenal gland. To locate one gland, a pair of curved forceps is used to spread the incision in the muscular layer. Using another pair of forceps the kidney is located. Once the kidney has been found, the gland is easily located. Pull the gland through the muscle incision while you hold it by the periadrenal adipose tissue. The gland should be removed by tearing the connecting blood vessels, thus crushing the vessels. This will lead to rapid coagulation and bleeding will be negligible.

On the right side, a liver lobe may obscure your view. The hole in the muscular layer should be made directly beside the spinal muscles at approximately one-fourth the way down this side of the rat and the liver lobe should be pushed aside.

The muscular layers only need to be sutured if the incision is larger than 5 mm. The skin is closed in the usual way.

References

Abad-Alegria, F. (1971) *Trab. Inst. Cajal Invest. Biol.* **63**, 103–124.

Abad-Alegria, F. (1973) *An. Anat. Zaragoza* **22**, 449–455.

Abad-Alegria, F. (1974) *An. Anat. Zaragoza* **23**, 157–161.

Abbott, C.P. and Lindsey, E.S. (1964) *Arch. Surg.* **89**, 645–652.

Acland, R.D. (ed.) (1980) *Microsurgery Practice Manual.* St Louis: C.V. Mosby.

Albe-Fessard, D., Stutinsky, F. and Libouban, S. (1966) *Atlas Stereotaxique du Diencephale du Rat Blanc.* Paris: Editions C.N.R.S.

Albe-Fessard, D., Libouban, S. and Stutinsky, F. (1971) *Atlas Stereotaxique du Diencephale du Rat Blanc.* Paris: Editions C.N.R.S.

Altman, J. and Bayer, S.A. (1994) *Atlas of Prenatal Rat Brain Development.* Boca Raton: CRC Press.

Anderson, R.M. and Romfh, R.F. (1980) *Technique in the Use of Surgical Tools.* New York: Appleton Century-Crofts.

Asimacopoulos, P.J., Molokhia, F.A., Pegg, A.S. and Norman, J.C. (1971) *Transplant. Proc.* **3**, 583.

Balabaud, C., Saric, L., Gonzalez, P. and Delphy, C. (1981) *Lab. Anim. Sci.* **31**, 273–275.

Bartels, H.L. (1979) *Biotechniek* **18**, 83.

Bito, L., Davson, H., Levin, E.M., Murray, M. and Snider, N. (1966) *J. Neurochem.* **13**, 1057–1067.

Bradfield, J.F., Schachtman, T.R., McLaughlin, R.M. and Steffen, E.K. (1992) *Lab. Anim. Sci.* **42**, 572–578.

Brown, M.R. and Hedge, G.A. (1972) *Neuroendocrinology* **9**, 158–174.

Buckingham, R.E. (1976) *J. Pharm. Pharmacol.* **28**, 459–461.

Bui-Mong-Hung and Vigano, M. (1966) *Presse Med.* **74**, 2047–2049.

Bunag, R.D. (1971) *J. Lab. Clin. Med.* **78**, 675–682.

Bunag, R.D., McCubbin, L.W. and Page, T.H. (1971) *Cardiovasc. Res.* **5**, 24–31.

Chipman, J.K. and Cropper, N.C. (1977) *Res. Vet. Sci.* **22**, 366–370.

Chisholm, B. and Singer, G. (1970) *Physiol. Behav.* **5**, 1069–1070.

Cocchetto, D.M. and Bjornsson, T.D. (1983) *J. Pharm. Sci.* **72**, 465–492.

Cunningham, M.G. and McKay, R.D. (1993) *J. Neurosci. Methods* **47**, 105–114.

Darracq, C., Conzalez, R. and Balabaud, C. (1980) *Physiol. Behav.* **25**, 327–329.

De Groot, J. (1959a) *Verh. K. Nederland. Akad. Wetenschap. Naturkunde.* **52**, 1–40.

De Groot, J. (1959b) *J. Comp. Neurol.* **113**, 389–400.

Dons, R.F. and Havlik, R. (1986) *Lab. Anim. Sci.* **36**, 544–547.

Enderlin, F.E. and Honohan, T. (1977) *Lab. Anim. Sci.* **27**, 490–493.

Ewing, A.G., Wightman, R.M. and Dayton, M.A. (1982) *Brain Res.* **249**, 361–370.

Faulkner, B.C., Gear, A.J.L., Hellewell, T.B., Mazzarese, P.M., Watkins, F.H. and Edlich, R.F. (1996) *J. Long-Term Effects Med. Implants* **6**, 169–179.

Fisher, B. and Vars, H.M. (1955) *Am. J. Med. Sci.* **222**, 116.

Gaddum, J.H. (1961) *J. Physiol.* **155**, 1–2.

Gonon, F.G., Buda, M., Cespuglio, R., Jouvet, M. and Pujol, J.F. (1980) *Nature* **268**, 902–904.

Greene, E.C. (1963) *Anatomy of the Rat.* New York: Hafner Publishing.

Grunden, L.R. and Linburn, G.E. (1969) *J. Pharm. Sci.* **59**, 182–183.

Hebel, R. and Stromberg, M.W. (1986) *Anatomy and Embryology of the Laboratory Rat.* Wörthsee: BioMed Verlag.

Heller, A., Hutchens, J.O., Kirby, M.L., Karapas, F. and Fernander, C. (1979) *J. Neurosci. Methods* **1**, 41–76.

Helman, A., Castaing, D., Morin, J., Pfister-Lemaire, N. and Assan, R. (1984) *Am. J. Physiol.* **246**, E544–E547.

Heron, I. (1971) *Acta Pathol. Microbiol. Scand.* **79**, 366–372.

Herr, N.G. (1971) *Bull. NY Acad. Med.* **47**, 1227.

Hoebel, B.G. (1964) *Electroenceph. Clin. Neurphysiol.* **16**, 399–402.

Hurt, G.A., Hanaway, J. and Netsky, M.G. (1971) *Confin. Neurol.* **33**, 93–115.

Hyun, S.A., Vanhoutte, G.V. and Treadwell, C.R. (1967) *Biochim. Biophys. Acta* **137**, 296–305.

Imperato, A. and Di Chiara, G. (1984) *J. Neurosci.* **4**, 966–977.

Jansco, G. and Kiraly, E. (1980) *J. Comp. Neurol.* **190**, 781–792.

Johnson, P. and Rising, P.A. (1978) *Xenobiotica* **8**, 27–36.

Khavari, K.A. (1970) *Physiol. Behav.* **5**, 1187–1189.

Kirk, R.M. (ed.) (1978) *Basic Surgical Techniques.* Edinburgh: Churchill Livingstone. London, New York.

Kline, J. and Reid, K.H. (1984) *Physiol. Behav.* **33**, 301–303.

Konertz, W. (1985) In: Thiede, A., Deltz, E., Engemann, R. and Mamelmann, H. (eds) *Microsurgical Models in Rats for Transplantation Research*, pp. 37–42. Berlin: Springer-Verlag.

Konig, J.F.R. and Klippel, R.A. (1963) *The Rat Brain. A Stereotaxic Atlas of the Forebrain and Lower Parts of the Brain Stem.* Baltimore: Williams & Wilkins.

Krieg, W.J.S. (1946a) *J. Comp. Neurol.* **84**, 221–275.

Krieg, W.J.S. (1946b) *J. Comp. Neurol.* **84**, 277–323.

Kuipers, F., Dijkstra, T., Havinga, R., van Asselt, W. and Vonk, R. (1985a) *Biochem. Pharmacol.* **34**, 1731–1736.

Kuipers, R., Havinga, R., Bosschieter, H., Toorop, G.R., Hindriks, F.R. and Vonk, R. (1985b) *Gastroenterology* **88**, 403–411.

Lambert, R. (1965) In: Lambert, R. (ed.) *Surgery of the Digestive System in the Rat*, pp. 113–168. Springfield, IL: Charles C. Thomas.

Lee, S., Willoughby, W.F., Smallwood, C.J., Dawson, A. and Orloff, M.J. (1970) *Am. J. Pathol.* **59**, 279.

Light, H.C., Witmer, C. and Vars, H.M. (1959) *Am. J. Physiol.* **197**, 1330–1332.

Marck, K.W. (1983) Longtransplantaie bij de rat, pp. 1–44. Thesis, University of Groningen.

Massopust, L.C. Jr (1961) In: Sheer, D.E. (ed.) *Electrical Stimulation of the Brain*, pp. 182–202. Austin: University of Texas Press.

Myers, R.D. (1963) *J. Appl. Physiol.* **18**, 221–223.

Myers, R.D. (1970) *Physiol. Behav.* **5**, 243–246.

Myers, R.D., Casady, G. and Holman, R.B. (1967) *Physiol. Behav.* **2**, 87–88.

Nicolaidis, S., Rowland, N., Meile, M.J., Marfaing-Jallat, P. and Pesez, A. (1974) *Pharmacol. Biochem. Behav.* **2**, 131–136.

Nieuwenhuys, R., Geeraedts, L.M. and Veening, J.G. (1982) *J. Comp. Neurol.* **206**, 49–81.

Ono, K. and Lindsey, E.S. (1969) *J. Thorac. Cardiovasc. Surg.* **57**, 225–229.

Paxinos, G. and Watson, C. (1982) *The Rat Brain in Stereotaxic Coordinates.* New York: Academic Press.

Paxinos, G. and Watson, C. (1986) *The Rat Brain in Stereotaxic Coordinates*, 2nd edn. New York: Academic Press.

Paxinos, G. and Watson, C. (1998) *The Rat Brain in Stereotaxic Coordinates*, Deluxe Fo, 4th edn. New York: Academic Press.

Paxinos, G., Watson, C., Pennisi, M. and Topple, A. (1985) *J. Neurosci Methods* **13**, 139–143.

Pellegrino, L.J. and Cushman, A.J. (1967) *A Stereotaxic Atlas of the Rat Brain.* New York: Appleton-Century-Crofts.

Pellegrino, L.J., Pellegrino, A.S. and Cushman, A.J. (1979) *A Stereotaxic Atlas of the Rat Brain.* New York: Plenum.

Pelzmann, K.S. and Havemeyer, R.N. (1971) *J. Pharm. Sci.* **60**, 331–332.

Peters, M. (1974) *Physiol. Behav.* **13**, 133–141.

Popovic, V., Kent, K.M. and Popovic, P. (1963) *Proc. Soc. Exp. Biol. Med.* **113**, 599–602.

Popp, M.B. and Brennan, M.F. (1981) *Am. J. Physiol.* **241**, H606–H612.

Prop, Jm., Nieuwenhuis, P. and Wildevuur, Ch.R.H. (1980) *Eur. Surg. Res.* **12** (suppl. 1), 80.

Prop, Jm. (1984) Lung allograft rejection in the rat. Thesis, University of Groningen.

Prop, Jm. and Marck, K.W. (1984) In: Olszewski, W.L. (ed.) *Handbook of Microsurgery*, Vol. II, pp. 493–509. Boca Raton: CRC Press.

Rath, L. and Hutchison, M. (1989) *Lab. Anim.* **23**, 163–168.

Remie, R. and Zaagsma, J. (1986) *Am. J. Physiol.* **251**, H463–H467.

Remie, R. Knot, H.J., Bos, E.A. and Zaagsma, J. (1988a) *Eur J. Pharmacol.* **157**, 37–43.

Remie, R., Knot, H.J., Kolker, H.J. and Zaagsma, J. (1988b) *Naunyn-Schmiedeberg's Arch. Pharmacol.* **338**, 215–220.

Remie, R., Coppes, R.P. and Zaagsma, J. (1989) *Br. J. Pharmacol.* **97**, 586–590.

Remie, R., Coppes, R.P., Meurs, H., Roffel, A.F. and Zaagsma, J. (1990a) *Br. J. Pharmacol.* **99**, 223–226.

Remie, R., Rensema, J.W., van Wunnik, G.H.J. and van Dongen, J.J. (1990b) In: van Dongen, J.J., Remie, R., Rensema, J.W. and van Wunnik, G.H.J. (eds) *Manual of Microsurgery on the Laboratory Rat*, pp. 11–15. Amsterdam: Elsevier Science.

Remie, R., Bertens, A.P.G.M., van Dongen, J.J., Rensema, J.W. and van Wunnik, G.H.J. (1990c) In: van Dongen, J.J., Remie, R., Rensema, J.W. and van Wunnik, G.H.J. (eds) *Manual of Microsurgery on the Laboratory Rat*, pp. 61–80. Amsterdam: Elsevier Science.

Remie, R., van Dongen, J.J., Rensema, J.W. and van Wunnik, G.H.J. (1990d) In: van Dongen, J.J., Remie, R., Rensema, J.W. and van Wunnik, G.H.J. (eds) *Manual of Microsurgery on the Laboratory Rat*, pp. 81–156. Amsterdam: Elsevier Science.

Remie, R., van Dongen, J.J. and Rensema, J.W. (1990e) In: van Dongen, J.J., Remie, R., Rensema, J.W. and van Wunnik, G.H.J. (eds) *Manual of Microsurgery on the Laboratory Rat*, pp. 159–170. Amsterdam: Elsevier Science.

Remie, R., Rensema, J.W., van Wunnik, G.H.J. and van Dongen, J.J. (1990f) In: van Dongen, J.J., Remie, R., Rensema, J.W. and van Wunnik, G.H.J. (eds) *Manual of Microsurgery on the Laboratory Rat*, pp. 201–212. Amsterdam: Elsevier Science.

Remie, R., Rensema, J.W., Havinga, R. and Kuipers, F. (1991) In: Siegers, C.-P. and Watkins III, J.B. (eds) *Progress in Pharmacology and Clinical Pharmacology*, pp. 127–145. Stuttgart: Gustav Fisher Verlag.

Robinson, T.E. and Justice, J.B. Jr (eds) (1991) *Microdialysis in the Neurosciences*, Amsterdam: Elsevier Science.

Rosenberg, R.S., Bergmann, B.M. and Rechtschaffen, A. (1976) *Physiol. Behav.* **17**, 931–938.

Russell, P.J.D. and Mogenson, G.J. (1975) *Am. J. Physiol.* **229**, 1014–1018.

Sable-Amplis, R. and Abadie, D. (1975) *J. Appl. Physiol.* **38**, 358–359.

Santiago, M. and Westerink, B.H.C. (1990) *Naunyn-Schmiedeberg's Arch. Pharmacol.* **342**, 407–414.

Sawyer, L. and Lepkovsky, S. (1934) *J. Lab. Clin. Med.* Oct, 958–963.

Scremin, O.U. (1970) *J. Comp. Neurol.* **139**, 31–52.

Sherwood, N.M. and Timiras, P.S. (1970) *A Stereotaxic Atlas of the Developing Rat Brain.* Berkeley: University of California Press.

Simson, E.L., Jones A.P. and Gold, R.M. (1981) *Brain Res. Bull.* **6**, 297–326.

Sloop, C.H. and Krause, B.R. (1981) *Physiol. Behav.* **26**, 529–533.

Smit, M.J., Tennerman, A.M., Havinga, R., Kuipers, F. and Vonk, R. (1990) *Biochem. J.* **269**, 781–788.

Steffens, A.B. (1969) *Physiol. Behav.* **4**, 833–836.

Strubbe, J.H. (1974) *Physiol. Behav.* **12**, 317–319.

Strubbe, J.H. (1975) Insulin, glucose and feeding behaviour in the rat: A reappraisal of the glucostatic theory, pp. 8–12. Thesis, University of Groningen.

Suzuki, T., Sattoh, Y., Isozaki, S. and Ishida, R. (1973) *J. Pharm. Sci.* **62**, 345–347.

Tera, H. and Åberg, C. (1976) *Acta Chir. Scand.* **142**, 1–7.

Thomas, D.W. and Mayer, J. (1968) *Physiol. Behav.* **3**, 499–500.

Tomita, F. (1966) *Sapporo Med. J.* **30**, 165.

Tomlinson, P.W., Jeffery, D.J. and Filer, C.W. (1981) *Xenobiotica* **12**, 863–870.

Tracy, D.L. (ed) (1994) In: *Mosby's Fundamentals of Veterinary Technology; Small Animal Surgical Nursing.* St Louis: Mosby Year Book.

Tse, F.L.S., Ballard, R. and Jaffe, L.M. (1982) *J. Pharmacol. Methods* **7**, 139–144.

Ungersted, U. (1984) In: Marsden, C.A. (ed) *Measurement of Neurotransmitter Release in vivo*, pp. 81–105. New York: John Wiley.

Ungerstedt, U. (1991) In: Robinson, T.E. and Justice, Jr, J.B. (eds) *Microdialysis in the Neurosciences*, pp 3–22. Amsterdam: Elsevier Science.

Valenstein, T., Case, B. and Valenstein, E.S. (1969) *Dev. Psychobiol.* **2**, 75–80.

Van Dongen, J.J., Van der Wal, J.C., Rensema, J.W., Eversden, M. and Remie, R. (1990) In: van Dongen, J.J., Remie, R., Rensema, J.W. and van Wunnik, G.H.J. (eds) *Manual of Microsurgery on the Laboratory Rat*, pp. 35–60. Amsterdam: Elsevier Science.

Vonk, R.L., van Doorn, A.B.D. and Strubbe, J.H. (1978a) *Clin. Sci. Mol. Med.* **55**, 253–259.

Vonk, R.L., Scholtens, E. and Strubbe, J.H. (1978b) *Clin. Sci. Mol. Med.* **55**, 399–406.

Waynforth, H.B. (1993) *Scand LAS* 43–46.

Weeks, J.R. and Jones, J.A. (1960) *Proc. Soc. Exp. Biol. Med.* **104**, 646–648.

Weis, E.E. and Barth, C.A. (1978) *J. Lipid. Res.* **19**, 856–862.

Westerink, B.H.C. and De Vries, J.B. (1988) *J. Neurochem.* **51**, 683–687.

Westerink, B.H.C. and Justice, Jr, J.B. (1991) In: Robinson, T.E. and Justice Jr, J.B. (eds) *Microdialysis in the Neurosciences*, pp. 23–43. Amsterdam: Elsevier Science.

Wind, G.G. and Rich, N.M. (eds) (1987) *Principles of Surgical Technique.* Baltimore: Urban & Schwarzenberg.

Wunscher, W., Schober, W. and Werner, L. (eds) (1965) *Architektonischer atlas vom hirnstamm der ratte.* Leipzig: S. Hirzel-Verlag.

Zetterström, T., Sharp, T., Marsden, C.A. and Ungerstedt, U. (1983) *J. Neurochem.* **41**, 1769–1773.

Zyll, A. van (1959) *S. Afr. Med. J.* **33**, 618.

CHAPTER 28

Necropsy Techniques with Standard Collection and Trimming of Tissues

Cynthia D Bono
Experimental Pathology Laboratories, Herndon, VA, USA

Michael R Elwell
Covance Laboratories, Vienna, VA, USA

Keith Rogers
Experimental Pathology Laboratories, Herndon, VA, USA

Introduction

The necropsy examination, including tissue collection and preservation, represents one of the most critical phases for the histopathological evaluation of animals from toxicity and carcinogenicity studies. Any potential errors identified in subsequent phases of the histopathological portion of the study (tissue trimming, slide preparation, microscopic diagnoses) can generally be corrected. However, failure to perform a thorough gross examination with accurate documentation, followed by careful collection and preservation of all required tissues and gross lesions can result in the irretrievable loss of potential treatment-related tissue effects. The purpose of this chapter is to provide details related to performance of necropsy examination, tissue collection and fixation. Instructions for standard trimming and blocking of the common protocol-required tissues for microscopic evaluation are also provided. Although, routine fixation methods will be briefly discussed, the reader is referred to Chapters 26 and 27 for more extensive information on perfusion fixation techniques.

Necropsy Preparation

Necropsy Room Requirements

Purpose-built necropsy facilities are designed with optimal air handling and individually ventilated workstations. Work areas are normally built of stainless steel or other impermeable surfaces which are easily cleaned and disinfected. Each workstation should be equipped with running water.

One popular concept is the downdraft workstation. This is a self-contained workstation with a perforated work surface through which fumes are drawn down and away from the work area. Beneath the removable work surface is a sink which facilitates easy clean-up. This type of workstation is commercially available from several sources or can be tailor-made to the individual laboratory requirements.

Within the necropsy room, all work area surfaces must be easy to clean. Balances to weigh both animals and organs should be in close access to the dissection area. Many facilities have computer stations for on-line collection of body/organ weights and necropsy data. If fixative containers are to be prepared in the necropsy area, it is necessary to consider ventilation for filling and storage, as well as adequate temporary space for the completed tissue containers during the necropsy.

Instruments and equipment

The choice of instruments for necropsy is generally a personal preference. Poor choice of instruments or instruments which are dull and unkempt will cause artifacts despite otherwise good dissecting technique. Below is a list of the essential requirements:

- *Scissors, large* Large enough to open the body cavities and cut through skin. Scissors 15–18 cm in length with sharp/blunt points provide the most leverage and flexibility for rats.
- *Scissors, small* For dissection of internal organs, scissors 10–13 cm in length with sharp/blunt points and the same length with curved-sharp/sharp points will be adequate. The curved points are indispensable for removing the eyes.
- *Scalpels* No. 11 or 22 blades for trimming tissues. Make it a practice to use a new scalpel blade for each rat. This will help to eliminate artifacts related to pressure or compression of tissues.
- *Spatulas* Helpful for lifting small organs, e.g. pituitary, from the surrounding tissue when forceps become impractical.
- *Bone cutters* For the skull and other bones.
- *Forceps* 'Rat toothed' for gripping surrounding tissues. The teeth can be very helpful for heavier tissues, but care must be taken not to grip tissues where histologic sections are to be taken.
- *Forceps* Straight-grooved for handling tissues. Again, when possible, handle sample area by the surrounding tissue to avoid creating artifacts.
- *Umbilical tape or heavy-duty thread* To ligate lungs or urinary bladder after perfusion. There are also plastic clips available which are quite convenient and easier to handle for this purpose.
- *Metric ruler* For measuring dimensions of lesions.

Other supplies

It is advisable to use a cutting board for the dissection. The board should be made of a hard plastic, which is easy to clean between animals. Cork boards can be used, but the cork surface easily stains and absorbs fluids, and therefore requires careful cleaning for storage.

In addition, it is necessary to have a labeled container of normal buffered saline to rinse tissues, such as stomach and cecum. A good light source is useful, especially for examining suspected lesions. It is also helpful to have a labeled container of water to rinse and hold instruments during the dissection.

An abundant supply of 2 × 2 gauze squares is useful for absorbing blood when exsanguinating the animal, as well as gentle blotting of tissues *in situ* to facilitate efficient identification and dissection.

Tissue cassettes to hold small organs or lesions/ masses, along with waterproof markers or pencils are essential.

A 5–10-mL syringe and needle is necessary for

infusion of the lungs and urinary bladder with formalin.

A clipboard is essential to keep documents such as individual animal necropsy records away from fixative and body fluids in the dissection work area and to facilitate writing.

As will be discussed later, it is preferable to have a shallow tray in the work area to hold the required tissues (in saline) until the dissection is completed. At that time, the collection of all tissues can be documented and the tissues placed into the labeled container of fixative.

Documentation

The extent to which the necropsy findings are documented will depend on the focus of the study. A pre-printed form (necropsy record) is useful for all situations where standard information is to be gathered.

Space should be devoted to areas for recording the following types of information:

- Study identification
- Animal identification
- Terminal body weight
- Time and date of necropsy
- Method of euthanasia
- Organ weights
- Necropsy observations
- Tissues/organs collected in fixative
- Signature of prosector (and others involved in the necropsy).

Many laboratories have computer systems for the on-line collection of data in such cases, much of the above information may be entered directly into the computer system.

Recent clinical and in-life observations (e.g. palpable masses) should be available at the time of necropsy.

Urine and Blood Collection, Exsanguination, and Bone Marrow Collection

Urine collection

Throughout the course of a toxicity study, urine sampling may be a requirement of the experimental protocol. During the in-life phase of the study, various types of metabolism cages can be used to collect urine in adequate volume to perform a complete evaluation of renal function and analysis of urine.

At the time of necropsy, urine can frequently be obtained by using a tuberculin syringe and needle to aspirate the contents of the urinary bladder. The obvious disadvantages are that this technique is not dependable for obtaining samples from all rats and the volume is usually very small (~ 0.1 mL). However, it is a potential method to obtain an aseptic sample of urine.

Blood collection

There are various standard methods and sites for blood collection from rats during the in-life phase. All require appropriate anesthesia and all have certain limitations, depending on volume requirements and type of analyses to be performed on the sample. At the time of scheduled sacrifice, blood samples may be easily obtained from rats under anesthesia and immediately prior to the necropsy examination and collection of other tissues. Typically, blood samples may be taken by syringe or Vacutainer™ tube from the abdominal aorta or vena cava of the anesthetized animal. Alternatively, the jugular vein, retroorbital vein or heart may be used; exsanguination is completed immediately following the blood sampling.

Exsanguination

Whether blood sampling at terminal sacrifice is a requirement or not, exsanguination is usually performed on all animals prior to the necropsy examination. Typically, the abdomen of the anesthetized rat is opened and the intestines are gently reflected to expose the abdominal aorta and vena cava. The aorta should be incised and gauze pads are applied over the area to absorb blood. The gauze is used primarily to prevent excessive blood staining and discoloration of surrounding tissues that might otherwise adversely affect the subsequent gross examination and tissue collection. The primary advantage of exsanguination is that after the removal of the majority of blood from tissues, there is a much better quality of tissue section for microscopic examination. More importantly, it has been shown that failure to exsanguinate rats will result in markedly increased organ weights, particularly in the liver and kidneys (Sullivan, 1985). Incomplete exsanguination of rats can result in highly variable, inaccurate organ weight data.

Bone marrow smears

Collection of bone marrow for smears should be performed as soon as practical after the animal has been exsanguinated. When bone marrow is required, it typically should be obtained from the sternum. A slide is labeled with the animal's identification. With a scalpel open one of the sternebrae, exposing the bone marrow. With the bone clippers grasp the end of the sternebrae and squeeze out a small droplet of bone marrow. Using a small paintbrush which has been dipped in albumin or calf serum, pick up marrow from the droplet. Create a very thin smear on the surface of the slide. The slide should be air-dried in a rack or slide box for future staining. It is important to note that slides for blood smears or bone marrow smears must be maintained as far from the formaldehyde fumes as possible because the fixative will affect the quality of the stain.

Euthanasia

Legal requirements regarding the euthanasia of animals must be taken into account. In many countries, live animals are not to be kept in the necropsy area. It is advisable to hold and euthanize animals in a separate room adjacent to the main necropsy area. This area can also be used for the collection of terminal blood samples (e.g. retroorbital, jugular) and body weights.

There are many acceptable methods of euthanasia. Once again, local laws and standard practices at the laboratory may prohibit certain methods. The method of euthanasia may also be influenced by the specific protocol for the study. The classic methods of euthanasia using chloroform and ether have largely been discontinued for safety reasons. Various anesthetic gases have been adopted, including methoxyflurane and halothane. They are expensive and require appropriately ventilated areas. Cervical dislocation may be an acceptable method for euthanasia of immature rats if special requirements in the protocol preclude more standard methods. This requires specific training and technical skills when used for euthanasia. On rare occasion, decapitation may be an alternative method of euthanasia. This method requires special equipment and personnel well-trained in performing the procedure (Sharp and La Regina, 1998). The following are two methods recommended for routine use.

Sodium pentobarbital anesthesia followed by exsanguination

This is the method of choice for many laboratories. It allows for excellent tissue retention with the minimum of retained blood in the tissues. Large volumes of blood may be collected from the heart or the abdominal aorta after suitable anesthesia.

Carbon dioxide asphyxiation

This is one of the simpler and more common methods of euthanasia. It is done in a closed tank with a supply of carbon dioxide gas. Animals are placed into the tank and the gas allowed to flow until the animal is anesthetized. As death follows in seconds, this method of euthanasia is not as effective as sodium pentobarbital for exsanguination.

Tissue Fixation

The chemical preservation of tissues (fixation) is a vast and complex subject. In this section, we will address the most common fixatives and some of the basic rules governing good fixation (Bancroft and Stevens, 1982). Most routine tissue fixation is done by immersion. That is to say, the tissues are placed whole or in part into the fixative solution and fixed from 'the outside in'. Perfusion is a much more effective method for rapid fixation. Perfusion may be done for selected organs of interest, or the whole body can be perfused. Normally, whole-body perfusion is done for neurotoxicity studies.

Sample size

Most routine tissue fixatives are slow to penetrate tissues. Formalin penetrates at the rate of approximately 1 mm per hour. In practical terms, this means that tissue samples need to be as thin as possible to allow penetration to be completed before significant autolysis occurs. In the rat, the only organs where this becomes an issue are liver, kidneys, lung and brain. Cuts are made in the liver and kidneys, opening the tissue to allow more rapid penetration to the interior of the organs. Lungs should be infused and inflated with fixative at the time of necropsy. It is not advisable to cut the brain prior to fixation. Immersion fixation is adequate in most instances; however, if the brain is the organ of special interest then perfusion is recommended.

Standard fixatives

A number of 'older' fixatives are no longer in common use due to the fact that many contained heavy metals and other hazardous chemicals. The fixatives detailed below are recommended for use in all 'routine' situations. Many others are commercially available when special circumstances dictate.

Fixation is a chemical reaction and as such is subject to the laws of chemistry. Heat and gentle agitation (automatic shaker) will speed up the process, and time is also an important factor. As a general rule, the volume of fixative required is ten times the volume of tissue preserved. Some fixatives continue to affect tissue after optimum fixation has occurred. In such cases, tissues can become hard and uncuttable if exposure to the fixative is allowed to continue.

Formaldehyde

Formaldehyde is the most widely used fixative in histology and is adequate for most routine methods in most tissues. This solution is commercially available at 35–40% of gas by weight. It is usually diluted 1 in 10 and is more commonly referred to as 10% formalin (a 4% solution of formaldehyde). The preferred method of preparation is in a phosphate buffer at a neutral pH to avoid the formation of formalin pigments (Table 28.1). Tissue preservation is generally good. It has the one merit that tissues may remain in formalin for long periods of time

without adverse effects. Some of the negative aspects of formalin are excessive shrinkage, poor cellular detail, loss of certain staining characteristics, etc. To some degree, these disadvantages may be overcome by post-treatment of specimens or by the use of different processing schedules. For example, many of the shrinkage artifacts after paraffin embedding of the testes are greatly diminished by using glycol methacrylate (GMA) embedding. Additionally, postfixation in picric acid fixatives (Bouin's) can restore many of the staining characteristics of these tissues.

Picric acid fixatives

There are a number of different formulae that use picric acid together with primary fixatives such as formaldehyde and alcohol. The most widely used is Bouin's fluid. This is a mixture of saturated picric acid, concentrated formaldehyde and glacial acetic acid (Table 28.1).

There are many disadvantages to the use of picric acid fixatives. In its dry form, picric acid is explosive. Bouin's fluid also stains tissue bright yellow which will be transferred to the processing solutions. Extended fixation in Bouin's fluid (more than 24 hours) will cause excessive shrinkage and 'dryness' of the tissues. This can be avoided by rinsing the tissues well in 70% alcohol after no more than 24 hours of fixation in Bouin's. Tissues can then be stored in 10% neutral buffered formalin for extended periods of time.

Table 28.1 Some commonly used fixatives

Fixative	Composition	Notes
Neutral buffered formalin	100 mL 35–40% formaldehyde 900 mL distilled or tapwater 4 g sodium phosphate monobasic, monohydrate 6.5 g sodium phosphate dibasic, anhydrous	Store at room temperature
Bouin's fluid	1500 mL saturated picric acid (21 g to 1 L) in distilled water 500 mL 35–40% formaldehyde 100 mL glacial acetic acid	Store at room temperature
Davidson's solution	330 mL 95% ethyl alcohol 220 mL formaldehyde (35–40% formaldehyde solution) 115 mL glacial acetic acid 335 mL distilled or tapwater	Store at room temperature

Bouin's fixation is advocated, in particular, for pancreas, testis and eyes. Although it is certainly superior to formalin, the authors recommend Davidson's solution for eye fixation.

Davidson's solution

This alcohol-based fixative is used almost exclusively for fixation of eyes (Table 28.1). Formalin-fixed rodent eyes are rarely well preserved. Retinal detachment and fragmentation combined with poor preservation of the cornea make it necessary to seek an alternative. Davidson's solution preserves the retina and other structures well, but has a tendency to harden the lens. Tissues are fixed for no more than 24 hours in Davidson's before transfer to 70% alcohol where they may be held prior to processing.

Necropsy Procedures

Only systematic necropsy techniques can ensure that all lesions and protocol-required tissues are examined, documented as appropriate, and collected for histologic examination (Experimental Pathology Laboratories, 1998). Improper or incomplete necropsy examination can seriously affect the overall evaluation of a study, thus potentially diminishing the value of results derived from many hours of effort and costly investment.

The quality of the histological section to be prepared is dependent on appropriate handling of tissues. Good techniques assure that tissues will be free of artifacts that may affect adversely the evaluation of microscopic changes.

The necropsy should be regarded as a team effort accomplished by the prosectors, assisting technicians and pathologists working together. The end result depends on how well the efforts of all are coordinated. Expertise as a necropsy specialist is maintained and perfected only by a constant awareness of the possible consequences of deviation from routine established procedures (Bono, 1994).

Preparation of work area

A copy of the Standard Operating Procedures for the necropsy requirements and a copy of the specific study protocol must be available in the necropsy area. An individual animal necropsy record is prepared for each animal along with a labeled container which holds an adequate amount of fixative. A copy of pertinent clinical observations (e.g. head tilt) and palpable masses noted in life should be included with the necropsy record for each animal.

Although careful dissection and complete collection of tissues is the goal, the quality of the necropsy is dependent on every phase of the procedure – from accurate animal identification and record-keeping to consistent procedures for weighing tissues.

The work area is organized to allow the dissection of tissues, weighing and fixation of the tissues for each rodent to be completed in an efficient and timely manner – within approximately 20 minutes from the time of death.

It has become common practice at many laboratories to retain the dissected tissues in compartmented trays or other similar holding containers until the dissection and organ weights are completed, and a full tissue collection can be verified. Divided trays are commercially available for this type of use. In the opinion of the authors it is very difficult to remember if each tissue has been placed into the fixative container as they are dissected during the necropsy. It is also cumbersome to interface with a computer requiring continual interruption of the dissection during the necropsy to record an entry as each tissue is saved. A tray with a small amount of saline solution to keep the tissues moist ensures complete collection of tissues (see Tissue accountability).

External examination

Before the examination and dissection can begin, it must be verified that the animal is in a deep state of anesthesia. This is accomplished by touching the eye and squeezing the paw for a reflex reaction. No response indicates that the animal is adequately anesthetized for euthanasia by exsanguination. Confirm the identification of the animal and compare to the worksheet and container label information.

Examine and palpate both the dorsal and ventral surfaces of the anesthetized animal for any abnormalities or masses that might be present on or beneath the skin surface. The presence or absence of the most recent gross observations should be confirmed and documented.

Examine the anus, perineum and the urethral orifice for blood, mucus or evidence of diarrhea. Both ears are examined for any exudate or ear tag lesions. Eyes are examined for corneal or lens opacities. The nose is checked for excess mucus, blood, or excess porphyrin tear staining of the hair. The oral cavity is checked for broken or misaligned teeth and lesions in the soft tissues of the mouth. All

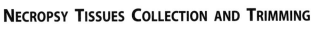

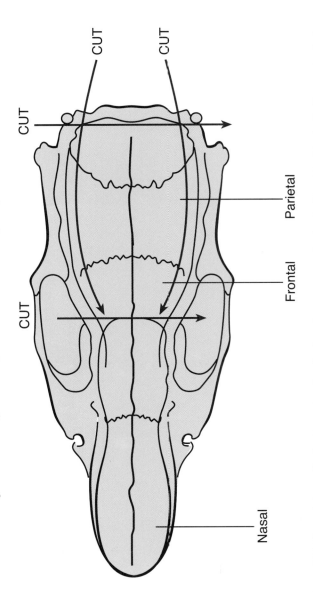

Globe of eye

Exorbital lacrimal gland

Harderian/ lacrimal gland

Nictitating membrane

Figure 28.1 Head (skin removed) showing anatomic relationship of glands to eye/orbit.

external gross lesions noted during this process are recorded on the necropsy record before proceeding with the dissection.

Note that if blood or urine collection is required, these procedures are to take place immediately prior to the internal examination and tissue collection.

Dissection procedures

Limited details of the gross anatomy as it pertains to the necropsy are provided in this chapter. For more extensive anatomic descriptions, the reader is referred to the anatomy section of this book or sources on gross anatomy of this section (Chiasson, 1988).

Eyes, optic nerves, Harderian/lacrimal glands

To begin, remove the skin below the ears. Note that if an ear tag has been used to identify the animal, the ear tag, with the pinna, is to be removed and saved in fixative. Below each ear is a round tan gland, the exorbital lacrimal gland. These glands may be left

attached to the head and saved *in situ* or removed and placed in a labeled cassette. Grasp the skin around the eye and trim from the head.

Remove the remaining adnexa (nictitating membrane) and skin from around the eyes. This procedure makes the periphery of the orbit visible. Then by grasping the conjunctiva with forceps, trim around the globe of the eye with curved scissors. Be careful not to puncture the globe. Remove the eyes from the orbit with the Harderian/lacrimal glands and optic nerve attached. The Harderian/lacrimal glands can be left attached with the eye for fixation. Figure 28.1 illustrates the relationship of the eye, orbit and these glands.

Brain

To prepare for collection of the brain, remove all of the remaining skin from the head to reveal the calvarium or the top of the skull. Note that the bones comprising the calvarium create landmarks, where cuts are made to expose the brain (Figure 28.2). These landmarks also show the boundaries of the nasal cavity which contains the fragile tissues of the nasal turbinates. Using bone clippers, follow these landmarks, making shallow cuts into the bones to detach the calvarium. If the cuts are made too deep, the points of the bone clippers may nick the brain surface, creating an artifact.

Once the shallow cuts have been completed, lift the calvarium, examine it for potential gross lesions and set it aside. (Note: The calvarium will fracture into pieces during this process if the cuts are not made completely around the landmarks described.)

CUT

CUT

CUT

CUT

Nasal

Frontal   Parietal

Figure 28.2 Dorsal view of calvarium showing landmarks to expose the brain. Nasal turbinate limits are shaded.

With the calvarium removed, the brain is exposed. Using a small spatula to sever the brainstem from the cervical spinal cord and the olfactory bulbs at the cranial end, the brain can be gently lifted up and out, beginning at the cranial end of the brain. Take care not to disturb the pituitary which lies beneath the brain. Tip the nose up vertically, and use the brain's weight to assist in its removal from the skull. One to two vertebral segments of the cervical spinal cord may be dissected to remain attached to the brain. Alternately, the cervical section can be dissected separately. In neurotoxicity studies, the olfactory bulbs are usually examined. In perfusion-fixed brain, these rarely remain attached to the brain when it is removed and must be dissected from their location posterior to the ethmoid bone.

Pituitary

With the brain removed, note the pituitary between the two large white trigeminal nerves. The pituitary is a very fragile organ and is often fixed in the skull before it is removed. If it must be weighed in a fresh state, it is removed from the head with the use of a scalpel blade and spatula. With the scalpel, cut around the lateral boundaries of the pituitary. Use the spatula to lift the pituitary from the base of the skull. If removed at necropsy, the pituitary is placed in a labeled cassette.

If the pituitary is not to be weighed or is to be

weighed after fixation, it is to remain in the skull. The entire head is placed into fixative with the pituitary intact for fixation. Removal of the head from the body is done at the end of the necropsy because there are other procedures to first be completed on the ventral side of the head.

Body cavities

Before opening the body cavities, any skin and subcutaneous masses which were identified during the palpation of the animal are collected. Masses are removed by cutting the muscle and the skin surrounding each mass. The masses are examined and described using the criteria discussed subsequently (Gross lesion descriptions). Depending on the size and number of masses, they are identified in labeled cassettes, labeled bags, or tagged in such a way to maintain identity as described. Larger masses should be incised at 1–2-cm intervals to ensure adequate fixation.

At this point, the dissection can proceed to the opening of the thoracic and abdominal cavities. Beginning above the urethral orifice, grasp the skin with the forceps. Make a V-shaped incision which extends from the tip of the forceps along the lateral sides of the rib cage to the tip of the mandible as shown in Figure 28.3.

This area of skin has mammary tissue but can be set aside if there is no special requirement for sampling of multiple mammary gland sites. Either cavity

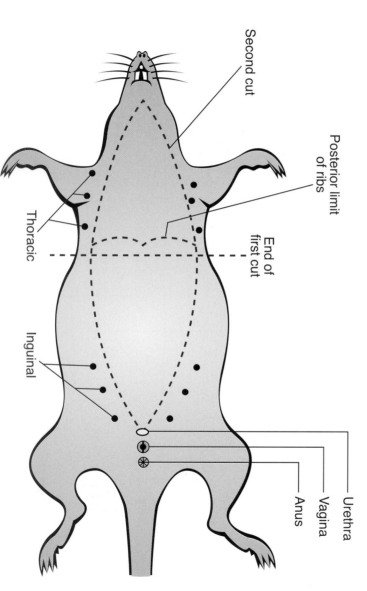

Thoracic

Inguinal

Second cut

Posterior limit of ribs

End of first cut

Urethra

Vagina

Anus

Figure 28.3 Ventral surface of thorax and abdomen showing pattern for initial incisions in relationship to nipples.

can be opened at this point depending on the type of study or the standard operating procedures of the laboratory. To open the abdomen, grasp the abdominal muscle in the same area near the urethra and make a 'V' cut to the edge of the ribs (as the first cut in Figure 28.3) and remove this muscle. The abdominal viscera and the diaphragm are now exposed. With an inhalation study, the thoracic cavity is often opened first to collect all required tissues, including mediastinal and/or bronchial lymph nodes.

Skin and mammary gland

The removal of the ventral skin provides an opportunity to collect the standard section of mammary gland. The mammary gland on the rodent is located lateral to the midline ventral surface from the inguinal to the cervical area, as shown in Figure 28.4. Two rows of nipples can also be identified in these areas. If the experimental design does not specify an area to collect, it is recommended that either the thoracic or inguinal skin and mammary gland be routinely collected from all animals. Once an area of mammary gland to be collected (e.g. inguinal) has been identified, use forceps and scissors to cut a portion (~2–3 cm square) of skin and subcutaneous tissue with gland from the animal. The skin is pinned to cork or cardboard with subcutis side out. The purpose of this procedure is to prevent the skin from folding with fixation, thus providing a more uniform histologic section of skin with mammary gland.

The thoracic cavity and cervical area

Removing the ventral thoracic skin from the posterior most ribs to the tip of the mandible exposes the thoracic and cervical area (second cut in Figure 28.3). When removing the skin in the cervical area, observe the salivary glands and lymph nodes which will be removed subsequently. Note that these tissues lie superficial to the sternohyoideus muscle as shown in Figure 28.5. This muscle, which also covers the trachea, should remain intact until the next step.

Remove the salivary glands and the submandibular lymph nodes together by grasping the fascial tissues surrounding the salivary glands at their caudal end.

With the forceps, grasp the xyphoid cartilage at the caudal end of the sternum and lift it to expose the diaphragm. Puncture the diaphragm and the lungs will collapse in the thorax of the animal. While holding the xyphoid cartilage, cut the ribs on each side of the sternum with scissors. The cut is to include the costochondral junction of the ribs. Observe the position of the lungs through the opening made in the diaphragm, so the lungs are not punctured as the cuts through the ribs are made. Cut to the cervical area and remove the sternum and ribs together. A length of 3–4 sternal segments should be trimmed of excess tissue and retained in fixative.

With the removal of the sternum, it is now possible to observe the tissues in the thoracic cavity and abdominal cavities. The organs which are visible are shown in Figure 28.6.

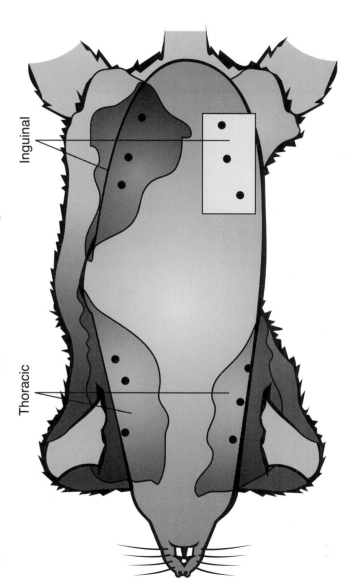

Inguinal

Thoracic

Figure 28.4 Ventral surface with skin partially reflected, showing distribution of mammary glands and standard section for collection.

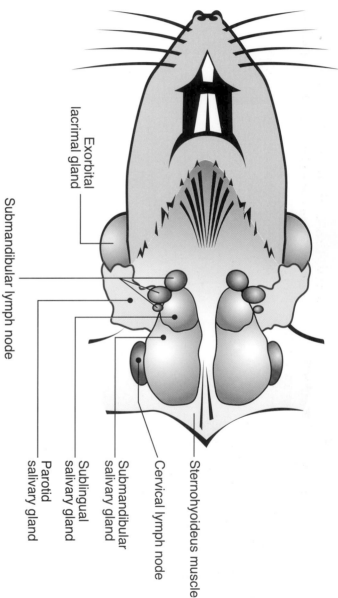

Figure 28.5 Ventral view of cervical area showing position of salivary glands and surrounding lymph nodes.

Exorbital lacrimal gland

Submandibular lymph node

Sternohyoideus muscle
Cervical lymph node
Submandibular salivary gland
Sublingual salivary gland
Parotid salivary gland

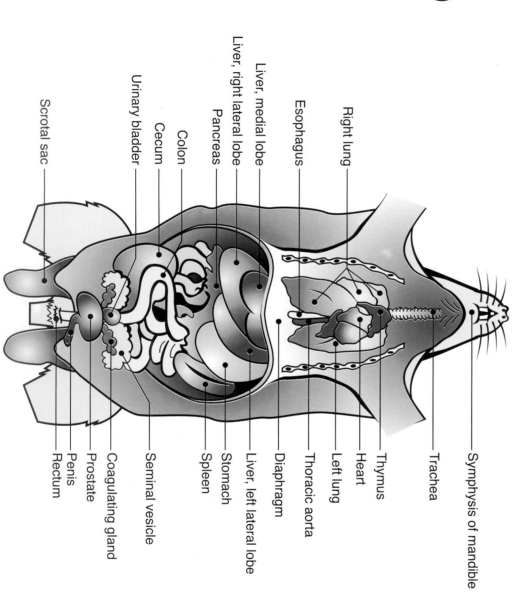

Figure 28.6 Thoracic and abdominal cavities with viscera *in situ*.

Scrotal sac
Urinary bladder
Cecum
Colon
Pancreas
Liver, right lateral lobe
Liver, medial lobe
Esophagus
Right lung

Rectum
Penis
Prostate
Coagulating gland
Seminal vesicle
Spleen
Stomach
Liver, left lateral lobe
Diaphragm
Thoracic aorta
Left lung
Heart
Thymus
Trachea
Symphysis of mandible

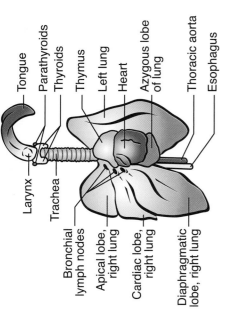

Tongue
Parathyroids
Thyroids
Thymus
Left lung
Heart
Azygous lobe of lung
Thoracic aorta
Esophagus
Larynx
Trachea
Bronchial lymph nodes
Apical lobe, right lung
Cardiac lobe, right lung
Diaphragmatic lobe, right lung

Figure 28.7 Thoracic 'pluck' removed from cavity.

Remove the muscle that covers the trachea, taking care not to cut through the trachea. Then, push the point of the scissors under the tip (symphysis) of the mandible on the midline and cut between the lower incisors.

Grasp the tongue and begin to cut the tissues which connect the tongue to the oral cavity, and the trachea, esophagus and lungs to the cervical and thoracic spinal column. Care should be taken not to stretch the trachea because this will cause an artifact in the mucosa. Note that the thoracic aorta is removed with this group of tissues.

At the diaphragm, cut across the esophagus and the thoracic aorta and remove the entire thoracic 'pluck' which is comprised of the tissues shown in Figure 28.7.

If any organ in the thoracic pluck is to be weighed, this group of tissues must be dissected. Remove the thymus first and place in a labeled cassette. In older rats, the thymus is variably atrophic and loses its shape and consistency. In older rats, the experimental design will usually require 'thymic area' which comprises brown fat and mediastinal tissue that usually contains remnants of thymus. The heart is removed by gently grasping the area of the aortic arch with forceps and making a cut in the mediastinal tissue near the forceps. As the heart is removed, take care not to cut through the bifurcation of the trachea because the lungs are to be perfused through the trachea. Remove the thoracic aorta from the dorsal side of the lungs. The esophagus is then removed from the dorsal aspect of the lower trachea before the lungs are weighed. Cut the trachea at a point midway between the larynx and the bifurcation of the lungs. The thyroids are frequently weighed after fixation and they should remain attached to the trachea. The

tongue, larynx, trachea, esophagus, thyroids and parathyroids can remain intact as a block of tissues for fixation.

To provide an ideal microscopic section, the lungs are perfused via the trachea with formalin after the tissue is weighed. A ligature is placed around the trachea no further down than the length of the perfusion needle used.

The needle is inserted into the trachea and the ligature is tightened around the needle. Formalin is gently injected (~3–5 mL, depending on the size of the animal) into the lung just until the margins of the lobes begin to fill. This procedure will inflate the alveoli and provide for optimal microscopic evaluation of the lung structure. Overinflation can tear the alveolar walls and distort the normal morphology of the lungs.

The abdominal cavity

The tissues visualized in the opened abdominal cavity are shown in Figure 28.8. The first tissue to be removed from the abdomen is the spleen. If the spleen is not being weighed, the pancreas can be left attached. Depending on the size of the spleen, several cuts perpendicular to the long axis are to be made through the capsule to provide for better fixation.

The next tissues removed are the kidneys and adrenals. The paired adrenals are situated cranial/medial to each kidney. The adrenals are partially embedded in the abdominal fat and can be removed by grasping the surrounding fat (see Figures 28.8, Figures 28.11 and 28.12).

If the adrenals are to be weighed, as much fat as possible is removed without damaging the adrenal itself. After both adrenals have been trimmed of fat, they can be weighed and then placed in a labeled cassette for fixation.

Before the kidneys are removed, both ureters are located and examined. A dilated ureter could indicate a lesion in the lower urinary tract or in the kidneys. Ureters are usually not required for microscopic examination unless there is a gross abnormality. If it is necessary that ureters be taken, they should be retained in a labeled cassette. Remove the kidney by grasping the fat above each kidney. If the kidneys are required to be weighed, all surface fat is removed to assure an accurate weight. During this process, maintain the identity of the kidney as to left and right. This is most easily done by incising the right kidney in a transverse section and the left kidney longitudinally. These cuts should start at the hilus so that orientation of the cut can be controlled. This will also allow formalin fixative to diffuse rapidly throughout the kidneys.

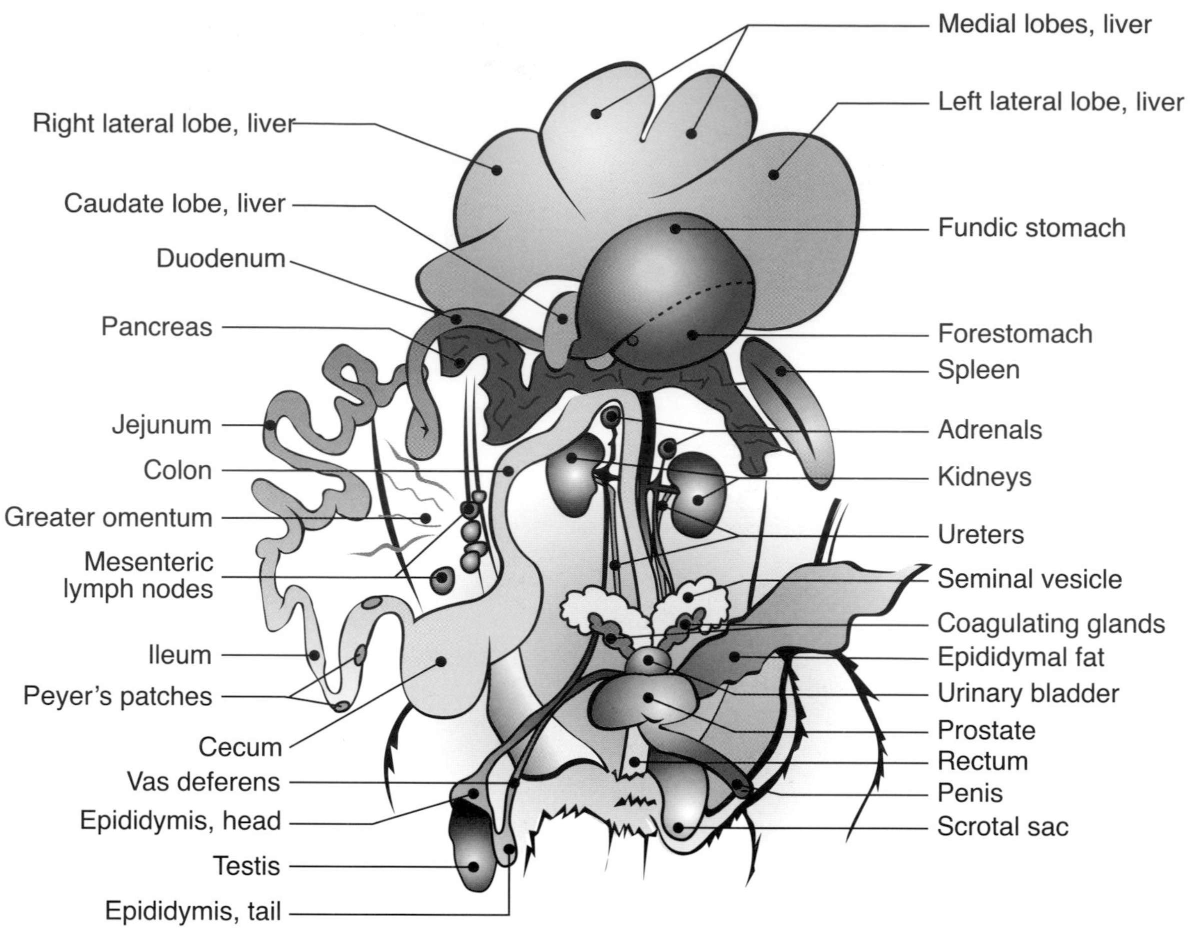

Gently detach the diaphragm from the abdominal wall. The liver is then removed with the diaphragm attached. The diaphragm can be used to handle the liver, preventing any artifacts that may be caused by grasping the liver directly. Trim off excess tissues such as the diaphragm or fat before weighing.

If there are gross lesions in the liver, their location should be noted at the time they are described. The lobes of the liver are identified in Figure 28.9. For more information on rat liver lobulation, see Chapters 13 and 15.

Before the liver is placed into fixative, each lobe of the liver is cut several times with a scalpel blade to ensure proper fixation. Next, the gastrointestinal tract is removed. Commonly required sites of the gastrointestinal tract and related tissues are identified in Figure 28.10.

The entire tract from stomach to colon (cut just before the rectum) is removed from the body as a block of tissue. Cut the mesentery which supports the intestines, so that the intestinal tract can be extended and examined.

The stomach is separated from the tract just below the pylorus. Open the stomach along its

Figure 28.8 Abdominal viscera with liver and stomach reflected anteriorly and intestines to the right.

Right lateral lobe, liver

Caudate lobe, liver

Duodenum

Pancreas

Jejunum

Colon

Greater omentum

Mesenteric lymph nodes

Ileum

Peyer's patches

Cecum

Vas deferens

Epididymis, head

Testis

Epididymis, tail

Medial lobes, liver

Left lateral lobe, liver

Fundic stomach

Forestomach

Spleen

Adrenals

Kidneys

Ureters

Seminal vesicle

Epididymal fat

Urinary bladder

Coagulating glands

Prostate

Rectum

Penis

Scrotal sac

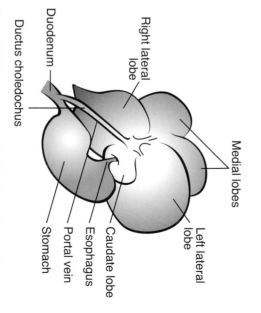

Figure 28.9 Ventral view of lobes of the liver, reflected cranially.

Right lateral lobe

Medial lobes

Left lateral lobe

Caudate lobe

Esophagus

Portal vein

Stomach

Duodenum

Ductus choledochus

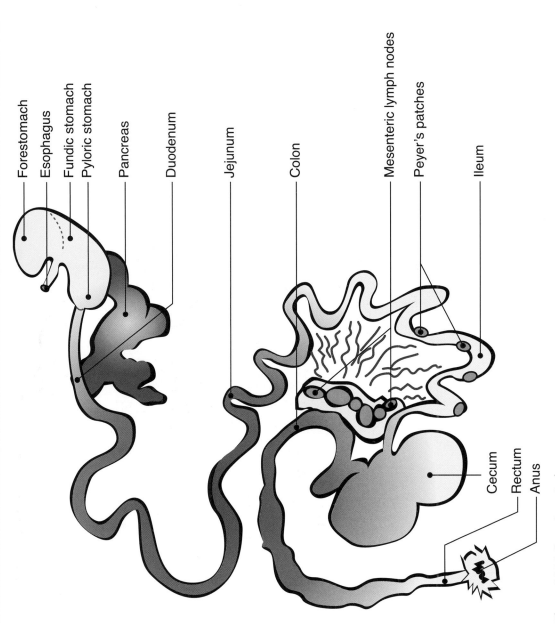

Figure 28.10 Gastrointestinal tract.

Forestomach
Esophagus
Fundic stomach
Pyloric stomach
Pancreas
Duodenum
Jejunum
Colon
Mesenteric lymph nodes
Peyer's patches
Ileum
Cecum
Rectum
Anus

greater curvature to expose all the regions of the stomach. The fundic region of the glandular mucosa is the darkest in color. The pylorus has a smooth mucosa like the small intestine. The cut made should continue to the duodenal valve. The stomach is rinsed so that any lesions on the mucosa can be visualized and may be pinned flat to a piece of cork or cardboard to prevent curling during fixation.

The duodenum extends on 2–3 cm from the duodenal valve. The section of the duodenum is to have a section of pancreas attached as a landmark for trimming. A separate larger section of pancreas should also be taken. The jejunum is the longest portion of the intestine. It will also be the only piece of intestine which will be saved with no landmark. The cecum, colon, ileum (with Peyer's patches) and mesenteric lymph node are to be maintained as a block of tissue. Alternatively, the mesenteric lymph

nodes can be placed in a labeled cassette. Open the cecum along its greater curvature, just as the stomach was, and rinse to remove any contents. The rectum will be removed with the urogenital tract.

Female urogenital tract

The organs of the female urogenital tract are shown *in situ* in Figure 28.11. Beginning at the caudal end, make a single cut through the pelvic symphysis on the midline. With the points of the scissors, spread the bones of the girdle until the vagina and rectum are visible. Grasp the caudal end of the rectum/anus and remove with the vagina, urinary bladder, uterus and ovaries attached.

The bladder may be empty (contracted) or distended with urine. For consistent sections, it should be infused for fixation. With a syringe, inject a small amount of formalin into the lumen of the bladder. If

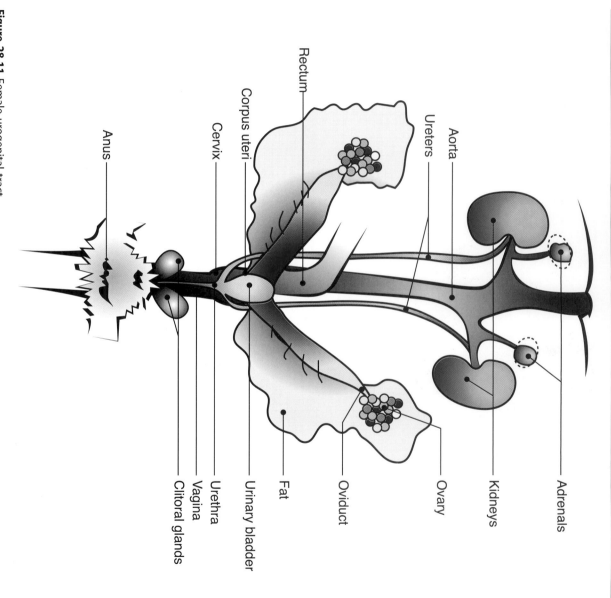

Figure 28.11 Female urogenital tract.

the ovaries are to be weighed, they are separated from the uterus and trimmed of excess fat. The ovarian bursa and oviducts are left attached to the ovary (unless weights are required for the ovaries).

Male urogenital tract

The organs of the male urogenital tract are shown *in situ* in Figure 28.12. Grasp the epididymal fat (panniculus adiposus) and pull the testis and epididymis from the scrotal sac. Cut the vas deferens and spermatic cord to separate the testes and epididymides from the body.

Beginning at the caudal end, make a single cut through the pelvic symphysis on the midline. With the points of the scissors, spread the bones of the girdle until the prostate and rectum are visible.

Grasp the caudal end of the rectum/anus and remove with the prostate, urinary bladder and seminal vesicles attached.

In most cases, the testis is weighed without the epididymis; therefore, the epididymis must be separated from the testis. Care should be taken not to cut through the wall of tunica albuginea, the thick capsule of the testes when removing the epididymides. If the seminal vesicle or prostate are to be weighed, the seminal vesicles are removed just caudal to the entrance of the ureter into the urethra, and the prostate begins just after this entrance. Otherwise, the prostate, seminal vesicles urinary bladder and rectum can be fixed as a block of tissue. The urinary bladder should be infused with fixative as discussed above for the female urogenital tract.

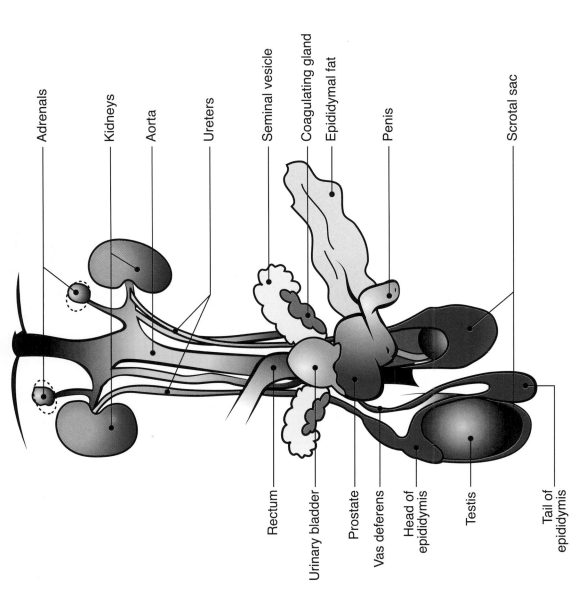

Figure 28.12 Male urogenital tract.

Adrenals

Kidneys

Aorta

Ureters

Seminal vesicle

Coagulating gland

Epididymal fat

Penis

Scrotal sac

Rectum

Urinary bladder

Prostate

Vas deferens

Head of epididymis

Testis

Tail of epididymis

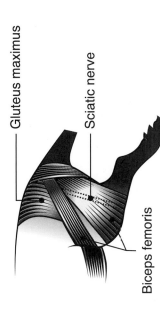

Gluteus maximus

Sciatic nerve

Biceps femoris

Figure 28.13 Sciatic nerve beneath biceps femoris dorsolateral view – hind limb.

Skeletal muscle and sciatic nerve

The sciatic nerve begins at the lumbosacral plexus and extends to the deep caudal muscles which are located more to the lateral side of the femur. The biceps femoris is the most lateral skeletal muscle in relation to the sciatic nerve. This muscle runs from the perianal area to the front of the tibia and distal end of the femur (Figure 28.13).

Using a scalpel, cut through the muscles in the inguinal area and disarticulate the hind leg at the hip. Remove the skin from the lateral surface of the leg. Take a block of muscle below the femur to include the biceps femoris with the sciatic nerve attached. A longitudinal and transverse section of muscle and nerve will be prepared from this block of tissue; therefore, include as much of the sciatic nerve as possible. Alternately, the entire leg (skin removed) may be saved, if the femur is a required tissue.

Spinal cord

The vertebral column is divided as follows: 8 cervical, 13 thoracic, 6 lumbar, 4 sacral and 27–30 caudal segments. It is important to note that the spinal cord extends caudally to a level between the fourth and fifth lumbar vertebrae. From this point, the spinal cord branches into the spinal nerves for the hind limbs and tail. This area can be identified by locating the lumbar vertebrae with their large transverse processes ('wings') which extend laterally out from the base of each vertebrae, the wide spinous process ('dorsal fin') and the sacral vertebrae which is four vertebrae fused into a flatten bone between the ilium bones of the pelvic girdle.

There are many approaches to collecting the spinal cord. It is the opinion of the authors that the spinal cord should not be removed from the vertebral column until after fixation is complete. As noted earlier, the first one or two segments of cervical cord may be taken with the brain. To facilitate thorough fixation *in situ*, the cervical, thoracic and lumbar regions of the vertebral column are dissected from the carcass and then divided into three sections. These sections are to be no longer than the limits of each level as described above. Remove the dorsal arches from the vertebrae in each section to expose the spinal cord within the column and place into fixative.

Nasal turbinates and Zymbal's glands

The nasal turbinates are located under the nasal and frontal bones of the skull. The brain and eyes have been removed at the start of the dissection. The head should now be detached from the spinal column. Turn the head with the hard palate up. Caudal to the hard palate is the soft palate which covers the nasopharynx. The nasopharynx opens into the back of the oral cavity.

To ensure that the nasal turbinates are adequately fixed for evaluation, use a syringe to inject formalin through the nasopharyngeal duct in the soft palate until the fixative flows from the nares. This will fill the nasal cavity with fixative prior to immersion.

Frequently, the Zymbal's gland is required by protocol. This gland is a modified sebaceous gland located at the base of the ear, below the ear canal, and is left *in situ* with the head for fixation. The actual dissection of the Zymbal's gland will be done prior to the decalcification of the head for sectioning of the nasal turbinates (see Standard trimming).

Tissue accountability

At this point, all of the required tissues have been removed from the animal. The carcass is not discarded until this checkout procedure is completed. One technician, usually the dissecting technician, will reconfirm the animal identification and container label and identify the tissues, one by one, as they are put into the necropsy container.

Any small organs such as pituitary, adrenal, ovaries, eyes, lacrimal glands, thymus and thyroid and parathyroids (if weighed) should have been placed in cassettes and labeled as to which tissues are in each cassette, along with the animal number. This will assist in retrieving these tissues at the time of gross trimming. The necropsy standard operating procedure should specify the routinely collected tissues to be placed in cassettes.

As each tissue is retrieved from the tissue collection tray to place in the fixative container, it is checked off on the necropsy form. This process continues until all tissues in the tissue tray have been placed into the necropsy container and until all tissues and gross lesions are accounted for.

The technicians sign and date the form, and the necropsy area should be cleaned of all debris before the next animal is necropsied. At completion of the checkout procedure, the carcass can be disposed of according to established laboratory procedures and local disposal laws.

Criteria for Gross Lesion Description

Introduction

In order to ensure that all histologic sections of gross lesions are prepared and presented to the pathologist, concise and complete descriptions of the observations must be recorded during the necropsy. These descriptions must be made as each lesion is observed, not at the end of the dissection. When numerous animals are dissected in one day by a technician, it s easy to overlook recording a lesion if an attempt is made to describe all gross observations at the completion of the necropsy.

It is the responsibility of the dissecting technician in concert with the pathologist to describe each lesion, creating a verbal picture of what was observed, without providing a diagnosis. Diagnostic terms such as neoplasm, hemorrhage and atrophy should not be used because they indicate a specific pathologic change. Frequently, the actual pathologic process is not evident until microscopic evaluation. Macroscopic observations should be described using the following general criteria:

location, number, size, distribution, color, characteristics, and consistency. The glossary associated with each criterion listed below provides some of the more commonly used terminology.

Location

The general location refers to the organ, body cavity or body region where a lesion is located. Specific location refers to more localized regions such as subcutaneous, right or left, or a specific lobe of an organ. Common terms for location are listed below:

- *Abdominal* The part of the body between the thorax and the pelvis. The anterior border is the diaphragm.
- *Anterior* In front of or in the front part of; sometimes used synonymously with ventral.
- *Axillary* Pertaining to the area beneath the shoulder joint.
- *Caudal* Referring to the tail or that part of the body closest to the tail.
- *Cervical* Pertaining to the neck region.
- *Cortex* The outer portion of an organ such as kidney; as opposed to the inner portion or the medulla.
- *Cranial* Pertaining to the skull or bones of the head collectively. Cranial can also be used to described a direction toward the head.
- *Cutaneous* Relating to the skin.
- *Distal* Indicating area farthest to the body or the point of origin.
- *Dorsal* Relating to the back (vertebral column); the opposite side of ventral.
- *Hilus* The part of an organ where the nerves and vessels enter.
- *Inguinal* Pertaining to the groin; the region at the caudal ventral abdomen; junction of the thigh and the abdomen.
- *Lateral* Pertaining to the side; that part farthest from the center (midline).
- *Lumbar* Relating to the loin or part of the back and sides between the ribs and the pelvis.
- *Lumen* The space in the interior of a tubular structure such as an artery or intestine.
- *Medial* Relating to the middle; that part nearer the midline.
- *Medulla* The inner portion of certain organs as opposed to the cortex.
- *Mucosa* Referring to the luminal epithelial lining of organs such as in the digestive system, respiratory system and urogenital system.
- *Palmar* Relating to the ventral portion of the front foot.
- *Peripheral* Relating to or situated at the edge.
- *Plantar* Relating to the ventral portion of the hind foot.
- *Posterior* Referring to the back; opposite of anterior.
- *Proximal* That area nearest to the body or the point of origin.
- *Sacral* Referring to the vertebral region around the pelvis; caudal to the lumbar region and cranial to the tail.
- *Serosa* The thin membranous surface (peritoneal) which covers all abdominal organs.
- *Subcutaneous* Beneath the skin; referring to the connective tissue beneath the epidermis and underlying muscle.
- *Superficial* On or near a surface.
- *Thoracic* The part of the body between the neck and abdomen. The posterior border is the diaphragm.
- *Ventral* Pertaining to the belly or abdomen; opposite of dorsal.

For application of this terminology, see Chapter 15.

Number

All lesions observed at necropsy should be recorded and sampled. When a tumor mapping system (numbered tumors observed during the in-life portion of the study) is used, tumors should be correlated to the tumor mapping for each animal and identified accordingly. When multiple lesions occur within an organ such as liver or intestine, the entire organ should be preserved. When multiple masses occur in the subcutis, skin or body cavities, representative samples of all masses observed should be described and collected or the entire carcass can be preserved.

Size

A decrease or increase in the size of a normal structure can be described with actual measurements or by using generally qualitative terms such as slight, minimal, moderate or marked. For example, measurements should be provided for readily quantifiable lesions, e.g. red area (3 mm diameter) on the liver capsule. However, in some instances, more general descriptive terms are preferable, e.g. pinpoint gray foci on corneal surface of left eye. Tissue masses should be individually described with three measurements. When more than five masses are present with similar characteristics, a size range should be used.

Distribution

A lesion may be focal, multifocal or diffuse. It may involve an entire organ or a specific portion.

Distribution may be a description of a pattern such as linear or circular. Common terms for distribution are listed below:

- *Area* A lesion usually characterized by a change (e.g., color) which is larger than 1 mm (or dimension specified by the laboratory SOP) in diameter.
- *Bilateral* Pertaining to both sides or paired organs.
- *Diffuse* Not definitely limited or localized; widely distributed.
- *Focal* Pertaining to a solitary lesion which is approximately 1 mm or less (or dimension specified by the laboratory SOP) in diameter.
- *Multifocal* Multiple lesions which are approximately 1 mm or less (or dimension specified by the laboratory SOP) in diameter.
- *Random* A distribution which possesses no characteristic pattern.
- *Symmetrical* A similar arrangement in form and relationship on each side of a plane of the body.
- *Unilateral* Affecting one side only.
- *Patchy* Multiple poorly delineated lesions with an irregular distribution.

Color

Color description is self-explanatory. Straightforward terms such as tan, red, black, white, etc. should be used.

Characteristics

The characteristics of a lesion describe the nature and conformation of the change, such as distention, nodule or mass. In addition, the demarcation between normal and abnormal may be either poorly or well circumscribed. Modifiers such as pedunculated, umbilicated or thickened (e.g. gastric mucosa diffusely thickened) may be used to describe the characteristics of a lesion. Common terms are listed below:

- *Autolysis* The spontaneous post mortem degeneration of tissues or cells.
- *Adhesion* A fibrous band or structure by which two structures abnormally adhere or stick together.
- *Circumscribed* Clearly bounded or limited; confined to a limited space.
- *Confluent* Becoming merged; not discrete.
- *Dilated* Enlargement of a space or lumen, such as seen in renal pelvis or heart chambers.
- *Distended* A term applied to hollow organs when the lumen has been expanded, such as seen in the urinary bladder.
- *Focus* A lesion usually observed as a color change which is 1 mm or less in diameter (plural: foci).

- *Lobulated* Made up of or divided into more or less well-defined portions demarcated by fissures or bands of tissue.
- *Mass* An abnormal piece of tissue which is generally separated from or well delineated from normal structures.
- *Mottled* Being irregularly spotted with patches of various colors.
- *Nodular* Characterized by many solid masses often becoming confluent.
- *Nodule* A firm, well-circumscribed piece of tissue within the parenchyma of an organ or associated with a surface.
- *Opaque* Impervious to light rays; neither transparent nor translucent.
- *Papule* A small, circumscribed superficial solid elevation of the skin.
- *Papillary* Characterized by a stem-like connecting part or stalk by which a growth is attached to the normal tissue.
- *Perforated* A hole completely through a part or substance.
- *Pitted* Characterized by multiple depressed foci.
- *Polypoid* Resembling a polyp or protruding growth from a mucous membrane.
- *Translucent* Transmitting light but diffusing it so that objects beyond are not clearly distinguished.
- *Transparent* Permitting the passage of rays of light so that objects may be seen through the substance.
- *Umbilicated* Characterized by depressed or sunken areas on an often smooth surface.

Consistency

Nodules and masses may be soft or firm and fluids may be gelatinous or watery. Changes in the consistency of normal structures should be noted, such as scaliness of the skin or the irregular, roughened surface of an organ. A few common examples are listed below:

- *Caseous* Resembling cheese or curd.
- *Flocculent* Containing flaky material.
- *Friable* Easily crushed or crumbled.
- *Frothy* Having a foamy or bubbly appearance.
- *Gelatinous* Jelly-like or fluctuant. Conveying a sensation of or exhibiting wave-like motion on palpation due to a liquid content.
- *Granular* Made up of or marked by the presence of small particles or granules.
- *Lamellar* Characterized by layered appearance.
- *Viscous* Pertaining to the fluid which is relatively thick.

Trimming of Fixed Tissues for Processing

Introduction

Good Laboratory Practice guidelines and regulations published by the US Food and Drug Administration (FDA), EPA and other regulatory authorities rarely give specific details for the histopathological examination of tissues. In most cases these guidelines recommend a list of tissues to be examined depending on the protocol and the purpose of the test. In certain protocols, there may be recommendations for specific trimming requirements, but these are rare. Typically, the laboratory makes the decision for tissue trimming based on established standard operating procedures.

It is important to be able to compare the results observed in one animal with those observed in others. The key to meaningful comparison is to be consistent in the collection and preparation of tissues. In this respect, it is necessary to consider the following aspects:

- Uniform sample size
- Sampling from the same area using landmarks
- Cutting in the same tissue in the same plane of section
- Maintaining natural borders/margin(s) of tissues
- Maintaining orientation
- Maintaining tissue identification (left and right organs where this is important and lymph nodes where lymph nodes are sampled from different areas).

Although there are many ways that tissues should not be trimmed, there are equally as many ways that will give acceptable results. The purpose of this section is to attempt to provide a degree of standardization and, at the same time, try to caution against some of the more obvious pitfalls of poor trimming technique.

One initial source of confusion in trimming is interpreting the definition of the 'plane of section'. Some of the many terms that have been used in study protocols include:

- Cross
- Longitudinal

Necropsy Techniques, Errors and Artifacts

Good necropsy technique is essential to facilitate accurate, reproducible tissue trimming. Below are examples of more common deficiencies in necropsy technique that can adversely affect trimming and subsequent histologic preparation:

- *Insufficient sample* The portion of an organ saved is too small to adequately represent the tissue or to obtain the required orientation.

- *Tissues cut in the opposite plane to the required plane of sectioning* A kidney scored transversely when a longitudinal section is required for histopathology.

- *Improper retention* The stomach not rinsed and pinned flat or infused with formalin (if not opened at necropsy) to permit correctly oriented sections.

- *Wrong portion of a tissue* A hip joint retained in place of stifle joint, or sacral spinal cord taken in place of lumbar at necropsy.

- *Tissues not collected* Usually the result of incorrect identification at necropsy, such as lymph node mistaken for adrenal gland.

- *Artifacts* Forceps marks and fragmentation can be introduced by poor handling. Autolysis of endocrine or weighed tissues will result from drying or delay in fixation.

- *Tissues not readily identified in fixative container* Left and right organs' identity should be maintained when required. Regional lymph nodes, depending upon necropsy technique, may change in appearance and otherwise not be identifiable among all tissues in fixative. Lymph nodes and small tissues, such as adrenals or pituitary, can maintain identity by placement in labeled cassettes. Maintaining an attachment to a regional organ, such as mesenteric lymph node to mesenteric fat or cecum, can also be used to help identify an organ in fixed tissue.

- *Noninfused lungs* Histology section is generally inadequate for evaluation if the lungs are not perfused with fixative at necropsy.

- *Number of samples from paired organs* The number of tissues sampled may depend on whether the paired organs were written in the plural or singular. (Why take two salivary glands when the protocol clearly states 'salivary gland?'). This problem can be resolved by clear instructions in the histology SOPs.

- Transverse
- Coronal
- Sagittal
- Frontal
- Diagonal
- Proximal
- Distal
- Whole
- Representative.

By far the most widely used and unclear term is 'cross-section'. The phrase 'cross-section' is usually intended to describe the action of cutting a section of tissue across its shortest dimension. All of the above become meaningless if the tissue retention at necropsy is not done correctly.

For the sake of consistency in this chapter, the following terms will be used for trimming discussions:

- Transverse – a section perpendicular to the long axis of the organ.
- Longitudinal – a midline section along the longest axis of the organ.
- Sagittal – a section (lateral to midline) parallel to the long axis of the organ.
- Distal – that area farthest from a body or point of origin.
- Proximal – that area nearest to the body or point of origin.

Trimming of routine protocol required tissues will be discussed in the next section.

Gross Lesions

Lesions such as tissue masses and nonprotocol tissues need to be sampled in a consistent manner. During the necropsy, a number of 'normal' findings may also have been recorded. These findings may be considered observations rather than lesions. It must be decided in advance of trimming if these tissues are to be sampled for all animals or not. Examples of such 'non' lesions are:

- Staining and discharge around the eyes, nose, mouth and urogenital region
- Crooked or maloccluded teeth
- Ear lesions due to ear tagging
- Autolysis.

Paired Organs

Lesions often occur in only one of a paired organ, e.g. enlarged left axillary lymph node. There are two possible approaches in this respect. Many prefer to take both organs of the pair for comparison. Others see this as processing of unnecessary tissues, particularly if the lesion in a paired tissue does not really require the other organ for comparison, e.g. black focus on right inguinal lymph node. Once again, it is important to take a reasoned and consistent approach, maintaining the same rule throughout the entire study.

Masses

Long-term carcinogenicity studies will generate a large number of masses; in turn, some of these masses may grow to a considerable size. While the mass is obviously an important tissue to sample, it should not be over- or undersampled. The center of a large mass may often consist of an area of necrotic tissue. The important areas of a mass to sample are junctions with skin or other surrounding tissue and areas of change of color or consistency. In this way, one or two blocks containing 1–3 sections per block will normally be sufficient to represent even the largest tissue masses.

Gross Lesion Sampling in Protocol-Required Tissues

Lesions, nodules and masses in protocol-required tissues are to be sampled with the routine section, when possible. The lesion should be trimmed so that it will readily appear in the plane of tissue section.

When extra tissue sections are taken to encompass a lesion, this increases the sample size taken for that animal and thus increases the amount of tissue being examined. This increase in sample size can bias the results by presenting more tissue for examination in only those animals that have lesions. For this reason, care should be taken not to oversample tissues with lesions, but rather take just as many sections necessary to represent the lesion and the routine tissue.

It is highly recommended that small focal lesions be sampled separately and placed in an additional block. This will isolate the small lesions, making it easier to locate during microtomy and include in the histologic section.

Photographs and Drawings

Many laboratories make extensive use of photographs and drawings to illustrate either routine trimming cuts for tissues or specific gross lesions. This is an invaluable tool for the trimming technician. Photographs taken at necropsy will easily show color changes and other subtle lesions that may be lost after fixation. Line drawings and diagrams can highlight specific landmarks for trimming and embedding orientation, helping to maintain a consistent sampling of all tissues.

Randomization

Individual technician trimming differences, processing artifacts and slide staining variation are three common areas where bias and artifacts can be introduced in the histology laboratory. These effects can be greatly reduced by randomization of animals.

Animals from a study are often processed in order by group and sex. This can allow mishaps to occur to only one of the dose groups in a study or allow the stain to be more intense in one or more groups compared to others. By randomizing the population of animals, in particular for processing and staining, these potential variations can be distributed across the dose groups and thus such an effect will be minimized.

Gross Trimming Artifacts

The gross trimming technician can inadvertently introduce artifacts into the tissues that will affect the final appearance of the microscope slides and possibly influence the pathological interpretation. More common artifacts are listed below.

Floaters

These are small pieces of material that are left on the cutting board becoming attached to or embedded in other tissues either from the same animal, or, worse still, from a completely different animal. Floaters can be pieces of organs, feces, or in some cases pieces of tumors. Tissues should be rinsed thoroughly before trimming to remove as much unwanted debris as possible. The cutting board should be wiped clean between trimming each tissue and rinsed under the tap between each animal and instruments should be kept as clean as possible during the trimming process.

At the very least consequence, floaters are an irritation to the pathologist and a reflection of poor technique. At the worst, the extraneous piece of tissue can adversely affect the interpretation of findings for an animal and the overall scientific quality of a study.

Crushed or fractured tissues

Poor trimming technique and the use of dull instruments will result in mechanical damage to the tissues. Scalpel blades should be changed frequently and correct cutting technique should be employed at all times. In this way, the tissue is cut rather than being squashed by applying unnecessary pressure. Particularly susceptible to damage are adrenals, eyes and testes. Mechanical damage can also be inflicted by the incorrect use of forceps in holding the tissues. This can result in depressions and condensed areas in the tissues, in particular lungs and other soft organs.

Dry tissues

Trimming a full screen of tissues from a rat may take up to an hour or more depending on the number of lesions present. During this time, the tissues will dry rapidly, especially in the high air flow of a trimming room. Once tissues become dry, the damage caused can be permanent. Dried tissues will not easily rehydrate and, in this state, the tissue processing will be poor. Physical dehydration (air drying) rather than chemical dehydration by the use of alcohol is not compatible with paraffin wax infiltration. For this reason, the tissues need to be kept in a moist environment during tissue trimming. It is advisable to keep the tissue cassettes slightly submerged in a shallow tray of water or saline. The top surface of both the trimmed and untrimmed fixed tissues can be lightly 'misted' with a spray of normal buffered saline to prevent the surface from drying during the trimming process.

Trimming of Protocol-Required Tissues

Some anatomical features essential for trimming are described with the organs below. More detailed descriptions can be found in the anatomy section of this book. For many rodent tissues, the size of the sample is dictated by the overall size of the tissue. Some tissues, however, do allow for size variation in sampling. Rat liver sections can be cut as long as the tissue cassette or trimmed to the size of an adrenal. It is important to submit a consistent, uniform section that is representative of the standard protocol-required tissue. The RITA (Registry of Industrial Toxicology Animal-data) guidelines for tissue trimming were designed to provide a standardized sampling and trimming procedure and to indicate alternate approaches for some tissues (Bahnemann et al., 1995). The guidelines presented here are generally similar to the RITA guidelines with a few exceptions.

Adrenal glands

The adrenal glands are bilateral organs that are essentially oval in shape. When making a cut through the longest plane of each adrenal gland, notice that there are two distinct zones – the center zone or medulla being the darker and the outer zone or cortex tan in color (Figure 28.14).

Sections of the adrenal glands should include the largest cut surface possible to include the cortex and medulla of each organ. Two-thirds of each organ should be embedded with the cut surface down in the block, so that the cut surface is microtomed first.

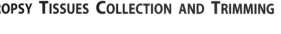

Figure 28.14 Adrenal gland. Transverse section with cortex and medulla.

— Cortex
— Medulla

Aorta

A transverse section of the aorta should be obtained from the midthoracic area. This section should be placed in the block perpendicular to the block face, maintaining the transverse orientation for microtoming.

Brain

The brain consists of two cerebral hemispheres joined by the corpus callosum, a band of white tracts between the hemispheres. The posterior brain consists of the convoluted lateral hemispheres of the cerebellum. Ventrally attached to the cerebellum is the medulla and pons. The medulla oblongata is the most caudal part of the brainstem which decreases in size and becomes the spinal cord. Routinely, the areas of interest which should be included in sections of the brain are: cerebral and cerebellar cortex, hippocampus, basal ganglia, thalamus, hypothalamus, midbrain, pons and medulla oblongata. Note that the proximal cervical spinal cord can be taken with the brain.

Three transverse sections through portions of these areas will provide an acceptable overview of any effects in the brain (Figure 28.15). The first section is cut at the level of the optic chiasma to include the cerebrum, the second at the level of the

base of the posterior hypothalamus at the widest part of the cerebrum, and the third to include a section through the midcerebellum, and pons/medulla oblongata. When olfactory bulbs are required for examination, they are usually not trimmed, but are embedded whole with the largest surface (lateral) down in the block.

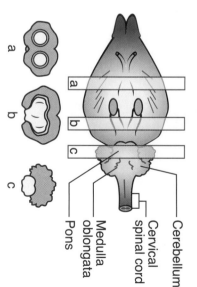

Figure 28.15 Brain. Transverse sections.

a
b
c

Cerebellum
Cervical spinal cord
Medulla oblongata
Pons

Epididymides

The epididymides consist of a coiled tubule situated around the lateral surface of the testes. There are three regions in the epididymides – the caput or head, cauda or tail, and the corpus or body which connects the head and tail. Generally, the epididymides are removed from the testes before weighing.

The standard section should include the head, tail and body of each epididymis in one longitudinal section. One side of the head and tail should be trimmed to allow the three regions to be embedded on the same level (Figure 28.16).

Eyes, optic nerves and Harderian glands

The rat eye is one of the more difficult organs to section due to the different consistency of the tissue

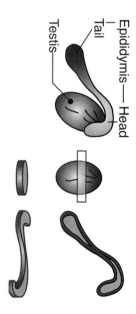

Figure 28.16 Epididymis and testis. Sectioning and orientation.

Testis —
Tail —
Epididymis — Head

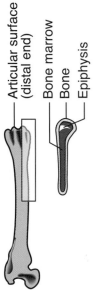

Figure 28.17 Eye and Harderian/lacrimal glands. Sagittal section.

types joined in close proximity. For instance, the lens is large compared to the size of the eye in general and is very firm. The suspensory fibers connecting the lens to the interior of the globe or sclera are quite fragile. When the lens is trimmed, it will break free and rotate, creating artifacts by displacing many of the small structures in the section. Also, the retina has a tendency to detach during fixation, due to the differential shrinkage between the different layers. In an effort to prevent some of these obvious trimming problems, an aerosol freezing/cooling media can be used. Before sectioning, the entire eye may be snap-frozen to harden all of the structures, and reduce damage.

The sagittal section should be taken to include cornea, iris, lens, suspensory fibers, ciliary muscles, sclera, retina and optic nerve (Figure 28.17). Care should be taken to include the optic nerve with each eye. It is necessary to trim at least one callotte from the lateral aspect of the eye to allow paraffin to adequately enter the globe to support the lens and other structures. The Harderian glands are wrapped around the eye deep in the eye socket. These glands can be sectioned with plane of the eye section (attached to the eye) or as a separate section. A separate section is preferable due to the fact that the gland obscures the position of the optic nerve when taken intact with the eye.

Femur and marrow

The standard section of femur should be made through the distal end to provide a suitable routine section. This end of the femur provides a large articular surface, the growth plate or physis, and if the tibia is included, the cartilage, ligaments and tendons surrounding the joint. The femoral shaft provides a histologic section of marrow.

After removing as much muscle as possible, place the entire bone into decalcification solution.

Depending on the solution used, this decalcification process can take from 8 to 24 hours to completely soften the bone. The decalcification will allow trimming to include the bone with marrow, articular surface and synovial space. The section will include a longitudinal section beginning at the midfemoral shaft, and preferably continuing through the knee joint to include the proximal tibia (Figure 28.18).

Gastrointestinal tract

The trimming of the gastrointestinal tract will be discussed as a unit covering esophagus, stomach, duodenum, pancreas, jejunum, ileum, cecum, colon, mesenteric lymph nodes and rectum. Generally, all of the intestines are cut into transverse sections approximately 3–4 mm in length. These sections can be embedded vertically in the block on either cut surface.

For the esophagus, a transverse section approximately 3–4 mm in length will provide a representative sample. Dependent on the necropsy technique used, the esophagus may be sectioned attached to the trachea and thyroids as a block of tissue. This trimming technique is useful in orienting the thyroids and parathyroids for a transverse section.

The stomach has two distinct regions – the forestomach (nonglandular) and the glandular stomach. The forestomach is characterized by a white smooth mucosa which lies in folds much like that of the esophagus. The fundus is the largest region of the glandular stomach with a thick mucosa. The fundic mucosa is darker in color than the other regions. The pyloric region near the distal end and adjacent duodenum has a smoother mucosa similar to the duodenum. The pyloric stomach and the duodenum are separated by a thick muscular sphincter.

The opened stomach, pinned to a piece of cork, will provide a flat section to work with at trimming. Two sections should be taken which will permit evaluation of all regions of the stomach. One section is taken longitudinally just off the midline through the lesser curvature to include forestomach, a small

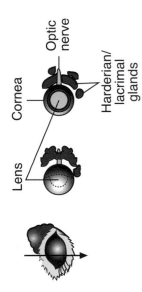

Figure 28.18 Femoral bone and marrow. Longitudinal sections of distal end.

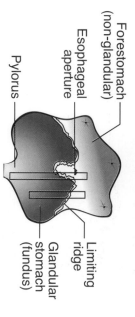

Figure 28.19 Stomach (pinned) showing mucosal surface. Two longitudinal sections.

fundic area and pyloric regions (when possible include the duodenum). The second section should be taken parallel and lateral to the first to include forestomach and greater representative portion of the fundus (Figure 28.19).

A transverse section should be made of the duodenum (with pancreas attached 1 cm from the stomach (Figure 28.20). A transverse section of jejunum should be made at a standard distance from the duodenum (e.g. 10 cm) and a transverse section of the ileum to include a Peyer's patch (GALT, gut-associated lymphoid tissue) should also be trimmed.

Typically, the Peyer's patch can be easily identified grossly throughout the small intestine and to a lesser extent in the cecum and colon/rectum. Usually, an attempt is made to include a representative sample of Peyer's patch with the standard section of ileum. If Peyer's patch is a separate protocol-required tissue for evaluation and is not grossly apparent in the ileum, a portion of Peyer's patch from jejunum or duodenum may be included to ensure accountability for this tissue.

The cecum is a large pouch-like portion of the large intestine located at the end of the ileum and beginning of the colon. Providing an exact transverse

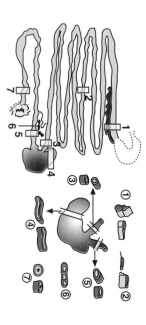

Figure 28.20 Gastrointestinal tract (without stomach). (1) Duodenum with pancreas, (2) jejunum, (3) ileum with Peyer's patch, (4) cecum, (5) colon, (6) mesenteric lymph nodes, (7) rectum.

section is sometimes difficult at the embedding phase of preparation. Trimming a section which includes a complete transverse 'ring' helps to eliminate most of this problem. The colon extends from the cecum to the rectum and should have a transverse section through the ascending colon segment. The rectum sample should be trimmed transversely within 1 cm from the anus.

The mesenteric lymph node is one of the more routinely collected lymph nodes for evaluation. These lymph nodes are located in the mesentery in the area where the ileum, cecum and colon join together. They are situated in a line of multiple nodes surrounded by fat at the 'hub' of the mesenteric strands. The section of mesenteric lymph nodes should include a longitudinal section through the line which includes a portion of one to several nodes.

Heart

The heart should be prepared with a frontal/longitudinal section to include both atria, ventricles and septum. Whenever possible, the proximal aorta and other vessels should remain as part of this section (Figure 28.21).

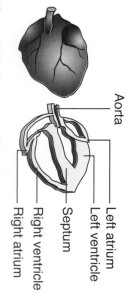

Aorta
Left atrium
Left ventricle
Septum
Right ventricle
Right atrium

Figure 28.21 Heart. Frontal/longitudinal section, to include both atria, ventricles and septum.

If the kidneys have been identified left and right, this differentiation should be maintained. It is common practice to mark the left kidney with a longitudinal cut and the right with a transverse cut. These cuts have served two purposes – identity as well as fixation of the interior of the organ. With the hilus in view, a longitudinal section of the left kidney and

Kidneys

The kidneys have a clearly defined outer layer or cortex and inner portion or medulla. The medulla (renal papilla) protrudes up into the space (renal pelvis) created by the ureter at the hilus. All of these structures should be present in each section of kidney, if possible.

Forestomach (non-glandular)
Esophageal aperture
Pylorus
Limiting ridge
Glandular stomach (fundus)

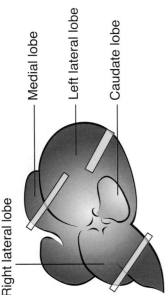

Figure 28.22 Kidneys. Right-transverse and left-longitudinal sections to include medulla, cortex and renal pelvis.

transverse section of the right should be taken (Figure 28.22).

Lacrimal glands

The lacrimal glands are located both intraorbital and exorbital. The intraorbital gland is usually quite small. Therefore, the exorbital glands are typically considered as the tissue for the protocol-required lacrimal gland. The section of intraorbital gland (if required) should include the entire gland intact or in conjunction with the Harderian gland (see Eyes, Figure 28.17). The exorbital lacrimal glands are large and a transverse section of each should be taken.

Larynx

The larynx is covered on its cranial end by the epiglottis, a leaf-like projection, and on its caudal limit is the cricoid cartilage. The cricoid cartilage forms a complete circle of cartilage around the base of the larynx and is followed by the incomplete rings of the trachea. For inhalation studies, three transverse sections of larynx are recommended: at the base of the epiglottis to include the beginning of the vocal cords, middle of the thyroid cartilage to include ventral diverticulum, and through the cricoid cartilage at the base of the larynx (Figure 28.23).

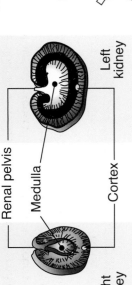

Figure 28.23 Larynx. Ventral frontal view.

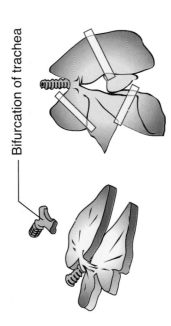

Figure 28.24 Liver. Transverse sections of the three largest lobes.

These sections should be embedded cranial side down in the block. If larynx is required for a noninhalation study, one section at the base of the epiglottis should be taken.

Liver

The liver consists of four lobes – left and right lateral lobes, the medial lobe which is bifurcated, and the small caudate lobe. For more details about the liver lobes see Chapters 13 and 15. There is no gall bladder in the rat. The common bile duct or ductus choledochus (ductus hepatoentericus) is the junction of many ducts from all liver lobes.

Sections of the liver should include transverse sections of the three largest lobes (left and right lateral and the medial lobe) (Figure 28.24).

Lungs

The rat lung has five separate lobes. The left lung consists of one lobe which extends the same length as the right, which has four lobes: apical (cranial), cardiac (middle), diaphragmatic (caudal) and azygous (accessory) lobes (see Chapters 13 and 15). There are numerous approaches to sectioning the lungs.

Inhalation studies obviously will require specific attention to the lung where a full frontal section is optimal (Figure 28.25). If this full frontal section is

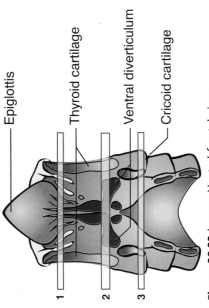

Figure 28.25 Lung. Left: Inhalation section. Right: Standard gross trimming.

too large to embed in one block of tissue, the left and right sides may be embedded separately by removing the lungs from the tracheal bifurcation. The bifurcation would be embedded as well. This frontal section provides maximum lung tissue, as well as much of the bronchial tree for examination. For noninhalation study, a transverse section of the left lobe and transverse sections of the apical (top) and diaphragmatic (bottom) lobes of the right lung is acceptable.

Lymph nodes

In most cases, lymph nodes can be sectioned through the longest axis of each node or smaller nodes can be embedded whole. Typically, mesenteric and mandibular lymph nodes are most often required. It also is commonly required to retain regional 'draining' lymph nodes for masses, and these are listed in Table 28.2.

Table 28.2 Regional lymph nodes required for masses

Regional lymph node	Tissue/region draining
Mandibular	Tongue, oral cavity, external ear, salivary gland, skin of rostral head region
Cervical	Floor of the oral cavity, tongue, pharynx, larynx, thyroid and parathyroid gland, initial part of esophagus
Axillary	Thoracic limb, skin of thoracic and lateral abdominal wall and neck region
Thoracic	Region of thoracic vertebral column and diaphragm
Mediastinal	Aortic arch, skin of ventral cervical region, mammary gland, heart, thymus, lung, dorsal thoracic cavity
Renal	Lateral abdominal wall, lumbar region, abdominal cavity, kidney, testes or ovaries, uterus, cervix
Iliac	Tail, sacral region, genital region, accessory sex glands, penis, vagina, rectum, anus
Mesenteric	Distal duodenum, ileum, cecum, ascending and transverse colon
Sacral hypogastricus	Pelvic limb, abdominal wall, tail, abdominal cavity, pelvic cavity, genital region, rectum, anus
Popliteal	Pelvic limb including the stifle joint, skeletal muscle, sciatic nerve, foot pad
Inguinal	Skin of thigh, lateral abdominal wall, genital region, base of tail

Mammary glands

The rat has six pairs of nipples with underlying mammary glands. There are three pairs in the thoracic/pectoral region and three pairs in the lower abdominal/inguinal region. In adult animals, the mammary glands in these two regions are joined unilaterally with no distinguishable separation from nipple to nipple. The largest area with little or no mammary gland is the mid-ventral abdomen.

Sections of mammary gland should be taken with associated nipple and skin (Figure 28.26). The inguinal area is the recommended area for harvesting mammary gland. The section should be taken in the direction of the lay of hair. Excess hair should be trimmed away from the skin. The section will be embedded on the cut edge so that the section reveals skin, subcutis and mammary gland.

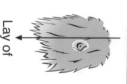

Lay of the hair

Nipple

Mammary gland

Subcutis

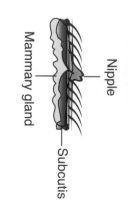

Figure 28.26 Mammary gland and associated skin, including the nipple. Longitudinal section with the lay of hair.

Nasal turbinates

The nasal passages are routinely taken in inhalation studies: a series from 3–6, but generally 4 sections are taken for examination of the entire nasal cavity. A procedure developed by Young (1981) has remained a standard for trimming the nose. It presents a reproducible procedure based on palatal landmarks for sections. In studies using other routes of administration, one or two sections (e.g. levels II and IV) may be required.

The Young procedure utilizes obvious landmarks on the surface of the hard palate as shown in Figure 28.27.

Ovaries and oviducts

Generally, the ovary and oviduct are collected together, unless weights are required for the ovaries.

The ovaries are processed whole and intact with the oviducts. The tip of the uterine horn may be left attached to assist with orientation of the oviducts. When embedding, the ovary and its oviduct are positioned on the same plane in the block (Figure 28.28).

Peripheral nerve and skeletal muscle

The sciatic nerve is generally collected for evaluation of a representative peripheral nerve. At necropsy, this nerve is collected attached to the muscles in the hind leg. The skeletal muscles in the hind leg provide a suitable section for evaluation. The biceps femoris is the largest muscle in the upper hind leg and the sciatic nerve lies on its full length from the inguinal area to its major branching near the distal end of the femur.

The nerve should be taken attached to the muscle section because this provides easier orientation of the nerve and prevents it from twisting during fixation (Figure 28.29). Transverse and longitudinal sections are taken of the muscle and nerve. The nerve in the longitudinal section should be trimmed at least 2 × the length of the transverse section. This will identify clearly the orientation for embedding.

Pituitary

The pituitary is best sectioned whole. The entire pituitary should be embedded with its pontal (dorsal) surface down in the block to provide the best representative transverse section (Figure 28.30).

Prostate

A transverse section through the dorsolateral and ventral lobes to include urethra should be presented. The dorsocranial lobes (coagulating glands) are included with the seminal vesicles (Figure 28.31).

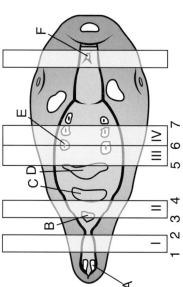

Figure 28.27 Ventral view of rat hard palate with the lower jaw removed, showing the four tissue slices I–IV, which will be embedded, anterior face down. The arabic numbers (1–7) indicate the levels of the seven cuts necessary to produce the four slices. (A) Upper incisor teeth, (B) incisive papilla, (C) first palatal ridge, (D) second palatal ridge, (E) first upper molar tooth, (F) posterior opening of the pharyngeal duct (nasopharynx).

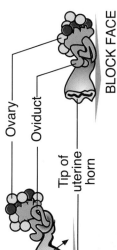

Figure 28.28 Ovary and oviduct with uterus showing embedding orientation.

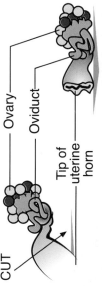

Figure 28.29 Skeletal muscle and sciatic nerve. Sections showing orientation of transverse and longitudinal embedding.

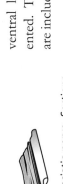

Figure 28.30 Pituitary showing embedding orientation on pontal surface.

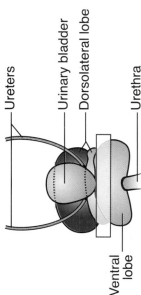

Figure 28.31 Ventral view of prostate showing lobes in relationship to bladder and urethra.

Rib

The section, if required, should include one rib with the costochondral junction (Figure 28.32). There should be an equal amount of bone and cartilage. This section will be embedded flat so that a longitudinal section with the junction of bone and cartilage is present in the section for evaluation. The rib section should also include bone marrow.

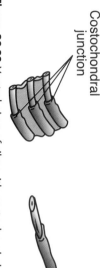

Routinely, a longitudinal section will be taken to include the submaxillary and sublingual salivary glands with submandibular lymph nodes attached (Figure 28.33). If the parotid is required, it can be taken as a separate longitudinal section.

Salivary glands

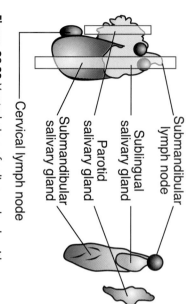

Costochondral junction

Figure 28.32 Ventral view of ribs with costochondral junction and section for evaluation.

Submandibular lymph node

Sublingual salivary gland

Parotid salivary gland

Submandibular salivary gland

Cervical lymph node

Figure 28.33 Ventral view of salivary glands with associated lymph nodes and longitudinal sections for evaluation.

Seminal vesicles

Sections of the seminal vesicles should include the adjoining coagulating gland (Figure 28.34). Take a transverse section in the middle of each lobe.

Skin

The skin is one of the more difficult tissues to section because of the various densities of epidermis and subcutis, and the coarseness of the hair follicles. If mammary gland is required, the skin section should be taken in the inguinal area in one section as described in the discussion of mammary gland.

If only skin is required, which is occasionally the case for males, abdominal skin will suffice. The skin should be cut parallel to the direction of the hair shaft pattern (see mammary gland, Figure 28.26). When the test material is applied to the skin surface or injected subcutaneously, treated and control areas must be sampled and appropriately identified for histopathology.

Spinal cord

Generally, cervical, thoracic and lumbar levels are requested (Figure 28.35). Transverse sections can be taken in the middle of each level required. Detection of lesions in the terminal portions of the long ascending sensory tracts requires examination of the first cervical segments (see the brain).

Spleen

A transverse section through the middle of the spleen should be taken for examination (Figure 28.36).

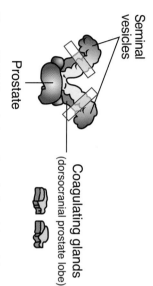

Seminal vesicles

Prostate

Coagulating glands (dorsocranial prostate lobe)

Figure 28.34 Ventral view of seminal vesicles with prostate and transverse sections for evaluation.

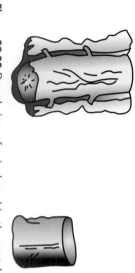

Figure 28.35 Dorsal view of spinal cord in the vertebrae and transverse section removed from bone.

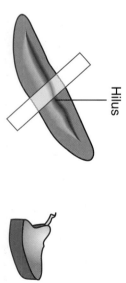

Hilus

Figure 28.36 View of spleen. Transverse section of midspleen.

Sternum with bone marrow

The sternum is used for the bone marrow section in most studies (Figure 28.37). A longitudinal section should be taken which includes at least two sternebrae with marrow.

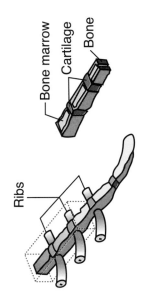

Figure 28.37 Dorsal view of sternum with ribs, longitudinal section of two segments with marrow exposed.

Testes

A transverse section of each testis is made at the greatest diameter (see epididymides, Figure 28.16).

Thymus

In the young animal, a section taken across the greatest dimension should be taken. In older animals, a representative section from the thymic area should be taken. This may contain atrophic thymic tissue, fat, nerves, and small lymph nodes.

Thyroids and parathyroids

The thyroid gland has two lobes which are positioned on each side of the trachea (Figure 28.38) at the level of the cricoid cartilage. The two lobes are connected by a thin strip of thyroid tissue called the isthmus. Near the cranial pole of each thyroid are the parathyroids. The parathyroids appear as white foci and are usually prominent enough to see macroscopically.

A transverse section can be taken at the level of the parathyroid to include thyroids, parathyroids, and trachea. Note that the esophagus is still attached to this group of tissues and can remain as part of this transverse section. Several levels of this tissue group can be taken at microtoming to assure the presence of the parathyroids for examination. If additional sections are prepared, it is important to prepare the same number for all animals.

If thyroid/parathyroid weights are required, the thyroid/parathyroid must be carefully trimmed from the trachea/esophagus. In this case, the two thyroid lobes with parathyroid are embedded flat for a longitudinal section.

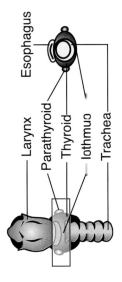

Figure 28.38 Ventral view of thyroid and associated structures. Transverse section shows esophagus on dorsal side of trachea.

Larynx
Parathyroid
Thyroid
Iothmuo
Trachea
Esophagus

Urinary bladder

The section should be longitudinal to include the neck of the bladder, as well as the ventral and dorsal walls (Figure 28.39).

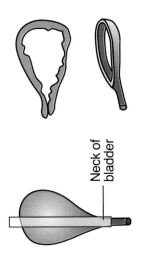

Neck of bladder

Figure 28.39 View of urinary bladder. Longitudinal section to include neck.

Uterus, cervix and vagina

Sections of these tissues can be achieved in three or four sections: a transverse section of each uterine horn, and one longitudinal section including the body of the uterus, cervix and vagina (Figure 28.40). Optionally, a separate transverse section of vagina can be submitted.

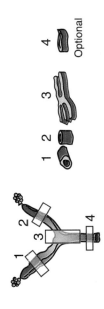

1 2 3 4
Optional

Figure 28.40 Female reproductive tract, uterine horns (1, 2), uterine body and cervix (3) (with vagina) and vagina (optional, 4).

Zymbal's glands

The Zymbal's glands are located at the base of the external ear. They are situated in a hollow surrounded by the muscle of the lower jaw and the skull. There are two methods for trimming the Zymbal's glands. One method involves removing the glands individually with a section of the outer ear canal (Figure 28.41). The skin is removed from the head along with the pinna. Starting behind the ear, make a cut toward the front, working the blade under the jaw muscle at a 45° angle. Turn the blade and scoop back, cutting deep into the muscle and as close to the bone as possible, then across the ear canal to include a circle of ear cartilage with Zymbal's gland attached. This method isolates the glands and requires no decalcification due to the lack of bone in the section.

The second method requires decalcification of the head. After the completion of decalcification, a transverse section through the head at the level of the ear canals will provide a section of the glands *in situ* along the canal at the point of the external opening of the ears.

Suggested Blocking Arrangement

It is common practice to multiple-embed rat tissues (two or more tissues per block). The efficiencies of multiple tissues in one block are numerous. For example, there will be fewer slides for the histology laboratory and pathologist to handle, a reduction in chemical and supply use, and a reduction in the space necessary for archiving slides.

The tissue/block arrangement shown in Table 28.3 is for suggestion only. Different tissues have been grouped in blocks based on microtoming characteristics that have provided consistent quality sections. These, of course, can be altered depending on individual laboratory preference. The general portioning or grouping of the tissues within a block can also be varied. Some laboratories embed tissues in the block in a straight line. Consistent tissue placement for all animals reduces the time requirement for the pathologist to move the slide to search for a particular tissue in a block that has multiple tissues embedded.

Generally, the blocking schemes are based on the

size and texture of the tissues required, to facilitate microtoming. A rat with a full screen of tissues (60–64 tissues) will usually have approximately 18–20 tissue blocks. Most laboratories develop a standard scheme which may adjust slightly with special study requirements.

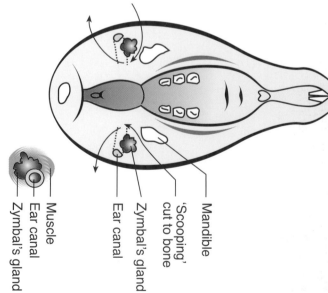

Figure 28.41 Ventral view of rat head showing 'scooping' cut to section individual Zymbal's gland.

Muscle
Ear canal
Zymbal's gland
Ear canal
Zymbal's gland
'Scooping' cut to bone
Mandible

References

Bahnemann, R., Jacobs, M. et al. (1995) *Exp. Toxicol. Pathol.* **47**, 247–266.

Bancroft, J.D. and Stevens, A. (eds) (1982) *Theory and Practice of Histological Techniques*, 2nd edn. Edinburgh: Churchill Livingstone.

Bono, C.D. (1994) *Necropsy of the Laboratory Rat*. Vienna, VI: D. Bono & Associates.

Chiasson, R.B. (1988) *Laboratory Anatomy of the White Rat*, 5th edn. William C. Brown.

Experimental Pathology Laboratories, Inc. (1998) Standard Operating Procedures SOP No. 14.2.

Sharp, P.E. and La Regina, M.C. (1998) *The Laboratory Rat*, pp. 124–127. Boca Raton: CRC Press.

Sullivan, D.J. (1985) *Toxicol. Pathol.* **13**, 229–231.

Young, J.T. (1981) *Fundam. Appl. Toxicol.* **1**, 309–312.

Table 28.3 Suggested tissue/block arrangements

	Tissues	No. of sections
Block 1	Brain	3
	Spinal cord	3
Block 2	Sciatic nerve	2
	Skeletal muscle	2
Block 3	Heart	1
	Aorta (thoracic)	1
	Thymus	1
Block 4	Lungs	2
Block 5	Liver	3
	Spleen	1
Block 6	Adrenals	2
	Pituitary	1
Block 7	Kidneys	2
Block 8	Salivary gland	1
	Submandibular lymph node	1
Block 9	Stomach	2
	Duodenum	1
	Pancreas	1
	Ileum	1
Block 10	Mesenteric lymph node	1
	Jejunum	1
	Cecum	1
	Colon	1
	Rectum	1
Block 11	Skin	1
	Mammary gland	1
Block 12	Eyes	2
	Optic nerves	2
	Harderian glands	2
	Intraorbital lacrimal glands	2
	Exorbital lacrimal glands	2
Block 13	Thyroids	2
	Parathyroids	2
	Esophagus	1
	Trachea	1
Block 14 (male)	Testis	1
Block 15 (malc)	Epididymis	1
	Testis	1
	Epididymis	1
Block 14 (female)	Ovaries	2
	Oviducts	2
Block 16 (male)	Prostate	1
	Seminal vesicles	2

Table 28.3 (continued)

	Tissues	No. of sections
Block 15 (female)	Urinary bladder	1
	Uterus	2
	Cervix	1
Block 17	Urinary bladder	1
	Femur	1
	Marrow	1
Block 18	Sternum	1
	Marrow	1
Block 19, 20 and as required	Gross lesions, optional sections of tissues such as Nasal turbinates, Rib, Tongue, Zymbal's glands etc, Vagina can be placed in female block 15	

Emerging
New Techniques

Contents

CHAPTER 29

Genetic Engineering and Molecular Technology

Brad Bolon
Amgen Inc., Thousand Oaks, CA, USA

Elizabeth Galbreath
Eli Lilly & Co., Indianapolis, IN, USA

Linda Sargent
National Institute of Occupational Safety and Health, Morgantown, WV, USA

Jürgen Weiss
University of Heidelberg, Heidelberg, Germany

Overview: Use of Genetic Methods in Vertebrate Biology

Scientists have been performing genetic manipulations and analyses since Mendel first reported the heritable nature of physical characteristics in pea plants in 1865. With respect to rats, experimental biologists who crossbred rat strains for a variety of traits (Chapter 1) were occasionally rewarded by the advent of an unexpected functional or structural phenotype. Such serendipitously acquired mutant lines, most of which result from a spontaneous mutation to a single gene, were often expanded and characterized to serve as animal models of human diseases. However, a large-scale random breeding program to produce new lines with novel mutations would be very costly in rodents, even if combined with treatments that accelerate the mutation rate (e.g. Kasarkis *et al.*, 1998). Furthermore, random breeding schemes and mutagenic agents cannot be employed effectively to produce defects in specific genes of interest.

Fortunately, the revolution in molecular biology of the past few decades has made possible the intentional engineering of rat models for many human diseases (Heideman, 1991; Paul *et al.*, 1994;

Tools for Exploring Interesting Genes

Charreau et al., 1996; Mullins and Mullins, 1996). The introduction of specific genes (and thereby new physiological properties) into the well-characterized biological backgrounds of common laboratory animals, including the rat, provides an in vivo means of examining the mechanisms by which the genes of interest control, and are regulated by, other molecules. The combined use of animals in which a gene has been either overexpressed, suppressed or deleted offers unique opportunities for basic researchers to dissect gene function at a fine level of detail. In addition, genetically engineered rats provide applied scientists with a new means of evaluating innovative therapeutic agents for potential efficacy, either by using rats in which human-like disease models have been engineered (e.g. hypertension (Paul et al., 1994); myelinopathy (Sereda et al., 1996)) or by creating rats in which one or more functional human genes have been introduced (arthritis (Hammer et al., 1990); gene therapy (Jaffe et al., 1992); lipoprotein metabolism (Swanson et al., 1992)). The trend in academia and industry is to establish research teams in which scientists with divergent fields of expertise collaborate in the production and analyses of such models using many different tools.

Genes of biological interest that may be evaluated using rat models can be classed into several categories. First, a gene and its product may have an endogenous and rat-specific function, but this normal rat expression may confound efforts to understand certain aspects of human biology. An example of such a gene is α_2-microglobulin, a hepatic protein which collects in rat (but not human) renal epithelium following exposures to certain rat-specific chemical carcinogens, but only in male rats of strains that express the gene (Dietrich and Swenberg, 1991). Gene targeting ('knockout') technology can be employed to investigate the nature of such rat genes by deleting the gene and examining the effects (if any) resulting from its absence. Second, genes and their products may be highly conserved across taxonomic groups so that characterization in rats will provide relevant data that can be extrapolated across many species. Many vertebrate genes have such properties, including growth hormone (Matsumoto et al., 1993), peripheral myelin protein 22 (Sereda et al., 1996) and renin (Mullins et al., 1990). Proteins derived from some conserved genes may exhibit biological activity in several species, while in other instances activity exists only in the species of origin (Ganten et al., 1992). Finally, genes may be inactivated or missing in rats but have an important function in another species. These latter two classes may be examined by transgenic technology through 'overexpression' of a foreign DNA fragment that has been incorporated into the rat genome.

Regardless of the ultimate application, genetically manipulated animals of any species are engineered and analyzed using comparable molecular techniques. A detailed technical consideration of these methods is beyond the scope of the current discussion. Therefore, we have chosen to focus on considerations that may affect the design, construction and interpretation of experiments in which genetically engineered rat models are employed. Where certain techniques have not yet been achieved in rats (e.g. 'knockouts'), we have extrapolated likely strategies from protocols used currently in mouse genetic engineering to provide background material for understanding their eventual application in rats.

The design of genetic engineering experiments in rats will benefit from thorough background information, which may be obtained from many sources. Genotypic (including data regarding the DNA sequence and/or the distribution and extent of gene expression at the mRNA and protein level) as well as phenotypic data (such as in vitro or in vivo functional assays) is determined within the home laboratory or is acquired through collaboration or from commercial sources. Additional information often may be located through citation databases (e.g. Medline [www.ncbi.nlm.nih.gov/PubMed/])[1] by searching with keywords relevant to the gene of interest. In our experience, categories of keywords for which citation data may exist include the common and abbreviated gene names, the gene or protein sequences, tissues in which the gene is expressed, and diseases (animal or human) in which the gene is postulated to have a role. Comparable searches performed on the Internet using a commercial

---

[1] For brevity the prefix 'http://' has been omitted from all Internet addresses (URLs) in the text. This prefix should be added when the URL is used to access the World Wide Web.

biology-based search engine (e.g. BioMedNet® [http://biomednet.com], Yahoo [www.yahoo.com/Science/Biology]) also may yield relevant information. However, in our experience random searches of the World Wide Web do not provide sufficient information to warrant their routine use. An exception would be participation in certain discussion groups (e.g. Embryo Mail [EmbryoMail@lpsi.bare.usda.gov]; Transgenic List [www.med.ic.ac.uk/db/dbbm/tglist.html]) that allow ongoing, real-time exchanges of text and pictorial data between researchers working with rats.

Bioinformatics melds data acquired from such diverse fields as biochemistry, experimental biology (animal, cellular and molecular), crystallography, and mathematics – to name a few – to find broad patterns within and among species that identify genes of interest. Specific branches of bioinformatic inquiry include **genomics** and **proteomics**, or the study of sequence and functional data for genes and proteins, respectively. While some questions in bioinformatics require formal training and very powerful (and expensive) computer platforms, a growing number of commercial software packages are available which can provide assistance to the general scientist. Examples of such applications include programs to compare a gene sequence with other gene sequences (e.g. BLAST and dbEST [both at www.ncbi.nlm.nih.gov]; GeneQuest® from DNASTAR, Madison, WI, USA); software to select molecular probes for genetic analyses (e.g. Oligo®, National Biosciences, Plymouth, MN, USA), and compilations describing protein structure and function (e.g. Swiss-PROT [www.genebio.com/sprot.html]). Large collections of molecular data representing the pooled efforts of many laboratories are increasingly available for comparison of gene and protein sequences both within a species (e.g. Rat Genetic Database [www.nih.gov/niams/scientific/ratgbase]; 'RatMap' Rat Genome Database [http:ratmap.gen.gu.se/]) and across several species (e.g. Whole Mouse Catalog [www.rodentia.com/wmc/] GenBank [www.ncbi.nlm.nih.gov/PubMed]; Mouse Genome Informatics [www.informatics.jax.org]; The Genome Database [www.gdb.org]). These resources provide cross-links to rat genetic data and provide an invaluable resource to researchers engaged in studies of the normal and genetically engineered rat genome. Finally, several databases are being compiled (chiefly for mice at present) that describe the traits of genetically engineered animals (e.g. Induced Mutant Resource Database [www.jax.org/ resources/documents/imr/]; Mouse Knock-Out and Mutation Database [http://biomednet.com/db/mkmd]; Transgenic and Targeted Mutation Database [www.jax.org/tbase]). As more genetically manipulated rat models are produced, we anticipate that relevant genetic and phenotypic data will be incorporated into these or comparable databases.

The Rat as a Species of Choice for Genetic Engineering

The mouse remains a preferred species for many transgenic applications. However, the rat is more suitable for many research questions. Desirable features of rat biology that would warrant their selection rather than a mouse model include more human-like physiological responses for some disease processes (e.g. arthritis (Greenwald and Diamond, 1988); cancer (Dycaico et al., 1994); hypertension (Paul et al., 1994; Charreau et al., 1996)), an extensive behavioral database, and larger size (better suited to surgical manipulation and repeated blood sampling; Gill et al., 1989). Even so, the relatively small size of rats removes many technical and financial drawbacks associated with breeding larger transgenic mammals, such as rabbits (Mullins and Mullins, 1996). Rats also share many useful traits with mice that are lacking in other laboratory animals of intermediate size (gerbil, guinea-pig, hamster, rabbit). These qualities include the availability of many normal and mutant strains, the presence of relatively homogeneous genetic backgrounds, and high fecundity (short gestation periods and good response to superovulation protocols; Robl and Heideman, 1994).

The successful production of transgenic rats was first described in the last decade (Hammer et al., 1990; Mullins et al., 1990). Since this time, new lines have been introduced rarely because few facilities routinely perform this technique in rats. Nevertheless, transgenic rat models provide essential mechanistic information that often assists in the biochemical dissection of human disease (e.g. chronic hypertension, autoimmune spondyloarthritides). In fact, rat models have often been proven to have a closer relationship to the human disease than do transgenic mice in which similar genetic material was inserted (reviewed in Charreau *et al.*, 1996). Genetic manipulation of rats will probably increase in the future where patent provisions for engineered animals (Lesser, 1995) promote such intellectually and economically profitable activities.

Several strains have been used successfully in the production of transgenic rats. Ideally, the use of genetically homogeneous inbred rat strains is preferable since variations in transgene expression or physiology arising from differences in genetic background can complicate the subsequent phenotypic analysis. Certain inbred strains, notably Fischer 344 (F-344) rats (Dycaico *et al.*, 1994; Veniant *et al.*, 1996; Lefevre *et al.*, 1997), have been used with success for genetic engineering. However, in practice most transgenic rats have been derived from outbred strains (e.g. Sprague-Dawley, Wistar) due to the ready availability of efficient superovulation protocols (Chapter 10; Mukumoto *et al.*, 1995) and the better reproductive performance of outbred rats (reviewed in Charreau *et al.*, 1996).

Genetic Manipulation of Rats

Equipment

A well-equipped molecular genetics facility contains dedicated laboratory areas for a variety of functions. The tasks to be performed in the production and analysis of genetically engineered rats will include recombinant DNA techniques (for generation of the transgene or targeting sequence as well as for analysis of the integration and expression of the inserted gene), cell culture, in-life and post-mortem assays of a transgene's effects on function and structure at the whole-animal and tissue levels, and photographic documentation. All instruments, reagents, and work areas for the molecular manipulations and cell culture activities must be separate from those used for in-life studies and post-mortem tissue processing. The specialized injection equipment used to transfer genetic material into single-celled (zygotes) or multicelled (blastocysts) embryos

(Figure 29.1) can be housed in any room with good lighting. However, for the practical purposes of proximity to the animal rooms and cleanliness, this equipment is often placed in a surgical suite located within the transgenic animal facility. Tissue harvests are typically performed in a room that is outside the barrier that protects the animal colonies. Deliberate physical isolation of these *in vitro* and *in vivo* activities — modeled after features of facilities designed to perform the sensitive DNA amplification technique, polymerase chain reaction

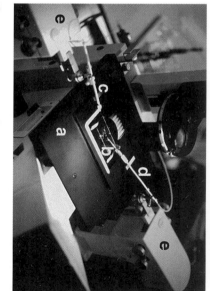
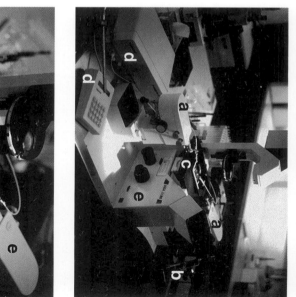

Figure 29.1 *Apparatus for pronuclear microinjection.* Introduction of transgenic DNA into rat zygotes (single-celled embryos) requires a suitable microscope (top panel) with servo-controlled pipettes for manipulating the cells (bottom panel). The layout of the injection station shown in panel A includes the micromanipulator controls for positioning the zygote (a), microliter pipette controls for introducing the DNA solution into a zygote (b), microscope stage (c), injector unit with keypad for controlling the delivery rate of the DNA solution (d), and microscope stage (e). In panel B, the microscope stage (a) supports a fluid-filled chamber (b) that contains suspended zygotes. The cells are immobilized with a holding pipette (c) and injected using a microinjection pipette (d). The placement of each pipette in three dimensions is controlled using the micromanipulator controls (e).

(Dieffenbach and Devksler, 1993) – will help to prevent spurious analytical results in molecular assays that result from contamination of samples with extraneous animal, microbial or recombinant DNA.

Transgenic Technology

Transgenic technology is the science (and art!) whereby foreign genetic material is introduced directly into the genome of an animal. In general, the procedures used to generate transgenic rats (Robl and Heidemann, 1994; Charreau et al., 1996) are comparable to those used in making transgenic mice (Hogan et al., 1994; Wassarman and DePamphilis, 1993). Two methods, pronuclear microinjection and systemic gene delivery, have been employed in the production of transgenic rat models.

Theory

Native rat genes contain alternating amino acid-encoding (exon) and noncoding (intron) regions controlled by various regulatory sequences (Figure 29.2). A typical transgene construct (Figure 29.3) consists of a gene's exons – often derived as a complimentary DNA (cDNA) sequence – flanked by a promoter (to control gene transcription) and a polyadenylation sequence (to enhance the stability of transgene messenger RNA). These three molecular elements need not be of rat origin, particularly where the structure and activity of the encoded protein products are conserved across species. Depending upon the nature of the scientific question, promoters are chosen based on their capacity to drive gene expression at high levels (Schmidt et al., 1990) or their ability to regulate gene expression in many tissues (e.g. actin; Qin and Gunning, 1997) or at specific sites (e.g. casein or lactalbumin in mammary gland; Hirabayashi et al., 1997).

During microinjection (see below), a few picoliters of solution containing about 100–200 copies of the transgene are introduced into a zygote (single-celled embryo, i.e. a fertilized ovum). Generally, integration of the transgenic DNA occurs randomly at a single site in the genome. Integration of the DNA may occur prior to DNA replication so that all cells of the rat, including the germline cells, will contain copies of the transgene. Alternatively, integration may occur after DNA replication is completed, resulting in the presence of the transgene in

some but not all of the rat's cells (yielding a mosaic pattern of gene expression). Because each integration site is different, the resulting genetic background of each founder rat is unique. Transgene copies often aggregate into repeating linear arrays known as **concatemers** (Brinster et al., 1985) either prior to injection of the foreign DNA or inside the rat pronucleus. Neither the number of copies in these concatemers nor their orientation during insertion can be controlled, and the number of copies often does not correlate with the degree of transgene expression. Instead, the extent of expression depends upon regulatory elements within the transgene construct; the location of transgene insertion (e.g. Clark et al., 1994) – particularly with respect to enhancer or repressor sequences in the genome (Blackwood and Kadonga, 1998; Ogbourne and Antalis, 1998); and the proper orientation of the open reading frame for transcription. Levels of expression will vary greatly between different lines that contain the same transgenic construct.

Additional factors have been described that may affect the presentation and complicate the analysis of phenotypes in transgenic rats. First, transgene integration into a critical locus of the genome can cause an insertional mutation that disrupts the normal function of one or more essential genes (e.g. Woychik et al., 1985). In such cases, the resulting effects of the induced mutation are superimposed on any changes associated with the expression of the transgene, and additional experiments will be required to fully separate the aspects of the genetic events. These unintended insertional mutations may have value as a guide to the genetic locus of an essential endogenous gene and, in some instances, as a novel model of a genetic disease. Insertional mutations are unique and occur in only a single animal line, while true transgenic phenotypes are comparable between all lines of transgenic mice established from different founders. Therefore, genesis of multiple lines derived from several different founder animals is a common research practice in order to confirm the presence of a true transgene-induced phenotype. Second, care must be given to controlling a variety of potential confounding conditions that may affect the severity of transgene-induced lesions. For example, the extent of arthritis and inflammatory bowel disease in rats transgenic for the human major histocompatibility complex antigen HLA-B27 is exacerbated by infection with intestinal or genitourinary tract bacteria but is ameliorated by preservation of a germ-free habitat

(a)

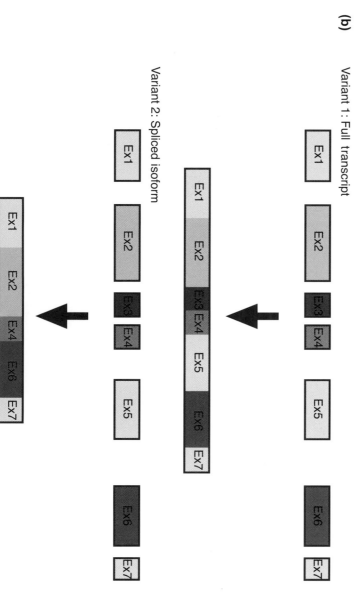

(b)

Variant 1: Full transcript

Variant 2: Spliced isoform

Figure 29.2 *Composition of a eukaryotic gene.* Mammalian genes often contain several regions including regulatory (R), promoter (P), signal (S), gene (G), and mRNA-stabilizing (A) sequences. Regulatory and promoter elements control gene transcription, the signal sequence indicates where transcription should be initiated, and the stabilizing sequence encodes the addition of a poly-adenosine (polyA) tail. (a) Most genes are divided into alternating amino acid-encoding regions: exon (Ex) sequences which are included in the mature RNA product, and intron (In) sequences that are transcribed but removed from the transcript as the exons are spliced together. (b) In some instances, alternative splicing during transcription of the exons yields different proteins. The lengths of the various genetic elements denote their relative number of nucleotides to indicate that not all exons are of the same size.

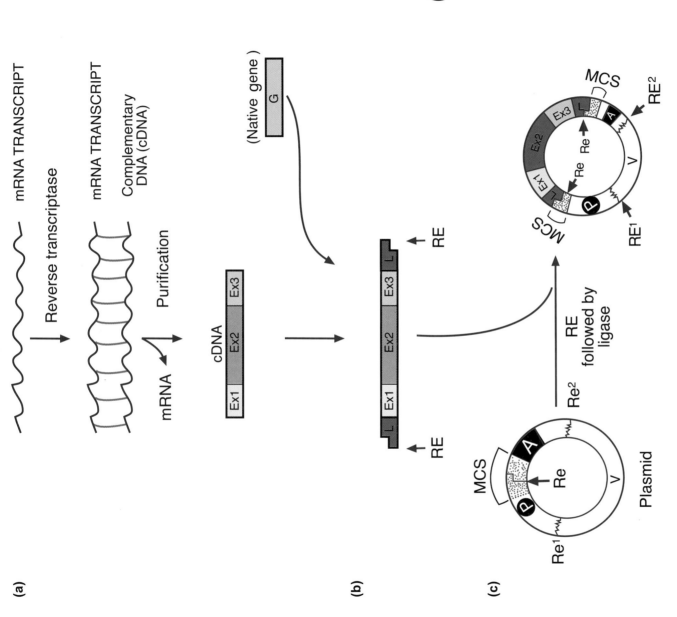

Figure 29.3 *Creating a transgenic construct.* (a) The DNA sequence of the gene of interest, or the complementary DNA (cDNA) representing the spliced exons (Ex) of the gene cloned from cellular mRNA, is the backbone on which the transgene is designed. In a series of steps, short sequences of linker nucleotides (L) containing sites for the action of a restriction enzyme (RE) are added to the ends of the DNA (b); different RE sites may be added to each end. When the DNA and the RE are mixed with a circular bacterial plasmid (the vector, V) containing a multiple cloning site (MCS; a region with cutting sites for several RE), the plasmid is cut and the DNA is inserted into the gap (c). Application of a ligase seals the DNA into the plasmid. Promoter (P) and mRNA stabilizing (A) sequences to direct the strength and location of transgene expression are added to (or already present in) the vector. The circular plasmid containing the transgene is introduced into bacteria to allow exponential amplification of the transgenic DNA. The bacteria are collected and treated with detergents to disrupt their membranes, and the plasmids are isolated by centrifugation. The plasmid is linearized using a different RE (d), and the vector (V) sequences are pruned with an additional RE to prevent possible deleterious effects of the vector sequences on expression of the transgene (e). The linearized construct is purified (f) prior to use.

(d)

(e)

(f)

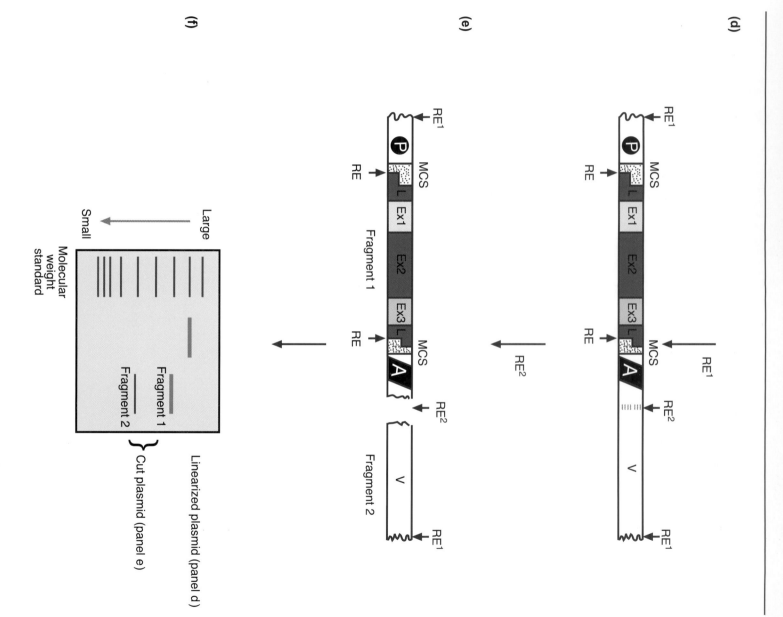

Linearized plasmid (panel d)

Cut plasmid (panel e)

(Taurog *et al.*, 1994). These confounding effects may require the investigation of apparent transgenic phenotypes under a variety of conditions.

Pronuclear microinjection

Most transgenic animals are created using pronuclear microinjection (Figure 29.4), a technique in which foreign DNA contained in a vector is injected into the pronucleus of a zygote isolated shortly after fertilization. The injected embryos are reimplanted in the oviduct of a recipient rat to yield potentially transgenic offspring (founders). For technical details of the superovulation and embryo transfer procedures in rats, see Chapter 10 or other reference materials (Pinkert, 1994).

(a) Embryo donation

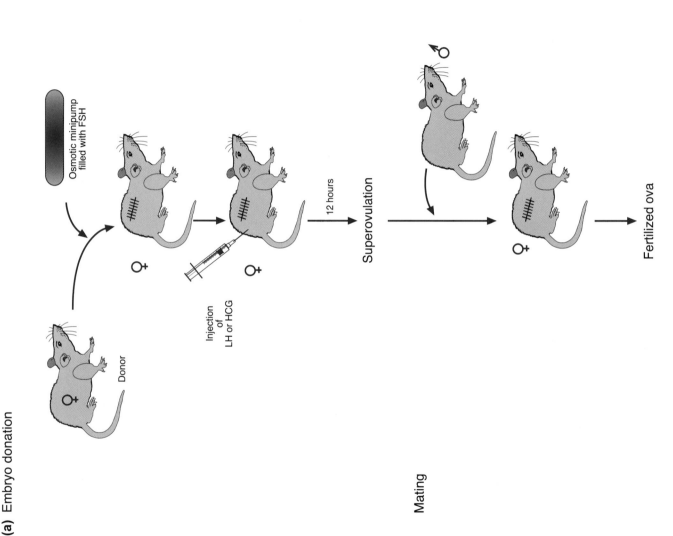

Figure 29.4 *Pronuclear microinjection technology.* The steps employed in microinjection protocols are superovulation, zygote isolation, microinjection, reimplantation and genotypic analysis of founders. First, embryo-donor females are treated with gonadotropic hormones to induce superovulation and then mated overnight with fertile males to produce fertilized ova (a). The oviducts are removed and flushed to gather the zygotes (single-celled embryos) (b). The outer cumulus layer is removed from each zygote by incubation in a protease solution (c). Zygotes with paired pronuclei are restrained with a holding pipette and then pierced with a microinjection pipette that contains the DNA solution (d). A few picoliters of DNA solution is introduced into one pronucleus, where one or more copies of the transgenic construct may be inserted at random into a break in the rat's genome. The embryos are reimplanted in the oviduct of a recipient female (e) to yield potentially transgenic offspring (founders). The genotype of each rat is determined by dissolving a tissue sample to isolate total genomic DNA, cutting the DNA with restriction enzymes, and then separating the DNA by electrophoresis (f). The probe detects a DNA sequence that is unique to the transgene. Once founder animals are established, PCR is often used to rapidly identify transgenic offspring.

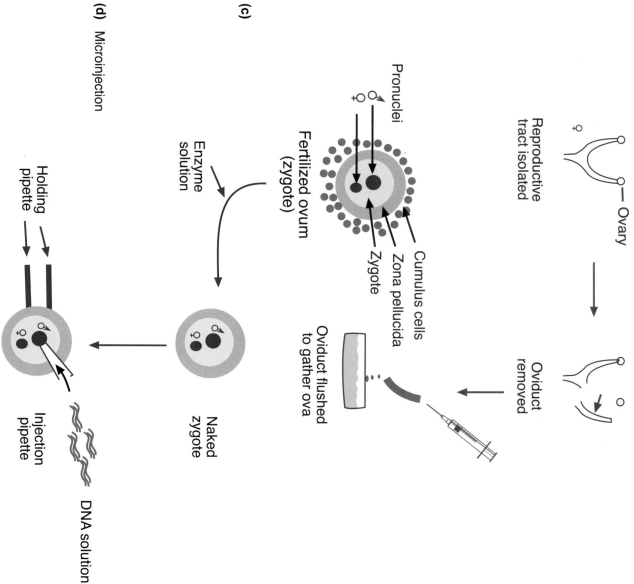

(b) Oocyte harvest

(c)

(d) Microinjection

Briefly, the sequential steps used in microinjection are superovulation, isolation of fertilized ova, micro-injection and reimplantation. First, large numbers of rat zygotes are obtained by timed administration of pituitary- or placenta-derived gonadotropic hormones to young adult, embryo-donor rats. Common inducing agents include mixtures of follicle-stimulating hormone (FSH) and luteinizing hormone (LH), human chorionic gonadotropin (HCG), and pregnant mare serum gonadotropin (PMSG; a single molecule with both FSH and LH activities). In rats, the usual protocol is continuous infusion of FSH (using a subcutaneously implanted minipump) followed by injection of LH or HCG (Chapter 10; James McCabe, personal communication). Ovulation will occur about 12 hours after the LH or HCG bolus. Treated donor females are mated overnight with fertile males to produce zygotes (fertilized ova). More zygotes per rat may be obtained if older animals (greater than 10 weeks of age) are used as donors (Mukumoto et al., 1995). In addition, the efficiency of fertile pairings may be increased by selecting female

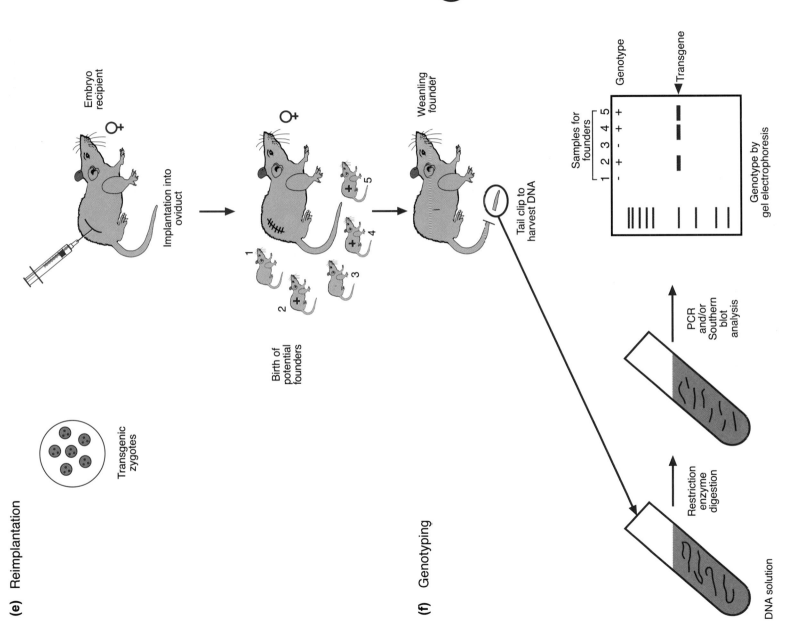

(e) Reimplantation

(f) Genotyping

rats in estrus based on the presence of cornified epithelial cells in vaginal swabs (Waynforth and Flecknell, 1992) or by measuring electrical conductivity from the vaginal mucosa using an impedance probe (e.g., Rat Estrus Cycle Monitor; Fine Science Tools, Foster City, CA, USA). Zygotes are gathered by flushing both oviducts (removed terminally under general anesthesia from copulation plug- or sperm-positive donor females) about 24 hours after the hormone injection. In outbred rats, typical superovulation protocols release from 20 to 80 ova per animal (Chapter 10; Robl and Heideman,

1994; Charreau et al., 1996). Enough donor females are treated (usually 8–12) so that batches of at least 200 ova are available for microinjection. Batch processing increases the efficiency of the laborious microinjection step.

Next, zygotes are prepared for microinjection. These steps are conducted in a sterile environment. Zygotes are incubated in a protease solution to remove the associated cumulus cell layer and are then washed in culture medium. Zygotes with paired pronuclei are selected for microinjection, restrained with a holding pipette and then pierced with a microinjection pipette that contains the DNA solution (Figures 29.4 and 29.5). The perforations will reseal themselves after the pipette is withdrawn. A good operator can inject 80–150 rat zygotes per hour. The proportion of rat zygotes that disintegrate soon after injection varies greatly between batches of ova, with ranges of between 10% and 50% reported for the Sprague-Dawley (SD) strain (Charreau et al., 1996).

After transgene injection, zygotes are reimplanted into the oviducts of female rats. Typically, females from outbred strains are chosen for their good maternal care and ready acceptance of cross-fostered pups. Embryo recipient females are often pseudopregnant animals obtained by mating with a vasectomized male (Chapter 10). As an alternative, pregnant females from a strain with pigmented hair (e.g. hooded rat) may be used as recipients for microinjected embryos from an albino strain (e.g. SD or F-344); at birth, the nontransgenic (colored) pups are culled (James McCabe, personal communication). Some investigators culture the microinjected zygotes overnight at 37°C to allow more accurate selection of viable (two-celled) embryos for reimplantation. Almost 80% of viable rat zygotes are reported to achieve the two-cell stage of embryonic development after this overnight incubation (Charreau et al., 1996). However, other workers have attained up to a three-fold higher rate of pregnancy when embryo transfer is completed immediately after microinjection (Charreau et al., 1996; James McCabe, personal communication).

Zygotes are reimplanted in batches of 20–25 into one oviduct of each pseudopregnant female, necessitating about 8–10 recipient females for each day of transfer. Again, some researchers (Charreau et al., 1996) describe a three-fold higher pregnancy rate for bilateral transfer procedures (using 10–12 zygotes per side), presumably because the embryos do not have to migrate from one uterine horn to the other. The transfer of uninjected ('carrier') zygotes along with microinjected ones, while a common practice in mice to ensure larger litter sizes and sustainable pregnancies, may result in large litters with fewer transgenic pups in rats (Canseco et al., 1994). The transfer of only microinjected zygotes routinely produces litters of normal size (e.g. 8–15 pups; Charreau et al., 1996).

The typical survival rate for microinjected rat zygotes in culture (as reviewed by Charreau et al., 1996) ranges between 30% and 40%, although higher rates of about 60% have been reported (Dycaico et al., 1994). This efficiency is about half of that (70–90%) reported for comparably derived mouse zygotes (Brinster et al., 1985; Taketo et al., 1991; Canseco et al., 1994). However, the proportion of microinjected rat zygotes that, upon return to a recipient rat's uterus, undergo implantation and yield live pups ranges between 15% and 30% for outbred donors and is about 4% in inbred strains (reviewed in Charreau et al., 1996). This outcome in rats is higher than the reimplantation efficiencies recorded for most inbred and outbred mice (5–8%; Brinster et al., 1985; Canseco et al., 1994) except for the favored FVB/N strain (23%; Taketo et al., 1991).

In special instances, in vitro fertilization and/or cryogenic storage may be used to continue or retain important rat lines (Chapter 10). The advantage of these two techniques is that the useful 'lifespan' of aging transgenic rats from poorly reproducing lines can be extended. This ability is particularly useful if the transgenic animal is male, due to the large number of ova that can be fertilized in vitro using sperm from a single individual. Typically the technique is employed only for critical lines because of the technical difficulties. Briefly, rats are treated with hormones to induce superovulation, and the unfertilized ova are collected. Ova are mixed with epididymal (mature) sperm and cultured for a variable length of time before being grouped in cryopreservation straws and frozen rapidly in liquid nitrogen. After thawing, fertilized ova are transferred into pseudopregnant recipient females. About 10% of the ova will yield living pups (Nakagata, 1993; Anzai et al., 1994). Another recent advance, intracytoplasmic injection of freeze-dried and water-reconstituted sperm nuclei (Wakayama and Yanagimachi, 1998), may provide a much less expensive means of retaining important lines as it avoids the need for liquid nitrogen and low-temperature storage facilities.

Any or all of these genetic engineering procedures may be obtained as services from commercial vendors of transgenic rats.

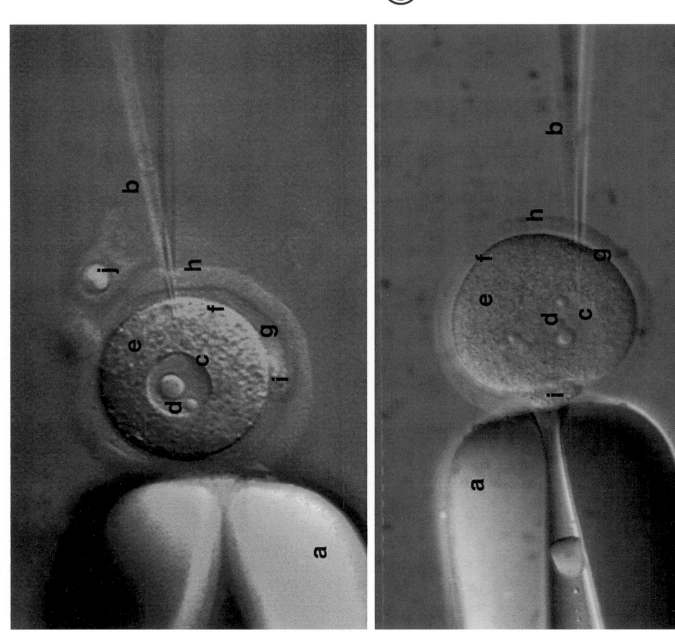

Figure 29.5 *Anatomy of rodent embryos during microinjection.* Zygotes (single-celled embryos) of the rat (upper panel) and mouse (lower panel) are immobilized by a holding pipette (a) while a microinjection pipette (b) is introduced into the large male pronucleus (c). The chief difference between the zygotes of these two species is that the rat cell has more flexible nuclear and plasma membranes, which renders penetration with the microinjection pipette more difficult. Nucleoli (d), cytoplasm (e), plasma membrane (f), perivitelline membrane (g), zona pellucida (h), polar body (i), and cumulus cells (j). Magnification, 490x.

Systemic gene delivery

The first genetically engineered animals were created by conveyance of transgenes using modified viral vectors. For this method, the vectors were engineered so that the host cells could not manufacture intact, infectious virus particles. The advantage of using viral vectors to deliver transgenes is that only a single transgene copy is integrated into the genome without the occurrence of transgene rearrangements or deletions that often arise during microinjection. The major disadvantage is that systemic gene delivery to multicelled organisms (adults or older embryos) typically does not lead to transgene integration in all cells, resulting in mosaic expression of the new gene. One of the most critical factors resulting from mosaic expression is the potential loss of a unique phenotype if the transgene is not transmitted to the germline cells of the transgenic animal. The lack of control over these essential factors is responsible for the shift to microinjection technology to produce transgenic animals in most facilities.

Nevertheless, systemic delivery systems may still have relevance in the exploration of those questions in which transgene expression in all cells is undesirable. For example, pronuclear microinjection with foreign DNA can induce a lethal phenotype in which the transgenic animal dies at some early stage of development, commonly before or shortly after birth. While such lethal events are interesting in and of themselves, the resulting inability to reproduce an adult disease model or establish a breeding colony may limit the utility of microinjection for such 'embryonic lethal' genes. In these cases, an alternative method is to introduce the transgene into the adult animal using a chemical (Simoes et al., 1998) or, more commonly, a viral vector (Robbins et al., 1998). In this manner, deleterious effects of the transgene to the developing embryo may be avoided. To our knowledge, this procedure has been reported only in mice (e.g. Sanes et al., 1986; Holzinger et al., 1995; Tsukui et al., 1996; Baldwin et al., 1997); however, implementation in the rat is feasible. Viral vector technology is described in more detail below in the section on Gene therapy.

Special methods in transgenic research

Modifications in the design of transgenic constructs have engendered several innovative ways to produce new and more finely controlled transgenic models.

While many of these techniques have been validated in mice, there is no theoretical barrier to their use in rats.

One exciting approach is the advent of conditional gene expression in transgenics (Figure 29.6). This tool regulates the onset of expression, providing another means of avoiding the adverse effects associated with constitutive transgene overexpression during early development. In addition to the usual elements (promoter, transgene, polyadenylation sequence), the construct for a conditional transgene includes a ligand-inducible control system (Kühn et al., 1995; Fishman, 1995). In this manner, gene expression will be essentially absent until activated by either the introduction (Passman and Fishman, 1994; Wang et al., 1997) or withdrawal (Gossen et al., 1995; Kistner et al., 1996) of an exogenous ligand. For example, in one system, the metallothionein (MT) promoter directs basal expression of certain endogenous genes at low levels in many tissues. If the MT promoter is joined to a transgene, addition of heavy metals to the animal's diet induces the MT promoter and drives an increase in hepatic expression of the transgene of up to 100-fold (Palmiter et al., 1983).

The main characteristics of an ideal conditional transgenic system would be low basal (no 'leakiness') and high peak activities, rapid induction upon administration of the ligand, and a single control protein (i.e. a simple signal transduction pathway). Some conditional gene expression systems require the engineering of two lines of transgenic animals: one carrying the gene of interest under the control of an inducible promoter and another expressing a -acting control protein (Byrne and Ruddles, 1989; Gardner et al., 1996). Mating of the two lines results in progeny that contain both constructs, allowing the -acting control protein to act as the inducing ligand for the promoter that controls the transgene of interest. An alternative is to create double transgenic animals in which both the transgene and control protein have been introduced in the same construct (Schultze et al., 1996). The best conditional gene expression systems have been engineered using nonmammalian control elements (e.g. Gossen et al., 1993) since promoters of mammalian origin (e.g. MT) can react in a physiological manner and, therefore, are both leaky and subject to endogenous regulatory systems (Yarranton, 1992; Fishman, 1995). Ligands that have been validated in transgenic mice produced by microinjection include tetracycline (Furth et al., 1994; Kistner et al., 1996; Schultze et al., 1996), the insect hormone

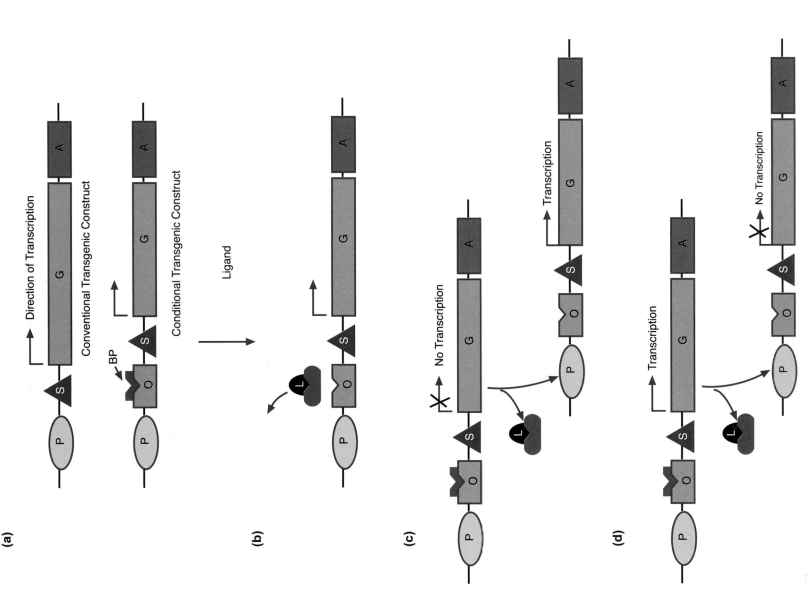

Figure 29.6 *Conditional gene expression.* Transgene expression may be controlled by the timed administration of an exogenous ligand. (a) In addition to the conventional elements in a transgenic construct (Figure 29.3), a conditional transgene includes an operator (O; a regulatory domain) with which the ligand-binding protein (BP) may interact. (b) Presence of the ligand (L) results in a conformational change in the ligand-binding protein, resulting in dissociation of the protein from the transgene. (c, d) Removal of this protein results in either initiation or cessation of the transgene's transcription. Notations for gene nomenclature are identical to those provided for Figure 29.2.

ecdysone (No et al., 1996), and the progesterone analog mifepristone (RU486; Wang et al., 1997). Conditional transgenic rats have been reported in which expression of marker genes injected directly into a specific organ of an adult was regulated using systemic administration of mifepristone (Oligino et al., 1998) or tetracycline (Fishman et al., 1994). To our knowledge, conditional transgenic rats have yet to be created by introduction of genetic material into embryos.

Another interesting possibility is the production of animals in which functional deficiencies have been imposed through the reduction of an endogenous gene's activity. Three methods have been described. First, the transgene product may act as a 'dominant negative' element with respect to the endogenous protein. In other words, the introduction of a single transgene allele can regulate a strong ('negative') function that reduces or cancels the normal ("positive') activity of an endogenous protein. An alternative possibility is that the transgene product binds and inactivates an endogenous protein. This latter paradigm has been employed in vitro and in vivo by the expression of transgenes that encode single-chain antibodies (scFv; Beerli et al., 1994; Deshane et al., 1997). Such transgenes are designed so that the protein product consists of the antigen-binding variable portion (Fv) of an antibody, directed against an intracellular antigen, but lacks a secretory tag. Expression of the scFv transgene results in manufacture and cytoplasmic retention of the scFv protein, leading to binding and inactivation of the antigen. Finally, a genetic ablation technique may be used to eliminate specific cell types by introducing a transgene that encodes a cytotoxic protein under the control of a tissue-specific promoter (Palmiter et al., 1987; Borrelli et al., 1988; Mintz and Klein-Szanto, 1992). Thus, all three schemes may yield functional phenotypes with features similar to those resulting from genotypic 'knockouts' produced by gene targeting. The main advantages of these three approaches are that this transgenic technology is usually simpler, less expensive, and more rapid than gene targeting.

Gene Targeting

A breakthrough approach in the manipulation of the mammalian genome was the isolation and culture of mouse embryonic stem (ES) cells, each of which is capable of contributing to the formation of all adult tissues. These cells were derived initially from the inner cell mass (representing the nascent embryo) of preimplantation blastocysts (Evans and Kaufman, 1981; Martin, 1981; Bronson and Smithies, 1994). At present, reliable ES cell lines have been obtained from only a few mouse strains. Development studies with ES cell cultures soon expanded to include successful germline transmission of genetic mutations introduced into mice by incorporation of recombinant DNA into cultured ES cells followed by introduction of the modified ES cells into the inner cell mass of blastocysts (Bradley et al., 1984; Gossler et al., 1986; Robertson et al., 1986). While mouse ES cells injected into rat morulae also yield viable interspecific chimeric finders, pluripotent rat ES cells have yet to be isolated (Iannaconne et al., 1994, with published erratum, 1997).

Recently, precise manipulation of the mouse genome has been accomplished through the gene targeting approach (Figure 29.7). Recent progress in rat ES cell biology (Charreau et al., 1996; Takahama et al., 1998) as well as the many similarities between mouse and rat reproduction suggest that gene targeting in rats will become feasible in the near future. Therefore, we believe that a discussion of this technology is appropriate here. First, recombinant DNA methods are used to alter the cloned sequence of a selected chromosome locus. This gene alteration is then transmitted into the genome of the ES cells through the process of homologous recombination (Smithies et al., 1985; Doetschman et al., 1987; Thomas and Capecchi, 1987; for reviews, see Capecchi, 1989, or Koller and Smithies, 1992). During homologous recombination (Figure 29.7), the introduced DNA will pair with the locus of endogenous DNA that possesses the complimentary nucleotide sequence. When the ends of the regions of nucleotide homology are cut, the DNA pieces are exchanged, and the transgene is incorporated into the genome (Folger et al., 1982). Thus, the engineered gene is switched with the endogenous copy and is automatically integrated at the specific and proper location in the genome. The orientation of the homologous regions in vector and chromosomal DNA will determine whether the engineered gene replaces the endogenous one or whether the entire vector is inserted into the genome (Hasty and Bradley, 1993).

The properties of the engineered gene determine what its functional significance to the animal might be. For example, one common scenario is to disrupt the normal coding sequence of the gene, thereby disturbing normal gene expression and creating a null mutation (i.e. a 'knockout'). A second paradigm

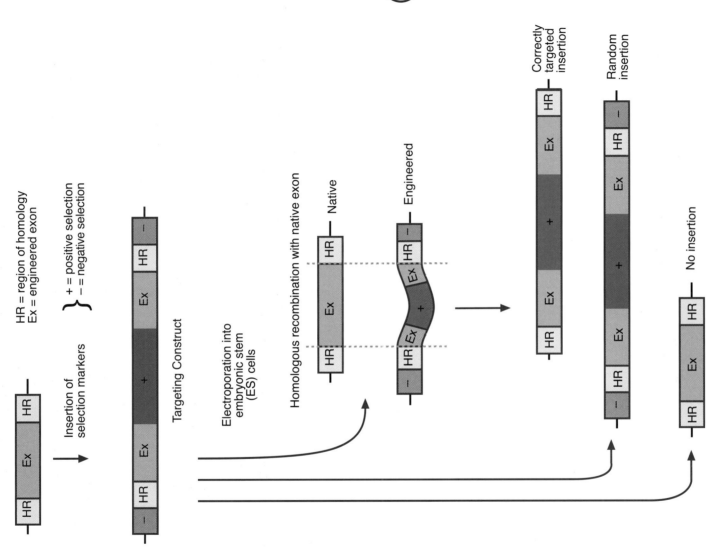

Figure 29.7 *Gene targeting technology.* The steps involved in targeting an endogenous gene with an engineered gene include design of the construct, selection of viable stem cell clones, injection of blastocysts, and reimplantation. (a) Commonly, the targeting construct consists of a plasmid containing the engineered gene linked to one or more additional genes that encode for xenobiotic selection markers. After amplification in culture, linearized plasmids are introduced into the embryonic stem (ES) cells. (b) The complimentary sequences of the endogenous gene and the plasmid-borne engineered gene align and are exchanged by homologous recombination. The ES cells are tested for the proper introduction of the engineered gene by addition of selection agents.

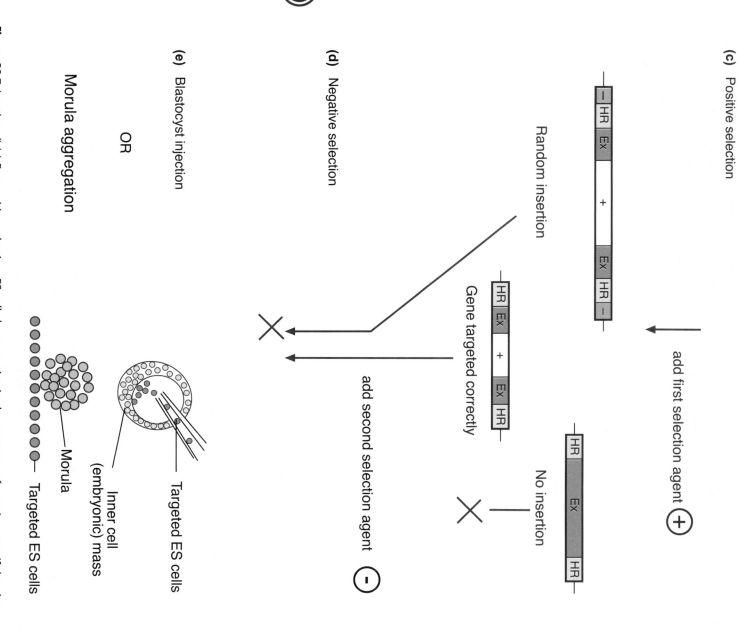

(c) Positive selection

Random insertion

Gene targeted correctly

No insertion

add first selection agent ⊕

add second selection agent ⊖

(d) Negative selection

(e) Blastocyst injection

OR

Morula aggregation

Targeted ES cells

Inner cell (embryonic) mass

Morula

Targeted ES cells

Figure 29.7 (continued) (c) For positive selection, ES cell clones survive in the presence of a toxic agent if they have incorporated correctly a targeting construct that includes an appropriate and functional copy of the toxin resistance gene. (d) Negative selection chooses ES cell clones with the appropriate integration of the targeting vector based on the loss of a toxin sensitivity gene and resistance of the ES cells to a toxic agent. When integration of the targeting vector occurs outside the region of homology, the sensitivity gene is retained, allowing the ES cells to die. (e) Cells from clones with the correctly targeted gene are expanded and then injected into the inner cell mass of a blastocyst or aggregated into a morula. The embryos are reimplanted in the oviduct of a recipient female. The resulting progeny are chimeric to variable degrees, depending upon the contribution of the ES cells to embryonic development. Note: In mice, the ES cells, the blastocyst or aggregation cells, and the recipient female are all derived from mouse lines with different coat colors, allowing for selection of chimeric progeny with the highest amounts of the targeted gene based on the greatest degree of coat color consistent with that of the animals from which the ES cells were established.

is to modify the targeting sequence into a constitutively activated form and insert it in place of the endogenous gene (a 'knockin'; Hanks et al., 1995). A loss or gain of gene function may result in functional or structural deficits of varying degrees. Alternatively, the introduced mutation may have no apparent effect, suggesting that proteins derived from endogenous genes are compensating for the engineered DNA defect.

An engineered gene is added to a bacterial plasmid to produce the targeting vector (Hasty and Bradley, 1993) (Figure 29.7). The targeting construct is introduced into ES cells by using chemicals or electrical current (electroporation) to create transient pores in the cellular membranes. The efficiency of gene entry is low, and only a few of the cells which pick up the vector will actually undergo homologous recombination to replace the targeted endogenous gene with the engineered DNA in an appropriate orientation. The majority of the targeting constructs insert randomly within the genome, or do not integrate at all. Therefore, to identify ES cells that contain the properly targeted gene, many targeting protocols include positive and/or negative selection steps (Wurst and Joyner, 1993). A positive selection (Figure 29.7) identifies ES cells that have incorporated a drug-resistance gene that was retained by being designed internal to the regions of homology on the targeting vector. Culture of the targeted ES cells in the presence of the drug results in death of all ES cells in which the proper genetic recombination did not occur. In contrast, negative selection (Figure 29.7) is carried out by incorporating a drug-sensitivity gene external to the regions of homology such that correct integration of the targeting vector results in loss of the sensitivity gene and resistance of the ES cells to the selection agent. Individual cells are cultured, and colonies are screened for proper orientation and integrity of the targeted mutant gene. Once correctly targeted ES cells are identified, they are expanded into large cultures, isolated by trypsinization, and added to cells of the inner cell mass of the preimplantation blastocyst by microinjection or coaggregation (Wood et al., 1993). At birth, the tissues of the progeny will be chimeras derived from both endogenous and engineered ES cells; extensive characterization then is required to select founders in which the engineered gene is transmitted through the germ line (i.e. in which the gene-targeted ES cells contributed to gonadal development) (Papaioannou and Johnson, 1993). However, a recent technical modification is the

production of animals (mice) in which the embryonic component is formed entirely by gene-targeted ES cells (www.mshri.on.ca/nagy/Tetraploid/Tetra.htm). This technique will greatly reduce the time required to obtain a gene-targeted line. In addition, the ability to intermingle embryonic and extraembryonic (placental) components between wild-type and gene-targeted embryos will aid greatly in differentiating between embryonic and placental mechanisms by which targeted genes may lead to embryonic lethality (Rossant et al., 1998).

Thorough screening of all ES cell cultures avoids the high labor, monetary and time costs associated with use of incorrectly targeted genes. In addition, ES cells should be surveyed for microorganisms to prevent introduction of pathogens into the breeding colony. In our experience, fewer than 3% of ES clones contain the engineered gene both in the correct orientation and with intact sequence. In mice, about 30% of injected embryos contain tissues that are derived from ES cells, and an even smaller fraction of these chimeric founders contain the engineered gene in their germ cells.

Special methods in gene targeting research

Two additional means of producing gene-targeted animals have been developed in recent years for use in research questions in which gene inactivation must be limited to selected times or tissues. The first procedure, administration of **antisense oligonucleotides,** is simple, relatively inexpensive, and can be used in rats at this time. In this method, large numbers of oligonucleotides are administered by intravenous injection (intra-amniotic microinjection for embryos; Chen and Hales, 1995). These agents are taken into cells, where they bind to mRNA molecules with complementary (sense) sequences. These duplexes are stable, so the protein cannot be made and the gene is effectively inactivated. However, the disadvantages of this technique include the variable extent of cellular uptake and the leakiness of the system resulting from incomplete mRNA binding.

An alternative protocol is the use of site-specific recombinases, including the Cre/loxP gene targeting strategy (Figure 29.8). The Cre recombinase, first identified in the bacteriophage P1, is a protein which excises any DNA sequence located between two loxP sites (a 34-bp (base pair) nucleotide sequence that has not been found in vertebrate

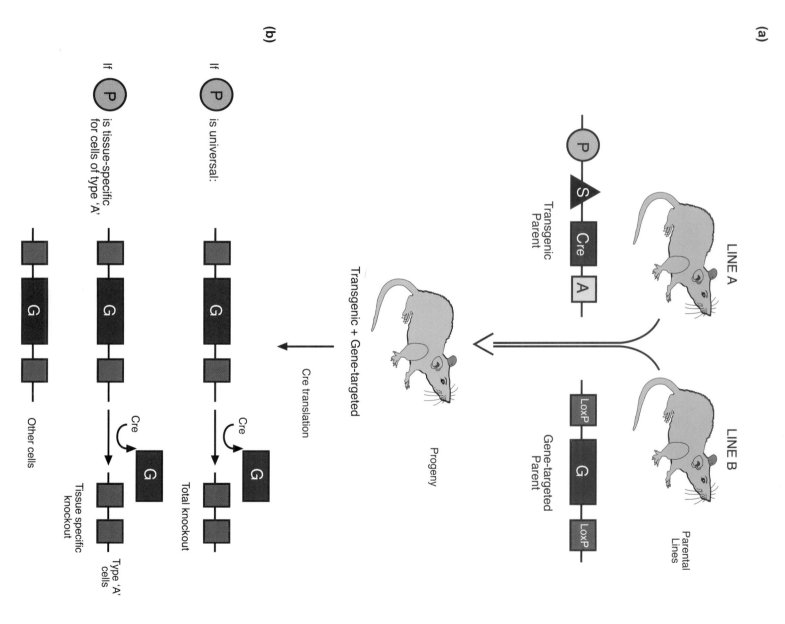

Figure 29.8 *Site-specific recombination: an alternative gene targeting strategy.* Microbial recombinase enzymes mediate the excision of genetic material located between adjacent loci of certain novel nucleotide sequences. This paradigm requires the creation of two genetically altered animal lines (a): a transgenic line incorporating a recombinase gene (e.g. the Cre protein) and a gene-targeted line in which the targeting construct contains a functional form of the endogenous gene of interest flanked by two recombinase recognition sites (e.g. the *loxP* locus, a unique 34-bp sequence recognized by Cre). The two parent lines of animals are normal, but crossing them results in progeny in which the *loxP*-flanked gene has been excised in cells that express the transgenic Cre protein (b).

genomes) (Sauer, 1993; Marth, 1996; Akagi et al., 1997). This paradigm requires the creation of two genetically altered animal lines: a gene-targeted line in which the engineered construct contains a functional form of the gene of interest flanked by two loxP sites (Gu et al., 1994; Kühn et al., 1995), and a second transgenic line incorporating the Cre gene under the control of a suitable promoter. The two parent lines of animals are normal, but crossing them results in progeny in which the loxP-flanked gene has been excised in cells that express the transgenic Cre protein. Gene inactivation can be limited to a single tissue by placing the Cre transgene under the control of a tissue-specific promoter (Orban et al., 1992; Gu et al., 1994; Rajewsky et al., 1996; Rohlmann et al., 1996; Tsien et al., 1996). In addition, Cre activity can be regulated by using a ligand-dependent conditional gene expression system to control Cre expression (Metzger et al., 1995). The novel yeast-derived Flp recombinase system has been employed in a comparable fashion (Dymecki, 1996). The recombinase approach should prove to be especially useful for studying the loss of developmentally essential genes in specific tissues of adult animals, particularly where a global gene knockout approach would result in embryonic lethality (Copp, 1995).

Gene Therapy

We have discussed above the production of transgenic rats by administration of foreign genetic material in a viral vector. While this method has been used successfully to engineer rat models in order to answer basic research questions, an even more important consideration may be the preclinical application of such technology in rats to assess risk-to-benefit ratios for potential human gene therapies, including such uses as tissue-specific transfer of a gene to replace a defective protein (perhaps to cure a lysosomal storage disease) or to deliver a therapeutic agent (such as a cytotoxic protein to kill cancer cells). Chemical (Simoes et al., 1998) and viral (Robbins et al., 1998) vehicles are now being tested as therapeutic paradigms in many acquired and inherited human diseases. Potential rate-limiting steps in achieving successful gene transfer are the low efficiency of gene integration into the patient's genome in the proper target tissue and the short duration of activity that may result as the body's defense system degrades the transgene or the

protein product. Such issues may be addressed using rat models of gene therapy.

Two basic approaches are used for gene therapy experiments. In the ex vivo method, host cells are removed from the animal, transfected while being cultured, and then reinserted into the same animal. The alternative in vivo technique requires the parenteral delivery of the genetic material, usually by intravenous (for systemic exposure) or targeted intravenous (for systemic exposure) or targeted (for local action) injection, or by inhalation (for airway expression). Delivery may be made to the entire adult (Jaffe et al., 1992), to a specific region (La Salle et al., 1993), or to the conceptus (Baldwin et al., 1997). In general, genes are delivered in viral vectors or in nonviral constructs; the latter systems may include the passive carriage of unmodified DNA (e.g. liposomes) or may involve the covalent modification of the transgene (e.g. chemical conjugates). The ideal system for gene therapy will yield efficient gene delivery, minimal pathogenicity (particularly immunogenicity), and stable and permanent integration of the transgene into the desired target tissue(s) and cells. Typically, viral vectors provide more effective gene incorporation but have greater liabilities with respect to immunogenicity and their innate pathogenicity toward the host. While several viral vectors are used commonly in animal studies and in human clinical trials, the most common are adenoviruses (with linear double-stranded DNA genomes) and retroviruses (with linear single-stranded RNA genomes).

Regardless of the viral type, certain aspects of gene therapy technology are universal. First, one or more viral genes are deleted (often by replacing them with the transgene DNA). Ideally, these truncated viral genomes can neither initiate viral reproduction in host cells (yielding a 'replication-defective' or 'replication-incompetent' vector) nor direct the production of viral proteins (thereby reducing its immunogenicity). However, compromises between the efficiency of gene transfer and the degree of viral pathogenicity must be balanced against the experimental question. For example, advantages of adenoviral vectors include their ability to infect many different cells (including nondividing ones), their high expression level in the host animal, and their high titer. However, the primary disadvantage is the transient expression of the transgene, which may result from two factors. One reason is the episomal (away from the chromosome) location of the transfected material, resulting in presence of the transgene for a short period in the cytoplasm rather than permanent integration in the animal's genome. The second factor is the host's immune response against cells that express these viral proteins. In contrast, retroviral vectors are inserted permanently into the genome without expressing any immunogenic proteins. Nevertheless, stable infection with retroviral-borne transgenes occurs only in dividing cells, and levels of the transgene product may be low. Rats are important animal models for the preclinical biology and toxicology phases of gene therapy trials, although mice may be preferable for some applications since their smaller body size would allow for use of smaller amounts of the vector.

Cytogenetics

Cytogenetic technology has made large contributions to understanding the physical structure of the rat (and human) normal genome as well as in characterizing the genetic alterations that occur in certain diseases, most notably neoplasia (Kerler and Rabes, 1994). Karyotypic analysis (Figure 29.9), the assessment of chromosome structure, has been used for years to define gross abnormalities such as nondisjunctions and translocations (Mitelman, 1983; Ichikawa et al., 1990; Montaudon et al., 1990). This evaluation is made on metaphase chromosomes (termed 'spreads') that have been obtained by treatment of cells with colchicine (to arrest mitosis) and hypotonic chemical solutions (to rupture the cell and nuclear membranes, thereby releasing the condensed chromosomes).

Dye banding techniques (e.g. Giemsa or acridine orange) have revealed fine defects in chromosomal structure by demonstrating alterations in the location or width of various bands associated with more subtle genetic defects (Kerler and Rabes, 1994; Sargent et al., 1996). Several standard dye-specific banding patterns have been described for the 21 pairs of rat chromosomes (Levan, 1974; Ronne et al., 1987; Satoh et al., 1989). These older, powerful methods of purely physical chromosomal analysis have been significantly enhanced by the recent advent of molecular techniques (e.g. fluorescent in situ hybridization (FISH), which assess the location of a specific DNA sequence (i.e. for a gene of interest) in conjunction with its chromosomal address. For example, FISH analysis performed with probes for at least two single-copy genes can determine the chromosomal location as well as the genetic distance between genes in metaphase spreads, in interphase (intact) nuclei, and in stretched DNA (Trask et al., 1989). The resolution of chromosome mapping ranges from approximately 3 megabases (Mb) in metaphase spreads to about 100kb in interphase nuclei, depending on the local chromatin structure (Lichter et al., 1990). Molecular techniques even allow site-specific engineering of chromosomes to assess the impact of gene heterozygosity and chromosomal abnormalities in animals (Ramirez-Solis et al., 1995).

Recently, the application of fluorescent cytogenetics technology has been extended from the mapping of single-copy genes with FISH to scans of the entire genome either by comparative genomic hybridization (CGH) or spectral karyotyping (Chang and Mark, 1997). In CGH (Parra and Windle, 1993), a global analysis of recurrent chromosomal defects (gains or losses of genetic material) is performed, usually by competitive hybridization of probes between differentially labeled normal (e.g. a green fluorochrome) and tumor-derived (e.g. red fluorochrome) DNA. The labeled probes are hybridized to metaphase spreads, and a comparison of the intensities of green and red fluorescence along the chromosomes reflects the relative abundance of normal gene sequences in the tumor. Regions of the DNA that are overexpressed in the tumor are seen as regions of high red intensity on the target chromosome. The difference can be quantified by digital imaging analysis, with current software (available for the rat, mouse and human) capable of detecting a change of 10Mb (Kallioniemi et al., 1992). DNA from formalin-fixed, paraffin-embedded archival tissues may be assessed by CGH. For example, a small locus can be dissected from the tissue block or a single section (Simone et al., 1998), and the DNA can then be amplified to examine genetic changes within a defined tissue or cell population (Speicher et al., 1996). The microdissection approach is a particularly useful method for examining the early, subclinical stages of chronic diseases such as neoplasia.

Spectral karyotyping (SKY) surveys all chromosomes in a cell population simultaneously for many major rearrangement events, a screen not possible with other cytogenetic techniques. All chromosomes are labeled with oligonucleotide probes that have been conjugated to different fluorochromes (Telenius et al., 1992; Liyanage et al., 1996); for example, all 23 human chromosomes can be uniquely labeled using a combination of only five fluorochromes. To date, this method has

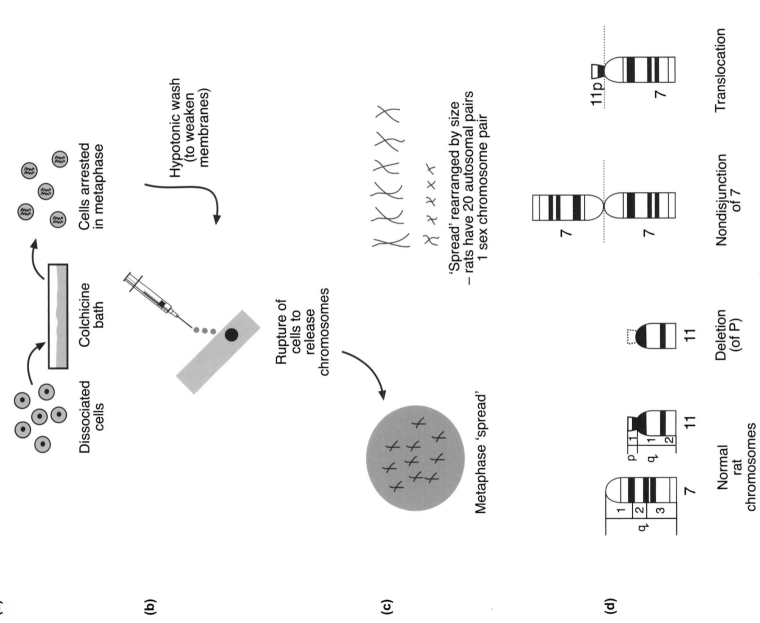

Figure 29.9 *Cytogenetic technology: karyotypic analysis.* Certain gross alterations in genomic DNA can be assessed by examining the structure of metaphase (condensed) chromosomes. (a) Dissociated cells are treated with colchicine to arrest mitosis at the metaphase stage. (b,c) Cells then are washed in hypotonic solutions to weaken the cellular membranes, and drops of the suspension are expelled onto glass slides to physically break the cells and release the condensed chromosomes. The chromosomes are stained and examined microscopically for major defects (d), such as deletions or nondisjunctions or translocations, as well as minor changes in the banding pattern (e). (f) These physical methods can be supplemented with fluorescent *in situ* hybridization (FISH), a molecular technique in which the chromosomal location of a specific DNA sequence can be determined by the use of an oligonucleotide probe conjugated to a fluorochrome. Banding pattern adapted from Kerler and Rabes (1994).

(e)

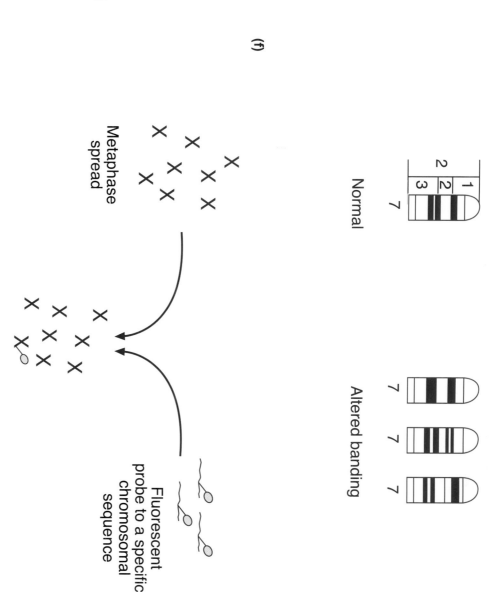

(f)

Normal

Altered banding

Metaphase spread

Fluorescent probe to a specific chromosomal sequence

been performed only for human and mouse cells, but further work with genetically engineered rats will likely result in the adaptation of this technology for use in this species.

Cloning

The ready availability of large numbers of genetically identical rats would facilitate research by greatly reducing the variation in physiological response that exists between subjects with different genetic backgrounds. In the past, the production of highly inbred rat strains removed much, but not all, of the genetic heterogeneity between individual animals (Chapter 1). Recently, cloning methods that allow the generation of genetically identical individuals have proven feasible in mammals (Campbell et al.,

1996; Wilmut et al., 1997; Wakayama et al., 1998). A cloned embryo is constructed by introduction of an intact diploid nucleus (in the quiescent (G0) stage of the cell cycle) into an enucleated oocyte (Figure 29.10). The isolated nucleus is joined to the oocyte either by electric fusion (Wilmut et al., 1997) or microinjection (Wakayama et al., 1998), and the genome is activated (to allow re-entry into the cell cycle) by electric pulses (Wilmut et al., 1997) or chemical media (Bos-Mikich et al., 1997). The cloned embryos are then implanted into the oviducts of recipient females. Primary cultures of embryonic, fetal or adult somatic cells have all been proven to work as sources for donor nuclei (Campbell et al., 1996; Wilmut et al., 1997), indicating that both partially and terminally differentiated genomes are capable of supporting the entire spectrum of development processes. In addition, adult cells have

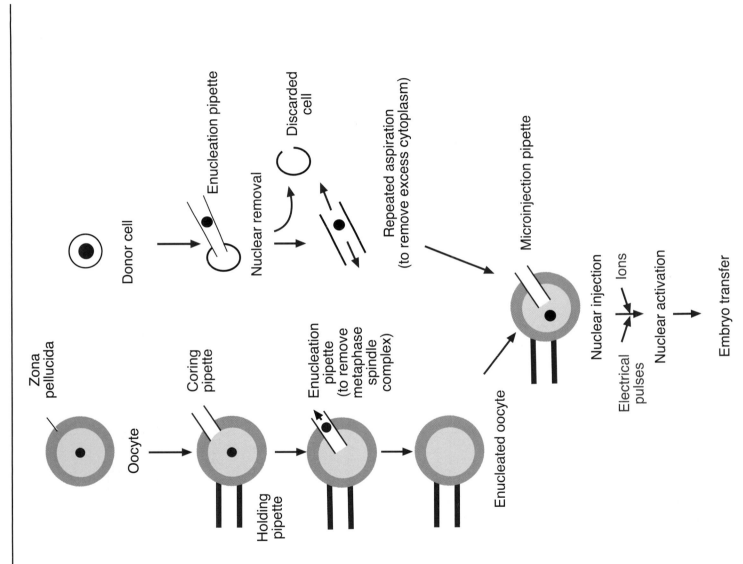

Figure 29.10 *Cloning.* A cloned embryo is constructed by introduction of an intact diploid nucleus (in the quiescent (G_0) stage of the cell cycle) into an enucleated oocyte. The isolated nucleus is joined to the oocyte by either electric fusion or microinjection, and the genome is activated (to allow re-entry into the cell cycle) by electric pulses or chemical media. The cloned embryos then are implanted into the oviducts of recipient females. Primary cultures of embryonic, fetal or adult somatic cells all have been proven to work as sources for donor nuclei. Adapted from Wakayama *et al.* (1998).

been shown to work without a passage in culture (Wakayama *et al*, 1998). Cloning of rats has not yet been reported. However, the recently described 'Honolulu technique' (Wakayama *et al*, 1998) has

been used to clone several generations of identical female mice at a relatively high efficiency (2–3% survival to term of implanted embryos). We believe that rat cloning will be described in the near future.

Genotypic Analysis of Engineered Rats – Detection of Gene Insertion

Techniques used to produce and characterize genetically engineered rats require a considerable degree of technical expertise. Fortunately, the widespread acceptance of these molecular procedures has resulted in the collection of many 'recipes' into manageable volumes of material (e.g. Sambrook et al., 1989; Brown, 1991; Ausubel et al., 1998).

The presence of foreign DNA in a genetically engineered animal may be checked in both qualitative and quantifiable manners using one or more molecular assays. Briefly, cells are harvested from the rat. Commonly, the tail tips of weanlings are removed for this purpose at the same time that the mice are given individual identification marks (by a coded sequence of clipped toes and/or ear punches, a metal ear tag, or an implanted microchip). However, tail clips or ear punch remnants may be taken at an earlier age, or oral washes may be gathered from neonates (Irwin et al., 1996), in order to expedite the genotyping process. The tissue specimens are dissolved in a buffered enzyme solution to release the total genomic DNA (with incorporated transgene). Next, DNA is purified using either a series of solvent extractions or by chromatographic separation. In many laboratories, each rat's genotype is checked first using the polymerase chain reaction (PCR). The exponential amplification offered by this technique can quickly differentiate between transgene-positive and non-transgenic animals. Typically, selecting several oligonucleotide primers that span both ends of the transgene increases the power of PCR. In this fashion, transcripts from transgenic and wild-type rats can be differentiated readily by sizing their distinct band migration patterns on an agarose gel. However, nonspecific annealing of oligonucleotide probes to DNA sites distant from the transgene may lead to false positive readings. For this reason, most laboratories confirm the PCR data by Southern analysis, in which unamplified DNA is separated on a gel. The omission of the enzymatic amplification step in this latter procedure prevents most erroneous results, but the trade-off is that the small quantity of unamplified transgenic DNA in the tissue sample may be difficult to detect. Interpretation of such faint bands is aided significantly by the use of restriction enzymes (specific for sites within the transgene). Digestion of transgenic and wild-type DNA strands results in restriction fragments of differing lengths, allowing detection of the two bands by their distinct gel migration patterns. Additional data obtained from the Southern blot are (1) confirmation that the founder rats have acquired the full-length transgene sequence without undergoing gene rearrangements or deletions, (2) information regarding the number of sites at which the transgene has been integrated, and (3) an estimate of the number of transgene copies that have been incorporated into the rat's genome. The multiplicity of integration sites is addressed by comparing the inherited bands of the founder with its progeny, and the bands of the offspring to possess the same integration site if the DNA bands resulting from restriction enzyme mapping of the transgenic DNA are identical.

An assessment of transgene copy number is performed by comparing the signal strength of the transgenic bands with a control lane containing a known amount (usually a single copy) of an endogenous gene. A comparable analysis may be used to determine whether the offspring of a heterozygous mating are heterozygous (one copy) or homozygous (two copies) for the transgene. Finally, fluorescent in situ hybridization (FISH) analysis using transgene-specific probes may be used in cytological preparations of interphase (intact) cells to determine whether or not nuclei contain one or two copies of transgenic DNA (Dinchuk et al., 1994; Nishino et al., 1995).

Phenotypic Analysis of Engineered Rats

Incorporation of foreign DNA does not necessarily lead to useful gene expression. Often, inserted DNA is not transcribed into stable full-length mRNA, or mRNA is not translated into a structurally or functionally active protein. Similarly, transgenic expression of a non-rat protein may not be associated with any physiological effect in the rat (Ganten et al., 1992). Ideally, a series of molecular biological and morphological assays may be performed to characterize both the presence and the effect of the transgene's product (e.g. Sereda et al., 1996). Again, protocols and application of these procedures within transgenic studies have been collected into reference manuals (Wassarman and DePamphilis, 1993; Hogan et al., 1994; Pinkert, 1994; Ausubel et al., 1998).

In general, gene expression is assessed by measuring either the DNA-derived message (mRNA) or, where possible, quantification of the presence or function of the ultimate transgene product (protein). Detection of the protein is usually preferable as high levels of mRNA often do not correlate with the quantity (or even capacity) for translation into protein. Furthermore, for some proteins the site of mRNA translation does not correlate with the ultimate site of protein activity. This circumstance is characteristic of tissues (e.g. brain) in which cell bodies contain RNA while the protein is transported to distant cellular processes, and of sites where the protein binds to receptors located on other cells or the extracellular matrix.

Quantitative Analysis of Gene Expression

Quantitative analysis is typically performed in homogenized tissues (for adult rats) or with pulverized conceptuses. Aliquots of homogenate are then purified to obtain the molecule to be assessed, either total RNA, mRNA or protein. The molecule is detected by hybridization with a single- or double-stranded nucleotide probe (for RNA) or binding of an antibody (for protein). These detection reagents are labeled with a radioisotope, a fluorochrome or an enzyme.

The analytical techniques of choice for RNA are the northern assay, reverse transcription polymerase chain reaction (RT-PCR), and the ribonuclease protection assay (RPA). Multiple probes may be readily prepared to interact with unique sequences that span both the gene-coding region, the promoter, and the flanking vector; the use of several probes may greatly increase the assay specificity. In methods employing electrophoresis, the identity of the molecule is verified by comparison to a standard (to evaluate size and migration characteristics) and, if necessary, by excising the band and sequencing the genetic material. Positive internal controls should be included in all assays, such as ubiquitously expressed

'housekeeping' genes (e.g. actin or glyceraldehyde-3-phosphate dehydrogenase, GADPH; Goldsworthy et al., 1993). The sensitivity and specificity of RPA and RT-PCR is increased over that of the northern assay because binding of the sense mRNA with a complementary probe occurs in the reaction buffer rather than on a solid membrane. In RPA, the generation of the double-stranded molecule is detected by the addition of a RNase with specificity for single-stranded nucleotides (RNA or DNA); the enzyme destroys all but the protected, hybridized message. The product of RT-PCR can be measured through detection of an appropriately sized molecule on a gel, or by real-time quantification of the hybridization reaction in solution using a luminescent detection system.

The quantifiable assays for the transgene-derived protein in tissues are the western analysis and enzyme biochemical procedures. The former technique measures the physical presence of the molecule, while the latter detects the presence and activity of the functional protein. In addition, secreted proteins encoded by transgenes may be detected in body fluids (e.g. serum) using enzyme-linked immunosorbent assays (ELISA) or enzyme kinetic tests to detect the physical or functional presence, respectively, of the protein. Multiple antibodies that interact with unique protein epitopes may be available. If a wild-type allele is replaced with a mutant allele or a marker gene, the use of probes with specificity for either the wild-type protein or the introduced molecule will increase the discriminating capacity of the assay.

Qualitative Localization of Gene Distribution

Once expression of the transgene has been confirmed in a genetically engineered line, a qualitative analysis to localize the RNA and/or protein is performed in tissues. These methods may detect molecules either in entire organs or embryos ('whole mount' procedures) or in tissue sections (slide-based procedures). If feasible, organs are preserved by fixation (usually by immersion in a dilute solution of buffered aldehyde) to preserve the overall tissue structure for subsequent analysis. However, in certain instances (e.g. proteins with delicate antigenic sites) the fresh tissues are embedded in mounting medium (e.g. O.C.T.; Miles Laboratories, Elkhart,

IN, USA) and flash-frozen in supercooled isopentane (2-methyl butane) to prevent degradation of the molecule while retaining acceptable tissue morphology. The analytical techniques used to localize sites of transgene expression are comparable to those described above for homogenized tissues. The principal method for demonstrating sense mRNA is *in situ* hybridization. Tissues are treated with a solution containing a complementary nucleotide probe labeled with an isotope, fluorochrome or enzyme. Next, multiple highly stringent washing steps (e.g. elevated temperature, low salinity) and a RNase bath are applied to remove nonspecifically bound probe. At present, isotopic methods are considered more sensitive, but it may be impossible to determine the exact cells in which transgenes are expressed. In contrast, probes conjugated to fluorochromes or enzymes often may be used to define the cellular and even subcellular distributions of mRNAs of interest. Protein products are defined by immunohistochemistry (Larsson, 1993; Osborn and Isenberg, 1994) and enzyme histochemistry (Chayen and Bitensky, 1994; Mercer, 1999). Again, the former method measures the physical presence of the transgene product, while the latter detects the presence and activity of the functional protein.

Antibodies are the main reagents used for immunohistochemistry. Anti-rat reagents may be available commercially for more common antigens (Weimer, 1996; Linscott, 1998); in addition, empirical testing may demonstrate the ability of antibodies directed against non-rat antigens to cross-react with rat molecules, thereby providing for their use in rat tissues (e.g. Smith, 1990). In many instances, however, antibodies must be made for the gene product of interest. Double-staining procedures to localize mRNA and protein simultaneously are possible by performing *in situ* hybridization and immunohistochemistry on the same sample. The mRNA method is commonly performed first because the nucleic acids are more vulnerable to the experimental conditions during this extended procedure.

Phenotypic Analysis

The two reasons for performing genetic engineering experiments are (1) to produce a rat model with specific biological features – often to generate an animal model of human disease – or (2) to introduce a gene sequence and to investigate the impact of altered gene expression *in vivo*. Regardless of the reason, engineered animals must be characterized fully to be of maximal use. Many different endpoints may be assessed, and the choice of which parameters to select often is dictated by the researcher's interests even more than the nature of any extraordinary findings. Two general categories to be evaluated are function and morphology of the rat. These features may be examined either in the intact animal *in vivo* or in relevant target tissues *in vitro*. Heterozygous animals should be included in the assessment of homozygous and control animals since partial penetrance (diluted intensity) of the transgene-induced phenotype may result from the reduced gene dosage (Lee et al., 1995; Langheinrich et al., 1996; Sereda et al., 1996). In addition, the generation of chimeras with different ratios of transfected ES cells will assist in the study of gene dosage in developing and adult animals, particularly where a homozygous mutation results in an embryonic lethal phenotype. Finally, sexual dimorphism with respect to gene expression and/or the severity of the phenotype may occur (e.g. Veniant et al., 1996; Cranston et al., 1997), so rats of both sexes should be assessed.

Function represents an important aspect of any evaluation. The battery of tests to be performed will depend upon the prior or predicted knowledge regarding a novel transgene's phenotype. For example, engineered genes with sequences that are homologous to members of a gene family or which are components of a specific biochemical pathway may be anticipated to have phenotypes comparable to other members of the group, so the battery of endpoints might concentrate upon confirming a known pattern of defects (e.g. Cacalano et al., 1998). In contrast, transgenes for which phenotypes have not been defined must be investigated using a more extensive regimen. Initial tests *in vivo* are made during the in-life portion of the experiment using behavioral and clinical endpoints. The data may be acquired repeatedly, are relatively noninvasive, and provide a dynamic assessment of a global physiological state. Transgene-induced behavioral alterations might only be manifested during a limited phase of the animal's life (e.g. the neonatal period, adulthood, senescence), or the effects may occur throughout life. For practical considerations (cost and time), many functional analyses are limited to neonatal and young adult animals. Conventional clinical pathology assays are performed on body fluids such as blood or urine and often include serum chemistry to assess organ function (chiefly for the kidney, liver and pancreas) as well as hematologic parameters to assess blood cell populations. Flow cytometric analysis (Camplejohn, 1994) of cell populations (e.g. blood cells, dissociated lymphoid organs and tumors) may also provide useful information regarding transgene-induced alterations. In addition, *in vitro* functional assays might evaluate cell culture (Sereda *et al.*, 1996) or tissue slice (e.g. Alger *et al.*, 1984) models using endpoints such as cytokine production (Shikishima *et al.*, 1997), electrophysiological properties (Sereda *et al.*, 1996), or metabolism (Yamaguchi *et al.*, 1992). Advantages of functional assays include the speed with which data may be gathered; the non-invasive nature of certain tests, which allows repeated measurements in the same animal; and the quantifiable nature of the results. The chief disadvantages will probably be the wide degree of biological variation between responses of individual rats, and between animals of different strains (Crawley *et al.*, 1997). The shifting nature of functional endpoints *in vivo* will often necessitate special experimental designs with larger numbers of animals to control for this variation. In all cases, data should be compared to the findings for normal rats, ideally using age-matched wild-type littermates as controls.

Morphology represents another element of the characterization process, and it often is used as the 'gold standard' for defining the effects of genetic manipulation. Initial clinical observations are gathered for the living rat, with subsequent macroscopic (gross) assessments of organ systems at necropsy. Specific endpoints that might be noted include alterations in the size (larger, smaller, absent), shape, color or location of organs, or the presence of aberrant elements (e.g. extra organs, tumors). Tissues then are fixed and processed for microscopic evaluation. If no obvious abnormalities are noted, and if an expected target organ is not known, a battery of organ systems is screened using a routine tissue stain (such as hematoxylin and eosin). Next, organs with confirmed transgene-induced lesions are subjected to more extensive analysis to define the biological mechanism. Techniques of value for such research might include electron microscopy, immunohistochemistry, *in situ* hybridization, magnetic resonance imaging (Lukkarinen *et al.*, 1997) and morphometry. The choice of methods is usually selected on a case-by-case basis.

The increasing use of genetic engineering technology has led to a rapidly growing list of genes that

have been shown to have a critical but previously unsuspected role in embryonic development. In many instances, alteration of these pathways during development announces its significance through the crude, but definitive, phenotype of embryonic lethality. Often, defining when and where the altered genes and their products exert their effects, as well as the mechanistic pathway involved, is extremely difficult. Initial attempts will probably include a sequential analysis of both gross and microscopic structure in the conceptus (and often the placenta). The goals at this stage are (1) to discover the developmental stage at which the lethal event is occurring and then (2) to find the target organ(s) in an earlier embryonic stage. The recent publication of several atlases describing prenatal development of rodents (Theiler, 1989; Kaufman, 1992; Altman and Bayer, 1995; Paxinos *et al.*, 1995) has greatly aided such investigations. Where feasible, insertion of a marker gene (Alam and Cook, 1990) in tandem with the transgene may provide a means of defining site(s) of early gene expression. Particular attention must be paid to ensure that any phenotype is the result of the desired genetic event and not an insertional mutation in an endogenous gene (Woychik *et al.*, 1985).

Disclaimer

The reference texts, software packages, and products mentioned in this chapter are included only for illustrative purposes. While these items have been used successfully by the authors, other products may serve the same purposes.

Acknowledgements

The authors thank John Kulik (Wyeth-Ayerst Research, Andover, MA, USA) for technical assistance, James McCabe (Amgen, Inc.) for editorial review, and Dr Georg Krinke (Novartis) for his assistance and patience in the writing process.

References

Akagi, K., Sandig, V., Vooijs, M. *et al.* (1997) *Nucleic Acids Res.* **25**, 1766–1773.

Alam, J. and Cook, J.L. (1990) *Anal. Biochem.* **188**, 245–254.

Alger, B.E., Dhanjal, S.S., Dingledine, R. et al. (1984) In: Dingledine, R. (ed.) Brain Slices, pp. 381–437. New York: Plenum Press.

Altman, J. and Bayer, S.A. (1995) Atlas of Prenatal Rat Brain Development. Boca Raton: CRC Press.

Anzai, M., Nakagata, N., Matsumoto, K., Takahashi, Y. and Miyata, K. (1994) Exp. Anim. 43, 247–250.

Ausubel, F.M., Brent, R., Kingston, R.E. et al. (1998) Current Protocols in Molecular Biology, Vols 1–3. New York: John Wiley.

Baldwin, H.S., Mickanin, C. and Buck, C. (1997) Gene Ther. 4, 1142–1149.

Beerli, R.R., Wels, W. and Hynes, N.E. (1994) J. Biol. Chem. 269, 23931–23936.

Blackwood, E.M. and Kadonga, J.T. (1998) Science 281, 60–63.

Borrelli, E., Heyman, R., His, M. and Evans, R.M. (1988) Proc. Natl Acad. Sci. USA 85, 7572–7576.

Bos-Mikich, A., Whittingham, D.G. and Jones, K.T. (1997) Dev. Biol. 182, 172–179.

Bradley, A., Evans, M., Kaufman, M.H. and Robertson, E. (1984) Nature 309, 255–256.

Brinster, R.L., Chen, H.Y., Trumbauer, M.E., Yagle, M. and Palmiter, R.D. (1985) Proc. Natl Acad. Sci. USA 85, 4438–4442.

Bronson, S.K. and Smithies, O. (1994) J Biol. Chem. 269, 27155–27158.

Brown, T.A. (1991) Essential Molecular Biology: A Practical Approach, Vols 1 and 2. Oxford: IRL Press.

Byrne, R.W. and Ruddle, F.H. (1989) Proc. Natl. Acad. Sci. USA 86, 5473–5477.

Cacalano, G., Fariñas, I., Wang, L.-C. et al. (1998) Neuron 21, 53–62.

Campbell, K.H.S., McWhir, J., Ritchie, W.A. and Wilmut, I. (1996) Nature 380, 64–66.

Campleiohn, R.S. (1994) J. Microsc. 176, 1–7.

Canseco, R.S., Sparks, A.E.T., Page, R.L. et al. (1994) Transgenic Res. 3, 20–25.

Capecchi, M.R. (1989) Science 244, 1288–1292.

Chang, S.S. and Mark, H.F. (1997) Cytobios 90, 7–22.

Charreau, B., Tesson, L., Soulillou, J.P., Pourcel, C. and Anegon, I. (1996) Transgenic Res. 5, 223–234.

Chayen, J. and Bitensky, L. (1994) In: Celis, J.E. (ed.) Cell Biology: A Laboratory Handbook, Vol. 2, pp. 245–252. San Diego: Academic Press.

Chen, B. and Hales, B.F. (1995) Biol. Reprod. 53, 1229–1238.

Clark, A.J., Bissinger, P., Bullock, D.W. et al. (1994) Reprod. Fertil. Dev. 6, 589–598.

Copp, A.J. (1995) Trends Genet. 11, 87–93.

Cranston, A., Bocker, T., Reitmar, A. et al. (1997) Nature Genet. 17, 114–118.

Crawley, J.N., Belknap, J.K., Collins, A. et al. (1997) Psychopharmacology 132, 107–124.

Deshane, J., Siegal, G.P., Wang, M. et al. (1997) Gynecol. Oncol. 64, 378–385.

Dieffenbach, C.W. and Devksler, G.S. (1993) PCR Methods Appl. 3, S2–S7.

Dietrich, D.R. and Swenberg, J.A. (1991) Fundam. Appl. Toxicol. 97, 749–762.

Dinchuk, J.E., Kelley, K. and Boyle, A.L. (1994) Bio Techniques 17, 954–959.

Doetschman, T., Gregg, R.G., Maeda, N. et al. (1987) Nature 330, 576–578.

Dycaico, M.J., Provost, G.S., Kretz, P.L. Ransom, S.L. Moores, J.C. and Short, J.M. (1994) Mutat. Res. 307, 461–478.

Dymecki, S.M. (1996) Proc. Natl Acad. Sci. USA 93, 6191–6196.

Evans, M.J. and Kaufman, M.H. (1981) Nature 292, 154–156.

Fishman, G.I. (1995) Trends Cardiovasc. Med. 5, 211–217.

Fishman, G.I., Kaplan, M.L. and Buttrick, P.M. (1994) J. Clin. Invest. 93, 1864–1868.

Folger, K.R., Wong, E.A., Wahl, G. and Capecchi, M.R. (1982) Mol. Cell. Biol. 2, 1372–1387.

Furth, P., St. Onge, L., Boger, H. et al. (1994) Proc. Natl Acad. Sci. USA 91, 9302–9306.

Ganten, D., Wagner, J., Zeh, K. et al. (1992) Proc. Natl Acad. Sci. USA 89, 7806–7810.

Gardner, D.P., Byrne, G.W., Ruddle, F.H. and Kappen, C. (1996) Transgenic Res. 5, 37–48.

Gill, T., Smith, G.J., Wissler, R.W. and Kuntz, H.W. (1989) Science 245, 269–276.

Goldsworthy, S.M., Goldsworthy, T.L., Sprankle, C.S. and Butterworth, B.E. (1993) Cell Prolif. 26, 511–517.

Gossen, M., Bonin, A.L. and Bujard, H. (1993) Trends Biol. Sci. 18, 471–475.

Gossen, M., Freundlieb, S., Bender, G., Müller, G., Hillen, W. and Bujard, H. (1995) Science 268, 1766–1768.

Gossler, A., Doetschman, T., Korn, R., Serfling, E. and Kemler, R. (1986) Proc. Natl Acad. Sci. USA 83, 9065–9069.

Greenwald, R.A. and Diamond, H.S. (1988) Handbook of Animal Models for Rheumatic Diseases, Vol. 1. Boca Raton: CRC Press.

Gu, H., Marth, J.D., Orban, P.C., Mossmann, H. and Rajewsky, K. (1994) Science 265, 103–106.

Hammer, R.E., Maika, S.D., Richardson, J.A., Tang, J. and Taurog, J. (1990) Cell 3, 1099–1112.

Hanks, M., Wurst, W., Anson-Cartwright, L., Auerback, A.B. and Joyner, A.L. (1995) Science 269, 679–682.

Hasty, P. and Bradley, A. (1993) In: Joyner, A.L. (ed.) Gene Targeting: A Practical Approach, pp. 1–31. Oxford: IRL Press.

Heideman, J. (1991) Bio/Technology 16, 325–332.

Hirabayashi, M., Takahashi, R., Sekiguchi, J. and Ueda, M. (1997) Exp. Anim. 46, 111–115.

Hogan, B., Beddington, R., Costantini, F. and Lacy, E. (1994) Manipulating the Mouse Embryo: A Laboratory Manual, 2nd edn. Cold Spring Harbor Press: Plainview, New York.

Holzinger, A., Trapnell, B.C., Weaver, T.E., Whitsett, J.A. and Iwamoto, H.S. (1995) *Pediatr. Res.* **38**, 844–850.

Iannacconne, P.M., Taborn, G.U., Garton, R.L., Caplice, M.D. and Brenin, D.R. (1994) *Dev. Biol.* **163**, 288–292. [Published erratum appears in *Dev. Biol.* **185**, 124–125 (1997)].

Ichikawa, T., Kyprianou, N. and Isaacs, J.T. (1990) *Cancer Res.* **50**, 6349–6357.

Irwin, M.H, Moffatt, R.J. and Pinkert, C.A. (1996) *Nature Biotechnol.* **14**, 1146–1148.

Jaffe, H.A., Daniel, C., Longenecker, G. *et al.* (1992) *Nature Genet.* **1**, 372–378.

Kallioniemi, A., Kallioniemi, O-P., Sudar, D. *et al.* (1992) *Science* **258**, 818–821.

Kasarkis, A., Manova, K. and Anderson, K.V. (1998) *Proc. Natl Acad. Sci. USA* **95**, 7485–7490.

Kaufman, M.H. (1992) *The Atlas of Mouse Development*, 2nd edn. San Diego: Academic Press.

Kerler, R. and Rabes, H.M. (1994) *Crit. Rev. Oncogenesis* **5**, 271–295.

Kistner, A., Gossen, M., Zimmermann, F. *et al.* (1996) *Proc. Natl Acad. Sci. USA* **93**, 10933–10938.

Koller, B.H. and Smithies, O. (1992) *Annu. Rev. Immunol.* **10**, 705–730.

Kühn, R., Schwenk, F., Aguet, M. and Rajewsky, K. (1995) *Science* **269**, 1427–1429.

Langheinrich, M., Lee, M.A., Boehm, M., Pinto, Y.M., Ganten, D. and Paul, M. (1996) *Am. J. Hypertension* **9**, 506–512.

Larsson, L.-I. (1993) *Appl. Immunohistochem.* **1**, 2–16.

La Salle, G.L.G., Robert, J.J., Berrard, S. *et al.* (1993) *Science* **259**, 988–990.

Lee, M.A., Boehm, M., Kim, S. *et al.* (1995) *Hypertension* **25**, 570–580.

Lefevre, P.A., Tinwell, H. and Ashby, J. (1997) *Mutagenesis* **12**, 45–47.

Lesser, W. (1995) In: Meyers, R.A. (ed.) *Molecular Biology and Biotechnology. A Comprehensive Desk Reference*, pp. 907–910. New York: VCH Publishers.

Levan, G. (1974) *Hereditas* **77**, 37–52.

Lichter, P., Chang, C.-J., Call, K. *et al.* (1990) *Science* **247**, 64–69.

Linscott, W.D. (1998) *Linscott's Directory of Immunological and Biological Reagents*, 10th edn. 4877 Grange Rd., Santa Rosa, CA.

Liyanage, M., Coleman, A., du Manoir, S. *et al.* (1996) *Nature Genet.* **14**, 312–315.

Lukkarinen, J., Groehn, O.H., Sinervirta, R. *et al.* (1997) *Stroke* **28**, 639–645.

Marth, J.D. (1996) *J. Clin. Invest.* **97**, 1999–2002.

Martin, G.R. (1981) *Proc. Natl Acad. Sci. USA* **78**, 7634–7638.

Matsumoto, K., Kakidani, H., Takahashi, T. *et al.* (1993) *Mol. Reprod. Dev.* **36**, 53–58.

Mercer, E. (1999) http://www.rodentia.com/wmc/;

Laboratory Section, Technical Guides and Protocols' sub-section/

Metzger, D., Clifford, J., Chiba, H. and Chambon, P. (1995) *Proc. Natl. Acad. Sci. USA* **92**, 6991–6995.

Mintz, B. and Klein-Szanto, A.J. (1992) *Proc. Natl Acad. Sci. USA* **89**, 11421–11425.

Mitelman, F. (1983) *Cytogenet. Cell Genet.* **36**, 1–515.

Montaudon, D., Benchekroun, M.N., Londos-Gagliardi, D. and Robert, J. (1990) *Anticancer Res.* **10**, 1667–1676.

Mukumoto, S., Mori, K. and Ishikawa, H. (1995) *Exp. Anim.* **44**, 111–118.

Mullins, L.J. and Mullins, J.J. (1996) *J. Clin. Invest.* **97**, 1557–1560.

Mullins, J.J., Peters, J. and Ganten, D. (1990) *Nature* **344**, 541–544.

Nakagata, N. (1993) *J. Reprod. Fertil. Steril.* **87**, 479–483.

Nishino, H., Herath, J.F., Jenkins, R.B. and Sommer, S.S. (1995) *BioTechniques* **19**, 587–588, 590, 592.

No, D., Yao, T.-P. and Evans, R.M. (1996) *Proc. Natl Acad. Sci. USA* **93**, 3346–3351.

Oligino, T., Poliani, P.L., Wang, Y. *et al.* (1998) *Gene Ther.* **5**, 491–496.

Orban, P.C., Chui, D. and Marth, J.D. (1992) *Proc. Natl Acad. Sci. USA* **89**, 6861–6865.

Ogbourne, S. and Antalis, T.M. (1998) *Biochem. J.* **331**, 1–14.

Osborn, M. and Isenberg, S. (1994) In: Celis, J.E. (ed.) *Cell Biology: A Laboratory Handbook*, Vol. 2, pp. 361–367. San Diego: Academic Press.

Palmiter, R.D., Norstedt, G., Gelinas, R.E., Hammer, R.E. and Brinster, R.L. (1983) *Science* **222**, 809–814.

Palmiter, R.D., Behringer, R.R., Quaife, C.J., Maxell, F., Maxwell, I.H. and Brinster, R.L. (1987) *Cell* **50**, 435–443.

Papaioannou, V. and Johnson, R. (1993) In: Joyner, A.L. (ed.) *Gene Targeting: A Practical Approach*, pp. 107–146. Oxford: IRL Press.

Parra, I. and Windle, B. (1993) *Nature Genet.* **5**, 17–21.

Passman, R. and Fishman, G.I. (1994) *J. Clin. Invest.* **94**, 2421–2425.

Paul, M., Wagner, J., Hoffman, S., Urata, H. and Ganten, D. (1994) *Annu. Rev. Physiol.* **56**, 811–829.

Paxinos, G., Ashwell, K.W.S. and Törk, I. (1995) *Atlas of the Developing Rat Nervous System*, 2nd edn. San Diego: Academic Press.

Pinkert, C.A. (1994) *Transgenic Animal Technology: A Laboratory Handbook*. San Diego: Academic Press.

Qin, H. and Gunning, P. (1997) *J. Biochem. Biophys. Methods* **36**, 63–72.

Rajewsky, K., Gu, H., Kühn, R. *et al.* (1996) *J. Clin. Invest.* **98**, 600–603.

Ramirez-Solis, R., Liu, P. and Bradley, A. (1995) *Nature* **378**, 720–724.

Robbins, P.D., Tahara, H. and Ghivizzani, S.C. (1998) *Trends Biotechnol.* **16**, 35–40.

Robertson, E., Bradley, A., Kuehn, M. and Evans, M. (1986) *Nature* **323**, 445–448.

Robl, J.M. and Heideman, J.K. (1994) In: Pinkert, C.A. (ed.) *Transgenic Animal Technology: A Laboratory Handbook*, pp. 265–278. San Diego: Academic Press.

Rohlmann, A., Gotthardt, M., Willnow, T.E., Hammer, R.E. and Herz, J. (1996) *Nature Biotechnol.* **14**, 1562–1565.

Ronne, M., Shibasaki, Y., Poulsen, B.S. and Andersen, O. (1987) *Cytogenet. Cell Genet.* **45**, 113–117.

Rossant, J., Spence, A. and Rossant, J. (1998) *Trends Genet.* **14**, 358–363.

Sambrook, J., Fritsch, E.F. and Maniatis, T. (1989) *Molecular Cloning: A Laboratory Manual*, 2nd edn. Cold Spring Harbor, New York: Cold Spring Harbor Laboratory Press.

Sanes, J.R., Rubenstein, J.L.R. and Nicolas, J.-F. (1986) *EMBO J.* **5**, 3133–3142.

Sargent, L., Dragan, Y., Xu, Y.H., Sattler, G., Wiley, J. and Pitot, H.C. (1996) *Cancer Res.* **56**, 2985–2991.

Satoh, H., Yoshida, M.C. and Sasaki, M. (1989) *Cytogenet. Cell Genet.* **50**, 151–154.

Sauer, B. (1993) *Methods Enzymol.* **225**, 890–900.

Schmidt, E.V., Christoph, G., Zeller, R. and Leder, P. (1990) *Mol. Cell. Biol.* **10**, 4406–4411.

Schultze, N., Burki, Y., Lang, Y., Certa, U. and Bluethmann, H. (1996) *Nature Biotechnol.* **14**, 499–503.

Sereda, M., Griffiths, I., Pülhofer, A. *et al.* (1996) *Neuron* **16**, 1049–1060.

Shikishima, H., Ikeda, H., Yamada, S. *et al.* (1997) *Leukemia* **11** (suppl. 3), 70–72.

Simoes, S., Slepushkin, V., Gaspar, R., deLima, M.C.P. and Duzgunes, N. (1998) *Gene Ther.* **5**, 955–964.

Simone, N.L., Bonner, R.F., Gillespie, J.W., Emmert-Buck, M.R. and Liotta, L.A. (1998) *Trends Genet.* **14**, 272–276.

Smith, R.A. (1990) *J. Histotechnol.* **13**, 255–269.

Smithies, O., Gregg, R.G., Boggs, S.S., Kordewski, M.A. and Kucherlapati, R.S. (1985) *Nature* **317**, 230–234.

Speicher, M.R., Gwyn-Ballard, S. and Ward, D.C. (1996) *Nature Genet.* **2**, 368–375.

Swanson, M.E., Hughes, T.E., Denny, I.S. *et al.* (1992) *Transgenic Res.* **1**, 142–147.

Takahama, Y., Ochiya, T., Sasaki, H. *et al.* (1998) *Oncogene* **16**, 3189–3196.

Taketo, M., Schroeder, A.C., Mobraaten, L.E. *et al.* (1991) *Proc. Natl Acad. Sci. USA* **88**, 2065–2069.

Taurog, J.D., Richardson, J.A., Croft, J.T. *et al.* (1994) *J. Exp. Med.* **180**, 2359–2364.

Telenius, H., Pelmear, A.H., Tunnacliffe, A. *et al.* (1992) *Genes, Chromosomes Cancer* **4**, 263–267.

Theiler, K. (1989) *The House Mouse: Atlas of Embryonic Development*. New York: Springer-Verlag.

Thomas, K.R. and Capecchi, M.R. (1987) *Cell* **51**, 503–512.

Trask, B., Pinkel, D. and van den Engh, G. (1989) *Genomics* **5**, 710–717.

Tsien, J.Z., Chen, D.F., Gerber, D. *et al.* (1996) *Cell* **87**, 1317–1326.

Tsukui, T., Kanagae, Y., Saito, I. and Toyoda, Y. (1996) *Nature Biotechnol.* **1**, 982–985.

Veniant, M., Menard, J., Bruneval, P., Morley, S., Gonzales, M.F. and Mullins, J. (1996) *J. Clin. Invest.* **98**, 1966–1970.

Wakayama, T. and Yanagimachi, R. (1998) *Nature Biotechnol.* **16**, 639–641.

Wakayama, T., Perry, A.C.F., Zuccotti, M., Johnson, K.R. and Yanagimachi, R. (1998) *Nature* **394**, 369–374.

Wang, Y., DeMayo, F.J., Tsai, S.Y. and O'Malley, B.W. (1997) *Nature Biotechnol.* **15**, 239–243.

Wassarman, P.M. and DePamphilis, M.L. (1993) *Guide to Techniques in Mouse Development*. San Diego: Academic Press.

Waynforth, H.B. and Flecknell, P.A. (1992) *Experimental and Surgical Techniques in the Rat*, 2nd edn. San Diego: Academic Press.

Weiner, R.V. (1996) *MSRS Catalog of Primary Antibodies*, 3rd edn. Birmingham, MI: Aerie [http:wwwantibodies-probes.com/1.

Wilmut, I., Schnieke, A.E., McWhir, J., Kind, A.J. and Campbell, K.H.S. (1997) *Nature* **385**, 810–813.

Wood, S.A., Allen, N.D., Rossant, J., Auerbach, A. and Nagy, A. (1993) *Nature* **365**, 87–89.

Woychik, R.P., Stewart, T.A., Davis, L.G., D'Eustachio, P. and Leder, P. (1985) *Nature* **318**, 36–40.

Wurst, W. and Joyner, A.L. (1993) In: Joyner, A.L. (ed.) *Gene Targeting: A Practical Approach*, pp. 33–61. Oxford: IRL Press.

Yamaguchi, T., Tokita, Y., Franco-Saenz, R., Mulrow, P.J., Peters, J. and Ganten, D. (1992) *Endocrinology* **131**, 1955–1962.

Yarranton, G.T. (1992) *Curr. Opin. Biotechnol.* **3**, 506–511.

Appendix 1   Table of Genetic Markers in the rat

Chromosome 1

Locus symbol	Previous symbol	RNO Location	Description	Mode	Status	Reference	HSA symbol	HSA Chr	MMU symbol	MMU Chr
Add3		1q55	Adducin gamma	D, S	P	94				
Adra2a		1	Adrenergic alpha 2A receptor, see also D1Smu2	–	P	66	ADRA2A	10q24–q-26	Adra2a	19
Adrb1		1	Adrenergic receptor beta 1, see also D1Arb28 and D1Smu1	–	C	15, 66				
Aldoa		1	Aldolase A fructose-bisphosphate, see also D1Arb19	–	C	15, 24, 31				
Ampd3		1q35–q36	Adenosine monophosphate deaminase 3	D	P	77				
Ap		1	Adrenomedullin precursor, see also D1Wox34	–	P	3, 98				
Atp1a3	Atpa1a3	1	ATPase, Na^+,K^+-transporting, alpha 3 subunit	–, S	C	31, 74, 104	ATP1A3	19q13.2	Atp1a3	7
Atp4a		1	ATPase, H^+,K^+-transporting, alpha / (gastric H,K-ATPase catalytic subunit)	–, S	C	13, 31, 89	ATP4A	19q13.1	Atp4a	7
Bax		1q31.2	Bcl2-associated X protein	D	P	58				
Bsis		1	Brain-specific identifier sequence	S	P	76				
Calca	Calc	1	Calcitonin/calcitonin-related polypeptide alpha, see also D1Smu11	–, S	C	3, 66, 92, 98	CALCA	11p15.2–p15.1	Calc	7
Calm3		1q22	Calmodulin III, see also D1Wox12 and D1Arb35	D, L, S	C	15, 23, 31, 62, 73, 76				
Cebpa	DBPCEP	1	CAAT/enhancer-binding protein, DNA-binding protein	S	C	76, 84	CEBPA	19q13.1	Cebpa	7

Cgm1		1	Carcinoembryonic antigen gene family (CGM1), see also D1Arb32 and D1Arb33	L	P	15				
Cgm3	Cea3	1	Carcinoembryonic antigen gene family (CGM3), GenBank no. M22228, J04626, see also D1Wox14 and D1Arb36	L, S	C	2, 15, 23, 78, 79, 105				
Cgm4	CGM4, Cear, Cea	1	Carcinoembryonic antigen gene family member 4 (carcinoembryonic antigen-related protein), see also D1Mgh5 and D1Wox15	L, S	C	2, 13, 15, 23, 31, 35, 68, 76				
Chrm1		1q43–q51	Acetylcholine receptor, muscarinic M1	D, S		38				
Ckm	Ckmm	1	Creatine kinase, muscle form, see also D1Kyo1	S	P	47	CKM	19q13.3	Ckmm	7
Cpbr	CARB07	1	Carboxypeptidase B-related, CARB07-related	L	P	24				
Cyp17		1q55	Cytochrome P450, 17	D	P	36				
Cyp2a1	Shdl	1	Cytochrome P450 IIA1 (hepatic steroid hydroxylase IIA1) gene, see also D1Wox16	L	C	3, 23, 31, 78, 79, 98				
Cyp2a2		1	Cytochrome P450 IIA2	L	P	31				
Cyp2a3a	Cyp2a3	1	Cytochrome P450, subfamily IIA (phenobarbital-inducible)/ (Cytochrome P450 IIA3)	L	C	3, 13, 31, 98				
Cyp2b1	Cypbe	1	Cytochrome P450, subfamily IIB (phenobarbital-inducible) (b, e)	L	C	72, 76, 101				
Cyp2b2	Cype	1	Cytochrome P450, subfamily IIB (phenobarbital-inducible) (b, e), see also D1Wox17	L	C	23, 31, 35, 71, 72, 74, 76, 78, 79, 101				
Cyp2b@		1	Cytochrome P450, subfamily IIB gene cluster							
Cyp2c12	P450pb1	1	Cytochrome P450 15-beta gene, see also D1Wox25	L	C	3, 23, 31, 74, 98				
Cyp2e1		1	Cytochrome P450, subfamily 2e1 (ethanol-inducible), see also D1Smu4	L	P	66				
Cyphp1		1	Hepatic cytochrome P450e-PB	S	P	33				
Dbp		1	D site albumin promoter-binding protein	S	P	84	DBP	19q13	Dbp	7
Esr		1q12	Oestrogen receptor	D	P	89				
Fgfr2		1	Fibroblast growth factor receptor 2, see also D1Smu5	Linkage	C	3, 66, 98				

Fut@		1q22–q31	Alpha-1,2-fucosyltransferase gene cluster	D		55				
Futa		1q22–q31	Alpha-1,2-fucosyltransferase a	D	P	55				
Futb		1q22–q31	Alpha-1,2-fucosyltransferase b	D	P	55				
Fz		1	Fuzzy (hair loss)	L	P	18, 29, 69				
Gabrb3		1	Gamma-aminobutyric acid receptor beta 3, see also D1Arb10	L	P	15	GABRB3	15q11.2–q12	Gabrb3	7
Gippr		1	Gastric inhibitory peptide receptor, see also D1Wox30	L	P	3, 98				
Got1	Aspat, Gaspat	1	Glutamic-oxaloacetic transaminase 1, soluble (aspartate aminotransferase, cytosolic), see also D1Mgh12	L, S	C	35, 103	GOT1	10q24.1–q25.1	Got1	19
Gpi		1	Glucose phosphate isomerase	S	P	106	GPI	19q13.1	Gpi	7
Grik5		1q21	Glutamate receptor, ionotropic, kainate 5	D, S	C	87, 89	GRIK5	19q13.2	Grik5	7
Grin2d		1	Glutamate receptor, ionotropic, N-methyl D-aspartate 2D	S	P	53			Grin2d	7
Grm1		1	Glutamate receptor, metabotropic 1, see also D1Mgh1	L, S	C	35, 53, 99				
Grm5		1	Glutamate receptor, metabotropic 5	S	P	53				
Gstp	GST-P, Gst3	1q43	Glutathione-S-transferase, placental enzyme pi type, see also D1Wox36	D, L, S	C	3, 39, 57, 59, 97, 98, 104	GSTP1	11q13	Hbb	7
H19		1q41–q42	H19 fetal liver mRNA	D	P	90				
Hbb		1q22	Haemoglobin beta	L	C	9, 15, 20, 64, 68, 76, 82				
He		1	Rat haematoma	L	P	16				
Hnf3g		1q21–q22	Hepatocyte nuclear factor 3 gamma	D	P	95				
Hras	HRAS1	1q41–q42	Harvey rat sarcoma viral (v-Ha-ras) oncogene homologue	S	C	17, 25, 91	HRAS1	11p15.5	Hras1	7
Hrev107		1	HRAS-revertant gene 107 (expression down-regulated in Hras-transformed rat 208F fibroblasts)	S	P	88				
Ic		1	Ichtyosis	L	P	42				

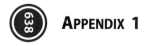

Igf2		1	Insulin-like growth factor II (somatomedin A), see also D1Mgh22, D1Wox22 and D1Arb24	L, S	C		IGF2	11p15.5	Igf2	7
Igf2r		1q11	Insulin-like growth factor 2 receptor	D	P	36				
Il4r		1	Interleukin 4 receptor, see also D1Smu6	L	P	66				
Inexa	Intlaa	1	Internexin alpha, see also D1Mgh13	L	P	35				
Ins1		1q54–q55	Insulin	D, S, L	C	2, 15, 22, 61, 68, 76, 82, 92			Ins1	19
Ins2		1q41	Insulin 2	D, S	C	82, 92	INS2	11p15.5	Ins2	7
Itgam		1	Integrin alpha-M, see also D1Smu10	L	C	3, 66, 98				
Jak2		1q51–q53	Janus kinase 2 (a protein tyrosine kinase)	D, L	C	71, 89				
Klk1	KAL	1	Kallikrein 1, renal/pancreas/salivary, see also D1Wox18	L, S	C	2, 7, 23, 31, 33, 52, 71, 74, 78, 79, 93	KLK1	19q13.3–q13.4	Klk1	7
Lap1		1	Leucine arylaminopeptidase 1	L	C	76, 96				
Ldha		1	Lactate dehydrogenase A	S	P	106	LDHA	11p15.1–p14	Ldh1	7
Ldr1		1	LDHA regulatory gene	L	P	83				
Lg		1	Grüneberg's lethal	L	P	30				
Lot1		1p	Lost on transformation 1	D	P	1				
Lpgp		1	Lipogenic protein S14, see also D1Arb38	L	P	15				
Mas1		1q11–q12	MAS1 oncogene	D	P	36	MAS	6p24–q27	Mas1	17
Mt1pa	Mtipa, D1Mtip9	1	Metallothionein 1, pseudogene A, see also D1Wox19	L	C	11, 31, 35, 68, 71, 74, 76				
Muc2	HH-Muc	1	Mucin 2	S	C	32, 40				
Myb		1	Avian myeloblastosis viral (v-myb) oncogene homologue	S	P	104				
Myl2	Mylpf, MLC2, Myolc1	1	Myosin, light polypeptide 3, alkali; ventricular, skeletal, slow, GenBank no: X00975, see also D1Mit13, D1Wox21, D1Arb18 and D1Wox32	L, S	C	3, 7, 15, 23, 24, 31, 33, 35, 71, 93, 98	MYL3	3p21.3–p-21.2		
Ngfg		1	Nerve growth factor, gamma polypeptide	S	P	104			Ngfg	7
Nras2		1	Neuroblastoma homologue 2 (v-ras)	L	C	51, 101				

Nrasp	*N12ep, Nras2*	1	N-*ras*1.2ep pseudogene, see also D1Wox33	L	C	3, 52, 98				
Oca2	*P*	1	Oculocutaneous albinism II (pink-eye dilution, murine), same as P	L	P	4, 64	OCA2	15q11.2–q12	*Pygm*	7
Oct1	*Roct1*	1q11–q12	Organic cation transporter	D	P	43, 44				
Omp		1	Olfactory marker protein, see also D1Mgh19	L	P	35	OMP	11q14–11-q21	*Omp*	7
Pbpc2		1	Prostatic binding protein C2, see also D1Wox23	D, L	C	2, 11, 23, 76, 107				
Pc		1q43	Pyruvate carboxylase	D	P	97				
Pdnpno		1p12	Phosphodiesterase/5'-nucleotidase gp130RB13-6	D	P	45				
Pepd		1	Peptidase D	S	P	106	PEPD	19q13.4	*Pkcc*	7
Pgy4	*Orfep*	1	P-glycoprotein 4, see also D1Mgh20	L	P	35				
Ppp1ca		1q43	Protein phosphatase type 1 alpha, catalytic subunit	D, S	C	75, 102				
Prkcb1	*Pkcb*	1	Protein kinase C beta, see also D1Smu9	L	C	3, 66, 98				
Prkcg	*PKC, Prkc*	1	Protein kinase C type I (gamma type), see also D1Wox11 and D1Arb31	L, S	C	2, 15, 23, 31, 33, 52, 73, 74				
Prt1	*Prt*	1	Protenase 1, submandibular gland protein	L	P	12, 101				
Prt2		1	Protenase 2, submandibular gland protein	L	P	12, 101				
Psbp1		1	Prostatic steroid-binding protein 1, see also D1Arb39	L	C	15				
Pth	*Pthr1, pth1*	1	Parathyroid hormone, see also D1Wox35	L, S	C	3, 24, 66, 71, 92, 98	PTH	11p15.2–p15.1	*Pth*	7
Pygm	*Muscpho*	1	Phosphorylase, glycogen; muscle (McArdle syndrome), see also D1Mgh11 and D1Wox28	L	C	3, 35, 98	PYGM	11q13.1	*Pygm*	19
R		1	Ruby or red eyed dilution	L	P	9				
Rrm1		1q34–q36	Ribonucleotide reductase 1	D, S	P	41				
Rt13	*GY1/34*	1	Cell surface alloantigen	L	P	6				
Rt4		1	Cell surface alloantigen	L	P	49				

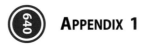

Rt6	Ag-F, Ly-2, PtaA, LY2, ART-2	1	Cell surface alloantigen, peripheral T-cell antigen	L	C	5, 14, 71, 100, 101	RT6	11q13	Rt6	7
Rw		1	Warfarin resistance	L	P	26–28			war	7
Sa		1	SsubA gene, GenBank no: U04637 o U04638	L, S	C	15, 19, 31, 48, 56, 66, 71, 85, 89				
Scnn1b		1q36–q37	Sodium channel, nonvoltage-gated 1, beta (epithelial), see also D1Smu8 and D1Smu7	D, L	C	3, 34, 50, 66, 70, 90, 98	SCNN1B	16p12.2–p12.1	Scnn1b	7
Scnn1g		1q36–q38	Sodium channel, nonvoltage-gated 1, gamma (epithelial)	D, L	C	34, 50, 70, 90	SCNN1G	16p12.2–p12.1	Scnn1g	7
Sct	Secr	1	Secretin	L, S	C	48, 76				
Shdl		1	Steroid hydroxylase, hepatic	S	P	76				
Slc6a3	Dat1	1	Solute carrier family 6 (neurotransmitter transporter, dopamine), member 3	L, S	C	79, 105				
Slc9a3	Nhe3	1p11	Solute carrier family 9 (sodium/hydrogen exchanger 3), antiporter 3, Na$^+$/H$^+$ (amiloride insensitive)	D, L, S	C	71, 86, 89	SLC9A3	5p15.3	Slc9a3	13
Smp2a		1	Rat senescence marker protein 2A gene, exons 1 and 2, see also D1Wox13	L	P	23				
Spe1		1	Salivary protein gene	L	P	81				
Spn	Lsn, Cd43	1	Sialophorin (gpL115, leukosianin, CD43), see also D1Wox20	L, S	C	7, 11, 22, 23, 31, 33, 35, 48, 56, 66, 71, 74, 76, 93	SPN	16p11–p-11.2	Spn	7
Srd5a1		1p11–q12	Steroid-5-alpha-reductase, alpha polypeptide 1 (3-oxo-5 alpha-steroid delta 4-dehydrogenase alpha 1)	D	P	89				
Sth1	St1	1q21.3–q22.1	Sulfotransferase hydroxysteroid gene 1	D	P	67				
Sth2	St2	1q21.3–q22.1	Sulfotransferase hydroxysteroid gene 2	D	P	67				
Stx2		1	Syntaxin 2, see also D1Arb21	L	P	15				

Tage4		1q22	Tumour-associated glycoprotein pE4	D	P	10				
Tal2		1	Tail anomaly lethal 2	L	P	63				
Tam1		1	Tamase, tosyl arginine methylesterase 1	L	P	60			TAm1	7
Tbm1		1	Tubular basement membrane antigen 1	L	P	60				
Tcp1		1q12	T-complex 1	D, L, S	C	2, 15, 68, 76, 89, 90, 104	TCP1	6q25–q27	Tcp1	17
Ten1		1	Thymus enlargement gene 1	L	P	65				
Th	The	1	Tyrosine hydroxylase, see also D1Smu3	L	P	66				
Tls1		1	Thymic lymphoma susceptible 1	L	C	80, 101				
Tnnt3	Tnt	1q41–q42	Troponin T, fast skeletal, see also D1Arb23	D, L	C	7, 15, 24, 73, 89, 93				
Ton		1	Tonin	L, S	C	2, 7, 33, 78, 79, 93				
Tp53l4	Trp53l4	1	Tumour protein p53-like 4	L	P	52				
Tpe1	Rtp2	1	Rat tear protein 2 (Tear protein 1 in mice)	L	C	46, 81				
Tph		1	Tryptophan hydroxylase	L, S	P	105				
Tsg101		1q22	Tumour supressor gene	D	P	90				
Tyr	C	1	Tyrosinase (albino coat colour)	L	C	7, 8, 20, 52, 64, 68, 71, 76, 81, 93				
Umod		1q36–q37	Urmodulin (Tamm–Horsfall protein)	D	P	21				
W		1	Waltzing	L	P	9, 37				
Yes1		1	Yamagichi sarcoma viral (v-yes-1) oncogene homologue 1	D	P	54				

References

1 Abdollahi et al. (1997) Cancer Res. **57**, 2029–2034.

2 Andoh et al. (1998) Mamm. Genome **9**, 287–293.

3 Bihoreau et al. (1997) Genomic Res. **7**, 434–440.

4 Brdicka (1968) Acta Univ. Carolinae Med. **14**, 93–98.

5 Butcher (1979) Transplant. Proc. **11**, 1629–1630.

6 Butcher (1996) Unpublished results.

7 Canzian (1996) Jpn. J. Cancer Res. **87**, 669–675.

8 Castle and King (1944) Proc. Natl Acad. Sci. USA **30**, 79–82.

9 Castle and King (1949) Proc. Natl Acad. Sci. USA **35**, 545–546.

10 Chadéneau et al. (1997) Mamm. Genome **8**, 157–158.

11 Chung et al. (1997) Genomics **41**, 332–344.

12 Deimling et al. (1982) Rat News Lett. **9**, 43.

13 Deng et al. (1994) Mamm. Genome **5**, 712–716

14   DeWitt and McCullough (1975) *Transplantation* **19**, 310–317.

15   Ding *et al.* (1996) *Genomics* **36**, 320–327.

16   Dunning and Curtis (1939) *Genetics* **24**, 70.

17   Fang *et al.* (1985) *Cytogenet. Cell Genet.* **40**, 627.

18   Ferguson *et al.* (1979) *Lab. Anim. Sci.* **29**, 459–465.

19   Frantz *et al.* (1996) *Mamm. Genome* **7**, 865.

20   French *et al.* (1971) *Biochem. Genet.* **5**, 397–404.

21   Fukuoka and Matsuda (1997) *Cytogenet. Cell Genet.* **79**, 241–242.

22   Galli *et al.* (1996) *Nature Genet.* **12**, 31–37.

23   Gauguier *et al.* (1996) *Nature Genet.* **12**, 38–43.

24   Goldmuntz *et al.* (1993) *Genomics* **16**, 761–764.

25   Gollahon and Aldaz (1992) *Cytogenet. Cell Genet.* **61**, 123–124.

26   Greaves and Ayres (1969) *Nature* **224**, 284–285.

27   Greaves and Ayres (1976) *Genet. Res.* **28**, 231–239.

28   Greaves and Ayres (1977) *Genet. Res.* **29**, 215–222.

29   Greaves and Ayres (1985) *Lab. Anim.* **19**, 145–147.

30   Grüneberg (1939) *Genetics* **24**, 732–741.

31   Gu *et al.* (1996) *J. Clin. Invest.* **97**, 777–788.

32   Hansson *et al.* (1994) *Biochem. Biophys. Res. Commun.* **198**, 181–190.

33   Hilbert *et al.* (1991) *Nature* **353**, 521–529.

34   Huang *et al.* (1995) *J. Hypertens.* **13**, 1247–1251.

35   Jacob *et al.* (1995) *Nature Genet.* **9**, 63–69.

36   Johansson *et al.* (1998) *Cytogenet. Cell Genet.* **81**, 217–221.

37   King (1936) *J. Mammal.* **17**, 157–163.

38   Klett *et al.* (1998) *Mamm. Genome* **9**, 476–478.

39   Klinga-Levan *et al.* (1993) *Hereditas* **119**, 285–296.

40   Klinga-Levan *et al.* (1996) *Mamm. Genome* **7**, 248–250.

41   Klinga-Levan *et al.* (1997) *Mamm. Genome* **8**, 47–49.

42   Knox and Lister-Rosenoer (1978) *J. Hered.* **69**, 391–394.

43   Koehler *et al.* (1996) *Mamm. Genome* **7**, 247.

44   Koehler *et al.* (1996) *Mamm. Genome* **7**, 638.

45   Koelsch *et al.* (1996) *Cytogenet. Cell Genet.* **73**, 228.

46   Kondo *et al.* (1987) *Transplant. Proc.* **19**, 3146–3147.

47   Kondo *et al.* (1993) *Mamm. Genome* **4**, 571–576.

48   Kovacs *et al.* (1997) *Biochem. Biophys. Res. Commun.* **235**, 343–348.

49   Kren *et al.* (1973) *Transplant. Proc.* **5**, 1463–1466.

50   Kreutz *et al.* (1997) *Hypertension* **29**, 131–136.

51   Kunieda *et al.* (1990) *Biochem. Genet.* **28**, 631–642.

52   Kunieda *et al.* (1995) *Exp. Anim.* **44**, 301–305.

53   Kuramoto *et al.* (1994) *Genomics* **19**, 358–61.

54   Levan *et al.* (1986) *Rat News Lett.* **17**, 3–8.

55   Liehr *et al.* (1997) *Mamm. Genome* **8**, 297–298.

56   Lindpaintner *et al.* (1993) *J. Hypertens.* **11**, 19–23.

57   Masuda *et al.* (1986) *Jpn. J. Cancer Res.* **77**, 1055–1058.

58   Matsuda *et al.* (1996) *Cytogenet. Cell Genet.* **74**, 107–110.

59   Matsumoto and Gasser (1983) *Biochem. Genet.* **21**, 1209–1213.

60   Matsumoto *et al.* (1984) *Immunogenetics* **20**, 117–123.

61   Mori *et al.* (1992) *Cytogenet. Cell Genet.* **59**, 31–33.

62   Mori *et al.* (1994) *Mamm. Genome* **5**, 824–826.

63   Morriss-Kay and Hunt (1986) *Rat News Lett.* **5**, 6–7.

64   Moutier *et al.* (1973) *Biochem. Genet.* **8**, 321–328.

65   Murakumo *et al.* (1996) *Mamm. Genome* **7**, 505–508.

66   Nabika *et al.* (1997) *Mamm. Genome* **8**, 215–217.

67   Nagai *et al.* (1996) *Cytogenet. Cell Genet.* **74**, 111–112.

68   National Institute of Arthritis and Musculoskeletal and Skin Diseases. The ARB Rat Genetic Database (http://www.nih.gov/niams/scientific/ratgbase/index.htm).

69   Palm and Ferguson (1976) *J. Hered.* **67**, 284–288.

70   Pravenec *et al.* (1996) *Folia Biol. (Praha)* **42**, 147–153.

71   Pravenec *et al.* (1996) *Mamm. Genome* **7**, 117–127.

72   Rampersaud and Walz Jr. (1987) *J. Biol. Chem.* **262**, 5649–5653.

73   Remmers *et al.* (1996) *Nature Genet.* **14**, 82–85.

74   Rubattu *et al.* (1996) *Nature Genet.* **13**, 429–434.

75 Saadat et al. (1995) Cytogenet. Cell Genet. **70**, 55–57.

76 Serikawa et al. (1992) Genetics **131**, 701–721.

77 Sermsuvitayawong et al. (1997) Mamm Genome **8**, 767–769

78 Shepel et al. (1998) Genetics **149**, 289–299.

79 Shepel et al. (1998) Mamm. Genome **9**, 622–628.

80 Shisa and Hiai (1985) Cancer Res. **45**, 1483–1487.

81 Shisa et al. (1997) Mamm. Genome **8**, 324–327.

82 Soares et al. (1985) Mol. Cell. Biol. **5**, 2090–2103.

83 Stolc and Gill III (1983) Biochem. Genet. **21**, 933–941.

84 Szpirer et al. (1992) Genomics **13**, 293–300.

85 Szpirer et al. (1993) J. Hypertens. **11**, 919–925.

86 Szpirer et al. (1994) Mamm. Genome **5**, 153–159.

87 Szpirer et al. (1994) Proc. Natl Acad. Sci. USA **91**, 11849–11853.

88 Szpirer et al. (1996) Mamm. Genome **7**, 701–703.

89 Szpirer et al. (1997) Mamm. Genome **8**, 657–660.

90 Szpirer et al. (1998) Mamm. Genome **9**, 721–734.

91 Szpirer et al. (1985) Somat. Cell Mol. Genet. **11**, 93–97.

92 Todd et al. (1985) Biochem. Biophys. Res. Commun. **131**, 1175–1180.

93 Toyota et al. (1996) Proc. Natl Acad. Sci. USA **93**, 3914–3919.

94 Tripodi et al. (1997) Biochem. Biophys. Res. Commun. **237**, 685–689.

95 Van Reeth et al. (1998) Cytogenet. Cell Genet. **81**, 174–175.

96 Van Zutphen et al. (1985) Biochem. Genet. **23**, 599–606.

97 Webb et al. (1997) Cytogenet. Cell Genet. **79**, 151–152.

98 The Wellcome Trust Centre for Human Genetics (http://www.well.ox.ac.uk/~bihoreau).

99 Whitehead Institute for Biomedical Research/MIT Center for Genome Research (http://www.genome.wi.mit.edu/rat/public).

100 Wonigeit (1979) Transplant. Proc. **11**, 1334–1336.

101 Yamada et al. (1994) Mamm. Genome **5**, 63–83.

102 Yamada et al. (1995) Mamm. Genome **6**, 308.

103 Yasue et al. (1991) Cytogenet. Cell Genet. **57**, 142–148.

104 Yasue et al. (1992) Genomics **12**, 659–664.

105 Yokoi et al. (1996) Mamm. Genome **7**, 71–73.

106 Yoshida (1984) Cytogenet. Cell Genet. **37**, 613.

107 Zhang et al. (1988) Cytogenet. Cell Genet. **48**, 121–123.

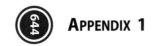
Chromosome 2

Locus symbol	Previous symbol	RNO Location	Description	Mode	Status	Reference	HSA symbol	HSA Chr	MMU symbol	MMU Chr
Acadm		2	Acyl-coenzyme A dehydrogenase, C-4 to C-12 straight-chain	S	**P**	47	*ACADM*	1p31	*Acadm*	3
Adh1		2	Alcohol dehydrogenase (class D, alpha polypeptide, GenBank no. U07347	L,S	**C**	9, 11, 15	*ADH1*	4q21–q23	*Adh1*	3H
Agtr1b		2q24	Angiotensin II receptor, type I (ATIB)	L, S, D	C	4, 10, 17, 30, 49, 52	*AGTR1B*	3q21–q25	*Agtr1b*	3
Ampd1		2	AMP deaminase 1, see also D2Wox37, GenBank no. M37940	L	P	4	*AMPD1*	1p13	*Ampd1*	3
Amy1		2	Amylase 1	L	P	41	*AMX1A*	1p21	*Amy1*	3
Arsb		2	Arylsulfatase B (MPS VI)	S		27	*ARSB*	5p11–q13	*As1*	13
Atp1a1		2q34	ATPase, Na$^+$K$^+$-transporting, alpha 1	L, S, D	C	4, 12, 18, 24, 36, 39, 50, 56, 58	*ATP1A*	1pl3	*Atp1a*	3
Bp6		2, near Cpb	Pulse pressure QTL in LH × LN F2 (LOD: 7.0)	L	P	13				
Bp 10		2, between Npr/Gca and D2N35 (= D2Nih4), i.e. near Atp1a1	Systolic blood pressure QTL in S × WKY and S × MNS F2s: (LOD = 5.66) (note: Atp1a1 has been reported to be mutated in S rats: Ruiz-Opazo et al., 1994) probably same as Bp14, Bp16, Bp19, Bp36	L	P	8, 10				
Bp 13		2, linked to D2Mit6 (and Cpb)	Systolic and diastolic blood pressure QTL in SHRSP × WKY F2 (LOD = 3.3–3.4); possibly same as Bp6	L	P	7				
Bp 14		2, between D2Mit14 and D2Mgh12	Blood pressure QTL in SHRSP × WKY F2 (LOD = 2.0–3. 1: suggestive); possible sex-specific effect (male); possibly same as Bp10, Bp16, Bp19	L	P	7				

Bp 16	2, near Atp1a1, between D2Wox23 (P9ka) and D2Mgh12	Blood pressure QTL in SHR × WKY F2 (LOD > 5); probably same as Bp10	L	P	39				
Bp 17	2, linked to D2N35	Diastolic pressure QTL in SHR × BN RI strains (p = 0.0008: suggestive linkage), linked to D2Nik4	L (RI-stains)	P	35				
Bp 18	2, close to Mtlpb and D2Mgh14	Salt-loaded systolic blood pressure QTL in SHR BN F2 (LOD: 3.0: suggestive), linked to D2Nik4	L	P	40				
Bp 19	2, between D2Mgh8 and Npr/Gca	Salt-loaded systolic blood pressure QTL in SHR × BN F2 (LOD: 6.3)	L	P	40				
Camk2d	2q43	Ca^{2+}/calmodulin-dependent protein kinase II, delta subunit	L, D	C	10, 12, 17, 44, 55, 50, 58				
Cd53	2q34–41	Leukocyte antigen, see also D2Wox27 (= Ox44)	L, S, D	C	2, 18, 51, 57	CD53	1p13	Cd53	3
Cp	2 (or 7?)	Ceruloplasmin	S, D	C	3, 32, 42	CP	3q23–q25	Cp	9D
Cpb	2	Carboxypeptidase B, see also D2Wox15	L, S	C	2, 5–7, 10, 12, 18, 20, 24, 36, 39, 53				
Dhfr1	2	Dihydrofolate reductase 1 (active)	S	P	19	DHFR	5q11.2–q13.2	Dhfr	13
Fg@	2q31–34	Fibrinogen gene cluster				FG@	4q28		
Fga	2q31–34	Fibrinogen alpha polypeptide, see also D2Mit19, D2Wox18	L, D	C	2, 6, 18, 24, 31, 36, 41, 53	FGA	4q28		
Fgb	2q31–34	Fibrinogen beta polypeptide	S, D	C	31, 45, 46	FGB	4q28	Fgb	
Fgg	2q31–34	Fibrinogen gamma polypeptide, see also D2Mit12, D2Wox17, D2Wox18	L, D	C	2, 4, 6, 10, 12, 18, 24, 31, 36, 41, 53, 58	FGG	4q28	Fgg	
Fim3	2	Friend murine leukaemia virus integration site 3 homologue	L	P	21	FIM3	3q26	Fim3	3

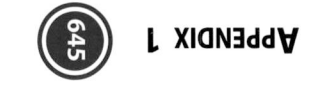

Fst		2	Follistatin, see also D2Wox13	L, S	C	2, 12, 18, 41				
Gstm1		2	Glutathione-S-transferase, mu type 1 (Ybl) (= Gsta3)	S	C	25, 34	GSTM1	1p13.3		
Gstm2		2	Glutathione-S-transferase, mu type 2 (Yb2) (= Gsta4)	S	C	34	GSTM2	1p13.3		
Hagh		2	Hydroxyacyl-glutathione-hydrolase	S	P	56	HAGH	16p13.3	Glo2	17
Hmgcs1		2	3-Hydroxy-3-methylglutaryl-coenzyme A synthase, mitochondrial, see also D2Mgh10	L	P	24	HMGCS1	1p13–p12	Hmgcs1	3
Hsc70ps 1		2	Heat shock cognate protein 70 pseudogene 1	S	P	38				
Hsd3b	Hsd1, RATH, SDI	2	Hydroxy-delta-5-steroid dehydrogenase, 3 beta- and steroid delta-isomerase, see also D2Wox25	L	C	2, 4, 10, 12, 18, 44, 58	HSD3B1	1p13.1	Hsd3b	3
Htr1a		2q16	S-Hydroxytryptamine (serotonin) receptor 1A, see also D2Wox11	L, D	C	12, 18, 22, 41, 42, 50	HTR1A	5cen–q11	Htr1a	13
Il6r		2	Interleukin 6 receptor	S	P	48, 55	IL6R	1q21	Il6r	3
Mcs1		2q1	Mammary cancer susceptibility gene, linked to D2Mit and D2Uwm1	L, S, D	C	22, 43				
Mcsp		2	Mitochondrial selenoprotein	S	P	1		1q21	Mcs	UN
Mlvi2		2	Moloney murine leukaemia virus (MoMuLV) integration site 2 homologue	L, S, D	C	12, 28, 37, 50, 54	MLVI2	5p14–p13	Mlvi2	15
Mme		2	Membrane metallo-endopeptidase/ neutral endopeptidase/enkephalinase (= Nep/CD10)	L	P	9, 10	MME	3q25.1–q25.2	Mme	3
Mt1pb		2	Metallothionein 1, pseudogene B, see also D2Mit3, D2Wox12	L, S	C	4, 6, 18, 24, 28, 41, 53				
Muc1		2	Mucin 1	S	P	26	MUC1	1q21–q23	Muc1	3
Ngfb		2	Nerve growth factor, beta polypeptide	S	C	29	NGFB	1p13	Ngfb	3
Nidd/gk2		2, linked to R8 (P9ka)	Noninsulin-dependent diabetes mellitus (same as Niddm2)	L	P	18				
Niddm2		2, linked to D2Mit14 and D2Mit15	Noninsulin-dependent diabetes mellitus (same as Nidd/gk2?)	L	P	16				

Npr1	Gca, Anpra	2q34	Natriuretic peptide receptor A/guanylate cyclase A, see also D2Mit21, D2Wox24 (= Anpra/Gca)	, D	C	7, 8, 10, 12, 17, 18, 22–24, 36, 39, 50	NPR1	1q21–q22	Npr1	3
Pflg		2	Profilagrin	S	P	41				
Pklr	PK1, PKL, Pklg	2	Pyruvate kinase, liver and RBC, see also D2Mit20, D2Wox19, 20–22		C	2, 6, 7, 14, 18, 20, 24, 36, 53, 58	PKLR	1q21	Pklr	3
Prlr		2	Prolactin receptor, see also D2Wox14	, S	C	2, 4, 6, 10, 12, 18, 28, 41, 42, 53	PRLR	5p14–q13	Prlr	
Rnu1a		2	Small nuclear RNA U1A (Ulb3)	D	P	29	RNN1A	1p36.1		
Slc16a1		2	Monocarboxylate transporter, see also D2Wox36, GenBank no. D63834 (= Mctl)		P	4	SLC16A1	1p13.2–p12	Slc16a1	UN
Tac3r		2	Tachykinin 3 (neuromedin KtNeurokinin B) 2 receptor (= Nmkr)	, S	C	2, 33, 41				
Uri	Uri	2	Uricase, see also D2Mgh13		P	24				

References

1 Adham et al. (1996) DNA Cell Biol. **15**, 159–166.
2 Andoh et al. (1998) Mamm. Genome **9**, 287–293.
3 Baranov et al. (1987) Chromosoma **96**, 60–66.
4 Bihoreau et al. (1997) Genomic Res. **7**, 434–440.
5 Brown et al. (1998) Mamm. Genome **9**, 521–530.
6 Canzian et al. (1996) Jpn J. Cancer Res. **87**, 669–675.
7 Clark et al. (1996) Hypertension **28**, 898–906.
8 Deng and Rapp (1992) Nature Genet. **1**, 267–272.
9 Deng et al. (1997) Hypertension **30**, 199–202.
10 Deng et al. (1994) J. Clin. Invest. **94**, 431–436.
11 Deng et al. (1994) Mamm. Genome **5**, 712–716.
12 Deng et al. (1997) Mamm. Genome **8**, 731–735.
13 Dubay et al. (1993) Nature Genet. **3**, 354–357.
14 Fulchignoni-Lataud et al. (1990) Cytogenet. Cell Genet. **53**, 172–174.
15 Fulchignoni-Lataud et al. (1992) Mamm. Genome **3**, 42–45.
16 Galli et al. (1996) Nature Genet. **12**, 31–37.
17 Garrett et al. (1998) Genome Res. **8**, 711–723.
18 Gauguier et al. (1996) Nature Genet. **12**, 38–43.
19 Hanson et al. (1990) Cytogenet. Cell Genet. **53**, 23–25.
20 Hilbert et al. (1991) Nature **353**, 521–529.
21 Hino et al. (1993) Proc. Natl Acad. Sci. USA **90**, 730–734.
22 Hsu et al. (1994) Cancer Res. **54**, 2765–2770.
23 Jacob et al. (1991) Cell **67**, 213–224.
24 Jacob et al. (1995) Nature Genet. **9**, 63–69.
25 Klinga-Levan et al. (1993) Hereditas **119**, 285–296.
26 Klinga-Levan et al. (1996) Mamm. Genome **7**, 248–250.
27 Kunieda et al. (1995) Genomics **29**, 582–587.
28 Kunieda et al. (1996) Mamm. Genome **7**, 924–925.
29 Levan et al. (1991) Genomics **10**, 699–718.

30 Lewis *et al.* (1993) *Biochem. Biophys. Res. Commun.* **194**, 677–682.

31 Marino *et al.* (1986) *Cytogenet. Cell Genet.* **42**, 36–41.

32 Miura *et al.* (1994) *Cytogenet. Cell Genet.* **65**, 119–121.

33 Mori *et al.* (1992) *Cytogenet. Cell Genet.* **60**, 222–223.

34 Muramatsu *et al.* (1993) *Cytogenet. Cell Genet.* **63**, 141–143.

35 Pravenec *et al.* (1995) *J. Clin. Invest.* **96**, 1973–1978.

36 Pravenec *et al.* (1996) *Mamm. Genome* **7**, 117–127.

37 Qiu *et al.* (1998) *Hereditas* **127**, 263–264.

38 Rothermel *et al.* (1995) *Mamm. Genome* **6**, 602–606.

39 Samani *et al.* (1996) *Hypertension* **28**, 1118–1122.

40 Schork *et al.* (1995) *Genome Res.* **5**, 164–172.

41 Serikawa *et al.* (1992) *Genetics* **131**, 701–721.

42 Shepel *et al.* (1997) *Cytogenet. Cell Genet.* **79**, 176–178.

43 Shepel *et al.* (1998) *Genetics* **149**, 289–299.

44 Shepel *et al.* (1998) *Mamm. Genome* **9**, 622–628.

45 Szpirer *et al.* (1987) *Cytogenet. Cell Genet.* **46**, 701.

46 Szpirer *et al.* (1988) *Cytogenet. Cell Genet.* **47**, 42–45.

47 Szpirer *et al.* (1989) *Cytogenet. Cell Genet.* **50**, 23–26.

48 Szpirer *et al.* (1991) *Genomics* **10**, 539–546.

49 Szpirer *et al.* (1993) *J. Hypertens.* **11**, 919–925.

50 Szpirer *et al.* (1998) *Mamm. Genome* **9**, 721–734.

51 Taguchi *et al.* (1993) *Cytogenet. Cell Genet.* **64**, 217–221.

52 Tissir *et al.* (1995) *Cytogenet. Cell Genet.* **71**, 77–80.

53 Toyota *et al.* (1996) *Proc. Natl Acad. Sci. USA* **93**, 3914–3919.

54 Tsichlis *et al.* (1985) *J. Virol.* **56**, 938–942.

55 Yamada *et al.* (1994) *Mamm. Genome* **5**, 63–83.

56 Yasue *et al.* (1991) *Cytogenet. Cell Genet.* **57**, 142–148.

57 Yokoi *et al.* (1996) *Mamm. Genome* **7**, 71–73.

58 Zha *et al.* (1993) *Cytogenet. Cell Genet.* **63**, 117–122.

Chromosome 3

Locus symbol	Previous symbol	RNO Location	Description	Mode	Status	Reference	HSA symbol	HSA Chr	MMU symbol	MMU Chr
A		3	Agouti (coat colour)	–	C	1, 7, 8, 13, 38, 43, 45, 54, 60, 68	ASIP	20q11.2–q12	a	2
Abl1		3q12	Abelson murine leukaemia viral (v-abl) oncogene homologue 1		C	67	ABL	9q34.1	Abl	2
Acp2		3	Acid phosphatase 2, lysozymal	S	P	75				
Ada		3	Adenosine deaminase	S	P	75	ADA	20q12–q13.1	Ada	2
Adra2b		3	Adrenergic, alpha2B, receptor class III, D3Mco1 and D3Mco2	S, L	C	3, 15, 21, 27, 33, 65	ADRA2B	2p13–q13	Adra2b	2
Ak1		3	Adenylate kinase 1	S	P	39	AK1	9q34.1–q34.2	Ak1	2
Aldr1p1		3	Aldehyde reductase (aldose reductase) (5.1 kb PstI fragment, probably pseudogene)	S	P	22				
Amd3		3	S-Adenosylmethionine decarboxylase 3	S	P	51				
Andpro		3	Androgen regulated 20 kDa protein, D3Wox17	L	P	3				
Avp		3q35 or 3q41–q42	Arginine vasopressin (diabetes insipidus), same as Di (conflicting physical mapping)	L, S, I	C	5, 30, 54, 60	AVP	20p13	Avp	2
B2m		3	Beta-2-microglobulin	S, L	C	2, 36, 41, 76	B2M	15q21–q22	B2m	2
Bcl2l		3q41.2	B cell lymphoma 2 like	I	P	42				
Bdnf		3	Brain-derived neurotrophic factor, GenBank no. D10938, D3Arb11	L	C	2, 78	BDNF	11p13	Bdnf	2
Bmyc		3	Avian myelocytomatosis viral (v-myc)-related oncogene	S	P	26				

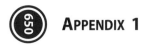

Bp15	3	Blood pressure 15 QTL (linked to D3Mgh16), possible sex specificity (male)	L	P	10, 11				
Bp20	3	Blood pressure QTL, LOD = 3.0, between D3Mgh2 and D3Mit2	L	P	55				
Bp37	3	Blood pressure QTL in F2 (Dahl salt sens. Dahl salt res.), LOD = 3.0 (peak at D3Mgh6)	L	P	18				
Calcrl	3	Calcitonin receptor-like receptor, D3Wox15	L	P	3				
Cat	3q32–q34	Catalase, GenBank no. M11670, M25669 and M23742, D3Mit7 and D3Arb10	I, L, S	C	2, 15, 24, 27, 41, 44, 47, 48, 78	CAT	11p13	Cas1	2
Cebpb	3	Liver-activating protein (LAP, also NF-IL6, nuclear factor-IL6, previously designated TCF5)	S	P	66	CEBPB	20q12–q-13.1	Cebp	2
Cel	3	Carboxyl ester lipase, D3Ucsf4	L	C	47, 49				
Chgb	3	Chromogranin B, parathyroid secretory protein	S	P	40				
Chole	3	Cholesterol esterase (pancreatic), D3Wox12, D3Wox13 and D3Wox26	L	C	3, 5				
Cst4	3	Cystatin S, D1Mgh18 (previously localized to RNO1)	L	I	3, 18, 27				
Cstrp1	3q41	Cystatin-related prostate protein gene 1	I, S	P	16				
Cstrp2	3q41	Cystatin-related prostate protein gene 2	I	P	16				
Edn3	3	Endothelin 3, D3Mco3 and D3Mgh10	L	C	2, 3, 10, 15, 20, 27, 29, 44, 47, 48	EDN3	20q13.2–q13.3	Edn3	2
F	3	Fawn (may not be located on RNO3)	L	P	8				
Fpgs	3	Folylpolyglutamate synthase	S	P	39	FPGS	9cen–q34	Fpgs	2
Gad1	3	Glutamate decarboxylase 1 (brain)	S	P	72	GAD1	2q31	Gad1	2
Ganc	3	Glucosidase, alpha; neutral C	S	P	75				
Gcg	3q22–q24	Glucagon, D3Mgh20	L, I	C	65				
Gnas	3	Guanine nucleotide-binding protein G-s, alpha subunit, GenBank no. U51565, D3Wox4	L	C	3, 29				
Gpd2	3q21–q23	Glycerol-3-phosophate dehydrogenase (mito-chondrial), D3Mgh21	L, I	C	5, 33, 65				

Grin1	3	Glutamate receptor, ionotropic, N-methyl D-aspartate 1	S	P	37	GRIN1	9q34.3	Grin1	2
Gstpl1	3q11–q12	Glutathione-S-transferase-like 1, pi type	S, I	C	31, 76				
Hao1	3	Hydroxyacid oxidase 1 (glycolate oxidase, Gox1)	L	C	13, 35, 36, 46, 47, 48, 50, 57, 70, 74			Hao1	2
Hdc	3	Histidine decarboxylase	S	P	61	HDC	15	Hdc	2
Hnf3b	3q41	Hepatocyte nuclear factor 3 beta	I	P	69				
Hoxd3	3	Homeobox gene D3	S	P	9	HOX@	2q31	Hox@	2
Il1a	3	Interleukin 1 alpha, D3Kyo4	S	P	34	IL1A	2q13	Il1a	2
Il1b	3	Interleukin 1 beta, D3M2Nds3	L, S	C	2, 34, 36, 44, 68	IL1B	2q13–q21	Il1b	2
Itga4	3	Integrin alpha 4	S	P	64	ITGA4	2q31–q32	Itga4	2
Itpa	3	Inosine trisphosphatase (nucleoside triphosphate pyrophosphatase)	S	P	75	ITPA	20p13	Itp	2
Ivd	3	Isovaleryl-coenzyme A dehydrogenase, microsatellite primer R53	S,	C	7, 36, 57, 63, 68				
Krt10l	3	K51 keratin-like locus	I	P	4				
Map1a	3q36	Microtubule-associated protein 1a	I	P	28				
Mdhl	3	Malate dehydrogenase-like enzyme	L	P	43				
Pax1	3	Paired box homeotic gene 1	L	P	46				
Pck1	3	Phosphoenolpyruvate carboxykinase, microsatellite primer R45 and R57, D3Mgh26	S, L	C	7, 17, 24, 36, 57, 68	PCK1	20q13.2	Pok1	2
Pe	3	Pearl (rat coat colour)	L	P	52				
Plcb1	3	Phospholipase C-beta1, D3Wox22	I, L	C	3, 6			Plcb	2
Plcb4	3	Phospholipase C (beta4), D3Wox21	L	P	3				
Prnp	3q35	Prion protein, structural, microsatellite primer prnpms	L, S, I	C	2, 36	PRNP	20pter–p12	Prn	2
Ptgs1	3	Prostaglandin G/H synthase I, RFLP marker	L	P	78	PTGS1	9	Ptgs1	2
Ptp	3	Protein-tyrosine phosphatase, microsatellite primer R156, D3Wox6	S, L	C	20, 29, 36, 57				
Rdy	3	Retinal dystrophy	L	P	38				

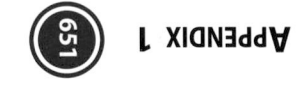

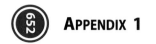

Rnr1	3	Ribosomal 18S and 28S RNA gene 1	I	C	53, 62				
Scn2a1	3	Sodium channel, voltage-gated, type II, alpha polypeptide, GenBank no. X03639, micro-satellite primer R69, D3Mit8, D3Wox9, D3Wox10, D3Wox14 and D3Arb7	S, L	C	2, 3, 7, 15, 20, 24, 27, 35, 44, 47–49, 57, 68, 73, 76, 78	*SCN2A1*	2q23	*Scn2a* 2
Sdc4	3	Ryudocan/syndecan 4, GenBank no. M81786, D3Wox5 and D3Arb12	L	C	2, 20, 78				
Slc12a1	3	Solute carrier family 12, member 1 (bumetanide-sensitive sodium-[potassium]-chloride cotransporter)	L	P	73				
Snap25	3	Synaptosomal-associated protein, 25 kDa, D3M2Mit28 and D3M2Nds33	L	C	36, 38, 78				
Sord	3	Sorbitol dehydrogenase	S	P	75				
Sp3	3q24–q31	*Trans*-acting transcription factor 3	I	P	56				
Stnl	3	Statin-like protein, GenBank no. M62752, D3Wox8 and D3Arb15	L	C	2, 3, 5, 20, 78				
Svp1	3	Seminal vesicle protein, secretion 1 (electrophoretic polymorphism of the protein), D3Wox7	L, S	C	1, 10, 13, 19, 20, 24, 29, 32, 36, 38, 45–48, 57, 70, 71, 74	*SEMG1*	20q12–q13.1	*Svp1* 2
Svp2	3	Seminal vesicle protein, secretion 2 (electrophoretic polymorphism of the protein)	L, S	C	2, 7, 46, 68, 71				
Svs2	3	Seminal vesicle protein, secretion 2, microsatellite marker, microsatellite primer R142, D3Arb13	L	C	24, 29, 35, 36, 41, 46, 57, 68, 78				
Svs4	3	Seminal vesicle protein 4, D3Mgh3	L	C	27, 32				
Tbm2	3	Tubular basement membrane antigen 2	L	P	23				
Wt1	3	Wilms' tumour 1	S	P	77	*WT1*	11p13	*Wt1* 2
Yy	3	Peptide tyrosine-tyrosine (YY), D3Wox23	L	P	3				
Zi	3	Zitter	L	C	36, 41, 57, 74				

References

1. Adams *et al.* (1984) *Biochem. Genet.* **22**, 611–629.
2. Andoh *et al.* (1998) *Mamm. Genome* **9**, 287–293.
3. Bihoreau *et al.* (1997) *Genome Res.* **7**, 434–440.
4. Biltueva *et al.* (1996) *Cytogenet. Cell Genet.* **73**, 209–213.
5. Brown *et al.* (1998) *Mamm. Genome* **9**, 521–530.
6. Calabrese *et al.* (1995) *Mamm. Genome* **6**, 549–550.
7. Canzian *et al.* (1996) *Jpn. J. Cancer Res.* **87**, 669–675.
8. Castle and King (1949) *Proc. Natl Acad. Sci. USA* **35**, 545–546.
9. Chung *et al.* (1993) *Mamm. Genome* **4**, 537–540.
10. Cicila *et al.* (1994) *J. Hypertens.* **12**, 643–651.
11. Clark *et al.* (1996) *Hypertension* **28**, 898–906.
12. Courvoisier *et al.* (1997) *Mamm. Genome* **8**, 282–283.
13. Cramer *et al.* (1986) *Biochem. Genet.* **24**, 217–227.
14. Dene *et al.* (1998) *Mamm. Genome* **9**, 517–520.
15. Deng *et al.* (1994) *J. Clin. Invest.* **93**, 2701–2709.
16. Devos *et al.* (1995) *Cytogenet. Cell Genet.* **68**, 239–242.
17. Fulchignoni-Lataud *et al.* (1992) *Mamm. Genome* **3**, 42–45.
18. Garrett *et al.* (1998) *Genome Res.* **8**, 711–723.
19. Gasser (1972) *Biochem. Genet.* **6**, 61–63.
20. Gauguier *et al.* (1996) *Nature Genet.* **12**, 38–43.
21. Ginn *et al.* (1994) *J. Hypertens.* **12**, 357–365.
22. Graham *et al.* (1991) *Gene* **107**, 259–267.
23. Guery *et al.* (1989) *Immunogenetics* **17**, 55–65.
24. Hilbert *et al.* (1991) *Nature* **353**, 521–529.
25. Hino *et al.* (1996) *Rat Genome* **2**, 6–9.
26. Ingvarsson *et al.* (1988) *Mol. Cell. Biol.* **8**, 3168–3174.
27. Jacob *et al.* (1995) *Nature Genet.* **9**, 63–69.
28. Johansson *et al.* (1998) *Cytogenet. Cell Genet.* **81**, 217–221.
29. Kato *et al.* (1996) *Mamm. Genome* **7**, 628–629.
30. Khegay (1996) *Mamm. Genome* **7**, 867.
31. Klinga-Levan *et al.* (1993) *Hereditas* **119**, 285–296.
32. Kobayashi (1992) *Biochem. Genet.* **30**, 339–346.
33. Koike *et al.* (1996) *Genomics* **38**, 96–99.
34. Kondo *et al.* (1993) *Mamm. Genome* **4**, 571–576.
35. Kuramoto *et al.* (1993) *Acta Histochem. Cytochem.* **26**, 325–332.
36. Kuramoto *et al.* (1994) *Biochem. Biophys. Res. Commun.* **200**, 1161–1168.
37. Kuramoto *et al.* (1994) *Genomics* **19**, 358–61.
38. LaVail (1981) *J. Hered.* **72**, 294–296.
39. Levan *et al.* (1986) *Rat News Lett.* **17**, 3–8.
40. Mahata *et al.* (1996) *Genomics* **33**, 135–139.
41. Maihara *et al.* (1995) *Transplant. Proc.* **27**, 1502–1504.
42. Matsuda *et al.* (1996) *Cytogenet. Cell Genet.* **74**, 107–110.
43. Matsumoto *et al.* (1982) *Biochem. Genet.* **20**, 443–448.
44. Matsumoto *et al.* (1998) *Mamm. Genome* **9**, 531–535.
45. Moutier *et al.* (1973) *Biochem. Genet.* **8**, 321–328.
46. Otsen *et al.* (1995) *Mamm. Genome* **6**, 666–667.
47. Pravenec *et al.* (1996) *Folia Biol. (Praha)* **42**, 147–153.
48. Pravenec *et al.* (1996) *Mamm. Genome* **7**, 117–127.
49. Pravenec *et al.* (1996) *Mamm. Genome* **7**, 559–560.
50. Prins *et al.* (1985) *Rat News Lett.* **15**, 19.
51. Pulkka *et al.* (1993) *Genomics* **16**, 342–349.
52. Robinson (1994) *J. Hered.* **85**, 142–143.
53. Sasaki *et al.* (1986) *Cytogenet. Cell Genet.* **41**, 83–88.
54. Schmale and Richter (1984) *Nature* **308**, 705–709.
55. Schork *et al.* (1995) *Genome Res.* **5**, 164–172.
56. Scohy *et al.* (1998) *Cytogenet. Cell Genet.* **81**, 273–274.
57. Serikawa *et al.* (1992) *Genetics* **131**, 701–721.
58. Shepel *et al.* (1998) *Mamm. Genome* **9**, 622–628.
59. Shisa *et al.* (1997) *Mamm. Genome* **8**, 324–327.
60. Stolc (1984) *Biochem. Genet.* **22**, 893–899.
61. Sullivan *et al.* (1991) *J. Biol. Chem.* **266**, 143–154.
62. Szabo *et al.* (1978) *Chromosoma* **65**, 161–172.
63. Szpirer *et al.* (1989) *Cytogenet. Cell Genet.* **50**, 23–26.

64   Szpirer *et al.* (1992) *Mamm. Genome* **3**, 685–688.

65   Szpirer *et al.* (1997) *Mamm. Genome* **8**, 586–588.

66   Szpirer *et al.* (1991) *Genomics* **10**, 539–546.

67   Takahashi *et al.* (1986) *Proc. Natl Acad. Sci. USA* **83**, 1079–1083.

68   Toyota *et al.* (1996) *Proc. Natl Acad. Sci. USA* **93**, 3914–3919.

69   Van Reeth *et al.* (1998) *Cytogenet. Cell Genet.* **81**, 174–175.

70   Van Zutphen *et al.* (1985) *Rat News Lett.* **15**, 19–20.

71   Van Zutphen *et al.* (1985) *Biochem. Genet.* **19**, 173–186.

72   Vassort *et al.* (1993) *Mamm. Genome* **4**, 202–206.

73   Wang *et al.* (1997) *Mamm. Genome* **8**, 379.

74   Yamada *et al.* (1989) *J. Hered.* **80**, 383–386.

75   Yasue *et al.* (1991) *Cytogenet. Cell Genet.* **57**, 142–148.

76   Yasue *et al.* (1992) *Genomics* **12**, 659–664.

77   Yeung *et al.* (1993) *Mamm. Genome* **4**, 585–588.

78   Zha *et al.* (1994) *Mamm. Genome* **5**, 538–541.

Chromosome 4

Locus symbol	Previous symbol	RNO Location	Description	Mode	Status	Reference	HSA symbol	HSA Chr	MMU symbol	MMU Chr
A2m		4	Alpha-2-macroglobulin (D4Mit20, D4Wox16)	S, L	C	18, 24, 33, 50, 51, 74				
Ad-cyap1r1		4	Rat pituitary adenylate cyclase-activating polypeptide 1 receptor	S	P	6				
Ad-cyap1r3		4	Rat pituitary adenylate cyclase-activating polypeptide 1 receptor	S	P	6				
Add2		4	Adducin beta	-	P	70	ADD2	2pter–2q-ter	Add2	6
Aldr1		4	Aldehyde reductase 1 (low K_m aldose reductase) (5.8 kb PstI fragment, probably the functional gene) (D4Mgh16, D4Arb10)	S	C	19, 20	ALDR1	7q35	Aldr1	3
Aldr1p2		4	Aldehyde reductase (aldose reductase) (7.5 kb PstI fragment, probably pseudogene)	S	P	20				
Ampp		4	Amplicon, Py-induced (D4Mit18, D4Wox17 and D4Arb16)	S	C	3, 9, 18, 33, 50, 52, 56, 68				
Apex2		4q12	Apurinic/apyrimidinic endonuclease 2	D	P	34				
Atp2b2		4q41.3–q42.1	ATPase isoform 2, Na$^+$,K$^+$-transporting, beta polypeptide 2	D	P	2	ATP2B2	3p26–p25	Atp2b2	6
Cacn-l1a1		4	Ca channel, L type, alpha 1(D4Arb4, D4Mgh30)	L	C	19, 52				
Cd4		4	CD4 antigen (p55)	L	P	14				
Cd8a		4	CD8 antigen, alpha chain	L	P	14				
Cd8b		4	CD8 antigen, beta chain	L	P	14				
Cd9		4	CD9 antigen (p24)	L	P	16				
Cd94		4	CD94 antigen (located within the rat natural killer gene complex)	L	P	17				

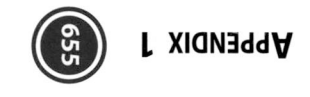

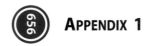

Cftr	4	Cystic fibrosis transmembrane conductance regulator	S	P	69	CFTR	7q31.3	Cftr	6
Cia3	4	Type II collagen-induced arthritis 3	L		21, 52				
Cpa1	4	Carboxypeptidase A1 (pancreatic) (D4Mit3)	L	C	15, 32	CPA1	7q32	Cpa	6
Cpa2	4	Carboxypeptidase A2 (pancreatic)	S, L	C	9, 56, 68				
Ddit1	4q31–q33	DNA damage-inducible transcript 1	D	P	59				
Dhfr2	4	Dihydrofolate reductase (probably pseudo-gene)	S	P	23				
Egr4l1	4	Zinc-finger transcription factor NGFI-C (early response gene), member of the GCGGGGGCG (GSG) element-binding protein family (D4Arb6)	L	P	19				
Eno2	4	Enolase 2, gamma, neuronal (D4Wox14, D4Wox15, D4Mit3, D4Mit31)	S, L, D	C	3, 14, 18, 19, 24, 33, 44, 50, 51, 59				
Fabp1	4	Fatty acid binding protein 1 liver (D4Mit12, D4Wox20, D4Arb21)	S, L	C	9, 18, 33, 52, 56, 68	FABP1	2p11	Fabp1	6
Gata2	4q34–q41	GATA-binding protein 2	D	P	46				
Grin2b	4	Glutamate receptor, ionotropic N-methyl D-aspartate 2B	S	P	38	GRIN2B	12p12	Grin2b	6
Grm3	4	Glutamate receptor, metabotropic 3	S	P	38				
Grpca	4q43–q44	Glutamine/glutamic acid-rich protein A	S, D	C	66				
Grpcb	4q43–q44	Glutamine/glutamic acid-rich protein B	S, D	C	66				
Hgf	4q12	Hepatocyte growth factor (scatter factor)	S, D	C	61, 71	HGF	7q21.1	Hgf	5
Hisr	4	Histamine receptor H1	S	P	42				
Hk2	4q34	Hexokinase	D	P	55				
Hoxa11	4	Homeobox gene A11	L	P	27				
Hoxa4	4	Homeobox gene A4	S	P	10				
Hoxa7	4	Homeobox gene A7	S	P	10				
Hoxa@	4	Homeobox A gene cluster region	S	P	10	HOXA@	7p15–p14	Hox@	6
Iapp	4	Islet amyloid polypeptide (D4Wox12, D4Arb1)	L	C	18, 19, 52	IAPP	12p12.3–p12.1	Iapp	6

Igk@		4	Immunoglobulin kappa chain gene cluster (D4Mit8)	D S, L	C	11, 32, 47	*IGK*	2p12	*Igk*	6
Igkc		4	Immunoglobulin kappa constant region	L, S	C	11, 32, 47				
Il6		4	Interleukin 6 (interferon beta 2) (D4Wox27, D4Arb14)	L, S	C	1, 3, 4, 9, 19, 30, 33, 44, 50, 51, 53, 56, 64, 67, 68	*IL6*	7p21–p15	*Il6*	5
Kap		4	Kidney androgen-regulated protein	L	P	16				
Kcna		4	Potassium (K+) channel protein, voltage-dependent	S	P	56	*KCNA1*	12q13	*Kcna1*	6
Klk1rs		4	Kallikrein-related sequence	L	P	50				
Klrb1@	*NKRP1*	4	Killer cell lectin-like receptor subfamily B, member 1 gene cluster	L	P	13, 16				
Kras2		4	Kirsten rat sarcoma viral oncogene homologue 2 (active)	S	P	63	*KRAS2*	12p21.1	*Kras2*	6
Ldhb		4	Lactate dehydrogenase B	S	P	80	*LDHB*	12p12.2–p12.1	*Ldh2*	6
Lxm		4	Polydactyly-luxate syndrome modifier gene	L	P	35				
Ly49		4	Lymphocye antigen 49 complex	L	P	16				
Mem1		4q34–q41	Maternal embryonic message 1	D	P	46				
Met		4q21	Met proto-oncogene	S, D	C	26, 71, 75	*MET*	7q31	*Met*	6
Mitf		4q34–q41	Microphthalmia-associated transcription factor	D	C	46, 62				
Nkrp2		4	NKR-P2, orthologue of human NKG2D	L	P	16				
Nos3		4q11	Endothelial nitric oxide synthase 3	S, L, D	C	30, 53, 59	*NOS3*	7q35–q36	*Nos*	5
Npy		4	Neuropeptide Y (D4Wox21, D4Hri1, D4Mgh4, D4Wox22, D4Arb7, D4Mit7, D4Mit23)	S, L	C	3, 18, 19, 27, 29, 32, 33, 50, 51, 56	*NPY*	7pter–7q-22	*Npy*	6
Pap1		4q33–q34	Pancreatitis-associated protein 1	D	P	58				
Pap2		4q33–q34	Pancreatitis-associated protein 2	D	P	58				
Pap3		4q33–q34	Pancreatitis-associated protein 3	D	P	58				
Pgy1		4q12	P-glycoprotein/multidrug resistance 1	S	C	22, 48	*PGY1*	7q21.1	*Pgy*	5
Pgy2		4q11–q12	P-glycoprotein 2/multidrug resistance 1b	D	C	48, 78			*Pgy2*	5

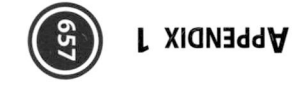

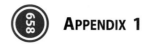

Pgy3	4q11–q12	P-glycoprotein 3/multidrug resistance 2	D	C	78				
Ppta3	4	?, see also D4Mgh31	L	C	32, 44				
Prpb	4	Proline-rich protein, salivary (D4Wox13 and D4Arb2)	S, L	C	18, 19, 67, 77				
Prss1	4	Trypsin 1 (D4Hri2, D4Wox24, D4Arb8 and D4Mgh32)	S, L	C	3, 9, 18, 19, 27, 29, 50, 51, 53, 56, 68				
Prss2	4	Pancreatic trypsin II (D4Wox23 and D4Arb9)	L	C	4, 19, 53, 67				
Pthlh	4q44	Parathyroid-like peptide (D4Wox11)	S, L, D	C	3, 9, 16, 18, 50, 51, 56, 59, 60, 68	*PTHLH*	12p12.1–p11.2	*Pthlh*	6
Ptn	4	Pleiotrophin (heparin-binding factor, Hbnf, in the mouse)	L	C	28				
Raf1	4q42	Murine leukaemia viral (v-*raf*-1) oncogene homologue 1 (3611-MSV)	S, D	C	26, 31, 79	*RAF1*	3p25	*Raf1*	6
Reg	4q33–q34	Regeneration protein, lithostatin, pancreatic stone protein (D4Wox28)	S, D	C	3, 4, 58, 67, 77				
Ret	4	Ret proto-oncogene (multiple endocrine neoplasia MEN2A, MEN2B and medullary thyroid carcinoma 1, Hirschsprung disease)	L	C	7–9, 68	*RET*	10q11.2	*R*	6
Rho	4	Rhodopsin (retinitis pigmentosa 4, autosomal dominant)	S	P	25	*RHO*	3q21.3–q-24	*Rho*	6
Rl	4q11.2	Reeler	D	P	41				
RT8	4	Cell surface alloantigen	L	C	1, 36, 37, 50				
Scnn1a	4q42	Sodium channel, nonvoltage-gated 1, alpha (epithelial)	–	P	59				
Sdf1	4q42.1	Stromal cell-derived factor 1	D	P	45				
Slc4a2	4q11	Solute carrier family 4, member 2, anion exchange protein 2 (D4Bro1)	L, D	C	1, 33, 51, 57				
Spr	4	Substance P receptor (D4Wox19, D4Mit23 and D4Mgh17 (exon 1))	S, D		18, 24, 50				

Tac1	4	Tachykinin (substance P, neurokinin A, neuropeptide K, neuropeptide gamma) (D4Mit1, D4Wox30)	L	C	4, 32, 67	NKNA	7q21.3-q-22.1	Tac1	6
Tac1r	4	Tachykinin 1 receptor (substance P receptor, neurokinin 1 receptor) (D4Mgh17)	L	C	3, 9, 24, 33, 43, 56, 68, 73				
Tbxas1	4q21–q22	Thromboxane synthase	D	P	65				
Tcp1l	4	T-complex 1-like 1	S	P	73, 74				
Tcrb	4	T-cell receptor, beta cluster (D4Mit4 and D4Arb12)	S, L	C	15, 19, 32, 40	TCRB	7q35	Tcrb	6
Tgfa	4	Transforming growth factor alpha (D4Wox18 and D4Arb5)	S, L	C	18, 19, 56, 75	TGFA	2p13	Tgfa	6
Tpi1	4	Triosephosphate isomerase 1	S	P	39	TPI1	12p13	Tpi	6
Vhl	4q41.3–q42.1	von Hippel–Lindau syndrome	D	C	2, 76				

References

1 Aitman et al. (1997) Nature Genet. **16**, 197–201.

2 Aldaz et al. (1995) Cytogenet. Cell Genet. **71**, 253–256.

3 Andoh et al. (1998) Mamm. Genome **9**, 287–293.

4 Bihoreau et al. (1997) Genomic Res. **7**, 434–440.

5 Brown et al. (1998) Mamm. Genome **9**, 521–530

6 Cai et al. (1995) Cytogenet. Cell Genet. **71**, 193–196.

7 Canzian et al. (1994) Xth International Workshop on Alloantigenic Systems in the Rat, Sapporo, Japan.

8 Canzian et al. (1995) Mamm. Genome **6**, 433–435.

9 Canzian et al. (1996) Jpn. J. Cancer Res. **87**, 669–675.

10 Chung et al. (1993) Mamm. Genome **4**, 537–540.

11 Collard et al. (1982) Cytogenet. Cell Genet. **32**, 257–258.

12 Dahlman et al. (1998) Eur. J. Immunol. **28**, 2188–2(196

13 Dissen and Fossum (1993) Intl. Workshop on Alloantipenic Systems in the Rat

14 Dissen and Fossum (1996) Immunogenet. **44**, 312–314.

15 Dissen et al. (1993) Immunogenet. **37**, 153–156.

16 Dissen et al. (1996) J. Exp. Med. **183**, 2197–2207.

17 Dissen et al. (1997) Eur. J. Immunol. **27**, 2080–2086.

18 Gauguier et al. (1996) Nature Genet. **12**, 38–43.

19 Goldmuntz et al. (1995) Mamm. Genome **6**, 459–463.

20 Graham et al. (1991) Gene **107**, 259–267.

21 Griffiths et al. (1996) XIth International Workshop on Alloantigenic Systems in the Rat, Toulouse, France.

22 Hanson et al. (1988) Bio-Science

23 Hanson et al. (1990) Cytogenet. Cell Genet. **53**, 23–25.

24 Hilbert et al. (1991) Nature **353**, 521–529.

25 Hino et al. (1993) Proc. Natl Acad. Sci. USA **90**, 730–734.

26 Hino et al. (1993) Proc. Natl Acad. Sci. USA **90**, 327–331.

27 Hornum and Markholst (1995) Mamm. Genome **6**, 559–560.

28 Hornum and Markholst (1996) Mamm. Genome **7**, 923.

29 Hornum et al. (1995) Mamm. Genome **6**, 371–372.

30 Hübner et al. (1995) Mamm. Genome **6**, 758–759.

31 Ingvarsson et al. (1988) Somat. Cell Mol. Genet. **14**, 401–405.

32 Jacob et al. (1992) Nature Genet. **2**, 56–60.

33 Jacob et al. (1995) Nature Genet. **9**, 63–69.

34 Johansson *et al.* (1998) *Cytogenet. Cell Genet.* **81**, 217–221.

35 Kren *et al.* (1990) *Transplant. Proc.* **22**, 2588–2589.

36 Kren *et al.* (1993) IXth International Workshop on Alloantigenic Systems in the Rat, Hannover, Germany.

37 Kren *et al.* (1993) *Transplant. Proc.* **25**, 2777.

38 Kuramoto *et al.* (1994) *Genomics* **19**, 358–361.

39 Levan *et al.* (1986) *Rat News Lett.* **17**, 3–8.

40 Levan *et al.* (1991) *Genomics* **10**, 699–718.

41 Matsuda *et al.* (1996) *Mamm. Genome* **7**, 468–469.

42 Moguilevsky *et al.* (1994) *Eur. J. Biochem.* **224**, 489–495.

43 Mori *et al.* (1992) *Cytogenet. Cell Genet.* **60**, 222–223.

44 National Institute of Arthritis and Musculoskeletal and Skin Diseases. The ARB Rat Genetic Database (http://www.nih.gov/niams/scientific/ratgbase/index.htm).

45 Nomura *et al.* (1996) *Cytogenet. Cell Genet.* **73**, 286–289.

46 Opdecamp *et al.* (1998) *Mamm. Genome* **9**, 617–621.

47 Perlmann *et al.* (1985) *Immunogenet.* **22**, 97–100.

48 Popescu *et al.* (1993) *Genomics* **15**, 182–184.

49 Pravenec *et al.* (1995) *J. Clin. Invest.* **96**, 1973–1978.

50 Pravenec *et al.* (1996) *Mamm. Genome* **7**, 117–127.

51 Pravenec *et al.* (1997) *Mamm. Genome* **8**, 387–389.

52 Remmers *et al.* (1996) *Nature Genet.* **14**, 82–85.

53 Rubattu *et al.* (1996) *Nature Genet.* **13**, 429–434.

54 Schork *et al.* (1995) *Genome Res.* **5**, 164–172.

55 Sebastian *et al.* (1997) *Cytogenet. Cell Genet.* **77**, 266–267.

56 Serikawa *et al.* (1992) *Genetics* **131**, 701–721.

57 Simon *et al.* (1996) *Mamm. Genome* **7**, 380–382.

58 Stephanova *et al.* (1996) *Cytogenet. Cell Genet.* **72**, 83–85.

59 Szpirer C. et al. (1998) *Mamm. Genome* **9**, 721–734

60 Szpirer *et al.* (1991) *Cytogenet. Cell Genet.* **56**, (193-)(195.)

61 Szpirer *et al.* (1992) *Genomics* **13**, 293–300.

62 Szpirer *et al.* (1997) 11th International Mouse Genome Conference, Florida, USA.

63 Szpirer *et al.* (1985) *Somat. Cell Mol. Genet.* **11**, 93–97.

64 Szpirer *et al.* (1991) *Genomics* **10**, 539–546.

65 Takeuchi *et al.* (1996) *Cytogenet. Cell Genet.* **76**, 47–48.

66 Ten Hagen *et al.* (1997) *Biochem. J.* **324**, 177–184.

67 The Wellcome Trust Centre for Human Genetics (http://www.well.ox.ac.uk/~bihoreau).

68 Toyota *et al.* (1996) *Proc. Natl Acad. Sci. USA* **93**, 3914–3919.

69 Trezise *et al.* (1992) *Genomics* **14**, 869–874.

70 Tripodi *et al.* (1995) *Gene* **166**, 307–311.

71 Wallenius *et al.* (1997) *Mamm. Genome* **8**, 661–667.

72 Whitehead Institute for Biomedical Research/MIT Center for Genome Research (http://www.genome.wi.mit.edu/rat/public).

73 Yamada *et al.* (1994) *Mamm. Genome* **5**, 63–83.

74 Yasue *et al.* (1992) *Genomics* **12**, 659–664.

75 Yeung *et al.* (1993) *Mamm. Genome* **4**, 585–588.

76 Yeung *et al.* (1993) *Proc. Natl Acad. Sci. USA* **90**, 8038–8042.

77 Yokoi *et al.* (1996) *Mamm. Genome* **7**, 71–73.

78 Zimonjic *et al.* (1996) *Mamm. Genome* **7**, 630–631.

79 Zullo and Upender (1995) *Genomics* **25**, 753–756.

80 Yasue *et al.* (1991) *Cytogenet. Cell Genet.* **57**, 142–148.

Locus symbol	Previous symbol	RNO Location	Description	Mode	Status	Reference	HSA symbol	HSA Chr	MMU symbol	MMU Chr
Aco1	Acon1	5	Aconitase 1, soluble	L	C	1–5	ACO1	2p22–q32	Aco1	4cen-C2
Ak2		5	Adenylate kinase 2	S	P	6, 7	AK2	1p34	Ak2	4
Aldh1	AHD2, Aldh2	5	Aldehyde dehydrogenase 2 (= aldehyde dehydrogenase 1 in other species)	L	C	3, 8	ALDH1	9q21	Aldh1	19
Aldob	LIV10	5	Aldolase B, fructose-biphosphate	S	P	9–11	ALDOB	9q22.3–q31	Aldo2	4
An	an-1	5	Anaemia	L	P	12–14			an	4
Bp7		5	Blood pressure 7, systolic pressure, QTL (possible candidate gene: Edn2). In an F2 (Dahl salt × sens. Dahl salt res.), LOD = 4.5 between D5Mit9 and D5Mco10 (peak at Edn2)	L	C	15, 16				
C8b		5	Complement component 8, beta polypeptide, see also D5Rhm3 and D5Rhm4	L	P	17	C8B	1p32	C8b	4
Cd30		5q36.2	Tumour necrosis factor superfamily, member CD30	A	P	18				
Cdkn2a	MTS1, INK4A	5q32–q34	Cyclin-dependent kinase inhibitor 2A (p16, inhibits CDK4)	A	P	19				
Cdkn2b		5q31–q33	Cyclin-dependent kinase inhibitor 2B (p15, inhibits CDK4)	A	P	19				
Cu1		5	Curly	L	P	13, 14				
Cyp4a11	Cyp4a2	5	Cytochrome P450, subfamily IVA, polypeptide 11, see also D5Mcw1, D5Wox12 and D5Wox2	L	C	20–24	CYP4B1	1p34–p12	Cyp4a10	4
Cyp4b1		5	Cytochrome P450, subfamily IVB, polypeptide 1, see also D5M4Rp1	S	P	10, 25				

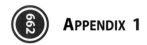

Dsi1		5	Moloney murine leukaemia virus integration site, rat homologure (David Steffen), see also D5Uwm5 and D5Wox14	S L	C	10. 25–27			*Dsi1*	4
Ece	*Ednce, Ednce1*	5	Endothelin-converting enzyme, see also D5Mco18	L	P	28	*ECE*	UN		
Edn2	*Et2*	5	Endothelin isopeptide 2, see also D5Mco19	S, L	P	15	*EDN2*	1p34	*Edn2*	UN
Ela2	*ELAII, Elaii1*	5	Elastase 2, pancreatic, GenBank no. L00118, see also D5Arb14	L	C	15, 24, 26, 29endash 32	*ELA2*	19p13.3	*Ela2*	UN
Eno1		5	Enolase 1 alpha	S	P	7, 33	*ENO1*	1p36	*Eno1*	4
Erk		5q36.13	ELK-related protein tyrosine kinase	A	P	34	*ERK*	1p36.1	*Erk*	4D2.2-3
Fuca		5	Fucosidase, alpha-L-1, tissue, see also D5Mco22	S, L	C	24, 29, 32, 35	*FUCA1*	1p35–p34	*Fuca*	4
Gdh		5	Glucose dehydrogenase	S	P	35	*GDH*	1p36		
Ggtb2		5	Glycoprotein-4-beta-galactosyltransferase 2	S	P	10, 25	*GGTB2*	9p21–p13	*Ggtb*	4
Gnb1		5	Guanine nucleotide-binding protein beta 1	L	P	36	*GNB1*	1p36–p31.2	*Gnb1*	4
Gstpl2	*GSTPL2*	5q13–q21	Glutathione-*S*-transferase-like 2, pi type	S, A	C	37, 38				
Hd		5	Rat hypodactyly	L	P	39				
Ifna		5q31–q33	Interferon alpha (leukocyte)	S, L, A	C	17, 40–42	*IFN1@*	9p22	*Ifa*	4C3-C6
Ifnb1		5q31–q33	Interferon beta 1, fibroblast	S	P	10, 25	*IFNB1*	9p22	*Ifb*	4C3-C6
In	*ia*	5	Incisorless	L	P	39, 43				
Je		5	Jerker, deafness locus	L	P	36			*je*	4
Jun		5q31–q33	Avian sarcoma virus 17 (v-*jun*) oncogene homologue	S, L	C	4, 8, 27, 44	*JUN*	1p32–p31	*Jun*	4
Lck	*Lck1, Lcktkr*	5	Lymphocyte-specific protein tyrosine kinase, see also D5Wox15	S, L	C	10, 17, 25, 45, 46	*LCK*	1p35–p34.3	*Lck*	4
Lepr	*Fa*	5	Leptin receptor (fatty)	L	C	17, 47			*db*	4
Mos		5	Moloney murine sarcoma viral (v-*mos*) oncogene homologue	S	C	10, 25, 41	*MOS*	8q11	*Mos*	4
Mup1	*A2UG*	5	Major urinary protein, alpha-2U-globulin, see also D5Wox9 and D5Wox13	L, A, S	C	3, 10, 20, 22, 25, 48–50			*Mup1*	4

Mycl1		5	Avian myelocytomatosis viral (v-myc) related oncogene homologue 1, lung carcinoma derived (L-myc)	S	P	51	MYCL1	1p32	Lmyc1	4
Nidd/gk4		5	Noninsulin-dependent diabetes mellitus (QTL)	L	P	22				
Nppa	ANF, ANP, Pnd	5	Natriuretic peptide precursor A, (pronatrio-dilatin, also Anf, Pnd), GenBank no. J03267 and K02062, see also D5Wox10	S, L	C	3, 8, 10, 15, 22, 24–26, 52	NPPA	1p36	Nppa	4
Nppb	Bnf	5	Brain natriuretic factor	L	P	26				
Oprd1		5	Opioid receptor	L	P	36	OPRD1	1p36.1–p34.3	Oprd1	4
Orm	AGP	5	Orosomucoid 1	S	P	10, 25	ORM1	9q32	Orm1	4C2-C7
Pbpc1		5q31	Prostatic-binding protein C1	A	P	53				
Pbpc3		5q21–q31	Prostatic-binding protein C3	A	P	53				
Pde4b		5q32	Phosphodiesterase 4B, cAMP-specific (dunce (Drosophila) homologue phosphodiesterase E4)	S, A	C	54, 55	PDE4B	1p31	Pde4b	4
Penk		5q13	Proenkephalin, see also D5Mgh2	L, A	C	20, 52, 56	PENK	8q11.23–q12	Penk	9
Pfkfb1l		5	6-Phosphofructo-2-kinase/fructose-2,6-bis-phosphatase 1-like (related) sequence	L	P	29				
Pgd		5	Phosphogluconate dehydrogenase	L, S	C	3, 7, 33, 57, 58	PGD	1p36.3–p36.13	Pgd	4
Pgm1		5	Phosphoglucomutase 1, see also D5Rhm1 and D5Rhm2	S, L	C	4, 6, 7	PGM1	1p22.1	PGM2	4C7
Pkdr1		5	Polycystic kidney disease rat 1	L	P	59				
Rtp1		5	Rat tear protein 1	L	P	60				
S		5	Silver	L	P	61				
Sai1		5	Transformation suppressor	C	P	40	SAI1	UN	Sai-1	4A4-C3
Sh		5	Shaggy	L	P	14				

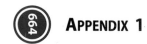

Slc2a1	*GLUTB, Glut1, Gtg3*	5q36.1	Solute carrier family 2 (facilitated glucose transporter) brain, GenBank no. M22061, see also D5Mit7, D5Wox11 and D5Arb7	S, L, A	C	3, 4, 10, 15, 17, 20, 22, 24, 29–32, 52, 56, 62	*SLC2A1*	1p35–p31.3	*Glut1*	4
Slc9a1	*Nhe1*	5	Solute carrier family 9 (sodium/hydrogen exchanger 1), antiporter, Na^+/H^+ (amiloride sensitive)	S	P	63	*SLC9A1*	1p36.1–p35	*Nhe1*	4
Sod2		5	Superoxide dismutase 2, mitochondrial	L	P	29, 32	*SOD2*	6q25.2	*Sod2*	17
Str2		5	Sensitivity to stroke (QTL) in a SHRSP × SHR F2, LOD = 4.7, peak at Anf	L	P	26				
Tubaps		5	Tubulin alpha, pseudogene, see also D5Arb10	L	C	29, 32				
Tyrp1	*B*	5q33	Tyrosine phosphatase 1, same as B (Brown)	L, S, A	C	2–4, 36, 50, 55, 62	*TYRP1*	9p23	*b=Tyrp*	4

References

1 Adams *et al.* (1984) *Biochem. Genet.* **22**, 611–629.

2 Cramer *et al.* (1986) *Biochem. Genet.* **24**, 217–227.

3 Serikawa *et al.* (1992) *Genetics* **131**, 701–721.

4 Pravenec *et al.* (1996) *Mamm. Genome* **7**, 117–127.

5 Shisa *et al.* (1997) *Mamm. Genome* **8**, 324–327.

6 Yoshida (1979) *Proc. Jpn. Acad.* **55**, 403–406.

7 Yoshida (1982) *Cytogenet. Cell Genet.* **32**, 330.

8 Kobayashi *et al.* (1994) *Mamm. Genome* **5**, 222–224.

9 Szpirer *et al.* (1987) *Cytogenet. Cell Genet.* **46**, 701.

10 Szpirer *et al.* (1990) *Genomics* **6**, 679–684.

11 Fulchignoni-Lataud *et al.* (1992) *Mamm. Genome* **3**, 42–45.

12 Castle and King (1941) *Proc. Natl Acad. Sci. USA* **27**, 394–399.

13 Castle and King (1944) *Proc. Natl Acad. Sci. USA* **30**, 79–82.

14 Castle and King (1947) *J. Hered.* **38**, 341–344.

15 Deng *et al.* (1994) *J. Clin. Invest.* **93**, 2701–2709.

16 Garrett *et al.* (1998) *Genome Res.* **8**, 711–723.

17 Truett *et al.* (1995) *Mamm. Genome* **6**, 25–30.

18 Satoh *et al.* (1996) *Gene* **182**, 155–162.

19 Laes *et al.* (1998) *Cytogenet. Cell Genet.* **81**, 290–291.

20 Jacob *et al.* (1995) *Nature Genet.* **9**, 63–69.

21 Stec *et al.* (1996) *Hypertension* **27**, 564–568.

22 Gauguier *et al.* (1996) *Nature Genet.* **12**, 38–43.

23 Courvoisier *et al.* (1997) *Mamm. Genome* **8**, 282–283.

24 Deng *et al.* (1997) *Mamm. Genome* **8**, 549–553.

25 Szpirer *et al.* (1989) 1087.

26 Rubattu *et al.* (1996) *Nature Genet.* **13**, 429–434.

27 Shepel *et al.* (1998) *Mamm. Genome* **9**, 622–628.

28 Deng and Rapp (1995) *Mamm. Genome* **6**, 759–760.

29 Goldmuntz *et al.* (1993) *Mamm. Genome* **4**, 670–675.

30 Canzian *et al.* (1996) *Jpn J. Cancer Res.* **87**, 669–675.

31 Toyota *et al.* (1996) *Proc. Natl Acad. Sci. USA* **93**, 3914–3919.

32 National Institute of Arthritis and Musculoskeletal and Skin Diseases. The ARB Rat Genetic Database (http://www.nih.gov/niams/scientific/ratgbase/index.htm).

33 Yoshida (1978) *Cytogenet. Cell Genet.* **22**, 606–609.

34 Saito *et al.* (1995) *Genomics* **26**, 382–384.

35 Yoshida (1984) *Cytogenet. Cell Genet.* **37**, 613.

36 Truett *et al.* (1996) *Mamm. Genome* **7**, 356–358.

37 Yasue *et al.* (1992) *Genomics* **12**, 659–664.

38 Klinga-Levan *et al.* (1993) *Hereditas* **1(19**,)285–296.

39 Moutier (1980) *J. Hered.* **71**, 129–130.

40 Islam *et al.* (1989) *J. Cell. Sci.* **92**, 147–162.

41 Hino *et al.* (1993) *Proc. Natl Acad. Sci. USA* **90**, 327–331.

42 Testa *et al.* (1992) *Cytogenet. Cell Genet.* **60**, 247–249.

43 Greep (1941) *J. Hered.* **32**, 397–398.

44 Szpirer *et al.* (1994) *Mamm. Genome* **5**, 361–364.

45 Bihoreau *et al.* (1997) *Genomic Res.* **7**, 434–440.

46 The Wellcome Trust Centre for Human Genetics (http://www.well.ox.ac.uk/ ~ bihoreau).

47 Truett *et al.* (1991) *Proc. Natl Acad. Sci. USA* **88**, 7806–7809.

48 Van Zutphen *et al.* (1981) *Biochem. Genet.* **19**, 173–186.

49 Kurtz (1981) *J. Mol. Appl. Genet.* **1**, 29–38.

50 Nikaido *et al.* (1982) *J. Hered.* **73**, 1(19–1)22.

51 Ingvarsson *et al.* (1987) *Somat. Cell Mol. Genet.* **13**, 335–339.

52 Andoh *et al.* (1998) *Mamm. Genome* **9**, 287–293.

53 Zhang *et al.* (1988) *Cytogenet. Cell Genet.* **48**, 121–123.

54 Szpirer *et al.* (1995) *Cytogenet. Cell Genet.* **69**, 11–14.

55 Tissir *et al.* (1996) *Mamm. Genome* **7**, 222–223.

56 Szpirer *et al.* (1998) *Mamm. Genome* **9**, 721–734.

57 Carter and Parr (1969) *Nature* **224**, 1214.

58 Koga *et al.* (1972) *Jpn. J. Genet.* **46**, 335–338.

59 Bihoreau *et al.* (1997) *Hum. Mol. Genet.* **6**, 609–613.

60 Kondo *et al.* (1987) *Transplant. Proc.* **19**, 3146–3147.

61 Castle (1953) *J. Hered.* **44**, 205–206.

62 Sjöling *et al.* (1996) *Mamm. Genome* **7**, 710–711.

63 Szpirer *et al.* (1994) *Mamm. Genome* **5**, 153–159.

Chromosome 6

Locus symbol	Previous symbol	RNO Location	Description	Mode	Status	Reference	HSA symbol	HSA Chr	MMU symbol	MMU Chr
Acp1		6	Acid phosphatase 1, soluble	S	P	48				
Akt		6q32	Murine thymoma viral (v-akt) oncogene homologue 1	A	P	4	AKT	14q32	Akt	12
Aldr1p3	ALR-P1, Alrp3	6	Aldehyde reductase (aldose reductase) (1.9 kb HindIII fragment, probably pseudogene)	S	P	17				
Cad		6	Carbamyl phosphatate synthetase	unpubl	P	10				
Calm1		6q31–q32	Calmodulin 1 (phosphorylase kinase delta)	A	P	30				
Calm2		6q11–q12	Calmodulin 2 (phosphorylase kinase delta)	A	P	30				
Cbg		6q32	Corticosteroid-binding globulin	A	P	21				
Chga		6	Chromogranin A, parathyroid secretory protein 1	S	C	27, 40	CHGA	14q32	Chga	12
Ckb	Ckbb, Ckbr	6q32	Creatine kinase, brain, GenBank no. M18668 and M26669, see also D6Mit6, D6Wox13, D6Wox15 and D6Arb1	S, L, A	C	6, 7, 15, 18, 20, 34, 43, 44	CKB	14q32.3	Ckb	12
Crip		6	Cysteine-rich intestinal protein, see also D6Wox21	L	P	7				
Ef1	Ef1 aa	6	Transcription factor EF1(a), see also D6Mgh2	L	P	20				
Esr2		6q24	Oestrogen receptor 2 (ER beta)	A	P	21				
Fkhr	Fkhl1	6	Forkhead-like transcription factor BF-1, GenBank no. M87634, see also D6Arb13	L	C	15				
Fos		6q21–q23	FBJ murine osteosarcoma viral (v-fos) oncogene homologue	A	P	26	FOS	14q24.3	FOS	12
Hnf3a		6q23–q24	Hepatocyte nuclear factor 3 alpha gene	A	P	45				
Iddm4		6	Insulin-dependent diabetes gene (QTL)	L	P	23				

Igh@	IGHE, Igca	6q32	Immunoglobulin heavy-chain gene cluster (V,D,J,C), see also D6Wox11 and D6Wox12	S, L	C	2, 3, 18, 20, 33, 34	IGH@	14q32.33		12
Igha	IHG1	6q32	Immunoglobulin heavy chain (alpha polypeptide)	L	P	2				
Ighe	IGH2	6q32	Immunoglobulin heavy chain (epsilon polypeptide)	S, CH, L	C	7, 18, 33, 34, 44				
Ighen		6	IGH 3' enhancer sequence, see also D14Mgh4 (previously localized to RNO14)	L	I	7, 20				
Ighg	IGH3	6q32	Immunoglobulin heavy chain (gamma polypeptide)	L	P	3				
Klkbp	Kbp	6	Kallikrein-binding protein (kallistatin), see also D6Elh1	L	P	9				
Kzf1		6	Kruppel-associated box (KRAB) zinc finger 1	S, L	P	5				
Mdg1		6q16-q23	Microvascular endothelial differentiation gene 1	A	P	35				
Mycn	Nmyc	6	Avian myelocytomatosis viral (v-myc) related oncogene, neuroblastoma derived (N-myc)	S	P	19	MYCN	2p24.1	Nmyc	12
Odc1		6	Ornithine decarboxylase, GenBank no. X07944	S	P	13	ODC1	2p25	Odc	12
Pi	AAT	6	Alpha-1-antitrypsin (protease inhibitor)	S	P	16	PI	14q32.1	Spi1(Aat)	12
Pomc2		6	Proopoimelanocortin beta (endorphin beta)	S	P	49				
Ppm1a	Pp2c1	6	Protein phosphatase type 1A (formerly 2C), Mg-dependent, alpha isoform	S	P	47				
Ppp1cd		6	Protein phosphatase type 1 delta	S	P	31				
Prkar2b		6	Type II beta regulatory subunit of cAMP-dependent protein kinase, GenBank no. M75151, see also D6Arb12	L	C	15				
Rnu1b		6q21	Small nuclear RNA, U1, class 11 gene (18-3A), see also D6Mit3	L,A	C	20				
Rnu1c		6	Small nuclear RNA, U1, 18-3A, see also D6Arb17	L	C	15				
Rrm2		6q16	Ribonucleotide reductase 2	S,A	P	22				
Slc10a1		6q24	Solute carrier family 10 (sodium/bile acid cotransporter family), member 1	A	P	11				

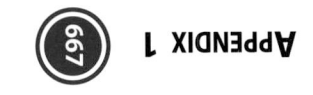

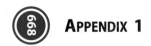
Sp4		6q23	*Trans*-acting transcription factor 4	A	P	37				
Spin2a	*SPI1, Spin1*	6	Serine protease inhibitor	S	P	32				
Spin2b	*SPI2, Spin2*	6	Serine protease inhibitor	S	P	32				
Spin2c	*SPI3, Spin3*	6	Serine protease inhibitor	S	P	32				
Sstr1	*Gpcrrna*	6	Somatostatin receptor subtype 1, see also D6Wox18	L	P	6				
Synd1		6	Syndecan	L	P	12	*SDC*	2p	*Synd1*	12
Vsnl1		6	Neural visinin-like protein 1, GenBank no. D10666, see also D6Arb7	L	C	15				
Yy1		6q32	YY1 transcription factor	A	P	8				

References

1 Andoh *et al.* (1998) *Mamm. Genome* **9**, 287–293.

2 Bazin *et al.* (1974) *J. Immunol.* **112**, 1035–1041.

3 Beckers and Bazin (1975) *Immunochemistry* **12**, 671–675.

4 Bellacose *et al.* (1993) *Oncogene* **8**, 745–754.

5 Bellefroid *et al.* (1998) *Biochim. Biophys. Acta* **1398**: 321–329

6 Bihoreau *et al.* (1997) *Genome Res.* **7**, 434–440.

7 Ganzian *et al.* (1996) *Jpn. J. Cancer Res.* **87**, 669–675

8 Chen *et al.* (1996) *Cytogenet. Cell Genet.* **74**, 277–280.

9 Chen *et al.* (1997) *Mamm. Genome* **8**, 701–703.

10 Chernova *et al.* (1995) *Trends Biochem. Sci.* **20**, 431–434.

11 Cohn *et al.* (1995) *Mamm. Genome* **6**, 60.

12 Cui *et al.* (1998) *Exp. Anim.* **47**, 83–88.

13 Deng *et al.* (1994) *Mamm. Genome* **5**, 712–716.

14 Deng *et al.* (1998) *Mamm. Genome* **9**(1): 38–43.

15 Du *et al.* (1995) *Cytogenet. Cell Genet.* **68**, 107–111.

16 Fulchignoni-Lataud *et al.* (1992) *Mamm. Genome* **3**, 42–45.

17 Graham *et al.* (1991) *Gene* **107**, 259–267.

18 Hilbert *et al.* (1991) *Nature* **353**, 521–529.

19 Ingvarsson *et al.* (1987) *Somat. Cell Mol. Genet.* **13**, 335–339.

20 Jacob *et al.* (1995) *Nature Genet.* **9**, 63–69.

21 Johansson *et al.* (1998) *Cytogenet. Cell Genet.* **81**, 217–221.

22 Klinga-Levan *et al.* (1997) *Mamm. Genome* **8**, 47–49.

23 Klöting *et al.* (1998) *Biochem. Biophys. Res. Commun.* **245**, 483–486.

24 Kondo *et al.* (1997) *Transplant. Proc.* **29**, 1766–1767.

25 Kuramoto *et al.* (1995) *Exp. Anim.* **44**, 119–125.

26 Li *et al.* (1989) *Cytogenet. Cell Genet.* **52**, 42–44.

27 Mahata *et al.* (1996) *Genomes Genomics* **33**, 135–139.

28 Maihara *et al.* (1995) *Transplant. Proc.* **27**, 1502–1504.

29 Matsumoto *et al.* (1998) *Mamm. Genome* **9**, 531–535.

30 Mori *et al.* (1994) *Mamm. Genome* **5**, 824–826.

31 Muramatsu *et al.* (1995) *Mamm. Genome* **6**, 307–308.

32 Pagés *et al.* (1990) *Gene* **94**, 273–282.

33 Pear *et al.* (1986) *Immunogenetics* **23**, 393–395.

34 Pravenec *et al.* (1996) *Mamm. Genome* **7**, 117–127.

35 Pröls *et al.* (1996) *Mamm. Genome* **7**, 867.

36 Serikawa *et al.* (1992) *Genet.* **131**, 701–721.

37 Scohy *et al.* (1998) *Cytogenet. Cell Genet.* **81**, 273–274.

38 Shepel *et al.* (1998) *Mamm. Genome* **98**, 662–628.

39 Shisa *et al.* (1997) *Mamm. Genome* **8**, 324–327.

40 Simon-Chazottes *et al.* (1993) *Genomics* **17**, 252–255.

41 Sverdlov *et al.* (1998) *Mamm. Genome* **9**, 243–245.

42 Szpirer *et al.* (1996) *Folia Biol. (Praha)* **42**, 175–226.

43 Szpirer *et al.* (1998) *Mamm. Genome* **9**, 721–734.

44 Toyota *et al.* (1996) *Proc. Natl Acad. Sci. USA* **93**, 3914–3919.

45 Van Reeth *et al.* (1998) *Cytogenet. Cell. Genet.* **81**, 174–175.

46 Van Zutphen *et al.* (1998) *Rat Genome* **4**, 43–50.

47 Yamada *et al.* (1994) *Mamm. Genome* **5**, 63–83.

48 Yasue *et al.* (1991) *Cytogenet. Cell Genet.* **57**, 142–148.

49 Yeung *et al.* (1993) *Mamm. Genome* **4**, 585–588.

50 Yokoi *et al.* (1996) *Mamm. Genome* **7**, 71–73.

Chromosome 7

Locus symbol	Previous symbol	RNO Location	Description	Mode	Status	Reference	HSA symbol	HSA Chr	MMU symbol	MMU Chr
Acr	Acro		Acrosin, see also D7Mgh2	L, S	C	1, 2	ACR	22q13–ter	Acr	15
Avpr1a			Vasopressin receptor V1a	I	P	42				
Bw/gk1			Body weight (same as Weight1?)	L	P	3				
Bzrp			Benzodiazepin receptor (peripheral), see also D7Mit12, D7Wox20	L	C	2, 4	BZRP	22q13.31–qter	Bzrp	15
Cia4			Type II collagen-induced arthritis 4, QTL	L	P	43				
Col6a			Collagen, type VI, alpha 1	S	P	6	COL6A1	21q22.3	Col6a1	10
Cyp11b1			Cytochrome P450, subfamily XIB, polypeptide 1 (steroid 11-beta-hydroxylase), see also D7Wox19	L, S	C	4, 7, 8	CYP11B1	8q21–q22	Cyp11b1	15
Cyp11b2			Cytochrome P450, subfamily XIB, polypeptide 2 (aldosterone synthase), see also D7Wox16	L, S	C	4, 7, 8	CYP11B2	8q21–q22	Cyp11b2	15
Cyp11-b@			Cytochrome P450, subfamily XIB gene cluster, see also D7Wox18	L, S	C	8				
Cyp2d2			Cytochrome P450, subfamily IID2, see also D7Wox21	L	P	44				
Cyp2d3			Cytochrome P450, subfamily IID3, see also D7Mgh3	L	P	2				
Cyp2d4			Cytochrome P450, subfamily IID4, see also D7Mit16	L	P	2				
Den			Dendrin	I	P	42				
Dia1	Nadhob5		Diaphorase (NADH) (cytochrome b-5 reductase), see also D7Wox30	L	P	44	DIA1	22q13–ter	Dia1	15
Dmo2			NIDDM (OLETF) QTL	L	P	45				
Ela1			Elastase 1, see also D7Mit26, D7Wox23	S	P	14	ELA1	12	Ela1	15

G22p1	Ku70	DNA-binding component of DNA-dependent protein kinase complex	I	P	40	G22P1	22q13	G22p1	15
H1fo		Histone H1°	S		15	H1FO	22q13.1	H1fv	15
Hoxc4	Hox3r3	Homeobox gene C4	S	P	16	HOXC4	12q12–q13	Hoxc4	15
Hoxc8	Hox3r4	Homeobox gene C8	S	P	16	HOXC8	12q12–q13	Hoxc8	15
Hoxc@	Hox3@	Homeobox C gene cluster region	S	P	16	HOXC@	12q12–q13	Hoxc	15F
Igf1		Insulin-like growth factor I, see also D7Mit23, D7Wox13	S	P	14	IGF1	12q22–q23	Igf1	10
Itga5		Integrin alpha 5 (fibronectin receptor alpha)	S	P	17	ITGA5	12q11–q13	Itga5	15
Lalba		Lactalbumin alpha, see also D7Mit19, D7Wox22	S	P	14	LALBA	12q13	Lalba	UN
Lck2		Lymphocyte tyrosine kinase 2	S	P	18, 19				
Lysz		Lysozyme, see also D7Mgh22	L	P	47	LYZ	12	Lysz	10
Mcs2		Mammary carcinoma susceptibility gene 2			46				
Mlvi4		Moloney murine leukaemia virus (MoMuLV) integration site 4 homologue	S	P	21	MLVI4	8q24	Mlvi4	15
Myc		Avian myelocytomatosis viral (v-myc) oncogene homologue, see also D7Arb5, D7Kyo1, D7Mit27, D7Wox14, D7Wox15, D7Wox29	CH, L, S	C	4, 11, 14, 23, 24, 41	MYC	8q24.12–q24.13	Myc	15D2-D3
Odf1		Sperm outer dense fibre major protein 1	S	P	25	ODF1	8q22	Odf1	15
Pah		Phenylalanine hydroxylase	S	P	26	PAH	12q22–q24.2	Pah	10
Pdgfb	SIS	Platelet-derived growth factor beta	S	P	27	PDGFB	22q12.3–q13.1	Pdgfb	15E
Pepb		Peptidase B	S	P	28	PEPB	12q21	Pep2	10
Pmch		Promelanin-concentrating hormone	S	P	29	PMCH	12q23–q24	Pmch	10

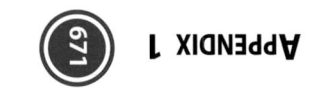

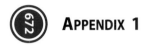

Prph	Perf	Peripherin, see also D7Mit9, D7Wox24	L, S	C	4, 14, 41	PRPH	12q12–q13	Prph	15
Pvt1	Mlvi1, Mis1	Pvt-1 (murine) oncogene homologue, MYC activator	S	C	24, 30, 31	PVT1	8q24	Pvt1	15D2-D3
Rarg		Retinoic acid receptor gamma	S	P	32	RARG	12q13	Rarg	15F
Sp1		Sp1 transcription factor	S	P	33	SP1	12q13	Sp1-1	15
Tbxa2r		Thromboxane receptor	I	P	34	TBXA2R	19p13.3	Tbxa2r	10
Tegt		Testis enhanced gene transcript	S	P	35, 39	TEGT	12q12–q13	Tegt	15
Tg		Thyroglobulin	S	P	36	TG	8q24	Tgn	15B3-ter
Vdr		Vitamin D (1,25-dihydroxyvitamin D3) receptor	S	P	33	VDR	12q12–q14		
Weight1		Body weight (same as Bw/gk1?)	L	P	37				
Wnt1	Int1	Wingless-type MMTV integration site 1, homologue, see also D7Kyo2	S	P	11	WNT1	12q13	Wnt1	15

References

1. Adham et al. (1991) Cytogenet. Cell Genet. **57**, 47–50.
2. Jacob et al. (1995) Nature Genet. **9**, 63–69.
3. Gauguier et al. (1996) Nature Genet. **12**, 38–43.
4. Pravenec et al. (1996) Mamm. Genome **7**, 117–127.
6. Hino et al. (1993) Proc. Natl Acad. Sci. USA **90**, 730–734.
7. Cicila et al. (1993) Nature Genet. **3**, 346–353.
8. Inglis et al. (1995) J. Mol. Endocrinol. **14**, 303–311.
9. Du et al. (1995) Mamm. Genome **6**, 295–298.
10. Hino et al. (1996) Rat Genome **2**, 6–9.
11. Kondo et al. (1993) Mamm. Genome **4**, 571–576.
13. Hilbert et al. (1991) Nature **353**, 521–529.
14. Serikawa et al. (1992) Genetics **131**, 701–721.
15. Walter et al. (1996) Cytogenet. Cell Genet. **73**, 136–139.
16. Chung et al. (1993) Mamm. Genome **4**, 537–540.
17. Szpirer et al. (1992) Mamm. Genome **3**, 685–688.
18. Szpirer et al. (1989) Cytogenet. Cell Genet. **51**, 1087.
19. Szpirer et al. (1990) Genomics **6**, 679–684.
21. Tsichlis et al. (1990) J. Virol. **64**, 2236–2244.
23. Sümegi et al. (1983) Nature **306**, 497–498.
24. Tsichlis P et al. (1985) J. Virol. **56**, 938–942.
25. Burfeind et al. (1993) Eur. J. Biochem. **216**, 497–505.
26. Fulchignoni-Lataud et al. (1990) Cytogenet. Cell Genet. **53**, 172–174.
27. Fang et al. (1985) Cytogenet. Cell Genet. **40**, 627.
28. Yasue et al. (1991) Cytogenet. Cell Genet. **57**, 142–148.
29. Nahon et al. (1992) Genomics **12**, 846–848.
30. Ingvarsson et al. (1987) Cytogenet. Cell Genet. **45**, 174–176.
31. Koehne et al. (1989) J. Virol. **63**, 2366–2369.
32. Mattei et al. (1991) Genomics **10**, 1061–1069.
33. Szpirer et al. (1991) Genomics **11**, 168–173.
34. Takeuchi et al. (1996) Cytogenet. Cell Genet. **73**, 79–80.
35. Walter et al. (1994) Mamm. Genome **5**, 216–221.

36 Brocas et al. (1985) Cytogenet. Cell Genet. **39,** 150–153.

37 Gall et al. (1996) Nature Genet. **12,** 31–37.

38 Pravenec et al. (1996) Folia Biol. **42,** 147–153.

39 Helou et al. (1966) Rat Genome **2,** 149.

40 Koike et al. (1996) Genomics **38,** 38–44.

41 Otsen et al. (1996) Genomics **37,** 289–294.

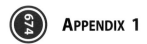

Chromosome 8

Locus symbol	Previous symbol	RNO Location	Description	Mode	Status	Reference	HSA symbol	HSA Chr	MMU symbol	MMU Chr
Acca	Kactap, PKATA	8q32	Acetyl-CoA acyltransferase, 3-oxo acyl-CoA thiolase A, peroxisomal, see also D8Wox10 and D8Arb22	D, L, S	C	2, 10, 17, 19, 22, 47, 53, 57, 68, 75				
Acat1		8q24.1	Acetyl-Co A acetyltransferase 1, mitochondrial		P	39				
Acpp	Acpp11	8	Prostatic acid phosphatase, see also D8Wox15	L	P	6, 67				
Acy1		8	Aminoacylase 1	S	P	21	ACY1	3p21.1	Acy1	9
Ad-cyap1r2		8	Rat pituitary adenylate cyclase activating polypeptide 1 receptor (2)	S	P	9				
Apeh	D3S48E, Rik, Acph	8	N-Acylaminoacyl-peptide hydrolase, see also D8Wox5 and D8Wox11	L, S	C	11, 16, 17, 20, 22, 47, 56	APEH	3p21.3–p21.2	Apeh	9
Apoa1		8q23–q24	Apolipoprotein A-I	D, L	C	18				
Apoa4		8	Apolipoprotein A-IV	L	P	18				
Apoc3	Apoc2	8q23–q25	Apolipoprotein C-III, see also D8Mit7 and D8Wox4	D, L, S	C	10, 17, 18, 26, 47, 49, 56, 68	APOC3	11q23–qter	Apoc3	9
Atm		8q24.1	Ataxia telangiectasia gene mutated in human beings		P	39				
Casp1	Il1bc, Ice	8	Interleukin 1beta-converting enzyme	L	P	51				
Ccnd3		8	Cyclin D3, see also D8Mgh14	L	P					
Cd24		8q13	CD24 antigen	D	P	23				
Chrna3		8	Acetycholine receptor alpha 3 (neuronal nicotine), see also D8Bord1	L	P	11				
Chrna5		8	Acetycholine receptor alpha 5, see also D8Bord1	L	P	11				
Chrnb4		8	Acetycholine receptor beta 4, see also D8Bord1	L	P	11				
Crabp1		8	Cellular retinoic acid-binding protein 1	L	P	49				

Cyp1a1	Cyp45c	8	Cytochrome P450, subfamily I (aromatic compound-inducible), member A1 (C6, form c), see also D8Mgh7	L, S	C	7, 22, 37, 46	CYP1A1	15q22–q24	Cyp1a1	9
Cyp1a2	P-450d	8	Cytochrome P450, subfamily I (aromatic compound-inducible), member A2 (Q42, form d), see also D8Wox5	L, S	C	6, 37, 67	CYP1A2	15	Cyp1a2	9
Cyp19		8q23–q24	Cytochrome P450, 19, aromatase	D	P	23				
Ddx6	Rck, Hlr2	8	D-E-A-D (aspartate-glutamate-alanine-aspartate) box polypeptide 6 (RNA helicase)	D	P	39				
Dop	Myh12, D	8	Dilute-opisthotonus	L	P	43				
Drd2		8q24	Dopamine receptor D2	D, L	C	33, 46	DRD2	11q22.2–q22.3	Drd2	9
Elnl1	Eln	8	Elastin-like 1	L	P	38, 69				
Epor		8	Erythropoietin receptor	S	P	75	EPOR	19p13.2	Epor	9
Es6		8	Esterase 6	L	C	26, 45, 47–49, 56				
Ets1	Tpl1, Ets-1, Etsoncb	8	E26 avian leukaemia oncogene-1, 5' domain (tumour progression locus 1), see also D8Wox17	L, S	C	4–6, 67	ETS1	11q23.3	Ets1	9
Glb1		8	Galactosidase beta 1	S	P	73	GLB1	3p22–p21.3	Bg1	9
Gpd1	Gdc1	8	Alpha-glycerophosphate dehydrogenase 1	L	P	56				
Grik4	KA1	8	Glutamate receptor, ionotropic, kainate 4	D, L, S	C	51, 62	GRIK4	11q23	Grik4	9
Grm2		8	Glutamate receptor, metabotropic 2	S	P	34				
Gsta1		8	Glutathione-S-transferase, alpha type (Ya)	D, S	C	25, 60, 72	GSTA2	6p12.2	Gsta	9
Gstpl3	GSTPL3	8q13–q21	Glutathione-S-transferase-like 3, pi type	D, S	C	25, 74				
Hexa		8	Hexose aminidase A (alpha polypeptide)	S	P	73	HEXA	15q23–q24	Hexa	9
Hnf6		8q24–q31	Hepatic nuclear factor 6	D, S	P	84				
Hsc70		8	Heat shock cognate protein 70	S	P	5, 45				
Htr1b		8q31	Serotonin (5-hydroxytryptamine (5HT)) receptor, type 1B	D	P	13				

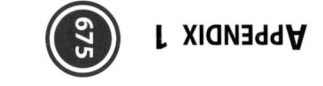

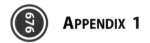

Kcnj1	Kcnj	8	Potassium inwardly rectifying channel, subfamily J	L	C	33, 46, 48, 51			
Lipc	Hpl	8	Lipase, hepatic	S	C	46, 48	LIPC	15q21–q23	HPL	9
Lx		8	Polydactyly-luxate syndrome	L	C	29, 33, 45, 47, 49, 50			
Matr1		8	Matrin F/G	L	P	38			
Me1		8	Malic enzyme 1, soluble	S	P	35	ME1	6q12	MOD1	9
Mll		8	Mixed-lineage leukaemia (also acute lymphocytic leukaemia 1 or tritorax *Drosophila* gene)	L	P	50			
Mobp	Mobp81p	8	Myelin-associated/oligodendrocytic basic protein 81, see also D8Wox13	L	P	6, 67			
Mpi		8	Mannose phosphate isomerase	S	P	76	MPI	15q22–qter	MPI	9
Mst1	D8h3f15s2	8	Macrophage-stimulating 1 (hepatocyte growth factor-like), see also D8H3F15S2	S	P	36, 75			
Myl3	Mylc1v	8	Myosin light chain, alkali, cardiac ventricles, see also D8Wox8 and D8Wox9	L, S	C	10, 17, 47, 56, 68	MYL3	3p21.3–p21.2	Mylc	9
Ncam	Cd56	8	Cell adhesion molecule, neural (CD56)	L, S	C	2, 26, 47, 49, 74	NCAM	11q23.1	Ncam	9
Pccb		8	Propionyl coenzyme A carboxylase, beta polypeptide	S	P	61			
Pgr		8q11	Progesterone receptor	D	P	23			
Plcd1	Plc1	8	Phospholipase C-delta1	S	P	24			
Plod2		8	Procollagen-lysine, 2-oxoglutarate 5-dioxygenase (lysine hydroxylase) 2	S	P				
Pthr	PTHrel	8	Parathyroid hormone/parathyroid hormone-related peptide receptor	L, S	I	44	PTHR	3p22–p21.1	Pthr	9
Rbp1		8	Retinol-binding protein 2	S	P	48			
Rbp2	Crbp	8q31	Retinol-binding protein 2, cellular, see also D8Mgh3, D8Wox6 and D8Arb17	D, L, S	C	2, 10, 17, 22, 47, 53, 56, 68	RBP2	3p11–qter	Rbp2	9

RT5		8	Cell surface alloantigen	L	C	29, 30, 47				
Scn2b	*vrSkM2*	8	Skeletal muscle voltage-sensitive sodium channel subtype 2, see also D8Wox12	L	P	6, 67				
Sm22	*Tagln*	8q24	Smooth muscle 22 protein, transgelin, see also D8Mcw1	L	P					
Tf		8	Transferrin	S	I	3, 65	*TF*	3q21	*Trf*	9
Thy1	*CD7*	8	Thymus cell surface antigen	L, S	C	2, 10, 31, 47, 49, 51, 68	*THY1*	11q22.3–q23	*Thy1*	9
Tpm1	*Tma2*	8	Tropomyosin 1 (alpha), see also D8Mgh5	L, S	C	7, 22, 47, 49, 56	*TPM1*	15q22	*Tpm1*	9
Vipr1		8	Vasopressive intestinal peptide receptor	S	P	15				

References

1 Adams *et al.* (1984) *Biochem. Genet.* **22**, 611–629.

2 Andoh *et al.* (1998) *Mamm. Genome* **9**, 287–293.

3 Baranov *et al.* (1987) *Chromosoma* **96**, 60–66.

4 Bear *et al.* (1989) *Proc. Natl Acad. Sci. USA* **86**, 7495–7499.

5 Bellacosa *et al.* (1994) *J. Virol.* **68**, 2320–2330.

6 Bihoreau *et al.* (1997) *Genomic Res.* **7**, 434–440.

7 Bottger *et al.* (1996) *J. Clin. Invest.* **98**, 856–862.

8 Brown *et al.* (1998) *Mamm. Genome* **9**, 521–530.

9 Cai *et al.* (1995) *Cytogenet. Cell Genet.* **71**, 193–196.

10 Canzian *et al.* (1996) *Jpn. J. Cancer Res.* **87**, 669–675.

11 Cook *et al.* (1997) *Mamm. Genome* **8**, 177–178.

12 Courvoisier *et al.* (1997) *Mamm. Genome* **8**, 282–283.

13 Courvoisier *et al.* (1997) *Mamm. Genome* **8**, 792–793.

14 Cui *et al.* (1998) *Exp. Anim.* **47**, 83–88.

15 Deng *et al.* (1994) *Mamm. Genome* **5**, 712–716.

16 Erlandsson *et al.* (1991) *Cytogenet. Cell Genet.* **57**, 149–150.

17 Gauguier *et al.* (1996) *Nature Genet.* **12**, 38–43.

18 Haddad *et al.* (1986) *J. Biol. Chem.* **261**, 13268–13277.

19 Hilbert *et al.* (1991) *Nature* **353**, 521–529.

20 Hino *et al.* (1993) *Proc. Natl Acad. Sci. USA* **90**, 327–331.

21 Hino *et al.* (1993) *Proc. Natl Acad. Sci. USA* **90**, 730–734.

22 Jacob *et al.* (1995) *Nature Genet.* **9**, 63–69.

23 Johansson *et al.* (1998) *Cytogenet. Cell. Genet.* **81**, 217–221.

24 Katsuya *et al.* (1992) *Biochem. Biophys. Res. Commun.* **187**, 1359–1366.

25 Klinga-Levan *et al.* (1993) *Hereditas* **119**, 285–296.

26 Kobayashi *et al.* (1992) *Mamm. Genome* **3**, 656–658.

27 Koike *et al.*(1998) *Mamm. Genome* **9**, 76–77.

28 Kondo *et al.* (1996) XIth International Workshop on Alloantigenic Systems in the Rat, Toulouse, France, 21–24 August, p. 79.

29 Kren (1975) *Acta Univ. Carolinae Med.* **68**, 1–103.

30 Kren *et al.* (1973) *Transplant. Proc.* **5**, 1463–1466.

31 Kren *et al.* (1993) IXth International Workshop on Alloantigenic Systems in the Rat, Hannover, Germany, 23–26 February, p. 27.

32 Kren *et al.* (1997) *J. Clin. Invest.* **99**, 557–581.

33 Krenova *et al.* (1996) XIth International Workshop on Alloantigenic Systems in the Rat, Toulouse, France, 21–24 August, p. 51.

34 Kuramoto *et al.* (1994) *Genomics* **19**, 358–361.

35 Levan *et al.* (1986) *Rat News Lett.* **17**, 3–8.

36 Levan *et al.* (1990) (S.J. O'Brien Ed.), Genetic Maps 1990 New York: Cold Spring Harbor Press.

37 Levan *et al.* (1991) *Genomics* **10**, 699–718.

38 Mathern *et al.* (1994) *Cytogenet. Cell. Genet.* **66**, 283–286.

39 Matsuda (1996) *Genomics* **34**, 347–352.

40 Moisan *et al.* (1996) *Nature Genet.* **14**, 471–473.

41 Nabika, T., (1997) *Mamm. Genome* **8**, 215–217.

42 National Institute of Arthritis and Musculoskeletal and Skin Diseases. The ARB Rat Genetic Database (http://www.nih.gov/niams/scientific/ratgbase/index.htm).

43 Ohno (1996) *Exp. Anim.* **45**, 71–75.

44 Pausova *et al.* (1994) *Genomics* **20**, 20–26.

45 Pravenec *et al.* (1987) *J. Immunogenet.* **14**, 313–316.

46 Pravenec *et al.* (1996) *Folia Biol. (Praha)* **42**, 147–153.

47 Pravenec *et al.* (1996) *Mamm. Genome* **7**, 117–127.

48 Pravenec *et al.* (1997) *Folia Biol. (Praha)* **43**, 97–99.

49 Pravenec *et al.* (1997) *Mamm. Genome* **8**, 455.

50 Pravenec *et al.* (1997) *Mamm. Genome* **8**, 625–626.

51 Pravenec *et al.* (1998) *Folia Biol. (Praha)* **44**, 107–109.

52 Rastegar *et al.* (1998) *Biochem. J.* **334**, 565–569.

53 Remmers *et al.* (1996) *Nature Genet.* **14**, 82–85.

54 Rothermel *et al.* (1995) *Mamm. Genome* **6**, 602–606.

55 Schork *et al.* (1995) *Genome Res.* **5**, 164–172.

56 Serikawa *et al.* (1992) *Genetics* **131**, 701–721.

57 Shepel *et al.* (1998) *Mamm. Genome* **9**, 622–628.

58 Shepel *et al.* (19??) *Genetics* **149**, 289–299.

59 Shisa *et al.* (1997) *Mamm. Genome* **8**, 324–327.

60 Sladka *et al.* (1992) *Folia Biol. (Praha)* **38**, 84–89.

61 Szpirer *et al.* (1989) *Cytogenet. Cell Genet.* **50**, 23–26.

62 Szpirer *et al.* (1994) *Proc. Natl Acad. Sci. USA* **91**, 11849–11853.

63 Szpirer *et al.* (1997) *Mamm. Genome* **8**, 707–708.

64 Szpirer *et al.* (1998) *Mamm. Genome* (submitted).

65 Szpirer *et al.* (1987) *Cytogenet. Cell Genet.* **46**, 701.

66 Szpirer *et al.* (1988) *Cytogenet. Cell Genet.* **47**, 42–45.

67 The Wellcome Trust Centre for Human Genetics (http://www.well.ox.ac.uk/~bihoreau).

68 Toyota *et al.* (1996) *Proc. Natl Acad. Sci. USA* **93**, 3914–3919.

69 Vorobieva *et al.* (1995) *Cytogenet. Cell Genet.* **68**, 91–94.

70 Whitehead Institute for Biomedical Research/MIT Center for Genome Research (http://www.genome.wi.mit.edu/rat/public).

71 Yamada *et al.* (1994) *Mamm. Genome* **5**, 63–83.

72 Yamada *et al.* (1992) *Cytogenet. Cell. Genet.* **61**, 125–127.

73 Yasue *et al.* (1991) *Cytogenet. Cell. Genet.* **57**, 142–148.

74 Yasue *et al.* (1992) *Genomics* **12**, 659–664.

75 Yeung *et al.* (1993) *Mamm. Genome* **4**, 585–588.

76 Yoshida (1978) *Cytogenet. Cell. Genet.* **22**, 606–609.

Chromosome 9

Locus symbol	Previous symbol	RNO Location	Description	Mode	Status	Reference	HSA symbol	HSA Chr	MMU symbol	MMU Chr
Adcyap1			Rat pituitary adenylate cyclase activating polypeptide 1	S	P	5				
Agxt	Spat	9	Alanine-glyoxylate aminotransferase (serine-pyruvate aminotransferase)	D, L	C	17, 29, 36				
Alpi	Alp1, Akp3, Akp-1, AKP1	9	Alkaline phosphatase 1, intestinal, defined by SSR, GenBank no. S51097	S, L	C	4, 6–10, 43				
Bp34		9	Blood pressure QTL in F2 (Dahl salt sens. × Dahl salt res.), LOD = 5.0, between D9Uia6 and D9Uia9 (peak close to Inha)	L	P	4				
C3		9	Complement component 3, see also C3 RFLP	S, L	C	11–13, 43	C3	19p13.3	C3	17
Chcg	Scg2	9	Chromogranin C (secretogranin II)	S	P	32, 43				
Cps1		9	Carboamyl-phosphate synthetase 1	S, D	C	14				
Cryg@	Len	9q34	Crystallin, gamma gene cluster, including A, B, C, D and E, see also D9Mit2, D9Wox8, R27 and R28	L	C	1, 2, 15–17, 43, 44	CRYG@	2q33–q35	Cryg	1
Cryga	Len, Cryg1	9	Crystallin, gamma polypeptide 1, see also D9Mit2, D9Wox8, R27 and R28	S, L	C	1, 10, 17–21				
Crygb	Len, Cryg2	9	Crystallin, gamma polypeptide 2, see also D9Mit2, D9Wox8, R27 and R28	S, L, D	C	1, 17–20, 22				
Crygc	Len, Cryg3, Cryg	9q32–q33	Crystallin, gamma polypeptide 3, see also D9Mit2, D9Wox8, R27 and R28	S, L, D	C	1, 17–20, 22, 23				
Crygd	Len, Cryg4	9q32–q33	Crystallin, gamma polypeptide 4, see also D9Mit2, D9Wox8, R27 and R28	S, L	C	17–20				
Cryge	Len, Cryg5	9	Crystallin, gamma polypeptide 5, see also D9Mit2, D9Wox8, R27 and R28	S, L	C	17–20				

Crygf	Len, Cryg6	9	Crystallin, gamma polypeptide 6, see also D9Mgh4	S, L	C	1, 17–20, 23				
Ercc5	Xpg	9	Excision repair cross-complementing rodent repair deficiency, complementation group 5 (xeroderma pigmentosum complementation group G (Cockayne syndrome))	D	P	24, 43, 44				
Gls	Glut	9q22.3	Glutaminase, see also D9Wox15	S, L, D	C	2, 15, 17, 21, 22, 25, 43	GLS	2q32–q34	Gls	1
Gnmt		9q31–q32	Glycine methyltransferase, see also D9Arb1	L	C	1				
Gsta2		9	Glutathione-S-transferase, alpha type (Yc?)	S	C	17, 26, 27				
Idh1		9	Isocitrate dehydrogenase 1, soluble	S	P	17, 28, 43	IDH1	2q32–qter	Idh1	9
Inha		9	Inhibin alpha, see also D9Wox10	S, L	C	1, 4, 10, 17, 21, 29, 30, 43	INHA	2q33–q34	Inha	1
Livtr		9	Liver-specific transporter, see also D9Uwm3	L	P	31				
Ncl		9	Nucleolin, see also D9Arb5	L	C	1				
Nramp1	Bcg, Itg, Lsh	9	Natural resistance-associated macrophage protein, see also D9Arb3	L	P	1, 16				
Slc4a3	Aep3, Ae3	9	Solute carrier family 4, member 3, anion exchange protein 3, see also D9Bro1	L, S, D	C	4, 9, 22, 23, 33, 34, 44				
Slc9a2	Nhe2	9q34	Solute carrier family 9 (sodium/hydrogen exchanger 2), antiporter 2, Na^+/H^+ (Na^+/H^+ exchanger 2)	S	P	35, 43	SLC9A2	2pter–2qter	Slc9a2	1
Slc9a4	Nhe4	9	Solute carrier family 9 (sodium/hydrogen exchanger), isoform 4	S	P	35, 43	SLC9A4	2pter–qter	Slc9a4	1
Stat1		9q22	Signal transducer and activator of transcription 1	D	P	22				
Tnp1		9q31–q32	Transition protein 1	S	P	17, 38, 43	TNP1	2q34	Tnp1	1
Tp53l1	Trp53l1	9	Tumour protein p53-like 1	S	P	17, 39, 43				
Ugt1a1		9	UDP-glucuronosyltransferase 1 family, member 1	D	P	40	UGT1A1	2q37	Ugt1a1	1
Vav1		9q35–q36	Vav oncogene	D	P	41	VAV	19p13.3	Vav	17

| Xrcc5 | Ku80, Kup80 | 9q11–q12 9q34 | X-ray repair cross complementation (double-strand-break rejoining; Ku autoantigen, 80 kDa) | D | P | 42 |
| Zap70 | Srk | 9q34–q36 | Syk-related protein tyrosine kinase | D | P | 37 |

References

1 National Institute of Arthritis and Musculoskeletal and Skin Diseases. The ARB Rat Genetic Database (http://www.nih.gov/niams/scientific/ratgbase/index.htm).

2 The Wellcome Trust Centre for Human Genetics (http://www.well.ox.ac.uk/~bihoreau).

3 Whitehead Institute for Biomedical Research/MIT Center for Genome Research (http://www.genome.wi.mit.edu/rat/public).

4 Rapp et al. (1998) Genomics 51, 191–196.

5 Cai et al. (1995) Cytogenet. Cell Genet. 71, 193–196.

6 Adams et al. (1984) Biochem. Genet. 22, 611–629.

7 Cramer et al. (1986) Biochem. Genet. 24, 217–227.

8 Pravenec et al. (1994) Genomics 19, 190–191.

9 Deng et al. (1994) Mamm. Genome 5, 712–716.

10 Pravenec et al. (1996) Mamm. Genome 7, 117–127.

11 Szpirer et al. (1987) Cytogenet. Cell Genet. 46, 701.

12 Szpirer et al. (1988) Cytogenet. Cell Genet. 47, 42–45.

13 Gulko et al. unpublished RFLP linkage data.

14 Helou et al. (1997) Mamm. Genome 8, 362–364.

15 Bihoreau et al. (1997) Genome Res. 7, 434–440.

16 Ge et al. (1996) Mamm. Genome 7, 856–857.

17 Yamada et al. (1994) Mamm. Genome 5, 63–83.

18 Donner et al. (1985) Biochem. Genet. 23, 787–800.

19 Den Dunnen et al. (1987) Exp. Eye Res. 45, 747–750.

20 Hilbert et al. (1991) Nature 353, 521–529.

21 Andoh et al. (1998) Mamm. Genome 9, 287–293.

22 Szpirer et al. (1998) Mamm. Genome 9, 721–734.

23 Jacob et al. (1995) Nature Genet. 9, 63–69.

24 Harada et al. (1995) Genomics 28, 59–65.

25 Mock et al. (1989) Genomics 5, 291–297.

26 Yamada et al. (1992) Cytogenet. Cell Genet. 61, 125–127.

27 Klinga-Levan et al. (1993) Hereditas 119, 285–296.

28 Yasue et al. (1991) Cytogenet. Cell Genet. 57, 142–148.

29 Serikawa et al. (1992) Genetics 131, 701–721.

30 Gauguier et al. (1996) Nature Genet. 12, 38–43.

31 Shepel et al. (1998) Mamm. Genome 9, 622–628.

32 Mahata et al. (1996) Genomics 33, 135–139.

33 Simon et al. (1996) Mamm. Genome 7, 380–382.

34 Ginn et al. (1994) J. Hypertens. 12, 357–365.

35 Szpirer et al. (1994) Mamm. Genome 5, 153–159.

36 Mori et al. (1992) Genomics 13, 686–689.

37 Saito et al. (1997) Mamm. Genome 8, 45–46.

38 Adham et al. (1991) Cytogenet. Cell Genet. 57, 47–50.

39 Yasue et al. (1992) Genomics 12, 659–664.

40 Nagai et al. (1995) Cytogenet. Cell Genet. 69, 185–186.

41 Johansson et al. (1998) Cytogenet. Cell Genet. 81, 217–221.

42 Koike et al. (1996) Genomics 38, 38–44.

43 Serikawa et al. (1998) Exp. Anim. 47, 1–9.

44 Brown et al. (1998) Mamm. Genome 9, 521–530.

Locus symbol	Previous symbol	RNO Location	Description	Mode	Status	Reference	HSA symbol	HSA Chr	MMU symbol	MMU Chr
Acly	Clatp	10	ATP citrate lyase, see also D10Wox19 and D10Arb16	L	C	7, 16, 45	ACLY	5q23–5q32		
Adra1b		10q21	Adrenergic, alpha 1B-, receptor, see also D10Wox8	S, L, D	C	16, 48, 54	ADRA1B	5q23–5q32	Adra1	W
Aldoc	F16dip7, RATALDCAA	10	Aldolase C, fructose-bisphosphate, see also D10Wox15 and D10Arb9	S, L	C	12, 14, 15, 16, 21, 29, 45	ALDOC	17pter–17qter	Aldo3	11
Asgr1	RATRHL1, ASGR, RHL1	10	Asialoglycoprotein receptor 1 (hepatic lectin), see also D10Wox14 and D10Mgh22	L, S	C	4, 16, 19, 29, 45, 58, 66	ASGR1	17p13–17p11	Asgr1	11
Atp1b2	Amog, ATPB2, RATATPB2S, ATPB2S	10	ATPase, Na$^+$,K$^+$-transporting, beta polypeptide 2	S, L	C	3, 29, 56, 63	ATP1B2	17pter–17qter	Atp1b2	11
Atps2		10	Aurothiopropanolsulfonate-induced auto-immune glomerulonephritis 2	L	P	22				
Brca1		10	Breast cancer 1	L	P	8	BRCA1	17q21–17q21	Brca1	11
Chrnb1	Acrb, RNACRB1	10	Acetycholine receptor beta	S, L	C	15, 29, 62, 63	CHRNB1	17p12–17p11	Acrb	11
Ciaa2		10	Type II collagen-induced arthritis antibody 1			17				
Dcp1	Ace, StsRR92	10	Dipeptidyl carboxypeptidase 1 (angiotensin I-converting enzyme), see also D10Mit1 and D10Wox18	S, L	C	13, 15, 19–21, 29, 32, 44	DCP1	17q23–17q23	Ace	11

Symbol	Alt symbol	Location	Name	Method	P/C	Refs	Human symbol	Human location	Mouse symbol	Mouse chr
Erbb2		10q32.1	Avian erythroblastosis viral (v-erb-B2) oncogene homologue 2 (neuro/glioblastoma-derived oncogene homologue)	S, L	C	25, 45, 55	ERBB2	17q11.2–17q12	Erbb2	11
Es13		10	Esterase 13	L	P	44				
Galk		10	Galactokinase	S	P	35	GALK1		Glk	
Gapd	Gapdh	10q12	Glyceraldehyde-3-phosphate dehydrogenase	N	P	53	GAPD	12p13–12p13	Gapd	6
Gcgr		10q32.3	Glucagon receptor, perhaps same as Niddm3, see also D10Mcw1	L, D	C	27, 61–63	GCGR	17q25–17q25	Gcgr	UN
Gfap		10	Glial fibrillary acidic protein, see also D10Kyo1	S, L	C	27, 61–63	GFAP	17q21–17q21	Gfap	
Gh	RNGHGP	10q32	Growth hormone 1, see also D10Wox22 and D10Mit12	S, L	C	2–4, 11, 19, 20, 28, 29, 32, 33, 42, 45, 56	GH1	17q22–17q24	Gh	11
Gludins	RATGLU-DINS	10	Glucose-dependent insulinotropic peptide, see also D10Wox23	L	P	3, 56				
Glut4		10	Glucose transporter 4, insulin-responsive, see also D10Uwm1	L	P	49				
Grin2a		10	Glutamate receptor, ionotropic, N-methyl-D-aspartate 2A	L	P	34	GRIN2A	16p13–16p13	Grin2a	16
Grin2c		10	Glutamate receptor, ionotropic, N-methyl-D-aspartate 2C	S	P	34	GRIN2C	17q25–17q25	Grin2c	11
Grm6		10	Glutamate receptor, metabotropic 6	L	C	12, 15, 34	GRM6			
Gspt1		10	G_1-to-S phase transition 1	L	C	62, 64	GSPT1	16p13.13–16p13.13		
Gstpl4	GSTPL4	10q31–q32	Glutathione-S-transferase-like 4, pi type	S, DNA-Annealing	C	23, 60				
Hoxb@	Hox2@	10	Homeobox B gene cluster region	S	P	1, 61	HOXB@	17q21–17q22	Hoxb	11

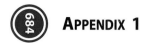

Hoxb7	Hox2r1b	10	Homeobox gene B7	S	Provisional	10	HOXB@	17q21–17q22	Hoxb	11
Hoxb8	Hox2r1a	10	Homeobox gene B8	S	P	10	HOXB@	17q21–17q22	Hoxb	11
Igfbp4	IGF-BP4	10	Insulin-like growth factor-binding protein	L	P	37	IGFBP4	17q12–17q21.1	Igfbp4	UN
Il3		10	Interleukin 3, see also D10Wox10	L	C	15, 31, 42, 62, 63	IL3	5q23–5q31	Il3	11
Il4	Il4e12	10	Interleukin 4, see also D10Mgh9 and D10Wox9	L	C	16, 21, 28	IL4	5q23–5q31	Il4	11
Il5		10	Interleukin 5 (colony-stimulating factor, eosinophil)	S	P	63	IL5	5q23–5q31	Il5	11
Il9r		10	Interleukin 9 receptor	L	C	62, 64	IL9R	Xq28–Xq28	Il9r	11
Impnb		10q32.1	Importin beta	D	P	38			Impnb	11
Irf1		10	Interferon regulatory factor 1	L	P	30	IRF1	5q23–5q31	Irf1	11
Kid1	Tcf17	10q21	Kidney 1	D, L	C	62, 63				
Mpg		10	N-Methylpurine-DNA glycocyclase	L	C	62, 64	MPG	16p13.3–16p13.3	Mpg	11
Mpo		10	Myeloperoxidase	S	P	61	MPO	17q21.3–17q23	Mpo	11
Mrp		10q11–q12	Multiple drug resistance-associated protein	D	P	62	MRP	16p13.1–16p13.1	Mdrap	16
Mtapt	pTau, RNPTAU	10	Tau microtubule-associated protein, see D10Wox21	L	P	3, 56			Mtapt	11
Myh11		10	Myosin heavy chain 11	L	C	62, 64	MYH11	16p13.1–16p13.1	Myh11	16
Myh3	Myhse, RNMHCG	10	Myosin, heavy polypeptide 3, skeletal muscle, embryonic, see also D10Mgh8 and D10Wox11	S, L	C	3, 5, 16, 19, 21, 29, 44, 45, 56, 57	MYH3	17pter–17p11	Myhse	11
Nat4		10q32.3	Serotonin N-acetyltransferase	D	P	65				

Nf1		10	Neurofibromatosis type 1	L	P	30	NF1	17q11.2	Nf1	11
Ngfr	RNNGFRR	10	Nerve growth factor receptor, fast, see also D10Wox16, D10Arb21 and D10Mit13	S, L	C	2, 4, 15, 16, 19, 29, 32, 45	NGFR	17q21–17q22	Ngfr	11
Nos2		10	Nitric oxide synthase 2, inducible, see also D10Mc038, D10Mco39, D10Mco40 and D10Wox24	S, L	C	3, 12, 14, 15, 29, 42, 56, 66	NOS2A	17q11–17q12	Nos2	11
Pkd1		10q12	Polycystic kidney disease 1	N	P	24	PKD1	16p13.3	Pkd1	17
Pld2	Pldc	10q23.3–q24	Phospholipase D gene 2	D	P	41				
Pmp22		10q22	Peripheral myelin protein	S, L	C	36, 61	PMP22	17p11.2	Pmp22	11
Pnmt		10	Phenylethanolamine N-methyltransferase	S, L	P	26	PNMT	9p21	Pnmt	UN
Polr2a	Rpo2-1	10	Polymerase (RNA II) (DNA-directed), large polypeptide	S	P	63	POLR2A	17p13.1		
Ppm1b	Pp2c2	10	Protein phosphatase type 1B (formerly 2C), Mg-dependent, beta isoform	S	P	40	PPM1B		Ppm1b	17
Ppp2ca	Pp2a1	10	Protein phosphatase 2 (formerly 2A), catalytic subunit, alpha isoform	S	P	40	PPP2CA	5q23–5q31		
Ppy		10	Pancreatic polypeptide, see also D10Wox17	L, S	C	2, 4, 5, 16, 21, 28, 32, 42, 44, 45, 48	PPY	17q21	Ppy	UN
Prkca	Pkca	10	Protein kinase C alpha	S	P	63	PRKCA	17q22–17q24	Pkca	11
Prm1		10q12	Protamine 1	S, L, D	C	1, 62, 63	PRM1	16p13.13	Prm1	16
Prr1		10q26–q31	Proline-rich polypeptide 1 (prostatic), see also D10Mgh21	D, L	C	53, 62, 63, 67	PRR1		Prp	6
Rara		10	Retinoic acid receptor alpha	S	P	39	RARA	17q12	Rara	11
Rfp2		10	Ret finger protein 2 (probably a pseudogene)	S	P	52				
Ril	H-Rev18	10	Reversion-induced LIM gene	S	P	52				
Scya2	Sigje	10	Small inducible gene JE, see also D10Kyo2	S	P	27			Scya2	11
Shbg	Abpa	10	Sex hormone-binding globulin or androgen-binding protein (other gene product from ABP gene), see also D10Wox12	S, L	C	3, 19, 29, 33, 44, 45, 49, 51, 63	SHBG	17pter–17p12	Shbg	11

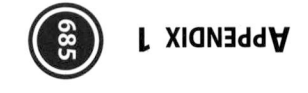

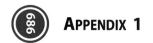

Slc4a1		10q32	Solute carrier family 4, member 1, anion exchange protein 1 (kidney band 3), see also D10Wox20	S, L, D	C	2, 4, 16, 28, 32, 33, 37, 42, 44, 48, 50, 53	SLC4A1	17q12– 17q21	Ae1	W
Sp2		10q31–q32.1	Trans-acting transcription factor 2	D	P	47	SP2	17		
Sparc		10	Secreted acidic cysteine-rich glycoprotein	L	C	62, 63	SPARC	5q31– 5q33	Sparc	11
Stat3		10q32.1	Signal transducer and activator of transcription 5a	D	P	54				
Stat5a		10q32.1	Signal transducer and activator of transcription 5a	D	P	9				
Stat5b		10q32.1	Signal transducer and activator of transcription 5a	D	P	54				
Syb2	Vamp2, SYB, RAT-VAMPB, RATVAMPIR	10q24	Synaptobrevin 2 (vesicle-associated membrane protein, VAMP-2), see also D10Mit8 and D10Wox13	L, S, D	C	2, 3, 5, 15, 16, 19, 21, 29, 32, 33, 44, 56, 57, 61	SYB2	17pter– 17p12	Syb2	11
Thra1	ERBA1	10	Thyroid hormone receptor alpha 1 (avian erythroblastic leukaemia viral (v-erb-a) oncogene homologue 1, formerly ERBA1)	S, L	C	55, 62, 63	THRA1	17q11.2– 17q12	Thra	11
Tk		10	Thymidine kinase 1, soluble	S	C	35, 63	TK1	17q23.2– 17q25.3	Tk1	11
Tm		10	Tremor	L	P	32				
Tnfaip1	Edp1	10	Tumour necrosis factor alpha-induced protein 1 (endothelial)	S	P	58, 63	TNFAIP1	17q22– 17q23	Tnfaip1	W
Tnp2		10	Transition protein 2	S, L	C	1, 62, 63	TNP2	16p13.13– 16p13.13	Tnp2	16
Tp53	p53, Trp53	10	Tumour protein p53 (Li–Fraumeni syndrome)	S, L	C	5, 6, 57, 58, 60, 63	TP53	17p13.1– 17p13.1	Trp53	11
Tsc2	Rc	10q12	Tuberous sclerosis 2 (renal carcinoma)	L, N	C	24, 62–64	TSC2	16p13.3– 16p13.3	Tsc2	17
Umph2		10	Uridine 5′-monophosphate phosphohydrolase 2	S	P	59	UMPH2	17q23– 17q25	Umph2	11

Whn	Rnu, Hfh, 11*rnu	10	Winged-helix nude or HNF-3/forkhead homologue 11 (rat athymic nude gene)	_	C	7, 33, 43, 58	WHN	17q11–q12	Hfh11	11
Wnt3	INT4	10	Wingless-type MMTV integration site 3, homologue	5, L	P	61–63	WNT3	17q21–17q22	Wnt3	11
Znf179	Bfb	10q22	Brain finger protein	C	P	38	ZNF179	17p11.2–17p11.2	Zfp179	11

References

1 Adham *et al.* (1991) *Cytogenet. Cell Genet.* **57**, 47–50.

2 Andoh *et al.* (1998) *Mamm. Genome* **9**, 287–293.

3 Bihoreau *et al.* (1997) *Genomic Res.* **7**, 434–440.

4 Brown *et al.* (1998) *Mamm. Genome* **9**, 521–530.

5 Canzian *et al.* (1996) *Jpn J. Cancer Res.* **87**, 669–675.

6 Canzian *et al.* (1996) *Mamm. Genome* **7**, 630.

7 Cash *et al.* (1993) *Mamm. Genome* **4**, 37–42.

8 Chen *et al.* (1996) *Carcinogenesis* **17**, 1561–1566.

9 Chen *et al.* (1996) *Cytogenet. Cell Genet.* **74**, 277–280.

10 Chung *et al.* (1993) *Mamm. Genome* **4**, 537–540.

11 Cooke *et al.* (1986) *Endocrinology* **119**, 2451–2454.

12 Deng and Rapp (1995) *J. Clin. Invest.* **95**, 2170–2177.

13 Deng and Rapp (1992) *Nature Genet.* **1**, 267–272.

14 Deng *et al.* (1994) *Mamm. Genome* **5**, 712–716.

15 Dukhanina *et al.* (1997) *Mamm. Genome* **8**, 229–235.

16 Gauguier *et al.* (1996) *Nature Genet.* **12**, 38–43.

17 Griffiths *et al.* (1996) XIth International Workshop on Alloantigenic Systems in the Rat, p. 57.

18 Hilbert *et al.* (1991) *Nature* **353**, 521–529.

19 Hilbert *et al.* (1991) *Nature* **353**, 521–529.

20 Jacob *et al.* (1991) *Cell* **67**, 213–224.

21 Jacob *et al.* (1995) *Nature Genet.* **9**, 63–69.

22 Kermarrec *et al.* (1996) *Genomics* **31**, 111–114.

23 Klinga-Levan *et al.* (1993) *Hereditas* **119**, 285–296.

24 Kobayashi *et al.* (1995) *Nature Genet.* **9**, 70–74.

25 Koelsch (1998) *Cytogenet. Cell Genet.* **81**, 182 .

26 Koike *et al.* (1995) *Hypertension* **26**, 595–601.

27 Kondo *et al.* (1993) *Mamm. Genome* **4**, 571–576.

28 Kovacs *et al.* (1997) *Biochem. Biophys. Res. Commun.* **235**, 343–348.

29 Kreutz *et al.* (1995) *Proc. Natl Acad. Sci. USA* **92**, 8778–8782.

30 Kubo *et al.* (1994) *Cancer Res.* **54**, 2633–2635.

31 Kunieda *et al.* (1992) *Mamm. Genome* **3**, 464–66.

32 Kuramoto *et al.* (1994) *Biochem. Biophys. Res. Commun.* **200**, 1161–1168.

33 Kuramoto *et al.* (1993) *Cytogenet. Cell Genet.* **63**, 107–110.

34 Kuramoto *et al.* (1994) *Genomics* **19**, 358–361.

35 Levan *et al.* (1986) *Rat News Lett.* **17**, 3–8.

36 Liehr and Rautenstrauss (1995) *Mamm. Genome*, **6**, 489.

37 Lorentzen *et al.* (1998) *Proc. Natl Acad. Sci. USA* **95**, 6383–6387.

38 Matsuda *et al.* (1996) *Genomics* **33**, 325–327.

39 Mattei *et al.* (1991) *Genomics* **10**, 1061–1069.

40 Muramatsu *et al.* (1994) *Mamm. Genome* **5**, 515–517.

41 Nakashima *et al.* (1997) *Cytogenet. Cell Genet.* **79**, 109–113.

42 National Institute of Arthritis and Musculoskeletal and Skin Diseases. The ARB Rat Genetic Database (http://www.nih.gov/niams/scientific/ratgbase/index.htm).

43 Nehls *et al.* (1994) *Nature* **372**, 103–107.

44 Pravenec *et al.* (1996) *Mamm. Genome* **7**, 117–127.

45 Remmers *et al.* (1992) *Genomics* **14**, 618–623.

46 Remmers *et al.* (1996) *Nature Genet.* **14**, 82–85.

47 Scohy *et al.* (1998) *Cytogenet. Cell Genet.* **81**, 273–274.

48   Serikawa *et al.* (1992) *Genetics* **131**, 701–721.

49   Shepel *et al.* (1998) *Mamm. Genome* **9**, 622–628.

50   Simon *et al.* (1996) *Mamm. Genome* **7**, 380–382.

51   Sullivan *et al.* (1991) *J. Biol. Chem.* **266**, 143–154.

52   Szpirer *et al.* (1997) *Cytogenet. Cell Genet.* **78**, 137–139.

53   Szpirer *et al.* (1997) *Mamm. Genome* **8**, 586–588.

54   Szpirer *et al.* (1998) *Mamm. Genome* **9**, 721–734.

55   Szpirer *et al.* (1991) *Oncogene* **6**, 1319–1324.

56   The Wellcome Trust Centre for Human Genetics
(http://www.well.ox.ac.uk/~bihoreau).

57   Toyota *et al.* (1996) *Proc. Natl Acad. Sci. USA* **93**, 3914–3919.

58   Yamada *et al.* (1994) *Mamm. Genome,* **5**, 63–83.

59   Yasue *et al.* (1991) *Cytogenet. Cell Genet.* **57**, 142–148.

60   Yasue *et al.* (1992) *Genomics* **12**, 659–664.

61   Yeung *et al.* (1993) *Mamm. Genome* **4**, 585–588.

62   Yeung *et al.* (1996) *Mamm. Genome* **7**, 425–428.

63   Yeung *et al.* (1993) *Proc. Natl Acad. Sci. USA* **90**, 8038–8042.

64   Yeung *et al.* (1994) *Proc. Natl Acad. Sci. USA* **91**, 11413–11416.

65   Yoshimura *et al.* (1997) *Cytogenet. Cell Genet.* **79**, 172–175.

66   Zha *et al.* (1995) *Mamm. Genome* **6**, 137–138.

67   Zhang *et al.* (1989) *Cytogenet. Cell Genet.* **52**, 197–198.

Chromosome 11

Locus symbol	Previous symbol	RNO Location	Description	Mode	Status	Reference	HSA symbol	HSA Chr	MMU symbol	MMU Chr
B1		10	Rat hepatocyte antigen	S	P	4				
Casr		11	Calcium-sensing receptor (hypocalciuric hypercalcaemia 1, severe neonatal hyper-parathyroidism)	S	P	5	CAST	3q13.3–q21	Casr	16
Comt		11	Catechol-O-methyltransferase, see also D11Mgh1, D11Mgh8 and D11Wox6	S, L, D	C	1, 3, 6–9, 11–13	COMT	22q11.2	Comt	16
Ets2		11q23	Avian erythroblastosis virus E26 (v-ets) oncogene homologue 2	S	P	12, 14	ETS2	21q22.3	Ets2	16
Fet	Pp63	11	Fetuin (phosphoprotein, 63 kDa, inhibits tyrosine kinase activity of the insulin receptor)	S	P	15				
Fgfl2		11	Fibroblast growth factor-like protein 2	L	P	10				
Igl@		11	Immunoglobulin light chain, lambda gene cluster	S	P	12, 16	IGLL@	22q11.2	Igl@	16
Kngk		11	K-kininogen, differential splicing leads to HMW Kngk, see also D11Elh1	L	P	17				
Kngt1	Tkg, Kng, Kngt	11	T-kininogen, see also D11Elh1 and D11Mit8	S, L, D	C	13, 17–21				
Mox2	Cspmo2, MRCOX2	11q23	Cell surface protein (thymocyte, antigen identified by monoclonal antibody MRC-OX2, see also D11Wox3, D11Arb6 and D11Mit6	S, L, D	C	1, 11, 19, 20, 22–25				
Mx1	IFI78	11q21–q22	Myxovirus (influenza) resistance, homologue of murine Mx (also interferon-inducible protein IFI78)	S	P	12, 26	MX1	21q22.3	Mx1	16
Odcp	Podca	11	Ornithine decarboxylase antizyme pseudo-gene, see also D11Wox9, D11Arb10	L, S	C	1, 3, 9, 27				
P2x6	Rnap2x6	11	P2X6 receptor, see also D11Wox5	L	P	3, 9				

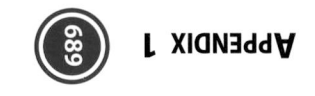

Prkcs	*PKCS*	11	Protein F1 (substrate of protein kinase C)	S	P	18				
Rnr2		11	Ribosomal 18s and 28s RNA	D, C	C	28, 29				
Siat1		11	Sialyltransferase 1 (beta-galactoside alpha-2,6-sialyltransferase), see also D11Mgh7	L	P	13				
Sod1		11	Superoxide dimutase 1, soluble	S	P	12, 30	*SOD1*	21q22.1	*Sod1*	16
Sst	*Smst*	11	Somatostatin, see also D11Wox2, D11Arb1, D11Mit7	S, L, D	C	1, 11–14, 18–21, 23, 24, 31, 32	*SST*	3q28	*Smst*	16
Vpreb1		11q23 11q23	Immunoglobulin lambda Vpreb1 chain	L	P	8, 12	*VPREB1*	22q11.2	*Vpreb*	16

References

1. National Institute of Arthritis and Musculoskeletal and Skin Diseases. The ARB Rat Genetic Database (http://www.nih.gov/niams/scientific/ratgbase/index.htm).
2. The Wellcome Trust Centre for Human Genetics (http://www.well.ox.ac.uk/~bihoreau).
3. Whitehead Institute for Biomedical Research/MIT Center for Genome Research (http://www.genome.wi.mit.edu/rat/public).
4. Perrotez *et al.* (1989) *Cytogenet. Cell Genet.* **52**, 154–156.
5. Janicic *et al.* (1995) *Mamm. Genome* **6**, 797–801.
6. Yeung *et al.* (1993) *Proc. Natl Acad. Sci. USA* **90**, 8038–8042.
7. Jacob *et al.* (1995) *Nature Genet.* **9**, 63–69.
8. Yeung *et al.* (1996) *Mamm. Genome* **7**, 246.
9. Bihoreau *et al.* (1997) *Genome Res.* **7**, 434–440.
10. Sverdlov *et al.* (1998) *Mamm. Genome* **9**, 816–821.
11. Szpirer *et al.* (1998) *Mamm. Genome* **9**, 721–734.
12. Serikawa *et al.* (1998) *Exp. Anim.* **47**, 1–9
13. Brown *et al.* (1998) *Mamm. Genome* **9**, 521–530.
14. Hino *et al.* (1993) *Proc. Natl Acad. Sci. USA* **90**, 730–734.
15. Falquerho *et al.* (1991) *Gene* **98**, 209–216.
16. Szpirer *et al.* (1988) *Curr. Topics Microbiol. Immunol.* **137**, 33–38.
17. Harris *et al.* (1997) *Mamm. Genome* **8**, 791–792.
18. Serikawa *et al.* (1992) *Genetics* **131**, 701–721.
19. Canzian *et al.* (1996) *Jpn. J. Cancer Res.* **87**, 669–675.
20. Toyota *et al.* (1996) *Proc. Natl Acad. Sci. USA* **93**, 3914–3919.
21. Andoh *et al.* (1998) *Mamm. Genome* **9**, 287–293.
22. Hilbert *et al.* (1991) *Nature* **353**, 521–529.
23. Du *et al.* (1994) *Cytogenet. Cell Genet.* **65**, 186–189.
24. Gauguier *et al.* (1996) *Nature Genet.* **12**, 38–43.
25. Borriello *et al.* (1998) *Mamm. Genome* **9**, 114–118.
26. Levan *et al.* (1991) *Genomics* **10**, 699–718.
27. Deng *et al.* (1994) *Mamm. Genome* **5**, 712–716.
28. Szabo *et al.* (1978) *Chromosoma* **65**, 161–172.
29. Sasaki *et al.* (1986) *Cytogenet. Cell Genet.* **41**, 83–88.
30. Yamada *et al.* (1992) Unpublished.
31. Yasue *et al.* (1992) *Genomics* **12**, 659–664.
32. Pravenec *et al.* (1996) *Mamm. Genome* **7**, 117–127.

Chromosome 12

Locus symbol	Previous symbol	RNO Location	Description	Mode	Status	Reference	HSA symbol	HSA Chr	MMU symbol	MMU Chr
Brca2		12	Breast cancer 2	L	P	27				
Epim		12q16	Epimorphin	D, S	P	34				
Epo		12q12–q13	Erythropoietin	D, L	C	23, 28	EPO	7q21.3–q22.1	Epo	5
fh		12	Flathead, an autosomal recessive mutation in Wistar rats at the University of Connecticut (WUC1) resulting in reduced brain growth	L	P	39				
Gusb		12	Glucuronidase beta	L, S	C	36, 28	GUSB	7q22	Gus-s	5
Hsp27		12	Heat shock 27 kDa protein	L	P	15				
Insr		12q12	Insulin receptor	D, L, S	C	20	INSR		Insr	
Irg2		12	Insulin-resistance gene 1, glucose uptake QTL in SHR WKY F2 (LOD = 6.3) and SHR × WKY backcross (LOD = 1.9), between D12Mit8 and D12Mgh1	L	P	26				
Lsn2	LSNR	12	Leukosianin-related, see also D12Wox9	L, S	C	2, 4, 5, 10, 11, 13, 30, 31				
Mdh2		12	Malate dehydrogenase 2, NAD (mitochondrial), see also D12Wox10	L, S	C	3, 7, 10, 11, 13, 28, 30, 31	MDH2	7p13–q22	Mor1	5
Muc3		12	Mucin 3	S	P	14	MUC3		Muc3	
Niddm5		12	Noninsulin-dependent diabetes mellitus QTL in 13M WKY F2, BMI (LOD = 5.07) plasma insulin concentration (LOD = 3.37), between D12Mit5 and D12Mgh6	L	P	29				
Nidd9/of		12	Suggestive QTL, fasting glucose level in (OLETF × F344)F2 (LOD = 3.87) in D12Mgh5	L	P	38				

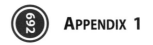

Nos1		12q16	Nitric oxide synthase 1 (neuronal), see also D12Mco2	D, L	C	9, 10, 21, 22, 32	NOS1	12q24.2–q24.3	Nos1	5
Pai1	Pai1aa, Planh	12q11–q12	Plasminogen activator inhibitor, see also D12Mit2, D12Wox11, D12Wox12 and D12Arb4	D, L, S	C	3, 7, 10, 11, 16, 17, 18, 24, 27, 32, 33	PAI1			
Pdx1		12	Pancreatic and duodenal homeobox gene 1	S	P	41	IPF1		Pdx1	
Pepckr2		12	Phosphoenolpyruvate carboxykinase-related sequence 2	L	P	18				
Plod3		12	Lysyl hydroxylase 3	S	P	40	PLOD3			
Pole		12	DNA polymerase epsilon	S	P	12	POLE			
Ppp1cc1		12	Protein phosphatase 1, catalytic subunit, gamma isoform 1 (possible existence of an alternative gene product, Ppp1cc2)	S	P	6	PPP1CC			
Ppp1cc2		12	Protein phosphatase 1, catalytic subunit, gamma isoform 2 (possible alternative product of Ppp1cc1 gene)	S	P	6	PPP1CC			
Rn5sp	Rn5s1	12	Ribosomal 5S RNA	D	C	4, 19				
Rnr3		12	Ribosomal 18S and 28S RNA	D	C	1, 2, 4	RNR3			
Sdh	Sdhe1	12	Serine dehydratase, see also D12Wox15 and D12Arb7	L	C	18, 21, 22, 33, 34				
Sercall		12	Sarco(endo)plasmic reticulum Ca^{2+}-dependent ATPase II	S	P	35				
Srb1	SR-B1	12q15–q16	Scavenger receptor class B type 1	D	P	25	SRB1			
Tcf1	Hnf1a, Lfb1	12	Transcription factor 1, hepatic; LF-B1, hepatic nuclear factor (HNF1): albumin proximal factor, also TCF1 and D12Mgh11	L, S	C	8, 28, 43	TCF1	12q24.3	Tcf1	5
Trela	Trela26, TRELA	12	Tropoelastin, see also D12Wox14, D12Mgh12 and D12Mgh13	L	P	21, 22, 43				

References

1 Kano *et al.* (1976) *Chromosoma* **55**, 37–42.

2 Sasaki *et al.* (1986) *Cytogenet. Cell Genet.* **41**, 83–88.

3 Serikawa *et al.* (1992) *Genetics* **131**, 701–721.

4 Szabo *et al.* (1978) *Chromosoma* **65**, 161–172.

5 Hilbert *et al.* (1991) *Nature* **353**, 521–529.

6 Muramatsu et al. (1994) *Cytogenet. Cell Genet.* **67**, 58–60.

7 Jacob et al. (1995) *Nature Genet.* **9**, 63–69.

8 Szpirer et al. (1992) *Genomics* **13**, 293–300.

9 Deng et al. (1995) *Mamm. Genome* **6**, 824.

10 Gauguier et al. (1996) *Nature Genet.* **12**, 38–43.

11 Pravenec et al. (1996) *Mamm. Genome* **7**, 117–127.

12 Szpirer et al. (1994) *Genomics* **20**, 223–226.

13 Yokoi et al. (1996) *Mamm. Genome* **7**, 71–73.

14 Klinga-Levan et al. (1996) *Mamm. Genome* **7**, 248–250.

15 Hamet et al. (1996) *Hypertension* **28**, 1112–1117.

16 Canzian et al. (1996) *Jpn. J. Cancer Res.* **87**, 669–675.

17 Toyota et al. (1996) *Proc. Natl Acad. Sci. USA* **93**, 3914–3919.

18 Mathern et al. (1993) *Biochem. Genet.* **31**, 441–448.

19 Frederiksen et al. (1997) *Cytogenet. Cell Genet.* **76**, 101–106.

20 Szpirer et al. (1997) *Mamm. Genome* **8**, 586–588.

21 Bihoreau et al. (1997) *Genomic Res.* **7**, 434–440.

22 The Wellcome Trust Centre for Human Genetics (rat map: http://www.well.ox.ac.uk/~bihoreau/).

23 Helou et al. (1997) *Rat Genome* **3**, 138–139.

24 Matsumoto et al. (1997) *Rat Genome* **3**, 156–164.

25 Johnson et al. (1998) *Endocrinology* **139**, 72–80.

26 Altman et al. (1997) *Nature Genet.* **16**, 197–201.

27 Yamada et al. (1997) *Mamm. Genome* **8**, 850–851.

28 Pravenec et al. (1997) *Mamm. Genome* **8**, 387–389.

29 Chung et al. (1997) *Genomics* **41**, 332–344.

30 Yamada et al. (1994) *Mamm. Genome* **5**, 63–83.

31 Andoh et al. (1998) *Mamm. Genome* **9**, 287–293.

32 Szpirer et al. (1998) *Mamm. Genome* **9**, 721–734.

33 National Institute of Arthritis and Musculoskeletal and Skin Diseases. The ARB Rat Genetic Database (http://waldo.wi.mit.edu/rat/public/).

34 Zha et al. (1996) *Genomics* **37**, 386–389.

35 Ohno et al. (1996) *Biochem. Biophys. Res. Commun.* **227**, 789–793.

36 Yasue et al. (1991) *Cytogenet. Cell Genet.* **57**, 142–148.

37 Wei et al. (1998) *Mamm. Genome* **9**, 1002–1007.

38 Kanemoto et al. (1998) *Mamm. Genome* **9**, 419–425.

39 Cogswell et al. (1998) *Neurosci. Lett.* **251**, 5–8.

40 Valtavaara et al. (1998) *J. Biol. Chem.* **273**, 12881–12886.

41 Yokoi et al. (1997) *Exp. Anim.* **46**, 323–324.

42 Whitehead Institute for Biomedical Research/MIT Center for Genome Research (http://www.genome.wi.mit.edu/).

43 Brown et al. (1998) *Mamm. Genome* **9**, 521–530.

44 The Rat Genome Database (http://ratmap.gen.gu.se/).

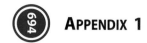

Chromosome 13											
Locus symbol	Previous symbol	RNO Location	Description	Mode	Status	Reference	HSA symbol	HSA Chr	MMU symbol	MMU Chr
A39		13	Hepatocyte antigen	S	P	32				
Abl2	*Abll*	13	Abelson murine leukaemia viral (v-*abl*) oncogene homologue 2 (Abelson-related gene)	S	P	54	*ABL2*	1q24–q25	*Abll*	1
Aldh	*Ahd-c, AHDC*	13	Aldehyde dehydrogenase (Ahd-c)	L	P	10, 22, 50	*ALDH1*	9q21.1	*Aldh1*	19
Atp1a2		13	ATPase, Na$^+$,K$^+$-transporting, alpha 2 polypeptide, see also D13Arb11 and D13Mgh17	S, L, D	C	7, 24, 29, 31, 37, 38, 41, 43, 46, 53	*ATP1A2*	1q21–q23	*Atp1a2*	1
Bcl2		13	B cell lymphoma 2-associated oncogene, see also D13Kyo4	L, S	C	23, 34	*BCL2*	18q21.33	*Bcl2*	1
Bp11		13	Blood pressure QTL, close to Ren (probably same as Bp5, Bp24, Bp25 and Bp31)	L	P	12				
Bp24		13	Blood pressure QTL (probably same as Bp5, Bp11, Bp25 and Bp31)	L	P	42				
Bp25		13	Blood pressure QTL between Syt2 and D13M1Mit108 (probably not the same as Bp5, Bp11, Bp24 and Bp31)	L	C	55				
Bp31		13	Blood pressure QTL in SHR × WKY F2, LOD = 5.75, close to D13Mit2 (perhaps more than one QTL in this region) (probably same as Bp5, Bp11, Bp24 and Bp25)	L	P	39				
Bp5		13	Blood pressure QTL in LH × LN F2, diastolic pressure LOD = 5.6, systolic pressure LOD = 3.4, close to Ren (probably same as Bp11, Bp24, Bp25 and Bp31)	L	P	13				

C4bp@		13	Complement component 4-binding protein gene cluster				C4BP@	1q32	C4b@	1
C4bpa	C4BP	13	Complement component 4-binding protein alpha	S	P	2		1q32		
C4bpb		13	Complement component 4 binding protein beta	S	P	2	C4BPB	1q32		
Dbi	Acoabp3	13	Diazepam binding inhibitor (GABA receptor modulator, acyl-coenzyme A-binding protein), see also D13Wox14	L, D	C	5, 43, 45	DBI	2q12–q21	Dbi	UN
Eag1 ·		13	Rat kidney endothelial antigen	L	P	9				
F5		13	Coagulation factor V (proaccelerin, labile factor)	S	P	11	F5	1q21–q25	Cf-5	1
Fcer1a	Iger01	13	Fc fragment of IgE, high affinity I, receptor for, alpha polypeptide, see also D13Wox17	L	P	5, 45	FCER1A	1q23	Fcer1a	1
Fh		13	Fumarate hydratase	L, S	C	1, 8, 9, 31, 34, 35, 37, 40, 48, 52	FH	1q42.1	Fh1	RE
Glul		13	Glutamine synthetase (glutamate-ammonia ligase)	S, D	C	17	GLUL	1q25		
Hsd11b1		13	Hydroxysteroid dehydrogenase, 11 beta type 1	D	P	43				
Mgd1		13	Methylglyoxal dehydrogenase 1	L	P	4, 34		3		16
Mpz		13	Myelin protein zero (Charcot-Marie-Tooth neuropathy 1B)	D	P	26	MPZ	1q22–q23	Mpz	1
Mr1		13	MHC class I-related gene	L	P	48	MR1	q25.3	Mr1	1H1
Pepc	PEP3	13	Peptidase C	L, S	C	10, 47, 49, 52	PEPC	1q25	Pep3	1D
Pfkfb2		13	6-Phosphofructo-2-kinase/fructose-2,6-bis-phosphatase 2 (heart) (conflicting physical mapping)	S, L, D	C	19, 30, 31, 37, 41, 43	PFKFB2	1q31	Pfkfb2	UN
Pigr	Pigr, RNPIGR2	13	Polymeric immunoglobulin receptor, see also D13Wox15	L	P	5, 45	PIGR	1q31–q41	Pigr	UN
Pla2a	Pla2p	13	Phospholipase A2 polypeptide a (pancreatic), see also D13Mgh7 and D13AT1	L	P	21	PLA2G1B	12q23–qter	Pla2g1b	UN

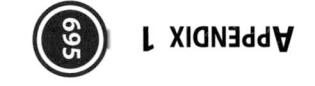

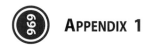

Pla2g4	*Pla2c, cPLA2*	13	Phospholipase A2, cytosolic	L	P	44	*PLA2G4*	1q24–q25	*Pla2g4*	UN
Ptprc	*T200, CD45, RT7, Lca, ART-1, Ly-2*	13	Protein tyrosine phosphatase, receptor-type, c polypeptide (antigen Cd45, leukocyte-common antigen/T200 glycoprotein) also RT7	S, L	C	15, 30, 31, 34, 36, 37, 40	*PTPRC*	1q31–q32	*Ptprc*	1
Rafas		13	Breakage region for raf-rearrangement	S	P	20				
Ren		13	Renin, see also D13Uwm1, D13Wox5 and D13Arb7	L, S	C	3, 5, 7, 12, 18, 21, 27, 29, 30, 31, 33, 34, 37, 38, 40, 43, 45, 46, 51, 55	*REN*	1q32	*Ren*	1
RT3	*Ag-D*	13	Cell surface alloantigen (= Ag-D)	L	Inc	6, 16, 25, 31, 37				
Syt2	*SYNII*	13	Synaptotagmin II, see also D13Wox6 and D13Arb8	L, D	C	14, 29, 38, 43, 55			*Syt2*	1
Ten2		13	Thymus enlargement gene 2	L	P	28				
Tnnt2	*Tnnt3, Ctt*	13	Troponin T, cardiac, see also D13Wox9 and D13Arb9	L, D	C	5, 14, 29, 38, 43, 45	*TNNT2*	1q	*Tnnt2*	UN
Trnegl	*Traggl*	13	Asp-, Gly-, Glu- and Leu-tRNAs cluster, see also D13Mgh8 and D13Arb12	S, L	C	5, 21, 29, 34, 38, 40, 45				

References

1 Adams *et al.* (1984) *Biochem. Genet.* **22**, 611–629.

2 Andersson *et al.* (1990) *Somat. Cell Mol. Genet.* **16**, 493–500.

3 Andoh *et al.* (1998) *Mamm. Genome* **9**, 287–293.

4 Bender *et al.* (1994) *Biochem. Genet.* **32**, 147–154.

5 Bihoreau *et al.* (1997) *Genomic Res.* **7**, 434–440.

6 Brdicka and Frenzl (1978) *Folia Biol. (Praha)* **24**, 381–382..

7 Canzian *et al.* (1996) *Jpn. J. Cancer Res.* **87**, 669–675.

8 Carleer and Ansay (1976) *Int. J. Biochem.* **7**, 565–566.

9 Cramer *et al.* (1985) *Biochem. Genet.* **23**, 623–629.

10 Cramer *et al.* (1986) *Biochem. Genet.* **24**, 217–227.

11 Dahlbäck *et al.* (1988) *Somat. Cell Mol. Genet.* **14**, 509–514.

12 Deng and Rapp (1992) *Nature Genet.* **1**, 267–272.

13 Dubay *et al.* (1993) *Nature Genet.* **3**, 354–357.

14 Gauguier *et al.* (1996) *Nature Genet.* **12**, 38–43.

15 Goldner-Sauve *et al.* (1991) *Biochem. Genet.* **29**, 275–286.

16 Hedrich and Reetz (1990) *Transplant. Proc.* **22**, 2559–2560.

17 Helou *et al.* (1997) *Mamm. Genome* **8**, 362–364.

18 Hilbert *et al.* (1991) *Nature* **353**, 521–529.

19 Hilliker *et al.* (1991) *Genomics* **10**, 867–873.

20 Ingvarsson *et al.* (1988) *Somat. Cell Mol. Genet.* **14**, 401–405.

21 Jacob *et al.* (1995) *Nature Genet.* **9**, 63–69.

22 Kobayashi *et al.* (1995) *Mamm. Genome* **6**, 889.

23 Kondo *et al.* (1993) *Mamm. Genome* **4**, 571–576.

24 Kunieda *et al.* (1992) *Mamm. Genome* **3**, 564–567.

25 Kunz and Gill III (1978) *J. Immunogenet.* **5**, 365–382.

26 Liehr *et al.* (1995) *Mamm. Genome* **6**, 824–825.

27 Mori *et al.* (1992) *J. Hered.* **83**, 204–207.

28 Murakumo *et al.* (1996) *Mamm. Genome* **7**, 505–508.

29 National Institute of Arthritis and Musculoskeletal and Skin Diseases. The ARB Rat Genetic Database (http://www.nih.gov/niams/scientific/ratgbase/index.htm).

30 Pape *et al.* (1996) *Mamm. Genome* **7**, 559.

31 Pape *et al.* (1996) XIth International Workshop on Alloantigenic Systems in the Rat, p. 55.

32 Perrotez *et al.* (1989) *Cytogenet. Cell Genet.* **52**, 154–156.

33 Pravenec *et al.* (1991) *Genomics* **9**, 466–472.

34 Pravenec *et al.* (1996) *Mamm. Genome* **7**, 117–127.

35 Pravenec *et al.* (1990) *Transplant. Proc.* **22**, 2555.

36 Prokop *et al.* (1993) *Transplant. Proc.* **25**, 2795–2796.

37 Prokop *et al.* (1997) *Transplant. Proc.* **29**, 1771.

38 Remmers *et al.* (1993) *Genomics* **18**, 277–282.

39 Samani *et al.* (1996) *Hypertension* **28**, 1118–1122.

40 Serikawa *et al.* (1992) *Genetics* **131**, 701–721.

41 Shepel *et al.* (1998) *Mamm. Genome* **9**, 622–628.

42 St Lezin *et al.* (1997) *J. Clin. Invest.* **97**, 522–527.

43 Szpirer *et al.* (1998) *Mamm. Genome* **9**, 721–734.

44 Tay *et al.* (1995) *Genomics* **26**, 138–141.

45 The Wellcome Trust Centre for Human Genetics (http://www.well.ox.ac.uk/~bihoreau).

46 Toyota *et al.* (1996) *Proc. Natl Acad. Sci. USA* **93**, 3914–3919.

47 Walker *et al.* (1996) *Mouse Genome* **94**, 149–151.

48 Walter and Günther (1998) *Immunogenetics* **47**, 477–482.

49 Womack and Cramer (1980) *Biochem. Genetics* **18**, 1019–1026.

50 Yamada *et al.* (1994) *Mamm. Genome* **5**, 63–83.

51 Yamada *et al.* (1992) Unpublished.

52 Yasue *et al.* (1991) *Cytogenet. Cell Genet.* **57**, 142–148.

53 Yasue *et al.* (1992) *Genomics* **12**, 659–664.

54 Yeung *et al.* (1993) *Mamm. Genome* **4**, 585–588.

55 Zhang *et al.* (1997) *Mamm. Genome* **8**, 636–641.

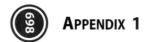

Chromosome 14

Locus symbol	Previous symbol	RNO Location	Description	Mode	Status	Reference	HSA symbol	HSA Chr	MMU symbol	MMU Chr
Add1		14	Adducin 1 alpha	Unpubl	P	45	ADD1	4p16.3	Add1	5
Adra2c		14	Adrenergic, alpha2C-, receptor class I	L	P	23	ADRA2C	4p16.3–p-15	Adra2c	5
Afp		14	Alpha-fetoprotein	L, S, D	C	1, 5, 7, 12, 13, 21, 24, 25, 43	AFP	4q11–q13	Afp	5
Alb	Albza	14	Albumin	Flow sorted chromo-somes, S, D, L	C	1, 5, 7, 13, 21, 24, 25, 27, 41–44	ALB	4q11–q13	Alb1	5
Camk2b	Ck2b	14	Ca^{2+}/calmodulin-dependent protein kinase II, beta subunit	S	P	40	CAMK2B	22q12	Camk2b	11
Cckar		14	Cholecystokinin A receptor	L	P	22	CCKAR	4	Cckar	5
Csn1	Csna, Casa	14	Casein alpha	L, S	C	1, 5, 7, 13, 21, 24, 25	CSN1	4q21.1	Csna	5
Ddc		14	Dopa decarboxylase (aromatic L-amino acid decarboxylase)	S	P	39				
Dmo3		14	Diabetes mellitus, OLETF type 3 (involved in plasma glucose homeostasis)	L	P	38				
Drd1B	Drd5	14	Dopamine receptor D5	L, S	C	1, 14, 23				
Egfr	ERBB1	14	Epidermal growth factor receptor, formerly avian erythroblastic leukaemia viral (v-erbB) oncogene homologue (Erbb1)	S	P	37	EGFR	7p12	Egfr	11
Gc	Vdbp	14	Group-specific component vitamin D-binding protein)	L, S	C	1, 2, 5, 6, 13, 28, 35, 36	GC	4q12–q13	Gc	5
Gck	GLUKA	14	Glucokinase, see also D14Arb12	L, S, D	C	1, 14, 28, 34				
Gfi1		14	Growth factor independent-1	D	P	33	GFI1	1p22	Gfi1	5

Gl1		14	Rat plasma protein	L	P	30, 32				
Gpx1		14	Glutathione peroxidase 1	S	P	31				
H		14	Hooded	L	C	21, 25, 27, 28, 29, 30				
Hm		14	Hooded modifier	L	P	26				
Ighen	Ighen	14	Immunoglobulin heavy chain 3 enchancer sequence	L	C	47				
Ibsp	Bsp	14	Integrin-binding sialoprotein (bone sialo-protein II)	L	C	1, 7, 14, 21, 25	IBSP	4q28–q31	Ibsp	5
Igfbp3	Igfbp	14	Insulin-like growth factor-binding protein (IGF-BP3)	S, L	C	1, 5, 7, 21–24	IGFBP3	7p13–p12	IGfbp3	11
Irjhm		14	Immune response to JHM	L	C	9, 20				
Mucsmg		14	Rat submandibular gland apomucin	S	P	19				
Nefh	Nfh	14	Neurofilament, heavy polypeptide	D	P	18	NFH	22q12.1–q13.1	Nfh	11
Nefml		14	Neurofilament protein-like	S	P	10				
Odb2		14	OLETF rat diabetogenic gene 2 (diabetes mellitus)	L	P	16, 17				
Peps		14	Peptidase S	S	P	15	PEPS	4p11–p12	Pep7	5
Pf4	Pf4a	14	Platelet factor 4	L	C	1, 2, 6, 14				
Pgam2	Pgmut	14q21-14q22	Phosphoglycerate mutase 2	L, D	C	12. 13	PGAM2	10q25.3		
Rrm1p		14	Ribonucleotide reductase 1 pseudogene	S, D	P	11				
Tp53	Trp53l2	14	Tumour protein p53-like 2	S	P	9, 10				
Ugt2b2		14	Androsterone UDP-glucuronosyltransferase	D	P	8				
Vcsa1	Smr1, Smr1g, Arp	14	Variable coding sequence A1 (androgen-regulated protein (SMR1) gene)	S, L, D	C	2, 4–7				
Vcsa2		14	Variable coding sequence A2	D	P	4				
Vcsb1		14	Variable coding sequence B1	S, L, D	P	4				
Vcsd1		14	Variable coding sequence D1	D	P	4				
Vcsd2		14	Variable coding sequence D2	D	P	4				
Vcsd@		14	Variable coding sequence gene cluster		P	4				

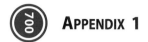
References

1 National Institute of Arthritis and Musculoskeletal and Skin Diseases. The ARB Rat Genetic Database (http://www.nih.gov/niams/scientific/ratgbase/index.htm).

2 The Wellcome Trust Centre for Human Genetics (http://www.well.ox.ac.uk/~bihoreau).

3 Whitehead Institute for Biomedical Research/MIT Center for Genome Research (http://www.genome.wi.mit.edu/rat/public).

4 Rosinski-Chupin et al. (1995) Mamm. Genome 6, 153–154.

5 Gauguier et al. (1996) Nature Genet. 12, 38–43.

6 Bihoreau et al. (1997) Genomic Res. 7, 434–440.

7 Andoh et al. (1998) Mamm. Genome 9, 287–293.

8 Satoh et al. (1993) Cytogenet. Cell Genet. 62, 49–51.

9 Yamada et al. (1994) Mamm. Genome 5, 63–83.

10 Yasue et al. (1992) Genomics 12, 659–664.

11 Klinga-Levan et al. (1997) Mamm. Genome 8, 47–49.

12 Szpirer et al. (1998) Mamm. Genome 9, 721–734.

13 Jacob et al. (1995) Nature Genet. 9, 63–69.

14 Remmers et al. (1993) Mamm. Genome 4, 90–94.

15 Yasue et al. (1991) Cytogenet. Cell Genet. 57, 142–148.

16 Hirashima et al. (1996) XIth International Workshop on Alloantigenic Systems in the Rat, Toulouse, France, 21–24 August, p. 48.

17 Hirashima et al. (1996) Rat Genome 2, 132–135.

18 Yeung et al. (1993) Proc. Natl Acad. Sci. USA 90, 8038–8042.

19 Albone et al. (1996) Glycoconjugate J. 13, 709–716.

20 Watanabe et al. (1987) Lab. Invest. 57, 375–384.

21 Canzian et al. (1996) Jpn. J. Cancer Res. 87, 669–675.

22 Hirashima et al. (1996) Rat Genome 2, 136–139.

23 Ginn et al. (1994) J. Hypertens. 12, 357–365.

24 Hilbert et al. (1991) Nature 353, 521–529.

25 Toyota et al. (1996) Proc. Natl Acad. Sci. USA 93, 3914–3919.

26 Stolc (1984) J. Hered. 75, 81.

27 Pravenec et al. (1996) Mamm. Genome 7, 117–127.

28 Serikawa et al. (1992) Genetics 131, 701–721.

29 Shumiya and Nagase (1988) Biochem. Genet. 26, 585–593.

30 Moutier et al. (1973) Biochem. Genet. 10, 395–398.

31 Hino et al. (1993) Proc. Natl Acad. Sci. USA 90, 730–734.

32 Palm (1971) Transplantation 11, 175–183.

33 Bell et al. (1995) Cytogenet. Cell Genet. 62, 49–51.

34 Sebastian et al. (1997) Cytogenet. Cell Genet. 77, 266–267.

35 Shisa et al. (1997) Mamm. Genome 8, 324–327.

36 Cooke et al. (1987) Cytogenet. Cell. Genet. 44, 98–100.

37 Szpirer et al. (1991) Oncogene 6, 1319–1324.

38 Kanemoto et al. (1998) Mamm. Genome 6, 419–425.

39 Vassort et al. (1993) Mamm. Genome 4, 202–206.

40 Levan et al. (1991) Genomics 10, 699–718.

41 Gal et al. (1984) Mol. Gen. Genet. 195, 153–158.

42 Sugiyama et al. (1984) Jpn. J. Genet. 59, 577–583.

43 Szpirer et al. (1984) Cytogenet. Cell Genet. 38, 142–149.

44 Collard et al. (1982) Cytogenet. Cell Genet. 32, 257–258.

45 Tripodi et al. (1995) Gene 166, 307–311.

46 Serikawa et al. (1998) Exp. Anim. 47, 1–9.

47 Brown et al. (1998) Mamm. Genome 9, 521–530.

Chromosome 15										
Locus symbol	Previous symbol	RNO Location	Description	Mode	Status	Reference	HSA symbol	HSA Chr	MMU symbol	MMU Chr
Apex1		15p14	Apurinic/apyrimidinic endonuclease 1	D	P	9	APE	14q11.2–q12	Apex	14
Ednrb	Etb, Ednra	15q21–q22	Endothelin receptor type B (D15Mco2)	S, L, D	C	4, 8, 14	EDNRB	13q22–q31	Ednrb	14
Egr3		15cen–q11	Early growth response 3	D	P	9				
Esd		15	Esterase D/formylglutathione hydrolase	L	P	12, 24				
Gnrh		15	Gonadotropin-releasing hormone (D15Mgh12)	L	P		GNRH	8p21–p11.2	Gnrh	14
Gucb2 Locus		15	Guanylate cyclase beta 2	S	P	26				
Lre3	Lin3A	15	LINE retrotransposable element 3 (D15Mgh1)	L	P	8				
Mlvi3		15	Moloney murine leukaemia virus (MoMuLV) integration site 3 homologue	S	P	21				
Nefm		15	Neurofilament protein, middle polypeptide	S	P	25			Nfm	14
Np		15	Nucleoside phosphorylase	S	P	24	NP1	14q11.2	Np	14
Ppp3ca		15	Calcineurin subunit A alpha	S	P	23				
Ppp3cb		15	Calcineurin subunit A beta	S	P	23				
Ptpg		15	Protein tyrosine phosphatase gamma (provisional HGM11 symbol)	S	P	26				
Rarb		15	Retinoic acid receptor beta	S	C	6, 7, 10	RARB	3p24.3–p24.2	Rarb	14
Rb1		15q12	Retinoblastoma 1 (including osteosarcoma)	S, D, L	C	13, 16, 22, 27	RB1	13q14.2	RB1	14
Retl2		15	Tyrosine kinase receptor ligand 2 (D15Wox6)	L	P	1, 15, 16, 19				
TEp1		15	Telomerase protein component 1	L	P	3	TEP	14q11.2	Tep1	14

| Thrb | 15 | Thyroid hormone receptor, beta (avian erythroblastic leukemia viral (v-*erb*-a) oncogene homologue 2) (D15Wox5) | S, L | C | 2, 5–7, 20 | *THRB* | 3p24.1–p22 | *Thrb* | un |
| Trpm2 | 15 | Testostrone-repressed prostate message 2 | S, L | C | 11 | | | | |

References

1 Bihoreau and Gauguier (1998) *Rat Genome* **4**, 60–62.

2 Bihoreau *et al.* (1997) *Genomic Res.* **7**, 434–440.

3 Brown *et al.* (1998) *Mamm. Genome* **9**, 521–530.

4 Deng *et al.* (1994) *J. Clin. Invest.* **93**, 2701–2709.

5 Goldner-Sauvé *et al.* (1991) *Biochem. Genet.* **29**, 275–286.

6 Hino *et al.* (1993) *Proc. Natl Acad. Sci. USA* **90**, 327–331.

7 Hino *et al.* (1993) *Proc. Natl Acad. Sci. USA* **90**, 730–734.

8 Jacob *et al.* (1995) *Nature Genet.* **9**, 63–69.

9 Johansson *et al.* (1998) *Cytogenet. Cell Genet.* **81**, 217–221.

10 Mattei *et al.* (1991) *Genomics* **10**, 1061–1069.

11 Moralejo *et al.* (1998) *Exp. Anim.* **47**, 141–142.

12 Moutier *et al.* (1973) *Biochem. Genet.* **9**, 109–115.

13 Ono and Yoshida (1993) *Jpn. J. Genet.* **68**, 617–621.

14 Pravenec *et al.* (1996) *Folia Biol. (Praha)* **42**, 147–153.

15 Szpirer *et al.* (1988) *Curr. Top. Microbiol. Immunol.* **137**, 33–38.

16 Szpirer *et al.* (1991) *Oncogene* **6**, 1319–1324.

17 Szpirer *et al.* (1996) *Folia Biol. (Praha)* **42**, 175–226.

18 Szpirer *et al.* (1998) *Mamm. Genome* **9**, 721–734.

19 Szpirer *et al.* (1987) *Cytogenet. Cell Genet.* **46**, 701.

20 The Wellcome Trust Centre for Human Genetics (http://www.well.ox.ac.uk).

21 Tsichlis *et al.* (1985) *J. Virol.* **56**, 938–942.

22 Yamada *et al.* (1997) *Mamm. Genome* **8**, 454–455.

23 Yamada *et al.* (1994) *Cytogenet. Cell Genet.* **67**, 55–57.

24 Yasue *et al.* (1991) *Cytogenet. Cell Genet.* **57**, 142–148.

25 Yasue *et al.* (1992) *Genomics* **12**, 659–664.

26 Yeung *et al.* (1993) *Mamm. Genome* **4**, 585–588.

27 Zullo and Upender (1995) *Genomics* **25**, 753–756.

Chromosome 16

Locus symbol	Previous symbol	RNO Location	Description	Mode	Status	Reference	HSA symbol	HSA Chr	MMU symbol	MMU Chr
Adrb3		16	Adrenergic receptor beta 3	L	P	10				
Atp4b		16	ATPase, H+,K+-transporting, beta (gastric H,K-ATPase beta subunit); defined by D16Mco8	S	P	13	ATP4B	13q34	Atp4b	8
Atp7b	Hts, Wd	16q12.2	ATPase, Cu2+-transporting, beta polypeptide (same as Wilson disease)	D, S, L	C	24	ATP7B	13q14.3–q21.1	Atp7b	8
Fnta		16	Alpha farnesyltransferase	L	P	10	FNTA	8p22–q11	Fnta	8
Glud1		16p16	Glutamate dehydrogenase; defined by D16Mgh3, D16Mco9	S, L, D	C	13, 15, 18	GLUD1	10q13.3	Glud1	14
Gstpl5	GSTPL5	16p11	Glutathione-S-transferase-like 5, pi type	S	C	19, 38				
Hgl		16	Heregulin; defined by D16Wox14 and D16Wox15	L	P	3, 33				
Jund		16	Jun D proto-oncogene	S	P	33	JUND	19p13.2	Jund	8
Klk3		16ql1	Kalpl Plasma kallikrein; defined by D16MghS and D16Wox13	L	P	3				
Lpl		16	Lipoprotein lipase	L	P	4, 26	LPL	8p22–q11		8
Mbpa		16	Mannose-binding protein A, serum, defined by D16Wox9	S, L, D	C	14, 16, 25, 26				
Ppp2cb	Pp2a2	16	Protein phosphatase 2 (formerly 2A), catalytic subunit, beta isoform	S	P	22				
Rbp3	Irbp	16	Retinol-binding protein 3, interstitial	S	P	39	RBP3	10q11.2	Rbp3	14
Sftp1	Sftpa	16	Surfactant-associated protein 1 (pulmonary surfactant protein, SP-A); defined by D16Mgh2	S, L, D	C	18, 39	SFTP1	10q21–q24	Sftp1	14
Tpm4		16	Tropomycin 4; defined by D16Mgh4, D16Wox10 and D16Wox11	L	C	14, 18				

References

1 Andoh et al. (1998) Mamm. Genome 9, 287–293.

2 Amarger et al. (1998) Genomics 52, 62–71.

3 Bihoreau et al. (1997) Genome Res. 7, 434–440.

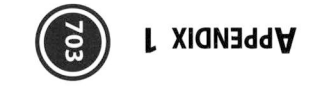

4   Bottger *et al.* (1996) *J. Clin. Invest.* **98**, 856–862.

5   Brown *et al.* (1998) *Mamm. Genome* **9**, 521–530.

6   Canzian *et al.* (1996) *Jpn. J. Cancer Res.* **87**, 669–675.

7   Canzian *et al.* (1996) *Mamm. Genome* **7**, 630.

8   Chung *et al.* (1997) *Genomics* **41**, 332–344.

9   Courvoisier *et al.* (1997) *Mamm. Genome* **8**, 282–283.

10 Cui *et al.* (1998) *Exp. Anim.* **47**, 83–88.

11 Deng *et al.* (1994) *Mamm. Genome* **5**, 712–716.

12 Du *et al.* (1996) *Genomics* **32**, 113–116.

13 Deng *et al.* (1998) *Mamm. Genome* **9**, 38–43.

14 Gauguier *et al.* (1996) *Nature Genet.* **12**, 38–43.

15 Helou *et al.* (1997) *Mamm. Genome* **8**, 362–364.

16 Hilbert *et al.* (1991) *Nature* **353**, 521–529.

17 Hino *et al.* (1996) *Rat Genome* **2**, 6–9.

18 Jacob *et al.* (1995) *Nature Genet.* **9**, 63–69.

19 Klinga-Levan *et al.* (1993) *Hereditas* **119**, 285–296.

20 Kuramoto *et al.* (1995) *Exp. Anim.* **44**, 119–125.

21 Larsson *et al.* (1998) *Mamm. Genome* **9**, 479–481.

22 Matsumoto *et al.* (1998) *Mamm. Genome* **9**, 531–535.

23 Muramatsu *et al.* (1994) *Mamm. Genome* **5**, 515–517.

24 Ono *et al.* (1995) *Jpn. J. Genet.* **70**, 25–33.

25 Pravenec *et al.* (1996) *Mamm. Genome* **7**, 117–127.

26 Pravenec *et al.* (1996) *Folia Biol. (Praha)* **42**, 147–153.

27 Sasaki *et al.* (1994) *Biochem. Biophys. Res. Commun.* **202**, 512–518.

28 Schork *et al.* (1995) *Genome Res.* **5**, 164–172.

29 Shepel *et al.* (1998) *Mamm. Genome* **9**, 622–628.

30 Ståhl *et al.* (1998) *Rat Genome* **4**, 111–1(19.

31 Ståhl and Levan (1996) *Rat Genome* **2**, 197–199.

32 Sverdlov *et al.* (1998) *Mamm. Genome* **9**, 816–821.

33 Szpirer *et al.* (1994) *Mamm. Genome* **5**, 361–364.

34 Szpirer *et al.* (1996) *Folia Biol. (Praha)* **42**, 175–226.

35 Szpirer *et al.* (1998) *Mamm. Genome* **9**, 721–734.

36 Tissir *et al.* (1998) *Rat Genome* **4**, 98–102.

37 Toyota *et al.* (1996) *Proc. Natl Acad. Sci. USA* **93**, 3914–3919.

38 Yasue *et al.* (1992). *Genomics* **12**, 659–664.

39 Yeung *et al.* (1993) *Mamm. Genome* **4**, 585–588.

40 Yeung *et al.* (1993) *Cytogenet. Cell Genet.* **62**, 149–153.

41 Yokoi *et al.* (1998) *Rat Genome* **4**, 84–97.

42 Yokoi *et al.* (1996) *Mamm. Genome* **7**, 71–73.

Chromosome 17

Locus symbol	Previous symbol	RNO Location	Description	Mode	Status	Reference	HSA symbol	HSA Chr	MMU symbol	MMU Chr
Agtr1a	At1, At1a	17p12	Angiotensin II receptor, type 1 (AT1A), see also D17Arb4	S, L, D	C	1–11				
Bp8		17	Blood pressure, QTL (localized near D17Mgh3). In an F2 (Dahl salt sens. Lewis), LOD = 2.2 between D17Mco3 and D17Mco10	L	C	2, 12				
Chrm3	ACRM, Acrm3	17q12.1	Cholinergic receptor, muscarinic 3, GenBank no. M16408, see also D17Mit4, D17Arb7, D17Wox12, D17Wox13 and D17Wox1	L, S, D	C	2, 3, 6, 7, 10, 13–18				
Csh1	Rhco1, Pl-I, Pl-Im	17	Chorionic somatomammotropin hormone 1; placental lactogen 1	S	P	19				
Csh1v	Pl-Iv	17	Chorionic somatomammotropin hormone 1 variant; placental lactogen 1	S	P	20				
Csh2	Pl2	17	Chorionic somatomammotropin hormone 2; placental lactogen 2	S	P	21	CSH2	17q22–q24	Pd2	13
Dmy		17	Demyelination	L	P	7				
Dprp	d/tPRP	17p12	Decidual prolactin-related protein	S, D	C	10, 22				
Drd1a	D1a	17p14	Dopamine-1A receptor, see also D17Mco4	L	C	2, 6, 8, 9, 18, 24	DRD1	5q34–q35	Drd1a	13
Edn1	Et1	17	Endothelin 1, see also D17Mco5	L, S	C	2, 6, 8, 9, 24, 25	EDN1	6p24.1	Edu1	13
Facc		17	Fanconi anaemia group C gene	S	P	26	FACC	9q22.3	Facc	13
Fbp1	Fdp	17p14	Fructose-1,6-biphosphatase, see also D17Mgh1	L, S, D	C	3, 10, 27				
Fgfr4		17p14	Fibroblast growth factor receptor 4	D	P	10				
Gad2		17	Glutamate decarboxylase 2 (islet)	S	P	28	GAD2	10p12–p11.2	Gad2	2
H1d	H14	17p12–p11	Histone 1d	L	P	29				

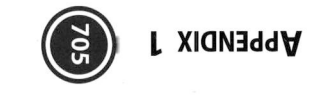

H1t		17	Testis-specific histone 1, probably same as Hh1tts	S	P	29				
Hh1tts	*H1th4c*	17	Testis-specific histone, H1t and H4t, see also D17Mgh3	S, L	C	2, 3, 7, 30				
Hk3		17q12	Hexokinase 3	D	P	31	*HK3*			
Nidd/gk6		17	Noninsulin-dependent diabetes mellitus (QTL)	L	P	6				
Ntrk2	*Tkrb*	17	Neural receptor protein-tyrosine kinase (trkB), see also D17Wox10	L	P	8, 9				
Plpa		17	Prolactin-like protein A	S	P	21				
Plpb		17	Prolactin-like protein B	S	P	21				
Plpc		17	Prolactin-like protein C	S	P	32				
Plpcv	*Plp-Cv*	17p12	Prolactin-like protein C variant	S, D	C	33, 10				
Prl	*Prol, PRLB*	17p12	Prolactin, GenBank no. J00766, see also D17Wox11 and D17Wox18	D, S, L	C	2, 6–11, 13, 14, 18, 34, 35	*PRL*	6p23–p22.3	*Prl*	13
Rfp1		17	Ret finger protein 1	S	P	36				
Rpl35p		17	Ribosomal protein L35a-related pseudogene	S	P	30				
Sca1		17	Spinocerebellar ataxia type 1, see also D17Wox16	L	P	8, 9				
Syk		17p14	Spleen tyrosine kinase	D	P	37				
Tcrg		17	T-cell receptor, gamma cluster	S	P	38	*TCRG*	7p15	*Tcrg*	13
Th2a		17	Testis-specific histone 2a	S	P	29				
Th2b		17	Testis-specific histone 2b	S	P	29				
Tpl2	*D17TPL2*	17q12	Tumour progression locus 2	D, S	P	39, 40	*TPL2*	10p11	*Tpl2*	18

References

1 Szpirer *et al.* (1993) *J. Hypertens* **11**, 919–925.

2 Deng *et al.* (1994) *J. Clin. Invest.* **93**, 2701–2709.

3 Jacob *et al.* (1995) *Nature Genet.* **9**, 63–69.

4 Tissir *et al.* (1995) *Cytogenet. Cell Genet.* **71**, 77–80.

5 Du *et al.* (1996) *Genomics* **32**, 113–116.

6 Gauguier *et al.* (1996) *Nature Genet.* **12**, 38–43.

7 Kuramoto *et al.* (1996) *Mamm. Genome* **7**, 890–894.

8 Bihoreau *et al.* (1997) *Genomic Res.* **7**, 434–440.

9 The Wellcome Trust Centre for Human Genetics (http://www.well.ox.ac.uk/~bihoreau).

10 Szpirer *et al.* (1998) *Mamm. Genome* **9**, 721–734.

11 Shepel *et al.* (1998) *Mamm. Genome* **9**, 622–628.

12 Garrett *et al.* (1998) *Genome Res.* **8**, 711–723.

13 Hilbert *et al.* (1991) *Nature* **353**, 521–529.

14 Pravenec *et al.* (1996) *Mamm. Genome* **7**, 117–127.

15 Canzian *et al.* (1996) *Jpn. J. Cancer Res.* **87**, 669–675.

16 Toyota *et al.* (1996) *Proc. Natl Acad. Sci. USA* **93**, 3914–3919.

17 Courvoisier *et al.* (1997) *Mamm. Genome* **8**, 282–283.

18 Andoh *et al.* (1998) *Mamm. Genome* **9**, 287–293.

19 Dai *et al.* (1996) *Endocrinology* **137**, 5020–5027.

20 Cohick *et al.* (1996) *Mol. Cell. Endocrinol.* **116**, 49–58.

21 Duckworth *et al.* (1993) *Sereno Symposia*, Springer-Verlag, p. 169-190.

22 Roby *et al.* (1993) *J. Biol. Chem.* **268**, 3136–3142.

23 Pravenec *et al.* (1996) *Folia Biol. (Praha)* **42**, 147–153.

24 National Institute of Arthritis and Musculoskeletal and Skin Diseases. The ARB Rat Genetic Database (http://www.nih.gov/niams/scientific/ratgbase/index.htm).

25 Cai *et al.* (1994) *Mamm. Genome* **5**, 594.

26 Wevrick *et al.* (1993) *Mamm. Genome* **4**, 440–444.

27 Fulchignoni-Lataud *et al.* (1992) *Mamm. Genome* **3**, 42–45.

28 Vassort *et al.* (1993) *Mamm. Genome* **4**, 202–206.

29 Walter *et al.* (1996) *Cytogenet. Cell Genet.* **75**, 136–139.

30 Serikawa *et al.* (1992) *Genetics* **131**, 701–721.

31 Sebastian *et al.* (1997) *Cytogenet. Cell Genet.* **77**, 266–267.

32 Deb *et al.* (1991) *J. Biol. Chem.* **266**, 23027–23032.

33 Dai *et al.* (1996) *Endocrinology* **137**, 5009–5019.

34 Cooke *et al.* (1986) Endocrinology **119**, 2451–2454.

35 Yamada *et al.* (1992) Unpublished.

36 Szpirer *et al.* (1997) *Cytogenet. Cell Genet.* **78**, 137–139.

37 Johansson *et al.* (1998) *Cytogenet. Cell Genet.* **81**, 217–221.

38 Yasue *et al.* (1992) *Genomics* **12**, 659–664.

39 Yeung *et al.* (1993) *Cytogenet. Cell Genet.* **62**, 149–152.

40 Yamada *et al.* (1994) *Mamm. Genome* **5**, 63–83.

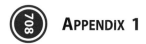

Chromosome 18

Locus symbol	Previous symbol	RNO Location	Description	Mode	Status	Reference	HSA symbol	HSA Chr	MMU symbol	MMU Chr
Adrb2		18	Adrenergic, beta 2, receptor, surface	L, S	C	3, 4, 7, 9, 17, 18, 20, 23, 24	ADRB2	5q31–q32	Adrb2	18
Apc		18	Adenomatosis polyposis coli, GenBank no. D38629	L, S	C	4, 23, 24, 27	APC	5q21–q22	Apc	18
Bp2		18	QTL Blood pressure between Ttr and Grl, possibly same as Bp41 and Bp46	L, S	P	10				
Bp41		18	QTL Blood pressure between Ttr and Grl, possibly same as Bp2	L	P	6				
Bp46		18	QTL Blood pressure between D18Mco3 and D18Mit1, possibly same as Bp2	L	P	15				
Bp47		18q	QTL Blood pressure between Grl and Gja1	L	P	15				
Bp48		18p	QTL Blood pressure between Olf and D18Mit9	L	P	15				
Camk4	Ccdpk	18	Calmodulin-dependent protein kinase IV	L	P	2	CAMK4	5q21–q23	Camk4	18
Csf1r		18	Colony-stimulating factor 1 receptor	L	P	18	CSF1R	5q33–q35	Csfmr	18D
Egr1		18q	Early growth response 1	S	P	27	EGR1	5q23–q31	Egr1	18
Gja1		18q	Gap junction protein, alpha 1, 43 kDa (connexin 43)	L, S	C	1, 3, 4, 7, 15, 18, 20, 23, 24	GJA1	6q21–q23.2	Gja1	10
Gnal	Olf, Golf	18	Olf-alpha protein (olfactory neuron-specific G protein	L, S	C	1, 4, 5, 7, 9, 15, 18, 20, 22, 24	GNAL	18p11.22–p11.21	Gnal	18
Grl	Gcr	18p	Glucocorticoid receptor	L, S	C	7–9, 11, 15, 17, 22	GRL	5q31–32	Grl1	18
Iddm3		18q	Insulin-dependent diabetes mellitus, around Olf in (BB/OK DA) and (BB/OK SHR) cross	L	P	13	IDDM6	18q21–q23		
Lox	Rrg1, H-ev142	18	Lysyl oxidase (an H-rev gene with its expression downregulated in HRAS-transformed rat 208F fibroblasts)	S	P	21	LOX	5q23.3–q31.2	Lox	18

Mbp		18	Myelin basic protein	L S	C	1, 8, 13, 14, 20, 26	*MBP*	18q23	*Mbp*	18
Mcc		18	Mutated in colorectal cancers	D	P	27	*MCC*	5q21–q22	*Mcc*	18
Myr 6		18	Myosin of the dilute-myosin-V family	L	P	29				
Ngfi	*Ngf1*	18	Nerve growth factor-induced gene	S	P	20				
Pcdh3		18	Cadherin-related protein, protocadherin 3	L	P	19	*PCDH3*		*Pcdh3*	
Pdgfrb		18p	Platelet-derived growth factor receptor beta	S	P	27	*PDGFRB*	5q33–q35	*Pdgfrb*	
Spink1	*Tilp*	18	Serine protease inhibitor, kanzal type 1/trypsin inhibitor-like protein, pancreatic	L S	C	1, 7, 15, 16, 18, 20	*SPINK1*	5q31–q33		
Tp53l3		18p	Tumour protein p53-like 3	S		25, 26				
Ttr		18p	Transthyretin (prealbumin, amyloidosis type I)	L S	C	1, 4, 7, 11, 15, 17, 18, 20, 23, 24	*TTR*	18q12.1	*Ttr*	18

References

1 Andoh *et al.* (1998) *Mamm. Genome* **9**, 287–293.
2 Bihoreau *et al.* (1997) *Genomic Res.* **7**, 434–440.
3 Brown *et al.* (1998) *Mamm. Genome* **9**, 521–530.
4 Canzian *et al.* (1996) *Jpn. J. Cancer Res.* **87**, 669–675.
5 Galli *et al.* (1996) *Nature Genet.* **12**, 31–37.
6 Garrett *et al.* (1998) *Genome Res.* **8**, 711–723.
7 Gauguier *et al.* (1996) *Nature Genet.* **12**, 38–43.
8 Goldner-Sauve *et al.* (1991) *Biochem. Genet.* **29**, 275–286.
9 Hilbert *et al.* (1991) *Nature* **353**, 521–529.
10 Jacob *et al.* (1991) *Cell* **67**, 213–224.
11 Jacob *et al.* (1995) *Nature Genet.* **9**, 63–69.
12 Kloting *et al.* (1998) *Biochem. Biophys. Res. Commun.* **245**, 483–486.
13 Klöting *et al.* (1998) *Rat Genome* **4**, 63–69.
14 Koizumi *et al.* (1991) *Cytogenet. Cell Genet.* **56**, 201.
15 Kovacs *et al.* (1997) *Biochem. Biophys. Res. Commun.* **235**, 343–348.
16 National Institute of Arthritis and Musculoskeletal and Skin Diseases. The ARB Rat Genetic Database (http://www.nih.gov/niams/scientific/ratgbase/index.htm).
17 Pravenec *et al.* (1996) *Mamm. Genome* **7**, 117–127.
18 Remmers *et al.* (1993) *Mamm. Genome* **4**, 265–270.
19 Sago *et al.* (1995) *Genomics* **29**, 631–640.
20 Serikawa *et al.* (1992) *Genetics* **131**, 701–721.
21 Szpirer *et al.* (1996) *Mamm. Genome* **7**, 701–703.
22 Szpirer *et al.* (1998) *Mamm. Genome* **9**, 721–734.
23 Toyota *et al.* (1995) *Mamm. Genome* **6**, 746–748.
24 Toyota *et al.* (1996) *Proc. Natl Acad. Sci. USA* **93**, 3914–3919.
25 Yamada *et al.* (1994) *Mamm. Genome* **5**, 63–83.
26 Yasue *et al.* (1992) *Genomics* **12**, 659–664.
27 Yeung *et al.* (1993) *Mamm. Genome* **4**, 585–588.
28 Yeung *et al.* (1993) *Proc. Natl Acad. Sci. USA* **90**, 8038–8042.
29 Zhao *et al.* (1996) *Proc. Natl Acad. Sci. USA* **93**, 10826–10831.

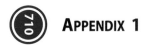

Chromosome 19

Locus symbol	Previous symbol	RNO Location	Description	Mode	Status	Reference	HSA symbol	HSA Chr	MMU symbol	MMU Chr
Agt	Ang	19	Angiotensinogen	D, L	C	1, 4, 23, 29, 31, 32, 37	AGT	1q42–q43	Agt	8
Bp32		19	Blood pressure QTL (systolic) in SHR × BN RI strains p = 0012, linked to D19Mit7	L	P	30				
Ctrb	Ctrpb	19	Chymotrypsin B, see also D19Mit6 and D19Wox7	S, L	C	1, 11, 15, 32	CTRB1	16q23–q24.1	Ctrb	8
Dia4		19	Diaphorase (NADH/NADPH)	S, L	I	3, 38, 47	DIA4	16q12–q22	Dia4	UN
Ednra	Eta	19	Endothelin receptor type A, GenBank no. M60786, see also D19Mco2	L	C	6, 7, 15, 31	EDNRA	4	Ednra	UN
Es1		19	Esterase 1, member of carboxylesterase cluster 2	L	C	2, 13, 25, 29, 33, 42				
Es2		19	Esterase 2, member of carboxylesterase cluster 1	L	C	4, 25, 29, 31, 32, 40, 42, 43				
Es3		19	Esterase 3, member of carboxylesterase cluster 1	L	C	29, 31, 32, 41, 42, 45				
Es4		19	Esterase 4, member of carboxylesterase cluster 1	L	C	4, 29, 31, 41, 45				
Es7		19	Esterase 7, member of carboxylesterase cluster 1	L	C	20, 29, 33				
Es8		19	Esterase 8, member of carboxylesterase cluster 1	L	C	4, 20, 29, 31				
Es9		19	Esterase 9, member of carboxylesterase cluster 1	L	C	24, 29, 33				
Es10		19	Esterase 10, member of carboxylesterase cluster 1	S, L	C	4, 29, 31				
Es14	Es-Si	19	Esterase 14, member of carboxylesterase cluster 2	L	C	4, 10, 13, 29, 31, 33, 44				
Es15		19	Esterase 15, member of carboxylesterase cluster 2	L	C	4, 13, 29, 31				
Es16		19	Esterase 16, member of carboxylesterase cluster 2	L	C	4, 29, 31, 44				

Es18		19	Esterase 18, member of carboxylesterase cluster 2	L	C	4, 17, 29, 31				
Es@1		19	Esterase cluster 1, including Es1, Es14, Es15, Es16, Es18			12			Es@1	
Es@2		19	Esterase cluster 1, including Es2, Es3, Es7, Es8, Es9, Es10			12			Es@2	
Hmox1	HEOXG, Heox, Hmox	19	Haem oxygenase, GenBank no. J02722	L, S	C	1, 6, 14, 31	HMOX1	22	Hmox1	UN
Hmox2		19	Haem oxygenase 2, GenBank no. M12129, see also D19Arb1	L	P	7	HMOX1	16p13.3		
Hp		19	Haptoglobin, see also D19Mgh5, D19Arb2 and D19Wox9	S, L	C	5, 7, 11, 15, 25, 32, 39	HP	16q22.2	Hp	8
Hsd11b2		19	Hydroxysteroid dehydrogenase, 11 beta type 2	D	P	37				
Itgb1		19	Integrin beta 1	S	P	35	ITGB1	10p11.2	Itgb1	UN
Junb		19	jun B proto-oncogene	S	P	36	JUNB	19q13.2	Junb	8
Lcat		19	Lecithin-cholesterol acyltransferase	L	P	4, 28	LCAT	16q22.1	Lcat	8
Lil1		19	Lipid level QTL in SHR BN.Lx, close to D19Mit2	L	P	4				
Mt		19	Metallothionein	S	P	22	MT1A	16q13	Mt1	8
Rb2		19	Retinoblastoma-related gene	S	P	48				
Rn5s	Rn5s2	19	Ribosomal 5S RNA	D	C	8, 34	RN5S1@	1q42.11–42.13	Rn5s	8E
Rrm2p		19	Ribonucleotide reductase 1 pseudogene	S, D	P	16				12
RT2	Ag-C	19	Cell surface alloantigen (= Ag-C)	L	C	18, 19, 21, 26, 27, 31, 33			Ea1	8
RT9		19	Cell surface alloantigen	L	P	19				
Tat		19	Tyrosine aminotransferase, see also D19Mgh2 and D19Wox4	L, S, D	C	1, 4, 5, 7, 9, 11, 14, 31, 37, 39	TAT	16q22.1	Tat	8E1-ter
Ucp	Uncp, Ucpa, Ucp1	19	Uncoupling protein, see also D19Mit9 and D19Wox8	L, S, D	C	1, 11, 14, 15, 25, 37	UCP	4q28-31	Ucp	8

References

1 Andoh et al. (1998) Mamm. Genome **9**, 287–293.

2 Augustinsson and Henricson (1966) Biochim. Biophys. Acta **124**, 323–331.

3 Bihoreau et al. (1997) Genomic Res. **7**, 434–440.

4   Bottger *et al.* (1996) *J. Clin. Invest.* **98**, 856–862.

5   Canzian *et al.* (1996) *Jpn. J. Cancer Res.* **87**, 669–675.

6   Deng *et al.* (1994) *J. Clin. Invest.* **93**, 2701–2709.

7   Du *et al.* (1996) *Genomics* **32**, 113–116.

8   Frederiksen *et al.* (1997) *Cytogenet. Cell Genet.* **76**, 101–106.

9   Fulchignoni-Lataud *et al.* (1990) *Cytogenet. Cell Genet.* **53**, 172–174.

10 Gasser *et al.* (1973) *Biochem. Genet.* **10**, 207–217.

11 Gauguier *et al.* (1996) *Nature Genet.* **12**, 38–43.

12 Hedrich and Deimling (1987) *J. Hered.* **78**, 92–96.

13 Hedrich *et al.* (1987) *Biochem. Genet.* **25**, 79–93.

14 Hilbert *et al.* (1991) *Nature* **353**, 521–529.

15 Jacob *et al.* (1995) *Nature Genet.* **9**, 63–69.

16 Klinga-Levan *et al.* (1997) *Mamm. Genome* **8**, 47–49.

17 Kluge *et al.* (1990) *Biochem. Genet.* **28**, 57–68.

18 Kunz and Gill III (1978) *J. Immunogenet.* **5**, 365–382.

19 Kunz *et al.* (1985) *J. Immunogenet.* **12**, 75–78.

20 Matsumoto (1980) *Biochem. Genet.* **18**, 879–885.

21 Misra *et al.* (1981) *J. Immunogenet.* **8**, 51–66.

22 Miura *et al.* (1994) *Cytogenet. Cell Genet.* **65**, 119–121.

23 Mori *et al.* (1989) *Cytogenet. Cell Genet.* **50**, 42–49.

24 Moutier *et al.* (1973) *Biochem. Genet.* **9**, 109–115.

25 Otsen *et al.* (1993) *J. Hered.* **54**, 149–151.

26 Owen (1962) *Ann. N Y Acad. Sci.* **97**, 37–42.

27 Palm (1962) *Ann. N Y Acad. Sci.* **97**, 57–68.

28 Pravenec *et al.* (1996) *Folia Biol. (Praha)* **42**, 147–153.

29 Pravenec *et al.* (1992) *Genomics* **12**, 350–356.

30 Pravenec *et al.* (1995) *J. Clin. Invest.* **96**, 1973–1978.

31 Pravenec *et al.* (1996) *Mamm. Genome* **7**, 117–127.

32 Serikawa *et al.* (1992) *Genetics* **131**, 701–721.

33 Shisa *et al.* (1997) *Mamm. Genome* **8**, 324–327.

34 Szabo *et al.* (1978) *Chromosoma* **65**, 161–172.

35 Szpirer *et al.* (1992) *Mamm. Genome* **3**, 685–688.

36 Szpirer *et al.* (1994) *Mamm. Genome* **5**, 361–364.

37 Szpirer *et al.* (1998) *Mamm. Genome* **9**, 721–734.

38 The Wellcome Trust Centre for Human Genetics (http://www.well.ox.ac.uk/~bihoreau).

39 Toyota *et al.* (1996) *Proc. Natl Acad. Sci. USA* **93**, 3914–3919.

40 Womack and Sharp (1976) *Genetics* **82**, 665–675.

41 Womack (1973) *Biochem. Genet.* **9**, 13–24.

42 Womack (1972) *Experientia* **28**, 1372.

43 Womack (1972) *J. Hered.* **63**, 41–42.

44 Yamada *et al.* (1980) *Biochem. Genet.* **18**, 433–438.

45 Yamori and Okamotu (1970) *Lab. Invest.* **22**, 206–211.

46 Yasue *et al.* (1991) *Cytogenet. Cell Genet.* **57**, 142–148.

47 Yeung *et al.* (1993) *Oncogene* **8**, 3465–3468.

Chromosome 20

Locus symbol	Previous symbol	RNO Location	Description	Mode	Status	Reference	HSA symbol	HSA Chr	MMU symbol	MMU Chr
Agl		20	Cell surface alloantigen	L	P	1, 2				
Amd1a		20	S-Adenosylmethionine decarboxylase 1A	S	P	3	AMD1	6		
Amd1b		20	S-Adenosylmethionine decarboxylase 1B	S	P	3				
Atps1		20	Aurothiopropanolsulfonate-induced auto-immune glomerulonephritis 1	L	P	4				
Bf		20	Properdin factor B, complement component	L	P	7	BF	6p21.3	Bf	17
C2		20	Complement component 2	L	P	8	C2	6p21.3	C2	17
C4		20	Complement component 4	L, S	C	7, 9–11	C4	6p21.3	C4	17
Cbs		20	Cystathionine beta synthase	S	P	10	CBS	21q22.3	Cbs	17
Cia1		20	Type II collagen-induced arthritis 1	L	C	124				
Ciaa1		20	Type II collagen-induced arthritis antibody 1	L	P	125				
Col11a2		20	Type XI collagen, alpha2 chain	P	P	12	COL11A2	6p21.3	Col11a2	17
Cryaa	Crya1, Acry-1	20	Crystallin, alpha polypeptide 1	L	P	13	CRYAA	21q22.3	Crya1	17
Ct		20	Cell surface alloantigen	L	P	2, 14				
Cth	H	20	CTL target antigen	L	P	32				
Cyp21	21-OH	20	Cytochrome P450, subfamily XXI (steroid 21-hydroxylase)	L	P	8	CYP21A1	6p21.3	Cyp21a1	17
D20H6S50E	G1	20	G1 protein	P	P	18	D6S50E	6p21.3	D17H6-S50E	17
D20H6S51E	G2, Bat2	20	DNA segment	P	P	18	D6S51E	6p21.3	D17H6-S51E	17
D20H6S53E	G4	20	DNA segment	P	P	18	D6S53E	6p21.3	D17H6-S53E	17
D20H6S58E	G9, Bat7	20	DNA segment	P	P	18	D6S58E	6p21.3	Bat7	17
D20H6S58-E-2	G9a, Bat8	20	G9a protein	P	P	18	D6S58E-2	6p21.3	Bat8	17

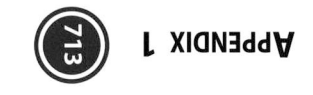

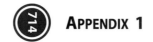

D20H6S59E	*G10*	20	DNA segment	P	P	18	*D6S59E*	6p21.3	*D17H6-S59E*	17
D20H6S81e	*Bat1*	20	Nuclear RNA helicase	I, P	C	5, 6, 134	*BAT1*	6p21.3	*Bat1*	17
D20H6-S111E	*Ring1*	20	RING finger protein	P	P	12	*D6S111E*	6p21.3	*D17H6-S111E*	17
D20H6-S112E	*Ring2, Ke6*	20	DNA segment, steroid and prostaglandin dehydrogenase-related protein	P	P	12	*D6S112E*	6p21.3	*D17H6-S112E*	17
D20H6-S209E	*G13*	20	Transcription factor	P	P	18	*D6S209E*	6p21.3	*D17H6-S209E*	17
D20H6-S211E	*G15*	20	DNA segment	P	P	18	*D6S211E*	6p21.3	*D17H6-S211E*	17
D20H6-S214E	*G18*	20	DNA segment	P	P	18	*D6S214E*	6p21.3	*D17H6-S214E*	17
Dw3		20	Body size (dwarf), Grc region	L	P	24, 25				
Fyn		20	Protooncogene	P	P	135	*FYN*	6q21	*Fyn*	10
Ft		20	Fertility, Grc region	L	P	25				
Ggt1		20	Gamma glutamyltransferase 1	L	P	15	*GGT1*	22q11.2–q12.1		
Glo1		20	Glyoxalase 1	L	C	26–28	*GLO1*	6p21.2–p21.1	*Glo1*	17
Glp1r		20	Pancreatic beta cell receptor for the gluco-incretin hormone glucagon-like peptide 1	L	P	126	*GLP1R*	6p21	*Glp1r*	17
Gna-rs1		20	Guanosine-triphosphate-binding protein	P	P	132	*GNL1*	6p21.3	*Gna-rs1*	17
Grc		20	Growth and reproduction complex	L, P	P	25, 29, 30				
Grm4		20	Glutamate receptor, metabotropic 4	S	P	31				
Hc		20	Anti-RT1a haemagglutinating antibody response	L	P	33				
Hk1		20	Hexokinase 1	P	P	127	*HK1*	10q22	*Hk1*	10
Hspa1a	*Hsp70-1*	20	Heat shock protein 70-1	I, L	C	11, 15, 17, 34, 35, 134	*HSPA1B*	6p21.3	*Hsp70-1*	17
Hspa1b	*Hsp70-2*	20	Heat shock protein 70-2	L	P	34, 35	*HSPA1A*	6p21.3	*Hsp70-3*	17
Hspa1l	*Hsp70-3*	20	Heat shock protein 70-1l	L	P	34, 35	*HSPA1L*	6p21.3	*Hsc70t*	17

Iddm2		20	Insulin-dependent diabetes mellitus 2	L	C	22, 36–38	IDDM1	6p21.3	Idd1	17
Lil3		20	Lipid level QTL	L	P	128				
Lmp2		20	Low molecular mass polypeptide 2	L	P	39, 40	LMP2	6p21.3	Lmp2	17
Lmp7		20	Low molecular mass polypeptide 7	L	P	40, 41	LMP7	6p21.3	Lmp7	17
Lta	Tnfb	20	Lymphotoxin B	P	P	122	LTA	6p21.3	Lta	17
Manb		20	Mannosidase, alpha B, lysosomal	L	P	42	MANB	19cen		
Mog		20	Myelin oligodendrocyte glycoprotein	L	P	43	MOG	6p22–p21.3	Mog	17
Mt2l		20	Metallothionein 2-like DNA	L	P	15				
Neu1		20	Neuraminidase 1	L	P	27, 42	NEU	6p21.3	Neu1	17
Oia1		20	Oil-induced arthritis QTL	L	P	129				
Olf89		20	Olfactory receptor 89	P	P	130	OLF89	6p21.3	Olf89	17
Pim1		20	Pim-1 oncogene	S	P	44	PIM	6p11–p21.1	Pim1	17
Pou5fl	Otf3	20	Transcription factor	P	P	132	POU5FL	6p21.3	Pou5fl	17
Pp		20	Pyrophosphatase, inorganic	S	P	28	PP	10q11.1–q24	Pyp	10
Prkacn2		20	cAMP-dependent protein kinase inhibitor 2	L	P	15			Prkacn2	10
Rcc		20	Resistance to chemical carcinogenesis, Grc region	L	P	45				
Rps2r1		20	Ribosomal protein S2	P	P	46, 47				
Rps2r2		20	Ribosomal protein S2 pseodogene	P	P	46, 47				
Rps2r3		20	Ribosomal protein S2 pseudogene	P	P	46, 47				
Rps18	Ke3	20	Ribosomal protein S18	I, P	P	48, 49, 134	RPS18	6p21.3	Rps18	17
RT1@	AgB, H1, R	20	Major histocompatibility locus	L	C	10	HLA	6p21.3	H2	17
RT1-A		20	RT1 region, class I	L	C	50, 51				
RT1-A		20	RT1 class Ia, locus A (A1)	L	C	52–59				
RT1-A2		20	RT1 class Ia, locus A2	L	P	58				
RT1A-1		20	RT1 class I gene		P	60				
RT1A-2		20	RT1 class I gene		P	60				
RT1A-4		20	RT1 class I gene		P	61				
RT1alc		20	NK cell target antigen	L	P	75, 76				

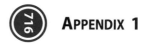

RT1-Aw2	*03-Jun*	20	RT1 class Ib gene	L	P	15, 53				
RT1-Aw3		20	RT1 class I gene		P	62				
RT1-B		20	RT1 region, class II	L, S	C	50, 51, 64				
RT1-Ba		20	RT1 class II, locus Ba	L	C	65–69	*HLA-DQA*	6p21.3	*H2-Aa*	17
RT1-Bb		20	RT1 class II, locus Bb	L	C	70–74	*HLA-DQB*	6p21.3	*H2-Ab*	17
RT1-C		20	RT1 region, class Ib	L	P	63				
RT1-C113	*11/3R*	20	RT1 class Ib gene	L	P	77				
RT1-Cl		20	RT1 class Ib gene	L	P	57				
RT1-Clw2	*LW2*	20	RT1 class Ib gene	L	P	78				
RT1-D		20	RT1 region, class II	L	P	79				
RT1-Da		20	RT1 class II, locus Da	L	C	80, 81	*HLA-DRA*	6p21.3	*H2-Ea*	17
RT1-Db1		20	RT1 class II, locus Db1	L	C	73, 82, 83	*HLA-DRB*	6p21.3	*H2-Eb*	17
RT1-Db2		20	RT1 class II, locus Db2	L	P	84	*HLA-DRB*	6p21.3	*H2-Eb*	17
RT1-DMa		20	RT1 class II, locus DMb	P	P	85	*HLA-DMA*	6p21.3	*H2-Ma*	17
RT1-DMb		20	RT1 class II, locus DMb	P	P	85	*HLA-DMB*	6p21.3	*H2-Mb*	17
RT1-DOa		20	RT1 class II, locus DOa	P	P	86	*HLA-DNA*	6p21.3	*H2-Oa*	17
RT1-DOb	*RT1.Bb2*	20	RT1 class II, locus DOb	L, P	P	87	*HLA-DOB*	6p21.3	*H2-Ob*	17
RT1-E		20	RT1 class I gene	L, P	C	62, 88–90				
RT1-F		20	RT1 class Ia gene	L	P	91, 92				
RT1-G		20	RT1 class Ib gene	L	P	93				
RT1-H		20	RT1 region, class II	L, P	C	64, 94–96				
RT1-Ha		20	RT1 class II, locus Ha	L, P	P	97	*HLA-DPA1*	6p21.3	*H2-Pa*	17
RT1-Hb		20	RT1 class II, locus Hb	L, P	P	97	*HLA-DPB1*	6p21.3	*H2-Pb*	17
RT1-K	*Pa*	20	Pregnancy-associated antigen	L	P	98–101				
RT1-Ke4	*Ke4*	20	Histidine-rich membrane protein	P	P	12	*KE4*	6p21.3	*H2Ke4*	17
RT1-Ke5	*Ke5*	20	Lymphoid cell-specific transcript	P	P	12		6p21.3	*H2Ke5*	17
RT1-L	*LH*	20	RT1 class Ib gene	L	P	102, 103				
RT1-M2		20	RT1 class 1b gene	L	P	43			*H2-M2*	17
RT1-M3		20	RT1 class Ib gene	L	P	43, 104			*H2-M3*	17
RT1-M4		20	RT1 class 1b gene	L, P	P	43			*H2-M4*	17
RT1-M5		20	RT1 class 1b gene	L, P	P	43			*H2-M5*	17
RT1-M6		20	RT1 class 1b gene	L, P	P	43			*H2-M6*	17

RT1-N1		20	RT1 class Ib gene, H2-TL-like, Grc region	L, P	C	15, 105				
RT1-N2		20	RT1 class Ib gene, H2-TL-like, Grc region	P	P	106				
RT1-N3		20	RT1 class Ib gene, H2-TL-like, Grc region	P	P	106				
RT1-O		20	RT1 class Ib gene, H2-Q-like, Grc region	P	P	108				
RT1-P		20	RT1 class Ib gene, H2-TLlike	L	P	107				
RT1-R	*RT1M*	20	RT1 class Ib gene	L	P	102				
RT1-S1		20	RT1 class Ib gene, H2-TL-like	P	P	46, 47				
RT1-S2		20	RT1 class Ib gene, H2-TL-like	P	P	46, 47				
RT1-U		20	RT1 class I gene	L	P	131				
RT1-V		20	RT1 class I gene	L	P	131				
RT1-Y		20	RT1 class I gene	L	P	131				
RT1-Z		20	RT1 class I gene	L	P	131				
RT(2.1)		20	RT1 class I gene	P	P	108				
RT11		20	Protein antigen of 29 kDa	L	P	11, 109				
RT12.5		20	RT1 class I gene	P	P	57				
RT21		20	RT1 class I gene		P	52				
RT44		20	RT1 class I gene		P	52				
RTA		20	RT1 class I gene		P	52				
RTBM1		20	RT1 class Ib gene		P	111, 112				
RTS		20	RT1 class I gene		P	52				
Rxrb		20	Retinoic acid receptor, beta	P	P	12	*RXRB*	6p21.3	*Rxrb*	17
S		20	Protein specifically expressed in the skin	P	P	132	*S*	6.p21.3	*S*	17
Sacm2l	*Are1*	20	Suppressor of actin mutation 2-like	P	P	133	*SACM2L*	6p21.3	*Sacm2l*	17
Sp		20	Serum protein (quantative level of C4-like protein)	L	P	113				
Tac2r		20	Tachykinin 2 (substance K) receptor	S	P	118	*TAC2R*	10		
Tap1	*Cim, mtp1*	20	Transporter associated with antigen processing, polypeptide	P	C	96, 114, 115	*TAP1*	6p21.3	*Tap1*	17
Tap2	*Cim, mtp2*	20	Transporter associated with antigen processing, polypeptide 2	P	C	96, 114–117	*TAP2*	6p21.3	*Tap2*	17
Tapbp		20	Tap-binding protein (tapasin)	P	P	133, 136	*TAPBP*	6p31	*Tapbp*	17

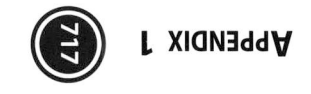

| Tnf | Tnfa | 20 | Tumour necrosis factor | I, L, P, S | C | 11, 15, 17, 19, 21, 119–123, 134 | TNF | 6p21.3 | Tnf | 17 |
| Vars2 | G7a, Bat6 | 20 | Valyl-tRNA synthetase 2 | P | P | 18 | VARS2 | 6p21.3 | Vars2 | 17 |

References

1 Lynch and DeWitt (1990) *J. Immunol.* **124**, 2247–2253.

2 Stephenson *et al.* (1985) *J. Immunogenet.* **12**, 101–114.

3 Pulkka *et al.* (1993) *Genomics* **16**, 342–349.

4 Kermarrec *et al.* (1996) *Genomics* **31**, 111–114.

5 Walter and Günther (1997) *Transplant. Proc.* **29**, 1660.

6 Lambracht *et al.* (1997) *Transplant. Proc.* **29**, 1665–1667.

7 Wurst *et al.* (1988) *Immunogenetics* **28**, 57–60.

8 Hassett *et al.* (1989) *Transplant. Proc.* **21**, 3244–3246.

9 Watters *et al.* (1987) *Immunogenetics* **25**, 204–206.

10 Locker *et al.* (1990) *Immunogenetics* **31**, 271–274.

11 Vardimon *et al.* (1992) *Immunogenetics* **35**, 166–175.

12 Walter *et al.* (1996) *Immunogenetics* **44**, 218–221.

13 Skow *et al.* (1985) *Immunogenetics* **22**, 291–293.

14 Marshak *et al.* (1977) *J. Exp. Med.* **146**, 1773–1790.

15 Remmers *et al.* (1995) *Immunogenetics* **41**, 316–319.

16 Pravenec *et al.* (1996) *Folia Biol. (Praha)* **42**, 147–153.

17 Pravenec *et al.* (1996) *Mamm. Genome* **7**, 117–127.

18 Lund *et al.* (1994) *Mamm. Genome* **5**, 282–287.

19 Kondo *et al.* (1993) *Mamm. Genome* **4**, 571–576.

20 Kuramoto *et al.* (1995) *Exp. Anim.* **44**, 119–125.

21 Jacob *et al.* (1995) *Nature Genet.* **9**, 63–69.

22 Jacob *et al.* (1992) *Nature Genet.* **2**, 56–60.

23 Otsen *et al.* (1996) *Genomics* **37**, 289–294.

24 Gill III and Kunz (1979) *Am. J. Pathol.* **96**, 185–202.

25 Kunz *et al.* (1980) *J. Exp. Med.* **152**, 1506–1518.

26 Stolc *et al.* (1980) *J. Immunol.* **125**, 1167–1170.

27 Gill III *et al.* (1982) *J. Immunogenet.* **9**, 281–293.

28 Yasue *et al.* (1991) *Cytogenet. Cell Genet.* **57**, 142–148.

29 Hassett *et al.* (1989) *J. Immunol.* **142**, 2089–2096.

30 Vincek *et al.* (1990) *Immunogenetics* **32**, 293–295.

31 Kuramoto *et al.* (1994) *Genomics* 358–61.

32 Davies *et al.* (1991) *J. Exp. Med.* **173**, 833–839.

33 Heslop and Jolly (1979) *Immunogenetics* **8**, 567–570.

34 Wurst *et al.* (1989) *Immunogenetics* **30**, 46–49.

35 Walter *et al.* (1994) *Immunogenetics* **40**, 325–330.

36 Colle *et al.* (1981) *J. Exp. Med.* **154**, 1237–1247.

37 Colle *et al.* (1986) *Diabetes* **35**, 454–458.

38 Günther *et al.* (1991) *J. Autoimmun.* **4**, 543–551.

39 Tamura *et al.* (1992) *J. Biochem.* **112**, 530–534.

40 Palmer *et al.* (1996) *Biochem. J.* **316**, 401–407.

41 Aki *et al.* (1992) *FEBS Lett.* **301**, 65–68.

42 VandeBerg *et al.* (1981) *J. Immunogenet.* **8**, 239–242.

43 Lambracht *et al.* (1995) *Immunogenetics* **42**, 418–421.

44 Yasue *et al.* (1992) *Genomics* **12**, 659–664.

45 Melhem *et al.* (1993) *Proc. Natl Acad. Sci. USA* **90**, 1967–1971.

46 Gill III *et al.* (1997) *Transplant. Proc.* **29**, 1657–1659.

47 Salgar *et al.* (1997) *Immunogenetics* **45**, 353–364.

48 Larsson *et al.* (1996) *Mamm. Genome* **7**, 90.

49 Walter and Günther (1994) *Transplant. Proc.* **27**, 1501.

50 Butcher and Howard (1977) *Nature* **266**, 362–364.

51 Stark *et al.* (1977) *Immunogenetics* **5**, 183–187.

52 Mauxion *et al.* (1989) *Immunogenetics* **29**, 397–401.

53 Rada *et al.* (1990) *Proc. Natl Acad. Sci. USA* **87**, 2167–2171.

54 Salgar *et al.* (1994) *Immunogenetics* **39**, 447.

55 Joly *et al.* (1995) *Immunogenetics* **41**, 326–328.

56 Walter *et al.* (1995) *Immunogenetics* **41**, 332.

57 Lambracht and Wonigeit (1995) *Immunogenetics* **41**, 375–379.

58 Joly *et al.* (1996) *J. Immunol.* **157**, 1551–1558.

59 Wang *et al.* (1996) *Immunogenetics* **43**, 318–320.

60 Kastern (1985) *Gene* **34**, 227–233.

61 Kryspin-Sorensen *et al.* (1991) *Immunogenetics* **33**, 213–215.

62 Salgar *et al.* (1995) *Immunogenetics* **42**, 244–253.

63 Kohoutova *et al.* (1980) *Immunogenetics* **11**, 483–490.

64 Fujii *et al.* (1991) *Transplantation* **52**, 369–373.

65 Wallis and McMaster (1984) *Immunogenetics* **19**, 53–62.

66 Barran and McMaster (1987) *Immunogenetics* **26**, 56–62.

67 Syha *et al.* (1989) *Nucleic Acids Res.* **17**, 3985.

68 Holmdahl *et al.* (1992) *Eur. J. Immunol.* **22**, 4(19–4)24.

69 Holmdahl *et al.* (1993) *Immunogenetics* **38**, 381.

70 Eccles and McMaster (1985) *Immunogenetics* **22**, 653–663.

71 Figueroa *et al.* (1988) *Nature* **335**, 265–267.

72 Fujii *et al.* (1991) *Immunogenetics* **33**, 399–403.

73 Chao *et al.* (1989) *Immunogenetics* **29**, 231–234.

74 Syha-Jedelhauser *et al.* (1991) *Biochim. Biophys. Acta* **1089**, 414–416.

75 Vaage *et al.* (1994) *J. Exp. Med.* **180**, 641–651.

76 Naper *et al.* (1996) *Int. Immunol.* **8**, 1779–1785.

77 Rothermel *et al.* (1993) *Immunogenetics* **38**, 82–91.

78 Walter *et al.* (1994) *Immunogenetics* **39**, 351–354.

79 Lobel and Cramer (1981) *Immunogenetics* **13**, 465–473, (1981).

80 Holowachuk (1985) *Immunogenetics* **22**, 665–671, (1985).

81 Holowachuk *et al.* (1987) *Nucleic Acids Res.* **15**, 10551–10567.

82 Robertson and McMaster (1985) *J. Immunol.* **135**, 4095–4099.

83 Syha-Jedelhauser and Reske (1990) *Nucleic Acids Res.* **18**, 4598.

84 Diamond *et al.* (1989) *J. Immunol.* **142**, 3268–3274.

85 Hermel and Monaco (1995) *Immunogenetics* **42**, 446–447.

86 Arimura *et al.* (1995) *Immunogenetics* **42**, 156–158.

87 Scholler and Lernmark (1985) *Immunogenetics* **22**, 601–608.

88 Kunz *et al.* (1982) *J. Immunol.* **128**, 402–408.

89 Hassett *et al.* (1986) *J. Immunol.* **137**, 373–378.

90 Kunz *et al.* (1993) *Transplant. Proc.* **25**, 2761–2762.

91 Misra *et al.* (1985) *J. Immunol.* **134**, 2520–2528.

92 Misra *et al.* (1990) *J. Immunogenet.* **17**, 109–121.

93 Kunz *et al.* (1989) *Immunogenetics* **30**, 181–187.

94 Watters *et al.* (1987) *Immunogenetics* **26**, 220–229.

95 Carter and Fabre (1991) *Immunogenetics* **33**, 202–205.

96 Carter *et al.* (1994) *Genomics* **22**, 451–455.

97 Arimura *et al.* (1995) *Immunogenetics* **41**, 320–325.

98 Ghani *et al.* (1984) *Transplantation* **37**, 187–194.

99 Radojcic *et al.* (1989) *Immunogenetics* **29**, 134–137.

100 Radojcic *et al.* (1990) *Immunogenetics* **31**, 326–332.

101 Vishteh *et al.* (1992) *Am. J. Reprod. Immunol.* **28**, 74–76.

102 Wonigeit and Hänisch (1991) *Transplant. Proc.* **23**, 468–470.

103 Lambracht *et al.* (1993) *Transplant. Proc.* **25**, 2766–2767.

104 Wang *et al.* (1995) *Immunogenetics* **42**, 63–67.

105 Kirisits *et al.* (1992) *Immunogenetics* **35**, 365–377.

106 Kirisits *et al.* (1994) *Immunogenetics* **39**, 301–315.

107 Matsuura *et al.* (1993) *Transplant. Proc.* **25**, 2754–2755.

108 Rushton *et al.* (1994) *Eur. J. Immunogenet.* **21**, 189–198.

109 Kunz *et al.* (1989) *Transplant. Proc.* **21**, 559–560.

110 Ho *et al.* (1989) *Transplantation* **48**, 123–130.

111 Parker *et al.* (1990) *Immunogenetics* **31**, 211–214.

112 Parker *et al.* (1991) *Immunogenetics* **34**, 211–213.

113 Cramer (1983) *Immunogenetics* **18**, 593–598.

114 Deverson *et al.* (1990) *Nature* **348**, 738–741.

115 Livingstone *et al.* (1991) *Immunogenetics* **34**, 157–163.

116 Powis *et al.* (1992) *Nature* **357**, 211–215.

117 Joly *et al.* (1994) *Immunogenetics* **40**, 45–53.

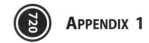
118 Mori *et al.* (1992) *Cytogenet. Cell Genet.* **60**, 222–223.

119 Shirai *et al.* (1989) *Agric. Biol. Chem.* **53**, 1733–1736.

120 Hilbert *et al.* (1991) *Nature* **353**, 521–529.

121 Serikawa *et al.* (1992) *Genetics* **131**, 701–721.

122 Kwon *et al.* (1993) *Gene* **132**, 227–236.

123 Kirisits *et al.* (1994) *Immunogenetics* **39**, 59–60.

124 Remmers *et al.* (1996) *Nature Genet.* **14**, 82–85.

125 Griffiths *et al.* (1996) XIth International Workshop on Alloantigenic Systems in the Rat, Toulouse, Abstract Book p. 57.

126 Bihoreau *et al.* (1997) *Genomic Res.* **7**, 434–440.

127 Sebastian *et al.* (1997) *Cytogenet. Cell Genet.* **77**, 266–267.

128 Bottger *et al.* (1996) *J. Clin. Invest.* **98**, 856–862.

129 Lorentzen *et al.* (1998) *Proc. Natl Acad. Sci. USA* **95**, 6383–6387.

130 Szpirer *et al.* (1997) *Cytogenet. Cell Genet.* **78**, 137–139.

131 Joly *et al.* (1997) *Rat Genome* **3**, 133–137.

132 Lambracht *et al.* (1997) *Transplant. Proc.* **29**, 1665–1667.

133 Walter and Günther (1998) *Genomics* **52**, 298–304.

134 Helou *et al.* (1998) *Immunogenetics* **47**, 166–169.

135 Johansson *et al.* (1998) *Cytogenet. Cell Genet.* **81**, 217–221.

136 Herberg *et al.* (1998) *Eur. J. Immunol.* **28**, 459–467.

Chromosome X

Locus symbol	Previous symbol	RNO Location	Description	Mode	Status	Reference	HSA symbol	HSA Chr	MMU symbol	MMU Chr
Agtr2		Xq34	Angiotensin receptor 2, see also DXWox27	I, L		18, 27	AGTR2	Xq22–q23	Agtr2	X
Amdp		X	S-Adenosylmethionine decarboxylase, pseudo-pene	S		22				
Ar	Andr, Tfm	X	Androgen receptor (testicular feminization), same as Tfm, see also DXWox9	I, L		1, 2, 6, 12, 18, 23	AR	Xql.2–q12	Ar	X
Atp7a	Mnk	X	ATPase, Cu^{2+}-transporting, alpha polypeptide (Menkes syndrome), see also DXWox23	I, L		18	ATP7A	Xql3.2–q13.3	Atp7a	X
Bp3	BP/SP2	X	Blood pressure 3, also called BP/SP2	L, S		7				
Cbpi		X	Calcium-binding protein, intestinal, vitamin D-dependent, see also DXWox7	L, S		2, 3, 6, 18, 23, 28	CALB3	Xp		
Chm		X	Choroideraemia, see also DXWox24 and DXWox25	I, L		18	CHM	Xp21.2		
Dmd		X	Dystrophin, GenBank no. X89427 and X89428, see also DXWox18 and DXWox19	I, L		18, 19	DMD	Xp21.3	Dmd	X
F9		X	Coagulation factor IX (plasma thromboplastic component, Christmas disease, haemophilia B), see also DXWox30	I, L		18	F9	Xq27.1	Cf9	X
Fmr1		X	Fragile X mental retardation 1	I		18	FMR1	Xq27.3	Fmrl	X
G6pd		X	Glucose-6-phosphate dehydrogenase	S		31	G6PD	Xq28	G6pd	XA6-A7
Gabra3		X	Gamma-aminobutyric acid (GABA) A receptor, alpha 3 see also DXWox31	I, L		18	GABRA3	Xq28	Gabra3	X
Gla		X	Galactosidase alpha	S		15	GLA	Xq21.3–q22	AGS	XF1
Glra2		X	Glycine receptor alpha 2 subunit (glycine receptor, neonatal), GenBank no. X57281	S, L		29	GLRA2	Xp22.1–p22	Glra2	X
Grpr		X	Gastrin-releasing peptide receptor, see also DXWox 17	I, L		18	GRPR	Xp22.2–p22.13	Grpr	X

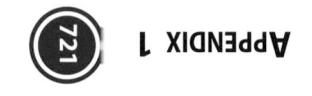

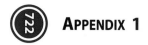

Gstpl6	*GSTPL6*	Xq22–q34	Glutathione-*S*-transferase-like 6, pi type	S	13, 29				
Hprt		X	Hypoxanthine phosphoribosyltransferase	I, L	18, 26, 31	*HPRT*	Xq26.1	*Hprt*	XA6
Hrasp	*HRAS2*	X	Harvey rat sarcoma viral (v-Ha-*ras*) oncogene homologue pseudogene	S	25	*HRASP*	Xp11.3–p11.23		
Hx		X	Histocompatibility X artigen	I	20			*Hxa*	X
L1cam	*Hsas, Hyd*	X	L1 cell adhesion molecule (hydrocephalus, stenosie of aqueduct of sylvius 1)	L, S	14	*L1CAM*	Xq28	*L1cam*	XA6-B
Lamp2		X	Lysosomal-associated membrane protein 2, see also DXWox28	I, L	18	*LAMP2*	Xq24	*Lamp2*	X
Mycs		X	Myc-like oncogene, s-*myc* protein, see also DXMit2 and DXWox5	I, L, S	2, 6, 12, 18, 21, 23				
Ocrl		X	Oculocerebrorenal syndrome of Lowe, see also DXWox29	I, L	18	*OCRL*	Xq25–q26.1		
Odbl		X	OLETF rat diabetogenic gene 1	L	10				
Pem		X	Homeabox gene Pem	S	17				X
Pfc		X	Properdin P factor, complement, see also DXWox21	I, L	18	*PFC*	Xp11.3–p11.23	*Pfc*	X
Pfkfl,Ol	*PFRX, PfkfbOl*	Xq22–q31	6-Phosphofructo-2-kinase/fructose-2,6-bisphosphatase I (liver and muscle), see also DXMgh5, DXArb5 and DXWox4	I, L, S	2–8, 12, 18, 28	*PFKFB1*	Xpter–Xqter		
Pgk		X	Phosphoglycerate kinase 1	S	15	*PGK1*	Xq13.3	*Pgk1*	XD-F1
Plp		X	Proteolipid protein (Pelizaeus–Merzbacher disease, spastic paraplegia 2, uncomplicated), see also DXWox26	I, L	18	*PLP*	Xq21.33–q22	*PLp*	X
Prps2		X	Phophoribosylpyrophosphate synthetase, subunit II, see also DXWox6	I, L, S	2, 5, 6, 11, 18, 23	*PRPS2*	Xp22.3–p22.2	*Prps2*	X
Rc		Xq11.1–q12	Regucalcin, see also DXWox11	I, L	2, 18, 24	*RC*	Xp11.3–p11.2		
Sts		Xq12–q14	Steroid sulfatase	I, L, S	16	*STS*	Xp22.32	*Sts*	XY
Syn1		X	Synapsin I, see also DXWox10	L	2, 18	*SYN1*	Xp11.23	*Syn1*	XA1-A4
Syp		X	Synaptophysin, see also DXMgh 1 and DXWox 12	L	2, 12, 18	*SYP*	Xp11.3–p11.22	*syp*	X

XK	X		Kell blood group precursor (McLeod phenotype), l, L		18	XK	Xp21.1	XK	X
			see also DXWox20						

References

1 Bardin et al. (1973) Recent Prog. Horm. Res. **29**, 65–109.
2 Bihoreau et al. (1997) Genome Res. **7**, 434–440.
3 Canzian et al. (1996) Jpn. J. Cancer Res. **87**, 669–675.
4 Darville et al. (1989) Arch. Int. Physiol. Biochem. **97**, B19.
5 Du et al. (1996) Genomics **32**, 113–116.
6 Gauguier et al. (1996) Nature Genet. **12**, 38–43.
7 Hilbert et al. (1991) Nature **353**, 521–529.
8 Hilliker et al. (1991) Genomics **10**, 867–873
9 Hino et al. (1996) Rat Genome **2**, 6–9.
10 Hirashima et al. (1995) Diabetes Res. Clin. Pract. **27**, 91–96.
11 Hirashima et al. (1996) Rat Genome **2**, 132–135.
12 Jacob et al. (1995) Nature Genet. **9**, 63–69.
13 Klinga-Levan et al. (1993) Hereditas **119**, 285–296.
14 Koto et al. (1987) Rat News Lett. **18**, 14–15.
15 Levan et al. (1986) Rat News Lett. **17**, 3–8.

16 Li et al. (1996) Genome **7**, 420–424.
17 Maiti et al. (1996) Genomics **34**, 304–316.
18 Millwood et al. (1997) Genomics **40**, 253–261.
19 Millwood et al. (1995) Mamm. Genome **6**, 668–669.
20 Mullen and Hilderman (1972) Transplantation **13**, 521–529.
21 Pravenec et al. (1996) Mamm. Genome **7**, 117–127.
22 Pulkka et al. (1993) Genomics **16**, 342–349.
23 Serikawa et al. (1992) Genetics **131**, 701–721.
24 Shimokawa et al. (1995) Mol. Cell. Biochem. **151**, 157–163.
25 Szpirer et al. (1985) Somatic Cell Mol. Genet. 11 :93–97.
26 Szpirer et al. (1984) Cytogenet. Cell Genet. **38**, 142–149.
27 Tissir et al. (1995) Cytogenet. Cell Genet. **71**, 77–80.
28 Toyota et al. (1996) Proc. Natl Acad. Sci. USA **93**, 3914–3919.
29 Yasue et al. (1992) Genomics **12**, 659–664.
30 Yokoi et al. (1996) Mamm. Genome **7**, 71–73.
31 Yoshida (1978) Cytogenet. Cell Genet. **22**, 606–609.

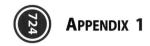

Chromosome Y

Locus symbol	Previous symbol	RNO Location	Description	Mode	Status	Reference	HSA symbol	HSA Chr	MMU symbol	MMU Chr
Bpy			Blood pressure on SHR Y	L		4				
Hy			Male histocompatability	L		3				
Smcy			Selected mouse cDNA on Y	D		1	SMCY	Y cen–q11.23	Smcy	Y
Tdy	Sry		Testis-determining – Y or sex-determining region on Y	D, L		1, 6	TDF	Y p11.3	Tdy	Y
Tspy			Testis-specific protein on Y	D		7		Y p	Tspy-ps	Y
Tty			Testosterone timing on Y	L	P	5				
Ube1y			Ubiquitin-activating enzyme E1 on Y	D		2			Ube1y1	Y
Zfy			Zinc finger protein on Y	D		1	ZFY	Y p11.3	Zfy1	Y

References

1 Affara *et al.* (1996) *Cytogenet. Cell Genet.* 73, 33–76.

2 Chang and Li (1995) *J. Mol. Evol.* 40, 70–77.

3 Dunn (1975) *Transplantation* 20, 142–149.

4 Ely and Turner (1990) *Hypertension* 16, 277–281.

5 Ely *et al.* (1994) *J. Hypertens.* 12, 769–774.

6 Griffiths and Tiwari (1993) *Mol. Ecol.* 2, 405–406.

7 Mazeyrat and Mitchell (1998) *Hum. Mol. Genet.* 7, 557–562.

Abbreviations: D, DNA-annealing (FISH); L, linkage; S, somatic cell hybridization; C, confirmed; P, provisional; I, inconsistent; U, unknown; HSA, human (homo sapiens); MMU, mouse (mus muscularis); RNO, (rattus norvegicus); Chr, chromosome.

Appendix 2 List of equipment suppliers/vendors by country

Contributors' and Editor's recommendations

The suppliers listed below are additional to those mentioned in the text.
This list is not intended to be comprehensive.

Czech Republic

AnLab Ltd.
142 20 Prague 4
Videnska 1083
Czech Republic

Health monitoring

Germany

Biodoc Hannover
Feodor-Lynen-Straße 23
30625 Hannover
Germany

Health monitoring (serology)

Great Britain

B&K Universal Ltd.
The Field Station
Grimston Aldbrough Hull
North Humberside
Hull 4QE
Great Britain

Rodents equipment

International Market Supply
Congleton, Cheshire
Great Britain

Equipment

The Microbiology Laboratories
56 Northumberland Road, North Harrow
Middlesex HA2 7RE
Great Britain

Health monitoring

Japan

Bio Research Center, Inc.
Yokota Building, 4th Floor
2–28–24 Izumi
Higashi-ku
Nagoya 461–0001
Japan

Research Instruments

Imamichi Institute for Animal Reproduction
1103 Fukaya, Kasumigaura
Niihari
Ibaraki 300–0134
Japan

Animals

Japan SLC, Inc.
3371–8 Kotou-cho
Hamamatsu
Shizuoka 431–1103
Japan

Nihon Nosan Kogyo Co., Ltd.
Landmark Tower, 46th Floor
2–2–1 Minatomirai
Nishi-ku
Yokohama 220–8146
Japan

Narishige Co., Ltd.
4–27–9 Minami-Karasuyama
Setagaya
Tokyo 157–0062
Japan

Muromachi Kikai Co., Ltd.
Ootsuji Building
4–2–1 Muromachi
Nihonbashi
Chuo-ku
Tokyo 103–0022
Japan

Teikoku Hormone Mfg. Co., Ltd.
2–5–1 Akasaka
Minato-ku
Tokyo 107–8522
Japan

Sweden

SVA-Statens Veterinärmedicinska Anstalt
Box 7073
S–750 07 Uppsala
Sweden

Switzerland

RCC Ltd.
Biotechnology and Animal Breeding Division
Wölferstraße 4
4414 Füllinsdorf
Switzerland

Animals

Animal food

Research instruments

Research instruments

Hormones and bioactive substances

Health monitoring

Health monitoring

USA

Anmed Biosafe, Inc.
7642 Standish Place
Rockville, Maryland 20855
USA

Health monitoring

Charles River Laboratories
251 Ballardvale Street
Wilmington, MA 01887
USA

Murine serologic reagents, diagnostic services, rodents, equipment

Harlan Sprague Dawley, Inc.
PO Box 29176
Indianapolis, IN 46229–0176
USA

Rats

Plastics One, Inc.
6591 Merriman Road, SW
Roanoke, VA 24018
USA

Research instruments

Research Animal Diagnostic and Investigative Laboratory (RADIL)
University of Missouri
1600 East Rollins Street
Columbia, Missouri 65211
USA

Health monitoring

Taconic
273 Hover Avenue
Germantown, NY 12526
USA

Rodents, transgenic services

Appendix 3 Societies Active in Laboratory Animal Science

Editor's Recommendations

LASA (Laboratory Animal Science Association)

PO Box 3993, Tamworth
Staffordshire B78 3QU
UK

GV-SOLAS (Gesellschaft für Versuchstierkunde
= Society for Laboratory Animal Science)

UNI Berlin, Zentrale Tierlaboratorien
Krahmerstrasse 6
D-12207 Berlin
FRG

NVP (Nederlandse Vereniging voor Proefdierkunde
= Dutch Association for Laboratory Animal Science)

Dienst voor Veiligheid en Milieu
Vrije Universiteit
Van der Boechorstraat 1
1081 BT Amsterdam
The Netherlands

SGV (Schweizerische Gesellschaft für Versuchstierkunde/
Société Suisse pour la Science des Animaux de Laboratoire
= Swiss Laboratory Animal Science Association)

Novartis Pharma AG
K 125.12.50
CH-4002 Basel
Switzerland

FELASA (Federation of European Laboratory
Animal Science Associations)

BCM Box 2989
London WC1N 3XX
UK

SECAL (Sociedad Espanola para las Ciencias del Animal
de Laboratorio = Spanish Society for Laboratory
Animal Science)

Faculdad de Medicine de la UAM
(Gabinete Veterinario)
c/Arzobispo Morcillo 4
28029 Madrid
Spain

AALAS (American Association of Laboratory Animal
Science)

70 Timber Creek Drive
Cordova, TN 38018
USA

AAALAC, International (Association for the Assessment
and Accreditation of Laboratory Animal Care, International)

11300 Rockville Pike
Suite 1211
Rockville, MD 20852-3035
USA

ACLAM (American College of Laboratory Animal Medicine)

200 Summerwinds Drive
Cary, NC 27511
USA

ANZCCART (Australia and New Zealand Council for the Care of Animals in Research and Teaching)

Australia:
The Executive Officer
PO Box 19
Glen Osmond
South Australia, 5064

New Zealand:
The Executive Officer
c/o The Royal Society of New Zealand
PO Box 598
Wellington
New Zealand

CALAS/ACTAL (Canadian Association for Laboratory Animal Science/L'Association Canadienne pour la Technologie des Animaux de Laboratoire)

CW 401 Biological Science Building
Bioscience Animal Service
University of Alberta
Edmonton
Alberta, T6G 2E9
Canada

ICLAS
(International Council for Laboratory Animals Science)

Department of Physiology
University of Kuopio
PO Box 1627
SF-70211, Kuopio
Finland

ILAR (Institute of Laboratory Animal Resources)

2101 Constitution Avenue, NW
Washington, DC, 20418
USA

JALAS
(Japanese Association for Laboratory Animal Science)

Central Institute for Experimental Animals
1430 Nogawa, Miyamae
Kawasaki 216
Japan

Journals

Editor's Recommendations

Contemporary Topics in Laboratory Animal Medicine
ILAR Journal
Journal of Experimental Animal Science
Lab Animal
Laboratory Animals
Laboratory Animal Science
Rat News Letter
Rat Genom

Glossary

Terms defined in the glossary are emboldened in the main text.

aberrant cell types: Morphology differing from the norm

abluminal: Release away from the lumen of a vessel

acariasis: Infestation with acarids or mites

acid detergent fibre: Fibre soluble in detergent under acid conditions

acidosis: Accumulation of acid in the blood

activated partial thromboplastin times: APTT – used to assess integrity of the intrinsic and final common clotting pathways

adjuvants: Non specific stimulator of immune response

airway resistance (r_{aw}): Functional measure of airway calibre

alleles: Alternative forms of a gene

alpha hemolysis: Greenish zone produced on blood agar dishes by certain bacteria e.g. pneumococci

androgenic: Producing masculine characteristics

anoxic artifacts: Artifacts produced by interrupting the oxygen supply

anthropomorphic: Applying human form or character to a non-human object

anticholinergics: Agents blocking parasympathetic nerves

antisense oligonucleotides: Structures which can bind to the normal or "sense" sequence in the RNA of a cell and inhibit its action

antithrombotic: Prevention of the formation of platelet aggregates

antrum: Cavity or chamber in anatomical nomenclature

apoproteins: The protein moiety of a conjugated protein or protein complex

aquaporin 1: Similar to bacteriorhodopsin with only 6 helices

arborized: Branching termination of processes

arthralgia: Pain in a joint

astrogliosis: See Gliosis

ataxia: Failure of muscular co-ordination

athymic nude mice: Lacking the thymus gland

athymic nude rats: Lacking the thymus gland

atresia: Congenital absence/closure of a normal orifice

autistic disorders: Preoccupation with inner thought, lacking connection with reality

autochthonous flora: Flora normally found in the animal

autoregulation: System exercised by negative feedback

autosomal recessive inheritance: Mode of inheritance in which two alleles have to be defective

autosomes: Any paired chromosomes except X and Y chromosomes

bacteremic: Bacteria in the blood causing illness

balanopreputial: Pertaining to the glans penis and the prepuce

baroreceptor: A type of interoceptor that is stimulated by changes in pressure

beta hemolysis: Clear zone produced on a blood agar plate by certain bacteria

blepharospasms: Producing almost complete closure of the eyelids

bolus: Ready-to-swallow rounded mass of food or drug

bradycardia: Slowness of the heartbeat

bronchiectasis: Chronic dilatation of the bronchi

bronchiolitis: Inflammation of the bronchioles

bronchiolitis obliterans: Closure of bronchiolar lumina by connective tissue ingrowth

carcinogen: Any cancer producing substance

carcinogenicity: The ability or tendency to produce cancer

cardiac tamponade: Pressure on the heart by surrounding fluid

centesis: Puncture of the bladder

cestodes: Tapeworm or platyhelminth/class Cestoidea

chief cells: Epithelial cells, either columnar or cuboidal, lining lower portions of gastric glands and secrete pepsin

chromodacryorrhea: Shedding of bloody tears

chronobiological rhythms: Relating to the effects of time on the biological rhythm

chylomicrons: A class of lipoproteins that transport oxogenous cholesterol and triglycerides from the small intestine to the tissues after meals

circular mating: Non-random breeding system (see Index)

circular pair mating system: Equal populations of males and females taken initially and repeated for the following generations

Clara cells: Nonciliated secretory epithelial cells of respiratory tract

coisogenic strain system: Strains of inbred animals bred to be genetically identical except for a difference at a single genetic locus

compliance: Yielding to pressure or force without disruption

concatemers: Repeating linear arrays formed by aggregation of transgene copies

conceptus: Sum of the derivatives of a fertilised ovum

cosomic: Strain used as starting material for a targeted recessive screen

coprophagy: Feeding on dung or faeces

countercurrent exchange: Flowing in the opposite direction

cretinism: Chronic condition due to cengenital lack of thyroid secretion

cyclical system: Breeding system

cystostomy: Direct puncture of the bladder through the abdomen

cytokines: Non antibody proteins released by one cell population

dark cell: May be an artifact resulting from the fixation process or metabolically altered

dissociative anesthetic: Breaks down into its individual components

distal axonopathy: Disorder disrupting normal functioning of axons starting at the periphery

diuresis: Increased excretion of urine

dysprea: Difficult/laboured breathing

ectopia (=heterotopia): Displacement or malpositioning of an organ or structure

eicosanoids: Any of the biological products derived from arachadonic acid e.g. prostaglandins and leukotrienes

electrolyte and water homeostasis: Balanced conditions

ELISA: Enzyme Linked ImmunoSorbent Assay

emphysema: Pathological accumulation of air in the tissue (lung)

enterocytes: Intestinal epithelial cells

enzootic: Present in an animal community at all times

enzootically infected: Disease of low morbidity constantly present

epizootic: Attacking many animals in any region at the same time

ethmoturbinates: Superior and middle nasal conchae

ethological: Scientific study of animal behaviour

euthanasia: Easy or painless death

euthymic mice: Possessing normal thymic activity

excipients: Inert substance added to a drug/vehicle

exencephaly: Brain lying outside the skull

exocytosis: Discharge from a cell of particles which are too large to diffuse through the wall

fecundity: Ability to produce offspring rapidly and in large numbers

Ferguson reflex: A neural reflex that involves the stimulation of oxytocin release as the fetus enters the cervical canal

fomites: Object able to harbour pathogenic micro-organisms

full-sib mated: Mated with true sibling

FRC: Functional residual capacity

gamma hemolysis: Absence of a zone around a bacterial colony on an agar plate

gavage administration: Force feeding via tube passed into the stomach

gemistocytic astrocytosis: Large round cells stuffed with fatty debris found in astrocytomas

gene therapies: Transfer of genes to an individual to correct defect

genetic contamination: Inadvertant introduction of foreign genes into an inbred strain by outcrossing

genetic loci: Known locations for genes

genomics: Study of sequence data for genes

germfree: Reared in a sterile environment

gestation: Period of development from fertilisation to birth

gliosis: An excess of astroglia in damaged area of the CNS

glycation reaction: The non-enzymatic reaction of glucose with amino groups of proteins – implicated as a cause of aging

gnotobiotic: Laboratory animal with known flora and fauna

gonadotroph: Any of the beta cells of the adenohypophysis

HAI: Hemagglutination inhibition assay

Han-rotation system: Used for breeding colonies (see Index)

hepatocytomegaly: Greatly enlarged liver cells

heterosomes: Sex chromosomes

heterozygous: Having two different alleles of a specified gene

homozygous: Possessing a pair of identical alleles of a specified gene

housekeeping genes: Ubiquitously expressed genes such as actin, GADPH etc.

hydraulic pressure: Utilising the potential energy of water (or another fluid) under pressure

hydrocephalus: Obstruction of the cerebrospinal fluid pathways

hyperpnea: Abnormal increase in respiratory movements

hyperpolarized: A negative shift in the resting potential of the cell

hypertensive rats: Rats bred or treated to give chronic raised blood pressure

hyphema: Suffused with blood

hypopyon: Accumulation of pus in the anterior chamber of the eye

hypovolemia: Abnormally decreased volume of circulating fluid in the body

IFA: Immunofluorescence Assay

immunodeficient: A deficiency of the immune response

impedance: Opposition to flow of an alternating current

inbred: Result of mating closely related individuals

incrosses: Mating of individuals homozygous for the same gene

integrin: One of the major classes of cell adhesion molecules

intercross: Mating of individuals heterozygous for the same gene

interstitial cells of Cajal: Network of astrocytes

intrinsic factor: A glycoprotein secreted by Parietal cells necessary for the absorption of B12

inward eutrophic remodelling: Remodelling of a vessel wall to the normal pattern

karyomegaly: Abnormal enlargement of the nucleus of a cell

"knock out": Deletion of a gene so as to study its function

latent infections: Dormant or quiescent infections

leptotene: Stage in meiosis when chromosomes are slender

linearized DNA: DNA that has been unfolded

lordosis: Anterior concavity in the curvature of the lumbar and cervical spine

lordosis quotient: Degree of curvature of the spine

luteolysis: Degeneration of the corpus luteum

M system: Layer of macrophage-like cells covering the Peyer's patches

MC: Multiplication colonies

meiosis: Cell division occurring during the maturation of gametes which results in a haploid genome

metritis: Inflammation of the uterus

MHC: Major histocompatibility complex

micelles: A colloid particle formed by an aggregation of small molecules

microcephaly: Abnormal smallness of the head

microsatellite marker: Marker with short repeated sequence containing a different no of copies (generally 4–40) mostly polymorphic

micturation: Artificial induction of urine production

minute ventilation: Total amount of gas (in litres) expelled from the lungs per minute

moist rales: Indicative of secretions in airways and lungs

morbidity: A diseased condition or state

MTD-maximum tolerated dose: Highest dose of a drug or chemical not inducing severe toxic effects

MUA: Multiple unit activity

myogenic reflex: Originating in myocytes or muscle tissue

5/6th nephrectomy model: Major removal of functional kidney

narcosis: A non-specific and reversible depression of function of the central nervous system

nasal turbinates: Turbinate bones of the nose

nephrocalcinosis: Deposition of calcium crystals in the kidney

nephropathy: A diet-related disease of the rat inducing kidney damage

neurobehavioural: Relating to neurological behaviour

neuroblasts: Any embryonic cell which develops into a nerve cell or neuron

neuroleptanalgesia: A state of quiescence etc. produced by a combination of a narcotic analgesic and a neuroleptic agent

neutral detergent fibre: Fibre soluble in detergent under neutral conditions

nociceptor impulses: Impulses received from the pain receptors

NOEL: Exposure level with No Observed Effect (Level)

non-gravid: Not pregnant

nucleus colonies (NC): Self-perpetuating system for maintaining an inbred strain

occult infections: Obscure or hidden infection

oncotic pressure: Osmotic pressure due to colloids in a solution

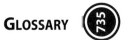

optochin inhibition test: Presumptive test used to identify strains of *Streptococcus peneumoniae*

organogenesis: The origin and development of organs

orphan: No known parent or related compound

osmotic pumps: Pumps designed to release their contents into the body by osmosis

otoscopic: Results from examining the ear with an otoscope

outcross: Bringing of new genetic material into a breeding programme

oxyuriasis: Infection with worms of the genus Oxyuris

pachytene: Stage in meoisis during which chromatids break up and material can be exchanged (crossing over)

paracrine modulator: Released hormone from endocrine cells binding to its receptor on nearby cells of a different type

parietal cells: Large spheroidal or pyramidal cells that are the source of gastric HCl and the site of intrinsic factor production

parotid: A gland situated near to the ear

pathognomonic: Specifically distinctive or characteristic of a disease or a pathological condition

PCR: Polymerase chain reaction

PEC: Pedigreed expansion colonies maintained by brother and sister mating

periventricular neuronal heterotopias: Displacement of neurons into periventricular region

pharmacokinetics: Fate of drugs in the body over a measured period of time

phonation: The utterance of vocal sounds

piloerection: Hair standing on end

pododermatitis: Dermatitis of the foot region

polytocous: Giving birth to several offspring at the same time

preleptotene: A stage in meiosis

primordial follicle: An ovarian follicle consisting of an egg surrounded by a single layer of cells

progenitor strains: Ancestral or parent strains

proteomics: Study of functional data for proteins

protooncogenes: A normal cellular gene which when altered, e.g. by mutation, becomes an oncogene

pulmonary resistance (R_L): See airway resistance

pulsatile flow: Pressure maintained on a push-release pattern

pyometra: An accumulation of pus in the uterus

recombinant inbred (IR) strains: Outcrossing followed by intercrossing

rederivation methods: For example, embryo transfer

resistance arteries: Regulators of peripheral resistance

resistive pressure: Degree of stiffness of lung and thorax

resorptions: Reabsorption of fluid, tissue, bone etc

retinopathy: Pathological damage to the retina of the eye

retroperitoneal space: Rear of the peritoneum

rotation breeding system: Subdivision of an outbred population into blocks, the total number of blocks being constant for all generations

RT-PCR: Reverse transcriptase PCR

salpingitis: Inflammation of the uterine tube

SDP: Strain distribution pattern

sentinel animals: Animals used to mark presence of infection in a colony

seroconversion: Change of a serological test from negative to positive

serrefine: a small spring forceps

SHR: Spontaneously hypertensive

Sialoadenitis: Inflammation of the salivary gland

slow-wave sleep: The dreamless period of sleep

somatotrophs: Alpha cells of the adenohypophysis which secrete growth hormone

speed congenics: Reduction in time for creating congenic strains using additional selection criteria

SPF: Specific pathogen free

strabismus: Deviation of the eye which the animal cannot overcome e.g. squinting

superovulation: Extraordinary increase in the number of cells in ovulation, usually hormone induced

synechia: Adhesion of parts e.g. iris to the cornea

systematic breeder rotation: System designed by Poiley which, however, leads to subline formation

TAL: Thick ascending limb of the Loop of Henle

telemetry: The making of measurements at a distance from the subject

teratogenic: Tending to produce anomalies of formation

teratology: Division of embryology and pathology which deals with abnormal development and congenital abnormalities

TGF: Tubuloglomerular feedback

The Rat Genome Database: Analysis of all the components of the rat genome allocating activities to each gene

thermal neutral zone: Range of temperatures within which the animal thrives normally

thermocauter: Hot wire or point used for cauterisation

thrombin: Enzyme which converts fibrinogen to fibrin

thrombocytopenia: Abnormally low blood platelet count

thyrotroph: Any of the beta cells of the adenohypophysis that secrete thyrotropin

TIDA system: Tuberoinfundibular dopaminergic system

tidal volume: Normal respiratory volume of the lung

toxicokinetics: Fate of toxins in the body over a measured period of time

transgenic strains: Pertaining to the experimental splicing of a segment of DNA from one genome on to the DNA of a different genome

transponders: Inserted measuring devices

tropic: Turning towards, changing

ultrafiltration coefficient (Kf): Rate measurement for urinary filtration

V2-receptors: Receptors in the lung relating to the control of respiration

vasculitis: Inflammation of a vessel

vector: a) Carriers of infectious disease b) constructs made to transport material into cells, e.g. plasmids

viral or non viral vectors: Vectors which may or may not be made from empty viral shells

virilization: Induction or development of male secondary sex characters

xenobiotics: Chemicals foreign to the biological system

zoonotic: Transmissible from animals to man under natural conditions

zygotene: In meiosis, the stage where the two leptotene chromosomes undergo pairing to give a bivalent structure

Index